CORE CONCEPTS IN HEALTH

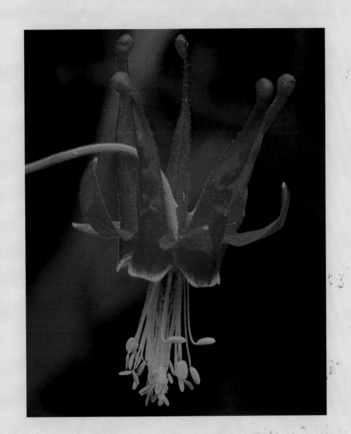

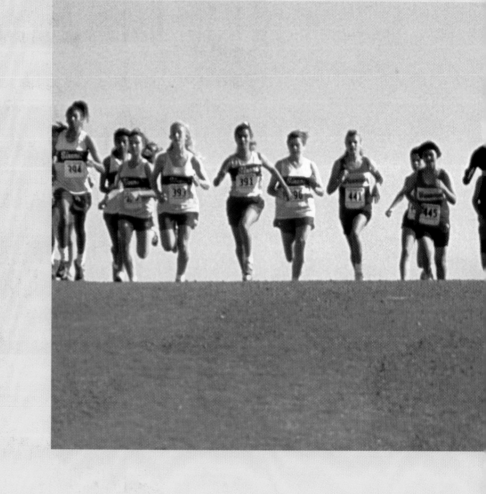

Core Concepts in Health

Seventh Edition

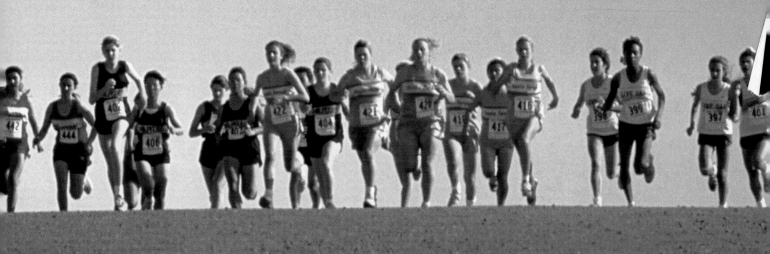

Paul M. Insel • Walton T. Roth
Stanford University

Mayfield Publishing Company
Mountain View, California
London • Toronto

Library of Congress Cataloging-in-Publication Data
Core concepts in health / (compiled by) Paul M. Insel, Walton T. Roth.
  — 7th ed.
    p.   cm.
  Optional package of supplementary teaching materials is available.
  Includes bibliographical references and index.
    ISBN 1–55934–210–2
    1. Health.   I. Insel, Paul M.   II. Roth, Walton T.
RA776.C83 1993
613—dc20   93–15380
                                                        CIP

Manufactured in the United State of America
10 9 8 7 6 5 4 3 2

Mayfield Publishing Company
1240 Villa Street
Mountain View, California 94041

Sponsoring editor, Erin Mulligan; *developmental editors,* Kirstan Price and Kathleen Engelberg; *production editor,* Carol Zafiropoulos; *manuscript editor,* Joan Pendleton; *art director and cover designer,* Jeanne M. Schreiber; *text designer,* Detta Penna; *illustrators,* Dale Glasgow, Robin Mouat, Kevin Somerville, Pamela Drury Wattenmaker; *photo researcher,* Melissa Kreischer; *cover photographer,* D. Lowe; *proofreader,* Carol Carter; *manufacturing manager,* Martha Branch. This text was set in 10.5/12 Berkeley Book by Graphic Typesetting Services and printed on 45# Chromatone LG by Banta Company.

Text and photo credits

Sources

Page 70, "Mind/Body Update" Copyright 1992 by Consumers Union of U.S., Inc., Yonkers, NY 10703-1057. Reprinted by permission from CONSUMER REPORTS ON HEALTH, August 1992.

Page 94, From *Secrets of Strong Families* by Nick Stinnett and John DeFrain. Copyright ©1985 by Nick Stinnett and John DeFrain. By permission of Little, Brown and Company.

Page 166, Copyright 1992 Time Inc. Reprinted by permission.

Page 192, "What's Lurking in Your Family Tree" Copyright 1992 by Consumers Union of U.S., Inc., Yonkers, NY 10703-1057. Reprinted by permission from CONSUMER REPORTS ON HEALTH, September 1992.

Page 345, Reprinted permission of the University of California at Berkeley Wellness Letter, ©Health Letter Associates, 1989.

Page 451, Reprinted permission of the University of California at Berkeley Wellness Letter, ©Health Letter Associates, 1987.

Page 496, Adapted from "Your Department of Defense." *Nutrition Action Healthletter,* August 1988.

Page 503, Reprinted permission of the University of California at Berkeley Wellness Letter, ©Health Letter Associates, 1992.

Page 656, Copyright 1992 Time Inc. Reprinted by permission.

Photo Credits

Chapter 1, pg. 1, © David Madison 1990; pg. 6, © Anthony Edgeworth/The Stock Market; pg. 10, © P. Davidson/The Image Works; p. 11, © Bill Horsman/Stock Boston; pg. 17, © Bob Dammrich/The Image Works; p. 20, © Sam Forencich

Chapter 2, pg. 25, © Bob Daemmrich/Stock Boston; pg. 27, © Tony Savino/The Image Works; pg. 30, © Bob Daemmrich/Stock Boston; pg. 31, © Stacy Pick/Stock Boston; pg. 36, © Suzanne Arms; pg. 37, Jim Weiner © 1985/Photo Researchers; pg. 38, © Tony Freeman/PhotoEdit; pg. 40, © Jeff Zaruba/The Stock Market

Chapter 3, pg. 49, © Jonathan A. Meyers/JAM Photography; pg. 53, © Suzanne Arms; pg. 55, © Elizabeth Crews; pg. 59, © Mark Antman/The Image Works; pg. 62, © Joel Gordon 1991; pg. 68, © Jim Harrison/Stock Boston; pg. 71, © 1992 B. Kramer/Custom Medical Stock Photo

Chapter 4, pg. 77, © Dorothy Littell Greco 1992/Stock Boston; pg. 80, © Frank Siteman/Stock Boston; pg. 84, © Lawrence Migdale/Stock Boston; pg. 85, © Joel Gordon 1990; pg. 89, © Suzanne Arms; pg. 92, © Phil Borden/PhotoEdit

Chapter 5, pg. 97, © Bob Daemmrich/Stock Boston; pg. 105, © Bob Daemmrich/The Image Works; pg. 108, © Suzanne Arms; pg. 115, © Elizabeth Crews; pg. 118, © Starr 1992/Stock Boston; pg. 121, © Joel Gordon 1992; pg. 124, © David R. Frazier/Photo Researchers

(Photo credits continue on p. 679, which constitutes a continuation of the copyright page)

Preface

Now in its seventh edition, *Core Concepts in Health* has maintained its leadership in the field of health education for nearly 20 years. Since we pioneered the concept of self-responsibility for personal health in 1976, hundreds of thousands of students have used our book to become active, informed participants in their own health care. Each edition of *Core Concepts* has brought improvements and refinements, but the principles underlying the book have remained the same. Our commitment to these principles has never been stronger than it is today.

OUR GOALS

Our goals in writing this book can be stated simply:

- To present scientifically based, accurate, up-to-date information in an accessible format
- To involve students in taking responsibility for their health and well-being
- To instill a sense of competence and personal power in students

The first of these goals means making expert knowledge about health and health care available to the individual. *Core Concepts* brings scientifically based, accurate, up-to-date information to students about topics and issues that concern them—exercise, stress, nutrition, weight management, contraception, intimate relationships, HIV infection, drugs, alcohol, and a multitude of others. Current, complete, and straightforward coverage is balanced with "user-friendly" features designed to make the text appealing. Written in an engaging, easy-to-read style and presented in a colorful, open format, *Core Concepts* invites the student to read, learn, and remember. Boxes, tables, artwork, photographs, and many other features highlight areas of special interest throughout the book.

The second of our goals is to involve students in taking responsibility for their health. *Core Concepts* uses innovative pedagogy and unique interactive features to get students thinking about how the material they're reading relates to their own lives. We invite them to examine their emotions about the issues under discussion, to consider their personal values and beliefs, and to analyze their health-related behaviors. Beyond this, for students who want to change behaviors that detract from a healthy lifestyle, we offer guidelines and tools, ranging from samples of health journals and personal contracts to detailed assessments and behavior change strategies.

Perhaps our third goal in writing *Core Concepts in Health* is the most important: to instill a sense of competence and personal power in the students who read the book. Everyone has the ability to monitor, understand, and affect his or her own health. Although the medical and health professions possess impressive skills and have access to a huge body of knowledge that benefits everyone in our society, people can help to minimize the amount of professional care they actually require in their lifetime by taking care of their health—taking charge of their health—from an early age. Our hope is that *Core Concepts* will continue to help young people make this exciting discovery—that they have the power to shape their own futures.

CONTENT AND ORGANIZATION OF THE SEVENTH EDITION

For this edition, all chapters were carefully reviewed, revised, and updated. The latest information from scientific and health-related research is incorporated in the text, and newly emerging topics and issues are discussed. The following list gives a sample of some of the current concerns addressed in the seventh edition:

- The changing profile of the epidemic of HIV infection and the latest approaches to treatment
- The new food labels and the Food Guide Pyramid
- The newest contraceptive methods, including the female condom, contraceptive implants, and Depo-Provera injections
- Effects of environmental tobacco smoke on nonsmokers
- Physician-assisted suicide
- Family violence
- Iron and cardiovascular disease
- The links between people's feelings and states of mind and their physical health
- Preconception care
- The rising incidence of tuberculosis
- Hostility and heart disease
- Nicotine replacement therapy
- Alzheimer's disease

Of all these current health concerns, the most pressing is HIV infection. Approximately half of Chapter 17 (Sexually Transmissible Diseases) is devoted to a discussion of this disease, and five boxes address related issues—"AIDS Milestones," "Who Needs an HIV Test?," "Changing Patterns of HIV Infection Around the World," "Preventing HIV Infection," and "Talking About Condoms and Safer Sex." Another box asks students to carefully examine their attitudes and behaviors to determine whether they are putting themselves at risk for HIV infection or another sexually transmissible disease. Another box on HIV in Chapter 18 (Infection and Immunity) explains how HIV infection affects the immune system.

An especially volatile current health concern is abortion. As in the previous two editions, we devote a separate chapter to abortion to reflect both the importance of this issue and our belief that abortion is not a form of contraception and should not be included in the chapter on that topic. As part of our balanced treatment of this controversial issue, we include statements representing opposing views on abortion, one by Kate Michelman of the National Abortion Rights Action League and the other by J. C. Wilke of the National Right to Life Committee. Also included in this chapter are a new box on adoption, an updated account of the latest legal rulings, a section on the "abortion pill" RU-486, and a sensitive discussion of the decision-making processes involved when abortion is being considered.

An area of particular concern and the subject of a great deal of recent research is cardiovascular disease, the number one killer of Americans. Chapter 15 reports the latest findings on the roles of hostility, cholesterol, iron, and a sedentary lifestyle in cardiovascular health and disease. Six new boxes address related topics, such as how to lower the risk of heart disease through diet.

Another area of great importance for college students is injuries, the leading cause of death for Americans under the age of 45. Chapter 23 (Injury Prevention and Control) has been completely revised and updated in light of current research on what factors cause injuries and how injuries can be prevented. The coverage of unintentional injuries has been expanded to include new information on safety belts and air bags, motorcycles and mopeds, bicycle and pedestrian safety, fire safety, and many other topics. Chapter 23 also covers the role of violence, which has recently been identified as an important public health problem. The goal of Chapter 23 is to make students more aware of why injuries happen and to give them concrete strategies for keeping themselves safe.

The seventh edition of *Core Concepts* also takes care to address the health issues and concerns of an increasingly diverse student population. While most health concerns are universal—we all need to eat well, exercise, and manage stress, for example—certain differences among people have important implications for health. These differences can be genetic or cultural, based on factors such as gender, socioeconomic status, age, and race or ethnicity. Where such differences are important for health, they are

discussed in the text or in a new kind of highlight box called Dimensions of Diversity (discussed in greater detail below). Examples of these discussions include the links between ethnicity and genetic diseases, special risks for women who smoke, and differences in alcohol metabolism based on gender and ethnicity. Throughout the text, box program, art, and photographs, *Core Concepts* presents health and wellness in ways that reflect America's ever-growing diversity.

Another important addition to *Core Concepts* is coverage of the 1991 *Healthy People 2000* report from the U.S. Surgeon General's Office. This report outlines health promotion and disease prevention goals and objectives for the United States to be achieved by the year 2000. In many ways, the principles and priorities of these national health goals parallel the personal health goals discussed in *Core Concepts*. The report itself is described in a highlight box in Chapter 1; specific objectives are discussed in later chapters where appropriate.

The health field is dynamic, with new discoveries, advances, trends, and theories reported every week. Ongoing research—on the role of a high-fat diet in certain cancers, for example, or on the genetic links in Alzheimer's disease—continually changes our understanding of the human body and how it works. For this reason, no health book can claim to have the final word on every topic. Yet within these limits, *Core Concepts* does present the latest available information and scientific thinking on innumerable topics.

In addition to being brought up-to-date for this edition, all chapters were reexamined for clarity and coherence. A number of chapters were completely reorganized to ensure that explanations and discussions were as clear as possible. The chapter outlines at the beginning of each chapter reflect this sharper focus.

The organization of this book as a whole remains essentially the same as in the sixth edition, with chapters divided into eight different parts. Part One, Establishing a Basis for Wellness, includes chapters on taking charge of your health, stress, and mental health. The division of topics in the chapters in Part Two, Understanding Sexuality, has been slightly revised. The part opens with an expanded exploration of intimate relationships, including friendship, intimate partnerships, marriage, and family (Chapter 4), and then moves on to discuss physical sexuality (Chapter 5). Other chapters in Part Two cover contraception, abortion, and pregnancy and childbirth. Part Three, Making Responsible Decisions: Substance Use and Abuse, deals with tobacco, alcohol, and other psychoactive drugs. Part Four, Getting Fit, covers nutrition, weight management, and exercise.

Part Five, Protecting Yourself from Disease, deals with the most serious health problems facing people today—cardiovascular disease, cancer, and sexually transmissible diseases—and with the body's impressive defense system against disease. Part Six, Accepting Physical Limits, explores aging and dying and death. Part Seven, Making Choices in Health Care, provides information about medical self-care and the health care system. And finally, Part Eight, Improving Your Chances: Personal Safety and Environmental Health, expands the boundaries of health care to include injury prevention and the effects of environment on personal health. Taken together, the parts of the book provide students with a complete guide to managing and protecting their health, now and through their entire lives, as individuals, as participants in a health care community and system, and as citizens of a planet that also needs to be protected if it is to continue providing human beings with the means to healthy lives.

A NEW LOOK

One thing that will be immediately apparent to past users of *Core Concepts* is that the book has a fresh and exciting new look. *Core Concepts* has always set the standard in the field for innovative graphics and illustrations, and this edition is no exception. A major part of this new look is the illustration program, which includes new renderings of the best art from the sixth edition and many new illustrations. Much of the anatomical art has been prepared by a medical illustrator in a dramatic new style that is both visually appealing and highly informative. These illustrations help students understand such important information as how blood flows through the heart; how the digestive system works; how the process of conception occurs; and how to use a condom. Many graphs, charts, and other illustrations have also been rendered in a dynamic, colorful, and appealing new style. These lively and abundant illustrations will particularly benefit those students who learn best from visual images.

The overall design of the book itself is also new—more dynamic, more colorful, and better able to catch and hold students' attention. A compelling photographic image appears at the opening of each chapter, suggesting an important theme of that chapter; the photos within the chapters are all in color and most are new. All the chapter elements have been designed and coordinated to make each page both visually appealing and easy for students to read and follow.

Taken together, these visual elements—new design, new illustrations, new photos—provide powerful pedagogical tools and create a colorful and inviting look.

FEATURES OF THE SEVENTH EDITION

This edition of *Core Concepts in Health* builds on the features that attracted and held our readers' interest in the previous six editions. One of the most popular features has always been the **boxes,** which allow us to explore a wide range of current topics in greater detail than is pos-

sible in the text itself. Over half the boxes are new to the seventh edition, and many others have been significantly revised or updated. A major change to the box program in this edition is the division of the boxes into six categories, each marked with a unique icon and label.

 Assess Yourself boxes give students the opportunity to examine their behavior and identify ways that they can change their habits to improve their health. By referring to these boxes, students can examine their eating habits to see what triggers their eating, for example; determine whether time pressure is a significant source of stress in their lives; discover if they are at increased risk for cancer or cardiovascular disease; evaluate their driving skills; examine their drinking behavior; and so on.

 Dimensions of Diversity boxes are part of our commitment to reflect and respond to the diversity of the student population. These boxes give students the opportunity to identify any special health risks that affect them because of who they are, as individuals or as members of a group. They also broaden students' perspectives by exposing them to a wide variety of viewpoints on health-related issues. The different dimensions reflected include gender, socioeconomic status, race or ethnicity, and age. The principles embodied by these boxes are described in the first box in the series, "Health Issues for Diverse Populations," which appears in Chapter 1. Topics covered in later chapters include ethnicity and genetic diseases, special cardiovascular disease risks for African Americans, exercise for people with disabilities, special risks for women who smoke, ethnic diets and cuisines, attitudes toward aging and the elderly, and links between poverty and cancer.

In addition, some of the Dimensions of Diversity boxes highlight health issues and practices in other parts of the world, allowing students to see what Americans share with people in other societies and how they differ. Students have the opportunity to learn about arranged marriages in India, laws and attitudes toward contraception and abortion in other countries, the pattern of HIV infection around the world, attitudes toward death among Mexicans and Mexican Americans, and other topics of interest.

 Sound Mind, Sound Body boxes explore the close connection between mind and body. Drawn from studies in psychoneuroimmunology, these boxes focus on total wellness by examining the links between people's feelings and states of mind and their physical health. By looking at these boxes, students can learn how stress affects the immune system, for example; the health benefits of intimate relationships; the links between hostility and cardiovascular disease; how exercise affects mood; and so on.

A Closer Look boxes highlight current health topics of particular interest to students. Topics include bicycle helmets, sleep, family violence, diabetes, preventive medicine for healthy adults, tuberculosis, testing for HIV infection, allergies and asthma, and physician-assisted suicide.

 Tactics and Tips boxes distill from each chapter the practical advice students need in order to apply information to their own lives. By referring to these boxes, students can easily find ways to reduce the amount of fat in their diets, to support their immune systems, to talk to sexual partners about condom use and STDs, to protect themselves from drunk drivers, to improve communication in their relationships, to use medications safely and effectively, and so on.

 Vital Statistics boxes, figures, and tables highlight important facts and figures in a memorable format that often reveals surprising contrasts and connections. From boxes, tables, and figures marked with the Vital Statistics label, students can learn about drinking among college students, health care costs in the United States, world population growth, trends in public opinion about abortion, the average American diet, cancer incidence and survival rates, and a wealth of other information. For students who grasp a subject best when it is displayed graphically, numerically, or in a table, the Vital Statistics feature provides alternative ways of approaching and understanding the text.

In addition to the new box program, the most popular and useful features of *Core Concepts* have been retained and revised for this edition. Each chapter opens with **Making Connections**, designed to facilitate learning by getting students personally involved in specific health-related issues. The Making Connections scenarios at the beginning of each chapter describe situations that involve concerns treated in the following pages. In each situation, someone has to make a decision, choose a course of action, or use information. We ask students to imagine themselves in the situation and consider what they would do, both before and after reading the chapter. The scenarios demonstrate ways students can use material in the chapter to address issues and solve problems in their lives.

Personal Insight is a revised and broadened version of Exploring Your Emotions, a feature that appeared in previous editions of *Core Concepts*. Each Personal Insight asks open-ended questions designed to encourage self-examination and heighten students' awareness of their feelings, values, beliefs, thought processes, and past experiences. These questions have been formulated in a nonjudgmental way to foster honest self-analysis, and they appear at appropriate points throughout the chapter.

Take Action, appearing at the end of every chapter, suggests hands-on exercises and projects that students can undertake to extend and deepen their grasp of the material. Suggested projects include interviews, investigations of campus or community resources, and experimentation with some of the behavior change techniques suggested in the text. Special care has been taken to ensure that the projects are both feasible and worthwhile.

New to the seventh edition is **Journal Entry**, a feature which also appears at the end of each chapter. These entries suggest ways for students to use their Health Journal (which we recommend they keep while using *Core Concepts*) to think about topics and issues, explore and formulate their own views, and express their thoughts in written form. They are designed to help students deepen their understanding of their own health-related behaviors.

Making wise choices about health requires students to sort through and evaluate health information. To help students become skilled evaluators, each chapter contains at least one **Critical Thinking** Journal Entry. These entries help students develop their critical thinking skills, including finding relevant information, separating fact from opinion, recognizing faulty reasoning, evaluating information, and assessing the credibility of sources. Critical Thinking Journal Entry questions do not have right or wrong answers; rather, they ask students to analyze, evaluate, or take a stand on a particular issue.

The **Behavior Change Strategies** that conclude many chapters offer specific behavior management/modification plans relating to the chapter's topic. Based on the principles of behavior management that are carefully explained in Chapter 1, these strategies will help students change unhealthy or counterproductive behaviors. Included are strategies for dealing with test anxiety, quitting smoking, developing responsible drinking habits, planning a personal exercise program, phasing in a healthier diet, and many other practical plans for change.

New and revised tables also add interest to the text. From the tables students can quickly learn about such topics as the effects of smoking, constructive and destructive aproaches to conflict resolution, infections and disorders commonly associated with HIV infection, and guidelines for cholesterol and blood pressure levels.

Also designed for quick reference are this edition's **appendixes.** An expanded version of the "The Facts About Fast Food," following Chapter 12 (Nutrition Facts and Fallacies), provides students with a handy guide to the nutritional content of the most commonly ordered menu items at seven popular fast food restaurants. Especially useful is the information about the fat and sodium content of each item and its proportion of fat calories to total calories. A "Red Cross First Aid Chart" appears inside the back cover of the text, providing information that can save lives. Revised and updated appendixes on self-care follow Chapter 21, titled "Self-Care Guide for Common Medical Problems," and "Resources for Self-Care." These guides offer students the kind of information they can keep and use for years to come.

LEARNING AIDS

Although all the features of *Core Concepts in Health* are designed to facilitate learning, several specific learning aids have also been incorporated into the text. **Chapter outlines** provide an overview of the contents of the following pages, orienting students at the outset of each new subject area. Important terms appear in boldface type in the text and are defined in a **running glossary**, helping students handle a large and complex new vocabulary.

Chapter summaries offer students a concise review and a way to make sure they have grasped the most important concepts in the chapter. Also found at the end of every chapter are **selected bibliographies** and annotated **recommended readings**, which have been expanded and carefully updated for this edition. Students can use these lists to extend and broaden their knowledge of particualr topics or pursue subjects of interest to them. A complete **index** at the end of the book includes references to glossary terms in boldface type.

TEACHING TOOLS

Available to qualified adopters of *Core Concepts in Health* is a comprehensive package of supplementary materials that enhance teaching and learning. Included in the package are the following items:

- Instructor's Resource Guide
- Examination questions
- Wellness Worksheets
- Student Study Guide
- Transparency acetates
- Videotapes
- Health Risk Appraisal software
- Nutrition Analysis software
- Brownstone Academic Management System

The **Instructor's Resource Guide** contains a variety of teaching aids, all revised and updated for the seventh edition: learning objectives for each chapter; extended chapter outlines; suggestions for student activities; listings of additional resources, including films, books, and periodicals; and health crossword puzzles. The guide also includes more than 70 transparency masters, providing additional lecture resources for instructors.

A complete set of **examination questions** provides instructors with 3,000 test questions to choose from when creating exams. The multiple choice and true/false questions have been carefully reviewed, and the answer keys list the page number in the text where the answer is found.

A set of 80 **Wellness Worksheets** helps students become more involved in their own health and be better prepared to implement successful behavior change pro-

grams. Most of the worksheets provide assessment tools that help students learn more about their health-related attitudes and behaviors. Some are strictly knowledge-based and help increase students' comprehension of key concepts. The Wellness Worksheets are available in an easy-to-use pad and in the student Study Guide.

The **Student Study Guide,** prepared by Thomas M. Davis of the University of Northern Iowa, is designed to help students understand and assimilate the material in the text. The guide includes learning objectives, key terms, major concepts, sample test questions, and the complete set of Wellness Worksheets.

The set of **transparency acetates,** many in full color, provides material suitable for lecture and discussion purposes. These acetates do not duplicate the transparency masters in the Instructor's Resource Guide, and many of them are from sources other than the text.

Our exciting **videotapes** give instructors the opportunity to illustrate and extend coverage of the most current and compelling health-related topics treated in the text. For information about the videos, instructors should contact their Mayfield representative or call 1-800-433-1279.

The computerized **Health Risk Appraisal software** package provides students with a self-assessment tool that alerts them to their personal risk areas and advises them on how to improve their risk profile. Designed for IBM-compatible computers, the program provides a detailed two-page report for each user.

The completely new **Nutrition Analysis software** package allows students to assess their current daily diet, evaluate menus, and compare their diets to current nutrition guidelines. Students receive a printout that includes an easy-to-understand scoring system and suggestions for improving food choices.

The **Brownstone Academic Management System** gives instructors a powerful, easy-to-use method of handling time-consuming tasks such as creating tests and calculating and entering grades. It is available for IBM-compatible and Apple computers. The Microtest program from the Chariot Software Group is available for Macintosh computer users.

A NOTE OF THANKS

The efforts of innumerable people have gone into producing this seventh edition of *Core Concepts in Health*. The book has benefited immensely from their thoughtful commentaries, expert knowledge and opinions, and many helpful suggestions. We are deeply grateful for their participation in the project.

Academic Contributors

Stephen Barrett, M.D., Consumer Advocate and Editor, *Nutrition Forum Newsletter*
The Health Care System

Roger Baxter, M.D., Internist and Infectious Disease Specialist, Kaiser Permanente Medical Center, Oakland, California
Immunity and Infection

Virginia Brooke, Ph.D., Intercollegiate Center for Nursing Education
Aging: A Vital Process

Boyce Burge, Ph.D., *Healthline*
Cancer

Thomas Fahey, Ed.D., California State University, Chico
Exercise for Health and Fitness

Michael R. Hoadley, Ph.D., University of South Dakota
Injury Prevention and Control

Paul Insel, Ph.D., Stanford University
Taking Charge of Your Health; Stress: The Constant Challenge; Toward a Tobacco-free Society; The Use and Abuse of Psychoactive Drugs; Cardiovascular Health

Bea Mandel, R.N., M.P.H., Executive Director, PRIDE, College of Health and Human Development, Pennsylvania State University
Sexually Transmissible Diseases

Joyce D. Nash, Ph.D., Pacific Graduate School of Psychology
Weight Management

David Quadagno, Ph.D., Florida State University
Sex and Your Body

Walton T. Roth, M.D., Stanford University School of Medicine
Mental Health

James H. Rothenberger, M.P.H., University of Minnesota
Environmental Health

Melinda J. Seid, Ph.D., MT (ASCP), CHES, California State University, Sacramento
"Chinese Herbal Medicine"

David Sobel, M.D., M.P.H., Director of Patient Education and Health Promotion, Kaiser Permanente Medical Care Program, Northern California Region
Medical Self-Care: Skills for the Health Care Consumer

Albert Lee Strickland and Lynne Ann DeSpelder, Cabrillo College
Dying and Death

Bryan Strong, Ph.D., University of California at Santa Cruz, and Christine DeVault
Intimate Relationships; Pregnancy and Childbirth

Jared R. Tinklenberg, M.D., Palo Alto Veterans Administration Medical Center and Stanford University
The Responsible Use of Alcohol

Mae V. Tinklenberg, R.N., N.P., M.S., Fair Oaks Family Health Center
Contraception; Abortion

Gordon Wardlaw, Ph.D., R.D., Ohio State University
Nutrition Facts and Fallacies

Academic Advisers and Reviewers

Lori J. Bechtel, Pennsylvania State University—Altoona Campus
Michael S. Davidson, Montclair State University
Thomas M. Davis, University of Northern Iowa
David F. Duncan, Brown University
R. Daniel Duquette, University of Wisconsin at La Crosse
Mary E. Etherington, California State University, Northridge
Jo Hill, New Mexico State University
Roberta B. Hollander, Howard University
Mark J. Kittleson, Southern Illinois University
Becky Kennedy Koch, Ohio State University
Beverly Saxton Mahoney, Pennsylvania State University
Anne Nadakavukaren, Illinois State University
James V. Noto, San Diego State University
Judy Oaks, Director, Center for Personal Recovery
Anne O'Donnell, Santa Rosa Junior College
Andrea Port Jacobs, Howard Community College
Bruce M. Ragon, Indiana University
Kerry J. Redican, Virginia Polytechnic Institute and State University
Janet Reis, University of Illinois at Urbana-Champaign
Mary Rose-Colley, Lock Haven University
James Rothenberger, University of Minnesota
John P. Sciacca, Northern Arizona University
Melinda Joy Seid, California State University, Sacramento
Philip A. Sienna, Mission College
David A. Sleet, Center for Injury Prevention and Control, Centers for Disease Control and Prevention
Thea Siria Spatz, University of Arkansas at Little Rock
Carol A. Wilson, University of Nevada, Las Vegas
Richard W. Wilson, Western Kentucky University

A special note of thanks is due to Bryan Strong and Christine DeVault, authors of Mayfield's new text, *Human Sexuality*, available for adoption as of January 1994.

Finally, the book could not have been published without the efforts of the staff at Mayfield Publishing Company and the *Core Concepts* book team: Erin Mulligan, Sponsoring Editor; Kirstan Price and Kate Engelberg, Developmental Editors; Linda Toy, Production Director; Carol Zafiropoulos, Production Editor; Jeanne M. Schreiber, Art Director; Pam Trainer, Permissions Editor; Melissa Kreischer, Photo Researcher; Martha Branch, Manufacturing Manager; Julie Wildhaber, Editorial Assistant; Larisa North, Production Assistant. To all, we express our deep appreciation.

Paul M. Insel
Walton T. Roth

Brief Contents

Contents

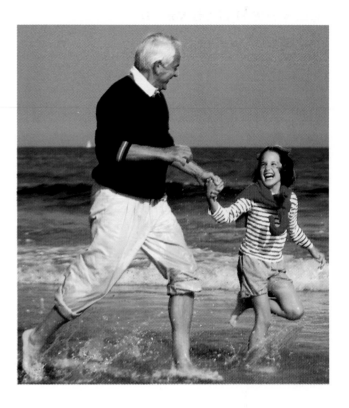

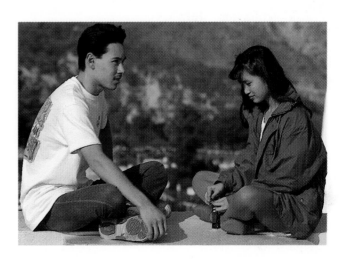

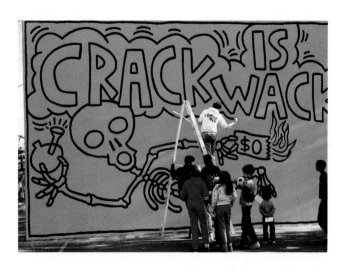

⟹ Part Three
Making Responsible Decisions:
Substance Use and Abuse

⮡ *Part Four   Getting Fit*

CHAPTER 12
NUTRITION FACTS AND FALLACIES   303

CHAPTER 13
WEIGHT MANAGEMENT   341

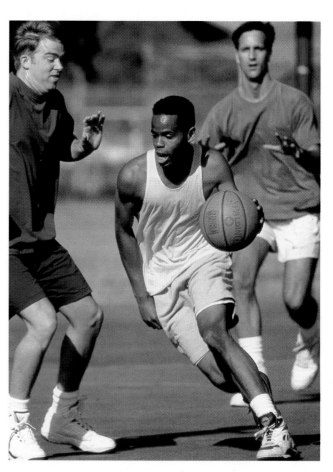

➠ *Part Five
Protecting Yourself from Disease*

CHAPTER 17
SEXUALLY TRANSMISSIBLE DISEASES 463

CHAPTER 18
IMMUNITY AND INFECTION 491

➠ *Part Six   Accepting Physical Limits*

CHAPTER 19
AGING: A VITAL PROCESS 515

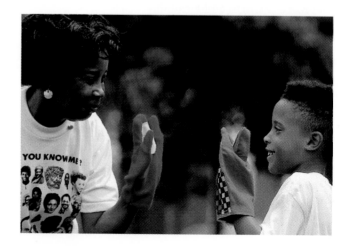

CHAPTER 20
DYING AND DEATH   537

➠ *Part Seven*
Making Choices in Health Care

CHAPTER 21
MEDICAL SELF-CARE: SKILLS FOR
THE HEALTH CARE CONSUMER   561

CHAPTER 22
THE HEALTH CARE SYSTEM   595

▥▶ **Part Eight**
Improving Your Chances: Personal Safety and Environmental Health

CHAPTER 23
INJURY PREVENTION AND CONTROL   615

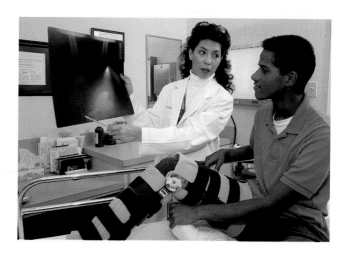

CHAPTER 24
ENVIRONMENTAL HEALTH   643

BOXES

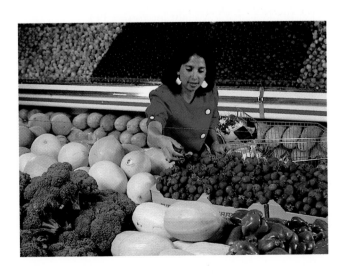

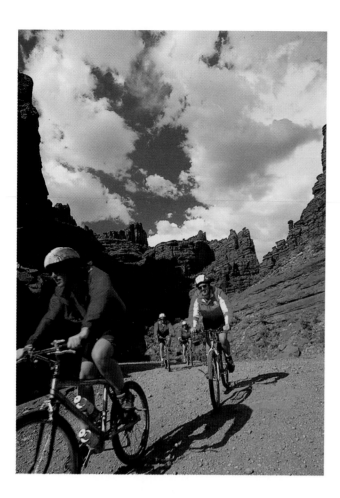

1

Taking Charge of Your Health

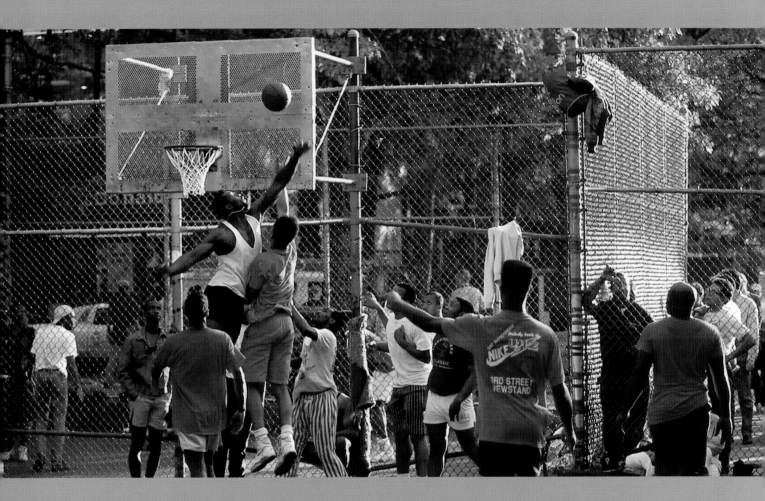

CONTENTS

You woke up early one morning to study and were surprised to run into one of your housemates just returning from a jog. You told her you liked jogging too but could never do it at that hour. She said she couldn't either if it weren't for her jogging buddy. "We agreed to jog together four days a week, and we make each other feel guilty if we miss a day. On days when it's still dark in the morning, we don't feel safe going alone, so if one of us doesn't show, the other one can't go at all. It's the buddy system—and it really works." Ordinarily you like jogging on your own, but lately you've been slacking off. Could the buddy system work for you?

One of your roommates never eats pizza when you all get together and order it for dinner, though she does join in the socializing. You thought she just didn't like it, but in the course of talking with her you found out otherwise. She mentioned that several members of her family died of colon cancer at an early age. "To help lower my risk of getting cancer, I try not to eat very many high-fat foods like cheese," she said. "That's why I usually don't eat pizza." You're a bit puzzled by her remarks—you thought no one knew exactly what caused cancer. And if cancer is inherited, what difference does it make what you eat? Is your roommate being an extremist, or does she know what she's talking about?

You started smoking as a sophomore in high school and finally managed to quit last summer. You'd like to convince your parents to stop smoking too, especially your dad, who's been smoking for 25 years and has a terrible cough. Armed with information about the hazards of smoking, you plan to mount a campaign over Christmas vacation to get them to quit. You tried to enlist your brother's help, but he says you'll never persuade them to change their ways, at least not just with facts. "Don't you think they know it's bad for them?" he asks you. Does he have a point? If so, what *can* you do?

College is great. The only thing is, your everyday routines have become haphazard as you've taken on new responsibilities. At first it was just a matter of skipping meals, staying up late, and procrastinating on homework, laundry, and housework. Now you've started sleeping through your alarm, missing your first class, and even forgetting assignments. You know you need to establish better habits, but you're not sure where to start. What can you do to get your life under control?

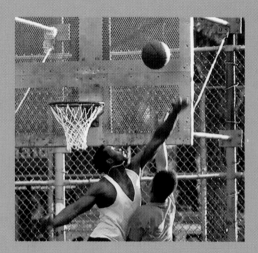

MAKING CONNECTIONS

Your experiences at college can present unique opportunities for change. Old routines are being discarded, and new patterns of behavior and thinking— some of which will become lifelong habits—are taking their place. The challenge is to make life-enhancing decisions and choices as you take charge of your health. In each of the health-related scenarios presented on this page, individuals have to use information, make a decision, or choose a course of action. What would you do in each of these situations? What response or decision would you make? This chapter provides information about health, wellness, and ways of changing behavior patterns that can be used in situations like these. After finishing the chapter, read the scenarios again. Has what you've learned changed how you would respond?

A sedentary college freshman begins riding his bike to class every day instead of driving. A hard-driving executive enrolls in a stress management course. A former smoker anticipates her impulse to backslide and joins a smoking-cessation support group. What do these people have in common? Each has made a commitment to take charge of his or her health.

Today, many people are striving for optimal health. A century ago, such a goal was unknown—people counted themselves lucky just to survive. A child born in 1890, for example, could expect to live only about 40 years. Killers such as polio, smallpox, diphtheria, measles, and mumps took the lives of a tragic number of infants and children in the days before vaccinations. Youngsters who escaped those threats still risked death from infectious diseases such as tuberculosis, typhus, or dysentery. In 1918 alone, 20 million people died in a flu epidemic. Millions of others lost their lives to common bacterial infections in the era before antibiotics. Environmental conditions—unrefrigerated food, poor sanitation, and air polluted by coal-burning furnaces and factories—contributed to the spread and the deadliness of these diseases.

The picture today is quite different. Over the past 100 years, life spans have nearly doubled. A sense of empowerment over our health has replaced the fatalism that prevailed in the last century. Today, our most serious health threats are chronic illnesses such as heart disease and cancer—diseases that we have the power to help prevent. Medical research has given us guidelines we can use to prolong our lives. Beyond that, it has provided us with information we can use to enjoy a quality of life unimagined by our grandparents.

The message of this book is that optimal health is something everyone can have. Achieving it requires knowledge, self-awareness, motivation, and effort; but the benefits last a lifetime. Optimal health comes mostly from a healthy lifestyle—patterns of behavior that promote and support your health now and as you get older. In the pages that follow, you'll find current information and suggestions about topics in health that you can use to build a better lifestyle. You'll also find tools for assessing yourself, for exploring your inner experiences, and for planning and carrying out specific behavior changes. You can use this book to take charge of your health and improve the quality of your life.

WHAT IS HEALTH?

What exactly is meant by the term *health?* The definition is influenced by how people lead their lives, and today's ideas about health are very different from those held in 1890. Let's look briefly at how the concept of health has evolved over a century.

Health as the Absence of Illness

In the past, a person who was free from pain, disability, and symptoms of disease was considered healthy. From the earliest times, epidemics of infectious diseases have periodically swept around the world, ravaging whole populations. The worst outbreak of bubonic plague took more than 25 million lives in Europe in the fourteenth century, but it was only one of more than 100 major outbreaks dating back to biblical times. Entire tribes of Native Americans were wiped out by infectious diseases brought to this country by European colonizers. No age was immune from the terrors of epidemic, whether of malaria, measles, syphilis, cholera, or some other contagious disease. No wonder health was defined as simply the absence of illness. Throughout history, this was the best one could hope for.

When medical science began to unravel the mystery of these diseases and bring them under control, life expectancies rose and death rates fell. (For a description of the important medical discoveries of the nineteenth and twentieth centuries, see the box "Ages of Health Advancement.") Notions about health changed, too.

Health as Longevity: Is Longer Better?

Once antibiotics were introduced for widespread use in the 1940s, people speculated that all diseases might soon be conquered by modern medicine. An age of medical miracles seemed just around the corner. Health began to be defined in terms of longevity—how long people could expect to live.

But as communicable disease yielded to antibiotics, vaccines, and public health campaigns, a different set of diseases emerged as a major health threat. A new pattern of death took shape. By the 1950s, degenerative diseases such as coronary heart disease, cancer, stroke, diabetes, atherosclerosis, and cirrhosis had replaced pneumonia and influenza as the leading causes of death in the United States.

Degenerative diseases spawned new treatments—open heart surgery, chemotherapy and radiation, organ transplants, and others—but they were less successful than earlier innovations had been. They were also enormously expensive and raised a new set of social and ethical questions. Many people began to question the value of some of the most advanced procedures, such as heart-lung transplants, which seem to lead to incapacitating strokes, and life-support systems, which sometimes are used to keep people alive in a permanent vegetative state. Merely being alive—with minimal physical and mental functions, supported by machines or in a coma—was now seen as a kind of living death.

It became apparent that quantity of life without quality of life is no blessing (Figure 1-1). It also became clear that the best treatment for the new killers is prevention—people taking care of their own bodies. A number of habits

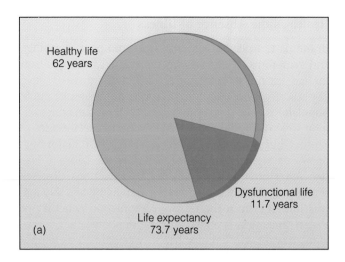

(a)

Healthy life
62 years

Dysfunctional life
11.7 years

Life expectancy
73.7 years

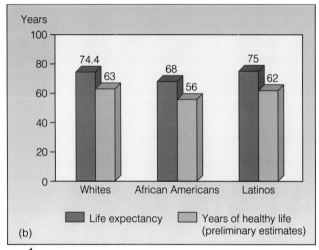

(b)

Life expectancy   Years of healthy life (preliminary estimates)

VITAL STATISTICS

Figure 1-1 *Quantity of life vs. quality of life.*
(a) Years of healthy life as a proportion of life expectancy, U.S. population.(b) Years of healthy life vs. life expectancy for whites, African Americans, and Latinos in the United States.
Adapted from Department of Health and Human Services. 1990. *Healthy People 2000: National Health Promotion and Disease Prevention Objectives.* Washington, D.C.: U.S. Government Printing Office. Publication No. (PHS)91-50212.

and behaviors were identified as culprits in the development of disease; others seemed to promote health. Many of these factors—diet, work, play, sexual and reproductive choices, and the environment in which we live—turned out to be things that individuals can themselves control. Health cannot be prescribed; physicians and the health establishment can do little more than provide information, advice, and encouragement—the rest is up to each individual.

TERMS

Wellness Optimal health and vitality, encompassing physical, emotional, intellectual, spiritual, interpersonal, social, and environmental well-being.
Vitality The ability of an organism to function with vigor.

Wellness: The New Health Goal

No longer do we consider health to be simply the absence of disease. Today we view it also as the presence of **vitality**—the ability to function with vigor and to live life actively, energetically, and fully. Vitality comes from **wellness**, a state of optimal physical, emotional, intellectual, spiritual, interpersonal, social, environmental, and even planetary well-being. At all ages and at all levels of physical and mental ability, people can increase their vitality and wellness.

Physical Health Optimal physical health requires eating well, exercising, avoiding harmful habits, making responsible decisions about sex, learning and watching for the symptoms of disease, getting regular medical and dental check-ups, and taking steps to prevent injuries at home, on the road, and on the job. The habits you develop and the decisions you make today will determine to a great extent not only how many years you will live but also the quality of life you will enjoy during those years.

Emotional Health Optimism, trust, self-esteem, self-acceptance, self-confidence, self-control, satisfying relationships, and an ability to share feelings are just some of the qualities and aspects of emotional wellness. Emotional health is a dynamic state that fluctuates with your physical, intellectual, spiritual, and interpersonal health. Maintaining emotional wellness requires monitoring and exploring your thoughts and feelings, identifying obstacles to emotional well-being, and finding solutions to emotional problems, with the help of a therapist if necessary.

Intellectual Health The hallmarks of intellectual wellness include an openness to new ideas, a capacity to question and think critically, and the motivation to master new skills. A sense of humor, creativity, and curiosity are others. An active mind is essential to overall wellness, for it is your mind that learns, evaluates, and stores health information. Your mind detects problems, finds solutions, and directs behavior. People who enjoy intellectual wellness never stop learning. They relish new experiences and challenges and actively seek them out.

Spiritual Health To enjoy spiritual health is to possess the capacity for love, compassion, forgiveness, altruism, joy, peace, and fulfillment. Spiritual wellness is a state of harmony and balance between oneself and others and between inner needs and the demands of the world. It is an antidote to cynicism, anger, bitterness, fear, anxiety, and pessimism. Organized religions help many people develop spiritual health. Many other people find meaning and purpose in their lives on their own, through nature, art, meditation, political action, or good works.

Ages of Health Advancement

A study of death rates over the last century illustrates the dramatic changes that have taken place in the nature of health problems and the solutions to these problems. The figure below shows overall death rates in the United States (age-adjusted) from 1885 to the present, with the times at which major medical innovations became available.

- Over 70 percent of the decline in death rate between 1885 and the present occurred *before* the most significant medical innovations were introduced, during a period dominated by improvements in the environment and in our public health policies.

- The discovery of antibiotics in the 1930s accelerated the decline in U.S. death rates for a period of about 20 years.

- The decline slid to a stop in the early 1950s as problems still responsive to antibiotics began to disappear. Over the next 20 years (early 1950s to early 1970s), there was almost no reduction in death rate or increase in life expectancy. Ironically, this is the period when many of our most expensive medical innovations were introduced.

- Death rates again began to decline in the early 1970s, due to a drop in deaths from heart attacks and strokes. This drop coincided with reduced rates of smoking, lower-fat diets, and increased exercise among American adults.

Adapted from D. M. Vickery. 1978. *Life Plan for Your Health* (Reading, Mass.: Addison-Wesley), pp. 17–18.

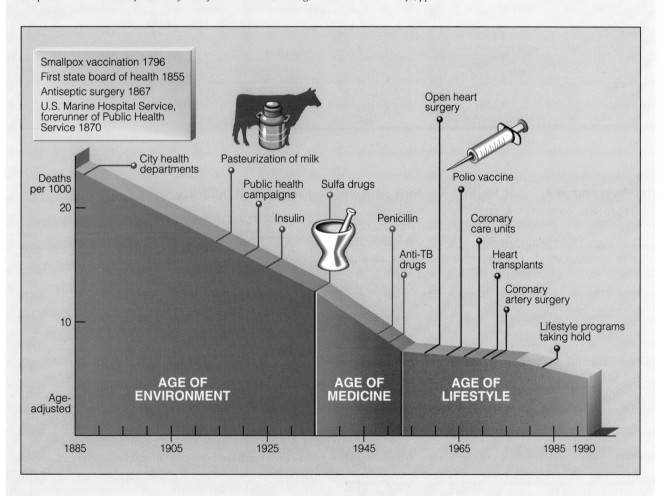

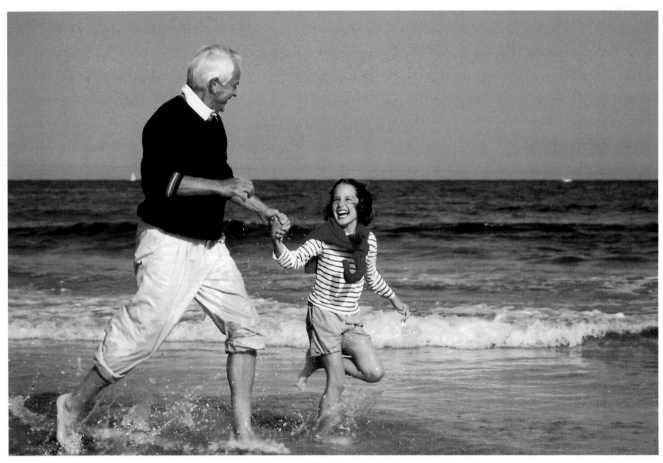

With wellness comes vitality, exuberance, a capacity for joy—and for fun. What makes you feel vital?

Interpersonal and Social Health Satisfying relationships are basic to both physical and emotional health. We need loving, supportive people in our lives. And we need to be needed by them. Developing interpersonal health means learning good communication skills, developing the capacity for intimacy, and cultivating a support network of caring friends or family members. Social health means participating in and contributing to your community, country, and world.

Environmental or Planetary Health Increasingly, personal health depends on the health of the planet. Wellness requires learning about and protecting yourself from environmental hazards—and doing what you can to reduce or eliminate them.

CHOOSING WELLNESS

This wellness model of health has a far-reaching effect on how we view ourselves and live our lives. We now have greater control over our health than human beings have ever had before—and greater responsibility for it as well.

Factors That Influence Wellness

Scientific research is continually revealing new connections between our habits and emotions and the level of health we enjoy. For example, heart disease, the nation's number one killer, is associated with cigarette smoking, high levels of stress, habitually hostile and suspicious attitudes toward the world and the people in it, a high-fat diet, and a sedentary way of life (Table 1-1). Other habits are beneficial. Regular exercise, for example, can help to prevent heart disease, high blood pressure, diabetes, osteoporosis, and depression and may reduce the risk of colon cancer, stroke, and back injury. As we learn more about how our actions affect our bodies and minds, we can make informed choices for a healthier life.

Of course, our behavior isn't the only factor involved in health. Our heredity, the environment we live in, and whether we have access to adequate health care are other important influences. These factors, which vary both for individuals and for groups, can interact in ways that produce either health or disease. (For a discussion of how different factors affect people as members of groups, see the box "Health Issues for Diverse Populations.") For example, a sedentary lifestyle combined with a genetic predisposition to diabetes can greatly increase an individual's

Rank	Cause of Death	Number	Percent of Total Deaths	Lifestyle Factors
1	Heart disease	718,090	33.2	D I S
2	Cancers	514,310	23.8	D S A
3	Strokes	144,070	6.7	D I S
4	Accidents	91,700	4.2	S A
	(Motor vehicle)	(45,240)	(2.1)	
	(All others)	(46,460)	(2.1)	
5	Chronic obstructive lung diseases	89,130	4.1	S
6	Pneumonia and influenza	74,980	3.5	S
7	Diabetes mellitus	49,980	2.3	D I
8	Suicide	30,200	1.4	A
9	AIDS	29,850	1.4	
10	Homicide	27,440	1.3	A
	All causes	2,165,000	100.0	

Key:
  D Cause of death in which diet plays a part.
  I Cause of death in which an inactive lifestyle plays a part.
  S Cause of death in which smoking plays a part.
  A Cause of death in which excessive alcohol consumption plays a part.

Source: National Center for Health Statistics. 1992. *Monthly Vital Statistics Report,* vol. 40, no. 13, 30 September.

risk of developing diabetes. If this person also lacks adequate health care, he or she is much more likely to suffer dangerous complications from diabetes and have a lower quality of life.

But in many cases, behavior can tip the balance toward health even where inheritance or environment are negative factors. For example, breast cancer can run in families, but it also may be associated with being overweight and having a sedentary lifestyle. A woman with a family history of breast cancer is less likely to develop the disease if she controls her weight, exercises regularly, does breast self-exams, and has regular mammograms taken.

Similarly, a young man with a family history of obesity can maintain a normal weight by being careful to balance calorie intake against activities that burn calories. If your life is highly stressful, you can lessen the chances of heart disease and stroke by learning ways to manage and cope with stress. If you live in an area with severe air pollution, you can reduce the risk of lung disease by not smoking. You can also take an active role in improving your environment. Behaviors like these allow you to make a difference in how great an impact heredity and environment will have on your health.

A Wellness Profile

What does it mean to be healthy today? A basic list of important behaviors and habits includes the following:

- Having a sense of responsibility for your own health and taking an active rather than passive stance toward your life

- Learning to manage stress in effective ways

- Maintaining high self-esteem and mentally healthy ways of interacting with other people

- Understanding your sexuality and having satisfying intimate relationships

- Avoiding tobacco and other drugs; using alcohol wisely, if at all

- Eating well, exercising, and maintaining normal weight

- Knowing when to treat your illnesses yourself and when to seek help

- Understanding the health system and using it intelligently

- Knowing the facts about cardiovascular disease, cancer, infections, sexually transmitted diseases, and injuries and using your knowledge to protect yourself against them

- Understanding the natural processes of aging and dying and accepting the limits of human existence

- Understanding how the environment affects your health and taking appropriate action to improve it

We Americans are a diverse people. Our ancestry is European, African, Asian, Pacific Islander, Latin American, and Native American. We live in cities, suburbs, and rural areas, working at every imaginable occupation, in luxury, comfort, and poverty. In no other country in the world do so many diverse people live and work together every day. And in no other country is the understanding and tolerance of differences so much a part of the political and cultural ideal. We are at heart a nation of diversity, and, though we often fall short of our goal, we strive for justice and equality among all people.

When it comes to health, most differences among people are insignificant—the majority of health issues concern us all equally. We all need to eat well, exercise, manage stress, and cultivate satisfying personal relationships. We need to know how to protect ourselves from heart disease, cancer, sexually transmitted diseases, and injuries. We need to know what to do when we're sick and how to use the health care system.

But some of our differences—differences among us both as individuals and as members of groups—do have important implications for health. Some of us, for example, have inherited predispositions to develop certain health problems, such as high cholesterol or osteoporosis. Some of us have grown up eating foods that raise our risk of heart disease or obesity. Some of us live in environments that increase the chances that we'll smoke cigarettes or abuse alcohol. These health-related differences among individuals and groups can be biological—determined genetically—or cultural—acquired as patterns of behavior through daily interactions with our families, communities, and society. Many health conditions are a function of biology and culture combined. A person can have a genetic predisposition to a disease, for example, but won't actually develop the disease itself unless certain lifestyle factors are present, such as stress or a poor diet.

When we talk about health issues for diverse populations, we face two related dangers. The first is the danger of stereotyping, of talking about people as groups rather than as individuals. It's certainly true that every person is an individual with his or her own unique genetic endowment as well as unique experiences in life. But many of these influences are shared with others of similar genetic and cultural background. Statements about these group similarities can be useful; for example, they can alert people to areas that may be of special concern for them and their families.

The second danger is that of overgeneralizing, of ignoring the extensive biological and cultural diversity that exists among peoples who are grouped together. Groups labeled Latino or Hispanic, for example, include Mexican Americans, Puerto Ricans, Cuban Americans, people from South and Central America, and other Spanish-speaking peoples. Similarly, the population labeled Native American includes hundreds of recognized tribal nations, each with its own genetic and cultural heritage. It's important to keep these considerations in mind whenever you read about different populations.

Health-related differences among groups can be identified and described along several different dimensions, including the following:

Gender. Men and women have different life expectancies, different reproductive concerns, and different incidences of many diseases, including heart disease, cancer, stroke, cirrhosis of the liver, and osteoporosis. Men are more likely to develop heart disease in middle age. Women are more affected by issues involving contraception and reproductive choices. They live longer than men. They have lower suicide rates. They are more likely to be poor.

Socioeconomic status. Many health differences in our society are related to income level. People with low income have higher rates of infant mortality, of traumatic injury and violent death, and of many diseases, including cancer, heart disease, tuberculosis, and HIV infection. They are more likely to eat poorly, be overweight, smoke, drink, and use drugs. They have less access to health care services and medical insurance. Poverty is a far more important predictor of poor health than is any factor of race or ethnicity. However, it is often mixed with other factors in a way that makes it difficult to distinguish what causes what. A factor that may be even more closely associated with health status is level of educational attainment.

Race/ethnicity. Some genetic diseases are concentrated in certain gene pools, the result of each ethnic group's relatively distinct history. Sickle-cell anemia occurs almost exclusively among people of African ancestry. Tay-Sachs disease afflicts people of Eastern European Jewish heritage. Cystic fibrosis is more common among Northern Europeans. In addition to biological differences, many cultural differences occur along ethnic lines. Ethnic groups may vary in their traditional diets; their patterns of family and interpersonal relationships; their attitudes toward tobacco, alcohol, and other drugs; and their health beliefs and practices, to name just a few differences.

Four broad racial/ethnic minority groups are usually distinguished in American society—African Americans or blacks; Latinos; Asian and Pacific Islander Americans; and Native Americans. Each has some special health concerns.

• African Americans are the largest minority group, making up 12 percent of the American population. Although African Americans are represented in every socioeconomic group, one-third live below the poverty line. This is a principal factor in the health status of African Americans, which lags behind that of the total population in several areas, including life expectancy, infant mortality, and incidence of chronic and infectious disease.

The leading causes of death among African Americans are the same as for the overall population, but African American men die from strokes at almost twice the rate of men in the total population. Strokes are related to high blood pressure, which is twice as common among blacks as among the total population. Also contributing to cardiorespiratory problems is sickle-cell anemia. Another special concern is cancer. African American men have a higher risk of cancer than do nonblack men, with a 25 percent higher risk for all cancers and a 45 percent higher risk for lung cancer. Diabetes is a special concern for African American women, especially those who are overweight.

• Latinos are the second largest and fastest growing minority group in the United States, making up about 8 percent of the total population. About two-thirds of the Latino population are of Mexican descent; 12 percent are Puerto Rican; 5 percent are Cuban American; and smaller proportions are of South or Central American or Caribbean background. There are many cultural and biological differences among the various Latino populations, but they are frequently grouped together, often under the umbrella term *Hispanic*. This label is somewhat misleading, since many Latinos are of mixed Spanish and American Indian descent, or of mixed Spanish, Indian, and African American descent. Nevertheless, *Hispanic* is the term most commonly used in studies and statistics to identify Latino populations.

Overall, Latinos tend to have lower rates of death from heart disease, stroke, and cancer than do non-Hispanic whites and African Americans. They also have lower incidences of high cholesterol, high blood pressure, and osteoporosis. Some special concerns are diabetes, gallbladder disease, and overweight, all probably related to American Indian descent. The birth rate among Latinos is higher than that of the total population, and the use of contraceptives is relatively low.

• Asian and Pacific Islander Americans, like Latinos, are characterized by diversity. The two oldest and largest groups are Japanese Americans and Chinese Americans. Other groups include Vietnamese, Laotians, Cambodians, Koreans, Filipinos, Asian Indians, Native Hawaiians, and other Pacific Islanders. Numbering over 11 million people, they speak more than 30 different languages and represent a similar number of distinct cultures.

Health differences also exist among these groups. For example, Southeast Asian men have higher rates of lung cancer and liver cancer than does the rest of the population, and Hawaiian women have higher than average rates of breast cancer. Diabetes is a concern among Asian Americans; its appearance may be triggered by the American diet. Among recent immigrants from Southeast Asia, tuberculosis and hepatitis B are serious health problems. Tobacco use is another concern; among some Southeast Asians, over 90 percent of the men smoke.

• Native Americans, also called American Indians and Alaska Natives, number about 1.6 million people. Most Native Americans embrace a tribal identity, such as Sioux, Navaho, or Hopi, rather than the identity of Native American.

Native Americans have lower rates of death from heart disease, strokes, and cancer than does the overall population, but they also have high rates of early death. For those under 45, causes of death include unintentional injuries (accidents), homicide, suicide, and cirrhosis; many of these problems are linked to alcohol abuse. Diabetes is very prevalent, occurring in over 20 percent of all adults in some tribes. Many Native Americans have limited access to health care services.

These are just some of the "dimensions of diversity"—differences among people and groups that are associated with different health concerns and problems. Other factors too, such as age or disability, are associated with particular health concerns. In this book, topics and issues in health that affect different American populations are given special consideration. Look for these discussions in boxes labeled "Dimensions of Diversity." Also discussed in these boxes are health issues and practices in other parts of the world. These explorations beyond the borders of the United States broaden our view, showing us both what we share with people in other societies and how we differ—our common concerns and our divergent solutions. All of these discussions are designed to deepen our understanding of the core concepts of health, vitality, and wellness in the context of ever-growing diversity.

This may seem like a tall order, and in a sense it *is* the work of a lifetime. But the habits that you establish now are crucial: They tend to set lifelong patterns. Some behaviors do more than set up patterns—they produce permanent changes in your health. If you become addicted to drugs or alcohol at age 20, for example, you may be able to kick the habit, but you will never again be a non-addict; you will always face the struggle of a recovered addict. If you contract gonorrhea, you may discover later that your reproductive organs were damaged without your realizing it, making you infertile or sterile. If you ruin your knees doing the wrong exercises or hurt your back in an automobile accident, you won't have them to count on when you're older. Some things just can't be undone.

> *Personal Insight* What sorts of health habits did your parents and other family members have when you were growing up? Were they active or sedentary? Did they smoke? What kind of foods did they eat? How have your own health habits been influenced by those of your family members?

GETTING DOWN TO BASICS: HOW DO YOU REACH WELLNESS?

Your life may not resemble that described by the Wellness Profile at all. You probably have a number of healthy habits and some others that place your health at risk. Maybe your life is more like this:

> It's Tuesday. Simon wakes up feeling blue, not really wanting to get out of bed. He wishes he knew what he wanted to do with his life. He wishes he'd meet someone new and fall in love. No time for breakfast, so he grabs a cup of coffee to drink during his first class. He hasn't done the reading and stares blankly at the teacher during the lecture. Later he goes to the student union and has a sugary doughnut and some more coffee; he lights up his first cigarette of the day. Lunch is a fast-food cheeseburger, french fries, and a shake. He spends the afternoon at the library desperately researching a paper that's due the next day, finally quitting at six o'clock and heading to the student union for a beer. He meets up with some buddies and joins them for pizza instead of having dinner at the dorm. By eleven he's tired, but he's written only one page, so he takes a little "speed" to keep going. It makes his heart race and floods his head with so many ideas he has difficulty sorting them all out. He works feverishly and finally finishes at four the next morning. Exhausted, he falls asleep in his clothes. The next thing he knows, it's Wednesday morning, time to start a new day.

This is hardly an ideal lifestyle, but it's not unusual. Simon functions okay, comes through on his commitments, and shows some self-discipline. On the other hand, time gets away from him, he doesn't get much exercise, doesn't eat as well as he could, and flirts with the dangers of taking drugs. Overall, he seems low on energy and has little control over his life. He could be living a lot better.

Simon isn't alone in neglecting or abusing his health; many people fall into a lifestyle that puts their health at risk. Some aren't aware of the damage they're doing to themselves; others are aware but aren't motivated or don't know how to change; and still others want to change but can't seem to get started. All of these are very real problems, but they're not insurmountable. If they were, there would be no ex-smokers, recovering alcoholics, or successful graduates of weight loss programs around. People can and do make difficult changes in their lives.

Taking big steps toward health may at first seem like too much work, but as you make progress toward wellness, it gets easier. At first you'll be rewarded with a greater sense of control over your life, a feeling of empowerment, higher self-esteem, and more joy in life. These benefits will encourage you to make further improvements. Over time, you'll come to know what wellness feels like—more energy; greater vitality; deeper feelings of curiosity, interest, and enjoyment; and a higher quality of life. To determine whether your current lifestyle promotes wellness, take the quiz in the box "Wellness: Evaluate Your Lifestyle."

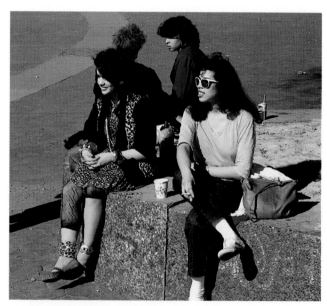

No facts, warnings, or advice from her friends or family will persuade this young woman to quit smoking until she decides to quit herself. Behavior changes, especially those involving powerful, long-standing habits, require self-examination and a deep personal commitment.

Taking Charge of Your Health: Knowledge, Motivation, Commitment, and Sense of Control

What makes you act the way you do? Countless factors come into play in determining your behaviors, both internal and external, both rational and irrational—knowledge, emotions, values, ideals, habit, circumstances, beliefs, and perceptions about yourself and the world.

Changing your behavior can be complicated by the many factors involved. To make good decisions, you need facts and information about topics and issues in health. To put those behavior changes into action, you also need knowledge about yourself—where you fit into the health picture and what strengths you can draw on to change your behavior and improve your health. Knowledge is a necessary ingredient, but knowledge alone isn't usually enough to make you act. For example, millions of smokers stick to their habit even though they know it's bad for their health.

Motivation is another prerequisite for change. Although some people are motivated by long-term goals, such as avoiding disease that may hit them in 20 or 30 years, most are more likely to be provoked to action by shorter-term, more personal goals. Looking better, being more popular with the opposite sex, doing better in school, getting a good job, improving at a sport, and gaining higher self-esteem are common sources of motivation.

Many behaviors involve making choices. For example, you might want to lose weight so you'll look good in a bathing suit next month. But you may also be sorely tempted by a hot fudge sundae right now. When the sundae is right in front of you, you'll probably choose immediate gratification over a long-term goal. Motivation alone is usually no more effective at breaking a long-standing habit than knowledge alone is.

What does it take? Motivation has to be built on commitment, the resolve to stick with a plan no matter what temptations you encounter. Commitment provides a turning point when you bring the full force of your resolve to change a particular situation. With deeply rooted habits, it often takes a while to build up to the level of commitment you need to conquer a habit. Many smokers, for example, don't succeed in quitting until their third or fourth try, when their commitment is fueled by frustration and disgust over earlier failures, anger at cigarette manufacturers, and a burning desire to succeed.

Whether you succeed in changing behaviors is rooted in how strongly you believe you will succeed, what you unconsciously intend, and the kind of support you can draw from family and friends. Perhaps the most crucial factor is how active or passive you want to be about your life. Who is controlling your life? Is it your parents, your friends, your school, circumstances, the stars? Or is it you? When you succeed in making changes, it is because *you* have taken charge of your life. You have come to see that what you do is within your control.

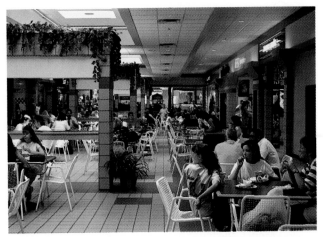

Many actions and behaviors are triggered by external stimuli, or cues in the environment. The sight and smell of this shopping mall restaurant court is a powerful stimulus, one that can lure people in for a meal whether or not they are really hungry. If these shoppers want to have more control over their eating in the future, they will probably have to avoid the restaurant court.

A Plan for Action: Behavior Self-Management

Most of your behaviors are habits you've learned. They may be deeply ingrained, long-standing habits; but they're still habits, and you can unlearn them the same way you learned them. The key is to approach them in a systematic way. The approach recommended in this book is based on principles of behavioral self-management that have proven effective in helping people make changes in their lives. As you read about different areas of health in the chapters that follow, you can apply the self-management model to your own behaviors to help you plan and carry out changes in your life.

The heart of the behavior self-management model is isolating a **target behavior** that you wish to change and identifying the circumstances that trigger it and the consequences that follow it. Once you know these, you can intervene to break the chain of habit.

Behaviors can be triggered or stimulated by many different circumstances. **External stimuli,** or cues, are events or sensations in the environment—the sound of your name being called in class, the smell of bacon cooking, the sight of a sexy person. **Internal stimuli** are thoughts, feelings, and other inner sensations and experiences that trigger an action—hunger, low levels of nicotine in the blood, exhaustion.

Target behavior   An isolated behavior selected as the object of a behavior change program.
External stimuli (cues)   Factors from outside the person that arouse activity.
Internal stimuli   Factors from within the person that arouse activity.

TERMS

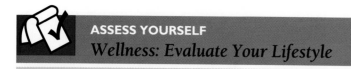

All of us want optimal health. But many of us do not know how to achieve it. That's what this brief test, adapted from one created by the U.S. Public Health Service, is all about. The behaviors covered in the test are recommended for most Americans. (Some of them may not apply to people with certain diseases or disabilities, or to pregnant women, who may require special advice from their physicians.) After you take the quiz, add up your score for each section.

Tobacco Use

If you never use tobacco, enter a score of 10 for this section and go to the next section.

	Almost Always	Sometimes	Never
1. I avoid using tobacco.	2	1	0
2. I smoke only low-tar-and-nicotine cigarettes, or I smoke a pipe or cigars, or I use smokeless tobacco.	2	1	0

Tobacco Score: _____

Alcohol and Other Drugs

1. I avoid alcohol, or I drink no more than 1 or 2 drinks a day.	4	1	0
2. I avoid using alcohol or other drugs as a way of handling stressful situations or problems in my life.	2	1	0
3. I am careful not to drink alcohol when taking medications, such as for colds or allergies, or when pregnant.	2	1	0
4. I read and follow the label directions when using prescribed and over-the-counter drugs.	2	1	0

Alcohol and Other Drugs Score: _____

Nutrition

1. I eat a variety of foods each day, including 5 or more servings of fresh fruits and vegetables.	3	1	0
2. I limit the amount of fat and saturated fat in my diet.	3	1	0
3. I avoid skipping meals.	2	1	0
4. I limit the amount of salt and sugar I eat.	2	1	0

Nutrition Score: _____

Exercise/Fitness

1. I engage in moderate exercise for 20 to 60 minutes, three to five times a week.	4	1	0
2. I maintain a healthy weight, avoiding overweight and underweight.	2	1	0
3. I do exercises to develop muscular strength and endurance at least twice a week.	2	1	0
4. I spend some of my leisure time participating in physical activities such as gardening, bowling, golf, or baseball.	2	1	0

Exercise/Fitness Score: _____

	Almost Always	Sometimes	Never

Emotional Health

	Almost Always	Sometimes	Never
1. I enjoy being a student and I have a job or do other work that I like.	2	1	0
2. I find it easy to relax and express my feelings freely.	2	1	0
3. I manage stress well.	2	1	0
4. I have close friends, relatives, or others I can talk to about personal matters and call on for help.	2	1	0
5. I participate in group activities (such as church and community organizations) or hobbies that I enjoy.	2	1	0

Emotional Health Score: _____

Safety

	Almost Always	Sometimes	Never
1. I wear a seat belt while riding in a car.	2	1	0
2. I avoid driving while under the influence of alcohol or other drugs.	2	1	0
3. I obey traffic rules and the speed limit when driving.	2	1	0
4. I read and follow instructions on the labels of potentially harmful products or substances, such as household cleaners, poisons, and electrical appliances.	2	1	0
5. I avoid smoking in bed.	2	1	0

Safety Score: _____

Disease Prevention

	Almost Always	Sometimes	Never
1. I know the warning signs of cancer, diabetes, heart attack, and stroke.	2	1	0
2. I avoid overexposure to the sun and use sunscreens.	2	1	0
3. I get recommended medical screening tests (such as blood pressure checks and Pap smears), immunizations, and booster shots.	2	1	0
4. I practice monthly breast/testicle self-exams.	2	1	0
5. I am not sexually active *or* I have sex with only one mutually faithful, uninfected partner *or* I always engage in "safer sex" (using condoms and a spermicide containing nonoxynol-9) *and* I do not share needles.	2	1	0

Disease Prevention Score: _____

What Your Scores Mean

Scores of 9 and 10   Excellent! Your answers show that you are aware of the importance of this area to wellness. More important, you are putting your knowledge to work for you by practicing good health habits. As long as you continue to do so, this area should not pose a serious health risk. It's likely that you are setting an example for your family and friends to follow. Since you earned a very high test score on this part of the test, you may want to focus on other areas where your scores indicate room for improvement.

Scores of 6 to 8   Your health practices in this area are good, but there is room for improvement. Look again at the items you answered with a "Sometimes" or "Almost Never."

What changes can you make to improve your score? Even a small change can often help you achieve better health.

Scores of 3 to 5   Your health risks are showing! You may need more information about the risks you are facing and about why it is important for you to change these behaviors. Perhaps you need help in deciding how to successfully make the changes you desire.

Scores of 0 to 2   Your answers show that you may be taking serious and unnecessary risks with your health. Perhaps you are not aware of the risks and what to do about them. You can easily get the information and help you need to improve, if you wish. The next step is up to you.

Behaviors can also have different kinds of consequences, or "payoffs." Consequences that tend to make you repeat a behavior are known as reinforcers. Some reinforcers, known as **positive reinforcers**, encourage you to repeat a behavior by adding something positive that makes you feel good. For example, drinking a few glasses of wine at a party may give you feelings of pleasure, excitement and fun, at least temporarily, and make it more likely you will drink again at the next party.

Other reinforcers, known as **negative reinforcers**, encourage a behavior by covering up or removing something unpleasant that was making you feel bad. When a person is addicted to nicotine, for example, smoking a cigarette removes the unpleasant feelings of nicotine craving. Both kinds of reinforcers help a behavior remain a habit, one by adding something and increasing your pleasure, the other by removing something and decreasing your discomfort. Sometimes a behavior is supported by both positive and negative reinforcers; for example, taking a drink makes you feel good and at the same time lowers your inhibitions and your anxiety around people. (Consequences that make a behavior less likely to happen are known as punishers, and for a variety of reasons they aren't effective in self-management programs.)

Intervening in the chain of events that occur before and after a behavior is the basis of behavior self-management. This approach provides surprisingly powerful tools that you can use to make the changes you want in your life. Let's consider now the actual steps involved in putting together a behavior management program.

Putting Together a Behavior Management Program

If your lifestyle is more like Simon's than the ideal, there may be several changes you can make to improve it. The worst thing you can do is to try to change everything at once—quit smoking, give up high-fat foods, eat a good breakfast, start jogging, do sit-ups, plan your study time better, avoid drugs, get enough sleep. Overdoing it leads to burnout. Concentrate on one behavior that you want to change and work on it systematically. To start with something simple, substitute margarine for butter in your diet, or skim milk for whole milk. Or you might concentrate on getting to sleep by 10 P.M. Working on even one behavior will make high demands on your energy. Once you've decided on a behavior you want to change, following the six steps we discuss next will help you succeed.

Your key to success is to be consistent and to persist. Don't skip steps or rush through the plan. You may think you know everything there is to know about your target behavior, but people are almost always surprised by patterns that emerge from carefully recorded daily accounts of their thoughts and actions.

1. *Monitor your behavior and gather data.* Begin your program by keeping careful records of the behavior you wish to change (your target behavior) and the circumstances surrounding it. You can keep these records in a health journal, a notebook in which you write the details of your behavior along with observations and comments. Note exactly what the activity was, when and where it happened, what you were doing, and what your feelings were at the time. In a journal for a weight loss program, for example, you would typically record how much food you ate, the time of day, the situation, the location, your feelings, and how hungry you were (Figure 1-2). Keep your journal for a week or two to get some solid information about the behavior you want to change.

2. *Analyze the data and identify patterns.* After you have collected data on the behavior, analyze the data to identify patterns in stimuli and responses. When are you most hungry? When are you most likely to overeat? What events seem to trigger your appetite? Perhaps you are especially hungry at midmorning or when you put off eating dinner until 9 P.M. Perhaps you overindulge in food and drink when you go to a particular restaurant or when you're with certain friends. Be sure to note the connections between your feelings and such external stimuli as time of day, location, situation, and the actions of others around you. Do you always think of having a cigarette when you read the newspaper? Do you always bite your fingernails when you're studying?

3. *Set specific goals.* Whatever your ultimate goal, it's a good idea to break it down into a few small steps, or "chunks." Your plan will seem less overwhelming and more manageable, increasing the chances that you'll stick to it. You'll also build in more opportunities to reward yourself (as discussed in step 5) as well as milestones you can use to measure your progress.

   If you plan to lose 30 pounds, for example, you'll find it easier to take off 10 pounds at a time. If you want to quit smoking, plan a series of steps that takes you to the day you'll quit, such as asking yourself how ready you are to quit, listing your reasons for quitting, looking at patterns from other times you tried to quit, then cutting your daily smoking in half, and, three days later, quitting altogether. Take the easier steps first and work up to the harder steps. If you think through your goals carefully, you'll probably succeed.

Time of day	M/S	Food eaten	Cals.	H	Where did you eat?	What else were you doing?	How did someone else influence you?	What made you want to eat what you did?	Emotions and feelings?	Thoughts and concerns?
7:30	M	1 C Crispix cereal 1/2 C skim milk coffee, black 1 C orange juice	110 40 — 120	3	dorm cafeteria	reading newspaper	eating w/ friends, but I ate what I usually eat	I always eat cereal in the morning	a little keyed up & worried	thinking about quiz in class today
10:30	S	1 apple	90	1	library	studying	alone	felt tired & wanted to wake up	tired	worried about next class
12:30	M	1 C chili 1 roll 1 pat butter 1 orange 2 oatmeal cookies 1 soda	290 120 35 60 120 150	2	cafeteria terrace	talking	eating w/ friends; we decided to eat at the cafeteria	wanted to be part of group	excited and happy	interested in hearing everyone's plans for the weekend
3:00	S	candy bar	250	1	hallway	waiting for next class	alone	wanted a break	bored	thinking about next class
6:30	M	4 oz roast chicken 3/4 C mashed potatoes 3/4 C peas 1/2 C ice cream 1 soda	205 150 90 125 150	3	student union	talking w/ friends	we all got ice cream for dessert	best thing available for dinner	relaxing w/friends	thinking about paper to write this evening
10:30	S	hot chocolate 1 C plain popcorn TOTAL FOR DAY	100 25 2230	1	living room	watch TV w/roommates	just went along with the group	it was already fixed	tired of studying; wanted a break	nothing in particular

M/S = Meal or snack   H = Hunger rating (0-3)

Figure 1-2 *Sample health journal.*

4. *Make a personal contract.* Once you have set your goals and developed a plan of action, make your plan into a personal contract. A serious personal contract clearly states your objective and your commitment to reach it. You may add details of your plan—the date you'll begin; the completed steps you'll use to measure your progress; the date you expect to reach your final goal; and perhaps the time, resources, and energy you've committed to the plan. The box "A Personal Contract for Change" gives more details. It often helps to have another person witness the contract, especially someone who may be actively involved in the behavior.

You can write a series of small contracts or one big one with a number of checkpoints. Either way, start by identifying your first goal and then lay out your subgoals to reach that goal. Be sure your first subgoal has a start and stop date and a clear description of what you hope to accomplish.

All of us are familiar with the power of signed contracts. Documentation that commits our word, money, and/or property carries a strong impact and results in a higher chance of follow-through than do casual, offhand promises. Contracts can be used to try to change a health behavior if they include the time, date, and details of the behavior change program. Some target behaviors, such as quitting smoking or giving up candy snacks, lend themselves to contracts with very specific goals. Often a witness is also asked to sign the contract; this helps to set in motion the support and encouragement of a social network. Contracts help prevent procrastination by specifying the dates and other details of the behavioral tasks and goals. They also act as reminders of a personal commitment to change.

Let's take the example of Michael, who wants to break a long-standing habit of eating candy and chips every afternoon and evening. Setting up a formal contract and program for giving up these snacks will help him succeed in changing his behavior.

Michael begins by keeping track of his snacking in a journal. He discovers that he always buys candy or a bag of chips at the snack bar on campus between two of his afternoon classes. In the evenings, he eats several candy bars or a large bag of chips while he studies at home.

Next, Michael sets specific goals for his program. He sets a start date for his program and decides to break it into two parts. He will begin by cutting out his afternoon snack of candy or chips. Once he successfully reaches this goal, he'll concentrate on his evening snacking. He decides to allow himself three weeks for each half of his behavior change program.

To help increase his chances of success, Michael decides to make several changes in his behavior to help control his urges to buy and eat candy and chips. He plans to bring a healthy snack, such as an apple or orange, to eat between his afternoon classes. He decides to avoid going near the snack bar; instead, he'll spend his between-class break taking a 15-minute walk around campus or reading in the student union. To help break his evening habit, he decides to try studying at the library instead of at home; when he's at home, he'll try studying in a different room. He also plans to stock the refrigerator with healthy snacks that he can have when he feels the urge to snack on candy or chips.

Finally, Michael decides on some rewards he'll give himself when he meets his goals, choosing things he likes that aren't too expensive. Now he's ready to create and sign a behavior change contract. He decides to enlist one of his housemates as a witness to his contract; he also asks his housemate to check on his progress and offer encouragement. (Contracts can be completed without a witness, but many people find that having another person involved in their program provides a motivational boost.)

Once Michael has signed his contract, he's ready to begin. He can increase his chances of success by continuing to monitor his behavior and his snacking urges in his health journal.

My Personal Contract for Giving Up Snacking on Candy and Chips

I agree to stop snacking on candy and chips twice every day. I will begin my program on __10/4__ and plan to reach my final goal by __11/15__. I have divided my program into two parts, with two separate goals. For each step in my program, I will give myself the reward listed.

1. I will stop having candy or chips for an afternoon snack on __10/4__.
(Reward: __new CD__)

2. I will stop having candy or chips for an evening snack on __10/25__.
(Reward: __Concert__)

My plan for stopping my snacking includes the following strategies:
1. __Avoid snack bar by taking a walk or reading at student union.__
2. __Eating healthy snacks instead of candy and chips.__
3. __Studying at the library instead of at home.__

I understand that it is important for me to make a strong personal effort to make this change in my behavior. I sign this contract as an indication of my personal commitment to reach my goal.

Witness: _Michael Cook_   9/28
          Katie Lim   9/28

5. *Devise a strategy or plan of action.* As you fill in your health journal, you gather quite a lot of information about your target behavior—the times it typically occurs; the situations in which it usually happens; the ways sight, smell, mood, situation, and accessibility trigger it. You can probably trace the chains of events that lead to the behavior, and you can probably also identify points along those chains where making a different choice means changing the behavior.

You can be more effective in modifying behavior if you control the environmental stimuli that provoke it. This might mean not having cigarettes or certain foods or drinks in the house, not going to parties where you're tempted to overindulge, or not spending time with particular people, at least for a while. If you always get a candy bar at a certain vending machine, change your route so you don't pass by it. If you always end up taking a coffee break and chatting with friends when you go to the library to study, choose a different place to study, such as your room.

It's also helpful to control other behaviors or habits that seem to be linked to the target behavior. You may give in to an urge to eat when you have a beer (alcohol increases the appetite) or when you watch TV. Try substituting some other activities for habits that seem to be linked with your target behavior, such as exercising to music instead of plopping down in front of the TV. Or, if possible, put an exercise bicycle in front of your TV and burn calories while you watch your favorite show.

You can change the cues in your environment so they trigger the new behavior you want instead of the old one. Put a picture of a gymnast on your refrigerator door or a picture of a cyclist speeding down a hill on your television set. Put a chart of your progress in a special place at home to make your goals highly visible and inspire you to keep going. When you're trying to change a strong habit, small cues can play an important part in keeping you on track.

A second very powerful way to affect your target behavior is by setting up a reward system that will reinforce your efforts. Most people find it difficult to change long-standing habits for rewards they can't see right away. Giving yourself instant, real rewards for good behavior along the way will help you stick with a plan to change your behavior.

Carefully plan your reward payoffs and what they will be. In most cases, rewards should be collected when you reach specific objectives or subgoals in your plan. For example, you might treat yourself to a movie after a week of avoiding extra snacks. Don't forget to reward yourself for good behavior that is consistent and persistent—if you simply stick with your program week after week. Decide on a reward

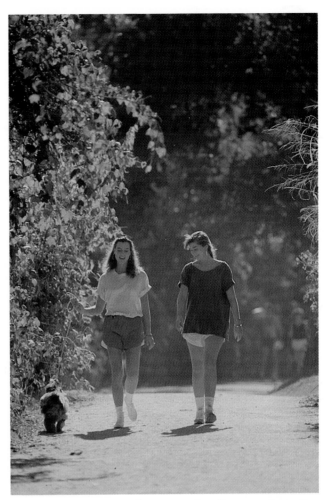

A beautiful day, a spectacular setting, a friendly companion—all conspire to make exercise a satisfying and pleasurable experience for these people. Choosing the right activity and doing it the right way are important elements in a successful health behavior management plan.

for yourself after you reach a certain goal or mark off the sixth week or month of a valiant effort, for example. Write it down in your health journal and remember it as you follow your plan—especially when the going gets rough.

Make a list of your activities and favorite events to use as rewards. They should be special, inexpensive, and preferably unrelated to food or alcohol. Depending on what you like to do, you might treat yourself to a concert, a ball game, a new CD, a long-distance phone call to a friend, a day off from studying for a long hike in the woods—whatever is rewarding to you. And don't forget to reward yourself with a pat on the back—congratulate yourself, notice how much better you look or feel, and feel good about how far you've come and how you've gained control of your behavior.

Rewards and support can also come from family and friends. Tell them about your plan and ask for their help. Get them to be active, interested participants. Ask them to support you when you set aside time to go running or avoid second helpings at Thanksgiving dinner. You may have to remind them not to do things that make you "break training" and not to be hurt if you have to refuse something when they forget. Getting encouragement, support, and praise from important people in your life can powerfully reinforce the new behavior you're trying to adopt.

6. *Keep track of your progress; revise your plan if necessary.* Use your health journal to keep track of how well you are doing in achieving your ultimate goal. Record your daily activities and any relevant details, such as how far you walked or how many calories you ate. Each week chart your progress on a graph and see how it lines up against the subgoals on your contract. You may want to track more than one behavior, such as the time you spend exercising each week and your weight.

If you don't seem to be making progress, analyze your plan to see what might be causing the problem. A number of possible barriers to success are listed in the section "Keeping on Track," along with suggestions for addressing them. Once you've identified the problem, revise your plan.

Making Sure You Succeed

Try one or more of these strategies to increase your chances of success.

- *Make your efforts time- and cost-effective.* Think about how to get the best return, the biggest health benefit, for your effort. Be sure that the new behavior you want has a real and lasting value for you personally. Then be realistic about the amount of time and energy you can put into it. The best program is usually one that you can keep following over a long time.

- *Find a buddy.* Ask around and you're likely to find someone who wants to make the same changes you do. Recruit one or more people to join your plan or join a formal program or group. Having social support makes it easier to stay with your program. You and your buddy can give each other encouragement, support, motivation, sympathy, and information. The fear of letting your buddy down makes it less likely that you'll take a day off. For some problems, the buddy system (used in Alcoholics Anonymous) is the most successful of all methods that have been tried.

- *Use a role model.* Find someone who reached the goal you're striving for. Once you start looking, you may

be surprised at the number of people you know who have stopped smoking, kept with a fitness program, lost weight, or broken a drug habit. Talk to them about how they did it. What strategies worked for them? What can you borrow from their experience?

- *Expect success.* What you expect can have a powerful effect on your behavior change program. Expect success and you will dramatically increase your chances of actually succeeding. Drop your old self-image and take on a new one. Picture yourself as a nonsmoker, a jogger, an A student, a thinner person. Monitor your "self-talk" and replace any negative, pessimistic comments with positive thoughts about your progress.

- *Realize that lasting change takes time.* Fad diets promise you'll lose weight instantly; but, in reality, weight loss and other major life changes are long-term projects that take weeks or months. They involve giving up a familiar and comfortable part of your life in exchange for something new and unknown. To be deep and long-lasting, changes have to take time. They happen one day at a time, with lots of ups and downs. At first you may notice a significant change, but then your progress levels off and you reach a plateau. Don't be discouraged—plateaus are natural. Be persistent and you'll work your way through the doldrums.

- *Forgive and forget.* When you slip, be easy on yourself. Feeling guilty, putting yourself down, and blaming yourself are all self-destructive and will work against you. Keeping up your self-esteem will help you stay with your plan; negative feelings will get in your way. Instead of berating yourself, try to discover what triggered the slip and decide how you'll deal with it next time.

One way to prevent slips is to rehearse what you would do differently in those situations where you know your target behavior will be triggered. If you don't want to drink too much at a party, decide on your drink limit ahead of time and switch to a soft drink when you hit your limit. If you want to go out to eat, decide ahead of time what you will order and stick to your decision once you're in the restaurant.

Keeping on Track: Some Troubleshooting Tips

As you continue with your program, don't be surprised when you run up against problems and obstacles—they're inevitable. In fact, it's a good idea to expect prob-

It takes motivation to change. But how do you get motivated? The following strategies may help:

- Write down potential benefits of the change. If you want to lose weight, your list might include increased ease of movement, energy, and self-confidence.

- Now write down the costs of not changing.

- Frequently visualize yourself achieving your goal and enjoying its benefits. If you want to manage time more effectively, picture yourself as a confident, organized person who systematically tackles important tasks and sets aside time each day for relaxation, exercise, and friends.

- Discount obstacles to change. Counter thoughts such as "I'll never have time to shop for and prepare healthy foods" with thoughts such as these: "Lots of other people have done it and so can I."

- Bombard yourself with propaganda. Subscribe to a self-improvement magazine. Take a class dealing with the change you want to make. Read books and watch talk shows on the subject. Post motivational phrases or pictures on your refrigerator or over your desk. Listen to motivational tapes in the car. Talk to people who have already made the change.

- Build up your confidence. Remind yourself of other goals you've achieved. At the end of each day, mentally review your good decisions and actions. See yourself as a capable person, one who is in charge of his or her health.

lems and to give yourself time out to step back, see how you're doing, and make some changes before going on again. If you find that your program is grinding to a halt, try to identify what it is that's blocking your progress. It may come from one of these sources.

- *Social influences.* Take a hard look at the reactions of the people you're counting on and see if they're really supporting you. If they come up short, try connecting and networking with others who will be more supportive.

   A related trap you should watch out for is trying to get your friends or members of your family to change *their* behaviors. The decision to make a major behavior change is something people come to only after intensive self-examination. You may be able to influence someone by tactfully providing facts or support, but that's all. Focus on yourself—if you succeed, you may become a role model.

- *Levels of motivation and commitment.* You won't make real progress until an inner drive leads you to make a personal commitment to the goal. If commitment is your problem, you may need to wait until the behavior you're dealing with makes your life more miserable; then your desire to change it will be stronger. Or you may find that changing your goal will inspire you to keep going. If you really want to change but your motivation comes and goes, look at your support system and at your confidence that you will succeed. Building these up may be the key to pushing past a barrier. Refer to the box "Motivation Boosters" for more ideas.

- *Choice of techniques and level of effort.* Your plan may not be working as well as you thought it would. Make changes where you're having the most trouble. If you've lagged on your running schedule, for example, maybe it's because you really don't like running. An aerobics class might suit you better. There are many ways to move toward your goal. Or you may not be trying hard enough. You do have to push toward your goal. If it were easy, you wouldn't need to have a plan.

- *Stress barrier.* If you've hit a wall in your program, look at the sources of stress in your life. If the stress is temporary, such as catching a cold or having a term paper due, you may want to wait until it passes before stepping up your efforts. If the stress is ongoing, try to find healthy ways to manage it. For example, taking a half-hour walk after lunch may help. You may even want to make stress management your highest priority for behavior change (see Chapter 2).

- *Games people play:* procrastinating, rationalizing, and blaming. Even when they want to change, people hold on fiercely to what they know and love (or know and hate). You may have very mixed feelings about the change you're trying to make, and your underlying motives may sabotage your conscious ones if you keep them hidden from yourself. Try to detect the games you might be playing with yourself so that you'll have the opportunity to change them.

   If you're procrastinating ("It's Friday already; I might as well wait until Monday to begin"), try breaking your program down into still smaller steps that you can knock off one day at a time. If you're rationalizing or making excuses ("I wanted to go swimming today, but I wouldn't have had time to wash my hair afterwards"), remember that the only

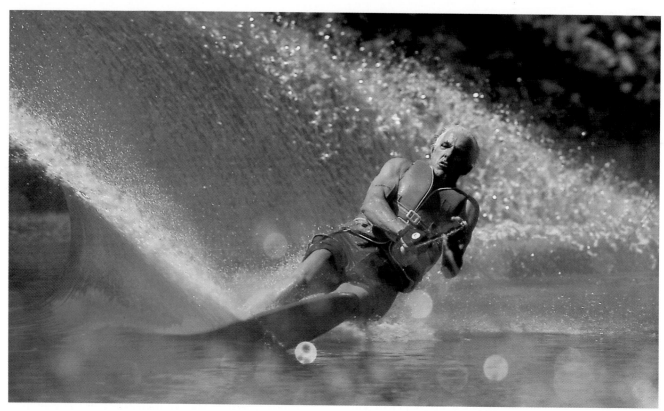

A 60-year-old man who water-skis like a 30-year-old gets his strength from years of vigorous activity. If you want to enjoy vigor and health in *your* middle and old age, begin now to make the choices that will give you lifelong vitality.

one you're fooling is yourself and that when you "win" by deceiving yourself, it's not much of a victory. If you're wasting time blaming yourself or others ("Everyone in that class talks so much that I don't get a chance to say my piece"), recognize that blaming is a way of taking your focus off the real problem and denying responsibility for your actions. Try refocusing by taking a positive attitude and renewing your determination to succeed.

Getting Outside Help

Outside help is often needed to change behavior that seems to be too deeply rooted for a self-management approach. Alcohol and other drug addictions, excessive overeating, and other conditions or behaviors that put you at a serious health risk fall into this category; so do behaviors that interfere with your ability to function. Many communities have programs to help with these problems; Weight Watchers, Alcoholics Anonymous, Smoke Enders, and Coke Enders are only a few of the better known ones.

On campus, you may find courses in physical fitness, stress management, and weight control. The student health center or campus counseling center may also be a source of assistance. Many communities offer a wide vari-

ety of low-cost services through adult education, school programs, health departments, and private agencies. Consult the yellow pages, your local health department, or the United Way; the latter often sponsors local referral services. Whatever you do, don't be stopped by a problem when you can tap into resources to help you solve it.

BEING HEALTHY FOR LIFE

Your first few behavior management projects may never go beyond the project stage. Those that do may not all succeed. But as you taste success and begin to see progress and changes, you'll start to experience new and surprising positive feelings about yourself. You'll probably find that you're less likely to buckle under stress. You may begin opening doors to different types of people and to a new world of enjoyable physical and social events. You may accomplish things you never thought possible—winning a race, climbing a mountain, breaking a nicotine habit, having a lean, muscular body. Being healthy takes extra effort, but the paybacks in energy and vitality are priceless.

Once you've started, don't stop. Assume health improvement is forever. Tackle one area at a time, but make a careful inventory of your health strengths and weaknesses and lay out a long-range plan. Take on the easier problems first and then use what you learned to attack more difficult areas. Look over your shoulder to make sure you don't fall into old habits. Keep informed about the latest health news and trends; research is constantly providing new information that directly affects daily choices and habits.

Making Changes in Your World

You can't completely control every aspect of your health. At least three other factors—heredity, health care, and environment—play important roles in your well-being. After you quit smoking, for example, you may still be inhaling smoke from other people's cigarettes. Your resolve to eat better foods may suffer a setback when you can't find any healthy choices in vending machines.

But you can make a difference—you can help create an environment around you that supports a healthy lifestyle. You can help support nonsmoking areas in public places. You can speak up in favor of more nutritious foods and better physical fitness facilities. You can include nonalcoholic drinks at your parties. You can vote for measures that improve access to health care for all people and support politicians who sponsor them.

You can also work on the larger environmental challenges facing us: air and water pollution, traffic congestion, overcrowding and overpopulation, depletion of the ozone layer of the atmosphere, toxic and nuclear waste disposal, and many others. These difficult issues need the attention and energy of people who are informed and who care about health. On every level, from personal to planetary, individuals can take an active role in shaping their environment.

What Does the Future Hold?

Sweeping changes in lifestyle have resulted in healthier Americans in recent years and could have even greater effects in the years to come (see box "Looking Toward the Year 2000"). Heart disease deaths, although still high, have dropped more than 40 percent since 1970. Stroke rates are down 50 percent. Average blood pressure and cholesterol levels have declined by small but significant amounts. Problems remain, of course—psychological, emotional, and learning disorders, along with hearing and speech impairments, are on the rise among children; access to health care is a critical problem; unacceptable disparities in health risks exist between races and ethnic groups; and **HIV infection** looms as an immense challenge for all of us. But all these problems can be addressed at least in part by individuals taking charge of their health and working to improve the health of the nation and the world.

In your lifetime, you can choose an active role in the movement toward increased awareness, greater individual responsibility and control, healthier lifestyles, and a healthier planet. Your choices and actions will have a tremendous impact on your present and future health. You have the opportunity to reach levels of wellness that your ancestors could only imagine. The door is open, and the time is now—you simply have to begin.

- A healthy lifestyle promotes optimal health. Through knowledge, self-awareness, motivation, and effort, everyone can achieve optimal health.

What Is Health?

- Ideas about health have changed over the years. Whereas once it was considered to be the absence of disease and disability, advances in medical science in the twentieth century led people to start thinking of health in terms of longevity.

- As chronic diseases such as coronary heart disease and cancer became the leading causes of death in the United States, people recognized that merely being alive is not the same as health.

- Today, health is perceived as a matter of *wellness*—having a sense of vitality and overall well-being in life. Health is dynamic and multidimensional; it incorporates physical, emotional, intellectual, spiritual, interpersonal, societal, and environmental factors.

Choosing Wellness

- People today have greater control over their health than ever before. Being responsible for one's health means making choices and adopting habits and behaviors that will ensure wellness.

- Scientific research regularly makes connections between wellness or disease and certain lifestyles or behaviors. Although heredity, environment, and health care all play roles in wellness and disease, behavior can mitigate their effects.

- Behaviors and habits that reinforce wellness include (1) taking an active, responsible role in one's health, (2) managing stress, (3) maintaining self-esteem and good interpersonal relationships, (4) understanding sexuality and having satisfying intimate relationships, (5) avoiding tobacco and other drugs and restricting alcohol intake, (6) eating well, exercising, and

HIV Infection   A chronic, progressive disease that damages the immune system; caused by the human immunodeficiency virus (HIV). Its most severe form, AIDS, is characterized by severe suppression of the immune system, leading eventually to death.

TERMS

We usually think of health and wellness as personal matters, things we deal with on our own—by exercising and managing stress, for example—or in conjunction with our physicians when we get sick. But did you know that the U.S. government has a vital interest in the health of all Americans? A healthy population is the nation's greatest resource, the source of its vigor and wealth. Poor health, in contrast, drains the nation's resources and raises national health care costs. As the embodiment of our society's values, the federal government also has a humane interest in people's health.

In 1990 the U.S. Department of Health and Human Services published a report entitled *Healthy People 2000: National Health Promotion and Disease Prevention Objectives.* The work of thousands of health professionals, this 700-page document sets forth health goals for the United States to be achieved by the year 2000. It also provides a framework within which individuals, communities, health care professionals, and government can work toward those goals. The broad national goals proposed by *Healthy People 2000* are the following:

- *To increase the span of healthy life for all Americans.* This means not only adding years to the life span but also enhancing the quality of life. Although the average American life span is about 74 years, a person may have a disabling stroke at 60, followed by 14 years of impaired life. The national goal is to increase years of healthy life for all Americans from 62 (the figure in 1980) to 65.

- *To reduce health disparities among Americans.* Many health problems disproportionately affect certain populations in the United States, including some age groups, people with low income, certain racial and ethnic minorities, and people with disabilities. For example, life expectancy for whites at birth has been gradually increasing for many years, but in 1986, 1987, and 1988 it actually decreased for African American males. *Healthy People 2000* calls for reducing, and finally eliminating, these disparities among groups, most of whom have historically been disadvantaged economically, educationally, and politically.

- *To secure access to preventive health services for all Americans.* Preventive services, such as prenatal care, nutritional counseling, and cancer screening, are the key to long-term improvements in national health. Because these services are usually offered in the course of

regular, basic care, this third goal means increasing the number of people who have a primary source of health care and adequate health insurance coverage.

These three goals—healthy lives for more Americans, elimination of disparities among groups, and access to necessary preventive services for everyone—are the broad aspirations of *Healthy People 2000* for American society. Giving substance to these broad goals are hundreds of specific objectives in many different "priority areas." These objectives are in the form of measurable targets for the year 2000—for example, to increase to at least 30 percent the proportion of people who engage in moderate daily physical activity, up from 22 percent in 1985.

The report groups these priority areas into three broad categories—Health Promotion, Health Protection, and Preventive Services. The first category, Health Promotion, encompasses areas involving individual actions and behaviors. Examples of these areas include physical fitness, nutrition, tobacco, alcohol and other drugs, family planning, and mental health. In these areas, health improvements will be made by educating people about healthy lifestyle choices and encouraging them to make those choices. The second category, Health Protection, encompasses areas involving environmental improvements—areas in which people's health needs to be protected on a wide scale. These areas include food and drug safety, protection from unintentional injuries (accidents), environmental health, and so on. The third category, Preventive Services, encompasses areas involving clinical services, such as prenatal care, childhood immunizations, and so on.

Healthy People 2000 takes special notice of a changing attitude among Americans that supports its aspirations—an emerging sense of personal responsibility as the key to good health. This new perspective is seen in the concern Americans have about smoking and drug abuse, for example; in our emphasis on physical and emotional fitness; in our interest in good nutrition; and in our concern about the environment. As you have seen in this chapter, personal responsibility—taking charge of your health—is the perspective upon which *Core Concepts in Health* is built. As you move on to other chapters, you will also see that the concerns encompassed in the various priority areas of *Healthy People 2000* are the principal topics covered in this book. In many ways, personal health goals are not different from national aspirations.

maintaining normal weight, (7) knowing about illnesses and how to treat them, (8) understanding and wisely using the health system, (9) knowing about diseases and accidents and protecting yourself against them, (10) understanding the processes of aging and dying, and (11) understanding the environment and its effects on your health and working to improve it.

Getting Down to Basics: How Do you Reach Wellness?

- Knowledge about topics in health and about oneself is necessary to achieve wellness.

- Motivation is one of the most important factors in behavior change. Most people are motivated most strongly by short-term, personal goals.

- Commitment is a third necessary factor in behavior change. It involves the full force of the resolve to change.

- The fourth and perhaps most important factor in behavior change is taking control of one's life, taking an active role in living and maintaining health. With motivation and commitment, habits that have been learned can be unlearned through behavioral self-management.

- Behavior can be traced to the circumstances that trigger it; the consequences of behavior can also be identified. The circumstances that trigger behavior include internal and external stimuli; the consequences of behavior can be positive and negative reinforcers. Reinforcers are the basis of behavior self-management.

- The best way to begin a behavior self-management program is to choose one target behavior and follow a systematic six-step program to change. Consistency and persistence are highly important.

- The six steps to behavior management are (1) monitoring behavior, often through a journal, (2) analyzing the recorded data, (3) setting specific goals, usually broken down into small steps, (4) making a personal contract, sometimes with a witness, (5) devising a strategy based on information gathered during the monitoring stage, and (6) keeping track of progress, constantly revising the strategy if barriers arise.

- Strategies for change include controlling environmental stimuli and setting up a reward system.

- Strategies for success include making your efforts time- and cost-effective, having a buddy help, looking for role models, expecting success, recognizing that change takes time, and learning to forgive oneself. Keeping up self-esteem helps; negative feelings undermine the plan.

- Obstacles sometimes come in the form of nonsupportive people, a low level of commitment, inappropriate techniques, too much stress, and procrastinating, rationalizing, and blaming.

- Taking advantage of outside sources and programs can help; some behavior is too deeply rooted to be changed by self-management techniques alone.

Being Healthy for Life

- Each small success in a behavior-management program leads to increased self-esteem and increased motivation to continue.

- Although people can't control every aspect of their health, individuals can make a difference in improving the environment—from insisting on nonsmoking areas in local restaurants to working on planetary issues like nuclear waste disposal and depletion of the ozone layer.

TAKE ACTION

1. Ask some older members of your family (parents and grandparents) what they recall about patterns of health and disease when they were young. Do they remember any large outbreaks of infectious disease? Did any of their friends or relatives die while very young or die of a disease that can now be treated? How have health concerns changed during their lifetime?

2. Choose a person you consider a role model and interview him or her. What do you admire about this person? What can you borrow from his or her experiences and strategies for success?

JOURNAL ENTRY

1. Purchase a small notebook to use as your health journal throughout this course. At the end of each chapter, we include suggestions for journal entries—opportunities to think about topics and issues, explore and formulate your own views, and express your thoughts in written form. These exercises are intended to help you deepen your understanding of health topics and your own behaviors in relation to them. For your first journal entry, make a list of the positive behaviors that enhance your health (such as jogging and getting enough sleep). Consider what additions you can make to the list or how you can strengthen or reinforce these behaviors. (Don't forget to congratulate yourself for these positive aspects of your life.) Next, list the behaviors that detract from wellness (such as smoking and eating a lot of candy). Consider which of these behaviors you might be able to change. Use these lists as the basis for self-evaluation as you proceed through this book.

2. *Critical Thinking:* Making smart choices about your health requires critical thinking. You have to sort through and evaluate the information you receive and then make intelligent decisions on the basis of what you've heard or read. Critical thinking involves

knowing where and how to find relevant information, how to separate fact from opinion, how to recognize faulty reasoning, how to evaluate information, and how to assess the credibility of sources. Consider, for example, the typical newspaper story describing new scientific findings about cholesterol, caffeine, or AIDS treatment. As a health consumer, you have to read the article critically to understand its implications. In evaluating such an article, remember that a single scientific study isn't sufficient to "prove" anything; results have to be repeated in other studies in order to be valid. Remember, too, that in their eagerness for news, the media often distort the meaning of studies. Wait and see how findings are interpreted by a number of experts. And don't forget to look askance at any findings cited in advertising; the motive, of course, is to persuade you to buy something.

In this book, a number of Journal Entry items are designed to help you sharpen your critical thinking skills. For your first Critical Thinking Journal Entry, write a short essay describing your sources of health information. Do you rely on newspaper or magazine articles? On television? On friends and family members? What criteria do you use to evaluate this information, to assess its credibility, and to make health decisions?

3. Think about what troubled you most during the past week. In your health journal, write down the names of three or four people who might be able to help you with whatever troubled you. If the problem persists, consider starting at the top of your list and talking to this person about it.

4. Think of the last time you did something you knew to be unhealthy primarily because those around you were doing it. How could you have restructured the situation or changed the environmental cues so that you could have avoided the behavior? In your health journal, describe several possible actions that will help you avoid the behavior the next time you're in a similar situation.

5. Make a list in your health journal of rewards that are meaningful to you. Add to the list as you think of new things to use. Refer to this list of rewards when you're developing plans for behavior change.

SELECTED BIBLIOGRAPHY

Barsky, A. J. 1988. *Worried Sick: Our Troubled Quest for Wellness.* Boston: Little, Brown.

Fries, J. F., and L. M. Crapo. 1981. *Vitality and Aging.* New York: W. H. Freeman.

Hiatt, H. H. 1987. *America's Health in the Balance: Choice or Chance?* New York: Harper and Row.

Justice, B. 1988. *Who Gets Sick: How Beliefs, Moods, and Thoughts Affect Your Health.* Los Angeles: Jeremy P. Tarcher.

National Center for Health Statistics. 1992. *Monthly Vital Statistics Report,* 40(13), 30 September.

Reader's Digest. 1988. *The Complete Manual of Fitness and Well-Being: A Lifetime Guide to Self-Improvement.* Pleasantville, N.Y.: Reader's Digest.

Samuels, M., and N. Samuels. 1988. *The Well Adult.* New York: Summit Books.

Travis, J., and R. S. Ryan. 1988. *Wellness Workbook.* Berkeley: Ten Speed Press.

U.S. Department of Health and Human Services. 1990. *Healthy People 2000: National Health Promotion and Disease Prevention Objectives.* Washington, D.C.: U.S. Government Printing Office, DHHS Pub. (PHS) 91-50213.

RECOMMENDED READINGS

The following are highly readable monthly or bimonthly newsletters and magazines filled with the latest research and thinking on health-related topics.

Consumer Reports on Health (101 Truman Avenue, Yonkers, NY 10703-1057)

Harvard Medical School Health Letter (P.O. Box 420300, Palm Coast, FL 32142-0300)

Health (formerly *Hippocrates* and *In Health*) (Hippocrates Partners, P.O. Box 56863, Boulder, CO 80322-6863)

Healthline (The C. V. Mosby Company, 11830 Westline Industrial Drive, St. Louis, MO 63146-3318)

Mayo Clinic Health Letter (Mayo Foundation for Medical Education and Research, P.O. Box 53889, Boulder, CO 80322-3889)

University of California at Berkeley Wellness Letter (P.O. Box 420148, Palm Coast, FL 32142)

2

Stress: The Constant Challenge

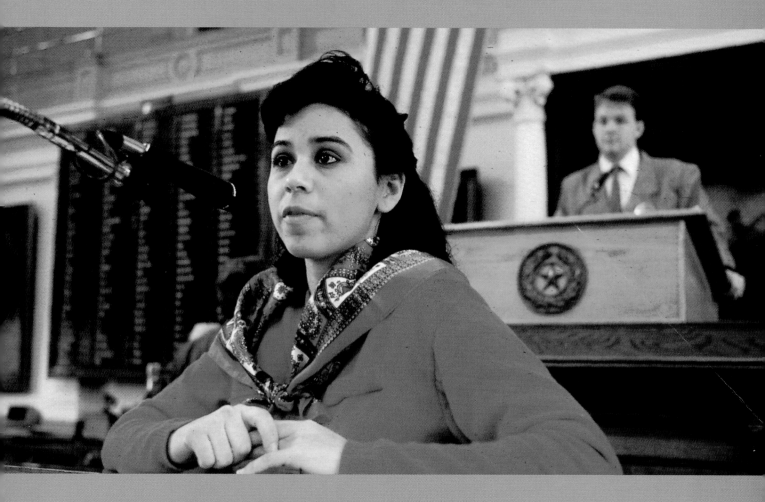

CONTENTS

- Yesterday you wrote a check for groceries—and put it in your pocket instead of giving it to the cashier. You've been forgetting other things, like locking your car, and you're having trouble concentrating when you study. You're also grouchy and getting a lot of headaches. You suspect the problem is that you're working many more hours this semester at your job in the campus bookstore than you did last term. Does the way you've been feeling mean you have to give up your job? Or do you just need a little more time to adjust to your new demands? How can you figure out what to do?

- Your mother recently achieved a goal she's dreamed of for years: starting her own business. To celebrate, she plans a huge party. You and your brothers and sisters all come home for the occasion. But you're surprised by how drained and even depressed your mother seems. She's gained a lot of weight and, worst of all, is smoking again after five years without cigarettes. What's going on? If this is what she's always wanted, why does she seem to be falling apart?

- Your new boss works long hours, usually skips lunch, always takes work home with him, and often comes in on weekends. He treats anyone who doesn't maintain the same pace as a freeloader. He is suspicious and hostile, and he seems to be angry at the world. When you described him to your mother on your last visit home, she commented, "He's digging his own grave." Was that more than a figure of speech?

- You complain about your insomnia to the resident adviser in your dorm. She recommends meditation. She says she used to have trouble sleeping, too, until she started meditating every afternoon for 20 minutes. She says it quiets her mind, relaxes her body, and gives her a feeling of being "centered." She also says she sleeps soundly now. Could a relaxation technique that you practice during the day really help you at night? Is it worth a try?

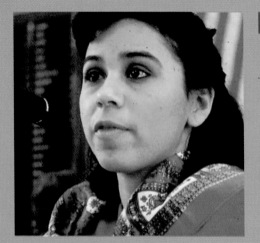

MAKING CONNECTIONS

People in our society face dozens of daily hassles, from finding car keys to finishing papers, as well as a lifetime of major changes: graduation and marriage, promotion and parenthood, mortgages and moves. Developing successful ways to cope with life's inevitable changes and challenges is an important task of adulthood—but one that many people fail to master. In each of the stress-related scenarios presented on this page, individuals have to use information, make a decision, or choose a course of action. How would you act in these situations? What response or decision would you make? This chapter provides information about stress that can be used in situations like these. After finishing the chapter, read the scenarios again. Has what you've learned changed how you would respond?

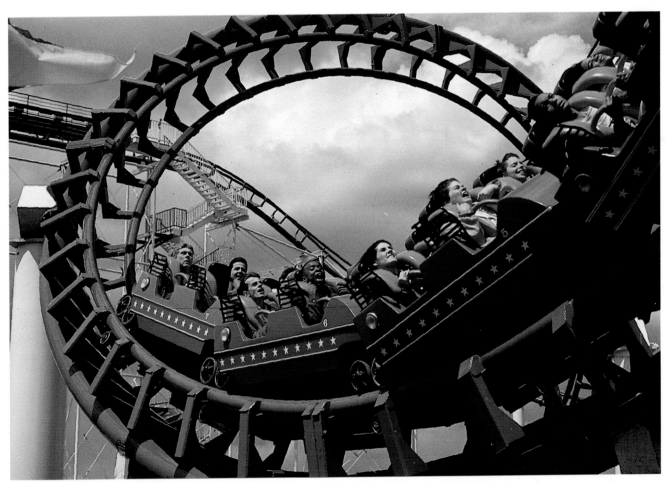

The experience of stress depends on many factors, including the nature of the stressor. Exciting experiences like this amusement park ride can produce a stimulating kind of stress known as eustress.

Everybody talks about **stress.** People say they're "over-stressed" or "stressed out." They may blame stress for headaches or ulcers, and they may try to combat stress with aerobics classes—or drugs. But what is stress? And why is it important to manage it wisely?

Most people associate stress with negative events: the death of a close relative or friend, financial problems, or other unpleasant life changes that create nervous tension. But stress isn't merely nervous tension. And it isn't something to be avoided at all costs. In fact, complete freedom from stress is death. Before we explore more fully what stress is, consider this list of common stressful situations or events:

Interviewing for a job

Running in a race

Being accepted to college

Going out on a date

Watching a basketball game

Getting a promotion

Obviously, stress doesn't arise just from unpleasant situations. Stress can also be associated with physical chal-

lenges and the achievement of personal goals. Physical and psychological stress-producing factors can be either pleasant or unpleasant. What's crucial is how the individual responds, whether in positive, life-enhancing ways or in negative, counterproductive ways.

As a college student, you may be in one of the most stressful periods of your life. You may be on your own for the first time, or you may be juggling the demands of college with the responsibilities of a job, a family, or both. Financial pressures may be intense. Housing and transportation may be sources of additional hassles. You're also meeting new people, engaging in new activities, learning new information and skills, and setting a new course for your life. Good and bad, all of these changes and challenges are likely to have a powerful effect on you, both

Stress   The sum of the physical and emotional reactions to any stimulus that disturbs the organism's homeostasis.

physically and psychologically. Respond ineffectively to stress, and eventually it will take a toll on your sense of well-being and overall health. Learn effective responses, however, and you will enhance your health and gain a feeling of control over your life.

How do you know when your stress level is getting dangerously high? How can you develop techniques to cope positively with the stress that is part of your life? This chapter will help you discover answers to these questions.

WHAT IS STRESS?

Just what is stress, if such vastly different situations can cause it? No one has explored the biochemical and environmental aspects of stress more thoroughly than Hans Selye, an endocrinologist and biologist. Selye defines stress as "the nonspecific response of the body to any demand." What is a "nonspecific response"? It's the body's total biological response, from sweating palms to a pounding heart to a stress-producing situation. What is "nonspecific" about this response? No matter what the specific stressful situation that provokes it—a date, a final

exam, or a flat tire—the physical response is the same. This response can vary in intensity—sometimes your heart races faster and your palms sweat more—but it is always limited to the same basic set of physical reactions.

In common usage, the word *stress* is used to refer to two different things: situations that trigger physical and emotional reactions and the reactions themselves. In this text, we'll use the more precise terms **stressor** to refer to situations that trigger physical and emotional reactions and the term **stress response** to refer to those reactions. A date and a final exam, then, are stressors; sweaty palms and a pounding heart are symptoms of the stress response. We'll use the term *stress* to describe the general physical and emotional state that accompanies the stress response. A person on a date or taking a final exam experiences stress.

Each individual's experience of stress depends on many factors, including the nature of the stressor. Stress triggered by a pleasant stressor, such as a date or a party, is called **eustress.** On the other hand, **distress** stems from an unpleasant stressor, such as a flat tire or a bad grade.

Physical Responses to Stressors: General Adaptation Syndrome

The light turns green and you step off the curb. Almost before you see it, you feel a car speeding toward you. With just a fraction of a second to spare, you leap safely out of harm's way. In that split second of danger, and in the moments following it, you have experienced a predictable series of physical reactions. Hans Selye termed this predictable pattern the **general adaptation syndrome (GAS).** Selye divided GAS into three distinct stages: alarm, resistance, and exhaustion.

GAS: Alarm   The instant you sense the oncoming car, an internal alarm sounds and the **sympathetic** branch of your **autonomic nervous system** takes command. For the most part, this part of your nervous system operates independently of conscious thought. It controls your heart rate, breathing, blood pressure, digestion, and hundreds of other functions you usually take for granted. It is also responsible for mobilizing your body for physical action in response to a stressor.

As the car travels toward you, you feel only fear. Your sympathetic nervous system, however, knows exactly what to do—and does it with breathtaking speed and efficiency. Its control center in the brain, the **hypothalamus,** orders the **pituitary gland** to release a chemical messenger called **adrenocorticotropic hormone (ACTH)** into the bloodstream. When ACTH reaches the **adrenal glands,** located just above the kidneys, it stimulates them to release **cortisol** and other key hormones into the bloodstream. Simultaneously, sympathetic nerves instruct your adrenal glands to release the hormones **epi-**

TERMS

Stressor   Any physical or psychological event or condition that produces stress.

Stress response   The physiological changes associated with stress.

Eustress   Stress resulting from pleasant stressors.

Distress   Stress resulting from unpleasant stressors.

General adaptation syndrome (GAS)   A pattern of stress responses described by Hans Selye as having three stages: alarm, resistance, and exhaustion.

Sympathetic nervous system   A division of the autonomic system that reacts to danger or other challenges by almost instantly putting the body processes in high gear.

Autonomic nervous system   The branch of the peripheral nervous system that, largely without conscious thought, controls basic body processes; subdivided into the sympathetic and parasympathetic systems.

Hypothalamus   A part of the brain that activates, controls, and integrates the autonomic mechanisms, endocrine activities, and many body functions.

Pituitary gland   The "master gland," closely linked with the hypothalamus, that controls other endocrine glands and secretes hormones that regulate growth, maturation, and reproduction.

Adrenocorticotropic hormone (ACTH)   A hormone, formed in the pituitary gland, that stimulates the outer layer of the adrenal gland to secrete its hormones.

Adrenal glands   Two glands, one lying atop each kidney, their outer layer (cortex) producing steroid hormones such as cortisol, and their inner core (medulla) producing the hormones epinephrine and norepinephrine.

Cortisol   A steroid hormone secreted by the cortex (outer layer) of the adrenal gland; also called *hydrocortisone*.

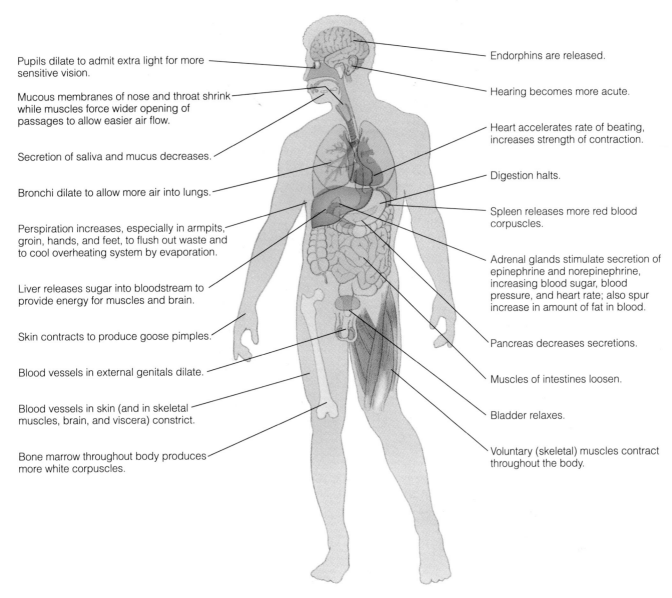

Pupils dilate to admit extra light for more sensitive vision.

Mucous membranes of nose and throat shrink while muscles force wider opening of passages to allow easier air flow.

Secretion of saliva and mucus decreases.

Bronchi dilate to allow more air into lungs.

Perspiration increases, especially in armpits, groin, hands, and feet, to flush out waste and to cool overheating system by evaporation.

Liver releases sugar into bloodstream to provide energy for muscles and brain.

Skin contracts to produce goose pimples.

Blood vessels in external genitals dilate.

Blood vessels in skin (and in skeletal muscles, brain, and viscera) constrict.

Bone marrow throughout body produces more white corpuscles.

Endorphins are released.

Hearing becomes more acute.

Heart accelerates rate of beating, increases strength of contraction.

Digestion halts.

Spleen releases more red blood corpuscles.

Adrenal glands stimulate secretion of epinephrine and norepinephrine, increasing blood sugar, blood pressure, and heart rate; also spur increase in amount of fat in blood.

Pancreas decreases secretions.

Muscles of intestines loosen.

Bladder relaxes.

Voluntary (skeletal) muscles contract throughout the body.

Figure 2-1 *The alarm reaction.*

nephrine, or adrenaline, and **norepinephrine,** which in turn trigger a series of profound changes as they circulate throughout your body (Figure 2-1). Your hearing and vision become more acute. Bronchi dilate to allow more air into your lungs. Your heart rate accelerates to pump more oxygen through your body. Your liver releases extra sugar into your bloodstream to provide an energy boost for your muscles and brain. Your digestion halts. You perspire more to cool your skin. **Endorphins** are released to relieve pain in case of injury. Blood cell production increases. These almost instantaneous changes give you the heightened reflexes and strength you need to dodge the car.

The alarm response, or **fight-or-flight reaction,** is a part of our biological heritage. It's a survival mechanism that has served humankind well. In modern life, however,

the alarm response is often absurdly inappropriate. It can be triggered by a party invitation, stumbling over a doorstep, or being insulted, as well as by physical threats like an out-of-control car. The alarm response prepares your body for physical action, regardless of whether

TERMS

Epinephrine   A hormone secreted by the medulla (inner core) of the adrenal gland; also called *adrenaline,* the "fear hormone."

Norepinephrine   A hormone secreted by the medulla (inner core) of the adrenal gland; also called *noradrenaline,* the "anger hormone."

Endorphins   Brain secretions that have pain-inhibiting effects.

Fight-or-flight reaction   A defense reaction that prepares the organism for conflict or escape by triggering hormonal, cardiovascular, metabolic, and other changes.

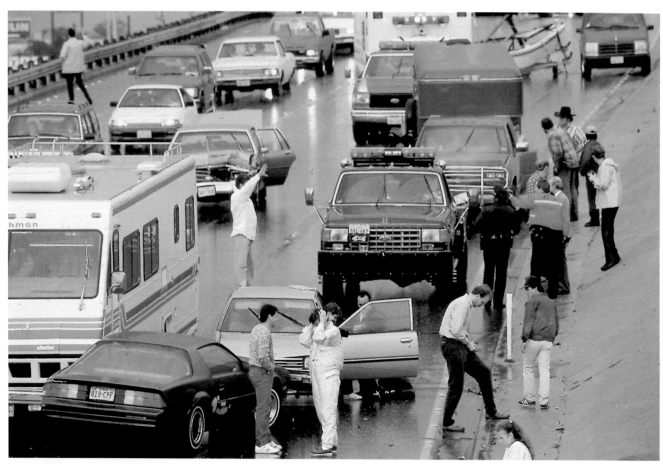

Heavy traffic on a rain-slicked highway is a recipe for stress. Some of the people involved in this series of collisions are still unnerved; others show signs of readjustment to normal functioning.

physical action is a necessary or appropriate response to a particular stressor.

GAS: Resistance Your body resists dramatic changes. Whenever normal functioning is disrupted, such as during the alarm reaction, your body strives for **homeostasis,** a state in which blood pressure, heart rate, hormone levels, and other vital functions are maintained within a narrow range of normal. Once a stressful situation ends, the **parasympathetic** branch of your autonomic nervous system takes command and halts the alarm reaction. It initiates the **adaptive reactions,** or adjustments, necessary to restore homeostasis. Your parasympathetic nervous system calms your body down, slowing rapid heartbeat, drying sweaty palms, and returning breathing to normal. Gradually, your body resumes its day-to-day "housekeeping" functions, such as digestion and temperature regulation. Damage that may have been sustained during the alarm reaction is repaired. The day after you narrowly dodge the car, you wake up feeling fine. The resistance phase of the GAS has enabled you to get on with your everyday life.

GAS: Exhaustion What if, instead of getting on with your everyday life, you found yourself confronted with a string of severe stressors? Your financial aid is cut, and you are forced to work more hours each week at your part-time job. Your bicycle is stolen. You do poorly in several courses and are placed on academic probation. You break up with the person you've been dating for the last six months. Your father suffers a heart attack. This group of events would cause your body to respond over and over with an alarm reaction. Some people in extreme circumstances—men and women who serve on the front lines in battle, hostages, prisoners of war, and victims of chronic domestic or neighborhood violence—are forced to confront life-and-death emergencies every day.

As you might imagine, both the mobilization of forces during the alarm reaction and the restoration of homeostasis during the resistance stage require a considerable amount of energy. If a stressor persists, or if a series of stressors occur in succession, readily available stores of energy can be depleted. Worse, reserves of **adaptive energy** can be drained as well. When these adaptive energy reserves are used up, general exhaustion results. This is not the sort of exhaustion people complain of after a long, busy day. It's a life-threatening type of physiological exhaustion characterized by such symptoms as distorted perceptions and disorganized thinking.

In laboratory experiments, Selye subjected rats to conditions that put them under extreme stress. He found that the rats responded with an alarm reaction when they first encountered a stressor. Over time, though, their nervous systems learned to view the stressor as normal and established a new homeostasis. However, the rats were able to sustain this resistance to the stressor for only a limited time. If the stressor continued, exhaustion eventually set in (Figure 2-2).

The Stress Response in Everyday Modern Life Few of us will suffer a string of disasters or endure combat in our homes or on a battlefield. But modern life, even when it's going well, consists of countless stressors. Some of them—noise, overcrowding, overwork, discrimination, competition, and economic pressures, for instance—go on not just for a few minutes but for days, weeks, months, or a lifetime.

Everyday stressors don't often lead to terminal exhaustion. But there is evidence that over the long term they can kill us just the same. Selye argues that cardiovascular disease, the leading cause of death in this country, is a "disease of adaptation"—a disease that results when the body is subjected too often to the drastic demands of the stress response. Selye also considers ulcers, some mental disorders, and possibly cancer as diseases of adaptation. These and other stress-linked diseases are discussed more fully later in the chapter.

GAS is a survival mechanism meant to mobilize us for fight or flight in rare life-and-death emergencies. Our bodies aren't designed to withstand its heavy demands on an ongoing basis. Ironically, the strains and hassles of life in a civilized world have transformed this life-saving mechanism into a potentially life-threatening one. How do you know if you're overstressed? Table 2-1 highlights some of the danger signals. Of course, you don't have to experience them all to realize you're encountering too many stressors too frequently. And some of the signals may be symptoms of a medical problem unrelated to stress. In general, though, such signals are distinct warn-

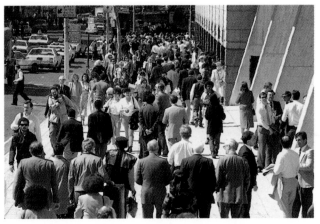

Cities, with their crowds, noise, dirt, and impersonality, offer an unrelentingly stressful environment to millions of people. Yet many individuals thrive there, finding excitement, challenge, and glamour. How do you react to cities?

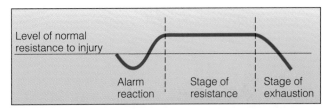

Figure 2-2 *General adaptation syndrome.*
In Selye's experiments, rats subjected to cold at first exhibited the hormonal changes typical of the alarm reaction but then adapted to life at lower temperatures. After several months, however, they lost their acquired resistance, and exhaustion set in.

ings about a problem that requires your attention. Ignoring or worrying about such symptoms will only add to the problem. If your body is trying to tell you something, it's important to listen. Methods for dealing with insomnia—one possible sign of excess stress—are described in the box "The Mystery of Sleep." Other actions you can take to relieve the discomfort of stress are described later in this chapter.

Emotional and Behavioral Responses to Stressors: Individual Variation

Physically, everyone responds to stressors in basically the same, predictable way. Emotionally and behaviorally, though, individuals may respond in very different ways. You may feel relaxed and confident about taking exams but be nervous about talking to members of the opposite sex, while your roommate may love challenging social situations but be very nervous about taking tests. A poor grade on a group project may prompt you to go for a 10-mile jog, while other members of your project team respond by eating chocolate or getting drunk. What accounts for these differences? Emotional and behavioral

What is sleep, and why do we need it? Surprisingly enough, the answers to these questions are not completely known. What is known is that all animal species sleep, and must sleep. The need to sleep has an awesome power over us. If deprived of sleep for long, we can't stay awake even to save our lives. The night workers at both Chernobyl and Three Mile Island were too sleepy to avert nuclear disasters. The operator of the *Exxon Valdez* couldn't maneuver the giant oil tanker because he was too sleepy to perform his job. And in many fatal car, truck, and train crashes, a major factor is sleep deprivation and fatigue.

We don't have to fall asleep at the wheel to know how much we need sleep. Without it, our mental and physical processes steadily deteriorate. We get headaches, feel irritable, are unable to concentrate, forget things, and may even become more susceptible to illness. Lack of sleep is a significant stressor; extreme sleep deprivation can lead to hallucinations and other psychotic symptoms. In contrast, sufficient sleep improves mood, fosters feelings of competence and self-worth, and supports optimal mental and emotional functioning.

Many experts believe that most Americans don't get enough sleep. Studies have shown that many people fall asleep in less than five minutes if stimulation is greatly reduced during the day, indicating that they are sleep-deprived. When these people are encouraged or allowed to sleep extra hours, their daytime alertness and their intellectual abilities improve significantly. Although sleep requirements vary among individuals, some adults need as much as nine hours of sleep to feel fully refreshed and alert.

Exactly what happens when we lie down to go to sleep? A healthy adult first drops off into a light, quiet sleep and then into successively deeper levels of sleep. This type of sleep is known as non-REM sleep, or non-rapid-eye-movement sleep. During non-REM sleep blood pressure, heart rate, body temperature, and breathing rate drop, release of growth hormone increases, and brain wave patterns become slow and even.

About an hour after falling asleep, the sleeper begins to move back upward from deep sleep and into REM sleep, or rapid-eye-movement sleep. During this type of sleep, when the eyes can be observed darting back and forth under closed eyelids, the person is dreaming, apparently continuously. Heart rate, blood pressure, and breathing rate increase and fluctuate. Muscles in the arms and legs relax completely, resulting in temporary paralysis, although some movement breaks through in twitches. The brain reaches its highest activity levels during REM sleep—higher than during waking consciousness—as it creates a complex dream world, responds to it, and then carefully blocks those responses at the level of the spinal cord so the body doesn't get up and act out the dream. The purpose of all this activity is still unknown.

The cycle of non-REM and REM sleep is repeated about five times during the night. Non-REM sleep becomes progressively lighter as the night goes on, and periods of REM sleep last longer, extending up to an hour by the last cycle. Most deep sleep occurs in the first half of the night.

Nearly everyone, at some time in life, has trouble falling asleep or staying asleep—a condition known as **insomnia.** Short-term insomnia can last anywhere from a few nights to a few weeks. Long-term insomnia can last for months or even years. The most common causes of insomnia are lifestyle factors, such as high caffeine or alcohol intake before sleep; medical problems, such as a breathing disorder; and psychological stress. Chronic sleep problems can themselves become a source of stress, as the person frets and worries about not getting enough sleep.

Most people can overcome insomnia by discovering the cause of poor sleep and taking steps to remedy it (see the tips below). Insomnia that lasts for more than six months and interferes with daytime functioning calls for consultation with a physician. Sleeping pills are not recommended for chronic insomnia because they can be habit-forming; they also lose their effectiveness over time.

If you're bothered by insomnia, here are some tips for getting a better night's sleep:

- Determine how much sleep you need to feel refreshed the next day and don't sleep longer than that (but do make sure you get enough).

- Go to bed at the same time every night and, more importantly, get up at the same time every morning, seven days a week, regardless of how much sleep you got. Don't nap during the day.

- Exercise every day but not too close to bedtime. Your metabolism takes up to six hours to slow down after exercise.

- Avoid tobacco (nicotine is a stimulant), caffeine in the later part of the day, and alcohol before bedtime (it causes disturbed, fragmented sleep).

- Have a light snack before bedtime—people sleep better if they're not hungry.

- Deal with worries before bedtime. Try writing them down, along with some possible solutions, and then allow yourself to forget about them until the next day.

- Use your bed only for sleep. Don't eat, read, study, or watch television in bed.

- Relax before bedtime with a warm bath (again, not too close to bedtime—allow about two hours for your metabolism to slow down afterward), a book, music, or some relaxation exercises. Don't lie down in bed until you're sleepy.

- If you don't fall asleep in 15 or 20 minutes, or if you wake up and can't fall asleep again, get out of bed, leave the room if possible, and do something boring until you feel sleepy.

- Keep a perspective on your plight. Losing a night's sleep isn't the end of the world. Getting upset only makes it harder to fall asleep. Relax and trust in your body's natural ability to drift off to sleep.

TABLE 2-1 Symptoms of Stress

Emotional Signs	Behavioral Signs	Physical Signs
Tendency to be irritable or aggressive	Increased use of alcohol, tobacco, or other drugs	Pounding heart
Tendency to feel anxious, fearful, or edgy	Excessive TV watching	Trembling, with nervous tics
Hyperexcitability, impulsiveness, or emotional instability	Sleep disturbances (e.g., insomnia) or excessive sleep	Grinding of teeth
Depression	Overeating or undereating	Dry mouth
Frequent feelings of boredom	Sexual problems	Excessive perspiration
Inability to concentrate		Gastrointestinal problems (diarrhea, constipation, indigestion, queasy stomach)
Fatigue		Stiff neck or aching lower back
		Migraine or tension headaches
		Frequent colds or low-grade infections
		Cold hands and feet
		Allergy or asthma attacks
		Skin problems (hives, eczema, psoriasis)

responses to stressor depend on a complex set of factors that includes temperament, health, life experiences, beliefs and ideas, and coping skills.

Common emotional responses to stressors include anxiety, depression, and fear. Although we often can moderate or learn to control them, emotional responses are determined in part by inborn personality or temperament. Some people seem to be born nervous and irritable, for example; others are innately calm and even-tempered. Scientists remain unsure just why this is or how the brain's complex emotional mechanisms work.

Our behavioral responses to stressors are controlled by the **somatic nervous system**, which manages our conscious actions. This means we can *choose* how we behave in response to the stressors in our lives. Depending on the stressor involved, effective behavioral responses may include crying, talking, or hugging; exercising, meditating, or laughing; or learning time management skills, finding a more compatible roommate, or looking for a different job. Inappropriate behavioral responses include overeating and using tobacco, alcohol, or other drugs. Effective behavioral responses promote mental and physical health and allow us to function at our best. Ineffective behavioral responses to stressors can harm our mental and physical health and can even become stressors themselves.

Let's consider the different emotional and behavioral responses of two students, Amelia and David, to a common stressor—the first exam of the semester. Both students feel anxious as the exam is passed out. Amelia relaxes her muscles and then starts by writing the answers she knows. On a second pass through the exam, she concentrates carefully on the wording of each question. Some material comes back to her, and she makes educated guesses on the remaining items. She spends the whole hour writing as much as she can and checking her answers. She leaves the room feeling calm, relaxed, and confident that she has done well on the exam.

David responds to his initial anxiety with more anxiety. He finds that he doesn't know some of the answers, and he becomes more worried. The more upset he gets, the less he can remember; and the more he blanks out, the more anxious he gets. He begins to imagine the consequences of failing the course and berates himself for not having studied more. David turns in his paper before the hour is up, without checking has answers or going back

Somatic nervous system The branch of the peripheral nervous system that governs motor functions and sensory information; largely under our conscious control.

Insomnia Inability to obtain adequate sleep.

TERMS

Several years ago, Herbert Benson developed a simple, practical technique for eliciting the relaxation response. Here's the basic procedure he recommends:

1. Pick a word, phrase, or object to focus on. If you like, you can choose a word or phrase that has a deep meaning for you, but any word or phrase will work. In Zen meditation, the word *mu* (literally, "absolutely nothing") is often used. Some meditators prefer to focus on their breathing.

2. Take a comfortable position in a quiet environment, and close your eyes if you're not focusing on an object.

3. Relax your muscles.

4. Breathe slowly and naturally. If you're using a focus word or phrase, silently repeat it each time you exhale. If you're using an object, focus on it as you breathe.

5. Keep your attitude passive. Disregard thoughts that drift in.

6. Continue for 10 to 20 minutes, once or twice a day.

7. After you've finished, sit quietly for a few minutes with your eyes first closed and then open. Then get to your feet.

Suggestions

Allow relaxation to occur at its own pace; don't try to force it. Don't be surprised if you can't tune your mind out for more than a few seconds at a time. It's nothing to get angry about. The more you ignore the intrusions, the easier doing so will get.

If you want to time your session, peek at a watch or clock occasionally, but don't set a jarring alarm.

The technique works best on an empty stomach—before a meal or about two hours after eating. Avoid times of day when you're tired—unless you want to fall asleep.

Although you'll feel refreshed even after the first session, it may take a month or more to get noticeable results. Be patient. Eventually the relaxation response will become so natural that it will occur spontaneously, or on demand, when you sit quietly for a few moments.

---

head and ending at your feet, contract and relax your other muscles. Repeat each contraction at least once, breathing in as you tense, breathing out as you relax. To speed up the process, tense and relax more muscles at one time—both arms simultaneously, for instance. With practice, you'll be able to relax very quickly and effectively by clenching and releasing only your fists.

Imagery   Imagery, or visualization, allows you to daydream without guilt. Elite athletes have found that the technique enhances sports performance, and visualization is even part of the curriculum at training camps for U.S. Olympic athletes. You can use the technique to help you relax, change your habits, or perform well, whether on an exam, a stage, or a playing field.

Next time you feel stressed, close your eyes. Imagine yourself floating on a cloud, sitting on a mountaintop, or lying in a meadow. What do you see and hear? Is it cold out? Or damp? What do you smell? What do you taste? Involve all your senses. Your body will respond as if your imagery were real. An alternative: Close your eyes and imagine a deep purple light filling your body. Now change the color into a soothing gold. As the color lightens, so should your distress. Imagery also can enhance performance. If you're worried about doing well at a task, visualize yourself performing it flawlessly.

Meditation   Meditation is a way of politely telling the mind to shut up for a while. The need to periodically stop the incessant mental chatter is so great that, from ancient times, hundreds of forms of meditation have developed in cultures all over the world. Because meditation has been at the core of many Eastern religions and philosophies, it has acquired an "Eastern" mystique that has caused some people to shy away from it. Yet meditation requires no special knowledge or background. We all know how to meditate; we need only discover that we do and then put our knowledge to use. Whatever philosophical, religious, or emotional reasons may be given for meditation, its power derives from its ability to elicit the relaxation response.

Meditation helps you to tune out the world temporarily, relieving you from both inner and outer stresses. It allows you to transcend past conditioning, fixed expectations, and the trivial pursuits of the psyche; it clears out the mental smog. The "thinker" takes time out to become the "observer"—calmly attentive, without analyzing, judging, comparing, or rationalizing. Regular practice of this quiet awareness will subtly carry over into your daily life, encouraging physical and emotional balance no matter what confronts you. See the box "Meditation and the Relaxation Response" for a step-by-step description of a meditation procedure.

Cognitive Techniques

Some stressors arise in our own minds. Ideas, beliefs, perceptions, and patterns of thinking can add to our emotional and physical stress responses and get in the way of effective behavioral responses. Each of the techniques de-

Like "planned spontaneity" or "intentional accident," "learned laughter" may sound like a contradiction. But according to William F. Fry, Jr., an emeritus professor of psychiatry at Stanford University and an authority on the physiology of mirth, you can teach yourself to laugh more. Fry, who calls himself a gelotologist (from the Greek root *gelos*, meaning laughter), says laughter defuses anger, lifts depression, increases alertness, enhances learning, promotes creativity and cooperation, fosters mental health, and may help prevent disease. It's also one of the most enjoyable ways to cope with stress.

Next time you're down or anxious, rent a Laurel and Hardy video or leaf through a book of *Far Side* cartoons. In his book *The Healing Power of Humor,* author Allen Klein also recommends these smile-inducing strategies:

- Collect silly props: clown noses, bubbles, "arrow" headbands. Put on the clown nose the next time you feel yourself getting anxious about an exam. Try blowing bubbles after an argument with your roommate.

- Have a punch line ready. When life deals you a blow—a bad grade, for example—try one of these widely applicable lines: "Oh, what an opportunity for growth and learning," "Take it back, it's not what I ordered," or "Beam me up, Scotty."

- Exaggerate to the point of absurdity. If you're having a bad day, pretend you're in the I-had-the-worst-day-in-the-world Olympics.

- Keep a photo of yourself laughing in a place where you can see it often.

- Smile when you feel down or tense. Sometimes mood follows facial expression.

- Identify traits you don't like in yourself and poke a little bit of fun at one of them at least once a day. Klein, who is bald, collects baldness jokes.

- Learn to view setbacks and annoyances as tests of your sense of humor.

For more information about the power of laughter, contact the American Association for Therapeutic Humor at 1163 Shermer Road, Northbrook, IL 60062 (708-291-0211) or the Humor Project at 110 Spring Street, Saratoga Springs, NY 12866 (518-587-8770).

---

scribed below can help you change unhealthy thought patterns to ones that will help you cope with stress. As with any skill, mastering these techniques takes practice and patience.

Worry Constructively   Worrying, someone once said, is like shoveling smoke. Think back to the worries you had last week. How many of them were needless? Worry only about things you can control. Try to stand aside from the problem, consider the positive steps you can take to solve it, and then carry them out. You've done what you can; you can quit worrying.

Moderate Expectations   Expectations are exhausting and restricting. The fewer expectations you have, the more you can live spontaneously and joyfully. The more you expect from others, the more often you will feel let down. Trying to meet the expectations others have of you is often futile as well. In fact, the surest road to failure is to try to please everyone around you. That's a road you can choose to bypass. As therapist Fritz Perls put it, "I don't exist to fulfill your expectations, and you don't exist to fulfill mine."

Monitor Self-Talk   If you catch your mind beating up on you—"Late for class again! You can't even cope with college! How do you expect to ever hold down a profes-

sional job?"—change your inner dialogue. Talk to yourself as you would to a child you love: "You're a smart, capable person. You've solved other problems; you'll handle this one. Tomorrow you'll simply schedule things so you get to class with a few minutes to spare."

Weed Out Trivia   You can burden your memory with too much information. A major source of stress is trying to "store" too much data. Forget unimportant details (they will usually be self-evident). Keep your memory free for essential ones.

Live in the Present   Do you clog your mind by reliving past events? Clinging to experiences and emotions, particularly unpleasant ones, can be a deadly business. Clear your mind of the old debris; let it go. Free yourself to enjoy what's happening now.

Cultivate Your Sense of Humor   When it comes to stress, laughter may be the best medicine. Even a fleeting smile produces changes in your autonomic nervous system that can lift your spirits. And a few minutes of belly laughing can be as invigorating as brisk exercise. Hearty laughter elevates your heart rate, aids digestion, eases pain, and triggers the release of endorphins and other pleasurable and stimulating chemicals in the brain. After a good laugh, your muscles go slack; your pulse and blood pressure dip below normal. You are relaxed. Ridicule, cynicism, and sarcasm don't have the same effects, however. Neither does gruesome or offensive black humor, which is an unconscious means of dealing with fears and anxieties. Therapeutic humor, in contrast, reflects a healthy appreciation of life's absurdities and paradoxes. Therapeutic humor gives you a break, even if a short one, from the hassles of daily life. It detaches you from both your situation and yourself. Cultivate the ability to laugh at yourself, and you'll have a handy and instantly effective stress reliever. Refer to the box "Laughing Matters" for some suggestions for adding more laughter to your life.

Go with the Flow Remember that the branch that bends in the storm doesn't break. Try to flow with your life, accepting the things you can't change. Be forgiving of faults, your own and others'. Instead of anticipating happiness at some indefinite point in the future, realize that pleasure is integral to being alive. You can create it every day of your life. View challenges as an opportunity to learn and grow. Be flexible. In this way you can make stress work for you rather than against you, enhancing your overall health.

CREATING A PERSONAL PLAN FOR MANAGING STRESS

What are the most important sources of stress in your life? Are you coping successfully with these stressors? There is no single strategy or program for managing stress that will work for everyone, but you can use the principles of behavior management described in Chapter 1 to create a program tailored specifically to your needs. The most important starting point for a successful stress management program is to learn to listen to your body. When you learn to recognize the stress response and the emotions and thoughts that accompany it, you'll be in a position to take charge of that crucial moment and handle it in a healthy way.

Identifying Stressors

Before you can learn to manage the stressors in your life, you have to identify them. A strategy many experts recommend is to keep a stress journal for a week or two. Each time you feel or display a stress reaction, record the time and the circumstances in your journal. Note what you were doing at the time, what you were thinking or feeling, and the outcome of your response.

After keeping your dairy for a few weeks, you should be able to spot some patterns. You may notice, for example, that mornings are usually the most stressful part of your day. Or you may discover that when you're angry at your roommate, you're apt to respond with behaviors that

only make matters worse. Once you've outlined the general pattern of stress in your life, you may want to focus in on a particularly problematic stressor or on an inappropriate behavioral response you've identified. Keep a stress log for another week or two that focuses just on the early morning hours, for example, or just on your arguments with your roommate. The more information you gather, the easier it will be to develop effective strategies for coping with the stressors in your life.

Designing Your Program

Earlier in this chapter, you learned about many different techniques for combating stress. Now that you've identified the key stressors in your life, it's time to choose the techniques that will work best for you and create an action plan for change. Finding a buddy to work on stress management with you can make the process more fun and increase your chances of success. Some experts recommend drawing up a formal contract with yourself like the one shown in Figure 2-3.

Whether or not you complete a contract, it's important to design rewards into your plan. You might treat yourself to breakfast in a favorite restaurant on the weekend if you eat a nutritious breakfast every weekday morning. If you practice your relaxation technique faithfully, you might reward yourself with a long bath or an hour of pleasure reading at the end of the day. It's also important to evaluate your plan regularly and redesign it as your needs change. Under times of increased stress, for example, you might want to focus on good eating, exercise, and relaxation habits. Over time, your new stress management skills will become almost automatic. You'll feel better, accomplish more, and reduce your risk of disease.

Getting Help

If the techniques discussed so far don't provide you with enough relief from the stress in your life, you might want to consult a peer counselor, join a support group, or participate in a few psychotherapy sessions. Your student health center or student affairs office can tell you whether your campus has a peer counseling program. Such programs are usually staffed by volunteer students who have received special training that emphasizes the preservation of confidentiality. Peer counselors can steer you to other campus or community resources, or simply provide you with an understanding ear.

Support groups are typically organized around a particular issue or problem. In your area, you might find a support group for first-year students; for reentering students; for single parents; for students of your race, ethnic group, religion, or national origin; for people with eating disorders; or for rape survivors. The number of such groups has increased in recent years, as more and more people discover how therapeutic it can be to talk with others who share the same situation.

Figure 2-3 *Sample contract for a stress management program.*

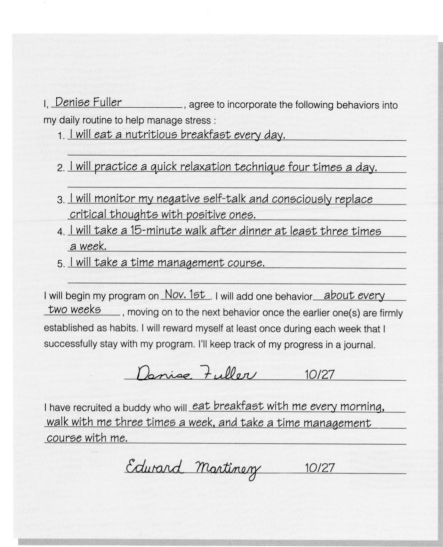

I, _Denise Fuller_, agree to incorporate the following behaviors into my daily routine to help manage stress :

1. _I will eat a nutritious breakfast every day._

2. _I will practice a quick relaxation technique four times a day._

3. _I will monitor my negative self-talk and consciously replace critical thoughts with positive ones._

4. _I will take a 15-minute walk after dinner at least three times a week._

5. _I will take a time management course._

I will begin my program on _Nov. 1st_. I will add one behavior _about every two weeks_, moving on to the next behavior once the earlier one(s) are firmly established as habits. I will reward myself at least once during each week that I successfully stay with my program. I'll keep track of my progress in a journal.

Denise Fuller   10/27

I have recruited a buddy who will _eat breakfast with me every morning, walk with me three times a week, and take a time management course with me._

Edward Martinez   10/27

Short-term psychotherapy can also be tremendously helpful in dealing with stress-related problems. Your student health center may offer psychotherapy on a sliding-fee scale; the county mental health center in your area may do the same. If you belong to any type of religious organization, check to see whether pastoral counseling is available. Your physician can refer you to psychotherapists in your community. Not all therapists are right for all people, so be prepared to have initial sessions with several. Choose the one you feel most comfortable with.

SUMMARY

Stress-creating situations can be physical or psychological, pleasant or unpleasant. How people respond to stress helps determine their sense of well-being and their feeling of control over their health and their lives.

What Is Stress?

- In Hans Selye's terms, stress is "the body's total biological response to any demand." Physically, everyone responds to stressors in generally the same way.

- The body's response to stress, or general adaptation syndrome (GAS), has three stages: alarm, resistance, and exhaustion. GAS is controlled by the autonomic nervous system.

- The alarm stage of GAS is the fight-or-flight reaction. The sympathetic nervous system stimulates the release of chemical messengers that trigger changes in the body that mobilize it for action.

- The resistance stage of GAS, controlled by the parasympathetic nervous system, allows the body to readjust; body systems are regulated, and any damage sustained is repaired. Both the alarm and the resistance stages require considerable energy.

- The exhaustion stage occurs only if the body's reserves of energy (including adaptive energy) are depleted in a stress response; the results are distorted perceptions, disorganized thinking, and—in extreme cases—death.

- Most stresses of modern life can't be handled with a physical response; moreover, many of them continue indefinitely. A person whose body is constantly mobilized against these stresses may become a victim of "diseases of adaptation."
- Emotional and behavioral responses to stressors vary among individuals based on factors such as temperament, past experiences, beliefs, and coping skills. Emotional responses can be moderated; behavioral responses can be controlled.

Stress and Disease

- The relationships between stress and disease is complex. Too many stressors or lack of coping skills can increase a person's risk of illness or disease.
- Stress can contribute to high blood pressure and atherosclerosis. People who tend to respond to stressors with anger and hostility are at increased risk for cardiovascular disease.
- Both emotional and physical stressors lead to a decline in the body's immune response; stress, therefore, affects our ability to fight infection.
- Stress can trigger or aggravate many other health problems, from asthma to post-traumatic stress disorder.

Techniques for Managing Stress

- Stressors from a variety of sources—the environment, social interaction, and our own bodies and minds— are an inevitable part of life. Appropriate responses to stressors offer protection against the damaging effects of stress.
- Emotional and social support systems help buffer people from the effects of stress and make illness and disease less likely.
- Exercise is a coping technique that reduces anxiety and increases energy.
- Good nutrition helps the body build an energy bank necessary for coping with stress.
- Time management is an effective coping technique for those who tend to procrastinate. Steps that can be taken include setting priorities, scheduling for peak efficiency, setting realistic goals, writing down goals, allowing enough time, and dividing long-term goals into short-term goals.
- The relaxation response is the opposite of the fight-or-flight response; techniques that trigger it counteract the physiological effects of chronic stress.
- Relaxation techniques include progressive relaxation, imagery, and meditation. Progressive relaxation involves tensing and then relaxing parts of the body; practice leads to the ability to quickly relax. The use

of imagery or visualization is a form of daydreaming or imagining; it aids not only in relaxing, but also in healing, changing habits, and improving performance. Through meditation, the world with all its stresses can be tuned out.
- There are many cognitive strategies that can help an individual cope with stress; these include worrying constructively, monitoring self-talk, and cultivating a sense of humor.

Creating a Personal Plan for Managing Stress

- People can create successful individualized programs for coping with stress. Stressors and inappropriate behavioral responses can be identified and studied with a stress journal or log. Completing a contract and recruiting a buddy can help a program succeed.
- Additional help in dealing with stress is available from peer counseling, support groups, and psychotherapy.

TAKE ACTION

1. Choose a friend or family member who seems to deal particularly well with stress. Interview that person about his or her methods of managing stress. What strategies does he or she employ? What can you learn from that person that can be applied to your own life?

2. Investigate the services available in your community to help people deal with stress, such as peer counseling, support groups, and time management classes. If possible, visit or gather information on one or more of them. Write a description and evaluation of their services, including your personal reactions.

3. Read through the stress management techniques described in the chapter and choose one to try for a week. If possible, select a behavior or strategy, such as regular exercise or systematic time management, that you've never tried before. After a trial period, evaluate the effectiveness of the strategy you chose. Did your stress level decrease during the week? Were you better able to deal with daily hassles and any more severe stressors that you encountered?

JOURNAL ENTRY

1. Watch for the physical changes of the stress response when you're in stressful situations. In your health journal, keep a stress log in which you note how many times in a day you experience the stress reaction to some degree. Also include a brief description of the circumstances surrounding your stress reaction. Is your life more or less stressful than you expected?

2. *Critical Thinking:* Some techniques for stress reduction, including meditation, imagery, and hypnosis, are considered strange or unscientific by some people. Find out more about one such stress reduction technique through library research. What evidence can you find to support or oppose the idea that the technique can help people manage stress? Based on your research, write a brief essay in your health journal that gives your opinion on the stress management technique you've chosen. As you consider the evidence, be sure to look closely at your sources of information.

3. Think about all the different environments in which you function, including your classrooms, the student union, the dorm, your house. Are some more stressful than others? Make a list of the environments ordered from the most stressful to the least stressful. Indicate next to each environment the reasons you think it is stressful or nonstressful. Now start at the top of your list and record three or more ways to reduce the stressful impact these environments have on you.

4. Make a list of daily hassles that you commonly encounter, such as being awakened early by loud neighbors, standing in long lines for lunch, or repeatedly misplacing your keys. Divide your list into two groups: those stressors you may be able to avoid and those that are inevitable. For each stressor that is potentially avoidable, describe a strategy for eliminating it from your life. For stressors that are inevitable, make a list of effective coping mechanisms.

5. Complete the "Time Stress Questionnaire" in this chapter to determine if you have difficulty with time-related stressors. If you do, review your responses and select the five most significant time-related stressors for you; record these in your health journal. Next, make a list of concrete steps you can take to deal with each of these key time-related stressors.

BEHAVIOR CHANGE STRATEGY

DEALING WITH TEST ANXIETY

Are you a person who doesn't perform as well as you should on tests? Do you find that anxiety interferes with your ability to study effectively before the test and to think clearly in the test situation? If so, you may be experiencing test anxiety. People suffering from test anxiety often see tests as threatening, feel inadequate to cope with them, concentrate on the negative consequences of doing poorly, and anticipate failure, which becomes a self-fulfilling prophecy. They often feel so helpless that they can't mobilize their resources to deal with the problem.

Test anxiety can be a serious problem, and it often gets worse rather than better with time. Typically, greater anxiety leads to a poorer performance, which leads to even greater anxiety, and so on. Sometimes the only solution the worried student can think of is to stop taking tests—that is, to drop out of school. Luckily, there are several ways to deal with test anxiety, some of which are also effective ways of dealing with anxiety in other forms, such as phobias and fear of public speaking.

Behavioral approaches to problems like this operate on the assumption that fear and anxiety are learned behaviors and that a person can unlearn them by following appropriate procedures. Test anxiety is an ineffective response to a stressful situation that can be replaced with more effective responses. Two methods that have proven effective in helping people deal with test anxiety are systematic desensitization and success rehearsal. Both can help people interrupt the vicious cycle of fear that prevents them from doing their best in stressful performance situations. If test anxiety is a problem for you, try implementing one of these programs before you take your next exam.

Systematic Desensitization

Systematic desensitization is based on the premise that you can't feel anxiety and be relaxed at the same time. The program described here has three phases—constructing an anxiety hierarchy, learning and practicing deep muscle relaxation, and carrying out the actual steps of the desensitization program.

Constructing an Anxiety Hierarchy Begin the first phase by thinking of 10 or more situations related to your fear, such as hearing the announcement of the test date in class, studying for the test, sitting in the classroom waiting to be handed an examination booklet, reading the test questions, and so on. Write each situation on an index card, using a brief phrase to describe it on one side of the card and on the other side listing several realistic details that will help you vividly imagine yourself actually experiencing the situation. For example, if the situation is "hearing that 50 percent of the final grade will be based on the two exams," the prompts might include such details as "sitting in the big lecture auditorium in Baily Hall," "taking notes in my blue notebook," "surrounded by many other students," and "listening to Professor Smith's voice."

Next, arrange your cards in order starting with the situation that causes the least anxiety and ending with the situation that causes the most anxiety. Rate each item to reflect the amount of anxiety you feel when you encounter it in the natural environment to make sure your hierarchy is accurate. Assign ratings on a scale of 0 to 100 and make sure that the distances between items are fairly small and approximately equal. When you're sure that your anxiety hierarchy is a true reflection of your feelings, number the cards.

Learning and Practicing Deep Muscle Relaxation

The second step of the program involves learning to relax your muscles and to recognize when they are relaxed. A very effective way to do this is through progressive relaxation, or deep muscle relaxation, which is described in this chapter. Basically, it consists of alternately tensing and relaxing your muscles, moving from one part of the body to another, while paying attention to the internal activities and sensations you are feeling at the time. Find a quiet, dimly lit setting where you won't be interrupted for 20 or 30 minutes and sit or lie on a comfortable couch or bed. It would be ideal to have instructions recorded on tape—such as "Make a fist with your left hand. Squeeze it as tightly as you can. (pause) Now relax it completely. Let your hand go limp. Notice how it feels. (pause)"—and listen to the tape the first several times you practice the relaxation procedure. As you become proficient at relaxing, you'll be able to relax without the tape and ultimately to skip steps and go directly to a deeply relaxed state within a few minutes. When you can do this, you're ready to go on to the next phase of the program.

Implementing the Desensitization Program   Use the quiet place where you practiced your relaxation exercises. Sit comfortably and place your stack of numbered cards within reach. Take several minutes to relax completely, and then look at the first card, reading both the brief phrase and the descriptive prompts. Close your eyes and imagine yourself in that situation for about 10 seconds. Then put the card down and relax completely for about 30 seconds. Look at the card again, imagine the situation for 10 seconds, and relax again for 30 seconds.

At this point, evaluate your current level of anxiety about the situation on the card in terms of the rating scale you devised earlier. If your anxiety level is 5 or below, relax for two minutes and go on to the second card. If it's higher than 5, repeat the routine with the same card until the anxiety decreases. If you have difficulty with a particular item, go back to the previous item and then try it again. If you still can't visualize it without anxiety, try to construct three new items with smaller steps between them and insert them before the troublesome item.

In general, you should be able to move through one to four items per session. Sessions can be conducted anywhere from twice a day to twice a week and should last no more than 20 minutes. Keep track of your progress by recording the names and numbers of the items you imagined successfully during each session, the number of times you imagined each one, and the anxiety rating of each item when you first prepared the hierarchy and after you desensitized yourself to it. It's helpful to graph your progress in a way that has meaning for you.

After you have successfully completed your program, you should be desensitized to the real-life situations that previously elicited anxiety. If you find that you do experience some anxiety in the real situations, take 30 seconds or a minute to relax completely, just as you did when you were practicing. Remember, fear and relaxation are incompatible; you can't experience them both at the same time. You have the ability to choose relaxation over fear.

Success Rehearsal

A variation on desensitization is the approach called success rehearsal. To practice this method, take your hierarchy of anxiety-eliciting situations and vividly imagine yourself successfully dealing with each one. Create a detailed scenario for each situation and use your imagination to experience genuine feelings of confidence. Recognize your negative thoughts ("I'll be so nervous I won't be able to think straight") and replace them with positive ones ("Anxiety will keep me alert so I can do a good job"). Proceed one step at a time, thinking of strategies for success as you go that you can later implement. These might include the following:

• Before the test, find out everything you can about it—its format, the material to be covered, the criteria used to grade essay answers. Ask the instructor for practice materials.

• Devise a study plan. This might include forming a study group with one or more classmates or outlining what you will study, when, where, and for how long.

• Once in the test situation, sit away from possible distractions, listen carefully to instructions, and ask for clarification if you don't understand a direction.

• During the test, answer the easiest questions first. If you don't know an answer and there is no penalty for incorrect answers, guess. If there are several questions you have difficulty answering, review the ones you have already handled. Figure out approximately how much time you have to cover each question or part of the test.

• For math problems, try to estimate the answer before doing the precise calculations.

• For true-false questions, look for qualifiers such as *always* and *never*. Such questions are likely to be false.

• For essay questions, look for key words in the question that indicate what the instructor is looking for in the answer. Develop a brief outline of your answer, sketching out what you will cover. Stick to your outline and keep track of the time you're spending on your answer. Don't let yourself get caught with unanswered questions when time is up.

• Remain calm and focused throughout the test. Don't let negative thoughts rattle you. If you start to become nervous, take some deep breaths and relax your muscles completely for a minute or so.

The best way to counter test anxiety is with successful test-taking experiences. The more times you succeed, the more your test anxiety will recede. If you find that these methods aren't sufficient to get your anxiety under control, you may want to seek professional help with the problem. But whether you use desensitization, success rehearsal, or another approach, it's wise to take action as early as possible to keep test anxiety from significantly interfering with your education plans and career goals.

SELECTED BIBLIOGRAPHY

American College of Sports Medicine. 1990. *The Recommended Quantity and Quality of Exercise for Developing and Maintaining Cardiorespiratory and Muscular Fitness in Healthy Adults.* Indianapolis: American College of Sports Medicine.

Benson, H., with W. Proctor. 1987. *Your Maximum Mind.* New York: Random House.

Borysenko, J. 1987. *Minding the Body, Minding the Mind.* Menlo Park, Calif.: Addison-Wesley.

Burka, J. B. 1990. *Procrastination: Why You Do It, What to Do About It.* Reading, Mass.: Addison-Wesley.

Cohen, S., and others. 1991. Psychological stress and susceptibility to the common cold. *New England Journal of Medicine* 325(9): 606–612.

Cooper, C. L. and R. Payne. 1988. *Causes, Coping, and Consequences of Stress at Work.* New York: John Wiley.

Girdano, D., and G. Everly. 1989. *Controlling Stress and Tension,* 3rd ed. Englewood Cliffs, N.J.: Prentice-Hall.

Hauri, P., and S. Linde. 1990. *No More Sleepless Nights.* New York: John Wiley.

Johansson, N. 1991. Effectiveness of a stress management program in reducing anxiety and depression in nursing students. *College Health* 40:125–129.

Karasek, R., and T. Theorell. 1990. *Healthy Work: Stress, Productivity, and the Reconstruction of Working Life.* New York: Basic Books.

Klein, A. 1989. *The Healing Power of Humor.* Los Angeles: Jeremy P. Tarcher.

Lambert, L. 1984. *The American Medical Association Guide to Better Sleep.* New York: Random House.

Lepore, S., and others. 1991. Dynamic role of social support in the link between chronic stress and psychological distress. *Journal of Personality and Social Psychology* 61(6): 899–909.

Martin, G., and J. Pear. 1988. *Behavior Modification: What It Is and How to Do It,* 3rd ed. Englewood Cliffs, N.J.: Prentice-Hall.

Miller, A. 1988. Stress on the job. *Newsweek,* 25 April, 40–45.

Mitler, E. A., and M. Merrill. 1990. *101 Questions About Sleep and Dreams.* Del Mar, Calif.: Wakefulness-Sleep Education and Research Foundation.

Ornstein, R., and D. Sobel. 1989. *Healthy Pleasures.* Reading, Mass.: Addison-Wesley.

Peterson, M. L., and others. 1991. Stress and pathogenesis of infectious disease. *Reviews of Infectious Diseases* 13:710–20.

Selye, H. 1976. *The Stress of Life,* rev. ed. New York: McGraw-Hill.

Selye, H. 1979. Stress: The basis of illness. In *Inner Balance: The Power of Holistic Health,* ed. E. M. Goldwag. Englewood Cliffs, N.J.: Prentice-Hall.

Smith, E. 1987. Meditation goes mainstream. *Washington Post Health,* 6 October.

Sweeney, D. R. 1989. *Overcoming Insomnia.* New York: G. P. Putnam's.

Wechsler, R. 1987. A new prescription: Mind over malady. *Discover,* February, 51–61.

RECOMMENDED READINGS

Antonovsky, A. 1990. *Learned Resourcefulness.* New York: Springer-Verlag. *Presents a variety of strategies for managing and coping with stress and increasing self-control and adaptive behavior.*

Cousins, N. 1989. *Head First: The Biology of Hope.* New York: E. P. Dutton. *An entertaining account of some of the scientific evidence for the view that positive emotions can help combat serious illness, drawn from the author's own experience of illness and his exchanges with many patients.*

Dement, W. C. 1992. *The Sleepwatchers.* Stanford, Calif.: Stanford Alumni Association. *An entertaining discussion of sleep and dreams by one of the world's foremost authorities on sleep.*

Farquhar, J. W. 1987. *The American Way of Life Need Not Be Hazardous to Your Health.* Reading, Mass.: Addison-Wesley. *Based on the research from the Stanford Heart Disease Prevention Program; describes effective stress management and encourages habits that will reduce the incidence of premature strokes and heart attacks.*

Hanson, P. G. 1986. *The Joy of Stress.* Kansas City: Andrews, McMeel and Parker. *Engagingly presented, compact, well-tested advice from a Canadian doctor who shows how to turn stress into an ally rather than an enemy.*

Justice, B. 1987. *Who Gets Sick?* Houston: Peak Press. *Explores current evidence suggesting that positive attitudes and beliefs can aid in health promotion and disease prevention.*

Lazarus, R. 1991. *Emotions and Adaptation.* New York: Oxford University Press. *Written by one of the foremost authorities on stress and adaptation, this book provides a theory of emotional processes that explains how different emotions are elicited and expressed and how the emotional range of an individual develops over his or her lifetime.*

Matheny, K. B., and R. J. Riordan. 1992. *Stress and Strategies for Lifestyle Management.* Atlanta: Georgia State University Business Press. *Includes practical and realistic insights into managing stress and changing maladaptive lifestyles. It contains separate chapters on stress inoculation and creating stress-free relationships.*

Schafer, W. 1992. *Stress Management for Wellness,* 2nd ed. Fort Worth: Harcourt Brace Jovanovich. *Presents basic information on stress and wellness and many different stress-management techniques; contains a separate chapter on college stress.*

3

Mental Health

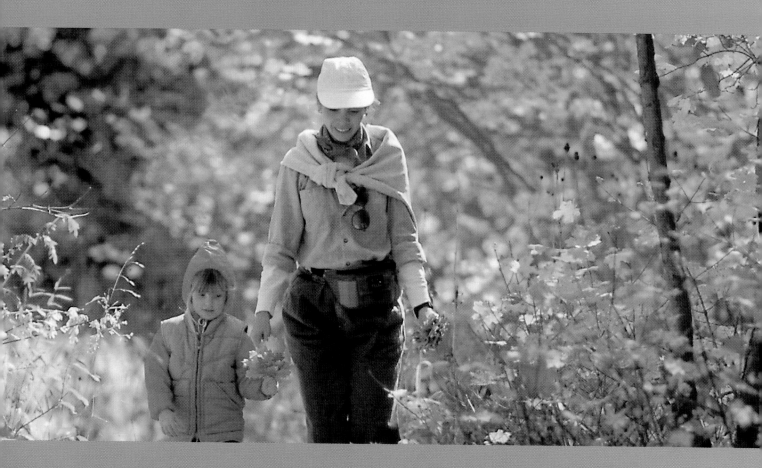

CONTENTS

⬧ You're intrigued by someone you know slightly at school. She's not particularly attractive, doesn't come from a wealthy or privileged background, and is just an average student. Yet she always seems confident, relaxed, and happy about who she is. It's fun to be around her because she's so energetic and unpretentious. You know a lot of people who have more going for them than she does but are filled with self-doubts. What's her secret, anyway? And how can you get to be as self-assured as she is?

⬧ Although you basically like your roommate, the two of you have very different ideas and habits and always seem to be at odds. You like to socialize at the student union and study in your room; your roommate prefers to study at the library and socialize in the room. You like to go to bed early; your roommate likes to stay up late listening to music. You're up at six o'clock and want to hear the news on your radio; your roommate wants to sleep till eight. You joked about it at first, but lately you've been getting on each other's nerves. In fact, you've stopped talking and started slamming doors. You don't want to spend the rest of the year with all this tension in the air. What can you do to improve the situation?

⬧ Things seemed to be going okay for you recently, but last week you had an unpleasant experience you can't understand. You suddenly felt terrified for no reason. You ran back to your room and stayed there until it passed. Now you're worried that it will happen again, and everything seems gray, gloomy, and threatening. You wonder if you're having an allergic reaction to something you ate, or if the medication you're taking for your skin could be causing these feelings. When you mentioned the incident to a friend, she suggested you see someone at the student health services. You're not so sure you want to tell anyone else about it. Should you?

⬧ You run into an old friend in a coffee shop and start talking about the "good old days." Things haven't been going too well for her lately, and in the course of the conversation she comments that her life isn't worth much. Then she remarks that people would be better off if she weren't around. When she says goodbye, she gives you a warm hug and is very emotional. You don't take her comments or behavior too seriously at the time, but later you keep thinking about them. Could she have been serious? Should you tell anyone or do anything? If so, what?

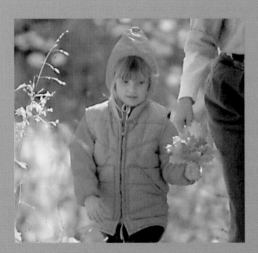

MAKING CONNECTIONS

Your overall health is powerfully influenced by some factors you may not be very aware of—your thoughts and beliefs about yourself, your habitual ways of handling your feelings, the patterns you've developed for interacting with other people. Looking more closely at these components of mental health can give you useful insights into yourself and lead to unexpected benefits. In the scenarios presented on these pages, each related to mental health, individuals have to use information, make a decision, or choose a course of action. How would you act in each of these situations? This chapter provides information about mental health, psychological problems, and getting help for psychological distress. After finishing the chapter, read the scenarios again. Have your responses changed?

What exactly is *mental* health? Some people justify their lifestyle by claiming that it promotes better mental health than others do, and they may even term those who refuse to accept the lifestyle as "sick" or "crazy." Mental health becomes the focus of battles in legislatures and courts, where expert witnesses contradict each other on whether defendants were mentally healthy enough to have been responsible for their acts or whether people are so mentally ill that they should be treated with medicine or hospitalized involuntarily. When the perpetrator of an especially heinous crime is found "mentally incompetent to stand trial" or "not guilty by reason of insanity," it's not unusual to hear mental illness declared a "myth" promoted by the mental health "establishment."

Is mental health a myth? We don't think so. We think there *is* such a thing as mental health just as there is physical health (and the two are intertwined). Just as your body can work well or poorly, giving you feelings of pleasure or pain, your mind can also work well or poorly, giving you happiness or unhappiness. If you feel pain and unhappiness rather than pleasure and happiness or if you sense that you could be functioning at a higher level, there may be ways you can help yourself, either on your own or with professional help. This chapter will explain how.

WHAT MENTAL HEALTH IS NOT

Mental health is not the same as mental **normality.** Being mentally normal simply means being close to average. You can define your normal body temperature because a few degrees above or below this temperature always means physical sickness. But your ideas and attitudes can vary tremendously without your losing efficiency or feeling emotional distress. And psychological diversity is valuable; living in a society of people with varied ideas and lifestyles makes life interesting. Such a society can respond creatively to unexpected challenges.

Conforming to social demands is not necessarily a mark of mental health. If you don't question what's going on around you, you're not fulfilling your potential as a thinking, questioning human being. For example, our society admires the framers of the U.S. Constitution and the abolitionists who rebelled against injustices. If conformity signified mental health, then political dissent would indicate mental illness by definition (and we have indeed seen that definition used by dictators in this century). Were such a definition valid, Galileo would have been mad for insisting that the earth went around the sun.

Never seeking help for personal problems also does not mean that you are mentally healthy, any more than seeking help proves that you are mentally ill. Unhappy people may not want to seek professional help because they don't want to reveal their problems to others, may fear what their friends might think, or may not know

whom to ask for help. People who are severely disturbed mentally may not even realize they need help, or they may become so suspicious of other people that they can be treated only against their will.

And we cannot say people are "mentally ill" or "mentally healthy" on the basis of symptoms alone. Life constantly presents problems. Time and life inevitably change the environment and change our minds and bodies, and changes present problems. The symptom of anxiety, for example, can help us face a problem and solve it before it gets too big. Someone who shows no anxiety may be refusing to recognize problems or refusing to do anything about them. A person who is anxious for good reason is likely to be judged more mentally healthy in the long run than someone who is inappropriately calm.

Finally, we cannot judge mental health from the way people look. All too often a person who seems to be OK and even happy suddenly takes his or her own life. Usually such people lack close friends who might have known of their desperation. We all learn early to conceal and "lie." We may believe that our complaints put unfair demands on others. True, suffering in silence can be a virtue sometimes, but it can also impede help.

WHAT MENTAL HEALTH IS

It is even harder to say what mental health *is* than what it is *not.* Mental health can be defined either negatively as the absence of sickness or positively as the presence of wellness. The narrower, negative definition has several advantages: It concentrates attention on the worst problems and on the people most in need, and it tends to avoid value judgments about which of the many ways we can lead our lives is best. However, if we consider everybody mentally healthy who is not severely mentally disturbed, we end up ignoring common psychological problems that can be addressed.

A positive definition—mental health as the presence of wellness—is a more ambitious way of looking at mental health. It tries to make you aware of human potential in yourself that you might want to develop. Freedom from psychological disorders is only one factor in mental wellness. Abraham Maslow, an American psychology professor, eloquently described an ideal of mental health in his book *Toward a Psychology of Being.* He was convinced that psychologists were too preoccupied with people who had failed in some way. He also did not like the way psychologists tried to reduce human striving to physiological

Normality   The mental characteristics attributed to the majority of people in a population at a given time.

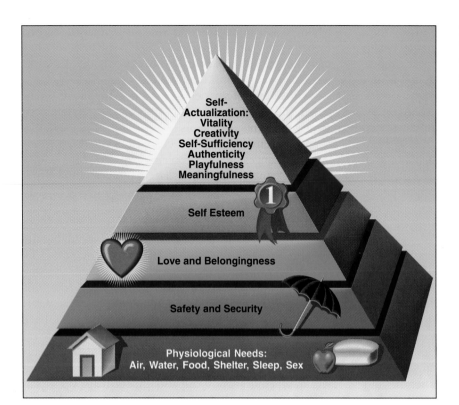

Figure 3-1 *Maslow's hierarchy of needs.*
Source: A. Maslow. 1970. *Motivation and Personality,* 2nd ed. (New York: Harper and Row).

needs or drives. According to Maslow, there is a *hierarchy of needs,* listed here in order of decreasing urgency: physiological needs, safety, being loved, maintaining self-esteem, and self-actualization (Figure 3-1). When urgent needs like the need for food are satisfied, less urgent needs take priority. Most of us are well fed and feel reasonably safe, so we are driven by higher motives. Maslow's conclusions were based on his study of a group of visibly successful people who seemed to be living at their fullest. Among them were historical figures such as Abraham Lincoln, Henry David Thoreau, and Ludwig van Beethoven; famous people then living, such as Eleanor Roosevelt and Albert Einstein; and some of his own friends and acquaintances. He called these people **self-actualized;** he thought they had fulfilled a good measure of their human potential and suggested that such people all share certain qualities.

TERMS

Self-actualized Describes a person who has achieved the highest level of growth in Maslow's hierarchy.

Self-esteem Satisfaction and confidence in oneself; the valuing of oneself as a person.

Self-concept The ideas, feelings, and perceptions one has about oneself.

Other-directed Guided in behavior by the values and expectations of others.

Inner-directed Guided in behavior by an inner set of rules and values.

Authenticity Genuineness.

Realism

Self-actualized people are able to deal with the world as it is and not demand that it be otherwise. If you are realistic, you know the difference between what is and what you want. You also know what you can change and what you cannot. Unrealistic people often spend a great deal of energy trying to force the world and other people into their ideal picture. Realistic people accept evidence that contradicts what they want to believe, and if it is important evidence, they modify their beliefs.

Acceptance

Mentally healthy people are able to largely accept themselves and others. Self-acceptance means that they have a positive **self-concept** or self-image, or appropriately high **self-esteem.** They have positive but realistic mental images of themselves and have positive feelings about who they are, what they are capable of, and what roles they play. People who feel good about themselves are likely to live up to their positive self-image and enjoy successes that in turn reinforce these good feelings. A good self-concept is based on a realistic view of personal worth—it does not mean being egocentric or "stuck on yourself."

Being able to tolerate our own imperfections and still feel positive about ourselves helps us tolerate the imperfections of others. Mentally healthy people tend to be optimistic about what they can expect from other people, until experience proves their optimism to be unrealistic. Acceptance means being willing to interact with people who are imperfect and unlikely to change.

Autonomy

Mentally healthy people are able to direct themselves, acting independently of their social environment. Autonomy is more than freedom from physical control by something or someone outside the self. Many people, for example, shrink from being themselves and from expressing their own feelings because they fear disapproval and rejection. They are unable to act freely and respond only to what they feel as outside pressure. Such behavior is **other-directed.** In contrast, **inner-directed** people find guidance from within, from their own values and feelings. They are not afraid to be themselves. Mentally free people act because they choose to, not because they are driven or pressured.

Being free can give healthy people certain childlike qualities. Very small children have a quality of being "real." They respond in a genuine, spontaneous way to whatever happens. Someone who is genuine needs no pretenses. Being free and genuine means not having to plan words or actions to get approval or to make an impression. It means being aware of feelings and being willing to express them; in other words, being unselfconsciously oneself, here and now. This quality is sometimes called **authenticity;** such people are *authentic,* the "real thing."

Capacity for Intimacy

Healthy people are capable of physical and emotional intimacy. They can expose their feelings and thoughts to other people. They are open to the pleasure of intimate physical contact and to the risks and satisfactions of being close to others in a caring, sensitive way. Intimate physical contact may mean "good sex," but it also means something more—intense awareness of both your partner and yourself in which contact becomes communication.

Chapters 4 and 5 discuss intimacy and sexuality in more detail.

Creativity

Mentally healthy people are creative and have a continuing fresh appreciation for what goes on around them. They are not necessarily great poets, scientists, or musicians, but they do live their everyday lives in creative ways: "A first-rate soup is more creative than a second-rate painting." Creative people seem to see more and to be open to new experiences; they don't fear the unknown. And they don't need to reduce uncertainty or to avoid it, but actually find it attractive.

How did Maslow's group achieve their exemplary mental health, and (more importantly) how can *we* attain it? Maslow himself did not answer that question, but we have a few suggestions. Undoubtedly it helps to have been treated with respect, love, and understanding as a child, to have experienced stability and to have been given a sense of mastery. As adults, since we cannot redo the past, we must concentrate on meeting current psychological challenges in ways that will lead to long-term mental wellness.

MEETING LIFE'S CHALLENGES

Life is full of challenges—large and small. Everyone, regardless of how fortunate in having the right genes and the right family, must learn to cope successfully with new situations and new people. To develop mental wellness, each of us must continue to grow psychologically, developing new and more sophisticated coping mechanisms to suit our current lives. We must develop an adult identity that enhances our self-esteem and autonomy. To interact

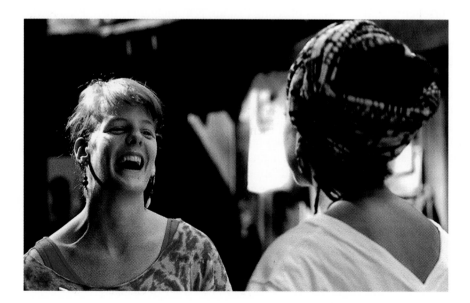

Self-actualized people respond in a genuine, spontaneous way to what happens around them.

TABLE 3-1 Erikson's Stages of Development

Age	Conflict	Important People	Task
Birth to 1 year	Trust vs. mistrust	Mother or other primary caregiver	In being fed and comforted, developing the trust that others will respond to your needs
1 to 3 years	Autonomy vs. shame and self-doubt	Parents	In toilet training, locomotion, and exploration, learning self-control without losing the capacity for assertiveness
3 to 6 years	Initiative vs. guilt	Family	In playful talking and locomotion, developing a conscience based on parental prohibitions that is not too inhibiting
6 to 12 years	Industry vs. inferiority	Neighborhood and school	In school and playing with peers, learning the value of accomplishment and perseverance without feeling inadequate
Adolescence	Identity vs. identity confusion	Peers	Developing a stable sense of who you are—your needs, abilities, interpersonal style, and values
Young adulthood	Intimacy vs. isolation	Close friends, sex partners	Learning to live and share intimately with others, often in sexual relationships
Middle adulthood	Generativity vs. self-absorption	Work associates, children, community	Doing things for others, including parenting and civic activities
Older adulthood	Integrity vs. despair	Humankind	Affirming the value of life and its ideals

Adapted from Erik Erikson. 1963. *Childhood and Society* (New York: W. W. Norton).

---

with others in a positive and meaningful way, we must also learn to communicate honestly and to avoid being defensive.

Growing Up Psychologically

Along the path from birth to old age, we are confronted with a series of challenges. How we respond to these challenges influences the development of personality and identity. Erik Erikson, a student of Freud with a broad social and cultural perspective, proposed that development proceeds through a series of eight stages, extending throughout the life span. Each stage is characterized by a major crisis or turning point, a time of increased vulnerability as well as increased potential for psychological growth (Table 3-1). For example, in the first stage, which lasts from birth to about one year, the conflict is between trust and mistrust—children learn how far they can trust their mothers (or other primary caregivers). In resolving this conflict, children develop enduring attitudes about how safe and giving the world is and about how worthy they are as individuals.

The successful mastery of one stage is a basis for mastering the next, so early failures can have repercussions in later life. Fortunately, life provides continuing opportunities to master these tasks. For example, although the de-

velopment of trust begins in infancy, it is refined as we grow older. We learn to trust people outside our immediate family and to limit our trust by identifying people who are untrustworthy.

A primary task beginning in adolescence is the development of an adult identity. A personal identity is a unified sense of self characterized by attitudes, beliefs, and ways of acting that are genuinely one's own. People who have developed identities know who they are, what they are capable of, what roles they play, and what their place is among their peers. They have a sense of their own uniqueness but also appreciate what they have in common with others. They view themselves realistically and can assess their own strong and weak points without relying on the opinions of others. Achieving an identity also means that one can form intimate relationships with others while maintaining a strong sense of self.

Our identities evolve as we interact with the world and make choices about what we'd like to do and whom we'd like to model ourselves after. Developing an identity is particularly challenging in a heterogeneous, secular, and relatively wealthy society like ours, in which many roles are possible, many choices are tolerated, and ample time is allowed for experimenting and making up one's mind.

Early identities are often modeled after parents—or the

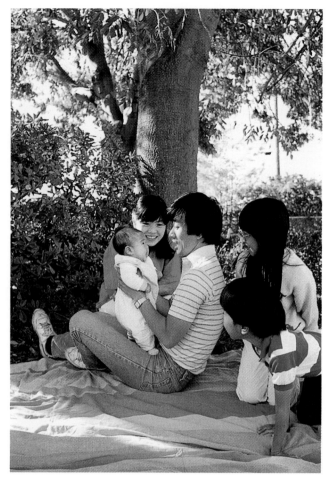

A positive self-concept begins in infancy. Knowing that she's loved and valued by her family gives this 3-month-old a solid basis for lifelong mental health.

opposite of parents, in rebellion from what they represent. Later, peers, rock stars, movie and sports heroes, and religious figures are added to the list of possible models. In high school and college, young people often join cliques that assert a certain identity—the "jocks," the "brains," the "stoners," or the "in-crowd." Although much of an identity is internal—a way of viewing oneself and the world—it can include things such as styles of talking and dressing, ornaments like earrings, and particular hairstyles.

Early identities are rarely permanent—a student who works for good grades and approval from parents and teachers one year can turn into a dropout devoted to hard rock and wild parties a year later. At some point, however, most of us adopt a more stable, individually tailored identity that ties together the experiences of childhood and the expectations and aspirations of adulthood. Erikson's theory does not suggest that suddenly one day we assume our final identity and never change after that. Life is more interesting for people who continue to evolve into more and more distinct individuals, rather than being rigidly controlled by their pasts. Identity reflects a lifelong

process, and it changes as a person develops new relationships and roles.

Developing an identity is an important part of mental wellness. Without an identity, we begin to feel confused about who we are—Erikson called this situation an *identity crisis*. Until we have "found ourselves," we cannot have much self-esteem because a self is not firmly in place.

How far have you gotten in settling on an identity? Try writing down a list of adjectives that you think a friend who knows you well would use to describe you. Rank them from the most to the least important. Your list might include elements such as gender, socioeconomic status, ethnic and religious identification, choice of college or major, parents' occupations, interests and talents, attitudes toward drugs and alcohol, style of dress, the kinds of people you typically associate with, expected niche in society, and characteristics of your personality. Which aspects of your identity do you feel are permanent and which do you think may change over time? Are there any adjectives missing from your list that you'd like to add?

Personal Insight   A task of adulthood is to redefine your relationship with your parents. Have your feelings and attitudes toward your parents changed? Does one or the other still treat you like a child? Do you react to them with childlike behavior? How can you change the relationship?

Achieving Realistic Self-Esteem

Positive self-esteem means regarding your self, which includes all aspects of your identity, as good, competent, and worthy of love. Ideally, a positive self-concept begins in childhood, based on experiences within the family and outside it. Children need to develop a sense of being loved and being able to give love and to accomplish their goals. If they feel rejected or neglected by their parents, they may fail to develop feelings of self-worth. They may grow to have a negative concept of themselves.

Another quality of the self-concept is its integration. An integrated self-concept is one that a person has made his or her own—it doesn't feel like someone else's mask or costume that doesn't quite fit. Important building blocks for the self-concept are personality characteristics and mannerisms of the parents, which children can take in uncritically without knowing they have done so. Later, they are surprised when they catch themselves acting like one of their parents, especially if they always objected to such behavior in that parent. Eventually, such building blocks should be reshaped and integrated into a new individual personality.

A further quality of the self-concept is its stability. Stability depends on the integration of the self and its freedom from contradictions. People who have received mixed messages about themselves from parents and friends may have contradictory self-images, which defy integration and which make them open to startling shifts of self-esteem. At times they regard themselves as entirely good, capable, and lovable—an ideal self—and at other times they see themselves as entirely bad, incompetent, and unworthy of love. While at the first pole, they may develop such an inflated ego that they totally ignore other people's needs and see others only as instruments for fulfilling their own desires. At the other pole, they may feel so small and weak that they run for protection to someone who seems powerful and caring. At neither extreme do such people see themselves or others realistically, and their personal relationships with other people are filled with misunderstandings and ultimately with conflict. The concepts people have about themselves and others are an important part of their personalities; all the qualities of the self-concept profoundly influence interpersonal relations.

As an adult, you sometimes run into situations that challenge your self-concept: People you care about may tell you they don't love you or feel loved by you, or your attempts to accomplish a goal may end in failure. You can react to such challenges in several ways. The best approach is to acknowledge that something has gone wrong and try again, adjusting your goals to your abilities without radically revising your self-concept. A less useful reaction is to deny that anything went wrong or to blame someone else. Assuming these attitudes preserves a good self-concept temporarily, but in the long run they keep you from mastering the challenge. The worst reaction is to develop a lasting negative self-concept in which you feel bad, unloved, and ineffective—in other words, become demoralized. Instead of coping, the demoralized person gives up, reinforcing the negative self-concept and setting in motion a vicious circle of bad self-concept and failure. In people who are biologically predisposed to depressions, demoralization can progress to additional symptoms, discussed later in the chapter.

One method for fighting demoralization is to recognize and test your negative thoughts and assumptions about yourself and others. The first step is to note exactly when an unpleasant emotion—feeling worthless, wanting to give up, feeling depressed—occurs or gets worse, to identify the events or daydreams that trigger that emotion, and to observe whatever thoughts come into your head just before or during the emotion. It is helpful to keep a systematic daily record of such events.

Let's consider the example of Jennifer, a student who went to the college counseling center because she had been feeling "down" lately. Her social life had not been going well, and she had begun to think that she was a boring, uninteresting person. Asked to keep a daily record, she wrote in it that she felt let down and discouraged

when a boyfriend who promised to meet her at 7:30 in the evening was 15 minutes late. The thoughts that occurred to her were "He's not going to come. It's my fault. He has more important things to do. Maybe he's with someone else. He doesn't like me. Nobody likes me because I don't have anything interesting to say. What if he got in a car accident?"

People who are demoralized tend to use all-or-nothing thinking: Things are either black or white, but never in between. They overgeneralize from negative events. They selectively see the negative and overlook the positive. They jump to negative conclusions. They minimize their own successes and magnify the successes of others. They take responsibility for unfortunate situations that are not their fault. The minute Jennifer's boyfriend was late, she jumped to the conclusion that he was not coming and blamed herself for it. From that point she jumped to more negative conclusions and more unfounded overgeneralizations.

Jennifer needs to develop more rational responses. For Jennifer, more rational thinking could be "He's a little late so I'll have time to reread the study questions." If he had not come after 30 minutes, she might have called him to see if something was holding him up, without jumping to any conclusions about the meaning of his lateness.

In your own fight against demoralization, it may be hard to figure out a rational response until hours or days after the event that upsets you, but once you get used to the way your mind works, you may be able to catch yourself thinking negatively and change the thought process before it goes too far.

This approach is not the same as positive thinking—substituting a positive thought for a negative one. Instead, you simply try to make your thoughts as logical and accurate as possible. If Jennifer continues to think she's boring, she should try to collect evidence to prove or disprove that. If she has exaggerated her dullness, as do many demoralized people, her investigations may prove her wrong. For example, she might ask her friends their candid opinions about her personality, and she can observe whether people seem interested in continuing a conversation with her. She might harbor the false assumption that if she's an interesting person, everyone must find her interesting. Following this assumption, if she could find one person who treated her as if she were boring, she could continue to believe that she isn't interesting. Demoralized people can be so tenacious about their negative beliefs that they make them come true in a self-fulfilling prophecy. Jennifer might conclude that she is so boring no one will like her anyway, so she need not bother to pay attention to what people say to her or to be involved in what is going on around her. This behavior could help her negative belief become a reality. Refer to the box "Realistic Self-Talk" for additional tips on how to change distorted, negative ways of thinking.

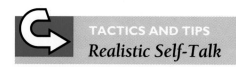

Do your patterns of thinking make events worse than they truly are? Do negative beliefs about yourself become self-fulfilling prophecies? Substituting realistic self-talk for negative self-talk can help you build and maintain self-esteem and cope better with the challenges in your life. Here are some examples of common types of distorted negative self-talk, along with suggestions for more accurate and rational responses.

Negative Self-Talk	Realistic Self-Talk
Focusing on negatives	
School is so discouraging—nothing but one hassle after another.	School is pretty challenging and has its difficulties, but there certainly are rewards. It's really a mixture of good and bad.
Expecting the worst	
Why would my boss want to meet with me this afternoon if not to fire me?	I wonder why my boss wants to meet with me. I guess I'll just have to wait and see.
Overgeneralizing	
(After getting a poor grade on a paper) Just as I thought—I'm incompetent at everything.	I'll start working on the next paper earlier. That way, if I run into problems, I'll have time to consult with the TA.
Minimizing	
I won the speech contest, but none of the other speakers was very good. I wouldn't have done so well against stiffer competition.	It may not have been the best speech I'll ever give, but it was good enough to win the contest. I'm really improving as a speaker.
Blaming others	
I wouldn't feel so lousy today if I hadn't had so much to drink at the party last night. Someone should have stopped me.	I overdid it last night. Next time I'll make different choices.
Expecting perfection	
I should have got 100 percent on this test. I can't believe I missed that one problem through a careless mistake.	Too bad I missed one problem through carelessness, but overall I did very well on this test. Next time I'll be more careful.
Believing you're the cause of everything	
Sarah seems so depressed today. I wish I hadn't had that argument with her yesterday; it must have really upset her.	I wish I had handled the argument better, and in the future I'll try to. But I don't know if Sarah's behavior is related to what I said, or even if she's depressed. In any event, I'm not responsible for how Sarah feels or acts—only she can take responsibility for that.
Thinking in black and white	
I've got to score 10 points in the game today. Otherwise, I don't belong on the team.	I'm a good player or else I wouldn't be on the team. I'll play my best—that's all I can do.
Magnifying events	
They went to a movie without me. I thought we were friends, but I guess I was wrong.	I'm disappointed they didn't ask me to the movie, but it doesn't mean our friendship is over. It's not that big a deal.

Adapted from W. Schafer. 1992. *Stress Management for Wellness*, 2nd ed. (Fort Worth: Harcourt Brace Jovanovich), pp. 227–31.

Being Less Defensive

Sometimes our wishes come into conflict with people around us or with our conscience, and we become frustrated and anxious. If we cannot resolve the conflict by changing the external situation, we try to resolve the conflict internally by rearranging our thoughts and feelings. Some standard ways that people defend themselves

TABLE 3-2 Defense and Coping Mechanisms

Mechanism	Description	Example
Projection	Reacting to unacceptable inner impulses as if they were from outside the self	A student who dislikes his roommate feels that the roommate dislikes him.
Repression	Expelling from awareness an unpleasant feeling, idea, or memory	The child of an alcoholic, neglectful father remembers him as a giving, loving person.
Regression	Acting in childish ways that used to be satisfying and acceptable	A person in line for movie tickets has a temper tantrum when told the movie is sold out.
Denial	Refusing to acknowledge to yourself what you really know to be true	A person believes that smoking cigarettes won't harm her because she's young and healthy.
Daydreaming	Escaping or finding fulfillment through fantasy	While waiting for midterms to be passed back, a student fantasizes that he receives the highest score in the class and the professor tells him he's very talented and offers to find him a high-paying job.
Idealization/denigration	Viewing others or self either as all good or all bad, often shifting from one to the other	A woman believes her husband is perfect and that he will love and care for her forever.
Passive-aggressive behavior	Expressing hostility toward someone by being covertly uncooperative or passive	A person tells a co-worker, with whom she competes for project assignments, that she'll help him with a report, but then never follows through.
Isolation of emotion	Detaching painful feelings from thoughts	A man feels no emotion when he recalls being beaten and robbed.
Displacement	Shifting of feelings about one person to another	A student who is angry with one of his professors returns home and yells at one of his housemates.
Reaction formation	Covering up a feeling by expressing its opposite	A young woman tells her roommate that she's a very nice person and a good friend, though in reality she thinks her roommate is inconsiderate.
Rationalization	Giving a false, acceptable reason when the real reason is unacceptable	A shy young man decides not to attend a dorm party, telling himself he'd be bored.
Avoidance/suppression	Deliberately avoiding tempting actions or thoughts that you think will have an undesirable outcome	A student decides to skip a fraternity party because he is worried he won't be able to withstand social pressure to drink.
Substitution	Deliberately replacing a frustrating goal with one that is more attainable	A student having a difficult time passing courses in chemistry decides to change his major from biology to economics.
Sublimation	Transforming aggressive or sexual impulses into socially approved forms	A man who is very angry with his brother goes for a five-mile jog.
Humor	Finding something funny in unpleasant situations	A student whose bicycle has been stolen thinks how surprised the thief will be when he or she starts downhill and discovers the brakes don't work.

against unacceptable thoughts or comfort themselves when under pressure are listed in Table 3-2. The drawback of many of these **defense mechanisms,** particularly those at the beginning of the list, is that although they succeed temporarily, they are dead ends that make finding ultimate solutions much harder. Projection, for example, distorts reality in a way that poisons interpersonal relationships. Repression or denial attempts to banish problems from our life that stubbornly return to haunt us. Daydreaming can be useful insofar as it is a rehearsal for

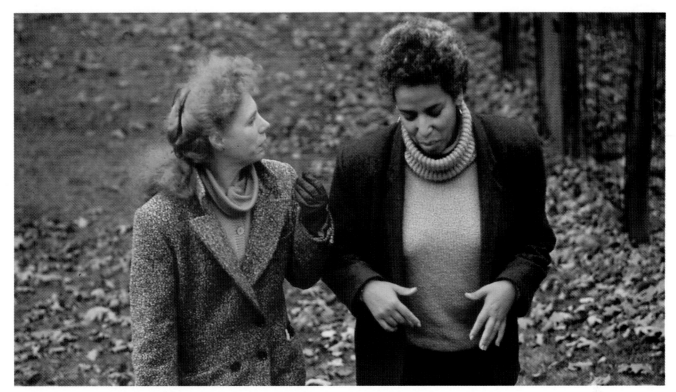

Communication is an important element in any interpersonal relationship. As these women express their thoughts and feelings to each other and listen attentively in response, they enhance their relationship, which in turn supports their psychological well-being.

future action, but as a substitute for action it quickly becomes unsatisfying and boring. The mechanisms at the end of the list—avoidance/suppression, substitution, sublimation, and humor—can be very useful for coping as long as they do not keep us from being what we want to be.

Recognizing your favorite mechanisms can be difficult, because they probably have become automatic habits, occurring outside of your conscious awareness. But lack of awareness is never complete—we each have some inkling about how our mind operates—and by remembering the details of conflict situations you have been in, you may be able to figure out which mechanisms you used in successful or unsuccessful attempts to cope. Try to look at yourself as an objective, outside observer would and analyze your thoughts and behavior in a concrete psychologically stressful situation from the past. Having insight into what defenses you typically use can lead to new, less defensive and more effective ways of coping in the future.

Personal Insight When you were a child, how were you taught to handle difficult feelings like anger, fear, and sadness? Do you still use the same methods? How are they working now?

Maintaining Honest Communication

Another important area of psychological functioning is relating to others and communicating honestly with them. It can be very frustrating for us and for people around us if we cannot communicate what we want and feel. Others can hardly respond to our needs if they don't know what those needs are. The first step is for us to realize what we want to communicate and then to express it clearly. For example, how do you feel about going to the party instead of to the movie? Do you care if your roommate types a paper late into the night? Some people know what they want others to do, but don't state it clearly because they are afraid that the request or they themselves will be rejected. Such people might benefit from **assertiveness** training. They need to learn to insist on their rights and to bargain for what they want. Assertiveness includes being able to say no or yes depending on the situation.

Because expressing feelings has become so central to pop psychology, many misconceptions have arisen. Neither "sharing" feelings with everyone on every occasion,

As a speaker . . .

- State your case as clearly as you can. Use "I messages." Ask for what you want directly, instead of hoping that the other person will read your mind. Say what you feel and what you want to have happen.

- Be specific about the particular behaviors that you like or don't like. Avoid generalizations such as, "You always . . ." and "You never . . ."

- Avoid blaming, accusing, and belittling. Even if you are 100 percent right, you have little to gain by putting the other person down. Studies have shown that when people feel criticized or attacked, they are less able to think rationally or solve problems correctly.

As a listener . . .

- Don't make assumptions about what the other person is saying. Ask for clarifications. Don't play "fill in the blanks."

- Develop the skill of reflective listening. Don't judge, blame, or evaluate. Remember, the person may just need to have you there in order to sort out feelings. By jumping in right away to "fix" the problem, you may actually be cutting off communication.

- When you listen, be sure you are *really* listening, not off somewhere rehearsing your reply! Try to tune in to the other person's feelings and check them out as well. Do let the other person know that you value what he or she is saying and want to understand. Respect for the other person is the cornerstone of clear communication.

---

nor letting feelings alone guide important decisions, are legitimate mental health goals. The word *feel* has at least two fairly distinct meanings in English. Compare "I feel sad" and "I feel that I should stay home tonight." The first sentence expresses an emotion; the second, a politely worded intention, or an intuition of need or duty. To tell people you are sad can imply various things and have various effects: They may feel closer to you and express an intimacy of their own, they may feel guilty because they may feel you are implying that they have caused your sadness, or they may feel angry because they feel forced to help cheer you up. Depending on your intention and prediction of how your statement will be taken, you may or may not want to make it. To say that you feel like staying home can also have a variety of implications according to the context. You may be politely saying "Don't bother me," opening a negotiation about what you will do with someone that evening, or expressing your demoralization. Good communication means saying things clearly when you intend to do so. You don't need any special psychological jargon to communicate clearly (see the box "Strategies for Clearer Communication").

PSYCHOLOGICAL DISORDERS

All of us have felt anxious, and in dealing with the anxiety have thought less rationally than when we were calm. Almost all of us have had periods of feeling down. Such feelings are normal responses to the ordinary challenges of life. But when emotions or irrational thoughts are strong enough to interfere with daily living, they can be regarded as symptoms of a psychological disorder.

Here we focus on anxiety disorders, mood disorders, and **schizophrenia**. Elsewhere in this book you can learn about other disorders—Alzheimer's disease in Chapter 19, disorders associated with psychoactive substances in Chapters 10 and 11, sexual disorders in Chapter 5, and eating disorders in Chapter 13.

Anxiety Disorders

Fear is a basic and useful emotion. Its value for evolutionary survival in prehistoric times cannot be overestimated; for modern humans it provides motivation for self-protection and learning to cope with new or potentially dangerous situations. Only when fear is out of proportion to real danger can it be considered a problem. Anxiety is another word for fear, referring especially to a feeling of fear that is not directed toward any definite threat. Only when anxiety is experienced almost daily or in life situations that recur and cannot be avoided, does it qualify anyone for a diagnosis of anxiety disorder.

The broad concept of anxiety disorders covers a variety of human problems. Here are the main types:

- *Simple phobia* is probably the most common and most understandable anxiety disorder, since many of us have a few specific fears—for example, fears of animals or certain locations. Typically feared animals are dogs, snakes, insects, and mice. Frightening locations are high places like tall buildings and closed places like airplanes. Sometimes these fears originate in bad experiences with the feared objects, but often there is no such explanation. People who are afraid of seeing blood or injuries are usually those who tend to faint in such situations.

Shyness is a form of social anxiety, a fear of what others will think of our behavior or appearance. Most people experience shyness in certain situations and are familiar with the telltale physical signs: pounding, rapid heartbeat; blushing; increased perspiration and clammy hands; butterflies in the stomach; trembling hands and legs; and a dry mouth. The accompanying feelings of self-consciousness, embarrassment, and unworthiness can be overwhelming. In order to escape these unpleasant feelings, a shy person may avoid volunteering or speaking up in public, refrain from making eye contact, and shun social gatherings and interpersonal interaction whenever possible.

Being shy is not the same thing as being introverted. Introverts prefer solitude to society, while shy people often long to be more outgoing. But it's often their own thoughts and beliefs that prevent shy people from enjoying the social interaction they crave. They dread being evaluated negatively by others, and, in anticipation of negative feedback, they become excessively self-conscious and self-critical. They resist positive feedback and tend to blame themselves for everything.

What causes people to become shy? Recent research indicates that the trait is at least partly inherited. Studies conducted by Harvard psychologist Jerome Kagan on children as young as 4 months showed that when faced with unfamiliar people or situations, shy infants and toddlers are frightened and upset and often withdraw. About 20 percent of children exhibit this type of response. At the other end of the spectrum, about 25 to 30 percent of children are consistently fearless, responding with calm or even delight to unfamiliar stimuli. These two temperaments remain fairly steady over time: Kagan's studies indicate that about half of the timid toddlers and 90 percent of the fearless ones will exhibit the same tendencies at age 7. Studies of identical twins also point to a genetic component in the development of shyness.

But for shyness as for many health concerns, biology is not destiny. About half of all shy children outgrow their shyness, just as others acquire it later in life. A variety of factors may be involved in the development of shyness in people who were not shy as infants. Possible culprits include stressors in the family environment, lack of support or emotional expressiveness in the family, or parental overemphasis on correct behavior. People may become shy as a result of one or more particularly negative social encounters or if they learn early to be uncertain about their intelligence or their appearance. Shyness can also occur if a person believes that he or she lacks the social skills needed for rewarding social interaction.

Approximately 30 to 40 percent of Americans think of themselves as shy, and about three-quarters of this group wish they weren't shy. For some, shyness is a serious problem, causing loneliness and depression. Because they have difficulty speaking up and believing in themselves, shy people are more likely to be underemployed. However, many shy people learn to work around their shyness. Some do better in structured rather than spontaneous settings and are able to experience positive social interaction through careful planning. About 20 percent of shy people are "shy extroverts"—people who, perhaps because of their shyness, have mastered ways to tell jokes or "work a crowd." Shyness may also have its upside: Shy people tend to be gentle, supportive, kind, and sensitive.

For people concerned about their own shyness or shyness in their children, several programs and strategies are available. Parents can help their shy children by accepting them as they are and by nurturing their self-esteem and sense of belonging. For shy adults, shyness classes, assertiveness training groups, and public speaking clinics offer training in social and cognitive skills, assertiveness, and changing negative self-perceptions. These programs are described in greater detail in the Behavior Change Strategy at the end of the chapter.

If you're worried about being shy, try to remember that shyness is widespread and that there are worse fates. The poet William Blake was so shy he could scarcely utter a sentence in public, so he made his pronouncements on paper. And they turned out just fine.

- *Social phobias* are similar to simple phobias, but they occur in interpersonal contexts. People with social phobias fear humiliation or embarrassment while being watched by others. Fear of speaking in public is perhaps the most common social phobia. Extremely shy people can have social fears that extend to almost all social situations (refer to the box "Shyness—The Discomfort of Social Anxiety" for more information).

- *Panic disorder* is characterized by sudden unexpected surges in anxiety, accompanied by symptoms such as rapid and strong heartbeats, shortness of breath, loss of physical equilibrium, and a feeling of losing mental control. Such attacks—the hallmark of **panic disorder**—usually begin in the early twenties and can lead to fear of being in crowds or closed places or of driving or flying. Sufferers fear that a panic attack will occur in a situation from which escape is difficult (as

Schizophrenia A mental disorder that involves a disturbance in thinking and in perceiving reality.

Panic disorder A syndrome of severe anxiety attacks accompanied by physical symptoms.

TERMS

in an elevator), where the attack could be incapacitating and result in dangerous loss of control (as in driving a car), or where no help was available if needed (as when a person is alone). People with this kind of phobia can often do what they would ordinarily avoid if a spouse or trusted companion accompanies them.

• *Obsessive-compulsive disorder* applies to people with obsessions or compulsions or both. **Obsessions** are recurrent, unwanted thoughts or impulses. For example, a parent may have impulses to kill a beloved child; a person may brood over whether he or she contracted HIV infection during a handshake; or a person may persistently wonder if he or she has done something unacceptable, such as having hit a pedestrian while driving. **Compulsions** are repetitive, difficult-to-resist actions associated with obsessions. A common compulsion is hand washing, associated with an obsessive fear of contamination by dirt. Other compulsions are counting or repeatedly checking if something has been done—for example, if a door has been locked or a stove turned off.

• *Post-traumatic stress disorder* is a reaction to severely traumatic events (events that produce a sense of terror and helplessness) such as physical violence to oneself or loved ones. Such traumas occur in personal assaults like rape or military combat, natural disasters like floods or earthquakes, and accidental disasters like fires, airplane crashes, and automobile accidents. Symptoms include repeated reexperiencing of the trauma in dreams and intrusive memories, efforts to avoid anything that is associated with the trauma, and a numbing of feelings. Sleep disturbances and other symptoms of anxiety and depression are also often present.

Therapies for anxiety disorders range from medication to psychological interventions that concentrate on a person's conscious or unconscious thoughts or on overt behavior. As we discuss later, different models of human nature lead to different ideas of causes and appropriate treatments.

Mood Disorders

Depression is the most common expression of a mood disorder. Depression comes in many kinds and degrees. Demoralization is usually part of any depression, but it's not

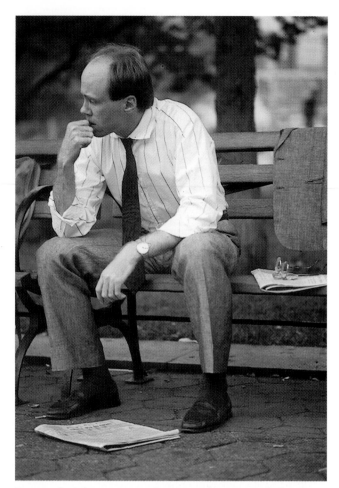

Having a bad day—or seriously depressed? Everyone feels dejected or defeated at times, but pervasive feelings of hopelessness, meaninglessness, or guilt signal deeper emotional problems. A person troubled by these feelings can often benefit from professional help.

the whole story. The following description of severe depression shows what it can include:

• A feeling of sadness and hopelessness
• Loss of pleasure in doing usual activities
• Poor appetite and weight loss
• Insomnia, especially early morning awakening
• Restlessness or, alternatively, lethargy
• Thoughts of worthlessness and guilt
• Inability to concentrate
• Thoughts of suicide

Not all these features are present in every depressive episode. Sometimes instead of poor appetite and insomnia, the opposite occurs—eating too much and sleeping too long. Amazingly, people can suffer the majority of symptoms of depression without feeling sad or hopeless or in a depressed mood, although they usually do experi-

TERMS

Obsession   Recurrent irrational, unwanted thoughts.
Compulsion   Irrational, repetitive, forced action, usually associated with an obsession.

Many popular statements made about suicide are false or true only in some cases. These statements may be false generalizations from a few atypical cases, wishful thinking, or just ignorance. People often conceal details about suicides, which promotes false assumptions such as the following:

Myth People who really intend to kill themselves do not let anyone know about it.

Fact This belief is a convenient excuse for doing nothing when someone says he or she might commit suicide. In fact, most people who eventually commit suicide *have* talked about doing it.

Myth People who made a suicide attempt but survived did not really intend to die.

Fact This may be true for certain people, but people who seriously want to end their life may fail because they misjudge what it takes. Even a pharmacist may misjudge the lethal dose of a drug.

Myth People who succeed in suicide really wanted to die.

Fact We cannot be sure of that either. Some people were trying only to make a dramatic gesture or plea for help but miscalculated.

Myth People who really want to kill themselves will do it regardless of any attempts to prevent them.

Fact Few people are single-minded about suicide even at the moment of attempting it. People who are quite determined to take their lives today may change their minds completely tomorrow.

Myth Suicide is proof of mental illness.

Fact Many suicides are committed by people who do not meet ordinary criteria for mental illness, although people with depression, schizophrenia, and other mental illnesses have a much higher than average suicide rate.

Myth Certain groups of the population are immune to suicide: alcoholics because they have alcohol as a crutch, elderly men because they have achieved a stable life adjustment, and black teenagers because they are not achievement-oriented.

Fact Certain groups do have low suicide rates, but not these—the first two groups mentioned have much higher than average suicide rates, and the suicide rate for black 15- to 24-year-olds is about the same as for whites of the same age.

Myth People inherit suicidal tendencies.

Fact Certain kinds of depression that lead to suicide can be inherited. But many examples of suicide running in a family can be explained by factors such as psychologically identifying with a family member who committed suicide, often a parent.

Myth All suicides are irrational.

Fact Maybe by some standards all suicides are "irrational." But many people find it at least understandable that someone might want to commit suicide, for example, when approaching the end of a terminal illness or when facing a long prison term.

---

ence a loss of interest or pleasure in things (see the box "Beck Depression Inventory"). In some cases, depression is a clear-cut reaction to specific events, such as the loss of a loved one or failing in school or work, while in other cases no trigger event is obvious.

One of the principal dangers of severe depression is suicide. Although suicide can happen unpredictably and even in the absence of depression, the chances of its happening are greater if the symptoms are numerous and severe. Additional danger signals of suicide include the following:

- Expressing the wish to be dead, or revealing contemplated methods
- Increasing social withdrawal and isolation
- A sudden, inexplicable lightening of mood (which can mean the person has finally decided to commit suicide)

Certain risk factors also increase the likelihood of suicide:

- A history of previous attempts

- A suicide by a family member or friend
- Readily available means, such as guns or pills
- Addiction to alcohol or drugs
- Serious medical problems

If you are severely depressed or know someone who is, expert help from a mental health professional is essential. Don't try to do it all yourself. If you suspect one of your friends is suicidally depressed, try to get him or her to see a professional.

Don't be afraid to discuss the possibility of suicide with people you fear are suicidal. You won't give them an idea they haven't already thought of (see the box "Myths About Suicide"). And asking direct questions is the best way to determine if someone seriously intends to commit suicide. Encourage your friend to talk and to take positive steps to improve his or her situation. If you feel there is an immediate danger of suicide, ensure that the person is not left alone, especially when he or she is emotionally upset and more likely to act impulsively. If you must leave your friend alone, have your friend promise not to do anything

This questionnaire contains groups of statements. Please read each group of statements carefully. Then pick out the *one* statement in each group that best describes the way you have been feeling the *past week, including today.* Circle the number beside the statement you picked. If several statements in the group seem to apply equally, circle the highest number. *Be sure to read all the statements in each group before making your choice.*

1. 0 I do not feel sad.
   1 I feel sad.
   2 I am sad all the time and I can't snap out of it.
   3 I am so sad or unhappy that I can't stand it.

2. 0 I am not particularly discouraged about the future.
   1 I feel discouraged about the future.
   2 I feel I have nothing to look forward to.
   3 I feel that the future is hopeless and that things cannot improve.

3. 0 I do not feel like a failure.
   1 I feel I have failed more than the average person.
   2 As I look back on my life, all I can see is a lot of failures.
   3 I feel I am a complete failure as a person.

4. 0 I get as much satisfaction out of things as I used to.
   1 I don't enjoy things the way I used to.
   2 I don't get real satisfaction out of anything anymore.
   3 I am dissatisfied or bored with everything.

5. 0 I don't feel particularly guilty.
   1 I feel guilty a good part of the time.
   2 I feel quite guilty most of the time.
   3 I feel guilty all the time.

6. 0 I don't feel I am being punished.
   1 I feel I may be punished.
   2 I expect to be punished.
   3 I feel I am being punished.

7. 0 I don't feel disappointed in myself.
   1 I am disappointed in myself.
   2 I am disgusted with myself.
   3 I hate myself.

8. 0 I don't feel I am any worse than anybody else.
   1 I am critical of myself for my weakness or mistakes.
   2 I blame myself all the time for my faults.
   3 I blame myself for everything bad that happens.

9. 0 I don't have any thoughts of killing myself.
   1 I have thoughts of killing myself, but I would not carry them out.
   2 I would like to kill myself.
   3 I would kill myself if I had the chance.

10. 0 I don't cry any more than usual.
    1 I cry more now than I used to.
    2 I cry all the time now.
    3 I used to be able to cry, but now I can't cry even though I want to.

11. 0 I am no more irritated now than I ever was.
    1 I get annoyed or irritated more easily than I used to.
    2 I feel irritated all the time now.
    3 I don't get irritated at all by the things that used to irritate me.

12. 0 I have not lost interest in other people.
    1 I am less interested in other people than I used to be.
    2 I have lost most of my interest in other people.
    3 I have lost all my interest in other people.

to harm himself or herself without first calling you. Get qualified help as soon as possible.

If your friend refuses help, you might try to contact your friend's relatives and tell them that you are worried. If the depressed person is a college student, you may need to let someone in your health service or college administration know your concerns. Finally, most communities have emergency help available, often in the form of a hotline telephone counseling service run by a suicide prevention agency (check the yellow pages).

Treatment for depression depends on its severity and on whether the depressed person is suicidal. The basic treatment is usually some kind of psychotherapy, which may be combined with drug therapy. "Uppers" such as amphetamines are not good antidepressants. More effective are special drugs that work over a period of two or more weeks. Therefore, when suicidal impulses are too strong, hospitalization for a week or so may be necessary. Electroconvulsive treatment is an effective therapy for severe depression when other approaches have failed.

Mania is a less common feature of mood disorder. People who are manic are restless, have a lot of energy, need little sleep, and often talk nonstop. They may devote themselves to fantastic projects and spend more money than they can afford. Many manic people swing between manic and depressive states, a syndrome called bipolar disorder because of the two opposite poles of mood. Tranquilizers are used to treat individual manic episodes,

13. 0 I make decisions as well as I ever could.
    1 I put off making decisions more than I used to.
    2 I have greater difficulty in making decisions than before.
    3 I can't make decisions at all anymore.

14. 0 I don't feel I look any worse than I used to.
    1 I am worried that I am looking old or unattractive.
    2 I feel that there are permanent changes in my appearance that make me look unattractive.
    3 I believe that I look ugly.

15. 0 I can work about as well as before.
    1 It takes an extra effort to get started at doing something.
    2 I have to push myself very hard to do anything.
    3 I can't do any work at all.

16. 0 I can sleep as well as usual.
    1 I don't sleep as well as I used to.
    2 I wake up 2–3 hours earlier than usual and find it hard to get back to sleep.
    3 I wake up several hours earlier than I used to and cannot get back to sleep.

17. 0 I don't get more tired than usual.
    1 I get tired more easily than I used to.
    2 I get tired from doing almost anything.
    3 I am too tired to do anything.

18. 0 My appetite is no worse than usual.
    1 My appetite is not as good as it used to be.
    2 My appetite is much worse now.
    3 I have no appetite at all anymore.

19. 0 I haven't lost much weight, if any, lately.
    1 I have lost more than 5 pounds.
    2 I have lost more than 10 pounds.
    3 I have lost more than 15 pounds.
    I am purposely trying to lose weight by eating less
    _____ yes _____ no

20. 0 I am no more worried about my health than usual.
    1 I am worried about physical problems such as aches and pains; or upset stomach; or constipation.
    2 I am very worried about physical problems, and it's hard to think about anything else.
    3 I am so worried about my physical problems that I cannot think about anything else.

21. 0 I have not noticed any recent change in my interest in sex.
    1 I am less interested in sex than I used to be.
    2 I am much less interested in sex now.
    3 I have lost interest in sex completely.

Add the numbers of the separate items selected. Do not score weight lost on purpose (Item 19). A score of 0–9 would be considered in the normal range, 10–15 would suggest mild depression, 16–23 would be consistent with moderate depression, and a score of 24 or more suggests marked depression.

Anyone who scores between 10 and 23 should repeat the test in two weeks. If the score is still between 10 and 23, and particularly if it has risen, a doctor should be consulted for an evaluation. If the score is greater than 23, a prompt evaluation is certainly indicated. If the score is less than 10 but other indications of depression exist, evaluation is also wise.

It is important not to depend too heavily on any one measure of depression. The subjective experience of depression is highly variable. Some people with normal scores on a depression questionnaire are severely depressed and respond dramatically to treatment.

Source: Beck, A. T., and R. W. Beck. 1972. "Screening Depressed Patients in Family Practice: A Rapid Technique." *Postgraduate Medicine* 52:81–85.

while special drugs like the salt *lithium carbonate* taken daily can prevent future mood swings.

Schizophrenia

Schizophrenia can be severe and debilitating or quite mild and hardly noticeable. Although people are capable of diagnosing their own depression, they usually don't diagnose their own schizophrenia, because schizophrenics often can't see that anything is wrong. This disorder is not rare; in fact, 1 out of 100 people has a schizophrenic episode sometime in his or her lifetime, most commonly starting in adolescence. However, because people who are directly or indirectly affected do not like to talk about

schizophrenia, its commonness is not generally appreciated. In addition, schizophrenics tend to withdraw from society when they are ill, another factor making it seem rarer than it is.

Some general characteristics of schizophrenia include the following:

- *Disorganized thoughts.* Thoughts may be expressed in a vague or confusing way that is hard for the listener to follow.

- *Inappropriate emotions.* Sometimes all emotion seems to be absent, and at other times emotions are strong but inappropriate.

- *Delusions.* People with delusions—firmly held false

beliefs—may think that their minds are controlled by outside forces, that people can read their minds, that they are great personages like Jesus Christ or the president of the United States, or that they are being persecuted by a group like the CIA.

- *Auditory hallucinations.* Schizophrenics may hear people talking about them and to them when no one is present.
- *Deteriorating social and work functioning.* Social withdrawal and increasingly poor performance at school or work may be so gradual that they are hardly noticed at first.

None of these characteristics is invariably present. Some schizophrenic people are quite logical except on the subject of their delusions. Others show disorganized thoughts or a lack of thoughts but no delusions or hallucinations.

A schizophrenic person needs help from a mental health professional. Suicide is a risk in schizophrenia, and expert treatment can reduce that risk and minimize the social consequences of the illness by shortening the period when symptoms are active. The keystone of treatment is regular medication. At times medication is like insulin for diabetes—it makes the difference between being able to function and not. Sometimes hospitalization is needed temporarily to relieve family and friends from responsibility for restraining erratic behavior.

> *Personal Insight* When you see people talking to themselves or acting strangely on the street, how do you feel? What do you do? Do you wonder what's going on in their mind? Do you label them as "sick"? What do you think causes them to act so strangely?

MODELS OF HUMAN NATURE AND THERAPEUTIC CHANGE

How people see the world is shaped largely by the model—the picture—of reality they carry in their minds. We will examine four of the most useful models of human nature: the biological, behavioral, cognitive, and psychoanalytic. As a way of understanding these models, let's consider the example of Rob.

Rob is a college student who finds himself so anxious whenever he's about to contribute to a class discussion that he can barely utter a word in class. In one month all students in this class are expected to make a brief oral presentation on a special topic. Rob's instructor is beginning to believe that Rob is either uninterested, not doing the assigned reading, or not bright enough for college. Rob has always been a shy person, but until recently he's been able to speak in public situations if he really tries. However, a few weeks ago when he began to answer a

question in class, he suddenly felt so nervous he couldn't continue. He started to sweat, lost his breath, and could feel his heart pounding in an alarming way. It was terribly embarrassing to have to stop speaking before he could complete his answer. Now he gets anxious just going into the classroom. All of this depresses him and makes him think about dropping out of school. Rob's mother was a school teacher until she died of heart disease a year ago. She was a strict person and often critical of her son. Rob's father is still living. He's an easygoing man who tends to drink a bit too much in the evenings and on weekends. We now present the four principal models, their views on psychological problems, and how they might approach Rob's case.

The Biological Model

The biological model emphasizes that the mind's activity depends completely on an organic structure, the brain, whose composition is determined by genes. The structure can be damaged by infectious agents, such as viruses or bacteria, or by physical trauma such as that which sometimes accompanies birth. Such damage can produce mental abnormalities. Chemical compounds introduced into the body can induce abnormal mental states that are similar to certain natural mental diseases; chemicals can also partially reverse such mental symptoms.

Certain differences among people in abilities and personality, just as in hair color, may stem from genetic differences. Evidence shows a link between genes and certain kinds of schizophrenia and depression. Studies of identical and fraternal twins, especially when they have been raised apart, have contributed to that evidence.

Genetic explanations of behavior, however, do not mean that the environment has no influence. Almost half of schizophrenic identical twins have a sibling who is not schizophrenic, although identical twins have exactly the same genes. Genes vary in what is called *penetrance,* the likelihood that their potential will actually be expressed in the individual. Environmental influences include events happening before birth, such as viral infections in the mother; events at the time of birth; and stresses in childhood, adolescence, and adulthood.

The biological model is used less in the mental health context than in the mental illness context. Schizophrenia and mood disorders have been of particular interest to biological psychiatrists. Chemists working for pharmaceutical firms have developed dozens of new antischizophrenic and antidepressant drugs; those that have shown effectiveness in patients without causing dangerous side effects receive Food and Drug Administration approval, which allows them to be prescribed by psychiatrists and other physicians. Recent investigations on panic disorder show that both antianxiety drugs and antidepressant drugs can sometimes block panic attacks.

What can a biological model say about our student

Rob? He is a shy person, a personality trait that usually begins in early childhood and has a basis in genetic differences. Taking an antianxiety drug before going to class might help him overcome his speech inhibitions, but the dose would have to be low or he might get sleepy and have trouble organizing his thoughts. He would have to be careful not to become dependent on such medicines since his father has tendencies toward alcoholism. If Rob inherited this tendency, he might be prone to addiction to tranquilizers. Since Rob had something like a panic attack when he tried to answer a question, he might be suffering from a form of panic disorder, in which case certain antidepressants might be advisable.

Although the evidence available today does not firmly prove the correctness of biological models for any mental health problem, such models have been useful in motivating scientists to develop new drugs for treating symptoms. These drugs have been immensely helpful, but it is important not to forget that all drugs have side effects, some of which are harmful. Thinking that focuses too narrowly on biology can result in the overprescribing of drugs. Opponents of the use of drugs in treating anxiety point out that although antianxiety drugs are seldom physically addicting, they can be a psychologically addictive substitute for more effective ways of dealing with anxiety.

The Behavioral Model

The behavioral model focuses on what people do—their overt behavior—rather than on brain structures and chemistry or thoughts and consciousness. This model regards psychological problems as "maladaptive behavior"—bad habits. When and how a person learned bad behavior in the past is less important than what makes it continue in the present. Behaviorists have built their treatment methods on studies of how animals learn and have verified the effectiveness of these methods in studies of humans. They analyze learning in terms of **stimulus, response,** and **reinforcement.**

The essence of behavior therapy is to analyze an undesirable behavior in terms of the reinforcements that keep it going and then try to alter those reinforcements. Clients are asked to keep a daily behavior journal to monitor the target behavior and events that precede and follow it. Chapter 1 uses snacking as an example and applies behavioral principles to overcoming it.

Rob might start a behavioral therapy program by writing down each time he makes a contribution to a classroom discussion and how many seconds he actually speaks. He should then develop concrete but realistic goals for increasing this amount each week and contract with himself to reward his successes by spending more time in activities he finds enjoyable. For example, his goals might first be to briefly contribute to class discussions, then to make longer statements, then to volunteer

to lead discussions, and finally to give a formal presentation. He can arrange for circumstances that make him more likely to speak—such as adequate preclass preparation or looking at a friendly classmate while speaking—to happen more frequently. Chapter 1 explains other useful measures such as developing social support for change and using role models.

Exposure is a primary therapeutic method in overcoming the fear of particular places and activities. The treatment program designed for Rob contained the essential ingredients of exposure—practice in speaking in the classroom arranged in assignments of gradually increasing difficulty. Further elements include staying in a feared situation until the fear has abated somewhat. Leaving when fear is still high causes immediate relief, which acts as a reinforcement of avoidance and escape. Exposure has proved particularly effective in treating people who have become afraid of going shopping because of panic attacks. The sequence of assignments might be (1) going into small stores with a friend, (2) going into small stores alone, (3) going into larger stores with a friend, (4) going into larger stores alone when they are not crowded, and finally (5) going into crowded stores alone. Therapists can have various roles: They help set up the assignments, accompany patients on their assignments, and organize groups of patients to do their assignments together.

Desensitization, which involves imagining the feared object or situation while maintaining relaxation, is another behavioral technique for overcoming fears. A model of a desensitization program is given in the Behavior Change Strategy for Chapter 2.

The Cognitive Model

The cognitive model emphasizes the effect of ideas on behavior and feelings. Human beings differ from other animals in thinking and expressing themselves in complex ways. In humans (according to the cognitive therapists), behavior results from complicated attitudes, expectations, and motives rather than from simple, immediate reinforcements. When behavioral therapies such as exposure work, it is because they change the way a person thinks about the feared situation and his or her ability to cope with it.

Stimulus Anything that causes an organism to respond.

Response An organism's reaction to a stimulus.

Reinforcement Increasing the future probability of a response by following it with rewards.

Exposure A therapeutic technique for treating fears in which the subject learns to come into direct contact with a feared situation.

Desensitization A therapeutic technique for treating phobias in which a phobic stimulus is vividly imagined while relaxation is maintained.

TERMS

One cognitive theory says that automatically recurring false ideas produce feelings such as anxiety and depression. Thus identifying and exposing these ideas as false should relieve these painful emotions. When people are anxious, the idea behind the anxiety is "Something bad is going to happen and I won't be able to handle it." Of course, each anxious person has his or her own versions of this basic idea. The therapist challenges such ideas in three ways: (1) showing that there isn't enough evidence for the idea, (2) suggesting different ways of looking at the situation, and (3) showing that no disaster is going to occur. The therapist does not just *state* his or her position, but encourages clients to examine the logic of their own ideas and then to test the truth of the ideas. "Of course, sometimes bad things do happen, and sometimes you can't handle them, at least alone. Life is not simple, and some fear is realistic."

Our student (Rob) who was afraid to speak up in class probably harbored ideas such as "If I begin to speak, I'll say something stupid; if I say something stupid, the teacher and my classmates will lose respect for me; and then I will get a low grade, my classmates will avoid me, and life will be hell. My heart's pounding; I could die at any minute of a heart attack like my mother." In cognitive therapy, Rob would be taught to examine these ideas critically. If he prepares for the presentation, how likely is it that he will sound stupid? Does Rob actually believe that everything he is going to say will be stupid, or is he really aiming for an impossible perfection, every sentence exactly correct and beautifully delivered? Will people's opinion of Rob be completely transformed by how he does in one presentation? Do his classmates even care that much about how well he does? And why does *he* care so much about what *they* think? Rob will be taught to notice thoughts that automatically attack him in feared situations and to substitute more realistic ideas for them. The therapist will advise him to speak in front of the class again and to test his assumptions.

The Psychoanalytic Model

The psychoanalytic model, like the cognitive model, emphasizes thoughts, but it says that false ideas cannot be fought directly because they are fed by other ideas that are **unconscious.** Sigmund Freud, a Viennese neurologist, developed these revolutionary theories around 1900. He discovered that certain paralyses that had no apparent physical basis and certain losses of sensory function (such as some cases of blindness) were better understood in terms of the patients' hidden (unconscious) wishes than

Unconscious   Whatever is in the mind but out of the awareness.

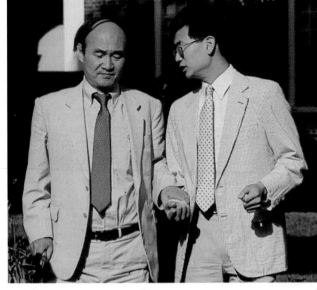

Developing a realistic view of one's parents is an important part of becoming a mentally healthy adult. This father and son have worked out an accepting and loving relationship with each other.

in terms of nerve pathways. The ideas that were disturbing behavior were at first hidden from both patient and therapist, but gradually surfaced in dreams, slips of the tongue, and the patient's behavior toward the therapist. Freud removed the moral stigma from such behavior by saying that patients had no conscious intention to deceive. In fact, such behavior was a medical disorder appropriately studied and treated by physicians. Freud also refused to make any sharp distinction between the mentally healthy and the mentally ill. We all have irrational ideas, which may emerge suddenly and demonstrate convincingly that we can't consciously control all of our own acts.

Therapies based on Freud's ideas do not take symptoms as isolated pieces of behavior but as results of a complex system of secret wishes, emotions, and fantasies hidden by active defenses that keep them unconscious. Defense mechanisms (see Table 3-2) operate unconsciously to conceal the truth so that people can both lie to themselves and conceal from themselves that they have lied. The concealed truth turns out to derive from wishes, often sexual or aggressive, that are unacceptable to society as well as to the individual's conscience.

The psychoanalytic model is often criticized nowadays for being unscientific and therapeutically ineffective. Yet certain of its basic ideas persist. One is that people will become more mentally healthy if they get to know themselves better, but that self-honesty can be painful. Another idea is that disclosure of one's fears and secrets to another person who can be trusted has therapeutic value. To encourage that, good therapists allow their clients to express themselves as freely as possible in therapy and do not try to impose their values on them.

If Rob received therapy inspired by this model, he would find a therapist interested not only in his problems in speaking but also in the totality of his personality—his most intimate wishes, hopes, and fears. Rob might learn some new and important things about himself. He would realize that his anxiety in speaking was part of a more general problem of shyness and low self-esteem. Standing up in front of others and letting them see him might make him feel as if he were under attack. For example, he might fear others will notice unpleasant traits he thinks he has. Finally, Rob might recall childhood experiences related to his current difficulties, such as being ridiculed by a parent for a stammer he had as a young child and might understand the impact of his critical mother and her recent death. In doing so, he might learn to distance himself from childish ways of thinking and reacting, such as a panicky avoidance of all public speaking.

Implications of the Four Models

The merits of these models are the focus of active debate. Behaviorists and cognitive therapists (usually psychologists) accuse supporters of the biological model (usually psychiatrists) of endangering patients with drug side effects and dependence. They attack psychoanalytically oriented psychotherapists for making a patient pay for endless, ineffective therapy. Psychoanalytically oriented therapists retaliate by accusing adherents of the other models of simplistic thinking, of regarding human beings as machines without rights or responsibilities.

The fact is that each model represents certain truths about human beings. Each model can help people dealing with specific types of human problems. When two therapies compete to solve the same problem, scientific studies should be conducted to measure rival claims. At present, strong evidence suggests that therapy is better than no therapy. Showing effectiveness is hardest for therapies that do not focus on specific problems or symptoms, because measuring the changes that occur is difficult, and differences in the therapists' skills may make the difference. There are important practical considerations too. Some people and some problems cannot wait long enough for slowly acting treatments to work.

Personal Insight   How do you react when you hear that someone is seeing a psychiatrist or is in therapy? Does it make a difference in how you feel about the person?

GETTING HELP

Knowing when self-help or professional help is required for mental health problems is usually not as difficult as knowing how to start or which professional to choose.

Self-Help

If you have a personal problem that you would like to solve, an intelligent way to begin is to find out what you can do on your own. Some problems are specifically addressed in this book. Behavioral and some cognitive approaches are especially useful for helping yourself. All of these involve becoming more aware of self-defeating actions and ideas and combating them in some way: being more assertive when you find yourself backing down; taking the risk of communicating honestly; improving your self-esteem by counteracting thoughts, people, and actions that undermine it; and confronting things you're afraid of rather than avoiding what you fear. Get more information about solving personal problems by seeing what books are available in the psychology or self-help sections of the library or bookstore. Be selective, however—watch out for self-help books making fantastic claims that deviate from the mainstreams of psychological thinking.

Expressing your feelings is important too. (See the box "Express Your Feelings.") Just being able to share what's troubling you with an accepting, empathetic person can bring relief. Comparing notes with people who have problems similar to yours can give you new ideas about coping. Many self-help groups work on the principle of bringing together people with similar problems to share their experiences and support each other. Some support groups are for the families of people with problems; Al-Anon, for the families of alcoholics, is an example.

For some people, religious belief and practice may promote psychological health. Religious organizations provide a social network and a supportive community, and religious practices, such as prayer and meditation, offer a path for personal change and transformation of the self.

Professional Help

Sometimes self-help or talking to nonprofessionals is not enough. More objective, more expert, or more discreet help is needed. Many people have trouble accepting the need for professional help to handle personal problems, and often the people who most need help are the most unwilling to get it. You may find yourself someday having to overcome your own reluctance toward seeking help or the reluctance of a friend for whom you want to get help.

In some cases, professional help is optional. Some people are interested in improving their mental health in a general way by going into individual or group therapy to learn more about themselves and how to interact with others. Certain therapies teach people how to adjust the effect of what they say and do on people around them. Clearly, seeking professional help for these reasons is a matter of individual choice. Interpersonal friction among family members or between partners often falls in the middle between necessary and optional. Successful help with such problems can mean the difference between painful divorce and a satisfying relationship.

Is it true that expressing your feelings is better for your health than keeping a stiff upper lip? Apparently it is. Numerous studies have suggested that people who hold in their feelings are more prone to illness. Now, researchers have reviewed a dozen experiments and concluded that expressing your emotions can help keep you healthy.

In the typical study design, half the subjects were randomly assigned to spend 15 to 20 minutes a day for several days reliving a traumatic experience, either by talking into a tape recorder or writing about it. The other subjects talked or wrote about more mundane subjects, such as their plans for the rest of the day.

After several weeks or months, the subjects who grappled with painful experiences reported fewer illnesses, had fewer visits to physicians, or had better immune function, in all but one of the studies. Why might expressing bottled-up emotions improve health? Researchers suggest that holding back emotions requires physical work that puts a chronic strain on the body.

As the studies illustrate, it doesn't take much talking or writing to have a beneficial effect. Nor do you have to reveal your deepest secrets to others—a notebook or tape recorder is audience enough.

Source: "Mind/Body Update," *Consumer Reports on Health,* August 1992.

Sometimes it is difficult to determine whether someone needs professional help, but it is important to be aware of behaviors that may indicate a serious problem (see the box "David: A True Story"). The following are some strong indications that you or someone else needs professional help:

- If depression, anxiety, or other emotional problems begin to interfere seriously with performance at school, work, or in getting along with other people
- If suicide is attempted or is seriously considered (refer to the danger signals listed in this chapter)
- If symptoms such as hallucinations, delusions, incoherent speech, or loss of memory occur
- If alcohol or drugs are used to the extent that they impair normal functioning during much of the week, if finding or taking drugs occupies much of the week, or if reducing their dose leads to psychological or physiological withdrawal symptoms

Mental health workers belong to several professions. *Psychiatrists* are medical doctors with five years of medical training after college, followed by three years of training in psychiatry. *Clinical psychologists* have usually completed a Ph.D. degree requiring at least five years of graduate work after college. *Social workers* typically have master's degrees requiring at least two years of graduate study. The requirements for licensed *counselors* varies from state to state. Some clergymen have special training in *pastoral counseling* in addition to their religious studies.

These professional groups differ somewhat in their roles. Only psychiatrists prescribe medications. They are experts in deciding whether a medical disease lies behind psychological symptoms. Psychiatrists are usually involved if hospitalization is required. All mental health professionals are trained to practice some kind of psychological therapy, but most restrict themselves to only one or two of the approaches described in this chapter. Psychologists have been important in developing behavioral and cognitive therapies and are often expert in these therapies or in psychoanalytically inspired therapies. Social workers have much experience in finding community support for the seriously ill. In hospitals and clinics, various mental health professionals join together in treatment teams. Psychiatric nurses often are important members of these teams.

Where do you actually find these professionals when you need them? College students are usually in a good position to find inexpensive mental health care. Larger colleges have both health services that employ psychiatrists and psychologists and counseling centers staffed by professionals and students (peer counselors). For less severe problems, psychology departments and education departments may offer student counselors. Student newspapers sometimes announce "sensitivity training groups" or other self-awareness groups sponsored by student organizations. Remember, though, that peer counselors are not professionals, and for problems of the kind listed earlier in this section it is better to go to someone with more training and experience. Self-awareness groups are also not really suitable for people who are in a crisis or not functioning.

Community mental health resources may include a school of medicine or teaching hospital with outpatient psychiatric clinics that offer psychological testing, diagnostic screening, and the ongoing services of psychiatrists, psychologists, and social workers. If you go first to an interdisciplinary team, you will find out whether your problems have physical origins, you will have access to professionals qualified to prescribe medication, and you

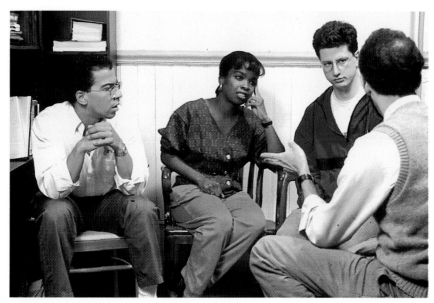

Group therapy is just one of many different approaches to psychological counseling. If you have concerns you would like to discuss with a mental health professional, shop around to find the approach that works for you.

will reap the benefits of several heads. Psychologists, counselors, or psychiatrists working in the community are listed in the local telephone book. Rather than choosing a name at random, get recommendations from a family physician, clergy, friends who have been in therapy, or community agencies.

Financial considerations are important. Be sure to check what kind of mental health benefits your personal health insurance or prepaid medical plan provides. At the time of this writing treatment by a psychiatrist in a private practice setting could cost $130 for a 45-minute session. Therapists in private practice charge more than those affiliated with centers or large institutions, and psychiatrists usually charge more than psychologists, who charge more than social workers or counselors. Group therapy is generally cheaper than individual therapy. Some therapists have a sliding-fee scale based on the client's income. If you are not adequately covered by a health plan, don't let that stop you from getting help; investigate low-cost alternatives. City, county, and state governments often support mental health clinics for those who can afford to pay little or nothing for treatment.

It will take a personal meeting to decide whether a therapist is right for you. Besides checking out a therapist's basic professional qualifications, you will need to know whether you feel comfortable with his or her personality, values and belief system, and psychological orientation. Does the therapist seem like a warm, intelligent person who would be able and interested in helping you? Is the therapist willing to talk about the techniques she or he uses? Does the therapist make sense to you? If the first

therapist you see seems all right, there is no need to look further; but if you feel at all uncomfortable, it's worthwhile setting up one-shot consultations with one or two others before you make up your mind. If you're not in need of emergency care, be prepared to spend as much time shopping for the right therapist as you would for anything else that is important to you. Of course, if you can afford only free or low-cost treatment, your options may be limited.

The number and frequency of sessions depends on the type of therapy. Psychological therapies focusing on specific problems may require eight or ten sessions at weekly intervals. Therapies aiming for psychological awareness and personality change can last months or years with one to four sessions per week. Treatment with medication usually starts with weekly sessions; after the best medication and optimal dose is found, the frequency of sessions is reduced. For schizophrenia or bipolar disorder, medication may have to be continued for years.

Whomever you choose to help you, respect your own judgment as to whether you are actually being helped. Although too much "shopping around" may be a way of avoiding the resolution of problems, you certainly have the right to change therapists if therapy is not helpful after a reasonable period of time. First, ask yourself whether you are displeased because your therapy is raising difficult, painful issues you don't want to deal with. Then express your dissatisfaction to your therapist and deal with it in your session. Finally, if you are convinced that your therapy isn't working or is harmful, find another therapist.

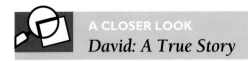
When a person begins to act strangely in public or when with friends or family, others rarely reach an immediate consensus about what this behavior means. Different observers form different opinions. These opinions do not just represent different levels of education or sophistication, because conflicts also occur between the best educated and most knowledgeable. Conflicts between models of mental health are not just theoretical but have practical results, as this true case history illustrates. Only his name and a few details have been changed to protect those involved.

David was a 20-year-old junior at a large and competitive university, majoring in humanities. He had been the best all-around student in his high school class. The principal of the high school remembered him as brilliant and caring. David had maintained his outstanding academic record. Students in his dorm said he was cheerful, outgoing, and "laid back." For six months he had been attending meditation classes, had become a vegetarian, and had started to jog daily. He avoided all drugs, including alcohol. Shortly before spring vacation, he told a friend he had been hearing voices and seeing "real" visions. He was convinced that the end of the world—the "Last Judgment"—was coming. He talked of taking his own life because he felt unworthy and said that his death would help humanity. In contrast to his usual cheerfulness, he became withdrawn and isolated. The worried friend called David's father, who lived far away from the university. The father talked to his son several times on the telephone and arranged to fly up to see him in a week. The day before they were to meet, David jumped off a high bridge and drowned.

How did different people make sense of what happened? In his father's opinion, David's suicide was a result of spiritual striving—a deep interest in Eastern religions—combined with a drive for perfection in everything he attempted. According to his father, David was totally committed in life and in death. The problem his son had faced was trying to live simultaneously in a world of reality and in a world devoted to spirituality.

His friend took a medical point of view. He thought David's visions and voices sounded schizophrenic. The father agreed only partially. From his telephone conversations,

he felt that something had temporarily snapped in David's mind. Perhaps a biochemical change had altered his mental state. But during the last telephone call, the day before the suicide, his son seemed to have become completely lucid and calm again. David assured him that he was OK now and that his father could stop worrying. They would see each other soon and be able to hold and love each other. His father found consolation in the thought that his son had found a kind of peace at the end. Yet to many who knew David, the story was only a tragedy—a talented, kind young person with most of his life in front of him died before the seriousness of his problems was recognized and treatment could be begun.

There is a strong temptation to lay blame here. Was his father spiritualizing a schizophrenic disorder? Of all people, the father, who had known his son for all of his 20 years, should have recognized that something was wrong. But his father lived far away and was merely empathetically supporting his son's spiritual quest. Religious impulses and spiritual crises are usually not crazy; they can have positive outcomes. And why did his friend not intervene more actively? He could have contacted a dean, faculty member, or someone at the student health service and insisted that someone in authority should step in. Perhaps his respect and admiration for David made him hesitate. David might have felt betrayed if he had been hospitalized. And what kind of university was it, where a student could become so troubled and so few people notice it? But many large universities do not watch students very closely, because they believe students should be treated as grown-ups, with rights to privacy and to living under a minimum of rules and social requirements. Troubled students often keep to themselves; it would be enforcing conformity not to allow them to do so.

Thus, we cannot convincingly lay blame, but we can hope that in the future better informed students, parents, and college administrators will be more sensitive to serious danger signs like the ones in this case: hearing voices and seeing visions, a major and sudden change in personality, suicidal thoughts, and the ominous false calm that can follow a firm decision to commit suicide.

Personal Insight If you were feeling depressed or anxious or were having trouble in your relationship, would you be tempted to see a counselor or therapist? If so, how would you choose among the various therapeutic types? What do you think is the basis for your choice?

SUMMARY

What Mental Health Is Not

- Mental health encompasses more than a single particular state of normality. Psychological diversity is valuable.

- Getting professional help does not necessarily indicate the presence of mental illness. Neither symptoms nor appearances are reliable indicators of an individual's mental health.

What Mental Health Is

- A definition of mental health as the absence of mental illness focuses attention on the most serious problems and the people in greatest need of help.
- Defining mental health as the presence of wellness means that to be healthy you must strive to develop your full potential.
- Maslow's definition of mental health centered on self-actualization, the highest level of his hierarchy of needs.
- Mentally healthy people are realistic and have high self-esteem, or a positive sense of self-worth.
- Being inner-directed is a sign of mental health; it signifies finding guidance from one's own values and feelings. A related quality is authenticity—being genuine and unselfconsciously oneself.
- Mentally healthy people are capable of emotional intimacy, interacting with others in ways that ensure good communication.
- Creativity and boldness are qualities that show an ability to deal with uncertainty and the unknown.

Meeting Life's Challenges

- A crucial part of mental wellness is to grow up psychologically. Erik Erikson viewed development as proceeding through eight stages; mastery of one stage is a basis for mastering the next.
- A personal identity—a sense of who you are and what you're capable of—develops as people interact with the world; an identity is necessary for the growth of self-esteem.
- A sense of self-esteem develops during childhood as a result of giving and receiving love and learning to accomplish goals. Someone with an unstable self-concept is unable to maintain consistency in relationships.
- Self-concept is challenged every day; healthy people adjust their goals to their abilities if they fail, but unhealthy people rely too much on defenses or become demoralized.
- Fighting demoralization requires recognizing and testing negative thoughts; keeping a daily record can help. Once unpleasant emotions and thoughts have been identified, it's possible to develop rational responses through practice in logical thinking.
- Using defense mechanisms to cope with problems can make finding solutions much harder. Analyzing thoughts and behavior can help people develop less defensive and more effective ways of coping.
- Honest communication requires recognition of what needs to be said and the ability to say it clearly. Assertiveness allows people to insist on their rights and to participate in the give-and-take of good communication.
- When people choose to express their feelings, they need to consider their intention and the way their statements will be taken.

Psychological Disorders

- People who suffer from psychological disorders have symptoms severe enough to interfere with daily living.
- Anxiety refers to a fear that is not directed toward any definite threat. Anxiety disorders include simple phobias, social phobias, panic disorder, obsessive-compulsive disorder, and post-traumatic stress disorder.
- Depression is a common mood disorder; loss of interest or pleasure in things seems to be its most universal symptom.
- Severe depression carries a high risk of suicide, and suicidally depressed people need professional help.
- Symptoms of mania include exalted moods with unrealistically high self-esteem, little need for sleep, and rapid speech. Elation gives way to depression in bipolar disorders.
- Schizophrenia is characterized by disorganized thoughts, inappropriate emotions, delusions, auditory hallucinations, and deteriorating social and work performance. Schizophrenia may be accompanied by depression, and suicide is a possibility.

Models of Human Nature and Therapeutic Change

- Theorists have attempted to understand and explain psychological development and problems by proposing different models of human nature.
- The biological model emphasizes that the mind's activity depends entirely on the brain, whose composition is genetically determined. Therapies based on this model focus on the use of psychiatric drugs.
- The behavioral model focuses on overt behavior and treats psychological problems as bad habits. Behaviorists teach new adaptive responses, partly by analyzing undesirable behavior in terms of the reinforcements that keep it going.
- Behavioral therapy uses the techniques of exposure and desensitization to treat phobias.
- The cognitive model considers how ideas affect behavior and feelings; behavior results from complicated attitudes, expectations, and motives—not just from simple reinforcements. Treatment focuses on changing the way a person thinks about situations and abilities.

- The psychoanalytic model asserts that false ideas are fed by unconscious ideas and cannot be attacked directly. Although many of this model's original tenets may have been repudiated, its basic ideas persist in many therapeutic practices.

- Each model represents certain truths about human behavior, and the most appropriate therapy depends upon the situation.

Getting Help

- Behavioral and cognitive approaches are useful in self-help. Books are available for guidance; talking to friends or relatives and joining self-help groups are ways to start treatment.

- Professional help is necessary if problems interfere with performance or interpersonal relationships; if suicide is considered or attempted; if hallucinations, delusions, memory loss, or other severe symptoms occur; or if alcohol or drug abuse impairs normal functioning.

- Mental health workers have various forms of training and play different roles in treatment. Several problems can probably be treated best by an interdisciplinary team. It helps to take time choosing a therapist and to continually review the benefits of therapy, changing therapists if necessary.

TAKE ACTION

1. Investigate the mental health services provided on your campus and in your community. What services are available? Think about which ones you would feel comfortable using, for either yourself or someone else, should the need ever arise.

2. Many colleges and communities have peer counseling programs, hot-line services (for both general problems and specific issues such as rape, suicide, drug abuse, parental stress, and so on), and other kinds of emergency counseling services. Some of these programs are staffed by volunteers trained in listening, helping, and providing information. Investigate such programs in your school (through the health clinic or student services) or community (look in the yellow pages), and consider volunteering for one. The training and experience can give you invaluable assistance in understanding both yourself and others.

3. Being assertive rather than passive or aggressive is a valuable skill that everyone can learn. To improve your ability to assert yourself appropriately, sign up for a workshop or class in assertiveness training on your campus or in your community.

JOURNAL ENTRY

1. Do you remember incidents or moments from childhood that stand out as wonderful or horrible? Write a short essay about two such incidents, including what your feelings were and what you think you learned from them. Then describe what you would do now in the same situations and why.

2. *Critical Thinking:* In the past, some political candidates have dropped out of a race or been defeated after it was revealed that they had undergone psychiatric treatment or some other form of mental health therapy. Do you think that a person who has been treated for a mental illness should be excluded from holding a public office or from any other profession? Why or why not? Does your position depend on the type of illness or the treatment the individual received? In your health journal, write a brief essay outlining your position.

3. Think about a person you admire. Describe that person in writing, listing the qualities that you admire in him or her. Do you have any of those qualities? What does your list say about the kind of person you want to be?

BEHAVIOR CHANGE STRATEGY

DEALING WITH SOCIAL ANXIETY

Everyone is lonely at times, but some people have a harder time meeting new people, initiating friendships, and establishing romantic or sexual relationships than others do. In some cases, the problem is social anxiety—also known as shyness, social inhibition, or interpersonal anxiety. Shyness is discussed in detail in a box in this chapter. This Behavior Change Strategy describes some of the ways the problem of social anxiety is approached in various programs.

Many programs focus on the variety of subtle social skills that are needed to initiate and sustain interpersonal relationships. These skills include appropriate eye contact, sense of humor, reflection, facial expression, initiating topics in conversation, maintaining the flow of conversation by asking questions, and so on. One general plan of treatment assumes a *skills-deficit perspective,* and it teaches college students how to use interpersonal skills to greater personal advantage by means of videotape feedback and modeling (practice exercises). Practice-dating

	DATE:	11/16	DATE:		DATE:	
	AM	PM	AM	PM	AM	PM
12		I,I,W				
1		AW				
2		S				
3		S				
4		S				
5		I,I				
6		W				
7		W				
8		S				
9		S,P,P				
10	I,I,S	S				
11	S	W				

Social Activity Journal
KEY
P = Social phone call
I = Social interaction (at least 5 minutes)
A = Social activity
S = Study time
W = Wasted time

programs in which both partners know that their interaction has been scheduled for practice and self-improvement help extend modeling well beyond the clinic into "real world" social settings.

A slightly different approach stems from the belief that people know well enough what to do to make and keep friends—the problem of social inhibition comes from the anxiety that reduces a person's ability to perform key social skills. Reduced performance produces even greater self-doubt and anxiety, which only interferes further with later performance to produce a vicious circle of damaging experiences. With this approach, people for whom anxiety plays a key role receive special training in relaxation skills and other stress management strategies—perhaps in conjunction with the more complex and time-consuming anxiety-reduction procedure known as *systematic desensitization.*

In most cases shyness and loneliness are not easily diagnosed as being only a problem of skills or only a problem of anxiety. Most programs assume that *both* skills and anxiety play a role, and these programs provide a comprehensive treatment that includes modeling, structural practice, and stress management components.

Programs usually begin with a self-monitoring phase in which all facets of a person's daily routine are noted in a journal format. The Social Activity Journal shows how a coding scheme (noted in the key) can be used to help keep track of the pattern of social contacts, the amount of time spent in effective studying, and the amount of time wasted each day. These patterns are monitored for at least one week so that general trends can be identified.

Depending on the particular program, the shy person is then told to make better use of "wasted time" and to begin to practice some of the skills he or she has learned in the class or clinic in the least troublesome (anxiety-producing) situations. This tactic might be translated into an assignment (and behavioral contract) to initiate brief, nonthreatening conversations with classmates on an academic topic (the upcoming midterm or the homework assignment, for example). Once these conversations are successfully accomplished, then the next phase of the program could encourage practice of discussions that involve more personal subjects (personal opinions about nonacademic topics). Later assignments might involve social gatherings. The individual steps would form a type of hierarchy, incorporating topics, people, and places, from least to most difficult.

The person would accomplish these steps by using a consistent theme of practice, modeling, and stress management skills while moving up the hierarchy. Using these techniques the person increases social skills and confidence levels, at the same time decreasing anxiety and feelings of insecurity, until social interactions can be sustained with comfort and enjoyment.

To evaluate your own level of social anxiety, examine the following list of statements made by college students identified as lonely in a study conducted at Stanford University. These students said that it was difficult for them to:

- Make friends in a simple, natural way
- Introduce themselves to others at parties
- Make phone calls to others to initiate social activity
- Participate in groups
- Get pleasure out of a party
- Get into the swing of a party
- Relax on a date and enjoy themselves

- Be friendly and sociable with others
- Participate in playing games with others
- Get buddy-buddy with others

These statements suggest a level of social anxiety and inhibition that interferes with dating and making friends. If they describe you, consider looking into a shyness clinic or treatment program on your campus. You have nothing to lose and everything to gain.

SELECTED BIBLIOGRAPHY

American Psychiatric Association. 1987. *Diagnostic and Statistical Manual of Mental Disorders*, 3rd ed., revised (DSM-III-R). Washington, D.C.: American Psychiatric Association Press.

Beck, A. T., A. J. Rush, B. F. Shaw, and G. Emery. 1987. *Cognitive Therapy of Depression: A Treatment Manual*. New York: Guilford Press.

Berger, P. A., and H. K. H. Brodie, eds. 1986. *American Handbook of Psychiatry*. Vol. 8, *Biological Psychiatry*. New York: Basic Books.

Cowley, G. 1991. The bold and the bashful: Even the terminally shy sometimes triumph on their own terms. *Newsweek Special Issue*, summer.

Duncan, D. D. 1987. Creativity and mental wellness. *Health Values* 2:3–7.

Erikson, E. 1963. *Childhood and Society*. New York: W. W. Norton.

Hatton, C. L., and S. M. Valente, eds. 1984. *Suicide: Assessment and Intervention*, 2nd ed. Norwalk, Conn.: Appleton-Century-Crofts.

Hersen, M., and A. S. Bellack, eds. 1985. *Handbook of Clinical Behavior Therapy with Adults*. New York: Plenum Press.

Hick, J. 1989. *An Interpretation of Religion: Human Responses to the Transcendent*. New Haven: Yale University Press.

Jacobson, L. F. 1985. The social disease called shyness. *Healthline*, July.

Kohut, H. 1971. *The Psychology of the Self*. New York: International Universities Press.

Lazare, A. 1973. Hidden conceptual models in clinical psychiatry. *New England Journal of Medicine* 288:345–51.

Maslow, A. H. 1968. *Toward a Psychology of Being*, 2nd ed. Princeton, N.J.: Van Nostrand Reinhold.

Newman, B. M., and P. R. Newman. 1991. *Development Through Life: A Psychosocial Approach*, 5th ed. Pacific Grove, Calif.: Brooks/Cole.

Nicholi, A. M., Jr. 1988. *The New Harvard Guide to Psychiatry*. Cambridge, Mass.: Harvard University Press.

Turner, S. M., K. S. Calhoun, and H. E. Adams, eds. 1992. *Handbook of Clinical Behavior Therapy*, 2nd ed. New York: John Wiley.

Vaillant, G. E. 1977. *Adaptation to Life*. Boston: Little, Brown.

Wenegrat, W. 1989. *The Divine Archetype: The Sociobiology and Psychology of Religion*. Lexington, Mass.: Lexington Books.

Winokur, G., and D. W. Black. 1992. Suicide—what can be done? *New England Journal of Medicine* 327:490–92.

RECOMMENDED READINGS

Agras, S. 1985. *Panic: Facing Fears, Phobias, and Anxiety*. San Francisco: W. H. Freeman. *This popular book explains the nature of fears and phobias and how to overcome them.*

Beck, A. T. 1989. *Love Is Never Enough*. New York: HarperCollins. *Subtitled "How couples can overcome misunderstandings, resolve conflicts, and solve relationship problems," this book was written by a pioneer in the field of cognitive psychotherapy for couples trying to maintain long-term relationships.*

Burns, D. D. 1989. *The Feeling Good Handbook*. New York: Penguin Books. *A self-help book with cognitive techniques for handling depression and anxiety.*

Davison, G. C., and J. M. Neale. 1990. *Abnormal Psychology*, 5th ed. New York: John Wiley. *This classic textbook is a good place to find more detailed descriptions of psychological disorders.*

Emery, G. 1988. *Getting Un-depressed: How a Woman Can Change Her Life Through Cognitive Therapy*. New York: Simon and Schuster. *Emery, a student of Beck, has written a self-help book specifically for depressed women.*

Gorman, J. M. *The Essential Guide to Psychiatric Drugs*, updated ed. New York: St. Martin's Press. *This authoritative guide is written for the layperson.*

Jeffers, S. 1987. *Feel the Fear and Do It Anyway*. New York: Fawcett Columbine. *This practical self-help book describes a variety of cognitive strategies and techniques for working through fears, irrational ideas, and self-defeating beliefs.*

Papolos, D. F., and J. Papolos. 1992. *Overcoming Depression*, rev. ed. New York: HarperCollins. *Its subtitle explains its contents: "For the millions who suffer depression and manic depression and for the families affected by these recurring disorders." The book's biological orientation is particularly appropriate for severe mood disorders.*

Patterson, C. H. 1990. *Theories of Counseling and Psychotherapy*, 4th ed. New York: Harper and Row. *This book summarizes the basic principles of a variety of psychological treatments.*

Sarason, I. G., and B. R. Sarason. 1989. *Abnormal Psychology: The Problem of Maladaptive Behavior*, 6th ed. Englewood Cliffs, N.J.: Prentice-Hall. *This up-to-date textbook is a good place to look for more detailed discussions of topics in this chapter.*

Torrey, E. F. 1988. *Surviving Schizophrenia: A Family Manual*, rev. ed. New York: Harper and Row. *This book is a detailed and intelligent account of what schizophrenia is and how to cope with it.*

Zimbardo, P. G. 1977. *Shyness—What It Is, What to Do About It*. Reading, Mass.: Addison-Wesley. *Students and their interpersonal problems are the focus of the research and therapy techniques reported in this book.*

4

Intimate Relationships

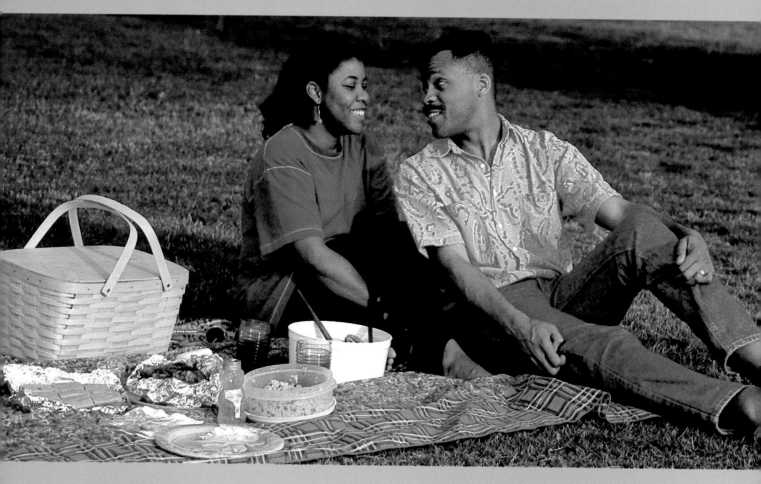

▶ You met someone quite different from yourself through a college club and have become seriously involved with him. You come from the South and have a European background; he's from New York City and has a Middle Eastern background. The two of you are intrigued by the differences in how you were brought up, how you express your feelings, and what you expect from life. Although you both identify with your backgrounds, it seems to be a case of opposites attracting. Both your parents and his, however, think you have too many differences. They say happy marriages are based on common backgrounds. They want you to date other people, preferably people more like yourselves. Are they being unreasonable, or do they have a point?

▶ A few months ago you fell in love with someone you met at a party. You were drawn to each other right away and soon were swept away on a flood of excitement, desire, and euphoria. You began spending practically all your time together, studying, eating, walking, and going to the beach; and when you weren't together you couldn't stop thinking about each other. It went on that way for several weeks, and then gradually the passion began to fade. Life began to seem ordinary again. You don't know what happened or what you ought to do. Is love over? Is this the way it always is? What happens now?

▶ You were surprised to discover that a couple you know are planning to get married. As long as you've known them, they've been unhappy together. They've even had affairs behind each other's backs. You contact them to offer your congratulations and find them completely immersed in planning an elaborate wedding. The man tells you that since they decided to get married, they've been too busy to fight. He says he's sure that any problems they have in their relationship will fade once they've made a formal commitment. Is he right that getting married can help solve problems in relationships? If you were asked, what advice would you give them?

▶ Your sister recently told you she's so frustrated with her husband she's considering separating from him. She says she's dissatisfied with their relationship but hasn't been able to talk to him about what's bothering her. Every time she brings something up, he gets uncomfortable and defensive. His goal seems to be to get things fixed as quickly as possible so the discussion can end. He says he doesn't think there's really anything to talk about. Are these two people incompatible? Are there things they can do to improve their relationship?

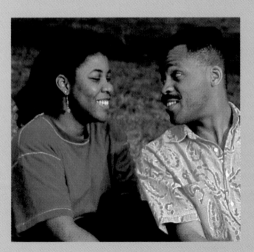

MAKING CONNECTIONS

Intimate relationships are an important part of wellness—people need to feel connected with others in order to function at their highest level. But intimacy and successful relationships are elusive for many people, as current divorce rates testify. In the scenarios presented on this page, each relating to intimacy, individuals have to use information, make a decision, or choose a course of action. What would you do in each of these situations? What response or decision would you make? This chapter provides information about forming intimate relationships, pairing and singlehood, marriage, and family life that can be used in situations like these. After finishing the chapter, read the scenarios again. Has what you've learned changed how you would respond?

Human beings need social relationships; people cannot thrive as solitary creatures. Nor could the human species survive if adults didn't cherish and support each other, if they didn't form strong mutual attachments with their infants, and if they didn't create families in which to raise children. Simply put, people need people.

Although people are held together in relationships by a variety of factors, the foundation of many relationships is love. Love in its many forms—romantic, passionate, platonic, parental—is the wellspring from which much of life's meaning and delight flows. In our culture, it binds us together as partners, parents, children, and friends. People devote tremendous energy to seeking mates, nurturing intimate relationships, keeping up friendships, maintaining marriages—all for the pleasure of loving and being loved.

Many human needs are satisfied in intimate relationships—needs for approval and affirmation, for companionship, for meaningful ties and a sense of belonging, for sexual satisfaction. Many of society's needs are fulfilled by relationships too, most notably the need to nurture and socialize children. Overall, intimate relationships are an important contributor to human well-being.

DEVELOPING INTIMATE RELATIONSHIPS

People who develop successful intimate relationships believe in themselves and in the people around them. They are willing to give of themselves—to share their ideas, feelings, time, needs—and to accept what others want to give them.

Self-Image and Self-Esteem

The principal thing that we all bring to our relationships is our *selves*. To have successful relationships, we must first accept and feel good about ourselves. A positive **self-image** and high **self-esteem** help us to love and respect others. How and where do we acquire a positive sense of self?

The roots of our sense of identity and self can be found in childhood, in the relationships we had with our parents and other family members. We're likely, as adults, to have a sense that we're basically lovable, worthwhile people and that others are trustworthy if, as babies and children, we felt loved, valued, and respected; if adults responded to our needs in a reasonably appropriate way; and if they gave us the freedom to explore and develop a sense of being separate individuals.

Our sense of personal identity isn't fixed or frozen. According to psychologist Erik Erikson, it continues to develop as we encounter and resolve various crises at each stage of life. The fundamental tasks of early childhood are the development of trust during infancy and of **autonomy** during toddlerhood. From these experiences and in-

teractions we construct our first ideas about who we are. (For a more detailed discussion of Erikson's theory, see Chapter 3.)

Another thing we learn in early childhood is **gender role**—the activities, abilities, and characteristics our culture deems appropriate for us based on whether we're male or female. In our society, men have traditionally been expected to work and provide for their families; to be aggressive, competitive, and power-oriented; and to use thinking and logic to solve problems. Women have been expected to take care of home and children; to be cooperative, supportive, and nurturing; and to approach the world emotionally and intuitively. Although more egalitarian gender roles are gradually emerging in our society, the stereotypes we absorb in childhood tend to be deeply ingrained and resistant to change.

Our ways of relating to others may also be rooted in childhood. Some researchers have suggested that our adult styles of loving may be based on the style of **attachment** we established in infancy with our mother, father, or other primary caregiver. According to this view, people who are secure in their intimate relationships may have had a secure, trusting, mutually satisfying attachment to their mother or other parenting figure. As adults they find it relatively easy to get close to others. They don't worry about being abandoned or having someone get too close to them. They feel that others like them and are generally well-intentioned.

People who are clinging and dependent in their relationships may have had an "anxious/ambivalent" attachment, in which their parent's inconsistent responses made them unsure that their needs would be met. As adults, they worry about whether their partners really love them and will stay with them. They tend to feel that others don't want to get as close as they do. They want to merge completely with another person, which sometimes scares others away.

People who seem to run from relationships may have had an "anxious/avoidant" relationship, in which their parent's inappropriate responses made them want to escape from his or her sphere of influence. As adults, they feel uncomfortable being close to others. They're distrustful and fearful of becoming dependent. Their partners usually want more intimacy than they do.

Even if people's earliest experiences and relationships

Self-image   The idea or conception one has of oneself or one's role.
Self-esteem   Feelings about one's own value and worth.
Autonomy   Independence; the sense of being self-directed.
Gender role   A culturally expected pattern of behavior and attitudes determined by whether a person is male or female.
Attachment   The emotional tie between an infant and his or her caregiver, or between two people in an intimate relationship.

TERMS

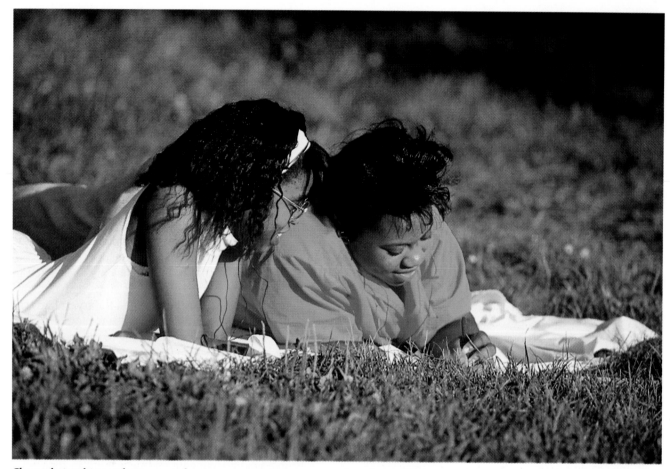

Close relationships without a sexual component are more common than those with sexual activity. Friendship satisfies the human needs for affection, affirmation, sharing, and companionship.

were less than ideal, however, they can still establish satisfying relationships in adulthood. Humans are resilient and flexible. They have the capacity to change their ideas, beliefs, and patterns of behavior. They can learn ways to raise their self-esteem; they can become more trusting, accepting, and appreciative of others; and they can acquire the communication and conflict resolution skills needed to maintain successful relationships. It helps to have a good start in life, but it may be more important to start from where you are.

Friendship

The first relationships we form outside the family are friendships. Whether with members of the same or the other sex, friendships give people the opportunity to share themselves and discover others. Friendships are reciprocal relationships between equals, held together with ties of respect, affection, trust, tolerance, and loyalty. Friends typically have interests and values in common, enjoy each other's company, and accept each other's individuality. When they are together, they feel comfortable, spontaneous, and authentic.

Friendship is like love in many ways, but love has additional characteristics. Love usually includes sexual desire, a greater demand for exclusiveness, and deeper levels of caring. But friendships are often seen as more stable and longer lasting than love relationships and less capable of "breaking up." Friends are more accepting and less critical than lovers, probably because their expectations are different. Like love relationships, friendships bind society together, providing people with emotional support and buffering them from stress.

Love, Sex, and Intimacy

Love is one of the most basic and profound human emotions. It is a powerful force in all our intimate relationships. Love encompasses opposites—affection and anger, excitement and boredom, stability and change, bonds and freedom. Love does not give us perfect happiness, but it does give our lives meaning.

In many kinds of adult relationships, love is closely intertwined with sexuality. In the past, marriage was considered the only acceptable context for sexual activities, but for many people today, premarital sex is legitimized by love. We now use personal standards rather than social norms to make decisions about sex. This trend toward personal responsibility results in even more of an emphasis on love than in the past.

For most people, love, sex, and commitment are closely linked ideals in intimate relationships. Love reflects the positive factors that draw people together and sustain them in a relationship. It includes trust, caring, respect, loyalty, interest in the other, and concern for the other's well-being. Sex brings excitement and passion to the relationship. It tends to intensify the relationship and add fascination and pleasure. Commitment, the determination to continue, reflects the stable factors that help maintain the relationship. Responsibility, reliability, and faithfulness are characteristics of commitment. Although love, sex, and commitment are related, they are not necessarily connected. One can exist without the others. Despite the various permutations of the three, most of us long for a special relationship that contains them all.

Other elements can be identified as features of love, such as euphoria, preoccupation with the loved one, idealization of the loved one, and so on, but these tend to be peripheral. As relationships progress, the central aspects of love and commitment become more characteristic of the relationship than the peripheral ones.

Another way of looking at love has been proposed by psychologist Robert Sternberg. He sees love as being composed of intimacy, passion, and decision/commitment. Intimacy refers to the feelings of warmth and closeness we have with someone we love. Passion refers to romance, attraction, and sexuality. Decision/commitment refers to both the short-term decision that you love someone and the long-term commitment to be in the relationship.

According to Sternberg, these three elements can be enlarged, diminished, or combined in different ways. Each combination gives a different kind of love:

- Liking (intimacy only)—the love between friends
- Infatuation (passion only)—an idealizing, obsessive, all-consuming love, characterized by a high degree of physical and emotional arousal; often unrequited; "love at first sight"
- Romantic (intimacy and passion)—commitment may develop in time
- Fatuous (passion and commitment)—deceptive love, the "whirlwind affair"; as passion fades, all that's left is commitment, but without time and intimacy, it's a poor foundation for an enduring relationship
- Empty (decision/commitment only)—dutiful love; also a poor foundation for a relationship
- Companionate (intimacy and commitment)— essentially a committed friendship; often begins as romantic love, but as passion diminishes and intimacy increases, it is transformed into companionate love

- Consummate (all three elements)—the love that dreams are made of; difficult to sustain

Men and women tend to have different views of the relationship between love (or intimacy) and sex (or passion). Numerous studies have found that men can separate love from sex rather easily, although many men find that their most erotic sexual experiences occur in the context of a love relationship. Women generally view sex from the point of view of a relationship. Some people believe you can have satisfying sex without love—with friends, acquaintances, or strangers. Although sex with love is an important norm in our culture, it is frequently disregarded in practice, as the high incidence of extrarelational affairs attests.

The Pleasure and Pain of Love The experience of intense love has confused and tormented lovers throughout history. They live in a tumultuous state of excitement, subject to wildly fluctuating feelings of joy and despair. They lose their appetites, can't sleep, and can think of nothing but the loved one. Is this happiness, misery, or both?

The contradictory nature of passionate love can be understood by realizing that human emotions have two components—physiological arousal and an emotional explanation for the arousal. (For a discussion of the biochemical and hormonal processes involved in arousal, see the description of the stress response in Chapter 2). Love is just one of many emotions accompanied by physiological arousal. Numerous unpleasant emotions can also generate physiological arousal, including fear, rejection, frustration, and challenge. Although experiences like attraction and sexual desire are pleasant, extreme excitement is similar to fear and is unpleasant. For this reason, passionate love may be too intense to enjoy. Over time the physical intensity and excitement tend to diminish. When this happens, pleasure may actually increase.

The Transformation of Love All human relationships change over time, and love relationships are no exception. At first, love is likely to be characterized by high levels of passion and rapidly increasing intimacy. In time, passion decreases as we become habituated to it and to the person. Generally, more time spent together does not increase arousal.

At the same time, the growth of intimacy slows and levels off. Sometimes intimacy is continuing to grow at a deeper, less conscious level; other times, people are drifting apart. Commitment isn't necessarily diminished or altered by time. It grows more slowly and is maintained as long as we judge the relationship to be successful. If the relationship begins to deteriorate, commitment usually decreases.

The disappearance of romance or passionate love is often experienced as a crisis in a relationship. If a more last-

Breaking Up Is Hard to Do

Even when they begin with the best of intentions, intimate relationships may not last. Sometimes a couple is mismatched to begin with; other times the relationship doesn't thrive and partners turn elsewhere for satisfaction. Ending an intimate relationship is usually difficult and painful. Both partners often feel attacked and abandoned, but feelings of distress are likely to be more acute for the rejected partner. If you are involved in a breakup, following a few simple guidelines can make the ending easier:

- Give the relationship the best chance you can before breaking up. If it still is not working, you'll know you did everything you could.

- Be fair and honest. If you are the one initiating the breakup, don't try to make your partner feel responsible.

- Be tactful and compassionate. You can leave the relationship without deliberately damaging your partner's self-esteem. Emphasize your mutual lack of fit and admit your own contributions to the problem.

- If you are the rejected person, give yourself time to resolve your anger and pain. You may go through a process of mourning the relationship, experiencing disbelief, anger, sadness, and finally acceptance. Despite all the romantic talk about your "one and only," remember that there are actually many potential candidates with whom you can have an intimate relationship.

- Find the value in the experience. Ending a close relationship can teach you valuable lessons about your needs, preferences, strengths, and weaknesses. Use your insights to increase your chances of success in your next relationship.

ing love fails to emerge, the relationship will likely break up and each person will search for another who will once again ignite his or her passion (for some tips on ending an intimate relationship, see the box "Breaking Up Is Hard to Do"). But love does not necessarily have to be passionate. When intensity diminishes, partners often discover a more enduring love. They can now move from absorption in each other to a relationship that includes external goals and projects, friends, and family. In this kind of intimate, more secure love, satisfaction comes not just from the relationship but also from achieving other creative goals, such as work or child rearing. The key to successful relationships isn't in love's intensity but in transforming passion into an intimate love, based on closeness, caring, and the promise of a shared future.

Personal Insight What are your expectations of love? How much are your expectations shaped by movies and magazines, by what your friends expect, by what you've observed of your parents' relationship? Are there any contradictions among these views? If so, can you reconcile them?

PAIRING AND SINGLEHOOD

Although most people eventually marry, all spend some time as singles, and nearly all make some attempt—conscious or unconscious—to find a partner. Intimate relationships are as important for singles as for couples.

Choosing a Partner

Most men and women select partners for stable relationships quite carefully and through a fairly predictable process. Although the pool of potential candidates appears huge, most people pair with someone who lives in the same geographical area and who is similar in racial, ethnic, and socioeconomic background, educational level, lifestyle, physical attractiveness, and other traits. In simple terms, people select partners like themselves.

First attraction is based on easily observable characteristics—looks, dress, social status, and reciprocated interest. Once the euphoria of romantic love winds down, personality traits and behaviors become more significant factors in how the partners view each other. Through sharing and self-disclosing, they gradually gain a deeper knowledge of each other. The emphasis shifts to basic values, such as religious beliefs, political persuasion, sexual attitudes, and future aspirations regarding career, family, and children. At some point, they decide whether the relationship feels viable and is worthy of their continued commitment. If they are compatible, many people gradually discover deeper, more enduring forms of love.

When people are choosing intimates, perhaps the most important question they can ask is, How much do we have in common? Although differences add interest to a relationship, similarities increase the chances of a relationship's success. If there are major differences, partners should ask, first, How accepting of differences are we? and second, How well do we communicate? Acceptance and communication skills go a long way toward making a relationship work, no matter how different the partners. Areas in which differences can affect the relationship in-

Arun Bharat Ram had come home to new Delhi after graduating from the University of Michigan when his mother announced she wanted to find him a wife. Her son was prime marriage material—27 years old, an heir to one of the largest fortunes in India, a sophisticated man who had gone to prep school with Rajiv Gandhi and who was soon to start work in the family's textile business. But Bharat Ram had dated American women in Ann Arbor, and the idea of entering into an arranged marriage, though expected in India, "did not seem quite right to me." He finally agreed to see a prospective bride so his mother would stop pestering him.

Manju, the prospect, was no less reluctant. She was 22, a recent graduate of a home economics college, from a conservative, middle-class family. She had always known that her marriage would be arranged, but she still shuddered when she remembered how a relative had been asked to parade before her future in-laws "like a girl being sold."

Arun and Manju met over coffee with their parents at a luxury hotel in New Delhi. Manju was so nervous that she dropped her cup, but everyone assured her this was a sign of good luck. Arun found Manju pretty and quiet; she was impressed that he didn't boast about his background. There were four more meetings, only one with the two alone. Then it was time to decide.

"If Arun wants to marry you," Manju's parents asked their daughter, "will you agree to marry him?" Manju had no major objections. She liked him, and that was enough. A few days later Arun's mother came to the house. "We want her," she said. Prime Minister Indira Gandhi and 1,500 others came to the wedding.

Few areas separate the East more from the West than their attitudes toward love, marriage, and sex. In India, sociologists estimate that 95 percent of all marriages are still arranged, including the majority of those among the educated middle class.

This is changing among the urban, westernized elite, but not entirely. An Indian man will still come home after years of dating American girlfriends to marry someone he hardly knows. The Sunday newspapers continue to be filled with pages of matrimonial ads. Many Indian college women still want their parents to find husbands for them, and they are so sure of the wisdom of their elders that some say yes to a prospective groom after a half-hour meeting. "Frankly, I don't think it's such a bad system," said Leila Seth, who is a high-court judge in India. As a socially progressive mother, Seth has told her daughter that she can make her own decision, but she will also help her find a husband if that's what she wants.

Since most Indian teenagers are still not allowed to date, parents think their children will be unprepared to make choices of their own. The big parental fear is that a daughter will fall for the first man who comes along. This kind of passion is considered dangerous. "I didn't love him," Manju recalled of the days after her engagement. "But when we talked, we had a lot of things in common." Arun said, "Obviously, I wasn't in love with her, but I was quite sure we would be interesting for each other. Whenever we met, we were comfortable. According to our tradition, that would lead to love." Today, almost 18 years and three children later, the Bharat Rams are a model of domestic contentment. "I've never thought of another man since I met him," Manju said. Arun added, "It wasn't something that happened overnight. It grew and became a tremendous bond. It's amazing, but in arranged marriages, people actually make the effort to fall in love with each other."

In the Indian view, American marriages fail because of the inevitable disappointment that sets in after the first few years of romantic love wear off. Most Indians believe that true love is a more peaceful emotion, based on long-term commitment and devotion to family. They also think they can "create" love between two people by arranging the right conditions for it, which is a marriage of common backgrounds and interests. In the West, love must come before marriage, but in India, it can only come after.

Indian girls are told from childhood that they will love the man their parents choose. Only in exceptional circumstances, like wife beating, will a mother listen to a daughter's complaints about her husband. Divorce has been legal since 1955, but it is still rare even among the urban elite. Most women say these customs suit them fine. And although exceptionally independent women (and men) do break away, that doesn't mean they reject arranged marriages for others.

Source: Associated Press. 30 December 1985.

---

clude values, religion, race, attitudes toward sexuality and gender roles, socioeconomic status, familiarity with the other's culture, and interactions with the extended family.

Dating

Every society has some rituals for pairing and finding mates. Parent-arranged marriages are still popular in many cultures. They are often very stable and permanent; divorce is unheard of, except for infertility. (For a closer look at arranged marriages, see the box "Love Comes Later: Arranged Marriages in India"). Although American culture emphasizes personal choice in courtship, the popularity of dating services (complete with personality tests and videotapes of prospects) suggests that many individuals do want assistance in finding suitable mates.

Most Americans—whether single, divorced, widowed, or gay—find romantic partners through some form of dating. They narrow the field through a process of getting to know each other. Dating often revolves around a mu-

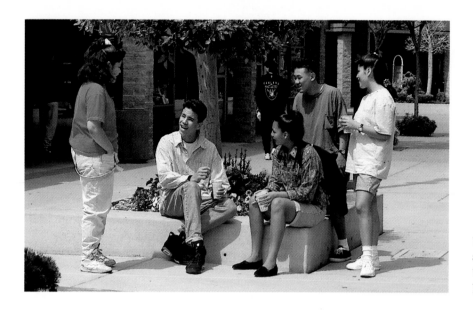

For many college students today, group activities have replaced dating as a way to meet and get to know potential partners.

tually enjoyable activity, such as seeing a movie or having dinner. In the traditional male-female dating pattern, the man takes the lead, initiating the date, while the woman waits to be called. In this pattern, casual dating might evolve into steady or exclusive dating, then engagement and finally marriage.

For many young people today, traditional dating has given way to a more casual form of "getting together." Greater equality between the sexes is at the root of this change. People may meet in groups rather than go out as couples, with each person paying his or her way. A man and woman may begin to spend more time together, but often in the group context. If sexual involvement develops, it is more likely to be based on friendship, respect, and common interests than on expectations related to gender roles. In this model, mate selection may progress from getting together to living together to marriage.

Living Together

According to the U.S. Census Bureau, over 2.9 million heterosexual couples (and 1.5 million gay and lesbian couples) were living together in the United States in 1990. Living together, or **cohabitation,** is one of the most rapid and dramatic social changes that has ever occurred in our society. It seems to be gaining acceptance as part of the normal mate selection process. By age 30, about half of all men and women will have cohabited. The only thing separating those who cohabit from those who don't is degree of religiousness. Several factors are involved in this change, including greater acceptance of premarital sex, increased availability of contraceptives, the tendency for people to wait longer before getting married, and a larger pool of single and divorced individuals.

Cohabitation is more popular among younger people than older, although a significant number of older couples live together without marrying because they would lose a source of income, such as Social Security benefits, if they were to marry. Cohabitation relationships usually end with the couple either splitting up or getting married; very few continue indefinitely. Whatever the reasons for choosing it, living together provides many of the benefits of marriage—companionship; a setting for an enjoyable and meaningful relationship; the opportunity to develop greater intimacy through learning, compromising, and sharing; and the development of a satisfying sex life.

For those who choose it, living together has certain advantages over marriage. For one thing, it can give the partners a greater sense of autonomy. They don't feel bound by the social rules and expectations that are part of the institution of marriage. They may find it easier to keep their identity and more of their independence, and they don't incur the same obligations that marriage brings. If things don't work out, they may find it easier and less complicated to leave a relationship that hasn't been legally sanctioned.

But living together has some liabilities, too. In most cases, the legal protections of marriage are absent; these include health insurance benefits and property and inheritance rights. These considerations can be particularly serious if the couple has children, from either former relationships or the current partnership. Since social acceptance of cohabitation is not universal, couples may feel pressure from family members or others to marry or otherwise change their living arrangements, especially if they have young children. The general trend, however, is toward legitimizing single relationships, whether gay or heterosexual. For example, some employers and communities now extend benefits to domestic partners.

Although many people choose cohabitation as a kind of trial marriage, there is little evidence as yet that people who live together before getting married have happier or longer-lasting marriages. Statistically, people who cohabit before marrying are just as likely to divorce as are those

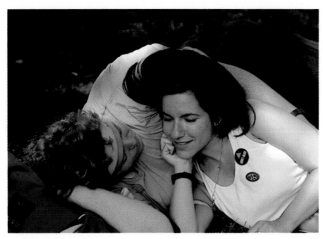

Greater openness has made gay men and lesbians more visible than they used to be, although they still constitute a minority of the population. Most gay men and lesbians have experienced at least one long-term relationship with a single partner.

who don't cohabit. One study found slightly less marital satisfaction among married couples who had cohabited. The researchers speculated that these people might have expected more out of marriage and been disappointed, or that people who cohabit might be less likely to adapt well to traditional marital roles. It may just be that whatever patterns are going to develop in the relationship, whether deeper intimacy or disillusionment, develop earlier than if the couple had not lived together before marriage.

Personal Insight How do you feel about cohabitation? Is it a choice you would make? What influences your attitude?

Gay and Lesbian Partnerships

Regardless of **sexual orientation,** most people are looking for love in a close, satisfying, committed relationship. Gay and lesbian (or **homosexual**) couples have many similarities with **heterosexual** couples (although they can't legally marry). According to one study, most gay men and lesbians have experienced at least one long-term relationship with a single partner. Like heterosexual relationships, gay and lesbian partnerships provide intimacy, passion, and security.

One difference among gay, lesbian, and heterosexual couples is that gay and lesbian couples tend to adopt "best friend" roles in their relationship rather than traditional gender roles. Domestic tasks are shared or split, and both partners usually support themselves. Another difference is that gay and lesbian couples often have to deal with societal hostility toward their relationships (in contrast to the approval given to heterosexual couples). Consequently, the community may be more important as a

source of identity and social support than it is for heterosexuals. Community support has been particularly important since the advent of the HIV/AIDS crisis. Gay men and lesbians have played an important role in the development of education and counseling programs, research foundations, and outreach programs for people infected with HIV.

Singlehood

Despite the prevalence and popularity of marriage, a significant proportion of adults in our society are unmarried. In 1990 nearly 79 million Americans were single. They are a diverse group, encompassing young people who have not married yet but plan to in the future, people who are living together, whether gay or heterosexual, and people of all ages who would like to marry but haven't found a suitable mate. In other words, the category includes people of all ages who are single both by choice and by chance.

Several factors contribute to the growing number of single people. One is the changing view of singlehood, which is increasingly being viewed as a legitimate option to marriage. Education and career are delaying the age at which young people are marrying. More young people are living with their parents as they complete their education, seek jobs, or strive for financial independence. Many other single people live together without being married. Gay people who would marry their partners if they were legally permitted to do so are counted among the single population. High divorce rates mean more singles, and people who have experienced divorce in their families may have more negative attitudes about marriage and more positive attitudes about singlehood.

Being single doesn't mean that people don't have close relationships, however. They may date, enjoy active and fulfilling social lives, and have a variety of sexual experiences and relationships. Other advantages of being single include more opportunities for personal and career development without concern for family obligations, greater variety in sexual partners, and more freedom and control in making life choices. Significant disadvantages of being single include loneliness and lack of companionship as well as economic hardships (mainly for single women). Single people, both male and female, experience some discrimination and often are pressured to get married.

Cohabitation   Living together in a sexual relationship without being married.
Sexual orientation   Sexual attraction to individuals of the opposite sex, same sex, or both.
Homosexual   Sexual orientation toward and preference for the same sex.
Heterosexual   Sexual orientation toward and preference for the opposite sex.

TERMS

Nearly everyone has at least one episode of being single in adult life, whether it's prior to marriage, between marriages, following divorce or the death of a spouse, or for the entire adult life span. How enjoyable and valuable this single time is depends on several factors, including how deliberately the person has chosen it; how satisfied the person is with social relationships, standard of living, and job; how comfortable the person feels when alone; and how resourceful and energetic the person is about creating an interesting and fulfilling life.

MARRIAGE

Although half of all marriages in our society now end in divorce, the popularity of marriage itself hasn't diminished. Marriage fulfills a number of basic needs. There are many important social, moral, economic, and political aspects of marriage, all of which have changed over the years. In the past, people married mainly for practical reasons, such as raising children or forming an economic unit. Today, people marry more for personal, emotional reasons. This shift places a greater burden on marriage to fulfill needs and expectations, sometimes unreasonably high ones. People may assume that all their emotional needs will be met by their partner, or they may think that fascination and passion will always remain at high levels, or they may simply expect to "live happily ever after." When people enter marriage with such preconceptions, it may be harder for them to appreciate the benefits that marriage really offers.

Personal Insight What are your ideas and beliefs about marriage? Do you think it should last forever? What influences your views of marriage?

Benefits of Marriage

The primary functions and benefits of marriage are those of any intimate relationship: affection, personal affirmation, companionship, sexual fulfillment, emotional growth. Marriage also provides a setting in which to raise children, although a growing number of couples choose to remain childless and people can also choose to raise children without being married. Marriage is also important for its provision for the future. By committing themselves to the relationship, people provide themselves with

lifelong companions as well as some insurance for their later years (see the box "Intimate Relationships Are Good for Your Health").

Issues in Marriage

Although we would all like to believe otherwise, love is not enough to make a successful marriage. Couples have to have strengths; they have to be successful in their relationship before marriage. Problems in relationships are magnified rather than solved by marriage. The following relationship characteristics appear to be the best predictors of a happy marriage:

- The partners have realistic expectations about their relationship.
- Each feels good about the personality of the other.
- They communicate well.
- They have effective ways of resolving conflicts.
- They agree on religious/ethical values.
- They have an egalitarian role relationship.
- They have a good balance of individual versus joint interests and leisure activities.

Once they're married, couples have a number of marital adjustment tasks to face. In addition to providing each other with emotional support, they have to negotiate and establish marital roles; establish domestic and career priorities; manage their budget and finances; make sexual adjustments; manage boundaries and relationships with their extended family; and participate in the larger community.

The area of marital roles and responsibilities has probably undergone the most change in recent years. Many couples no longer accept traditional assumptions about roles, such as that the husband is solely responsible for supporting the family and the wife is solely responsible for domestic work. Today, many husbands share domestic tasks and many wives work outside the home. In fact, over 50 percent of married women are in the labor force, including women with babies under one year of age. Although women still take most of the responsibility for home and children even when they work, and although men still suffer more job-related stress and health problems than women do, the trend is toward an equalization of duties and responsibilities.

Coping with all these challenges requires that couples be committed to remaining married through the inevitable ups and downs of the relationship. They will

TERMS **Communication** The process by which we establish contact and exchange information with others.

Personal Insight What do you think are appropriate roles and activities for husbands and wives? If both husband and wife work full time, do you think they should share housework and child care equally? What influences your views?

Intimate Relationships Are Good for Your Health

Alone on the banks of Walden Pond, Henry David Thoreau enjoyed a life of simplicity and solitude. But is the solitary lifestyle healthy? Recent research indicates that it's not. Studies underscore the importance of strengthening your family and social ties to help maintain your mental and physical health. Living alone, or simply feeling alone, can have a negative effect not only on your state of mind but on your physical health as well.

Two studies published in the January 1992 issue of the *Journal of the American Medical Association* showed that social isolation is a risk factor for people with heart problems. The first study looked at the effects of living alone on people who had had a heart attack. Those living alone had a 15.8 percent chance of having a second serious nonfatal or fatal heart attack, compared to 8.8 percent for those not living alone. The second study looked at people with severe narrowing of at least one major heart vessel. Those who were unmarried and without one close friend or confidant were "over three times more likely to die of a heart problem within five years than married patients or unmarried patients who did report having a confidant."

Similar evidence has been found for people with cancer. A long-term study of over 6,000 adults in California showed that women who had no or few social contacts were twice as likely to die of cancer. These women also were more than five times as likely to die of smoking-related cancers.

Another study at Stanford University Medical Center was conducted to evaluate the psychological effect of emotional support groups on cancer patients. Eighty-six women who were receiving treatment for breast cancer were randomly divided into two groups. One group took part in weekly discussions in which they shared their feelings and learned simple techniques to reduce stress. After a year, the women in the support group were less depressed, felt less pain, and had a more positive outlook than did the women who received only conventional treatment. To the surprise of the researchers, the women in the support group also survived nearly twice as long as the women in the control group. Researcher David Spiegel said, "Believe me, if we'd seen these results with a new drug, it would be in use in every cancer hospital in the country today."

What is it about social relationships that supports people's health? Researchers aren't sure, but they suggest that intimate relationships, and especially living with a loving partner, have both physical and emotional benefits. When you're sick, a partner can cook, bring you food, and make your life easier and more comfortable. Partners encourage and reinforce healthy habits, such as eating well, smoking and drinking less, and taking fewer risks. (Women generally have healthier lifestyles than men, so when people marry, men's health improves more significantly than women's.) Partners also help identify problems and encourage each other to rest, treat illnesses, see a physician, and so on. These are probably some of the reasons that married people live longer, have fewer illnesses, and report a higher sense of well-being than do their unmarried peers.

But it's not just the physical support that helps people get and stay well. Although married people have better emotional health than unmarried people, this is true only if the marriage is happy. Unhappily married people have *more* emotional distress than unmarried people. And when partners are unsupportive or unfair, sick people often feel depressed or demoralized.

Clearly, emotional support is a crucial element in physical health. When someone cares and listens, it helps reduce depression, anxiety, and other psychological problems. Feeling loved, esteemed, and valued brings comfort at a time of vulnerability. Being connected with others helps mitigate the damaging effects of stress. In general, improved emotional well-being improves physical health and survival ability.

Although solitude may have helped Thoreau achieve his purposes (he returned to life in Boston after two years at Walden Pond), prolonged isolation is a strain for most human beings. To protect your health over your whole life span, stay connected with people, maintain your social ties, and take good care of your intimate relationships.

Adapted from "Living Alone," *Mayo Clinic Health Letter,* September 1992; and P. Jaret, "Mind over Malady," *Health,* November/December 1992.

need to be tolerant of each other's imperfections, keep their sense of perspective and their sense of humor, and put energy into retaining sufficient levels of intimacy, sexual satisfaction, and commitment. The most important skills they bring to these challenges are their communication and conflict resolution skills.

Communication Skills

The key to developing and maintaining an intimate relationship is good **communication.** Most of the time, we

don't think about communicating—we simply talk and act in natural ways. But when problems arise—when we feel others don't understand us or when someone accuses us of not listening—we become aware of our limitations or, more commonly, what we think are other people's limitations. Miscommunications create frustration and distance us from our friends and partners.

As much as 65 percent of face-to-face communication is nonverbal. Even when we're silent, we're communicating. We send messages when we look at someone or look away, lean forward or sit back, smile or frown. Especially

- Face your partner and maintain eye contact. Provide appropriate nonverbal feedback (nodding, smiling, and so on).

- When your partner is speaking, don't interrupt.

- Don't offer unsolicited advice, comments, or criticism.

- Clarify your understanding of what your partner is saying by restating it in your own words and asking if your understanding is correct.

- When you're speaking, take responsibility for your messages by using "I" statements and avoiding statements beginning with "You."

- Make constructive requests that seek to change the way you interact with your partner. Begin your requests with "I would like . . ."

- Ask for actions ahead of time, not after the fact.

- Be respectful and polite.

- Respond to your partner's requests, and praise your partner for fulfilling your requests.

- Offer ongoing positive feedback, keeping the relationship open to positive change.

Adapted from R. B. Stuart. 1983. *Improving Communication.* Champaign, Ill.: Research Press.

important forms of nonverbal communication are touch, eye contact, and proximity. If someone we're talking to touches our hand or arm, looks into our eyes, and leans toward us when we talk, we get the message that the person is interested in us and cares about what we're saying. If a person keeps looking around the room while we're talking or takes a step backward, we get the impression that the person is uninterested or wants to end the conversation. The ability to interpret nonverbal messages correctly is important to the success of relationships. It's also important, when sending messages, to make sure our body language agrees with our words. When our verbal and nonverbal messages are incongruent with each other, we send a confusing mixed message.

Three keys to good communication in relationships are self-disclosure, listening skills, and feedback. Self-disclosure involves revealing personal information that we ordinarily wouldn't reveal because of the risk involved. It usually increases feelings of closeness and allows the relationship to move to a deeper level of intimacy. Friends often disclose the most to each other, sharing feelings, experiences, hopes, and disappointments; married couples sometimes share less because they think they already know everything there is to know about each other.

Listening is the second component of good communication, and it is a rare skill. Good listening skills require that we spend more time and energy trying to fully understand another person's "story" and less time judging, evaluating, blaming, advising, analyzing, or trying to control. Empathy, warmth, respect, and genuineness are qualities of skillful listeners. Attentive listening encourages friends or partners to share more and, in turn, to be attentive listeners. To connect with other people and develop real emotional intimacy, listening is essential.

Self-disclosing and good listening both build trust in a relationship. The third component of good communication is feedback—a constructive response to another's self-disclosure. Giving positive feedback means acknowledging that the friend's or partner's feelings are valid—no matter how upsetting or troubling—and offering self-disclosures in response. If, for example, your partner discloses unhappiness about your relationship, it is more constructive to say that you're concerned or saddened by that and want to hear more about it than to get angry, to blame, to try to inflict pain, or to withdraw. Self-disclosure and feedback can open the door to change, where other responses block communication and change. (For tips on how to have better communication skills, see the box "Improving Communication in Your Relationship.")

Some of the difficulties people encounter in relationships can be traced to common gender differences in communication. Many authorities believe that, because of the way they've been raised, men as a group and women as a group approach conversation and communication differently. (This doesn't mean that there aren't individual exceptions.) According to this view, men tend to use conversation in a competitive way, perhaps hoping to establish dominance in relationships. When male conversations are over, men often find themselves in a one-up or a one-down position. Women tend to use conversation in a more **affiliative** way, perhaps hoping to establish friendships. They negotiate various degrees of closeness, seeking to give and receive support. Men tend to talk more—though without disclosing more—and listen less. Women tend to use good listening skills like eye contact, frequent nodding, focused attention, and relevant questions.

Although these are generalized patterns, they can translate into problems in specific conversations. Even

TERMS

Affiliative Relating to connections, associations, or relationships.

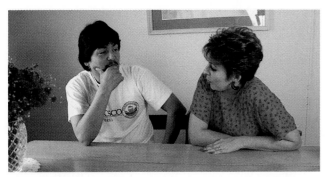

Conflict is an inevitable part of any intimate relationship. Couples need to develop constructive ways of resolving conflicts to maintain a healthy relationship.

when a man and a woman are talking about the same subject, their unconscious goals may be very different. The woman may be looking for understanding and closeness while the man may be trying to demonstrate his competence by giving advice and solving problems. Both styles are valid; the problem comes when differences in styles result in poor communication and misunderstanding.

Sometimes communication is not the problem in a relationship—the partners understand each other all too well. The problem is that they're unable or unwilling to change or compromise. Good communication can't salvage a bad relationship, but it does allow people to see their differences and make more informed decisions.

Conflict and Conflict Resolution

Conflict is natural in intimate relationships. No matter how close two people become, they still remain separate individuals with their own wants, needs, past experiences, and ways of seeing the world. In fact, the closer the relationship, the more differences will be discovered and the more opportunities for conflict will arise. Conflict itself isn't dangerous to intimate relationships; it may simply indicate that the relationship is growing. But if it isn't handled in a constructive way, it will damage—or destroy—the relationship.

Conflict is often accompanied by anger, a natural enough emotion but one that can be difficult to handle. If we vent anger, we run the risk of creating distrust, fear, and distance; if we act it out without thinking things through, we can cause the conflict to escalate; if we suppress it, it turns into resentment and low-level hostility. The best way to handle anger in a relationship is to recognize it as a symptom of something that requires attention and needs to be changed. When they are angry, the partners should back off until they calm down, then come back to the issue later and try to resolve it rationally. Negotiation will help to dissipate anger so that the conflict can be resolved.

Sources of conflict for couples change over time but revolve mainly around the basic task of living together—how housework is divided, how much time and attention are given to each other, how money is handled. Sexual interaction is a source of disagreement for many couples.

Although there are many theories on and approaches to conflict resolution, there are some basic strategies that are generally useful in successfully negotiating with a partner:

- Clarify the issue. Take responsibility for thinking through your feelings and discovering what is really bothering you. Agree that one partner will speak first and have the chance to speak fully while the other listens. Then reverse the roles. Try to understand the other's position fully by repeating what you've heard and asking questions to clarify or elicit more information. Agree to talk only about the topic at hand and not get distracted by other issues. Sum up what your partner has said.

- Find out what each person wants. Ask your partner to express his or her desires. Don't assume you know what your partner wants and speak for him or her. Clarify and summarize.

- Identify various alternatives for getting each person what he or she wants. Practice brainstorming to generate a variety of options.

- Decide how to negotiate. Work out some agreements or plans for change, such as agreeing that if one partner will do one task, the other will do another task or that a partner will do a task in exchange for being able to do something else he or she wants.

- Solidify the agreements. Go over the plan verbally and write it down if necessary to ensure that you both understand and agree to it.

- Review and renegotiate. Decide on a time frame for trying out the new plan and set a time to discuss how it's working. Make adjustments as needed.

To resolve conflicts, partners have to feel safe in voicing disagreements. They have to trust that the discussion won't get out of control, that they won't be abandoned by the other, and that the partner won't take advantage of their vulnerability. Partners should follow some basic ground rules when they argue, such as avoiding ultimatums, resisting the urge to give the silent treatment, refusing to "hit below the belt," and not using sex to smooth over disagreements. Table 4-1 shows some differences between constructive and destructive approaches to conflict resolution.

Personal Insight How did your parents resolve conflict when you were growing up? How effective were their methods? Has their model influenced the approach to conflict resolution you use in your relationships?

TABLE 4-1 Constructive and Destructive Approaches to Conflict Resolution

	Constructive Approach	Destructive Approach
Issues	Raise and clarify issues	Bring up old issues
Feelings	Express both positive and negative feelings	Express only negative feelings
Information	Provide complete and honest information	Provide selective information
Focus	Focus is on issue rather than person	Focus is on person rather than issue
Blame	Accept mutual blame	Blame other person(s)
Perception	Focus is on similarities	Focus is on differences
Change	Prevent stagnation by facilitating change	Increase conflict and minimize change
Outcome	Both win	One wins and one loses, or both lose
Intimacy	Resolving conflict increases intimacy	Escalating conflict decreases intimacy
Attitude	Trust	Suspicion

Source: D. Olson and J. DeFrain. 1994. *Marriage and Family*. Mountain View, Calif.: Mayfield.

Separation and Divorce

The high rate of divorce in the United States doesn't indicate that Americans don't believe in marriage any more. Instead, it reflects our extremely high expectations for emotional fulfillment and satisfaction in marriage. It also indicates that we no longer believe in the permanence of marriage.

The process of divorce usually begins with an emotional separation. Often one partner is unhappy and looks beyond the relationship for other forms of validation. Dissatisfaction increases until the unhappy partner decides that he or she can no longer go on. Physical separation follows, although it may take some time for the relationship to be over emotionally.

Except for the death of a spouse, divorce is the greatest stress-producing event in life. Both men and women experience turmoil, depression, and lowered self-esteem during and after divorce. People experience separation distress and loneliness for about a year and then enter on a one- to three-year-long recovery period. During this time they gradually construct a postdivorce identity along with a new pattern of life. Most people are surprised by how long it takes to recover from divorce. Children are especially vulnerable to the trauma of divorce, and sometimes counseling is appropriate to help them adjust to the changes in their lives.

Despite the distress of separation and divorce, the negative effects are usually balanced sooner or later by the possibility of finding a more suitable partner, constructing a new life, and developing new aspects of the self.

About three-quarters of all people who divorce remarry, often within five years. One result of the high divorce and remarriage rate is a growing number of stepfamilies (also known as "blended" families), a trend discussed in the next section.

FAMILY LIFE

American families are very different today than they were even a few decades ago (see the box "The Changing American Family"). Currently, about 50 percent of all families are based on a first marriage; 25 percent are headed by a single parent; 17 percent are remarriages; and 8 percent involve some other arrangement. Despite the tremendous variation apparent in American families, certain patterns can still be discerned.

The family life cycle usually begins with marriage. This first stage, when newlyweds are learning how to live together, ends abruptly with the arrival of a baby. New parents have a new set of responsibilities, and their roles change profoundly and irreversibly—no more spontaneous outings to see a movie or leisurely Sunday mornings sipping coffee and browsing through the paper. The third member of the family, the new infant, demands round-the-clock attention.

Becoming a Parent

Few new parents have any preparation for the job of parenting, yet they have to assume that role literally

- About 95 percent of all Americans marry at some time in their lives.

- About 5 percent of all Americans never marry.

- The median age for first marriage is 25.5 for bridegrooms and 23.3 for brides, according to the U.S. Census Bureau.

- Forty-one percent of marriageable adults (15 and older) are single, according to the U.S. Census Bureau. The rise of singlehood among those in their twenties and thirties has led family demographers to predict that the percentage of individuals who will never marry may double to 10 percent by the year 2,000.

- People marrying today have a 50–55 percent chance of divorcing.

- Generally, whites are less likely to divorce than blacks; older individuals are less likely to divorce than younger individuals; and those who marry in their twenties are less likely to divorce than those who marry while in their teens.

- Most divorces involve children; and more than one million children are affected by divorce each year in the United States.

- Mothers are awarded custody of the children in 9 out of 10 divorce cases. Joint custody, however, is now legal in 28 states and is favored by many.

- Most divorced individuals eventually remarry; for younger divorced individuals, this remarriage occurs within five years of the divorce. Men are slightly more likely to remarry than women and remarriage is more likely for younger divorced individuals than for older divorced individuals. Blacks are more likely than whites to remain separated without legally divorcing and are less likely than whites to remarry after divorce.

Changes in Marriage and Family, 1960 to 1990

	1960	1990
Percent of childbirths outside of marriage	5	25
Percent of teenage mothers who are unmarried	15	64
Divorced individuals per 1,000 married individuals	35	130
Percent of children living with only one parent	9	25
Percent of adult life spent with spouse and children	62	43

Source: D. Olson and J. DeFrain. 1994. *Marriage and Family.* Mountain View, Calif.: Mayfield.

overnight. They have to learn quickly how to hold a baby, how to change it, how to feed it, how to interpret its cries. No wonder the birth of the first child is one of the most stressful transitions for any couple.

Even couples with an egalitarian relationship before their first child is born find that their marriage becomes more traditional with the arrival of the new baby. The father becomes the principal provider and protector, and the mother becomes the primary nurturer. Most research indicates that mothers have to make greater changes in their lives than fathers do. Although men today spend more time caring for their infants than ever before, women still take the ultimate responsibility for seeing that the baby is fed, clean, and comfortable. In addition, women are usually the ones who make job changes; they may quit working or reduce their hours in order to stay home with the baby for several months or more, or they may try to juggle the multiple roles of mother, home-maker, and employee and feel guilty that they never have enough time to do justice to any of these roles.

Not surprisingly, marital satisfaction often declines after the birth of the first child. The wife who has stopped working may feel that she is cut off from the world; the wife who is trying to fulfill duties both at home and on the job may feel overburdened and resentful. The husband may have a hard time adjusting to having to share his wife's love and attention.

But marital dissatisfaction after the baby is born is not inevitable. Couples who successfully weather the stresses of a new baby seem to have three characteristics in common: They had developed a strong relationship before the baby was born; they had planned to have the child and want it very much; and they communicate well about their feelings and expectations.

Parenting and the Life Cycle of the Family

Sometimes being a parent is a source of unparalleled pleasure and pride—the first smile (at you), the first word, the first home run. But at other times, parenting can seem like an overwhelming responsibility. How can you be sure that you're not making some mistake that will stunt your child's physical or emotional growth? Child-rearing experts all seem to agree that (1) it's virtually impossible to stop a child's physical growth and development and (2) children's emotional health and self-esteem depend above all on their feeling that their parents want them, accept them, and love them, although there's no one right way to raise children that will ensure that they will become happy and productive adults.

At each stage of the family life cycle, the relationship between parents and children changes. And with those changes come new challenges. The parents' primary responsibility to a small, helpless baby is to ensure its physical well-being round the clock. As babies grow into toddlers and begin to crawl and walk and talk, they begin to be able to take care of some of their own physical needs. For parents, the challenge at this stage is to strike a balance between giving their children the freedom to explore and setting limits that will keep their children safe and secure. As children grow toward adolescence, parents need to allow them increasing independence and finally be willing to let them risk success or failure on their own.

Marital satisfaction for most couples is low while their children are in school. There are several reasons, including the financial and emotional pressures of a growing family and the increased job and community responsibilities for parents in their thirties, forties, and fifties. Once the last child has left home, marital satisfaction usually increases because the couple have time to enjoy each other once more.

Single Parents

Chances are good that you know a number of families who haven't followed the traditional family life cycle. In 1985, according to U.S. Census Bureau statistics, one out of every four families with children under 18 was a one-parent family. And more than one-third of women who were in their late twenties in 1984 could expect to be single parents at some point in their life. Their mothers and grandmothers had probably followed the traditional pattern of marriage, motherhood, and widowhood. But today the family life cycle for many women is marriage, motherhood, divorce, single parenting, remarriage, and widowhood.

In some single-parent families, the traditional family life cycle is reversed and the baby comes before the marriage. In these families, the single parent is usually a teenage mother; she may very well be African American or Latina; and she may never get married or may not marry for a number of years. In single-parent families that

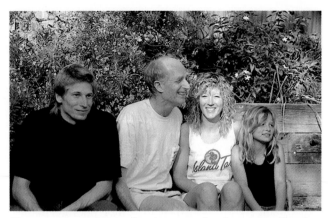

Almost one out of every five American families is a stepfamily, in which parents bring children from a previous marriage into a new family unit.

are the result of divorce, the mother usually has custody of the children, but a little over 10 percent of single-parent families are headed by fathers.

Economic difficulties are the primary problem for single mothers, especially for unmarried mothers who have not finished high school and have difficulty finding work. Divorced mothers usually experience a sharp drop in income the first few years on their own, but if they have job skills or education, they are usually eventually able to support themselves and their children adequately. Other problems for single mothers are the often-conflicting demands of playing both father and mother and the difficulty of filling their own needs for adult companionship and affection.

Financial pressures are also a complaint of single fathers, but they do not experience them to the extent that single mothers do. Because they are likely to have less practice than mothers in juggling parental and professional roles, they often worry that they do not spend enough time with their children. Because single fatherhood is so rare, however, the men who choose it are likely to be stable, established, and strongly motivated to be with their children.

Research on the effect on children of growing up in a single-parent family is not conclusive; however, evidence seems to indicate that children from single-parent families tend to have less success in school and in their careers than do children from two-parent families. Nevertheless, two-parent families are not necessarily better if one of the parents spends little time relating to the children or is physically or emotionally abusive.

Stepfamilies

Single-parenthood is usually a transitional stage; about three out of four divorced women and about four out of five divorced men will ultimately remarry. Overall, almost half of the marriages in the United States are remarriages

A sad fact about intimate relationships is that any form of intimacy increases the potential for violence. American families are the scene each year of uncountable violent acts, including stabbings, shootings, and sexual assaults. Violence within families may be seen on a continuum, with spanking and slapping—considered to be "normal" abuse in many families—on one end and murder on the other.

Violence against wives, or battering, occurs at every level of society but is more common at lower socioeconomic levels. It also occurs more frequently in marriages with a high degree of conflict—and an apparent inability to resolve arguments through negotiation and compromise. There are no figures on how many battered women there are in the United States, but battering is probably one of the most common and underreported crimes in the country.

In these relationships, the man usually has a history of violent behavior, traditional beliefs about gender roles in the family, and problems with alcohol abuse. He has low self-esteem and seeks to raise it by dominating and imposing his will on another person. Research has revealed a three-phase cycle of battering, consisting of a period of increasing tension, a violent explosion and loss of control, and a period of contriteness, in which the man begs forgiveness and promises it will never happen again. The batterer is drawn back to this cycle over and over again, but he never succeeds in changing his feelings about himself.

Battered women often stay in violent relationships for years. They may be economically dependent on their husbands, believe their children need a father, or have low self-esteem themselves. They may love or pity their husbands, or they may believe they'll eventually be able to stop the violence. They usually leave the relationship only when they become determined that the violence must end. Battered women's shelters offer them physical protection, counseling,

support, and various types of survival assistance.

Many battering husbands are arrested, prosecuted, and imprisoned. Treatment programs for men are helpful in some cases, but not all. Programs focus on stress management, communication and conflict resolution skills, behavior change, and individual and group therapy. A crucial factor in changing men's violent behavior seems to be their partners' adamant insistence that the abuse stop.

Family violence is also directed against children. At least 1 million American children are physically abused by their parents every year. Parental violence is one of the five leading causes of death for children aged 1 to 18.

Parents who abuse children tend to have low self-esteem, to believe in physical punishment, to have a poor marital relationship, and to have been abused themselves (although many people who were abused as children do not grow up to abuse their own children). Poverty, unemployment, and social isolation are characteristics of families in which children are abused. Single parents, both men and women, are at especially high risk for abusing their children. Very often one child, whom the parents consider different in some way, is singled out for violent treatment.

When government agencies intervene in child abuse situations, their goals are to protect the victims and to assist and strengthen the families. The most successful programs are those that stress education and early intervention, such as home visits to high-risk first-time mothers. Educational efforts focus on stress management, money management, job-finding skills, and information about child behavior and development. Parents may also receive counseling and be referred to alcohol or drug abuse programs. Support groups like Parents Anonymous are effective for parents committed to changing their behavior.

---

for the husband, the wife, or both. If either brings children from a previous marriage into the new family unit, a stepfamily is formed.

Stepfamilies are significantly different from intact families and should not be expected to duplicate the emotions and relationships of an intact family. Research has shown that healthy stepfamilies are less cohesive and more adaptable than healthy intact families; they have a greater capacity to allow for individual differences and accept that biologically related family members will have emotionally closer relationships. Stepfamilies gradually gain more of a sense of being a family as they build a history of shared everyday experiences and major life events.

Successful Families

Family life can be extremely challenging. A strong family isn't a family without problems; it's a family that copes

successfully with stress and crisis. (For a look at unsuccessful responses to stress, see the box "Family Violence.") Although there is tremendous variation in American families, researchers have proposed that six major qualities or themes appear in strong families.

- *Commitment.* The family is very important to its members; sexual fidelity between partners is included in commitment.

- *Appreciation.* People care about one another and let one another know it. The home is a positive place.

- *Communication.* People spend time listening to one another and enjoying one another's company. They talk about disagreements and attempt to solve problems.

- *Time together.* People do things together, often simple activities that don't cost money.

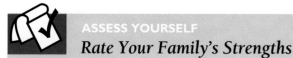
Rate Your Family's Strengths

This Family Strengths Inventory was developed by researchers who studied the strengths of over 3,000 families. To assess your family (either the family you grew up in or the family you have formed as an adult), circle the number that best reflects how your family rates on each strength. A 1 represents the lowest rating and a 5 represents the highest.

	1	2	3	4	5
1. Spending time together and doing things with each other	1	2	3	4	5
2. Commitment to each other	1	2	3	4	5
3. Good communication (talking with each other often, listening well, sharing feelings with each other)	1	2	3	4	5
4. Dealing with crises in a positive manner	1	2	3	4	5
5. Expressing appreciation to each other	1	2	3	4	5
6. Spiritual wellness	1	2	3	4	5
7. Closeness of relationship between spouses	1	2	3	4	5
8. Closeness of relationship between parents and children	1	2	3	4	5
9. Happiness of relationship between spouses	1	2	3	4	5
10. Happiness of relationship between parents and children	1	2	3	4	5
11. Extent to which spouses make each other feel good about themselves (self-confident, worthy, competent, and happy)	1	2	3	4	5
12. Extent to which parents help children feel good about themselves	1	2	3	4	5

Scoring   Add the numbers you have circled. A score below 39 indicates below-average family strengths. Scores between 39 and 52 are in the average range. Scores above 53 indicate a strong family. Low scores on individual items identify areas that families can profitably spend time on. High scores are worthy of celebration but shouldn't lead to complacency. Like gardens, families need loving care to remain strong.

Source: N. Stinnet and J. DeFrain. 1986. *Secrets of Strong Families.* Boston: Little, Brown, pp. 167–169.

- *Spiritual wellness.* The family promotes sharing, love, and compassion for other human beings.

- *Coping with stress and crisis.* When faced with illness, death, marital conflict, or other crisis, family members pull together, seek help, go with the flow, and use other coping strategies to meet the challenge.

It may surprise some people that members of strong families are often seen at counseling centers. They know that the smartest thing to do in some situations is to get help. Many resources are available for individuals and families seeking counseling; people can turn to physicians, clergy, marriage and family counselors, psychologists, or other trained professionals. To assess your own family, see the box "Rate Your Family's Strengths."

Families—and intimate relationships of all kinds—are essential to our health and well-being. A fulfilling life nearly always involves other people. Whether we're single or married, young or old, heterosexual or gay, we continue to need meaningful relationships throughout life.

SUMMARY

- Intimate relationship are important to people's health and well-being. Many intimate relationships are held together by love.

Developing Intimate Relationships

- Successful relationships begin with a positive sense of self and reasonably high self-esteem. Personal identity, gender roles, and styles of attachment are all rooted in childhood experiences.

- Friendships are reciprocal relationships between equals, held together by common interests, mutual acceptance, and feelings of respect and affection.

- Love, sex, and commitment are closely linked ideals in intimate relationships. Love includes trust, caring, respect, and loyalty. Sex brings excitement, fascination, and passion to the relationship. Commitment reflects the stable factors that help maintain the relationship.

- Sternberg sees love as composed of intimacy, passion, and decision/commitment. He defines seven types of love based on various combinations of these elements, ranging from friendship to consummate love.

- Intense love is usually accompanied by physiological arousal, a state that may be too extreme to be enjoyed. Familiarity gradually diminishes excitement.

- Love changes over time, with passion decreasing, intimacy increasing and then leveling off, and commitment increasing or decreasing. The disappearance of passion is often experienced as a crisis, but partners may then discover a more lasting love.

Pairing and Singlehood

- People usually choose partners like themselves. If partners are very different, acceptance and good communication skills are necessary to maintain the relationship.
- Most Americans find partners through dating or through "getting together."
- Cohabitation is a growing social pattern that allows partners to get to know each other intimately without being married. It has both advantages and disadvantages. People who live together before they're married have about the same level of marital satisfaction as those who don't cohabit.
- Gay and lesbian partnerships are similar to heterosexual relationships, with some differences. Partners are technically single, since they're not allowed to marry legally; they don't follow traditional gender roles; and they often experience hostility rather than approval toward their partnerships from society.
- Singlehood is a growing option in our society. Advantages include greater variety in sexual partners and more freedom in making life decisions; disadvantages include loneliness and possible economic hardship, especially for single women.

Marriage

- Marriage fulfills many functions for individuals and society. It can provide people with affection, affirmation, and sexual fulfillment; a setting for child rearing; and the promise of lifelong companionship.
- Love isn't enough to ensure a successful marriage. Partners have to be realistic, feel good about each other, have communication and conflict resolution skills, share values, and have a balance of individual and joint interests.
- Marital tasks include providing each other with emotional support, establishing domestic and career priorities, managing finances, making sexual adjustments, managing boundaries with parents and extended family, and participating in the community. The most rapidly changing area is martial roles, which are tending to become more egalitarian.
- Communication skills are essential to successful relationships. A great deal of communication is nonverbal. The keys to good communication in relationships are self-disclosure, listening skills, and feedback.
- Differences in how men and women have learned to communicate in our society can create misunderstandings and frustration in relationships.

- Conflict is inevitable in intimate relationships; partners need to have constructive ways to negotiate their differences.
- When problems can't be worked out, people often separate and divorce. Divorce is traumatic for all involved, especially children. The negative effects are usually balanced in time by positive ones. About three-quarters of all people who divorce remarry.

Family Life

- The family life cycle usually begins with marriage; the next stage begins with the arrival of a baby. Becoming a parent profoundly changes the relationship between the partners.
- At each stage of the family life cycle, relationships change. Marital satisfaction is often low during the child-rearing years and higher later.
- Many families today are single-parent families. Problems for single parents include economic difficulties, conflicting demands, and time pressures.
- Stepfamilies are formed when single or divorced people remarry and form new family units. Stepfamilies gradually gain more of a sense of being a family as they build a history of shared everyday experiences.
- Important qualities of successful families include commitment to the family, appreciation of family members, communication, time spent together, spiritual wellness, and effective methods of dealing with stress. Strong families use outside resources when they need help dealing with problems.

TAKE ACTION

1. Take an informal survey among your friends of what they find attractive in a member of the opposite sex and what they look for in a romantic partner. Are there substantial differences among different people? Do men and women look for different things?
2. Ask your parents what their experiences of dating and courtship were like. How are they different from your experiences? What do your parents think of current customs?

JOURNAL ENTRY

1. What are you looking for in an intimate relationship? In your health journal make a list of the needs you would like to have met by a partner. Are they needs that you can realistically expect to have satisfied in a relationship?

2. *Critical Thinking:* What approach do you take when it comes to communicating your feelings and needs to others? Think of a particular issue that has been bothering you and write down the statements you would make if you were discussing it. Examine your statements to see if unrelated feelings or issues are coming through in them. Devise a strategy for dealing with the issue, using the guidelines given in this chapter on conflict resolution.

SELECTED BIBLIOGRAPHY

Arond, M., and S. L. Panker. 1987. *The First Year of Marriage.* New York: Warner Books.

Bader, E., R. Riddle, and C. Sinclair. 1981. *Family Therapy News.* Washington, D.C.: American Association for Marital and Family Therapy.

Borcherdt, B. 1989. *Think Straight! Feel Great!* Sarasota, Fla.: Professional Resource Exchange.

Crosby, J. 1991. *Illusion and Disillusion.* Belmont, Calif.: Wadsworth.

DeMaris, A. and G. Leslie. 1984. Cohabitation with the future spouse: Its influence upon marital satisfaction and communication. *Journal of Marriage and the Family* 46(1): 77–84.

Fehr, B. 1988. Prototype analysis of the concepts of love and commitment. *Journal of Personality and Social Psychology* 55(4): 557–79.

Gelles, R. J., and J. R. Conte. 1991. Domestic violence and sexual abuse of children: A review of research in the eighties. In *Contemporary Families: Looking Forward, Looking Back,* ed. A. Booth. Minneapolis: National Council on Family Relations.

Gelles, R. J., and C. P. Cornell. 1990. *Intimate Violence in Families,* 2nd ed. Beverly Hills, Calif.: Sage.

Levine, L., and L. Barbach. 1983. *The Intimate Male.* New York: Signet.

Lewis, R. A., E. B. Kozac, R. M. Milardo, and W. A. Grosnick. 1981. Commitment in same-sex love relationships. *Alternative Lifestyles* 4(1): 22–42.

Lips, H. 1992. *Sex and Gender,* 2nd ed. Mountain View., Calif.: Mayfield.

Olson, D., and J. DeFrain. 1994. *Marriage and Family.* Mountain View, Calif.: Mayfield.

Olson, D., H. McCubbin, H. Barnes, A. Larsen, A. Muxem, and M. Wilson. 1983. *Families: What Makes Them Work?* Beverly Hills, Calif.: Sage.

Peplau, Letitia. 1988. Research on homosexual couples. In *Gay Relationships,* ed. J. DeCecco. New York: Haworth Press.

Raschke, H. 1987. Divorce. In *Handbook of Marriage and the Family,* ed. M. Sussman and S. Steinmetz. New York: Plenum Press.

Rice, F. P. 1993. *Intimate Relationships, Marriages, and Families,* 2nd ed. Mountain View, Calif.: Mayfield.

Shaver, P., and others. 1988. Love as attachment: The integration of three behavioral systems. In *The Psychology of Love,* ed. R. Sternberg and M. Barnes. New Haven: Yale University Press.

Stein, P., and M. Fingrud. 1985. The single life has more potential for happiness than marriage and parenthood for both men and women. In *Current Controversies in Marriage and the Family,* ed. H. Feldman and M. Feldman. Beverly Hills, Calif.: Sage.

Sternberg, R., and M. Barnes, eds. 1988. *The Psychology of Love.* New Haven; Yale University Press.

Stinnett, N., and J. DeFrain. 1986. *Secrets of Strong Families.* Boston: Little, Brown.

Strong, B., and C. DeVault. 1992. *The Marriage and Family Experience.* St. Paul, Minn.: West.

———. 1994. *Human Sexuality.* Mountain View, Calif.: Mayfield.

Stuart, R. B. 1983. *Improving Communication.* Champaign, Ill.: Research Press.

U.S. Bureau of the Census. 1991. Marital and living arrangements: March 1990. *Current Population Reports.* Series P-2. Washington, D.C.: U.S. Government Printing Office.

———. 1991. *Statistical Abstract of the Untied States,* 111th ed. Washington, D.C.: U.S. Government Printing Office.

Vaughan, D. 1986. *Uncoupling: Turning Points in Intimate Relationships.* New York: Oxford University Press.

Walker, L. 1979. *The Battered Woman Syndrome.* New York: Harper and Row.

RECOMMENDED READINGS

Alberti, R. E., and Emmons, M. L. 1983. *Your Perfect Right: A Guide to Assertive Living.* San Luis Obispo, Calif.: Impact. *This effective guide is designed to help individuals develop their assertiveness skills.*

Buscaglia, L. F. 1984. *Loving Each Other: The Challenge of Human Relationships.* Thorofare, N.J.: Charles B. Slack. *A university professor and popular public speaker, Buscaglia is witty and energetic on his favorite topic, the nature of love.*

DeFrain, J., J. Fricke, and J. Elmen. 1987. *On Our Own: A Single Parent's Survival Guide.* Lexington, Mass.: D.C. Heath. *This practical guide is based on interviews with 900 single parents from around the country.*

Hochshild, A. 1989. *The Second Shift.* New York: Viking. *The author, a sociologist, describes the dilemma of women who work outside the home and find themselves still putting in a "second shift" of spousal, parental, and household duties in the evening.*

Lerner, H. G. 1985. *The Dance of Anger.* New York: Harper and Row. *In this best-selling book, the author describes different styles of handling anger and suggests ways that people can balance them in their relationships.*

Strong, B., and C. DeVault. 1994. *Human Sexuality.* Mountain View, Calif.: Mayfield. *A comprehensive, up-to-date textbook covering all aspects of love, intimacy, and sexuality.*

Tannen, D. 1990. *You Just Don't Understand: Women and Men in Conversation.* New York: William Morrow. *This discussion of gender differences in language shows how men and women use language differently; it also provides many helpful ideas about how to improve communication in relationships.*

5

Sex and Your Body

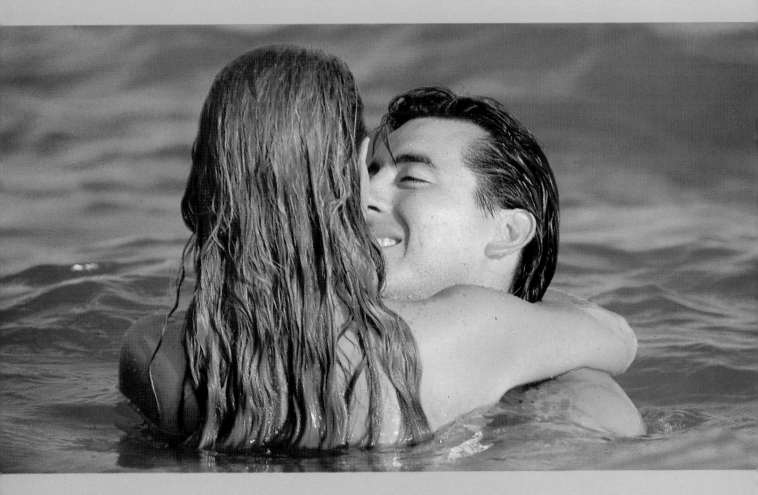

CONTENTS

◗ Everyone you know is circumcised, but one of your teammates on the soccer team isn't. He's from another country, and he says most males aren't circumcised there. In fact, he tells you that circumcision is commonly performed only in the United States and a few other countries. Most of the male population of the world isn't circumcised, he says. You find this hard to believe. He assures you it's true. "There aren't any medical reasons to do it," he says. "It's just a custom." Is he right?

◗ You recently had a troubling experience that you can't stop thinking about. You accepted a date with an attractive man from one of your classes. He took you to dinner at a fancy restaurant, ordered expensive food and wine, and charmed you with his sophisticated conversation. Afterwards you went back to his apartment and had some more wine. Then he began to make sexual advances, persisting even though you told him you weren't ready to go that far with him. The more you resisted, the more forceful he became, finally succeeding in having sex with you. Afterwards he said you led him on by going out to dinner with him and then back to his apartment. He said any man would have interpreted your actions the way he did. You're not sure why you went to his apartment, but you do know that you feel confused, guilty, and violated. Was what happened your fault? How can you make sure it doesn't happen again?

◗ An old friend recently called to tell you she's pregnant. She had been trying to conceive ever since she was married about two years ago. She says she got pregnant after her husband stopped wearing jockey briefs and started wearing boxer shorts. Is she putting you on?

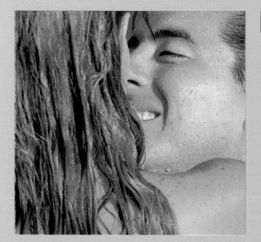

MAKING CONNECTIONS

Sexuality is an important part of being human. Sexuality develops and changes throughout life, and people have many choices about how they express their sexuality. Most adults are still learning about their sexuality and trying to link what they've heard and read with their own experiences. In each of the scenarios presented on this page, all related to sexuality, individuals have to use information, make a decision, or choose a course of action. How would you act in each of these situations? What response or decision would you make? This chapter provides information about sexual anatomy, functioning, and behavior that can be used in situations like these. After finishing the chapter, read the scenarios again. Has what you've learned changed how you would respond?

Human beings are sexual beings. Sexual activity is the source of our most intense physical pleasures, a central ingredient in many of our intimate emotional relationships, and, of course, the key to the reproduction of our species.

Sexuality is more than just sexual behavior. It includes sex (the quality of being biologically male or female), gender (masculine and feminine behaviors people take on), sexual anatomy and physiology, sexual functioning and behaviors, and social and sexual interactions with others. Our individual sense of identity is powerfully influenced by our sexuality—we think of ourselves in very fundamental ways as male or female; as heterosexual or homosexual; as single, attached, married, or divorced. Sexuality is a complex and interacting group of inborn, biological characteristics and acquired behaviors people learn in the course of growing up in a particular family, community, and society.

Sexuality arouses intense feelings, making communication about sexuality highly emotionally charged. And because of its basic role in human life, sexual expression is usually regulated with restrictions and taboos—written and unwritten laws specifying which functions and behaviors are acceptable and "normal" and which are unacceptable and "abnormal." Young people growing up in the United States are bombarded with conflicting messages about sex from television, movies, magazines, and popular music. The media suggest that the average person is a sexual athlete who continually jumps in and out of bed without using contraception, producing offspring, or contracting disease. Parents, educators, and other responsible adults give a more balanced picture but often convey their own hidden messages as well. Ignorance, confusion, and fear are often the result.

Basic information about the body and about sexual functioning and behavior are vital to healthy adult life (to assess your current level of knowledge, see the box "Test Your Sexual Knowledge"). Once we understand the facts, we have a better basis for evaluating all the messages we get and for making informed, responsible choices about our sexuality. If you have questions about aspects of your physical sexuality, this chapter will provide you with some answers.

SEXUAL ANATOMY

In spite of their different appearance, the sexual organs of men and women arise from the same structures and fulfill similar functions. Each person has a pair of **gonads**; ovaries are the female gonads, testes are the male gonads. The gonads produce **germ cells** and **sex hormones**. The female germ cells are ova (eggs); the male germ cells are sperm. Ova and sperm are the basic units of reproduction; their union can lead to the creation of a new life.

Female Sex Organs

The external sex organs, or genitals, of the female are called the vulva ("covering") and are illustrated in Figure 5-1a. The mons pubis, a rounded mass of fatty tissue over the pubic bone, becomes covered with hair during puberty. Below it are two paired folds of skin called the labia majora (major lips) and the labia minora (minor lips). Enclosed within are the **clitoris** and its **prepuce** (foreskin), the opening of the urethra, and the opening of the vagina. The clitoris is highly sensitive to touch and plays an important role in female sexual arousal and orgasm in many women. The clitoris, like the penis, consists of a shaft, glans, prepuce (also called the clitoral hood), and spongy tissue that fills with blood during sexual excitement. The glans is the most sensitive part of the clitoris and is covered by the clitoral hood, which is formed from the upper portion of the labia minora.

The female's urethra leads directly from the urinary bladder to its opening between the clitoris and the opening of the vagina; it conducts urine from the bladder to the outside of the body. Unlike the male's urethra, it is independent of the genitals.

The vaginal opening is partially covered by the hymen. This membrane can be stretched or torn during athletic activities or when a woman has sexual intercourse for the first time. The idea that an intact hymen is the sign of a virgin is a myth.

The vagina is the passage that leads to the internal reproductive organs (Figure 5-1b). It is the female organ for sexual intercourse and serves as the birth canal during childbirth. Its soft, flexible walls are normally in contact with each other. A cylinder of muscles surrounds the vagina. During sexual excitement, the tension in these muscles increases and the walls of the vagina swell with blood.

Projecting into the upper part of the vagina is the neck of the uterus, called the cervix. It is inside the pear-shaped uterus, which slants forward above the bladder, that the fertilized egg is implanted and grows into a fetus.

The pair of fallopian tubes (or oviducts) leads out from

Sexuality A dimension of personality shaped by biological, psychosocial, and cultural forces and concerning all aspects of sexual behaviors.

Gonads Primary reproductive organs that produce germ cells and sex hormones; ovaries and testes.

Germ cells Sperm and ova.

Sex hormones Chemical substances that stimulate and promote the development of sexual characteristics.

Clitoris Highly sensitive, erectile female genital structure.

Prepuce Foreskin of the penis or clitoris.

TERMS

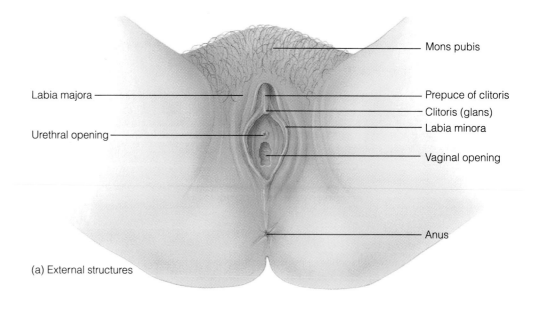

Mons pubis

Labia majora

Prepuce of clitoris

Clitoris (glans)

Labia minora

Urethral opening

Vaginal opening

Anus

(a) External structures

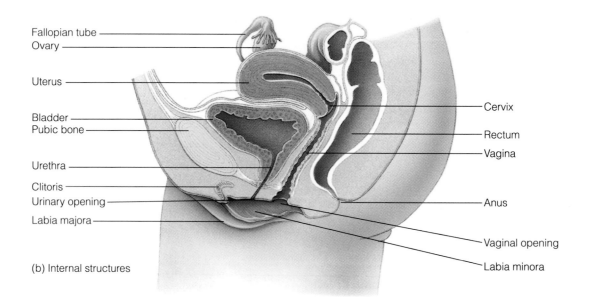

Fallopian tube
Ovary

Uterus

Bladder
Pubic bone

Urethra

Clitoris
Urinary opening
Labia majora

Cervix

Rectum

Vagina

Anus

Vaginal opening

Labia minora

(b) Internal structures

Figure 5-1 *Female sex organs.*

the top of the uterus. The fringed end of each tube surrounds an ovary and guides the mature ovum down into the uterus after the ovum bursts from its follicle on the surface of the ovary.

Male Sex Organs

A man's external sexual organs, or genitals, are the penis and the **scrotum** (Figure 5-2a and 5-2b). The penis consists of spongy tissue that becomes engorged with blood during sexual excitement, causing the organ to enlarge and become erect. The scrotum is a pouch that contains a

pair of testes. The purpose of the scrotum is to maintain the testes at a temperature approximately 5° F below that of the rest of the body—that is, at about 93.6° F. The process of sperm production is extremely heat-sensitive. In hot temperatures the muscles in the scrotum relax, and the testes move away from the heat of the body. Conversely, in cold temperatures the muscles of the scrotum contract, and the testes move upward toward the body, where they can maintain their 5-degree temperature difference. Even the increase in temperature caused by wearing tight "jockey type" underwear in the summer can interfere with normal sperm production.

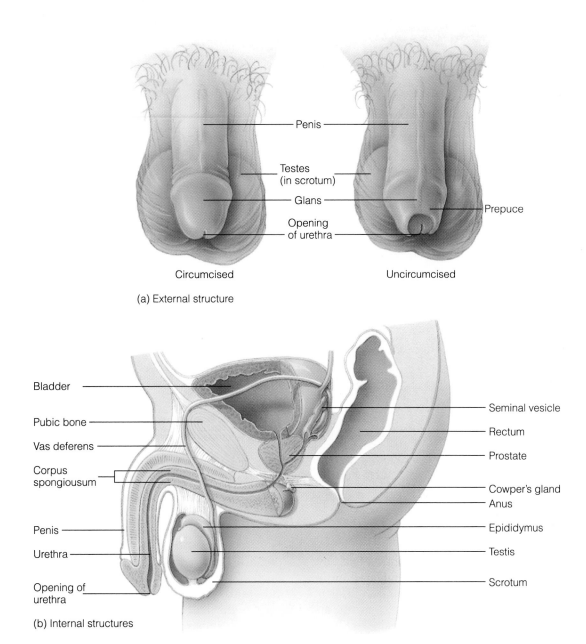

Penis

Testes
(in scrotum)

Glans

Opening
of urethra

Prepuce

Circumcised

Uncircumcised

(a) External structure

Bladder

Pubic bone

Vas deferens

Corpus
spongiousum

Penis

Urethra

Opening of
urethra

Seminal vesicle

Rectum

Prostate

Cowper's gland

Anus

Epididymus

Testis

Scrotum

(b) Internal structures

Figure 5-2 *Male sex organs.*

The smooth, rounded tip of the penis is the **glans** penis. It is a sensitive part of the penis and an important source of sexual arousal. It is partially covered by the foreskin, or prepuce, a retractable fold of skin that is removed by circumcision in about 60 percent of newborn males in the United States. Circumcision is performed for cultural, religious, and hygienic reasons, and rates of circumcision vary widely among different groups (see box "Circumcision: Standard Medical Procedure or Cultural Practice?").

Through the entire length of the penis runs a passage called the urethra, which can carry both urine and semen to the opening at the tip of the glans. Although urine and

semen share a common passage, they are prevented from mixing together by muscular sphincters that control their entry into the urethra.

The testes contain tightly packed seminiferous ("sperm-bearing") tubules within which sperm are pro-

Scrotum   The loose sac of skin and muscle fibers that contains the testes.

Glans   Rounded head of the penis or of the clitoris.

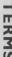

How much do you know about sexuality? When 2,000 Americans were asked a series of questions by the Kinsey Institute, only 45 percent of the respondents answered more than half the questions correctly. See how you do on this sample of true-or-false questions. (Answers are given at the bottom of the box and are discussed in this and other chapters of *Core Concepts in Health*.)

	T or F
1. The average American first has sexual intercourse at about 16 or 17 years of age.	_____
2. About 6 to 8 out of every 10 American women has masturbated.	_____
3. Most women have orgasms from penile thrusting alone.	_____
4. All men like large female breasts.	_____
5. People usually lose interest in sexual activities after age 60.	_____
6. Masturbation is physically harmful.	_____
7. The average length of a man's erect penis is 5 to 7 inches.	_____
8. Impotence usually cannot be treated successfully.	_____
9. Petroleum jelly, Vaseline Intensive Care, and baby oil are not good lubricants to use with a diaphragm or condom.	_____
10. Most women prefer a sexual partner who has a large penis.	_____
11. A woman cannot get pregnant if she has sex during her menstrual period.	_____
12. A woman cannot get pregnant if the man withdraws his penis before ejaculating.	_____

Answers: 1. T; 2. T; 3. F; 4. F; 5. F; 6. F; 7. T; 8. F; 9. T; 10. F; 11. F; 12. F.

Adapted from J. M. Reinisch and R. Beasley. 1990. *The Kinsey Institute New Report on Sex* (New York: St. Martin's Press).

duced. These tubules end in a maze of ducts that flow into a single storage tube called the epididymis, on the surface of each testis. This tube leads to the vasa deferentia (singular: vas deferens), two tubes that rise into the abdominal cavity and, inside the prostate gland, join the ducts of the two seminal vesicles, whose secretions provide nutrients to semen. The prostate gland produces some of the fluid in semen that nourishes and transports sperm. The tubes of the seminal vesicle and the vas deferens on each side lead to the ejaculatory duct, which joins the urethra. The Cowper's glands (bulbourethral glands) are two small structures flanking the urethra. During sexual arousal, these glands secrete a clear, mucuslike fluid that appears at the tip of the penis. The purpose of this preejaculatory fluid is not known, but it may contain a few sperm in some men. Withdrawal of the penis before ejaculation is therefore not a reliable form of birth control.

TERMS

Endocrine glands   Glands that produce hormones.

Androgens   Male sex hormones produced by the testes in males and by the adrenal glands in both sexes.

Estrogens   A class of female sex hormones, produced by the ovaries, that bring about sexual maturation at puberty and maintain reproductive functions.

Progestins   A class of female sex hormones, produced by the ovaries, that sustain reproductive functions.

Adrenal glands   Endocrine glands, located over the kidneys, that produce androgens (among other hormones).

Pituitary gland   An endocrine gland at the base of the brain that produces gonadotropic (FSH and LH) and other hormones.

Hypothalamus   A region of the brain above the pituitary gland whose hormones control the secretions of the pituitary and that is also involved in the nervous control of sexual functions.

Personal Insight   Do you ever wonder if you're sexually "normal"? Do you worry about the size, shape, or appearance of any part of your body? Where do you think your ideas of "normal" come from?

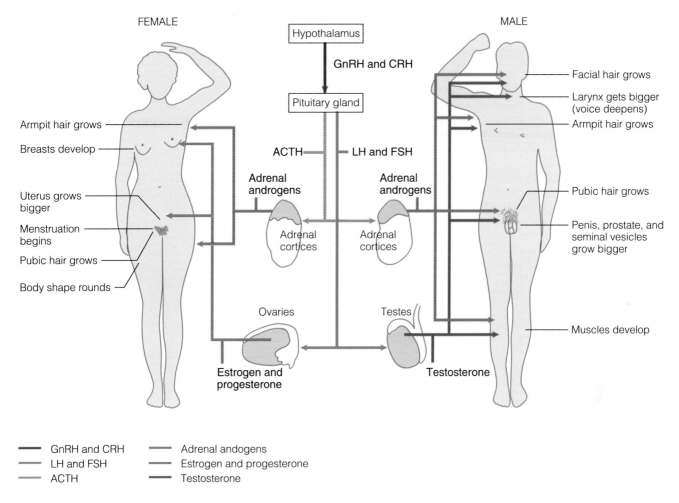

FEMALE

MALE

Hypothalamus

GnRH and CRH

Pituitary gland

ACTH — LH and FSH

Armpit hair grows

Breasts develop

Uterus grows bigger

Menstruation begins

Pubic hair grows

Body shape rounds

Adrenal androgens

Adrenal cortices

Adrenal androgens

Adrenal cortices

Facial hair grows

Larynx gets bigger (voice deepens)

Armpit hair grows

Pubic hair grows

Penis, prostate, and seminal vesicles grow bigger

Muscles develop

Ovaries

Testes

Estrogen and progesterone

Testosterone

--- GnRH and CRH
--- LH and FSH
--- ACTH
--- Adrenal androgens
--- Estrogen and progesterone
--- Testosterone

Figure 5-3 *Effects of hormones on physical development and sexual maturation at puberty.*
GnRH and CRH released from the hypothalamus stimulate the pituitary gland to release ACTH, LH, and FSH. ACTH stimulates the release of androgens from the adrenal cortices; LH and FSH stimulate the release of estrogen and progesterone from the ovaries (for females) and testosterone from the testes (for males). Together, adrenal androgens, estrogen, progesterone, and testosterone are responsible for most of the physical changes that occur at puberty.

HORMONES AND THE REPRODUCTIVE LIFE CYCLE

There are many powerful cultural and personal factors that help to shape the expression of your sexuality. But biology also plays an important role, particularly through the action of hormones, chemical messengers that are secreted directly into the bloodstream by **endocrine glands.** The sex hormones produced by the ovaries and testes have a major influence on the development and function of each individual's reproductive system throughout life.

The sex hormones made by the testes are called **androgens,** the most important of which is testosterone. The female sex hormones, produced by the ovaries, belong to two groups—**estrogens** and **progestins,** the most

important of which is progesterone. The cortex of the **adrenal glands** (located at the top of the kidneys) also produces androgens in both sexes.

The hormones produced by the testes, the ovaries, and the adrenal glands are regulated by the hormones of the **pituitary gland,** located at the base of the brain. This gland in turn is controlled by hormones produced by the **hypothalamus** in the brain (Figure 5-3). Sex hormones exert their primary developmental influences first in the embryo stage and later during adolescence.

Differentiation of the Embryo

The sex of an individual—male or female—is determined by the fertilizing sperm at the time of conception. All human cells normally contain 23 pairs of **chromosomes.** In 22 of the pairs, the two partner chromosomes match. But

Circumcision: Standard Medical Procedure or Cultural Practice?

Many people think of circumcision—the surgical removal of the foreskin of the penis—as a standard medical procedure, but it is equally a cultural practice, varying among different national, ethnic, and religious groups, among people of different educational and income levels, and even from one historical period to another.

Worldwide, groups who circumcise their males have always been in the minority. It is estimated that only about 15 percent of the world's population practices circumcision. Most groups do not, including most Europeans, Asians, South and Central Americans, and Africans. Jews and Muslims are the major groups who circumcise for religious reasons. For both groups, the practice derives from the biblical account of Abraham's "covenant" with God to have all his male descendants circumcised.

In the United States, circumcision was widely accepted from the early 1940s to the mid-1970s as a routine procedure that promoted hygiene and prevented genital disease. Educated middle-class parents almost always had their newborn sons circumcised. In the late 1960s, however, the practice began to be questioned, and in 1971 the American Academy of Pediatrics (AAP) took a stand against it as an unnecessary procedure. A strong anticircumcision movement grew, led by the same kind of affluent, well-educated, suburban parents who had originally supported the practice.

Between 1974 and 1984, the rate of circumcision in the United States fell from 85 to 70 percent. By 1990 it was estimated at about 60 percent, with the highest rates (about 70 percent) in the Midwest and the lowest (less than 50 percent) on the West Coast. California has the lowest rate of any state, partly because of active anticircumcision groups and partly because of large populations of Asians and Hispanics, groups in which circumcision is not traditionally practiced.

Ironically, as public sentiment against circumcision has grown over the last 20 years, evidence of its medical benefits has mounted. In 1988 the AAP reconsidered the issue and took a neutral position on circumcision, stating that it does carry some risks but also has some benefits.

What are the advantages and disadvantages of this five-minute procedure, and why is it so variable across cultures? Proponents of circumcision advocate it for several reasons, the two most notable being cleanliness and disease prevention. Bacteria and secretions can be trapped under the foreskin, and uncircumcised boys have to be taught good hygiene to prevent infection. Circumcision removes this potential source of trouble. Men who develop infection or inflammation of the penis sometimes have to be circumcised later in life, when the operation is more difficult.

Recently, evidence has indicated that uncircumcised infants have a much higher incidence of urinary tract infections, which can lead to very serious kidney damage. These are the findings that led the AAP to adopt its current neutral position on routine circumcision. There is also some evidence that circumcision may help reduce the spread of sexually transmitted diseases, including HIV infection, among young men. Finally, circumcised men are less likely to develop cancer of the penis, a rare disease that occurs almost exclusively in uncircumcised men. At one time it was thought that the female sexual partners of uncircumcised men had a higher risk of developing cervical cancer, but new findings indicate that the incidence of cervical cancer depends on many factors.

Opponents of routine circumcision point to its medical disadvantages, which include pain to the infant, the possibility of irritation of the penis, and the risk of complications and surgical errors. They assert that circumcision is the "leading unnecessary surgery" performed in the United States.

Although discussions of circumcision tend to focus on its medical advantages and disadvantages, most parents make their decision about circumcision mainly for social or cultural reasons. Fathers want their sons to look like them and their peers. Concern about the emotional impact of "being different" apparently outweighs any medical or health concerns. In many parts of the world, parents simply follow their traditional practices. In a country with wide cultural and socioeconomic differences like the United States, there is likely to be variation from one group to another and even from one family to another. Some parents don't hesitate to have their sons circumcised, while others decide against it. Although circumcision is still the majority practice in most parts of the United States, either decision may be the right one for a particular family, depending on a variety of religious, social, personal, and medical factors.

Adapted from Edgar J. Schoen. 1990. "The Status of Circumcision of Newborns." *The New England Journal of Medicine* 322(18): 1308–11.

in the twenty-third pair, the **sex chromosomes,** two configurations are possible. Individuals with two matching X chromosomes are female, and individuals with one X and one Y chromosome (a much shorter chromosome carrying specialized genes) are male. At the time of conception, each germ cell (sperm and ovum) contributes one sex chromosome to the fertilized egg. Germ cells from females, with their XX configuration, all contain an X chromosome. In males, with their XY configuration, some germ cells will contain an X chromosome and some will contain a Y. Thus, if the fertilizing sperm carries an X chromosome, the baby will be a girl (XX), and if it carries a Y chromosome, the baby will be a boy (XY).

Until the sixth week of embryonic life, the reproductive systems of both sexes are alike. If the undifferentiated reproductive system continues to develop without the in-

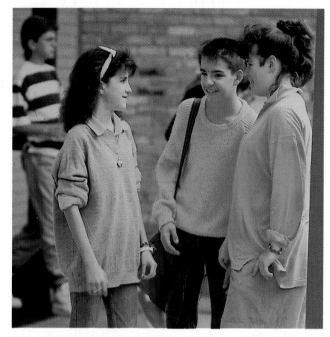

The physical changes of puberty usually begin between the ages of 8 and 13 for girls and 10 and 14 for boys. Once they reach puberty, these adolescents are biologically adults; however, it will take another five to ten years for them to become adults in social and psychological terms.

fluence of sex hormones, it develops into the normal female system, regardless of the fetus's genetic sex. The specialized genes on the Y chromosome, however, intervene to change this course of events. They influence the undifferentiated gonads to develop instead into testes. The embryonic testes in turn produce hormones, including testosterone, that lead to further development of male reproductive organs. The end result is a normal set of male genetic organs.

The common embryonic origin of male and female systems means that every structure in one sex has its developmental counterpart in the other. Thus, the penis corresponds to the clitoris, the scrotal sac to the labia major, and so on.

Female Reproductive Maturation

Although human beings are fully sexually differentiated at birth, the differences between males and females are accentuated at **puberty.** The reproductive system matures, secondary sexual characteristics develop, and the bodies of males and females come to appear more distinctive. The changes of puberty are initiated by the hypothalamus, which releases gonadotropin-releasing hormone (GnRH) and corticotropin-releasing hormone (CRH). Under the influence of GnRH, the anterior pituitary gland increases the production of two **gonadotropic hormones—follicle-stimulating hormone (FSH)** and **luteinizing hormone (LH).** CRH stimulates the pituitary

to release adrenocorticotropin (ACTH), which causes the adrenal cortex to release adrenal androgens (see Figure 5-3).

Physical Changes   The first sign of female puberty is breast development, followed by a rounding of the hips and buttocks. As the breasts develop, hair appears in the pubic region and later in the underarms. Shortly after the onset of breast development, girls show an increase in growth rate. Generally speaking, breast development begins at about age 8 to 13, and the time of rapid body growth occurs between 9 and 15 years of age. Estrogens and progestins from the ovaries as well as androgens from the adrenal glands are responsible for the physical changes that occur in the female at puberty.

The Menstrual Cycle   A major landmark of puberty among females is the onset of the **menstrual cycle,** the monthly ovarian cycle that leads to menstruation (loss of blood and tissue lining the uterus) in the absence of pregnancy. The first menstrual period, or menarche, occurs at the average age of 12.8 years in the United States, but it may also normally start several years earlier or later.

The menstrual cycle can be divided into four phases: (1) menses, (2) the estrogenic phase, (3) ovulation, and (4) the progestational phase (Figure 5-4). Day 1 of the cycle is considered to be the day of the onset of bleeding. For the purposes of our discussion, a cycle of 28 days will be used; however, normal cycles vary in length.

During the menses, characterized by the menstrual flow, hormones from the ovaries and anterior pituitary gland are found in relatively low amounts. This phase of the cycle usually lasts from day 1 to about day 5.

The estrogenic phase of the cycle begins when the menstrual flow ceases, and the anterior pituitary gland begins to produce increasing amounts of FSH and LH. Under the influence of FSH, an egg-containing ovarian

Chromosomes   The threadlike bodies into which the genetic material within the cell nucleus is organized.

Sex chromosomes   The X and Y chromosomes, which determine the sex of the individual.

Puberty   The period of biological maturation during adolescence.

Gonadotropic hormones   Follicle-stimulating hormone (FSH) and luteinizing hormone (LH), produced by the pituitary gland in both sexes.

Follicle-stimulating hormone (FSH)   The pituitary hormone that stimulates maturation of the ovum in the female and sperm production in the male.

Luteinizing hormone (LH)   The pituitary hormone that causes ovulation and stimulates the production of progestins in the female and androgens in the male.

Menstrual cycle   Monthly ovarian cycle controlled by pituitary and ovarian hormones; in the absence of pregnancy, menstruation occurs.

TERMS

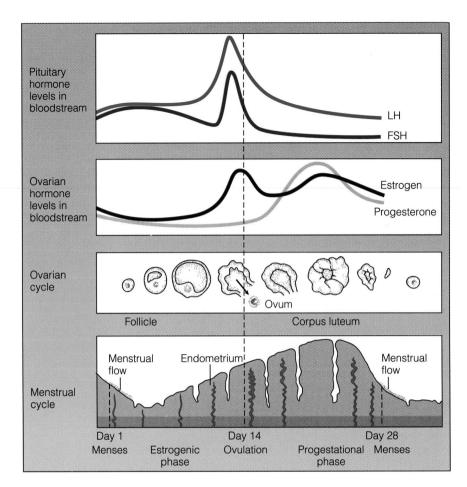

Figure 5-4 *The menstrual cycle.*
The anterior pituitary releases FSH and LH, which stimulate the ovarian follicle to develop and release a mature egg. The ovarian follicle releases estrogen and progesterone, which stimulate the endometrium to continue to develop so that it will be ready to receive and nourish a fertilized egg. Unless pregnancy occurs, ovarian hormone levels fall and the endometrium sloughs off (menses).

follicle begins to mature and to produce increasingly higher and higher amounts of estrogens. Stimulated by estrogen, the uterine lining, called the endometrium, thickens with large numbers of blood vessels and uterine glands.

A surge of a potent estrogen called estradiol from the follicle causes the anterior pituitary gland to release a large burst of LH and a smaller amount of FSH. The high concentration of LH stimulates the developing follicle to release its ovum. This event is known as ovulation. After ovulation, the follicle is transformed into the **corpus luteum,** which produces progesterone and estrogen. Ovulation usually occurs about 14 days prior to the onset of menstrual flow, a fact that can be used to predict the most fertile time during the menstrual cycle, useful in both fertility treatment and natural family planning methods (see Chapter 6).

During the progestational phase of the cycle, the amount of progesterone secreted from the corpus luteum increases and remains high until the onset of the next menses. Under the influence of estrogen and progesterone, the endometrium continues to develop, readying itself to receive and nourish a fertilized ovum. When pregnancy occurs, the fertilized egg produces a hormone called human chorionic gonadotropin (HCG), which maintains the corpus luteum. Thus, levels of ovarian hormones remain high and the uterine lining is preserved, preventing menses.

If pregnancy does not occur, the corpus luteum degenerates and levels of estrogen and progesterone gradually fall. Below certain hormonal levels, the endometrium can no longer be maintained, and it begins to slough off, initiating menses. As the levels of ovarian hormones fall, a slight rise in LH and FSH occurs, and a new menstrual cycle begins.

Menstruation is a normal biological process, but it may cause distressing physical or psychological symptoms in some women. Two common problems are dysmenorrhea and premenstrual tension. Dysmenorrhea ("painful menstruation") is characterized by cramps in the lower abdomen, backache, a bloated feeling, nausea, vomiting, diarrhea, and loss of appetite. Some of these symptoms can be attributed to uterine muscular contractions (spasms),

TERMS

Corpus luteum   The part of the ovarian follicle left after ovulation, which secretes hormones during the second half of the menstrual cycle.

Premenstrual syndrome (PMS)   A disorder characterized by physical discomfort, psychological distress, and behavioral changes that begin after ovulation and cease when menstruation begins.

Premenstrual syndrome (PMS) is characterized by a diverse group of physical, emotional, and behavioral symptoms that occur after ovulation but usually cease before menstruation. Many women experience mild physical and emotional changes prior to their menstrual periods, but a few—about 10 percent of menstruating women—experience more severe symptoms. Sufferers have reported a wide variety of symptoms associated with PMS, including tension, fluid retention, breast swelling and tenderness, constipation, craving for sweets or salty foods, dizziness, fainting spells, headache, joint pain, sensitivity to light and noise, increased appetite, anxiety, depression, decreased self-esteem, and sleep disturbances. Some women with PMS become virtually incapacitated for several days or weeks each month. For a woman with severe PMS, the physical and emotional symptoms that precede menstruation may dominate her life, leading her to plan her activities around the time she knows she'll be experiencing them.

Despite decades of study, researchers still don't understand exactly what causes PMS or why some women are more vulnerable to it than others. Research has focused on a variety of substances in the body that may fluctuate with the menstrual cycle, including progesterone, prostaglandins, certain vitamins and minerals, and a naturally occurring opiate known as beta-endorphin. Researchers have found that blood levels of beta-endorphin dropped sharply in the majority of women with PMS during the week preceding menstruation; women without PMS symptoms were found to maintain consistently high levels of beta-endorphin. It's possible that social or psychological factors may also be important in the development of PMS in women with a biological predisposition.

There are no proven therapies for PMS, but many different treatments are under investigation: oral contraceptives; light therapy (exposing women to fluorescent lights for several hours each day prior to menstruation); antidepressants; antianxiety agents; antiprostaglandins; drugs that elevate levels of beta-endorphin; and other drugs that improve mood and diminish appetite. Over-the-counter medications for PMS commonly contain a diuretic (to compensate for water retention), an analgesic (for pain), and an antihistamine; women with mild PMS may obtain relief from some of their symptoms by using these medications.

PMS is under intensive study by the National Institute of Mental Health (NIMH) and many other agencies and research centers, so it may be just a matter of time before the mystery of this syndrome is unraveled and effective treatments are made available. In the meantime, women can take a few behavioral steps to treat the symptoms of PMS: Eat a nutrient-rich diet; get adequate sleep; decrease intake of alcohol, caffeine, nicotine, sugar, and salt to lessen nervousness, depression, and bloating; and increase exercise to stimulate relaxation. This approach is sensible and safe and may relieve the discomfort of PMS.

---

which are caused by chemicals called prostaglandins that are released from the uterine lining as it is shed during menstruation. Any drug such as aspirin or ibuprofen that blocks the effects of prostaglandins will usually be effective in alleviating some of the symptoms of dysmenorrhea.

Premenstrual tension involves negative mood changes and physical symptoms associated with the time before the onset of menses (hence the name "premenstrual"). A more serious condition, **premenstrual syndrome (PMS),** is experienced by a smaller number of women (see the box "Premenstrual Syndrome: Still a Mystery").

Male Reproductive Maturation

Reproductive maturation of boys lags about two years behind that of girls and usually begins at about 10 or 11 years of age. Physical changes include enlargement of the testes, development of pubic hair, growth of the penis, the onset of ejaculation (usually at about age 11 or 12), deepening of the voice, the appearance of facial hair, and a period of rapid growth. The hormonal basis for physical changes in the male at puberty is quite similar to that of the female (see Figure 5-3). Hypothalamic hormones trigger the anterior pituitary to produce gonadotropins. FSH promotes the maturation of sperm; LH stimulates testicular cells to produce testosterone, which brings about most of the male changes of puberty.

Personal Insight   Think back to adolescence and try to recall your feelings about your sexuality as you went through puberty. Did you feel anxious or overwhelmed by the changes in your body or any emotions—worry, guilt, excitement—you felt about your sexuality? Do you still have any of the feelings about your sexuality that you had then? Are you satisfied with the adjustment to sexuality that you've made so far in your life?

Aging and Human Sexuality

Changes in hormone production and sexual functioning occur as we age. As a woman approaches age 50, her ovaries gradually cease to function and she enters the

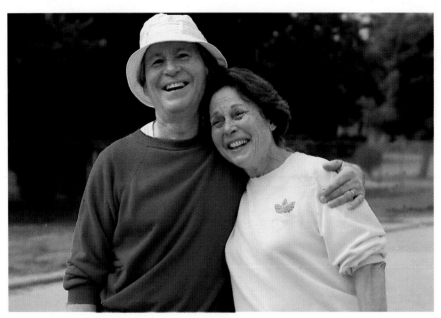

Although sexual physiology changes as people get older, many men and women readily adjust to these alterations. Sexual activity can continue throughout life for individuals like this healthy and vigorous couple in their middle sixties.

menopause (cessation of menstruation). For some women, the associated drop in hormone production causes a set of symptoms that are troublesome.

Among the most common physical symptoms of menopause are hot flashes (or flushes), consisting of a sensation of warmth rising to the face from the upper chest with or without perspiration and chills. Other symptoms include headaches, dizziness, palpitations, and joint pains. Osteoporosis can develop (that is, bones can become more porous), making older women more liable to suffer fractures (see Chapter 12). Some menopausal women become moody, even markedly depressed, and they may also complain of tiredness, irritability, and forgetfulness. Estrogen replacement therapy significantly improves most of these symptoms, but it may increase some women's risk of gallbladder disease and certain types of cancer.

As a result of the decrease in estrogen production, the vaginal walls thin and lubrication in response to sexual arousal diminishes. As a result, **sexual intercourse** may become painful. Hormonal treatment or the use of lubricants during intercourse eliminates these problems.

Some women have a difficult time making the psychological adjustment to this stage of life, associating it with a loss of youth and sexual attractiveness. Others welcome it as a time of increased personal freedom, when the responsibilities of child rearing are over and sexuality can be enjoyed without fear of pregnancy. Today, with longer life expectancies, many women are rejecting the view that the childbearing years are the central period of female life, flanked by youth and old age. Instead, they see three equally important periods characterized by different concerns—a time of growing and learning, a time of childbearing and nurturing (or creative expression), and a time of inner growth and repose. Menopause is seen as signaling the end of one phase of life and the beginning of another, equally meaningful one.

In men, testosterone production declines gradually with age. As they get older, men depend more on direct physical stimulation for sexual arousal. They take longer to get an erection and find it more difficult to maintain; orgasmic contractions are less intense.

Many men go through a period of reassessment and readjustment in middle age (sometimes popularly referred to as "midlife crisis"), which may have repercussions for their sexuality. As with women, sexual activity can continue to be a source of pleasure and satisfaction for men as they grow older. When problems do arise, they are more often due to psychological reactions to bodily changes than to the physical changes themselves.

Personal Insight Many people in their sixties, seventies, and eighties continue to enjoy sex as a vital part of their lives. What are your attitudes toward older people and sex? Where do you think your ideas come from?

Various manufacturers of perfumes and colognes claim to sell fragrances that will attract members of the opposite sex. The substance in the fragrance that does the "attracting" is called a pheromone. But do pheromones really exist? Do they actually attract members of the opposite sex?

Biologists use the term *pheromone* to refer to chemical substances secreted by one member of the species that influence the biology and/or behavior of another member of the same species. For example, female silk moths release a sex attractant pheromone that drifts on the wind and attracts males. Males will fly to the substance even in the absence of females. In the rhesus monkey, the female vaginal secretions contain a very potent pheromone that attracts males. The pheromone is abundant during the middle of the female monkey's menstrual cycle, when she is ovulating. The pheromone makes the male more attracted to the female at the time that fertilization of an egg is most likely to occur.

Do pheromones exist in humans? Human females who are not using oral contraceptives produce the same chemical identified as the male-attracting pheromone in the rhesus monkey. It is also produced during the middle of the menstrual cycle! Does it attract males? In a very clever study designed to answer this question, researchers prepared a "synthetic" mixture of this potential pheromone and recruited 62 young married couples to participate. Each couple received a set of coded containers, each with one of four different so-lutions: A mixture of the potential pheromone in alcohol, plain alcohol, plain water, or an inexpensive perfume.

It was predicted that, if the potential pheromone really worked, a husband would be more sexually attracted to his wife when she was "wearing" the potential pheromone, and sexual activities would be increased at this time. Each wife was told to rub the contents of an individual container between her breasts at bedtime (neither the wife nor the husband knew the contents of the individual containers). Results: The potential pheromones had no apparent effect on sexual arousal or activity.

A pheromone-related phenomenon that *has* been substantiated in a number of studies is menstrual synchrony, a decrease in time differences between the beginning of menstrual periods among women who live together or spend a lot of time together. Experiments have shown that exposure to perspiration from the underarms of certain "donor" women produced menstrual synchrony in other women. In this situation the women did not know or ever see the "donor"; these studies seem to argue for the existence of a human pheromone that can in fact change the biological functioning of other individuals.

Adapted from D. Quadagno. 1987. "Pheromones and Human Sexuality." *Medical Aspects of Human Sexuality* 21:149–54.

SEXUAL FUNCTIONING

In this section, we discuss sexual physiology—how the sex organs function during sexual activity—and problems that can occur with sexual functioning. Sexual activity consists of a stimulus and a response. Erotic stimulation leads to sexual arousal (excitement), which may culminate in the intensely pleasurable experience of **orgasm.** But sexual activity should not be thought of only in terms of the sex organs. Responses to sexual stimulation involve not just the genitals but the entire body—and the mind as well.

Sexual Stimulation

Sexual excitement can come from many sources, both physical and psychological. Although physical stimuli have an obvious and direct effect, some people believe psychological stimuli—thoughts, fantasies, desires, perceptions—are even more powerfully erotic. Regardless of the source of erotic stimuli, all stimulation has a physical basis, which is given meaning by the brain.

Physical Stimulation Physical stimulation comes through the senses: People are aroused by things they see, hear, taste, smell, and feel. It has even been suggested that they may be attracted and aroused by molecules of specific chemicals, called **pheromones,** that are produced by other people's bodies to create sexual excitement. (See the box "Pheromones and Human Sexuality.") Most often, sexual triggers come from other people, but they may come from books, photographs, paintings, songs, films, or other sources.

The most obvious and effective physical stimulation involves touching. Even though culturally defined practices vary and individual people have different preferences, most sexual encounters eventually involve some form of touching with hands, lips, and body surfaces.

Menopause   Cessation of menstruation in middle-aged women.

Sexual intercourse   Sexual relations involving genital union; coitus; also called "making love."

Orgasm   Discharge of accumulated sexual tension with characteristic genital and bodily manifestations and a subjective sensation of intense pleasure.

Pheromones   Chemical substances produced by animals that are released into the environment and stimulate other animals of the same species; presence in humans is uncertain.

TERMS

Kissing, caressing, fondling, and hugging are as much a part of sexual encounters as they are of expressing affection.

The most intense form of stimulation by touching involves the genitals. The clitoris and glans penis are particularly sensitive to such stimulation. Other highly responsive areas are the vaginal opening, the nipples, the breasts, the insides of the thighs, the buttocks, the anal region, the scrotum, the lips, and the earlobes.

Such sexually sensitive areas, or **erogenous zones,** are especially susceptible to sexual arousal for most people, most of the time. Often, though, it's not *what* is touched but how, for how long, and by whom that determines the response. Under the right circumstances, touching any part of the body can arouse someone sexually.

Psychological Stimulation   Sexual arousal also has an important psychological component, regardless of the nature of the physical stimulation. Fantasies, ideas, memories of past experiences, general "mood"—all can generate excitement. Erotic thoughts may be linked to an imagined person or situation or to a sexual experience from the past. Fantasies often involve activities a person doesn't actually wish to experience in reality, usually because they're dangerous, frightening, or forbidden.

Arousal is also powerfully influenced by emotions. How you feel about a person and how the person feels about you matters tremendously in how sexually responsive you are likely to be. Even the most direct forms of physical stimulation carry emotional overtones. Kissing, caressing, and fondling express affection and caring. The emotional charge they give to a sexual interaction is at least as significant to sexual arousal as the purely physical stimulation achieved by touching.

Historically, there have always been people interested in enhancing sexual stimulation through aphrodisiacs—substances believed to increase sexual desire, prolong sexual activity, intensify sexual sensations and responses, or improve sexual performance. Few, if any, substances have ever been shown to have these effects, a fact that underscores the important role played by psychological and emotional factors in arousal. Despite the lack of evidence for their effectiveness, aphrodisiacs are sought by some people in our society in drugs and alcohol. A list of drugs and their supposed and actual effects on sexual functioning is given in Table 5-1.

Sexual Response

Noted sex researchers William Masters and Virginia Johnson were the first to describe in detail the human sexual response cycle. Men and women respond physiologically with a predictable set of reactions (Figure 5-5), regardless of the nature of the stimulation—fantasy, masturbation, sexual intercourse, or some other form of sexual activity.

Two physiological mechanisms explain most genital and bodily reactions of men and women during sexual arousal and orgasm. These mechanisms are **vasocongestion** and **myotonia.** Vasocongestion is the engorgement of tissues that results when more blood flows into an organ than is flowing out. Thus, the penis becomes erect on the same principle that makes a garden hose become stiff when the water is turned on. Myotonia is increased muscular tension, which culminates in rhythmical muscular contractions during orgasm.

Four stages characterize the sexual response cycle. In the *excitement phase,* the penis becomes erect as its tissues become congested with blood. The testes expand and are pulled upward within the scrotum. In women, the clitoris and the labia are similarly congested with blood, and the vaginal walls become moist with lubricant fluid.

The *plateau phase* is an extension of the excitement stage. Reactions become more marked: In men, the penis becomes harder, and the testes larger. In women the lower part of the vagina swells, while its upper end expands and vaginal lubrication increases.

In the *orgasmic phase,* rhythmical contractions occur along the man's penis, urethra, prostate gland, seminal vesicles, and muscles in the pelvic and anal regions. These involuntary muscular contractions lead to ejaculation of semen, which consists of sperm cells from the testes and secretions from the prostate gland and seminal vesicles. In women, contractions occur in the lower part of the vagina and in the uterus, as well as in the pelvic region and the anus.

In the *resolution phase,* all the changes initiated during the excitement phase are reversed. Excess blood drains from tissues, the muscles in the region relax, and the genital structures return to their unstimulated state.

More general bodily reactions accompany the changes in the genital organs in both sexes. Beginning with the excitement phase, the nipples of both sexes become erect, the woman's breasts begin to swell, and in both sexes the skin of the chest becomes flushed; all these changes are more marked among women. The heart rate doubles by the plateau phase, and respiration becomes faster. During orgasm, breathing becomes irregular and the person may moan or cry out. A feeling of warmth leads to increased sweating during the resolution phase. Deep relaxation and a sense of well-being pervade the body and the mind.

Male and female reactions during the sexual response cycle differ somewhat. Generally, the male pattern is more uniform, whereas the female pattern is more varied. For

TERMS

Erogenous zones   Regions of the body highly responsive to sexual stimulation.

Vasocongestion   Accumulation of blood in tissues and organs.

Myotonia   Increased muscular tension.

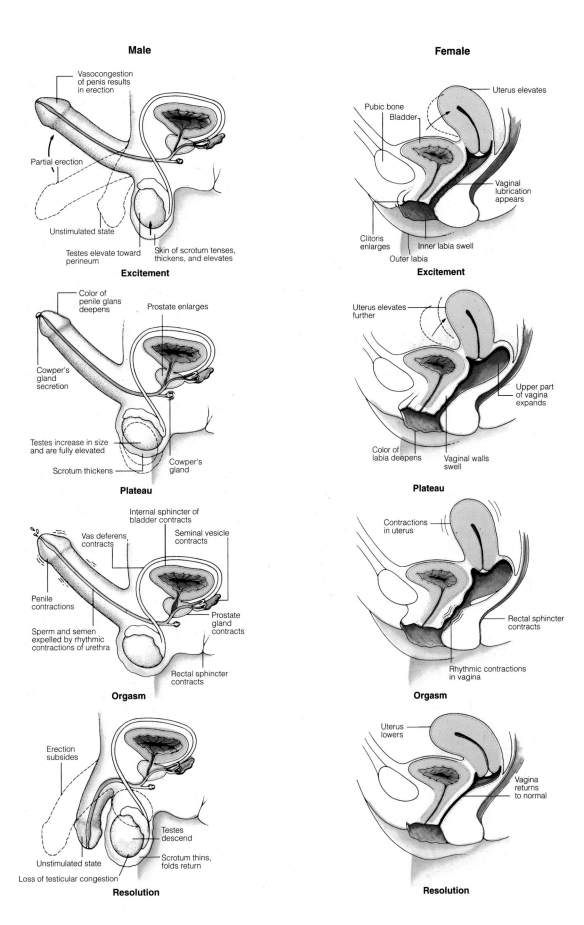

Figure 5-5 *Stages of sexual response.*

TABLE 5-1 Supposed and Actual Effects of Drugs on Sexual Functioning

Substance	Supposed Effect	Actual Effect
Alcohol	Stimulates sexual desire and sexual activity	In small amounts, reduces inhibitions and increases sexual desire; with increased consumption, decreases sexual response and sensations from the genitals.
Cocaine ("coke")	Enhances sexual desire and performance	Durng early use, some people report enhancement of sexual activities, others poor sexual performance. Chronic abuse frequently leads to diminished sexual desire.
Marijuana ("pot")	Increases sexual desire and performance	Reduces inhibitions. Actual influence varies from decreased to improved desire and performance.
LSD and other hallucinogens such as mescaline and psilocybin	Increase sexual desire and heighten sexual response	No physiological effect on reproductive system, but subjective experience of sexual desire and response may be enhanced or diminished.
Cantharis ("Spanish fly")	Increases desire for sexual activities	Acts as a powerful irritant; burns lining of bladder and urethra, mimicking sexual stimulation of genitals (causes erection in male, vasocongestion of clitoris, labia, and vagina in female).
Amyl nitrate ("snappers" or "poppers")	Increase pleasure of orgasm	Dilate (open) blood vessels in genital area and may enhance sensations or perceptions of orgasm. Can produce fainting, headaches, or dizziness.
Amphetamines ("uppers")	Increase sexual desire	Small doses may enhance sexual desire and response; larger doses lead to sexual dysfunctions.
Barbiturates ("downers")	Increase sexual desire and performance	In low doses, reduce inhibitions; in larger doses, inhibit sexual arousal and functioning.
Antihypertensives (blood pressure medication)	Control high blood pressure	Can negatively affect sexual function in men and women, partly because of inhibition of sympathetic nerves of genital region and psychological effects of being treated for high blood pressure

Source: C. Byer and others. 1988. *Dimensions of Human Sexuality.* (Dubuque: Wm. C. Brown); J. Cocores and M. Gold. 1989. "Substance Abuse and Sexual Dysfunction." *Medical Aspects of Human Sexuality* 23:22–31.

instance, the female excitement phase may lead directly to orgasm, or orgasmic and plateau phases may be fused.

Male orgasm is marked by the ejaculation of semen. After ejaculation, men enter a *refractory period* during which they cannot be restimulated to orgasm. Women do not have a refractory period; immediate restimulation is possible.

Sexual stimulation relies on the same set of sensory nerves that transmit other impulses from the body's surface. No special nerves are set aside for conveying sexual sensations. However, specialized nerve centers in the lower portions of the spinal cord regulate the mechanisms of erection and ejaculation. Their actions are **reflexive;** they do not need to be learned (although learned responses may inhibit them).

The ultimate control of sexual functions rests in the brain. As in the lower spinal centers, specific regions in the **limbic system** of the brain control sexual arousal and orgasm. We understand little about how the brain regulates the subjective experience of sexual arousal and the state of altered consciousness experienced during orgasm.

Sexual Disorders and Dysfunctions

Both psychological and physical problems can interfere with normal sexual functioning. If you are not in good physical health, for example, or if you are experiencing high levels of stress or anxiety, your sexual functioning might very well be negatively affected. Sexual problems caused mainly by biological or physical conditions are referred to as **sexual disorders**; problems of psychological origin are called **sexual dysfunctions**.

Common Sexual Disorders   Sexual disorders may be physiological in origin, but they may also be the result of infections, which can be prevented. Sexual disorders that affect women include the following:

- *Vaginitis* is inflammation of the vagina and can be caused by a variety of organisms, including *Candida* (yeast infection), *Trichomonas* (trichomoniasis), and *Gardnerella* (nonspecific vaginitis). The symptoms include a vaginal discharge, vaginal irritation, and pain during intercourse. Vaginitis is easily treated with various medications. In the case of trichomoniasis, both partners must be treated, as the organism can also be harbored in the male genital tract. (See Chapter 17 for a more detailed discussion of trichomoniasis.)

- *Endometriosis* is the growth of endometrial tissue (tissue normally found lining the uterus) outside of the uterus. It occurs most often in women of childbearing age, and pain in the lower abdomen and pelvis is the most common symptom. Painful intercourse may occur during the premenstrual phase of the cycle. Endometriosis can cause serious problems if left untreated because the endometrial tissue can scar and partially or completely block the oviducts, causing infertility (difficulty in conceiving) or sterility (inability to conceive). Endometriosis is treated with hormone therapy and/or surgery.

- *Pelvic inflammatory disease* (PID) is an infection of the uterus, oviducts, or ovaries and is caused when microorganisms spread to these areas from the vagina. Approximately 50 to 75 percent of PID is caused by sexually transmitted organisms associated with diseases such as gonorrhea and *Chlamydia* infections.

PID can cause scarring of the oviducts, resulting in infertility or sterility. Symptoms include pain in the abdomen and pelvis, fever, and possibly pain during intercourse. The treatment involves bed rest and antibiotic therapy. Prompt treatment lessens the chances of infertility and sterility. (Sexually transmitted diseases are discussed in detail in Chapter 17.)

Sexual disorders among men include the following:

- *Prostatitis* is inflammation or infection of the prostate gland. The symptoms include fever, chills, pain in the region of the genitals, frequent urination, and, in some cases, painful ejaculation. This disorder is more common in men over 40 and is treated with antibiotics.

- *Testicular cancer* occurs most commonly in men in their twenties and thirties. It is a rare cancer and has a very high cure rate if detected early. A testicular self-exam done after a hot bath or shower should be done on a regular basis (see Chapter 16 for more information). If any lumps are felt, a physician should check the suspected growth.

Sexual Dysfunctions   The term *sexual dysfunction* encompasses disturbances in sexual desire, performance, or satisfaction. Although a wide variety of physical conditions and drugs may interfere with sexual functions (for instance, diabetes may interfere with the blood and nerve supply to the sex organs), sexual dysfunctions more often result from psychological causes and problems in intimate relationships. The same two mechanisms—vasocongestion and myotonia—that are the basis of the sexual response cycle are also at the root of the main forms of sexual disturbance: inability to become aroused and problems with orgasm.

Common Sexual Dysfunctions   Common sexual dysfunctions in men include **erectile dysfunction** (previously called impotence), which is the inability to have or maintain an erection that is sufficient for sexual intercourse; **premature ejaculation,** which is ejaculation be-

---

Reflexive   Involving an involuntary response elicited by a specific stimulus.

Limbic system   A set of structures in the brain regulating motivational-emotional behaviors, including some aspects of sexual activity.

Sexual disorders   Disturbances in sexual desire, performance, or satisfaction having physical origins.

Sexual dysfunction   Disturbances in sexual desire, performance, or satisfaction having psychological origins.

Erectile dysfunction   Inability to have or maintain an erection.

Premature ejaculation   Involuntary orgasm before or shortly after the penis enters the vagina; ejaculation that takes place sooner than desired.

TERMS

fore or just on penetration of the vagina; and **retarded ejaculation,** the inability to ejaculate once an erection is achieved. Many men will experience occasional difficulty in achieving an erection or ejaculating because of excessive alcohol consumption, fatigue, or stress. In fact, it is estimated that 50 percent of all men in the United States experience occasional bouts of erectile dysfunction and retarded ejaculation. Usually, the dysfunction disappears when the interfering factor is removed. Because of the powerful effect of psychological factors on sexual behavior, especially anxiety about performance, an understanding attitude on the part of the sexual partner is an important component in restoring sexual functioning.

Two sexual dysfunctions in women are **vaginismus,** in which the woman experiences painful involuntary muscular spasms when sexual intercourse is attempted, and **orgasmic dysfunction,** which is the inability to experience orgasm. Vaginismus is a conditioned reflex probably related to fear of intercourse. Orgasmic dysfunction has been the subject of a great deal of discussion over the years as people debated the nature of the female orgasm and what constitutes dysfunction in women. Many women experience orgasm but not during intercourse, or they experience orgasm during intercourse only if the clitoris is directly stimulated at the same time. Do these patterns of response reflect normal female sexual functioning, or are they forms of orgasmic dysfunction? In general, the inability to experience orgasm under certain circumstances is a problem only if the woman considers it so. If she believes that she has a problem—for example, if she has never experienced orgasm under any circumstances—then she is considered to have orgasmic dysfunction.

Treating Sexual Dysfunction   Most forms of sexual dysfunction can be treated. The first step is to treat any underlying medical condition. Diabetes and heart disease, for example, may cause erectile dysfunction. Medications and drugs, especially depressants such as alcohol, may also inhibit sexual responses. Anyone experiencing sexual difficulties should have a thorough physical examination.

If no physical problem is found, the problem may be psychosocial in origin. Psychosocial causes of dysfunction include troubled relationships, lack of sexual skills, irrational attitudes and beliefs, anxiety, and psychosexual trauma, such as sexual abuse or rape. Many sexual myths can interfere with the sexual performance or satisfaction of people who believe them. Through their difficulties, their partners are affected as well. Like other skills, sexual competence is learned. We learn what makes us and others feel good by talking with them about sex, reading about it, watching films, and experimenting. Many people, however, do not acquire sexual skills because they lack the opportunity to experiment or because their cultural background causes even the thought of sexual behavior to create overwhelming anxiety for them.

Many of these problems can be addressed by sex therapy methods that seek to modify the behavior patterns that are interfering with satisfactory sexual relationships. The behavioral treatment of sexual dysfunction concentrates on reducing performance anxiety, changing self-defeating expectations, and learning sexual skills. Many sex therapists use techniques pioneered by Masters and Johnson in the 1960s. The therapy program usually includes "bibliotherapy" (reading self-help sex manuals) and learning new patterns of sexual behavior.

For example, a man experiencing erectile dysfunction learns to relax and receive sexual stimulation. He and his sexual partner first massage each other without touching the genitals, using verbal instructions and guiding each other's hands to communicate. Genital touching follows after a few sessions. The partners follow a gradual series of sexual activities that alleviates performance anxiety and ultimately ends in intercourse. Masters and Johnson report that erectile dysfunction has been reversed in 72 percent of the couples they have treated with this method. Premature ejaculation, another common problem, is often treated by the "squeeze technique," in which the tip of the penis is squeezed when the man feels he is about to ejaculate. This technique is reported to be effective in 90 percent of the men treated.

Women who seek treatment for orgasmic dysfunction often have not had the chance to learn through trial and error what types of stimulation will excite them and bring them to orgasm. Most sex therapists prefer to treat this problem with **masturbation.** Women are taught about their own anatomy and sexual responses and then are encouraged to experiment with masturbation until they experience orgasm. Once they can masturbate to orgasm, they may need additional treatment to transfer this learning to sexual intercourse with a partner.

Although sex therapy techniques may seem to focus narrowly on physiological responses, they actually highlight the fact that sex is not merely a mechanical body response. Sexual problems are closely tied to emotional and psychological concerns and with a person's thoughts, perceptions, beliefs, values, and relationships with others. The same can be said for all sexual functioning.

SEXUAL BEHAVIOR

Many behaviors stem from sexual impulses, and sexual expression takes a variety of forms. Probably the most basic aspect of sexuality is reproduction, the process of producing offspring. Sexual behaviors related to reproduction include sexual intercourse, contraception, pregnancy, childbirth, and breastfeeding. As important as reproduction is, the intention of creating a child accounts for only a small measure of sexual activity; most people have sex for other reasons as well.

Sexual excitement and satisfaction are aspects of sexual

behavior separate from reproduction. The intensely pleasurable sensations of arousal and orgasm are probably the strongest motivators for human sexual behavior. People are infinitely varied in the ways they seek to experience erotic pleasure. In this section, we'll examine how sexual behavior develops and take a closer look at different sexual behaviors.

The Development of Sexual Behavior

Sexual behavior is a product of many factors, including genetics, physiology, psychology, and social and cultural forces. Our behavior is shaped by the interplay of our biological predispositions and our learning experiences throughout life.

Gender Roles and Gender Identity   The term *gender* is usually used to refer to the state of being male or female; people often use the word *sex* to mean the same thing. Strictly speaking, *sex* refers only to being biologically male or female, while *gender* encompasses both your biological sex and your masculine or feminine behaviors. As mentioned in Chapter 4, your **gender role** is everything you do in your daily life that expresses your maleness or femaleness to others. Your **gender identity** is your personal, inner sense of your gender role as male or female. Gender role and gender identity are usually in agreement, but a few individuals experience conflict between the two. A male who feels trapped in the body of a male and who wants to be a female may exhibit the gender role of male, but his gender identity is that of a female (see the description of transsexualism later in this chapter).

Some gender characteristics are determined biologically, such as the genitals a person is born with and the secondary sex characteristics that develop at puberty. Others are defined by society and learned in the course of growing up. From birth, children are encouraged to behave in ways their culture deems appropriate for one sex or the other. In our society, parents usually give children gender-specific names, clothes, and toys; and children may model their own behavior after their same-sex parent. People are far more likely to tell a boy why the car is accelerating, and a girl why the cookies aren't chewy. Family and friends create an environment that teaches the child whether to become a woman or a man and how to act appropriately. Teachers, television, books, and even strangers model these gender roles.

Gender roles vary from one society to another and from one time to another. In the United States today, for example, many women shave their legs and wear makeup; in Muslim countries, women wear robes and veils that conceal their faces and bodies. Each set of behaviors expresses some learned aspect of the female gender role in that society, and each set would be inappropriate in the other society.

Historically, gender roles have tended to highlight and

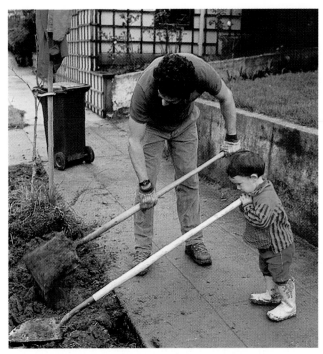

Hormones affect what we do in some ways, but our sense of gender identity and many of our behaviors are overwhelmingly influenced by cultural factors. This little boy is learning "male" behaviors by imitating his dad.

emphasize the differences between males and females, but new gender roles are emerging in our society that reflect more of a mix of male and female characteristics and behaviors. This tendency toward **androgyny** greatly broadens the range of experiences available to both males and females. Many educators, parents, and others have attempted to erase the lines between stereotypically masculine and feminine behaviors for children in hopes of freeing them from the constraints of inflexible gender roles.

Androgynous adults are less stereotyped in their thinking, in how they look, dress, and act, in how they divide work in the home, in how they think about jobs and careers, and in how they express themselves sexually.

Retarded ejaculation   Inability to ejaculate when one wishes to during intercourse.

Vaginismus   Painful, involuntary muscular contractions in the vagina that occur when sexual intercourse is attempted.

Orgasmic dysfunction   The inability to experience orgasm.

Masturbation   Self-stimulation to obtain sexual arousal and orgasm.

Gender role   The different behaviors and attitudes our society expects of women and men.

Gender identity   A person's personal, internal sense of maleness or femaleness.

Androgyny   A blending of male and female characteristics and roles, especially a lack of sex-typing with respect to roles.

TERMS

Women today are able and even expected to be much more assertive, competitive, ambitious, and powerful than they were allowed to be in the past, and men are able to be more sensitive, articulate, nurturing, and emotionally expressive. Children who are exposed to androgynous models are likely to have more choices when they grow up, although many learned gender-role behaviors are so subtle that it's virtually impossible to escape them.

Childhood Sexual Behavior   The capacity to respond sexually is present at birth. Ultrasound studies suggest that boys experience erections in the uterus. After birth, both sexes have the capacity for orgasm, though many babies may not experience it. As people grow, many discover this capacity through self-exploration. Sexual behaviors gradually emerge in childhood in the form of self-stimulating play. Self-exploration and touching the genitals are common forms of play, observed among infants as young as 6 months. They gradually lead to more deliberate forms of masturbation with or without orgasm.

Children often engage in sexual play with playmates by exploring each others' genitals. These activities are often part of games like "playing house" or "playing doctor." By age 12, 40 percent of boys have engaged in sex play; the peak exploration age for girls is age 9, by which time 14 percent have had such experiences. Although parents and teachers actively teach and socialize children, in our culture they largely avoid the task of sexual education or carry it out indirectly.

Adolescent Sexuality   A person who has experienced puberty is biologically an adult. But in psychological and social terms, human beings need five to ten more years to attain full adult status. This discrepancy between biological and social maturity creates considerable confusion over what constitutes appropriate sexual behavior during adolescence.

Sexual fantasies and dreams become more common and explicit in adolescence than at earlier ages, often as an accompaniment to masturbation. About 80 percent of teenage boys and 55 percent of teenage girls masturbate more or less regularly. Once puberty is reached, orgasm among boys is accompanied by ejaculation. Teenage boys also experience **nocturnal emissions** ("wet dreams"). Some girls also have orgasmic dreams. In general, mas-

turbation does not carry the social stigma and imagined perils of former times, but adolescents—and many adults as well—are often still embarrassed by it.

Sexual interaction in adolescence usually takes place between peers in the context of dating, which fulfills a variety of other social functions as well. Sexual intimacy is usually expressed in such relationships through petting and necking, which may involve kissing, caressing, and stimulating the breasts and the genitals. These activities lead to sexual arousal but may not culminate in orgasm.

Many American teenagers now also engage in premarital sexual relations (sexual intercourse before marriage). Recent surveys indicate that the average age of first sexual intercourse is about 16.2 years for girls and 15.7 years for boys; 50 percent of females between the ages of 15 and 19 and 70 percent of males between the ages of 17 and 21 report that they have had sexual intercourse. Rates for premarital sex vary considerably from one group to another, however, based on ethnic, educational, religious, geographic, and other factors. Engaging in sexual intercourse for the first time is affected by these same factors plus psychological readiness, fear of consequences, being in love, going steady, peer pressures, and the need to act like an adult, gain popularity, or rebel, among other factors. Some people thoughtfully weigh decisions and others plunge recklessly. Teenagers who engage in sexual intercourse or are close to doing so generally value personal independence, have loosened family ties in favor of more reliance on friends, and are more apt to experiment with drugs or alcohol and to engage in political activism than their contemporaries.

Adolescent sexual behaviors are not confined to **heterosexual** relationships. Beginning in childhood, sex play involves members of one's own sex as well as of the opposite sex. **Homosexual** attractions, with or without sexual encounters, are likewise common in adolescence. For many these are youthful experiments and don't mean that participants will ultimately be homosexual. For a minority they may be a factor in adult **sexual orientation.** Most adult gay men and women trace their preferences to their early years.

Adult Sexuality   Early adulthood is a time when people make important life choices, a time of increasing responsibility in terms of interpersonal relations and family life. In recent years, both in the United States and abroad, there has been a definite trend toward marriage at a later age than in past decades. And before marriage, more young adults are driven by an internal need to become sexually knowledgeable. Today more people in their twenties believe that becoming sexually experienced rather than preserving virginity is an important prelude to selecting a mate. According to psychologist Erik Erikson, developing the capacity for intimacy is a central task for the young adult.

Adult sexuality can include any of the sexual behaviors

TERMS

Nocturnal emissions   Orgasm and ejaculation (wet dream) during sleep.

Heterosexual   Sexual attraction toward people of the other sex.

Homosexual   Sexual attraction toward people of the same sex.

Sexual orientation   Sexual attraction to individuals of the other sex, same sex, or both.

Bisexual   Sexually attracted to people of both sexes.

Homophobia   Fear or hatred of homosexuals.

and practices described in this chapter. In mature love relationships, people ideally are able to integrate all the aspects of intimacy—physical, sexual, emotional—so that sexuality is a deeply meaningful part of how they express love. People can continue to enjoy sexual activities throughout their entire lives, varying and expanding the scope of their experiences as they gain more understanding of their own and their partners' needs and desires.

> ***Personal Insight*** What sexual practices are acceptable to you and what ones are unacceptable? What influences your feelings about them? Are there sexual practices that you object to but find arousing anyway? Remember, there's a big difference between what you think and what you do.

Sexual Orientation

Sexual orientation refers to the choice of sexual partners. An individual may be sexually attracted to members of the other sex (heterosexual), the same sex (homosexual), or both sexes (**bisexual**). The terms *straight* and *gay* are often used to refer to heterosexuals and homosexuals respectively, and female homosexuals are sometimes called *lesbians*. Researchers estimate that about 75 to 85 percent of the American adult population is exclusively heterosexual; about 1 to 3 percent of the female population and 3 to 16 percent of the male population is exclusively homosexual. The number of people who have had bisexual experiences is estimated to be about 4 to 11 percent of the female population and 9 to 32 percent of the male population.

Heterosexuality The great majority of people are heterosexual, sexually attracted to and satisfied by members of the other sex. The heterosexual lifestyle usually includes all the behavior and relationship patterns that were described in Chapter 4—dating, engagement, and/or living together, and marriage. Legally recognized and binding marriage is available in our society only to heterosexual couples.

Homosexuality People who are homosexual are sexually and romantically attracted to and satisfied by members of their own sex. Homosexuality exists in almost all cultures. Although homosexual couples cannot legally marry, many do form long-lasting close and stable ties with one partner (some religious organizations do solemnize gay and lesbian unions). The lifestyle of a homosexual depends in great part on whether an individual is an overt or covert homosexual. Those who feel forced to be secretive may lead double lives, one public and one private. Those who have "come out" participate more actively in gay activities and organizations.

The sexual practices of homosexuals resemble those of their heterosexual counterparts except for sexual intercourse. Before the AIDS epidemic, research indicated that most homosexual men had more sex partners than did most heterosexual men. More recent studies indicate that homosexual men have reduced the number of their sexual contacts, presumably because the risk of HIV infection rises with the number of sexual partners.

Some people are threatened or upset by homosexuality, perhaps because homosexuals are viewed as different or because no one is sure how sexual orientation develops. The "gay liberation" movements of the 1970s and 1980s helped to dispel some of the historical prejudice against gays and lesbians, but homosexuality still has not received widespread societal approval. In extreme cases, irrational fear or hatred of homosexuals (**homophobia**) causes people to discriminate against or even attack homosexuals.

Bisexuality Some bisexuals are involved with partners of different sexes at the same time, while others may alternate between same-sex partners and partners of the opposite sex ("serial bisexuality"). HIV infection is a risk associated with bisexuality, particularly in cases where bisexual men don't disclose their sexual orientation to their female partners. The largest group of bisexuals are married men who have secret sexual involvements with men but who rarely have female sexual contacts outside marriage.

The Origins of Sexual Orientation Many theories have been proposed to account for the development of sexual orientation. Biological theories have focused on genetic and hormonal influences. One recent study found structural differences between homosexual and heterosexual men in the brain region that controls sexual behavior. It remains unclear, however, whether this anatomical variation represents a cause or a result of sexual orientation.

Many psychological theories have also been proposed. According to Freud's theory of the Oedipus complex, children are romantically and sexually attracted to the parent of the other sex during the stage of psychosexual development that occurs between the ages of 3 and 5, but fear of punishment leads the child to renounce the attraction and identify with the parent of the same sex. This identification changes to a heterosexual orientation in adolescence and adulthood (and failure to resolve the Oedipal issues, according to Freud, results in a homosexual orientation). Although many psychologists accept the role of Oedipal relationships in personality development, they question the role of these relationships in the development of sexual orientation.

According to learning theory, behaviors that are rewarded increase in frequency and behaviors that are punished decrease in frequency. Negative experiences with

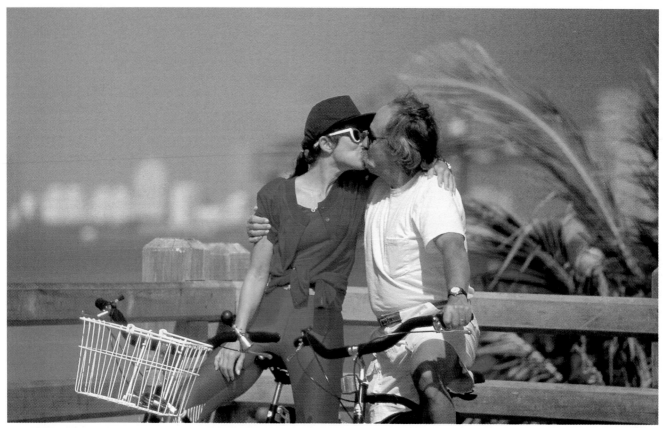

Human sexuality is not just a matter of bodies responding to each other. This couple's physical experiences together will be powerfully affected by their emotions, ideas, and values and by the quality of their relationship.

heterosexuality or positive experiences with homosexuality might cause someone to become homosexual. Other research, however, has indicated that sexual orientation has its origin outside of family communication patterns and is not shaped by learning.

The timing of puberty is another factor that has been proposed as an important influence on the development of sexual orientation. It is suggested that individuals who are just beginning to have erotic feelings are most likely to focus their erotic responses on the people with whom they are currently interacting. According to this theory, if individuals mature early, they are more likely to have erotic feelings when they are still interacting primarily with same-sex friends; thus, they develop a homosexual orientation. Research into this theory has yielded mixed results.

Most experts agree that a complicated series of interactions, both biological and psychosocial, go into producing sexual orientation.

Varieties of Human Sexual Behavior

Most people express their sexuality in a variety of ways. Some sexual behaviors are **autoerotic**—aimed at self-stimulation only, such as masturbation—while other practices involve social interaction in behaviors such as kissing and coitus. Some people choose not to express sexuality and practice celibacy instead.

Celibacy   Continuous abstention from sexual activities with others is the practice of **celibacy.** Celibacy can be a conscious and deliberate choice or it can be necessitated by circumstances. Health considerations—concerns about recurring vaginal infections, sexually transmitted diseases, and particularly the spread of AIDS—may contribute to a decision to practice celibacy. Religious and moral beliefs may lead some people to celibacy, particularly until marriage or until an acceptable partner appears.

Sexual abstention can be practiced temporarily or on a periodic basis, often for years, and sometimes for a lifetime. Some celibates masturbate; others engage in no sexual activities at all. A disadvantage of the celibate life is that it may lack physical contact and affection.

Autoeroticism and Masturbation   The most common autoerotic sexual activity is **erotic fantasy,** mental experiences that arise in the imagination and range from fleeting thoughts to elaborate scenarios. Fantasies may be replays of past sexual experiences, or they may be fabrications based on unfulfilled wishes or drawn from books, drawings, or photographs.

Masturbation typically involves manually stimulating the genitals, rubbing them against objects (such as a pillow), or using stimulating devices such as vibrators. Although commonly associated with adolescence, masturbation remains a sexual outlet for many throughout adult life. It may be used as a substitute for coitus and other sociosexual behaviors or as part of sexual activity with a partner. Masturbation gives a person control over the pace, time, and method of sexual release and pleasure. Most men and women masturbate. On average, two of three college students masturbate a few times a week, others do it more or less frequently, and some don't do it at all.

Touching and Foreplay Tactile stimulation—touching—is integral to sexual experiences, whether in the form of massage, kissing, fondling, or holding. The entire body surface is a sensory organ, and touching almost anywhere can enhance intimacy and sexual arousal. Some body areas, known as erogenous zones, are much more sensitive to touch as a sexual stimulus than others; lips, genitals, and nipples in particular are generously endowed with sensory nerve endings. Touching can convey a variety of messages, including affection, comfort, and a desire for further sexual contact.

During arousal many men and women manually and orally stimulate each other by touching, stroking, and caressing their partner's genitals. Men and women vary greatly in their preferences for the type, pacing, and vigor of such **foreplay**. Working out the details to accommodate each other's pleasure is a key to enjoying these activities. Direct communication about preferences can enhance sexual pleasure and protect both partners from physical and psychological discomfort.

Oral-Genital Stimulation **Cunnilingus** (the stimulation of the female genitals with the lips and tongue) and **fellatio** (the stimulation of the penis with the mouth) are quite common practices. A survey of several thousand college students in sexuality classes spanning 15 years revealed that approximately 89 percent of women and 82 percent of men had both administered and received oral-genital stimulation (although prevalence varies in different populations). Oral sex may be practiced either as part of arousal and foreplay or as a sex act culminating in orgasm. Like all acts of sexual expression between two people, oral sex requires the cooperation and consent of both partners. If they disagree about its acceptability, they need to discuss their feelings and try to reach a mutually pleasing solution.

Anal Intercourse Another practice, less common but well known, is anal stimulation and penetration by the penis or a finger. About 10 percent of heterosexuals and 50 percent of homosexual males regularly practice anal intercourse. In a study of married couples, 25 percent indicated that they had engaged in anal intercourse at some time. The receiver does not usually reach orgasm from anal intercourse, though men usually experience orgasm while penetrating. Many people have strongly negative attitudes toward anal sex because they consider it unclean, unnatural, or unappealing. Because the anus is composed of delicate tissues that tear easily under such pressure, anal intercourse is one of the riskiest of sexual behaviors associated with the transmission of HIV disease, the gonorrhea bacterium, and the syphilis organism. Routine use of condoms is recommended for anyone engaging in anal sex. Special care and precaution should be exercised if anal sex is practiced—cleanliness, lubrication, and gentle entry at the very least. Anything that is inserted into the anus should not subsequently be put into the vagina unless it has been thoroughly washed. Bacteria naturally present in the anus can cause vaginal infections.

Sexual Intercourse For most adults, most of the time, sexual intercourse is the ultimate sexual experience. Men and women engage in coitus—make love—to fulfill both sexual and psychological needs. The most common practice involves the man placing his erect penis into the woman's dilated and lubricated vagina after sufficient arousal.

Much has been written on how to enhance pleasure through various coital techniques, positions, and practices. For a woman, the key factor in physical readiness for coitus is adequate vaginal lubrication, and in psychological readiness, it is to be aroused and receptive. For a man, conditions and the partner must arouse him to attain and maintain erection. Personal preferences vary, but most people prefer a safe, private setting. Candlelight and music, for example, can enhance the mood of the occasion. Psychological factors and the quality of the relationship are more important to overall sexual satisfaction than sophisticated or exotic sexual techniques.

Problematic and Coercive Sexual Behaviors

In our society, a wide variety of sexual behaviors are accepted. However, some types of sexual expression are

---

Autoerotic behavior Activities aimed at sexual self-stimulation.

Celibacy Continuous abstention from sexual activities.

Erotic fantasy Sexually arousing thoughts and daydreams.

Foreplay The kissing, touching, and other oral-genital contact that stimulates people toward intercourse.

Cunnilingus Oral stimulation of the female genitals.

Fellatio Oral stimulation of the penis.

TERMS

considered unacceptable or harmful. The term **sexual variations** refers to less common types of sexual behaviors that are usually considered undesirable by others. These include adult behaviors such as exhibiting one's genitals in public, peeping uninvited into strangers' homes, child sexual abuse, and rape. The effects of these behaviors on others range from minor upset to serious physical and emotional harm. The use of force and coercion in sexual relationships is one of the most serious problems in human interactions. The most extreme manifestation of **sexual coercion**—forcing a person to submit to another's sexual desires—is rape, but sexual coercion occurs in many more subtle forms, including sexual harassment.

A person who repeatedly and persistently prefers certain unusual behaviors for sexual gratification is classified as a **sex offender** if his or her sexual activity violates moral and legal codes, offends the public sense of decency, or threatens others. Almost all sex offenders are men, though occasionally a woman is cited for sexual harassment or sexual abuse of children.

The search for genetic and hormonal causes for sexual variations has been inconclusive. Psychoanalytic theory explains them as unresolved immature sexual impulses from childhood. Other theorists explain these behaviors as products of social learning.

Paraphilias   Some atypical sexual behaviors can be partially explained by the concept of a **paraphilia,** a condition in which a person's sexual arousal and gratification depend on an unusual object or act. From a mental health perspective, however different, odd, or unusual a sexual behavior may be, even if it appears to be paraphilial, it is not considered pathological so long as it injures no one and involves only consenting adults. But because paraphilias are often accompanied by a thinly veiled hostile element, they become vehicles for more aggressive aspects of sexuality, male sexuality in particular. The most common paraphilias are listed below.

Voyeurism is the practice of watching others engage in sexual activities, usually without their knowledge or consent.

Exhibitionism, also known as exposing or "flashing," involves exhibiting the genitals to an involuntary observer. Usually the exhibitionist masturbates during or after the act, drawing sexual pleasure from the observer's shocked reaction.

Fetishism involves becoming sexually aroused by an inanimate object or a part of the human body, such as hair, feet, or a pair of pantyhose or underpants.

Pedophilia is sexual attraction to children.

Transvestism, or cross-dressing, involves repeatedly wearing the clothes of the opposite gender for the purpose of sexual arousal. *Transsexualism,* a gender disorder, is to be distinguished from transvestism: A transsexual wishes to be a member of the opposite sex and to have an anatomical gender change. Transsexuals also cross-dress, not for sexual arousal but for a sense of emotional completeness.

Sexual sadism involves sexual gratification through inflicting psychological and physical suffering on another person. *Masochism* is the erotic enjoyment of one's own suffering. Sadomasochism clearly demonstrates that dominance and aggression can play a role in sexual arousal.

Child Sexual Abuse   Children are vulnerable to sexual abuse, which is a sexual act imposed on a minor. Adults and older adolescents are able to coerce a child into sexual activity because of their authority and power over children; threats, force, or the promise of friendship or material rewards may be used to manipulate a child. Sexual contacts are typically brief and consist of genital manipulation; genital intercourse is much less common.

Sexual abusers are usually male, heterosexual, and known to the victim. The abuser may be a relative, a friend, a neighbor, or another trusted adult acquaintance. Child abusers are often pedophiles with poor interpersonal and sexual relations with other adults. They may also feel socially inadequate and inferior. One highly traumatic form of sexual abuse is **incest**, which is defined as sexual activity between persons too closely related to legally marry. The most common forms of incest are father-daughter (including stepfather-stepdaughter) abuse, brother-sister abuse (usually an adolescent boy abusing a preadolescent girl), and uncle-niece abuse; mother-son sexual activity is rare. Adults who commit incest may be pedophiles, but very often they are simply sexual opportunists or people with poor impulse control and emotional problems.

Most sexually abused children are between 8 and 12 years of age when the abuse first occurs. More girls are sexually abused than boys. The degree of trauma for the child can be very serious, but varies with the types of encounters, their frequency, the child's age and relationship

TERMS

Sexual variations   Atypical sexual behaviors considered undesirable by others.

Sexual coercion   Use of physical or psychological force or intimidation to force a person to submit to sexual demands.

Sex offender   One who engages in sexual behaviors prohibited by law.

Paraphilia   Variant choice of sexually arousing activities or partners.

Incest   Sexual activity between close relatives, such as siblings or parents and their children.

Sexual harassment   Sexual pressuring of someone in a vulnerable or dependent position, such as a youth, student, or employee.

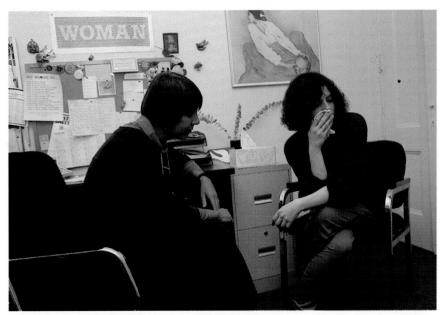

Victims of acquaintance rape usually don't suffer physical injury, but the psychological pain may be severe. Professional counseling may help this young woman overcome the shock, anxiety, depression, and feelings of self-blame typically experienced by victims of rape.

to the abuser, and the parents' response. Father-daughter abuse may be the most traumatic form of sexual abuse, in part because it is a violation of the basic parent-child relationship and because the abuse tends to be more frequent.

Sexual abuse is often unreported. Recent surveys suggest that as many as 27 percent of women and 16 percent of men were sexually abused as children. Child sexual abuse can leave lasting scars, and adults who were abused as children are more likely to suffer from low self-esteem, depression, anxiety, eating disorders, self-destructive tendencies, sexual problems, and difficulties in intimate relationships.

If you were a victim of sexual abuse as a child and feel it may be interfering with your functioning today, you may want to address the problem. A variety of approaches may help, such as joining a support group of people who have had similar experiences, confiding in a partner or friend, or seeking professional help. Some people have experienced tremendous relief by confronting the person who abused them years earlier, but the possible consequences of this course of action have to be carefully considered, preferably with the help of a counselor or therapist.

Sexual Harassment　　Sexual pressuring of someone in a vulnerable or dependent position—a youth, employee, or student, for example—is termed **sexual harassment.** Employers, professors, or other people in authority may use their ability to control or influence jobs or grades to coerce people into sexual relations, or to punish them if

they refuse. In extreme cases, a person may be threatened with being fired or being given a bad grade if he or she will not submit to the harasser's demands. Men are usually, but not always, the offenders, partly because they are more often in positions of power.

Sexual harassment can take a variety of forms, including verbal abuse, sexual remarks about clothing or appearance, unnecessary touching or pinching, and demands for sexual favors. It may be accompanied by implied or overt threats concerning the victim's job or grades. Victims often do not report the abuse, in part because they may fear they will be ignored or blamed. In a recent survey of 17,000 federal employees, 42 percent of women and 15 percent of men reported being sexually harassed.

If you have been the victim of sexual harassment, you can take action to stop it. Be assertive with anyone who uses language or actions you find inappropriate. If it's emotionally possible for you, confront your harasser either in writing, over the telephone, or in person, informing him or her that the situation is unacceptable to you and you want the harassment to stop. If that doesn't work, assemble a file or log documenting the harassment, noting the details of each incident along with any witnesses who may be able to support your claims. You may discover others who have been harassed by the same person, which will strengthen your case. Then file a grievance with the harasser's supervisor or employer, such as someone in the dean's office if you are a student or someone in the personnel office if you are an employee.

If your attempts to deal with the harassment internally

To reduce the risk of being raped, try not to let yourself get into vulnerable situations; specifically

- Avoid dark, lonely city streets or parks.

- Stay aware of your surroundings and notice if anyone is following you.

- Have your keys out in your hand as you approach your car or house so you can get inside quickly, and lock the door behind you.

- Avoid showing that you are alone in a house or apartment.

- Find out with certainty who is at the door before opening it.

- Try to look confident, strong, and purposeful when you're out by yourself.

- Try to remain as cool as possible in all situations.

- Think out in advance what you would do if you were threatened with rape.

When asked what to tell women who found themselves facing a rapist, an experienced counselor responded:

Please be very careful about giving specific advice on what to do. There is great disagreement on the subject. Some rapists say that if a woman had screamed or resisted loudly, they'd have run; others report they'd have killed her. Self-defense training is valuable in that it helps a woman feel and act more assertively, but it is risky in that none of us really knows how we would use it when scared to death—and badly or ineffectively used active self-defense could get us killed. Some say it is best to seem to give in quietly so as to avoid being injured or killed, and to try to calm the rapist, to win time, so that escape is more likely should the opportunity arise. The trouble with telling a woman she *should* resist and yell is that she adds to her already large burden of guilt if she does not do so, and it plays into the hands of prosecutors and those who insist (against the law) that a woman isn't really raped unless she is beaten up or

shows signs of struggle. I think it is best to give various options and then say that each woman and each rapist and each situation are unique, and the woman should respond in whatever way she thinks best.

If you are threatened by a rapist and decide to fight back, here is what Women Organized Against Rape (WOAR) recommends:

- *USE YOUR VOICE!* Yell and keep yelling. (This may sound obvious but you would be surprised how few people have ever really yelled. It takes practice and you should do it today.) Yelling will clear your head and start your adrenalin going. It may scare your attacker and also bring help.

- If you just throw your hands out for striking, they can be grabbed by an attacker and used to get you down.

- If an attacker grabs you from behind, use your *elbows* for striking the neck or his sides, or even his stomach to take him by surprise.

- Don't forget that a rapist also feels pain and is also afraid of pain, plus he is afraid of getting caught. Try to use this weakness to get away.

- Your legs are the strongest part of your body—they have been carrying you around all of your life. Your kick is longer than his reach and a series of hard, fast kicks should keep him away from you. Always kick with your rear foot and with the toe of your shoe. Aim low to avoid losing your balance.

- His most vulnerable spot is his *knee;* it's low, difficult to protect, and easily knocked out of place. The most effective kick is a glancing one across his kneecap.

- Don't try to kick a rapist in the crotch. He has been protecting this area all of his life. In addition, he may grab your foot, knocking you off balance.

- Trust your gut feelings. If you feel you are in danger, don't hesitate to run and scream. It is better to feel foolish than to be raped. In any situation, screaming and a general uproar are strongly recommended.

TERMS

Sexual assault   Use of force to gain sexual access to someone.

Rape   Coercing a person into sexual relations by threats or use of force.

Statutory rape   Sexual interaction with someone below the legal age of consent.

Acquaintance or date rape   Sexual assault by someone the victim knows or is dating.

aren't successful, you can file an official complaint with your city or state Human Rights Commission or Fair Employment Practices Agency or with the federal Equal Employment Opportunity Commission. You may also wish to pursue legal action under the Civil Rights Act or under local laws prohibiting employment discrimination. Very often the threat of a lawsuit or other legal action is enough to stop the harasser.

- Remember that ordinary rules of behavior don't apply. It's OK to vomit, act "crazy," or claim to have a sexually transmissible disease.

- When you do decide to fight, always accompany it with a strong bellowing war cry.

- Don't ever expect a single blow to end the fight. Don't give up, keep fighting. Your objective is to get away, and to get away as soon as you can.

- If a rapist is carrying a weapon, you shouldn't fight unless absolutely necessary.

If you are raped, WOAR gives the following advice:

- Tell what happened to the first friendly person you meet.

- Call the police. Use the emergency number. Give your location and tell them you were raped.

- Try to remember as many facts as you can about your attacker: clothes, height, weight, age, skin color, etc. Try to remember his car, license number, the direction in which he went, etc. Write all this down right away.

- *Don't* wash or douche before the medical exam, or you destroy important evidence. *Don't* change your clothes, but bring a new set with you if you can.

- At the hospital you will have a complete exam, including a pelvic exam. Show the doctor any bruises, scratches, etc.

- Tell the police simply but exactly what happened. Try not to get flustered. Have a friend or relative accompany you if possible. Be honest and stick to your story.

- If you do not want to report the rape to the police, see a doctor as soon as possible. Make sure you are checked for pregnancy and venereal disease.

- Contact an organization with skilled counselors so you can talk about the experience. Look in the telephone directory under "Rape" or "Rape Crisis Center" for a hotline number to call or a local chapter of WOAR.

To avoid date rape:

- Believe in your right to control what you do. Set limits and communicate these limits clearly, firmly, and early. Say "no" when you mean "no."

- Be assertive with someone who is sexually pressuring you. Often men interpret passivity as permission.

- Remember that some men assume sexy dress and a flirtatious manner mean a desire for sex.

- Remember that alcohol and drugs interfere with clear communication about sex.

- Use the statement that has proven most effective in stopping date rape: "This is rape and I'm calling the cops."

Guidelines for men:

- Be aware of social pressure. It's OK not to "score."

- Understand that "no" means "no." Don't continue making advances when your date resists or tells you she wants to stop. Remember that she has the right to refuse sex.

- Don't assume sexy dress and a flirtatious manner are invitations to sex, that previous permission for sex applies to the current situation, or that your date's relationships with other men constitute sexual permission for you.

- Remember that alcohol and drugs interfere with clear communication about sex.

Adapted from D. Goleman. 1989. "When the Rapist Is Not a Stranger." *New York Times,* 29 August, B1, B11; and M. S. Calderone and E. W. Johnson. 1989. *The Family Book About Sexuality.* (New York: Harper and Row), pp. 176–77.

Sexual Assault: Rape Sexual coercion that relies on the threat and use of physical force or takes advantage of circumstances that render a person incapable of giving consent (such as when drunk) constitutes **sexual assault** or **rape.** When the victim is younger than the legally defined "age of consent," the act constitutes **statutory rape,** whether or not coercion is involved. Coerced sexual activity in which the victim knows or is dating the rapist is often referred to as **acquaintance** or **date rape.**

Any woman—or man—can be a rape victim. It is conservatively estimated that at least 3.5 million females are raped annually in the United States. Some men are raped by other men, perhaps 10,000 annually—and not all of these rapes are committed in prison.

Rape victims suffer both physical and psychological injury. For most, physical wounds are not severe and heal

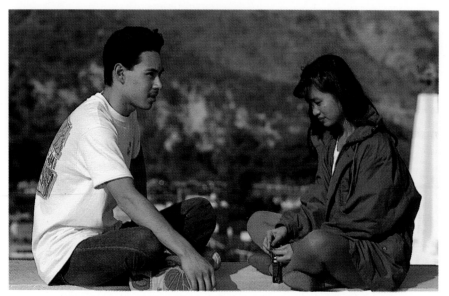

Sexual activity carries many consequences, including pregnancy, disease, and emotional changes in the relationship between partners. Honest communication is a crucial part of responsible sexual behavior.

within a few weeks. Psychological pain may endure and be substantial. Even the most physically and mentally strong are likely to experience shock, anxiety, depression, shame, and a host of psychosomatic symptoms after being victimized. These psychological reactions following rape are called rape trauma syndrome, which is characterized by fear, nightmares, fatigue, crying spells, and digestive upset. Self-blame is very likely; society has contributed to this tendency by perpetrating the myths that women can actually defend themselves and that no one can be raped if she doesn't want to. Fortunately, these false beliefs are dissolving in the face of evidence to the contrary.

Men who commit forcible rape may come from any social class and be any age. Some rapists are exploiters in the sense that they rape on the spur of the moment and mainly want immediate gratification. Some attempt to compensate for feelings of sexual inadequacy and inability to obtain satisfaction otherwise. Others are more hostile and sadistic and are primarily interested not in sex but in hurting and humiliating a particular woman or women in general.

Sometimes husbands rape wives. Strong evidence suggests that one of every seven American women who have ever married has been raped by her husband or ex-hus-

band. One study found that 60 percent of 430 battered women had been raped by their husbands. There is little evidence that mates rape because wives have refused reasonable sexual requests. Rather it appears that the husbands liked violent sex and used physical force to intimidate and control the wives. In some cases the situation grows out of a relationship characterized by poor communication and verbal and sometimes physical violence. A charge of mate rape can now be taken to court in over half the states.

Most women are in much less danger of being raped by a stranger than of being sexually assaulted by a man they know or date. Surveys suggest that as many as one woman in four has had experiences in which the man she was dating persisted in trying to force sex on her despite her pleading, crying, screaming, or resisting. One of every 6 to 15 women has been raped by a man she knew or was dating. Most cases of date rape are never reported to the police, partly because of the subtlety of the crime. Usually no weapons are involved and direct verbal threats may not have been made. Rather than being terrorized, the victim usually is attracted to the man at first. Victims of date rape tend to shoulder much of the responsibility for the incident, questioning their own judgment and behavior rather than blaming the aggressor.

One factor in date rape appears to be the double standard about appropriate sexual behavior for men and women. Although the general status of women in society has improved, it is still a commonly held cultural belief that nice women don't say yes to sex (even when they want to) and that real men don't take no for an answer.

There are also widespread differences between men

TERMS

Pornography   Explicit depiction of sexual activities; made to sell.

Erotica   Sensual depictions of adults engaging in sexual activities.

and women in how they perceive romantic encounters and signals. In one study, researchers found that men tend to interpret women's actions on dates, such as smiling or talking in a low voice, as indicating an interest in having sex, while the women interpreted the same actions as just being "friendly." Men's thinking about forceful sex also tends to be unclear. One psychologist reports that men find "forcing a woman to have sex against her will" more acceptable than "raping a woman," even though the former description is the definition of rape.

Aside from the double standard and unclear perceptions and thinking about sex, men who rape their dates tend to have certain attributes, including hostility toward women, a belief that dominance alone is a valid motive for sex, and an acceptance of sexual violence. They may feel that force is justified in certain circumstances, such as if they are sexually involved with a woman and she refuses to "go all the way," if the woman is known to have slept with other men, or if the woman shows up at a party where people are drinking and taking drugs. The man often primes himself to force himself sexually on his date by drinking, which lowers his ordinary social inhibitions. Many college men who have committed date rape tried to seduce their dates by plying them with alcohol and marijuana first.

Date rape is largely a result of sexual socialization in which the man develops an exaggerated sexual impulse and puts a premium on sexual conquests. Sex and violence are linked in our society, and coercion is accepted by some adolescents as an appropriate form of sexual expression. Both males and females can take actions that will reduce the incidence of date rape in our society; see the box "Dealing with Rape" for specific guidelines and suggestions.

The Role of Pornography The question of whether **pornography** contributes to rape and other acts of violence against women has been investigated in recent years. Many educators, social scientists, and feminists distinguish between "soft porn" or **erotica**—the explicit or implicit depiction of sexual activities in which mutual empathy and enjoyment are reflected—and "hard porn"—the explicit depiction of sexual activities involving violence, exploitation, and degradation of victims. People use soft porn to learn about different sexual behaviors and to become sexually aroused; heavy exposure to it seems to lead to satiation and boredom rather than to changes in sexual behavior. Hard porn, on the other hand, with its focus on violence and dominance, is associated with aggressive feelings and antisocial attitudes, especially toward women. But it appears to be the violence itself, not the sexual content of pornography, that stimulates aggression. Furthermore, there is no reliable evidence that pornography by itself causes men to rape women.

Responsible Sexual Behavior

Healthy sexuality is an important part of adult life. It can be a source of pleasurable experiences and emotions and an important part of intimate partnerships. But sexual behavior also carries many responsibilities, and you need to make choices about your sexuality that contribute to your well-being and your partner's well-being. Sexual responsibility includes the following:

- Open, honest communication about intentions. Each partner needs to clearly indicate what sexual involvement means to him or her. Does it mean love, fun, a permanent commitment, or something else?

- Sexual activities that both partners agree upon and are comfortable with. No one should pressure or coerce a partner. Sexual behaviors should be consistent with the sexual values and preferences of both partners. Everyone has the right to refuse sexual activity at any time.

- The use of contraception during sexual intercourse (if partners wish to avoid pregnancy). Both partners need to take responsibility for protecting against unwanted pregnancy. Partners should discuss contraception before sexual involvement begins. (See Chapter 6 for more information on contraception.)

- The use of safer sex practices to guard against HIV infection and other sexually transmissible diseases (STDs). Many sexual behaviors carry the risk of STDs, including HIV infection. Partners should be honest about their medical condition and work out a plan for protecting themselves from STDs. Behaviors that carry no risk of HIV infection are those that don't involve the exchange of bodily fluids (blood, semen, and vaginal secretions). A person not in a mutually monogamous relationship with an uninfected partner who wishes to engage in other sexual behaviors should always use a condom to help protect against STDs. (See Chapter 17 for more information on STDs and safer sex practices.)

- Taking responsibility for the consequences of sexual behavior. Everyone should be aware of the physical and emotional consequences of their sexual behavior and accept responsibility for them. These consequences include pregnancy, STDs, and emotional changes in the relationship between partners.

SUMMARY

Sexual Anatomy

- Female external sex organs are called the vulva; the clitoris plays an important role in sexual arousal and orgasm. The vagina leads to the internal sex organs, including the uterus, oviducts, and ovaries.

- Male external sex organs are the penis and the scrotum; the glans penis is an important source of sexual arousal. Internal sexual structures include the testes, vasa deferentia, seminal vesicles, and prostate gland.

Hormones and the Reproductive Life Cycle

- The testes and adrenal glands produce androgens; the ovaries produce estrogens and progestins.
- The fertilizing sperm determines the sex of the individual. Specialized genes on the Y chromosome initiate the process of male sexual differentiation in the embryo.
- Hormones initiate the changes that occur during puberty: The reproductive system matures, secondary sexual characteristics develop, and the bodies of males and females become more distinctive.
- Breast development is the first sign of puberty in the female, followed by rapid body growth.
- The menstrual cycle is divided into four phases: menstruation (the flow of blood and tissue from the uterus), the estrogenic phase (when the egg develops and endometrium is built up), ovulation (the release of the mature egg from the ovarian follicle), and the progestational phase (when the endometrium increases).
- Some females experience physical or psychological symptoms before or during menstruation.
- The reproductive system of boys matures later than that of girls; testosterone brings about most of the male changes of puberty.
- Ovaries cease to function as women approach 50, and they enter menopause. The pattern of male sexual responses changes with age, and testosterone production gradually decreases.

Sexual Functioning

- Sexual activity consists of a stimulus and a response. Stimulation may be physical or psychological.
- Vasocongestion and myotonia are the primary physiological mechanisms of sexual response.
- The sexual response cycle has four stages: excitement, plateau, orgasm, and resolution. Specific genital changes accompany each stage, as do more general body reactions.
- Specific regions in the limbic system of the brain control arousal and orgasm.
- Physical and psychological problems can both interfere with sexual functioning.
- Sexual disorders include vaginitis, endometriosis, and pelvic inflammatory disease in women and prostatitis and testicular cancer in men.

- In men, dysfunctions include erectile dysfunction, premature ejaculation, and retarded ejaculation. Dysfunction in women includes vaginismus and orgasmic dysfunction.
- Treatment for sexual dysfunction first addresses any underlying medical conditions and then looks at psychosocial problems. Sex therapy can help teach new patterns of sexual behavior.

Sexual Behavior

- Some gender characteristics are determined biologically and others are defined by society. Children learn traits and behaviors traditionally deemed appropriate for one sex or the other. Today gender roles are emerging that reflect a mix of male and female characteristics and behaviors.
- The ability to respond sexually is present at birth. Sexual behaviors emerging in childhood include self-exploration, perhaps leading to masturbation.
- Puberty indicates biological adulthood, but people need five to ten additional years to reach social maturity. Sexual fantasies and dreams and nocturnal emissions are characteristic of adolescence.
- Developing the capacity for intimacy and becoming sexually experienced now seem to be important tasks of young adults.
- A person's sexual orientation can be heterosexual, homosexual, or bisexual. A variety of theories have been proposed to explain the development of sexual orientation; possible factors include genetics, hormonal influences, experiences of early childhood, and the timing of puberty.
- Human sexual behaviors include celibacy, erotic fantasy, masturbation, touching, cunnilingus, fellatio, anal intercourse, and coitus.
- Some sexual variations can be explained by the concept of paraphilia, a condition in which a person's sexual arousal and gratification depend on an unusual object or act.
- Child sexual abuse often results in serious trauma for the victim; usually the abuser is a relative, friend, or other trusted adult acquaintance.
- Sexual harassment is sexual pressuring of someone in a vulnerable position.
- Rape victims suffer both physical and psychological pain. Most rape victims are women and most know their attackers.
- Responsible sexuality includes open, honest communication about intentions; sexual activities both partners agree upon; the use of contraception; safe sex practices; and taking responsibility for the consequences of sexual behavior.

1. There are many reputable self-help books about sexual functioning available in libraries and bookstores. If you're not satisfied with your level of knowledge and understanding, consider doing some reading.

2. If you have an intimate sexual relationship with a regular partner, think honestly about what is satisfying about it and what you would like to change. Is there anything you want to discuss with your partner but have been afraid to bring up? Take a chance and talk with your partner about it.

3. Investigate the resources on campus and in your community that deal with acquaintance rape. Are any education programs offered to help prevent acquaintance rape? What types of services are available for victims of acquaintance rape?

JOURNAL ENTRY

1. Sexual myths and misconceptions are common in our culture. In your health journal, make a list of statements about sexuality that you've heard but are not sure are accurate. Find out the facts by consulting books and pamphlets mentioned here or available through your school health center or library.

2. *Critical Thinking:* Many states have laws prohibiting certain sexual behaviors. How much control do you think society should have over an individual's sexual practices? What types of behaviors do you think should be regulated and why? What behaviors should be left up to the discretion of the individual? Write an essay outlining your position; be sure to explain your reasoning.

3. If you think you may have PMS, keep a diary of any physical, emotional, or behavioral symptoms that seem to fluctuate monthly (see the box in the chapter for a list of some possible symptoms of PMS); also keep track of when your period occurs. If you notice a definite cyclical character to your symptoms, consider taking some of the steps suggested in the box.

SELECTED BIBLIOGRAPHY

American Academy of Pediatrics. 1989. Report of the task force on circumcision. *Pediatrics* 84:388–91.

American Psychiatric Association. 1987. *Diagnostic and Statistical Manual of Mental Disorders,* 3rd ed., revised (DSM-III-R). Washington, D.C.: American Psychiatric Association Press.

Berkow, R. 1987. *The Merck Manual.* Rahway, N.J.: Merck.

Block, A. 1990. Rape trauma syndrome as scientific expert testimony. *Archives of Sexual Behavior* 19:309–23.

Chuong, C., and W. Gibbons. 1990. Premenstrual syndrome: Update on therapy. *Medical Aspects of Human Sexuality* 24:58–66.

Cocores, J., and M. Gold. 1989. Substance abuse and sexual dysfunction. *Medical Aspects of Human Sexuality* 23:22–31.

Craig, E., S. Kalichman, and D. Follingstad. 1989. Verbal coercive sexual behavior among college students. *Archives of Sexual Behavior.* 18:421–34.

Dickson, A. 1989. *The Mirror Within: A New Look at Sexuality.* New York: Quartet Books.

Jackson, J., and others. 1990. Young adult women who report childhood intrafamilial sexual abuse: Subsequent adjustment. *Archives of Sexual Behavior* 19:211–21.

Klinger, E. 1990. *Daydreaming: Using Waking Fantasies and Imagery for Self-Knowledge and Creativity.* New York: Jeremy P. Tarcher.

Kravis, D., and M. Molitch. 1990. Endocrine causes of impotence. *Medical Aspects of Human Sexuality* 24:62–67.

LeVay, S. 1991. A difference in hypothalamic structure between heterosexual and homosexual men. *Science* 253:1034–37.

Lizza, E., and R. Cricco-Lizza. 1990. Impotence—Finding the cause. *Medical Aspects of Human Sexuality* 24:30–40.

Masters, W. H., and V. E. Johnson. 1986. *Human Sexual Response.* Boston: Little, Brown.

Muehlenhard, C., and L. Hollabaugh. 1988. Do women sometimes say no when they mean yes? The prevalence and correlates of women's token resistance to sex. *Journal of Personality and Social Psychology* 54:872–79.

Quadagno, D. M. 1987. Pheromones and human sexuality. *Medical Aspects of Human Sexuality* 12:149–54.

Quadagno, D. M., and others. 1991. The menstrual cycle: Does it affect athletic performance? *The Physician and Sports Medicine* 19:121–24.

Reinisch, J. 1990. *The Kinsey Institute: New Report on Sex.* New York: St. Martin's Press.

Risman, B., and P. Schwartz. 1988. Sociological research on male and female homosexuality. *American Review of Sociology* 14:125–47.

Romberg, R. 1985. *Circumcision: The Painful Dilemma.* South Hadley, Mass.: Bergin and Garvey.

Rosen, R., and G. Beck. 1989. *Patterns of Sexual Arousal.* New York: Guilford Press.

Rubin, L. 1990. *Erotic Wars.* New York: Farrar, Straus and Giroux.

Spector, I., and M. Carey. 1990. Incidence and prevalence of the sexual dysfunctions: A critical review of the empirical literature. *Archives of Sexual Behavior* 19:389–408.

Wells, J. 1989. Sexual language usage in different interpersonal contexts: A comparison of gender and sexual orientation. *Archives of Sexual Behavior* 18:127–43.

Wilson, C., and W. Kaye. 1992. Premenstrual syndrome. In *Pediatric and Adolescent Gynecology,* ed. S. Carpenter and A. Rock. New York: Raven Press.

RECOMMENDED READINGS

Borhek, M. 1983. *Coming Out to Parents: A Two-Way Survival Guide for Lesbians and Gay Men and Their Parents.* New York: Pilgrim Press. *Discusses the concerns and fears of gays as they tell their parents about their homosexuality. The book also describes parents' reactions and provides the reader with suggestions for dealing with the coming-out process.*

Boston Women's Health Book Collective. 1992. *The New Our Bodies, Ourselves.* New York: Simon and Schuster. *A very readable book concerned with all aspects of female sexuality.*

Calderone, M. S., and E. W. Johnson. 1989. *The Family Book About Sexuality.* Rev. ed. New York: Harper and Row. *A comprehensive guide to the development of sexuality throughout life, appropriate for a family reference book. The authors present both sides of controversial issues and stress the importance of sex education. This edition sensitively addresses teenage sex, pregnancy, homosexuality, and sexuality in the elder years.*

Denney, N., and D. Quadagno. 1992. *Human Sexuality.* 2nd ed. St. Louis: Times-Mirror Mosby. *A human sexuality textbook with a complete discussion of all of the biological aspects of human sexuality that are presented in this chapter.*

The Diagram Group. 1983. *Man's Body.* New York: Bantam Books.

————. 1978. *Woman's Body.* New York: Bantam Books. *While these books are relatively old, they are still an excellent source of information about male and female sexuality.*

Greenberg, D. 1988. *The Construction of Homosexuality.* Chicago: University of Chicago Press. *An interesting and enlightening historical and cross-cultural analysis of society's treatment of homosexuality.*

Hay, L. 1988. *You Can Heal Your Life.* New York: Hay House. *A self-help book designed to promote, among other things, good sexual functioning.*

Leiblum, S., and R. Rosen. 1989. *Principles and Practice of Sex Therapy.* New York: Guilford Press. *Timely, up-to-date information on the treatment of sexual dysfunctions.*

Strong, B., and C. DeVault. 1994. *Human Sexuality.* Mountain View, Calif.: Mayfield. *A comprehensive introduction to human sexuality based on current research.*

6

Contraception

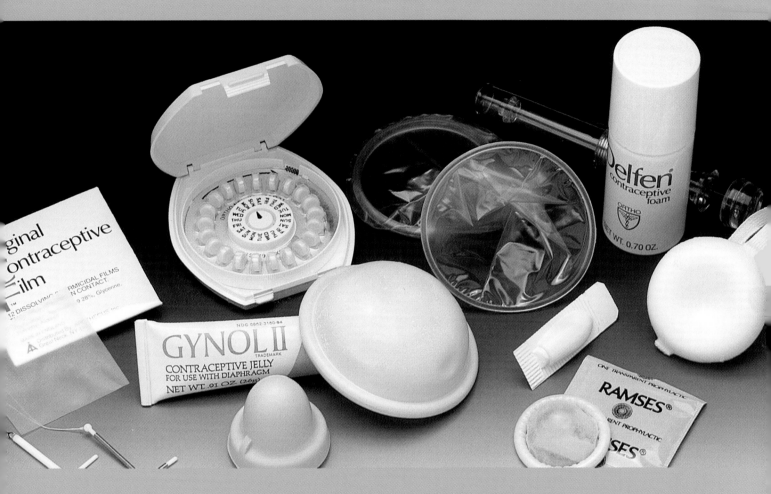

CONTENTS

You're talking to a friend about contraception and are surprised to learn that she became pregnant while using a diaphragm. That's the method you use, and you've always considered it to be very reliable. You'd like to continue to use the diaphragm because it fits your lifestyle and you feel comfortable with it. Just how reliable is a diaphragm? Is there anything you or your partner can do to make it more effective?

When you went home for Thanksgiving, you accidentally left your birth control pills at school. You missed three days, but started taking them again as soon as you got back, five days ago. Are your birth control pills providing you with effective contraception right now?

After a romantic evening with a man you've been dating for a few months, you and he go back to his room with the intention of having sex. Once you get there, you find he doesn't have any condoms. He assumed you had a diaphragm or took the pill. In fact, he says, "It's your responsibility—you're the one who could get pregnant." Is he right? Who is responsible? Is it up to you to get some contraceptives for future occasions?

You want to use Vaseline to lubricate your condom before you make love, but your girlfriend says it's too risky. She claims that oil makes latex condoms break. You've never heard that and in fact often use Vaseline or an oil-based hand lotion as lubrication. Is she wrong, or are you taking a big chance?

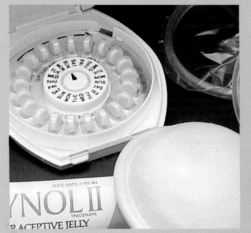

MAKING CONNECTIONS

Probably no single behavior has more potential for upsetting a person's life plans than unprotected sexual activity. Yet many people leave contraception up to chance. More than a million unplanned teenage pregnancies in the United States every year testify to the confusion and ambivalence surrounding contraceptive use in our country. In each of the contraception-related scenarios presented on these pages, individuals have to use information, make a decision, or choose a course of action. How would you act in each of these situations? What response or decision would you make? This chapter provides information about contraceptive principles, methods, and issues that can be used in situations like these. After finishing the chapter, read the scenarios again. Has what you've learned changed how you would respond?

According to the World Health Organization, every day there are at least:

100 million	acts of sexual intercourse
910,000	conceptions
365,000	cases of sexually transmissible diseases
150,000	abortions performed, resulting in the deaths of
500	women because of unsafe conditions

Source: WHO Report. *Reproductive Health, A Key to a Brighter Future* (quoted in *Time*, 6 July 1992).

In her lifetime, the ovaries of an average woman release over 400 eggs, one a month for about three and a half decades. Each is capable of developing into a human being if fertilized by one of the millions of sperm a man produces in every ejaculate. Furthermore, unlike most other mammals, human beings are capable of sexual activity at any time of the month or year. These facts help explain why people have always had a compelling interest in controlling fertility and in preventing unwanted pregnancies. Historical writings dating back to the fourth century B.C. mention the use of douches, sponges, and crude methods of abortion. Other materials mentioned as potential contraceptives include lemon juice, parsley, seaweed, olive oil, camphor, and opium. The underlying principle of these trial-and-error methods, although not clearly understood at the time, was basically the same as that of the **contraceptives** used today: The female's ovum (egg) was blocked from uniting with the male's sperm (**conception**), thereby preventing pregnancy.

Fortunately, modern contraceptive methods are much more predictable and effective than were those used in the past. Today, people have many choices when they're making decisions about sexual and contraceptive behavior. And because the prevention of unintended pregnancies and **sexually transmissible diseases (STDs)** is such a crucial element in lifelong health and well-being, these decisions are among the most significant people can make (Table 6-1). However, because these decisions are also emotional, complex, and difficult, they are often avoided or dealt with in ineffective ways.

While biological, social, and media pressures often encourage sexual activity at ever-younger ages, few forces in the United States support a factual, realistic discussion of the importance of either postponing sexual intercourse or using contraception when intercourse is chosen. Our present superficial approaches to education are clearly ineffective: The United States has one of the highest teen pregnancy rates of all developed nations. Because many of

women's changing roles are hampered severely by unplanned child rearing and the option of turning to abortion is becoming more restricted, the problem is even worse than the numbers show.

This chapter provides basic information on the various contraceptive methods, including their advantages and disadvantages for different individuals. The issues raised in the chapter should encourage you to think about your own beliefs and attitudes about sexual behavior and contraception and to discuss them with others. The most critical decisions for you will involve the time and type of sexual involvement best for you and the commitment to always protect yourself against unwanted pregnancy and STDs.

PRINCIPLES OF CONTRACEPTION

A variety of approaches has proven effective in preventing conception; these approaches are based on different principles of birth control. Barrier methods work by physically blocking the sperm from reaching the egg. Diaphragms, condoms, and several other methods are based on this principle. Hormonal methods alter the biochemistry of the woman's body, preventing ovulation and producing changes that make it more difficult for the sperm to reach the egg if ovulation does occur. Birth control pills operate on this principle. A variety of so-called natural

Contraceptive Any agent that can prevent conception. Condoms, diaphragms, intrauterine devices, and oral contraceptives are examples.

Conception The fusion of ovum and sperm, resulting in a zygote (fertilized egg).

Sexually transmissible diseases (STD) Any of several contagious diseases such as chlamydia and gonorrhea contracted through intimate sexual contact.

TERMS

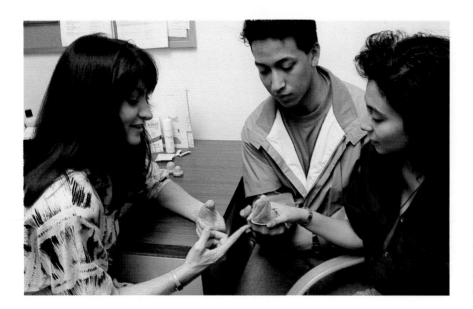

To be effective, contraceptives should be used in exactly the right way. A careful explanation by a health care professional will help this couple use condoms more effectively.

methods of contraception are based on the fact that egg and sperm have to be present at the same time if fertilization is to occur. Finally, surgical methods—female and male sterilization—more or less permanently prevent transport of the sperm or eggs to the site of potential conception.

All the contraceptive methods have advantages and disadvantages that make them appropriate for some people but not for others or at one period of life but not at another. Factors that affect the choice of method include effectiveness, convenience, cost, reversibility, side effects and risk factors, and protection against STDs. Later in this chapter, we help you sort through these factors to decide on the method that's best for you if you are sexually active. (See the box "Myths About Contraception" to make sure you're not basing your choice on common misinformation.)

Effectiveness, one of the factors listed above, requires further explanation. Contraceptive effectiveness is partly determined by the reliability of the method itself—the failure rate if it were always used exactly as directed. This rate cannot be accurately measured, but it can be inferred from studying the most successful users. Effectiveness is also determined by characteristics of the user, including fertility of the individual, frequency of intercourse, and, more importantly, how consistently and correctly the method is used. Because the "method" and "user" variables are difficult to separate out, one overall failure rate reflecting all variables is generally used. This **contraceptive failure rate** is based on studies that directly measure the percentage of women experiencing an accidental pregnancy in the first year of contraceptive use. Another measure of effectiveness is provided by the **continuation rate**—the percentage of people who continue to use the method after a specified period of time. This measure is important because many unintended pregnancies occur when a method is stopped and not immediately replaced with another. Thus, a contraceptive with a high continuation rate would be more effective at preventing pregnancy than one with a low continuation rate.

We turn now to a description of the various contraceptive methods, discussing first those that are reversible and then those that are permanent.

REVERSIBLE CONTRACEPTIVES

Reversibility is an extremely important consideration for young adults when they choose a contraceptive method, since most people either plan to have children or at least want to keep their options open until they're older. In this section we discuss the reversible contraceptives, beginning with the hormonal methods, then moving to the barrier methods, and finally covering the natural methods.

Oral Contraceptives—The Pill

A century ago or more, a researcher made a key observation: **Ovulation** does not occur during pregnancy. Further research brought to light the hormonal mechanism: During pregnancy, the **corpus luteum** secretes **progesterone** and **estrogen** in amounts high enough to suppress ovulation. (Refer back to Chapter 5 for a complete discussion of the hormonal control of the menstrual cycle.) **Oral contraceptives** (OCs), or birth control pills, prevent ovulation by mimicking the hormonal activity of the corpus luteum. The active ingredients in OCs are estrogen and progestins, laboratory-made compounds that are closely related to progesterone.

In addition to preventing ovulation, the birth control pill has other backup contraceptive effects. It hampers the movement of sperm by thickening the cervical mucus, alters the rate of ovum transport by means of its hormonal

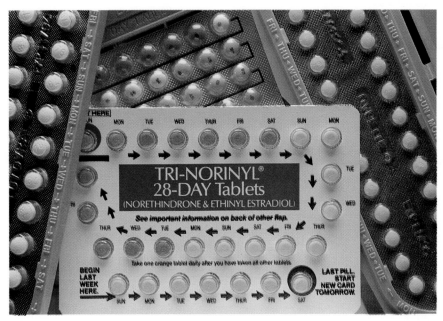

Oral contraceptives are the most popular reversible method of birth control among American women. When used correctly, oral contraceptives are highly effective.

effects on the oviducts, and may inhibit implantation by changing the lining of the uterus, in the unlikely event that a fertilized ovum reaches that area.

Today, the birth control pill is the most widely used form of contraception among unmarried women and is second only to sterilization among married women. The most common type of pill is the combination pill. Each one-month packet contains three weeks of pills that combine varying types and amounts of estrogen and progesterone. Most packets also include one week of inactive pills to be taken following the hormone pills; others instruct the woman to simply take no pills at all for one week before starting the next cycle. During the week in which no hormones are taken, a light menstrual period occurs. Many different types of combination pills are available today, and if minor problems occur with one brand, women can switch to another. The overall trend has been toward lower-dose pills (those with 50 micrograms or less of estrogen), which offer the same high effectiveness rate with fewer unwanted side effects.

A second, much less common type of OC is the "minipill," a small dose of a synthetic progesterone taken every day of the month. Because the minipill contains no estrogen, it has fewer side effects and health risks, but it also carries a higher risk of pregnancy and irregular bleeding.

Users must start the first cycle of the birth control pill with a menstrual period to increase effectiveness and eliminate the possibility of unsuspected pregnancy. Users must take each month's pills completely and according to instructions. A few pills taken before sexual relations will not prevent pregnancy.

Hormonal adjustments that occur during the first cycle or two may cause slight bleeding between periods. This spotting is considered normal. Full effectiveness cannot be guaranteed during the first month because maximal levels of hormones haven't yet been reached. A backup method such as foam and/or condoms is recommended during this time. After the first month, pregnancy is practically impossible if a pill is taken every day according to instructions. If a user forgets to take any pills, effectiveness decreases and a backup method should be used throughout the remainder of the cycle.

Pill use in the United States reached an all-time high in the mid-1970s and then declined rather rapidly between

---

TERMS

Contraceptive failure rate   The percentage of women using a particular contraceptive method who experience an accidental pregnancy in the first year of use.

Continuation rate   The percentage of women who continue to use a particular contraceptive after a specified period of time.

Ovulation   The release of the egg (ovum) from the ovaries.

Corpus luteum   A gland in the ovary that forms after ovulation; secretes progesterone. If the ovum is not fertilized, the corpus luteum degenerates each month, which causes the shedding of the uterine lining (menstruation).

Progesterone   A hormone produced by the corpus luteum and, during pregnancy, by the placenta. Used in oral contraceptives to prevent ovulation.

Estrogen   A hormone produced by the ovaries. An active ingredient in birth control pills.

Oral contraceptive (OC)   Any of various hormone compounds in pill form taken by mouth. Oral contraceptives prevent conception by preventing ovulation.

Myth Taking borrowed birth control pills for a few days before having sexual relations gives reliable protection against pregnancy.

Fact Instructions for taking birth control pills must be followed carefully to provide effective contraception. With most pills, this means starting them with a menstrual period and then taking one every day.

Myth Pregnancy never occurs when unprotected intercourse takes place just before or just after a menstrual period.

Fact Menstrual cycles may be irregular, and ovulation may occur at unpredictable times.

Myth During sexual relations, sperm enter the vagina only during ejaculation and never before.

Fact The small amounts of fluid secreted before ejaculation may contain sperm.

Myth If semen is deposited just outside the vaginal entrance, pregnancy cannot occur.

Fact Although sperm usually live about 72 hours within the woman's body, they can live up to six or seven days and are capable of traveling through the vagina and up into the uterus and oviducts.

Myth Douching immediately after sexual relations can prevent sperm from reaching and fertilizing an egg.

Fact During ejaculation (within the vagina), some sperm begin to enter the cervix and uterus. Since they are no longer in the vagina, it is impossible to remove them by douching after sexual relations. Douching may actually push the sperm up farther.

Myth A woman who is breastfeeding does not have to use any contraceptive method to prevent pregnancy.

Fact Frequent and regular breastfeeding may at times prevent ovulation, but does not do so in a consistent, reliable fashion. Ovulation and pregnancy may occur before the first period after birth.

Myth Women can't become pregnant the first time they have intercourse.

Fact *Any time* intercourse without protection takes place, sperm may unite with an egg to begin a pregnancy. There is nothing unique about first intercourse to prevent this.

1975 and 1977, following intense publicity regarding possible increased risks of heart attacks and strokes. In recent years, however, many of those risks have been reduced by using lower-dosage pills and by clarifying the personal factors that place a specific woman in a high-risk category. Currently, use of oral contraceptives is the most popular method of contraception among couples in whom neither partner has been sterilized.

Advantages The main advantage of the oral contraceptive is its high degree of effectiveness in preventing pregnancy. Nearly all unplanned pregnancies result because the user did not take the pill as directed. The pill is relatively simple to use and does not require any interruptions that could hinder sexual spontaneity. Most women also enjoy the predictable regularity of periods, as well as the decrease in cramps and blood loss. For young women, its reversibility is especially important; **fertility** (ability to reproduce) returns after the pill is discontinued, although not always immediately. The medical advantages include a decreased incidence of the following conditions: benign breast disease, iron-deficiency anemia, pelvic inflammatory disease (PID), ectopic pregnancy, endometrial cancer (of the lining of the uterus), and ovarian cancer. Women who have never used the pill are twice as likely to develop endometrial or ovarian cancer as are users who have taken it for at least 12 months.

Disadvantages Oral contraceptives give no known protection against HIV infection or other STDs. Regular condom use is recommended for an OC user unless she is in a long-term, mutually monogamous relationship with an uninfected partner.

The hormones in birth control pills influence all tissues of the body, and they can lead to a variety of minor disturbances. Symptoms of early pregnancy—morning nausea, weight gain, and swollen breasts, for example— may appear during the first few months of oral contraception. They usually disappear by the fourth cycle. Other complaints include depression, nervousness, changes in the sex drive, dizziness, generalized headaches, migraine headaches, bleeding between periods, and changes in the lining of the walls of the vagina, with an increase in clear or white discharge from the vagina. Chloasma, or "mask of pregnancy," sometimes occurs, causing brown "giant freckles" to appear on the face. Acne may develop or worsen, but in most women, using the pill causes acne to clear up, and it is sometimes pre-

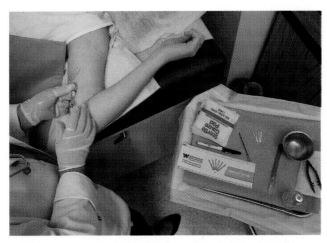

Contraceptive implants, filled with synthetic hormones and inserted under the skin on the arm or leg, can provide five years of protection against pregnancy.

scribed for young women for that purpose. Treatable yeast infections are also more common among women who are taking oral contraceptives.

Serious side effects of pill use have been reported in a small number of women. These include blood clots, stroke and heart attack, concentrated mostly in older women who smoke or have a history of circulatory disease. Pill users also show a slight increase in the incidence of high blood pressure, which is usually quickly reversed on discontinuation of the pill, and of benign tumors that may bleed and rupture.

Much research has been done to investigate possible links between oral contraceptive use and breast cancer. The results of these studies are not clear. Some women may be at higher risk of breast cancer due to OC use; these include women who started the pill before the age of 25 or before their first full-term pregnancy and those who had used the pill for five or more years. Further studies are needed to clarify whether or not these groups of women are actually at greater risk. However, young women who have been on the pill for some time may want to consider another method when lifestyle permits.

Recent evidence has also shown an increased risk of cervical cancer for oral contraceptive users, a risk that rises with increased duration of OC use. Other behaviors linked to cervical cancer include sexual relationships at an early age, sexual relationships with many partners, and smoking. Regular Pap smears for the detection of early cervical changes are especially important in pill users. Also, because other temporary cervical changes found in some women on OCs may contribute to an increased susceptibility to the STDs chlamydia and gonorrhea, regular screening for those diseases is also recommended, especially when condoms aren't being used.

In trying to decide whether to use oral contraceptives, each woman needs to weigh the benefits against the risks. To make an informed decision, she should seek the help of a health care professional in evaluating the risk variables that are known and that apply to her. A woman can take a number of steps to lower her risk from OC use:

- Request a low-dosage pill.
- Stop smoking.
- Follow the pill-taking instructions carefully and consistently.
- Be alert to preliminary danger signals (severe headaches, problems with vision, severe pain in the abdomen, chest, or legs).
- Have regular checkups of her blood pressure, weight, and urine and have an annual examination of the thyroid, breasts, abdomen, and pelvis.

For most women, the known, directly associated risk of death from use of the pill is much lower than the risk of death from pregnancy. Conditions that indicate a woman should not take oral contraceptives (or should take them with ongoing medical supervision) are listed in Table 6-2.

Effectiveness As explained earlier, the effectiveness of a contraceptive is determined by user failures as well as true method failures. Therefore, the commonly used figures represent the failure rate experienced by average people under average circumstances; they include pregnancies that result from erratic pill taking, as well as those that occur when a woman stops taking pills and she and her partner fail to use another method of contraception. Effectiveness will vary substantially among users because it depends so greatly on individual factors. A typical first-year failure rate is 3 percent. The continuation rate for OCs also varies from one group of users to another, with the range being 50 to 75 percent after one year.

Norplant Implants

A contraceptive implant, another method of hormonal birth control for women, was recently approved by the FDA and is now becoming widely available in the United States. This implant was developed in 1974 by researchers at the New York-based Population Council and given the trade name Norplant. This and other similar implants have been used for more than a decade in various countries, including several in South America, Asia, and Scandinavia.

Norplant consists of six flexible, matchstick-sized capsules, each containing progestin, a synthetic progesterone, released in steady doses for up to five years. The capsules are placed under the skin, usually on the inside

Fertility Ability to reproduce.

TERMS

TABLE 6-2 Risk Factors for Oral Contraceptives

Use of oral contraceptives is not recommended for women who have or have had any of the following conditions:	Use of oral contraceptives is questionable and ongoing medical evaluation is recommended for women who have any of the following conditions:
1. Blood clots	1. Severe headaches, especially migraines
2. Heart disease or stroke	2. High blood pressure
3. Any form of cancer or liver tumor	3. Gallbladder, kidney, or liver disease or acute mononucleosis
	4. Major surgery planned in next four weeks, especially surgery requiring immobilization, or major injury to lower leg
	5. Being 35 years of age or older and currently a heavy smoker.
	6. Diabetes or strong family history of diabetes.
	7. Sickle cell disease
	8. Vaginal bleeding from unknown causes
	9. Family history of death from heart attack before age 50, especially in a mother or sister
	10. Family history of high blood levels of cholesterol

Adapted from R. A. Hatcher and others. 1990. *Contraceptive Technology, 1990–92* (New York: Irvington), p. 247.

of a woman's upper arm in a fan-shaped configuration. The procedure can be done in less than 15 minutes, with a local anesthetic and only one very small incision. No stitches are required.

The progestin in Norplant has several contraceptive effects: Hormonal shifts may inhibit ovulation; thickening of cervical mucus hampers the movement of sperm; and transport of the egg through the tubes may be slowed.

More than 500,000 American women have had Norplant capsules implanted since the method became available. This method seems especially suited for women who wish to have continuous and long-term protection against pregnancy.

Advantages Norplant is the most effective reversible method of contraception now available. After insertion of the implants, no further action is required for up to five years of protection; at the same time, contraceptive effects are quickly reversed upon removal. Because Norplant, unlike the combination pill, contains no estrogen, it carries a lower risk of certain side effects, such as blood clots and other cardiovascular complications, and has fewer contraindications. In addition, the progestin is released at a steady rate, in smaller quantities than are found in oral contraceptives.

Disadvantages As with the pill, Norplant gives no protection against HIV infection and other STDs. Although the implants are barely visible, their appearance may be

bothersome to some women. The initial cost of Norplant can be high; however, this one-time fee can give contraceptive protection for five years and may be reduced in subsidized clinics. Both insertion and removal of implants are procedures that can be done only by specially trained practitioners.

The most common side effects of Norplant use are menstrual irregularities, including longer menstrual periods, spotting between periods, or having no bleeding at all. The menstrual cycle usually becomes more regular after one year of use. Less common side effects include headaches, weight gain, breast tenderness, nausea, acne, and mood swings.

The more serious health concerns are similar to those associated with the oral contraceptive, but they are less common with Norplant. The absolute contraindications are also similar, but fewer. They include a history of heart attack, stroke, or blood clots; acute liver disease; jaundice; and unexplained vaginal bleeding. Other health factors may also be important, and a complete medical history should be reviewed with a clinician before implants are used.

Effectiveness Typical failure rates are 0.04 percent in the first year of use, increasing slowly to about 1.1 percent in the fifth year of use. Some studies have shown slightly higher failure rates for women who weigh more than 154 pounds. A key factor contributing to Norplant's high effectiveness is its steady release of progestin, allow-

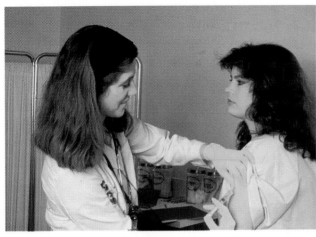

Depo-Provera contraceptive injections contain a long-acting progestin that protects against pregnancy for about 12 weeks.

ing for a more constant hormone level than results from pill taking, especially when pills are forgotten. The continuation rate after one year of use is about 85 percent.

Depo-Provera Injections

A contraceptive injection utilizing a long-acting progestin has also received recent approval for use in the United States. This mode of contraception was developed in the 1960s and is currently being used in at least 80 countries throughout the world. The injectable contraceptive available in the United States is marketed under the name Depo-Provera.

Injected in the arm or buttocks, Depo-Provera is usually given every 12 weeks, although it actually provides effective contraception for a few weeks beyond that. As another progestin-only contraceptive, it prevents pregnancy in the same ways as Norplant.

Advantages　The advantages of Depo-Provera are similar to those of Norplant: It is highly effective, requires little action on the part of the user, and has no estrogen-related side effects. In addition, Depo-Provera requires only periodic injections, rather than the minor surgical procedures of implant insertion and removal. Because the injections leave no trace and involve no ongoing supplies, they allow women almost total privacy in their decision to use contraception.

Disadvantages　Depo-Provera gives no protection against HIV infection and other STDs. Its users must visit a health care facility every three months to receive the injections. Its side effects are similar to those associated with Norplant use; menstrual irregularities are the most common complaint. After one year of using Depo-Provera, many women have no menstrual bleeding at all. After discontinuing use of Depo-Provera, women often experience infertility for up to 12 months. (It does not

lead to permanent infertility.) Other side effects include weight gain, headaches, depression, and dizziness. Contraindications for Depo-Provera are also similar to those for Norplant. Although early animal studies indicated that Depo-Provera increases the risk of breast and other cancers, the FDA has concluded that worldwide studies and years of human use have shown the risk of cancer in humans "to be minimal, if any."

Effectiveness　Typical failure rates reported with Depo-Provera have been under 1 percent.

The "Morning After" or Postcoital Pill

A much less commonly used hormonal method of contraception is the "morning after" or postcoital pill. Postcoital contraceptives work primarily by preventing uterine implantation of a fertilized egg, should one be present. They cause decreased production of progesterone by the corpus luteum, which may alter the uterine lining, and cause other disruptive effects. The uterine lining is shed rather than sustained for pregnancy, and menstruation occurs. Tubal transport of the fertilized egg may also be affected.

One type of pill, which contained large doses of a synthetic preparation of estrogen called **diethylstilbestrol (DES)**, was approved by the FDA in the mid-1970s as a postcoital contraceptive. Its approval was rescinded, however, because DES was linked to cervical and vaginal cancers in daughters of women who had taken the drug to avoid miscarriage, a common practice from 1945 to 1960. (When used shortly after sexual intercourse, DES prevents implantation; once pregnancy is established, however, the hormonal effects of DES are different.)

Another "morning after" pill, a combination of estrogen and progesterone, has been approved in western Europe for emergency situations such as rape. This same pill, although approved by the FDA as a prescription drug for other uses, has not been approved specifically for postcoital purposes in the United States. (There is opposition to the use of postcoital pills because they may act as **abortifacients** if used during a cycle in which fertilization has taken place.) However, once a drug has been approved for one purpose in the United States, physicians may legally prescribe it for others. Because of this regulation, many hospital emergency rooms now offer this drug to rape victims. Several college health services, family planning clinics, and private physicians also make this pill available in certain circumstances.

Diethylstilbestrol (DES)　A synthetic hormone that produces the effects of natural estrogen. DES is not approved for contraceptive use.

Abortifacient　Agent or substance that induces abortion.

TERMS

This "morning after" pill is actually not one pill but a series that must be started within 72 hours (preferably within 12–24 hours) after unprotected sexual intercourse. Studies regarding effectiveness have reported a wide range of results, partly because it is difficult to estimate the number of pregnancies that would have occurred without the pill's use. One overall analysis of the data concludes that the expected risk of pregnancy is reduced by more than 75 percent.

RU-486, the so-called abortion pill (see Chapter 7), is also being studied for use as a postcoital pill. Research thus far shows it to be very effective when taken within 72 hours after intercourse. Further investigation is under way.

The Intrauterine Device (IUD)

The **intrauterine device (IUD)** is a plastic device that is placed in the uterus as a contraceptive. At the height of its popularity in the early 1970s, about 10 percent of all women using contraceptives in the United States were using an IUD. In the late 1970s, however, IUD use began to decline, mostly due to the publicity about the increased risk of serious infections associated with the popular Dalkon Shield and its withdrawal from the market. Soon companies making other popular IUDs also stopped U.S. distribution, not because of new findings of increased medical risk with their products, but because of the financial risk of ongoing lawsuits. Today, only two IUDs are available in the United States: The hormone-releasing Progestasert, which requires replacement every year, and the newer Copper T-380A (also known as the ParaGard), which gives protection for up to eight years. In 1988, only about 2 percent of all American women who used contraception had IUDs.

No one knows exactly how IUDs work. They may cause biochemical changes in the uterus, such as the production of specific cells that destroy the egg and/or sperm; they may immobilize sperm in the uterus or shorten the normal travel time of the egg in the fallopian

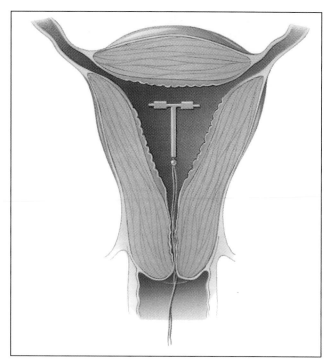

Figure 6-1 *An IUD (Progestasert) properly positioned in the uterus.*
The attached threads that protrude from the cervix into the upper vagina allow the woman to check to make sure that the IUD is in place.

tube; or they may interfere with the implantation of eggs in the uterus. Progestasert acts primarily by slowly releasing very small amounts of progesterone, which makes the uterine lining unsuitable for implantation. In the T-380A, a small amount of copper surrounding its T-shaped arms and leg seems to facilitate the contraceptive biochemical changes in the uterus.

An IUD can be inserted at any time during the menstrual cycle, as long as pregnancy has been ruled out. It is threaded into a sterile inserter, which is then introduced through the cervix until it reaches the lowermost portion of the uterus. The plunger pushes the IUD into the uterus, and the inserter is withdrawn. The threads protruding from the cervix are trimmed so that only 1 to 1½ inches remain in the upper vagina. These are usually not noticeable during coitus (Figure 6-1).

IUDs with nylon threads can usually be removed by pulling on the threads. Only a trained professional should undertake this process, however, because the cervix might have to be expanded, or dilated.

Advantages Intrauterine devices are highly reliable and are simple and convenient to use, requiring no attention except for a periodic check of the string position. They do not require the user to anticipate or interrupt sexual activity. Usually IUDs have only localized side effects, and in the absence of complications, their effects are considered fully reversible. In most cases fertility resumes as soon as

TERMS

Intrauterine device (IUD) A plastic device inserted into the uterus as a contraceptive.

Pelvic inflammatory disease (PID) An infection that progresses from the vagina and cervix and eventually moves into the pelvic cavity.

Spontaneous abortion A miscarriage; the premature expulsion of a nonliving fetus.

Condom A sheath, usually made of thin rubber, designed to cover the penis during sexual intercourse. Used for contraception and to prevent disease.

Barrier method A contraceptive that acts as a physical barrier, blocking the sperm from uniting with the egg.

Ejaculation An abrupt discharge of semen from the penis after sexual stimulation.

the IUD is removed. While the initial cost of IUD insertion may be substantial, the long-term expense is low.

Disadvantages Most side effects of IUD use are limited to the genital tract. By far the most common complaint is abnormal menstrual bleeding. The menstrual flow tends to appear sooner, last longer, and become heavier after insertion of an IUD. Bleeding and spotting between periods may also occur. Another common complaint is pain, particularly uterine cramps and backache, side effects that seem to occur most often in women who have never been pregnant.

Spontaneous expulsion of the IUD happens in 5 to 10 percent of all users within the first year after insertion, most commonly during the first months after insertion. For this reason, it is important to check occasionally that the device is in place by locating the threads, particularly prior to sexual activity. The older the woman is and the more children she has had, the less likely she is to expel the device.

A serious complication sometimes associated with IUD use is **pelvic inflammatory disease (PID).** Most pelvic infections among IUD users are relatively mild and can be treated successfully with antibiotics. However, early and adequate treatment is critical, for a smoldering infection can lead to tubal scarring and subsequent infertility. Infections are usually limited to the first four months after IUD insertion and to women exposed to STDs. There appears to be no increased risk of infection and infertility when a woman has a mutually faithful sexual relationship with only one partner, a situation in which exposure to the leading causes of PID, chlamydia and gonorrhea, is unlikely (see Chapter 17 for more information on PID). Some experts see the IUD as an ideal and underused method for many older women who fall into this category. IUDs offer no protection against STDs.

In about 1 of 2,000 insertions, the IUD punctures the wall of the uterus and migrates into the abdominal cavity. No evidence has been found that IUDs cause cancer in women, but the long-term effects are not well known.

Most physicians advise against the use of IUDs by young women who have never been pregnant because of the increased incidence of side effects in this subgroup and the risk of infection with the possibility of subsequent infertility. The IUD is not recommended for women of any age who have a history of pelvic infection, suspected pregnancy, large tumors of the uterus or other anatomical abnormalities, irregular or unexplained bleeding, history of ectopic pregnancy, rheumatic heart disease, or diabetes.

Early IUD danger signals that the user should be alert to are abdominal pain, fever, chills, foul vaginal discharge, irregular menstrual periods, and other unusual vaginal bleeding. An annual checkup is important and should include a Pap smear and a blood check for anemia if menstrual flow has increased. (And in the case of Pro-

gestasert use, the IUD must be replaced every 12 months.)

Effectiveness The typical failure rate of IUDs during the first year of use is 3 percent. Many of these pregnancies are due to undetected partial or complete expulsion of the device. The failure rate tends to decline rapidly after the first year. Because most pregnancies occur in the first few months after IUD insertion, some physicians advise using an additional method of contraception during that time. Regular checking of the cervix to verify the presence of thread and absence of the IUD stem is also recommended.

Pregnancy may occur with the device in place. If the woman wishes to maintain the pregnancy, the IUD should be removed. Following removal, there is a slightly increased incidence of a **spontaneous abortion** (miscarriage). Birth defects are no more common among babies born of such pregnancies than among other babies. Pregnancies with an IUD left in place may lead to fatal infection or bleeding, and they have a 50 percent chance of ending in miscarriage.

The continuation rate of IUDs is about 75 percent after one year of use.

Condoms

The **condom** is a thin sheath, usually made of latex, designed to cover the penis during sexual intercourse. It prevents sperm from entering the vagina and provides protection against disease. Condoms are the most widely used **barrier method** and the third most popular of all birth control methods used in the United States, exceeded only by the pill and sterilization.

Sales of condoms have increased dramatically in recent years, primarily because condom use provides some protection against all STDs and is the only method that gives substantial protection against HIV infection (see nearby box). At least one-third of all condoms are bought by women. This figure will probably increase as more women become aware of the serious risks associated with STDs and assume the right to insist on condom use. Women are more likely to contract an STD from an infected partner than vice versa. Women also face additional health risks from STDs, including cervical cancer, pelvic inflammatory disease, ectopic pregnancy (which is potentially life-threatening), and tubal infertility. (See Chapter 17 for more information on STDs.)

The user or his partner must put the condom on the penis before it is inserted into the vagina, because the small amounts of fluid that may be secreted unnoticed prior to **ejaculation** often contain sperm capable of causing pregnancy. The rolled-up condom is placed over the head of the erect penis and unrolled down to the base of the penis, leaving a half-inch space (without air) at the tip to collect semen (Figure 6-2). Some brands of condoms

Worldwide, more than 40 million couples use condoms for contraception. Two-thirds of them live in developed countries, with Japan accounting for about 25 percent of all condom sales. In the United States, women now purchase about 40 percent of all condoms sold. Condoms are recommended for a number of reasons:

• They are readily accessible and can be purchased without a prescription in drugstores, convenience stores, supermarkets, campus dormitories, student unions, hotels, and so on.

• They are relatively inexpensive compared with the pill, the IUD, and the diaphragm.

• They are moderately effective when used correctly as a contraceptive, especially in conjunction with spermicide. Effectiveness can be increased if condoms are combined with another method, such as the diaphragm.

• They help prevent the transmission of HIV infection and other STDs, especially if they're lubricated with nonoxynol-9 (latex condoms only). They are not 100 percent effective (only abstinence is), but they improve your chances of avoiding disease.

• They may slow or reduce the development of cervical abnormalities that could lead to cancer.

Despite their growing popularity, many people, especially teenagers, continue to view the use of condoms as an intrusion into their sexual activity, interfering with spontaneity. This attitude—that intercourse must be sponta-neous to be an expression of love—needs to be replaced with more practical and realistic ideas. Condoms don't have to interfere with sexual arousal or pleasure. They come in an array of styles, shapes, colors, thicknesses, and textures, and their use can be integrated into sexual activities before intercourse. Use them properly by following these guidelines:

• Buy latex. If you're allergic to rubber, try wearing a lambskin condom under a latex one.

• Buy fresh. Don't use it if it's more than a year old (most have a date stamped near the rim). Don't remove the condom from its individual sealed wrapper until you're ready to use it. Don't use it if it's gummy, dried out, or discolored.

• Store it right. Too much heat or cold can damage a condom. Don't leave it in your wallet longer than overnight.

• Practice. Condoms aren't hard to use, but practice helps. Take one out of its wrapper—examine it and stretch it to see how strong it is. Practice by yourself and with your partner.

• If you use a lubricant, choose one that is water-based, preferably one that also contains nonoxynol-9.

• Use it right (see Figure 6-2). Air bubbles and insufficient lubrication are the biggest reasons why condoms break. Use a new condom every time you have intercourse.

Adapted from Bernard Goldstein. 1989. "Condoms—On a Roll!" *Healthline*, August; and San Francisco AIDS Foundation. 1990. *The Condom Buyer's Guide*. San Francisco: Impact AIDS, Inc.

have a reservoir tip designed for this purpose. If the user has not been **circumcised,** he must first pull back the foreskin of the penis. He and his partner must be careful not to damage the condom with fingernails, rings, or other rough objects.

Some condoms are sold already lubricated. If the users wish, they can lubricate their own condoms with contraceptive foam, creams, or jelly or water-based preparations such as K-Y Jelly. All products that contain mineral oil—including baby oil, Vaseline Intensive Care lotion, Nivea hand lotion, and regular Vaseline petroleum jelly—should never be used; studies have shown that they cause latex condoms to begin to disintegrate within 60 seconds, thereby markedly increasing their chances of breaking.

Vegetable-based cooking oils—including Mazola and Wesson oils, as well as olive oil, Crisco, and butter—are also damaging.

When the man loses his erection after ejaculating, the condom loses its tight fit. To avoid spilling semen, the condom must be held around the base of the penis as the penis is withdrawn. If any semen is spilled on the vulva, the sperm may find their way to the uterus.

Prelubricated condoms are now available containing nonoxynol-9, the same spermicidal agent found in many of the contraceptive foams and creams that women use. Since the **spermicide** kills many of the sperm soon after ejaculation, its addition may significantly decrease contraceptive failure associated with breakage and the spilling of semen. Nonoxynol-9 also provides additional protection against STDs, including HIV infection.

Advantages Condoms are easy to purchase and are available without prescription or medical supervision. They are simple to use and allow increased male participation in contraception. Condoms do not require daily

TERMS

Circumcise To remove the foreskin of the penis.
Spermicide An agent that kills sperm.

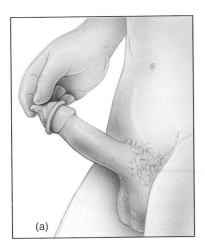

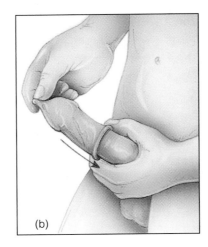

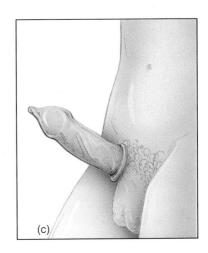

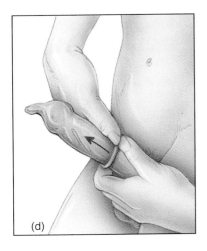

Figure 6-2 *Use of the condom.*
(a) Place the rolled-up condom over the head of the erect penis. Hold the top half-inch of the condom (with air squeezed out) to leave room for semen. (b) While holding the tip, unroll the condom onto the penis. Gently smooth out any air bubbles. (c) Unroll the condom down to the base of the penis. (d) To avoid spilling semen after ejaculation, hold the condom around the base of the penis as the penis is withdrawn. Remove the condom away from your partner, taking care not to spill any semen.

use during intervals of sexual inactivity, and their effects are immediately and completely reversible. In addition to being free of medical side effects (other than occasional allergic reactions), condoms made of rubber (not the lambskin type) help to protect against STDs and related consequences. Except for abstinence, condoms offer the most reliable protection available against transmission of HIV infection.

Disadvantages The two most nearly universal complaints about condoms are that they diminish sensation and interfere with spontaneity. Although some people find these drawbacks serious, others consider them only minor disadvantages. It is hard to think of a human activity in which losing sensation and spontaneity would be less welcome than in coitus. Many couples, however, learn to creatively integrate condom use into their sexual activities. Indeed, it can be a way to improve communication and add shared responsibility to the relationship. Condoms are now available in different sizes, textures, and flavors.

Effectiveness In actual use, the failure rate of condoms varies considerably. First-year rates among typical users average about 12 percent. At least some of these pregnancies happen because the condom is carelessly removed after ejaculation. Some may also happen because of a break or a tear, which is estimated to occur once in every 150 to 200 instances. Because heat destroys rubber, condoms should not be stored for long periods in a wallet or in the glove compartment of a car. Some consumer advocates have suggested that if kept away from heat and light, condoms will remain safe from three to five years. Manufacturers of condoms in the United States recently agreed to put expiration dates on their products and are in the process of determining what a safe "shelf life" would be.

If a condom breaks or is carelessly removed, the risk of pregnancy can be reduced somewhat by the immediate use of a vaginal spermicide. The use effectiveness of the condom can be greatly improved and approaches that of oral contraceptives if a spermicidal foam is also inserted just *before* intercourse.

The most common cause of pregnancy with condom

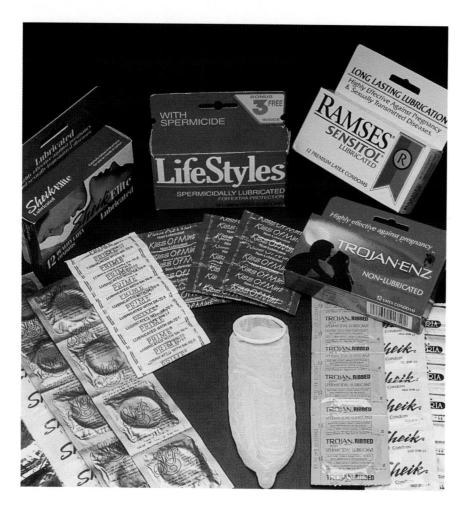

Condoms come in a variety of sizes, textures, and colors; some brands have a reservoir tip designed to collect semen. Used correctly and in conjunction with a spermicide containing nonoxynol-9, condoms provide the most reliable protection available against HIV infection for sexually active people.

users is "taking a chance"—that is, occasionally not using a condom at all—or waiting to use it until after preejaculate fluid (which may contain some sperm) has already entered the vagina.

Female Condoms

A female condom is a latex or polyurethane pouch that a woman or her partner inserts into her vagina. One brand, Reality, was approved in May 1993 for use in the United States. Reality is a disposable device that comes in one size and consists of a soft, loose-fitting polyurethane sheath with two flexible rings (Figure 6-3). The ring at the closed end is inserted into the vagina and placed at the cervix much like a diaphragm. The ring at the open end remains outside the vagina. The walls of the condom protect the inside of the vagina. It can be inserted well before intercourse, and should be used with the supplied lubricant or a spermicide to prevent penile irritation.

Another brand of female condom, Women's Choice, is made of increased-strength latex (30 percent thicker than male condoms) and is inserted like a tampon with a reusable plastic applicator. A third vaginal condom currently under preliminary study is in essence a latex bikini with a built-in rolled pouch that can be pushed into the vagina before intercourse. This device covers the entire genital area and should provide maximum protection against all STDs.

Advantages For many women, the greatest advantage of the female condom is the control it allows them to have over contraception and STD prevention. Female condoms can be inserted before intercourse and are thus less disruptive than male condoms. Because the outer part of the condom covers the area around the vaginal opening as well as the base of the penis during intercourse, it offers potentially better protection against genital warts or herpes. The pouch made of polyurethane can be used by people who are allergic to latex. In addition, because

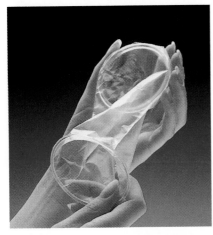

The Reality brand female condom is a polyurethane sheath about 6½ inches long. It is held in place by two flexible rings, a closed one that is placed at the cervix and an open one that hangs outside the body.

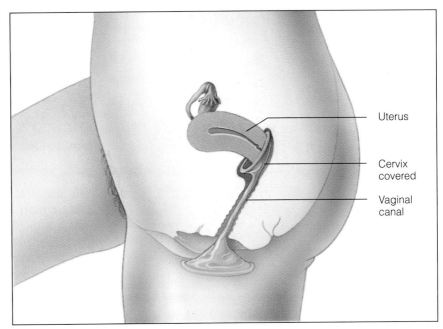

Uterus

Cervix covered

Vaginal canal

Figure 6-3 *Female condom.*

polyurethane is thin and pliable, there is little loss of sensation.

Disadvantages As with the traditional condom, interference with spontaneity is likely to be a common complaint. The outer ring, which hangs visibly outside the vagina, may be bothersome during foreplay; if so, couples may choose to put the device in just before intercourse. During coitus, both partners must take care that the penis is inserted in the pouch, not outside it, and that the device does not slip inside the vagina. For many couples, initial awkwardness and difficulty is largely eliminated after a few weeks' use. Female condoms, like male condoms, are made for one-time use and will probably cost about three times as much.

Effectiveness Preliminary studies indicate that the female condom is less effective than the male condom at protecting against pregnancy and STDs.

The Diaphragm and Jelly

Before oral contraceptives were introduced, about one-fourth of all American couples who used any form of contraception relied on the **diaphragm.** Many former diaphragm users have been won over to the pill or to IUDs, but the diaphragm continues to offer advantages that are important to certain couples. About 5.7 percent of all women who use contraception use diaphragms.

The diaphragm is a dome-shaped cup of thin rubber stretched over a collapsible metal ring. When correctly used with spermicidal cream or jelly, the diaphragm covers the cervix, blocking sperm from entering the uterus.

Diaphragms can be obtained only by prescription. Because of individual differences in women, a diaphragm must be carefully fitted to ensure that it will be both effective and comfortable, and only a trained person can make these adjustments. The fitting should be checked with each routine annual medical examination, as well as after childbirth, abortion, or a weight change of more than 10 pounds.

Before inserting the diaphragm, the woman should spread about a tablespoon of spermicidal jelly or cream over the surface of the dome that will be against the cervix and around the rim. The diaphragm is easiest to insert if the user squats, lies down, or stands with one foot raised. The user squeezes the diaphragm into a long narrow shape with one hand. She holds the labia apart with the other hand and pushes the diaphragm up along the back wall of the vagina as far as it will go, keeping it behind the cervix. She then tucks the front rim up behind the pubic bone (Figure 6-4). Because the vagina tilts backward, a user who inserts the diaphragm while she is standing up must insert it almost horizontally.

After the diaphragm is inserted, its position should be checked. The cervix should be located and felt through the dome of the diaphragm to make sure that it is completely covered and that the front rim of the diaphragm is pushed up behind the pubic bone.

> **Diaphragm** A contraceptive device consisting of a flexible, dome-shaped cup that covers the cervix. The diaphragm prevents sperm from entering the uterus.

TERMS

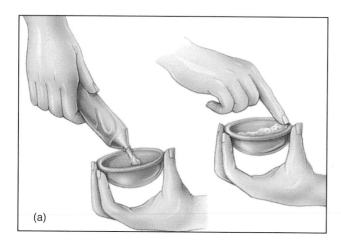

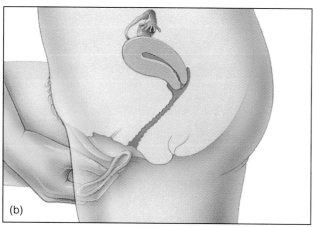

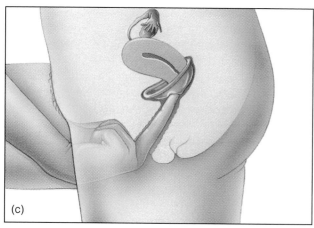

Figure 6-4 *Use of the diaphragm.*
(a) Place about one tablespoon of spermicidal jelly in the concave side of the diaphragm and spread it around the inside of the diaphragm and around the rim. (b) Press the diaphragm firmly between the thumb and forefinger and insert it in the vagina; push it along the back wall of the vagina as far as it will go. (c) Check the position of the diaphragm to make sure that the cervix is completely covered and that the front rim of the diaphragm is tucked behind the pubic bone.

The diaphragm must not be inserted more than six hours before intercourse. If the time between insertion and coitus is longer than six hours, an applicatorful of spermicide should be inserted into the vagina, or the diaphragm should be taken out and spermicide freshly applied before it is reinserted. Additional cream or jelly should also be inserted into the vagina before any additional act of coitus. The diaphragm must be left in place for at least six hours after the last act of coitus to give the spermicide enough time to kill all the sperm.

To remove the diaphragm, the user simply hooks the front rim down from the pubic bone with one finger and pulls it out. After the diaphragm is removed, it should be washed with mild soap and water, rinsed, and patted dry. It should then be examined for holes or cracks. Defects are most likely to develop near the rim, and can be spotted by looking at the diaphragm in front of a bright light. After the diaphragm is inspected, it can be dusted with cornstarch (*not* talcum powder, which may damage it and irritate the vagina) and stored in its case.

Advantages Diaphragm use is less intrusive than condom use because a diaphragm can be inserted up to six hours before intercourse. Its use can be limited to times of sexual activity only, and it allows for immediate and total reversibility. The diaphragm is free of medical side effects (other than rare allergic reactions). When used along with spermicidal jelly or cream, it offers significant protection against gonorrhea and perhaps chlamydia, STDs that are transmitted only by semen and for which the cervix is the sole portal of entry. Diaphragm use can also protect the cervix from semen infected with the human papillomavirus, which has been implicated as an important factor in cellular changes in the cervix that can lead to cancer. However, the diaphragm is unlikely to protect against STDs that can be transmitted through vaginal or vulvar surfaces (in addition to the cervix)—these include HIV infection, genital herpes, and syphilis.

Disadvantages Diaphragms must always be used with a spermicide, and therefore a user must keep both of these somewhat bulky supplies with her whenever she anticipates sexual activity. Diaphragms require extra attention, since they must be cleaned and stored with care to preserve their effectiveness. Some women cannot wear a diaphragm because of their vaginal anatomy. In other women, diaphragm use can cause an increase in bladder infections and may need to be discontinued if repeated infections occur. It has also been associated with a slightly increased risk of **toxic shock syndrome (TSS),** an occasionally fatal bacterial infection. To diminish the risk of TSS, women should wash their hands carefully with soap and water before inserting or removing the diaphragm, should not use the diaphragm during menstruation or whenever there is an abnormal discharge, and should never leave the device in place for more than 24 hours.

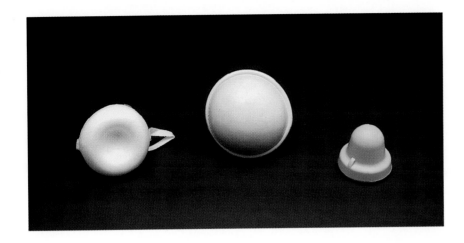

The sponge, diaphragm, and cervical cap work by covering the mouth of the cervix, blocking sperm from entering the cervix. The sponge can be purchased without a prescription. The diaphragm and cervical cap require professional fitting.

Effectiveness The effectiveness of the diaphragm is highly dependent on user factors. In actual practice, women rarely use the diaphragm correctly every time they have intercourse. Typical failure rates for the diaphragm are 18 percent during the first year of use. The main causes of failures are incorrect insertion, inconsistent use, and inaccurate fitting. Sometimes, too, the vaginal walls expand during sexual stimulation, allowing the diaphragm to be dislodged. This displacement seems to happen most commonly with the woman-on-top position.

The Cervical Cap

The **cervical cap** is another barrier device. It consists of a thimble-shaped rubber or plastic cup that fits snugly over the cervix and is held in place by suction. The cap comes in various sizes and must be fitted by a trained clinician. It is used in a manner similar to the diaphragm, a small amount of spermicide being placed in the cup before each insertion. Use of the cervical cap in the United States has increased recently, along with its availability, but still remains well below the level of diaphragm use.

Advantages Advantages of the cervical cap are similar to those associated with diaphragm use and include partial STD protection. In addition, it can be used as an alternative for women who have anatomical features that preclude diaphragm use, such as very lax vaginal tone, pressure discomfort, or recurrent urinary infections with diaphragm use. It may be left in place for up to 48 hours, compared with 24 hours for the diaphragm; and because the cap fits tightly, it does not require reintroduction of spermicide with repeated intercourse.

Disadvantages Along with most of the disadvantages associated with the diaphragm, difficulty with insertion and removal is a more common problem for cervical cap users. In addition, some studies have indicated that women who use the cap rather than the diaphragm initially have a higher rate of abnormal Pap smears. In most cases these result from inflammation or infections of the cervix, conditions that are easily treatable. As a safety precaution, the FDA has stated that the cap should be prescribed only for women with *normal* Pap smears and that a repeat test should be done after *three months* of use to confirm that no changes have occurred. Because there may be a slightly increased risk of TSS with prolonged use, the cap should not be left in place for more than 48 hours.

Effectiveness Studies completed thus far indicate that cervical cap effectiveness is about 18 percent, similar to that of the diaphragm.

The Sponge

The **sponge,** a more recent addition to the barrier methods, is a round, absorbent device about 2 inches in diameter with a polyester loop on one side (for removal) and a concave dimple on the other side, which helps it fit snugly over the cervix. Most sponges are made of polyurethane and are presaturated with the same spermicide that is used in contraceptive creams and foams. The spermicide is activated when moistened with a small amount of water just before insertion. The sponge, which can be used only once, acts as a barrier, as a spermicide, and as a seminal fluid absorbent.

Toxic shock syndrome (TSS) A disease whose major symptoms include high fever, vomiting, diarrhea, headache, sore throat, and rash. Although primarily associated with menstruating women who use tampons, the disease has also been reported in men. It is usually caused by the bacterium Staphylococcus aureus. Mortality rate has decreased from 10–15 percent to 3 percent or less due to earlier recognition and treatment.

Cervical cap A thimble-shaped cup that fits over the cervix, to be used with spermicide.

Sponge A contraceptive device about 2 inches in diameter that fits over the cervix and acts as a barrier, spermicide, and seminal fluid absorbent.

TERMS

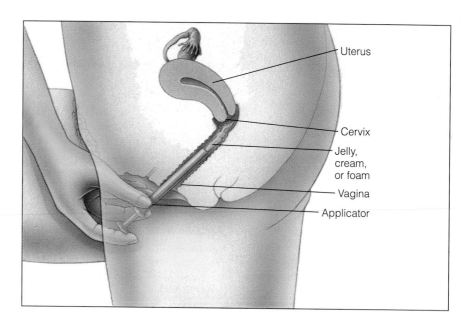

Figure 6-5 *Application of spermicide.*

Uterus

Cervix

Jelly, cream, or foam

Vagina

Applicator

Advantages The sponge offers advantages similar to those of the diaphragm and cervical cap, including partial STD protection. In addition, sponges can be obtained without a professional fitting, and they may be safely left in place for 24 hours without the addition of spermicide for repeated intercourse.

Disadvantages Reported disadvantages include difficulty with removal and an unpleasant odor if left in place for more than 18 hours. Allergic reactions, such as irritation of the labia, are more common with the sponge than with other spermicide products, probably because the overall dose contained in each sponge is significantly higher than that used with the other methods. (It contains 1 gram of spermicide compared to the 60–100 mg present in one application of other spermicidal products.) Because the sponge has also been associated with toxic shock syndrome, the same precautions must be taken as described for diaphragm use. A sponge user should be especially alert for symptoms of TSS when the sponge has been difficult to remove or was not removed intact. We do not know how much spermicide is absorbed through the vaginal walls with this device, or what possible effects are caused by recurring, extended exposure.

Effectiveness The use effectiveness of the sponge is similar to that of the diaphragm (18 percent failure rate during the first year of use) for women who have never experienced childbirth. For women who have had a child, however, sponge effectiveness is significantly lower than diaphragm effectiveness. One possible explanation is that the one size now marketed may be insufficient to adequately cover the cervix after childbirth. To ensure effectiveness, the user should carefully check the expiration date on each sponge, as shelf life is limited.

Vaginal Spermicides

In recent years spermicidal compounds developed for use with a diaphragm have been adapted for use without a diaphragm by combining them with a bulky base. Foams, creams, jellies, and vaginal suppositories are all available. Foam is sold in an aerosol bottle or a metal container with an applicator that fits on the nozzle. Creams and jellies are sold in tubes with an applicator that can be screwed onto the opening of the tube (Figure 6-5).

Foams, creams, and jellies must be placed deep in the vagina near the cervical entrance and must not be inserted more than one-half hour before intercourse. After an hour, their effectiveness is drastically reduced, and a new applicatorful must be inserted. Another application is also required before each repeated act of coitus. If the woman wants to **douche**, she should wait for at least eight hours after the last coitus to make sure that there has been time for the spermicide to kill all the sperm.

In recent years the spermicidal suppository has become widely marketed and publicized in the United States. It is small and easily inserted like a tampon. Because body heat is needed to dissolve and activate the suppository, it is important to wait at least 10 minutes after insertion before having intercourse. The suppository's spermicidal effects are limited in time, and coitus should take place within one hour of insertion. An additional suppository is required for each additional act of intercourse.

The latest addition to the vaginal spermicides is the vaginal contraceptive film (VCF) a paper-thin 2-inch square of film that incorporates the same spermicide as the methods already discussed. It is folded over one or two fingers and placed high in the vagina, as close to the cervix as possible. In about 10 minutes the film dissolves into a gel that exerts a contraceptive effect against sperm

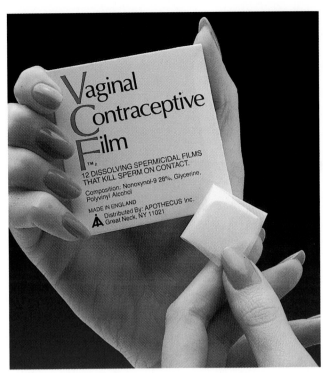

The vaginal contraceptive film shown here is a paper-thin square of film containing spermicide that is folded and placed high in the vagina.

for about 1½ hours. An additional film must be inserted each time intercourse is repeated.

Advantages The use of vaginal spermicides is relatively simple and can be limited to times of sexual activity. They are readily available in most drugstores and do not require a prescription or a pelvic examination. Spermicides allow for complete and immediate reversibility; the only known medical side effects are occasional allergic reactions. Vaginal spermicides may offer limited protection against some STDs, but should never be used instead of condoms for reliable protection, especially when there is a risk of HIV infection.

Disadvantages When used alone, vaginal spermicides must be inserted shortly before intercourse, so their use may be seen as an annoying disruption. Some women find the slight increase in vaginal fluids after spermicide use unpleasant. Spermicides can alter the balance of bacteria in the vagina by inhibiting certain bacteria while allowing others to grow. Because this may increase the risk of urinary tract infections, women who are especially prone to these infections may want to avoid spermicides. Potential risks of long-term spermicide use and spermicide use around the time of conception are currently being investigated.

Effectiveness The reported effectiveness rates of vaginal spermicides cover a wide range, again depending partly on how consistently and carefully instructions are followed. The typical failure rate is about 21 percent during the first year of use. Of the various types of spermicides, foam is probably the most effective, because its effervescent mass forms a more dense and evenly distributed barrier to the cervical opening. Creams and jellies give only minimal protection unless used with diaphragms or cervical caps. Vaginal spermicides are used by many couples in combination with condoms or as a backup with other birth control methods.

> **Personal Insight** How do you feel about buying contraceptives at the drugstore? About asking for a prescription contraceptive at your health clinic or from your physician? Why do you feel the way you do? Have your feelings changed as you've grown older?

Abstinence, Fertility Awareness, and Withdrawal

Millions of people throughout the world do not use any of the methods we have described. Either they will not because of religious conviction or cultural prohibitions or they cannot because of poverty or lack of information and supplies. If they use any method at all, they are likely to use one of the following relatively "natural" methods of attempting to prevent conception.

Abstinence The decision not to engage in sexual intercourse for a chosen period of time, or **abstinence**, has been followed by human beings throughout history for a variety of reasons. Until relatively recently, many people abstained because they had no other birth control measures. Today, with other methods available, about 5 percent of all American women who use birth control rely on periodic abstinence as a birth control method. To some of them, all other methods simply seem unsuitable. Concern regarding possible side effects, STDs, and unwanted pregnancy may be factors. Abstinence or remaining in a monogamous relationship with an uninfected partner is the only sure way to avoid HIV infection and other STDs. Even consistent condom use many fail because condoms can break and they may not always cover all infected surfaces, particularly in cases of herpes or genital warts. Intercourse may also be temporarily avoided because of medical reasons such as recent illness or surgery. In other

Douche To apply a stream of water or other solutions to a body part or cavity such as the vagina; not a contraceptive technique.

Abstinence Avoidance of sexual intercourse. This is one method of birth control.

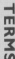

TERMS

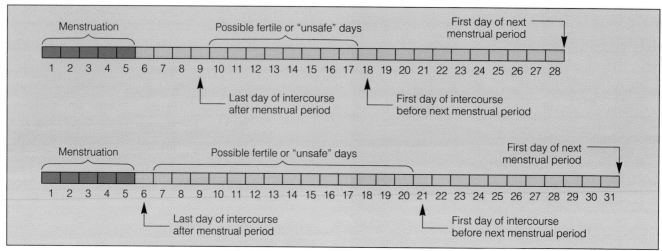

Figure 6-6 The Fertility Awareness Method of contraception, showing the safe and unsafe days for a woman with a regular 28-day cycle (top), and a woman with an irregular cycle, ranging from 25 to 31 days (bottom).

cases, abstinence may be seen as the wisest choice in terms of personal emotional needs. A period of abstinence may be chosen as a time to focus energies on other aspects of interpersonal or personal growth. Religious and cultural beliefs are sometimes motivating factors. For a variety of reasons, what may seem "right" and highly desirable for one person may be unacceptable for another. External pressure alone, either from individuals or from society at large, is being recognized as an unsatisfactory reason to engage in intercourse. Programs that focus on assertiveness and communication skills have been created for students at a variety of grade levels, from junior high to college.

Many couples who do choose to abstain from sexual intercourse in the traditional sense turn to other mutually satisfying alternatives. When open communication between partners exists, many new avenues may be explored. These may include dancing, massage, hugging, kissing, petting, mutual masturbation, and oral-genital sex. Sexual feelings and intimacy may be expressed and satisfied through a wide range of activities.

Fertility Awareness Method (FAM) The basis for **FAM** is abstinence from coitus during the fertile phase of a woman's menstrual cycle. Ordinarily only one egg is released by the ovaries per month, and it lives about 24 hours unless it is fertilized. Sperm deposited in the vagina are apparently on the average capable of fertilizing an egg for about six to seven days; so conception theoretically can only occur during eight days of any cycle. Predicting *which* eight days these are is difficult. It is done either by the calendar method or by the temperature method. Information on cyclical changes of the cervical mucus has also been helpful in determining the time of ovulation.

The *calendar method* is based on the knowledge that the average woman releases an egg 14 to 16 days before her next period begins. Few women menstruate with complete regularity, so a record of the menstrual cycle must be kept for 12 months, during which time some other method of birth control must be used. The first day of each period is counted as Day 1. To determine the first fertile, or "unsafe" day of the cycle, subtract 18 from the number of days in the shortest cycle. To determine the last unsafe day of the cycle, subtract 11 from the number of days in the longest cycle. The calendar method is illustrated in Figure 6-6.

The *temperature method* is based on the knowledge that a woman's body temperature drops slightly just before ovulation and rises slightly after ovulation. A woman using the temperature method records her basal, or resting, body temperature (BBT) every morning before getting out of bed and before eating or drinking anything, since the activities may alter the results. Once the temperature pattern can be seen (usually after about three months), the period unsafe for coitus can be calculated as the interval from Day 5 (Day 1 is the first day of the period) until three days after the rise in BBT. To arrive at a shorter unsafe period, some women combine the calendar and the temperature methods, calculating the first unsafe day from the shortest cycle of the calendar chart and the last unsafe day as the third day after a rise in the BBT.

The *mucus method* is based on changes in the cervical secretions throughout the menstrual cycle. During the estrogenic phase, cervical mucus increases and is clear and slippery. At the time of ovulation some women can detect a slight change in the texture of the mucus and find that it is more likely to form an elastic thread when stretched between thumb and finger. After ovulation these secretions become cloudy and sticky and decrease in quantity. Infertile, safe days are likely to occur during the relatively

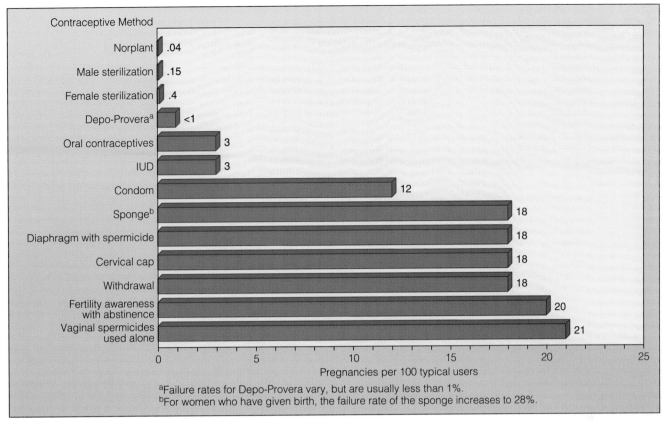

Contraceptive Method

Method	Pregnancies per 100 typical users
Norplant	.04
Male sterilization	.15
Female sterilization	.4
Depo-Provera[a]	<1
Oral contraceptives	3
IUD	3
Condom	12
Sponge[b]	18
Diaphragm with spermicide	18
Cervical cap	18
Withdrawal	18
Fertility awareness with abstinence	20
Vaginal spermicides used alone	21

Pregnancies per 100 typical users

[a]Failure rates for Depo-Provera vary, but are usually less than 1%.
[b]For women who have given birth, the failure rate of the sponge increases to 28%.

Figure 6-7 *Failure rates of contraceptive methods during first year of use.*

dry days just before and after menstruation. This is also called the **Billings method.** These additional clues have been found helpful by some couples who rely on the Fertility Awareness Method. One possible problem that may interfere with this method is that vaginal infections or vaginal products or medication can also change cervical mucus.

FAM is not recommended for women who have very irregular cycles—about 15 percent of all menstruating women. Any woman for whom pregnancy would be a serious problem should not rely on FAM alone, because the failure rate is high—approximately 20 percent among typical users during the first year of use.

Withdrawal Probably the oldest known method of contraception is **withdrawal.** In this method, the male removes his penis from the vagina just before he ejaculates. Withdrawal has three advantages: It is free, it requires no preparation, and it is always available. For many people, these advantages are far outweighed by the disadvantages: The male has to overcome a powerful biological urge. A man may also have difficulty judging when to withdraw. The fear that withdrawal may be too late can detract from sexual pleasure for both partners. Also, since many women take longer than men do to reach orgasm, with-

drawal before the woman's orgasm is likely and can leave the couple frustrated if she relies on coitus for satisfaction. The typical failure rate for withdrawal is 18 percent during the first year. One key factor in the high failure rate is the degree of self-control necessary. In addition, preejaculatory fluid, which may contain viable sperm, is commonly secreted unnoticed before actual ejaculation occurs.

Figure 6-7 summarizes the use effectiveness of eight reversible contraceptive methods.

Combining Methods

Couples can choose to combine the preceding methods in a variety of ways, both to add STD protection and/or to

---

Fertility Awareness Method (FAM) A method of preventing conception based on avoiding coitus during the fertile phase of a woman's cycle.

Billings method A method of predicting the fertile period in a woman's cycle by means of the texture, color, and amount of cervical mucus.

Withdrawal Purposely interrupting sexual intercourse by withdrawing the penis before ejaculation (to avoid conception).

TERMS

About half of all the world's couples of reproductive age currently use some form of contraception. Worldwide, sterilization is the most commonly used method followed by IUDs, oral contraceptives, condoms, and natural family planning methods. But striking differences exist from one country to another in both the rates of contraceptive use and method chosen. These differences reflect a variety of factors, including the following:

• *Access to services.* How far people have to travel for contraceptive services and how long they have to wait once they get there are important factors in contraceptive use. Geographical barriers can be significant, particularly in developing countries or isolated rural areas. For example, a study of contraceptive use in rural Bangladesh revealed that the presence of paved roads was as much a factor as the location of facilities.

• *Availability.* Not all methods are available in every country. In the United States, for example, access to IUDs is limited, and Norplant and Depo-Provera have only recently become available. IUDs and injectables are more available—and more widely used—in Mexico than in the United States. In Japan, oral contraceptives are available only in high dosages and only for a few women; this may be one reason why condom use is high there.

• *Cost.* Studies have shown that people are willing to pay moderate amounts for contraceptive supplies; but for many people, the price threshold is fairly low. Furthermore, many methods have hidden costs, such as the purchase of spermicide for use with a diaphragm.

Methods that require the replenishing of supplies are less likely to be used in developing nations.

• *Political, cultural, and religious factors.* Government policies can have a strong impact on contraceptive use. The Chinese government limits family size to one child and penalizes families who have additional children. China has one of the highest rates of contraceptive use in the world. Cultural influences are important too. A woman seeking contraceptives may encounter opposition from her peer group, husband, or extended family. A large family may be valued as a source of labor, a symbol of virility or fertility, or a form of "social security" in old age. In some countries, religious traditions and doctrines prohibit contraceptive use. Roman Catholics have opposed national family planning efforts in Mexico, Kenya, and the Philippines. Muslim fundamentalists have done the same in Iran, Egypt, and Pakistan.

Although Americans tend to think of contraceptive use as a matter of personal choice, it is clearly bounded by numerous physical and cultural constraints, even in the United States. In many societies, most individuals may have very little choice in which, if any, contraceptive they use. On a worldwide scale, lack of contraceptive use is associated with rapid population growth, poverty, and high mortality rates from unsafe conditions of childbirth, risky illegal abortions, and sexually transmissible diseases. This is why family planning is sure to be one of the most pressing—and complex—issues that nations will face in the twenty-first century.

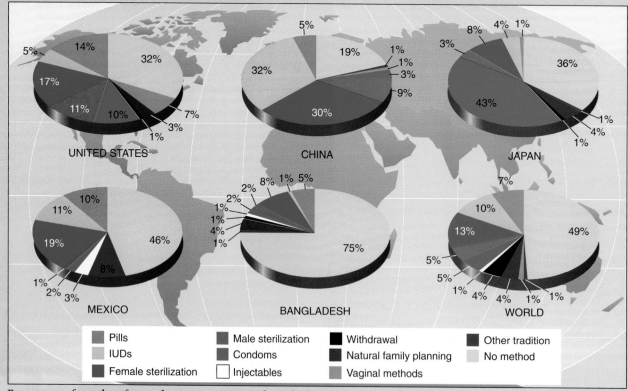

Percentage of couples of reproductive age using each method.

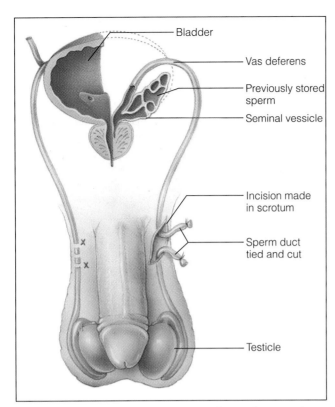

Figure 6-8   Vasectomy is a comparatively simple surgical procedure.

Labels in figure:
- Bladder
- Vas deferens
- Previously stored sperm
- Seminal vessicle
- Incision made in scrotum
- Sperm duct tied and cut
- Testicle

increase contraceptive effectiveness. For example, condoms are strongly recommended along with pill use whenever there is a risk of STDs. Foam may be added to condom use to increase protection against both STDs and pregnancy. For many couples, and especially for many women, the added benefits will far outweigh the extra effort and expense.

PERMANENT CONTRACEPTION— STERILIZATION

Sterilization is permanent, and it provides complete protection. For these reasons, it is becoming an increasingly popular method of birth control. At present it is the most commonly used method in the United States and in the world (see box "Contraceptive Use Around the World"). It is especially popular among couples who have been married 10 or more years, as well as among couples who have had all the children they intend. Sterilization provides no protection against STDs.

An important consideration in choosing sterilization is that, in most cases, it cannot be reversed. Although the chances of restoring fertility are being increased by modern surgical techniques, such operations are costly and pregnancy can never be guaranteed. Some couples choosing male sterilization are using sperm banks as a way of extending the option of childbearing.

Some recent studies have indicated that male sterilization is preferable to female sterilization in a variety of ways. The overall cost of a female procedure is about four times that of a male procedure, and women are much more likely than men to experience both minor and major complications following the operation. Furthermore, regret seems to be somewhat higher in women than in men after sterilization.

Although some physicians will perform surgery for sterilization on request, most require a thorough discussion with both partners before the operation. Most physicians also recommend that people who have religious conflicts, psychiatric problems related to sex, or unstable marriages not be sterilized. Young couples with one or two children, who might later change their minds and want more, are also frequently advised not to undergo sterilization.

Male Sterilization—Vasectomy

The procedure for male sterilization, **vasectomy,** involves severing the **vasa deferentia,** two tiny ducts that transport sperm from the testicles to the seminal vesicles. The testicles continue to produce sperm, but the sperm are absorbed into the body. Since the testicles contribute only about one-tenth of the total seminal fluid, the actual quantity of ejaculate is only slightly reduced. Hormone output from the testicles continues with very little change, and secondary sex characteristics are not altered.

Vasectomy is ordinarily done in the physician's office and takes about 30 minutes. A local anesthetic is injected into the skin of the scrotum and near the vasa. Small incisions are made at the upper end of the scrotum where it joins the body, and the vas deferens on each side is exposed, severed, and tied off or coagulated with electrocautery. The incisions are then closed with sutures, and a small dressing is applied (Figure 6-8). Pain and swelling are usually slight and can be relieved with an ice bag, aspirin, and use of a scrotal support. Bleeding and infection occasionally develop but in most cases are easily treated. Most men are ready to return to work in two days.

Men can have sex again as soon as they feel no further discomfort; for most men this means after about a week. Another method of contraception must be used for the first few weeks after vasectomy, however, because sperm produced before the operation may still be present in the semen. To make sure that sperm are no longer in the ejac-

Sterilization   Surgically altering the reproductive system to prevent pregnancy. Vasectomy is the procedure in males, tubal sterilization or hysterectomy in females.

Vasectomy   Surgical severing of the ducts that carry sperm to the ejaculatory duct.

Vasa deferentia   (Vas deferens, singular form) The two ducts that carry sperm to the ejaculatory duct.

TERMS

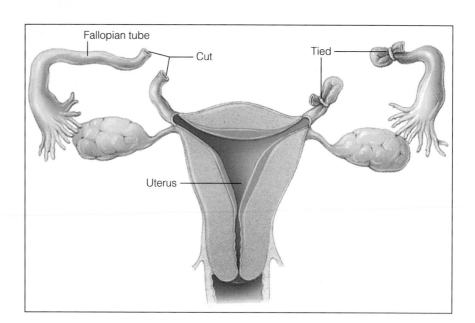

Figure 6-9 Tubal sterilization is more complex than vasectomy.

ulate and that another method of contraception is no longer necessary, a semen specimen should be examined under a microscope.

A new procedure, called the no-scalpel vasectomy, has been used extensively in China and is now being performed by some American physicians. With this technique, a tiny midline puncture, rather than incisions, is made in the scrotal skin. The puncture is stretched open slightly with a special instrument, and each vas deferens is located in turn and lifted out with a forceps. After the vas has been tied off or coagulated, it is allowed to slip back into the scrotum. There is no need for sutures, and less bleeding and fewer infections occur than with conventional vasectomy. This no-scalpel procedure is harder to learn, however, and identification of the sperm ducts is more difficult.

Research into possible links between vasectomy and cardiovascular disease and cancer have been inconclusive. Some studies have found an association between vasectomy and higher rates of disease, while others have found lower death rates among men who have had vasectomies.

Vasectomy is highly effective. In a small number of vasectomies, a severed vas rejoins itself, and sperm can again travel up through the duct and be ejaculated in the semen. Some physicians advise that a semen sample be examined yearly to check for this possibility. The overall failure rate for vasectomy is 0.15 percent.

Although some surgeons report pregnancy rates of about 80 percent for partners of men who have their vasectomies reversed within 10 years of the original procedure, most studies report figures in the 50 percent range. In at least half of all men who have had vasectomies, the process of absorbing sperm (instead of ejaculating it) results in antisperm antibodies that may interfere with later fertility. Other factors, such as length of time between the vasectomy and the reversal surgery, may also be important predictors of reversal success.

Female Sterilization

The most common method of female sterilization involves severing or in some manner blocking the oviducts, thereby preventing the egg from reaching the uterus and the sperm from entering the tubes. Ovulation and menstruation continue, but the unfertilized eggs are released into the abdominal cavity and absorbed. Although progesterone levels in the blood may decline slightly, in general hormone production by the ovaries and secondary characteristics are not affected.

One method of **tubal sterilization** is accomplished by making a small incision in the abdominal wall, locating each oviduct, bringing it into view, severing it, removing a small section, and tying or stapling shut the two ends (Figure 6-9). Another method involves making the incision through the vaginal wall, an approach that leaves no visible scar but is associated with a higher complication rate. Either a regional or a general anesthetic can be used with these two types of tubal sterilization, and the operation takes about 30 minutes. If no complications occur, many hospitals allow the patient to return to her home the same day. The operation can be performed shortly after a normal delivery, or in the case of cesarean section immediately after the incision in the uterus is repaired.

Female sterilization by the standard abdominal or vaginal procedure is riskier than male sterilization. About 7 percent of the patients experience problems after the operation. Such problems arise mainly from wound infection or bleeding. Serious complications are rare, and the death rate is low—especially when regional rather than general anesthesia is used.

An increasing number of tubal sterilizations are being

done by a method called **laparoscopy**. A laparoscope, which is a tube containing a small light, is inserted through a small abdominal incision, and the surgeon looks through it to locate the oviducts. Instruments are passed either through the laparoscope or through a second small incision, and the two oviducts are cauterized (sealed off) by electrocautery. Either a regional or general anesthetic can be used, but a general anesthetic is more common. The operation takes 15 minutes and can be done without overnight hospitalization. Most women leave the hospital two to four hours after surgery. Complications, such as bowel injury and hemorrhage, occur in 0.1 to 7 percent of laparoscopic sterilizations. This figure varies widely depending on the experience of the surgeon and type of equipment available. The mortality rate is low.

Laparoscopy has approximately the same failure rate as standard tubal ligations: about 4 out of every 1,000 cases. When pregnancies do occur, an increased percentage of them are ectopic. All women who undergo tubal sterilization should be alerted to this fact. Reversibility rates are 50–70 percent for all methods.

Complaints of long-term abdominal discomfort and menstrual irregularity have been reported following female sterilization, but these have been difficult to interpret. Most women are satisfied. The number of women who feel regret varies in follow-up studies, and this fact, too, is difficult to interpret. Regret, when it does appear, seems to be related to previous difficulties, initial doubts and reservations, feelings of being pressured by the spouse, or changes in marital and family circumstances.

Hysterectomy, removal of the uterus, is the preferred method of sterilization for only a small number of women, usually women with preexisting menstrual problems. Because of the risks involved, hysterectomy is not recommended unless the patient has serious gynecologic problems, such as disease or damage of the uterus, and future surgery appears inevitable.

NEW METHODS OF CONTRACEPTION

Even with all the improvements of recent years, the best of the present methods of contraception have drawbacks. The search still continues for the ideal method, the one that will be more effective, safer, cheaper, easier to use, more readily available, easily reversible, and acceptable to more people.

Many people place a high priority specifically on an increase in contraceptive alternatives for males. Throughout history, the responsibility for birth control has been assumed predominantly by women, partly because women have greater personal investment in preventing pregnancy, with its many risks, and childbearing, with the many demands that fall mostly on women. Some women

in some settings see complete control as crucial. More birth control options have been available for female use, because there are more ways to intervene in the female reproductive system. Another factor may be the continuing underrepresentation of women in medicine, scientific research, pharmaceutical management, the FDA, and other political forces. Participation by women and an emphasis on their needs regarding birth control has been limited in these areas.

After years of diminishing contraceptive choice in the United States, several new methods have recently been approved and are now being marketed. Many new birth control methods are used widely in other countries long before they become available in the United States. This delay is due in part to higher costs of preclinical safety testing in the United States, greater liability risk for manufacturers, and lower levels of government funding for contraceptive research. Some of the newest methods that are being studied are listed below:

• *Biodegradable implants.* As with Norplant capsules, these implants filled with progestin are inserted under the skin. They provide long-term, effective contraception. Unlike Norplant, the capsules dissolve over time, eliminating the need for surgical removal.

• *Vaginal ring.* The vaginal ring resembles the rim of a diaphragm and is molded with a mixture of progestin and estrogen. The woman inserts the ring herself and wears it for three weeks, during which time the hormones are absorbed into her bloodstream, preventing ovulation. Menstruation follows removal, and then a new ring is inserted.

• *Chemical contraceptives for men.* Male and female hormones can interfere with sperm development in the male in a way similar to ovulation suppression in the female. However, effectiveness of these hormones is often unpredictable, and side effects may include weight gain, acne, and perhaps a long-term risk of heart disease. In addition, weekly injections are usually required.

  Gossypol, a derivative of cottonseed oil, used for several years in China, also results in very low sperm counts. Reported side effects include disturbances in potassium metabolism and general weakness. Also, animal studies in the United States indicate that it may be carcinogenic.

• *Injectable microspheres.* A solution containing tiny clusters of molecules, each cluster filled with

---

Tubal sterilization   Severing or in some manner blocking the oviducts. This prevents ova (eggs) from reaching the uterus.

Laparoscopy   Examining the internal organs by inserting a tube containing a small light through an abdominal incision.

Hysterectomy   Total or partial surgical removal of the uterus.

hormones, is injected into the body. Over a period of one to six months, these particles release a fairly constant dose of hormones. This method is being studied with various hormones for use in both men and women.

- *Contraceptive immunization.* Immunity to fertility has—rarely—occurred because a man has been (nonexperimentally) sensitized to his own sperm cells. He then produces antibodies that inactivate sperm as if they were a disease. In theory, a woman could be purposely sensitized against her own egg cells or against her partner's sperm cells. Experimentally, at least, the theory works, but widespread human testing cannot begin until several questions have been answered. How long the immunity would last and how to control it are not yet known, and serious allergic reactions could be a life-threatening problem.

- *Reversible sterilization.* Present methods of sterilization of both men and women are reversible 50–70 percent of the time. Several new techniques of sterilization are being studied in the hope that restoring fertility can be made easier and more predictable.

Female sterilization has been attempted by injecting liquid silicone into the fallopian tubes, where it solidifies and forms a plug. In animal experiments, however, such plugs have been readily dislodged by normal muscle activity, so this method is not likely to be very effective.

In men, totally blocking sperm flow with removable clips and with various plugs has been tried, but both clips and plugs damaged the vasa, making restoration of fertility less likely. Recanalization of the vas, a phenomenon in which the sperm make a new path around the plug, has also occurred with plugs. Some of the plugs tested contain a tiny valve that can be opened manually or magnetically.

Even when tissue damage and recanalization can be prevented, researchers face another problem: Some men who have had vasectomies develop antibodies to their sperm, which may persist after vasectomy reversal.

- *Prostaglandins.* A new and promising use of **prostaglandins** is their application to tampons, which are inserted to bring on menstruation shortly after a period is missed. Prostaglandin tampons used regularly at the end of each cycle could induce menstruation each time whether or not the cycle had been fertile.

TERMS

Prostaglandins   Naturally occurring chemicals that stimulate uterine muscle and result in cramping.

- *Luteinizing hormone-releasing hormone (LHRH).* A naturally occurring compound in both men and women, LHRH acts on the pituitary gland, triggering the release of its hormones, which in turn play an essential role in sperm formation and ovulation. Synthetic analogs of LHRH, which are over 100 times as powerful as natural LHRH, are currently available. After these analogs are administered, the levels of pituitary hormones rise sharply, followed by a drop to subnormal levels, probably because the pituitary gland is overstimulated and exhausted. Once the low levels are established, it appears that in women (on whom most of the studies thus far have been completed) the pituitary-ovary cycle is effectively disrupted, and ovulation and menstruation stop temporarily. No immediate side effects have been detected. However, many questions regarding this complex interaction and its long-term effects remain, and any possible clinical application is undoubtedly several years away.

ISSUES IN CONTRACEPTION

The subject of contraception is closely tied to several issues that are currently receiving much attention in the United States—issues like premarital sexual relations, gender differences, and sex education for teenagers.

When Is It OK to Begin Having Sexual Relations?

One issue that strongly affects a society's approach to contraception is the question of when to begin having sexual relations. Opinions on this issue often determine one's views on sex education and contraception accessibility. A wide range of responses to this question can be found in the United States: Only after marriage, when 18 years or older, when in a loving, stable relationship, when the partners have completed their education and/or could support a child, and whenever both partners feel ready and are using protection against pregnancy and STDs.

Opinions on sexual behavior shift from one decade to another. Although attitudes toward sexual relations became more liberal through the 1960s and 1970s, people started holding more restrictive views as the 1980s passed. Current public opinion is almost evenly divided, with about half of Americans thinking premarital sex is wrong and about half finding it acceptable. The most common reasons given by individuals for their disapproval are moral or religious beliefs, risk of STDs, and risk of pregnancy.

Closely related to the issue of beginning sexual relations is the more personal question, What would you consider the ideal amount of previous sexual experience for you and your spouse at the time of your marriage? Again, the views on this vary, especially in terms of what

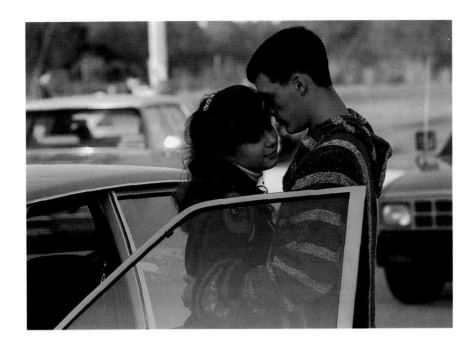

How old should people be when they become sexually active? The answer to this question depends on the personal values, beliefs, and experiences of the individuals involved.

is desirable for men and for women. While limited experience is still more commonly deemed desirable for women, being "sexually experienced" is often valued more highly for men.

As more women consider careers for themselves and therefore often delay childbearing and even marriage, the likelihood of sexual activity and the critical need for pregnancy and STD prevention only increase. As a result, making decisions about sexual activity and contraception becomes even more important to those starting college or a career. Unfortunately, however, many individuals in this age group, even those who protect their health in all other areas of their life, do end up taking high risks in their sexual behavior. Ambivalence and lack of communication about who will "take charge" is common and is partly due to the denial and hypocrisy regarding sexual behavior in our society.

Contraception and Gender Differences

A second issue, one all couples must confront, is the differing significance of contraception to women and men; the consequences of not using contraception are markedly different for men and women. In past years, women have accepted the primary responsibility of contraception, along with related side effects and health risks, partly because of the wider spectrum of birth control methods available to them. Men still have very few contraceptive options, with condoms being the only nonpermanent method. Recently, however, their participation has become critical, since condom use is central to "safer sex," even when OCs or other female methods are being used.

Although dependent primarily on cooperation of the man, condom use and the prevention of STDs has poten-

tially greater consequences for the woman. While men may suffer only local and short-term effects from the most common diseases (not including HIV infection), women face an increased risk of serious long-term effects, such as cervical cancer and/or pelvic infection with associated infertility, from these same prevalent STDs. In addition, women are more likely to contract HIV infection from an infected partner than vice versa. In other words, although dependent on the male, condom use is clearly a more important issue for women. The female condom may offer a helpful alternative, but cooperation of the male partner is still needed to ensure correct use.

Similarly, the experience of an unintended pregnancy is very different for the two involved partners. While men do suffer emotional stress from such an unexpected occurrence (and sometimes share financial and/or custodial responsibilities), women are much more intimately affected, simply by the natural, biological processes of the pregnancy and the outcome, whether abortion, adoption, or parenting. In addition, our societal attitudes are more severely punitive toward the woman and place much greater responsibility and blame on her when an unintended pregnancy occurs; the focus is almost entirely on the "girl who got into trouble" or the "unwed mother," with no mention of the "unwed father." With the current trend of cutting welfare support for single mothers, this growing number of young women and their children will live with even greater disadvantages.

Fortunately, there is a growing interest in the roles and responsibilities of men in family planning. For example, an American Public Health Association (APHA) Task Force on Men in Family Planning and Reproductive Health recently completed a review of available resources in this area. This group concluded that there is a serious

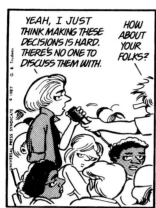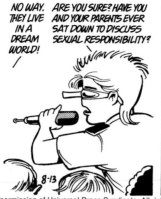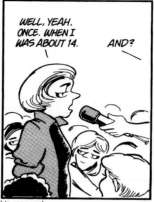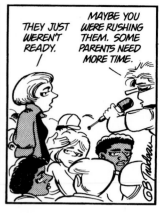

lack of both educational materials and clinical programs that focus on male contraception and reproductive health. Men can increase their participation in contraception by initiating and supporting communication regarding contraception and STD protection; buying and using condoms whenever indicated; assisting in payment of contraceptive expenses; and being available for shared responsibility in the resolution of an unintended pregnancy, should one occur.

Sex and Contraceptive Education for Teenagers

A third controversial question focuses on the best approach for sex education and pregnancy prevention programs for teenagers. Again, opinion in the United States is sharply divided. Certain religious groups express concern that more sex education, and especially the availability of contraceptives, will lead to more sexual activity and promiscuity. They maintain that greater access to improved contraception was a key factor contributing to the "sexual revolution" in the 1960s and that the ensuing liberal sexual attitudes have been generally more destructive than helpful. They point to an increase in divorces, a dramatic rise in STDs, and a general breakdown in morality as related negative effects.

Many in this group urge that educational responsibility be emphasized in the home, where parents can instill moral values, including premarital abstinence. According to some in this group, young people should primarily be taught and assisted to "just say no." They see most public education about contraception, and especially facilities that make supplies available, as only increasing the problem.

Other groups in the United States argue that encouraging public availability of contraceptive information and supplies does not necessarily result in an increase in promiscuous sexual behavior and point to the fact that many young teens are already pregnant when they first visit a health care facility. These groups assert that parents today aren't dealing effectively with the issue of sexuality and related problems and that a broader, coordinated approach involving public institutions, such as the school,

is needed, along with parental input. Many currently used programs focus on postponing sexual involvement as a central theme, but also emphasize contraceptive use for individuals who are sexually active. Increased availability of contraceptive information and the methods themselves is seen as a necessary and realistic part of this approach.

Proponents of sex and contraceptive education for teenagers point to countries like the Netherlands that have a far lower incidence of teenage pregnancy than does the United States (1.8 percent and 12.8 percent, respectively). Teenagers in the Netherlands are about as likely as American teens to engage in sexual intercourse, but they are far more likely to be using contraception. In the Netherlands, sex and contraceptive education are extensive and quite explicit in radio and television programming, and national health insurance and state-financed clinics provide and fund contraception. (For information on one organization's worldwide educational programs, see the box "Planned Parenthood.")

While sexual and contraceptive education in public facilities remains a volatile issue, there is overall growing support for such programs. Many studies do seem to show that sexually active students who receive sex education are more likely to use contraceptives and that those who are not sexually active are not encouraged to initiate such behavior. However, these programs are receiving increasing support mainly because of the prevalent fear of HIV infection and other STDs. In fact, in some cases the focus of "sex ed" is almost exclusively on disease prevention. Although not as deadly as the AIDS epidemic, the more than 1 million teen pregnancies that occur each year in the United States is a serious public health problem and warrants much greater national attention than it has received in the past.

> **Personal Insight** Did your parents tell you anything about contraception? Are your ideas and needs different from their expectations for you? What will you tell your children about contraception?

"Every child a wanted child": Since its stormy beginnings more than 60 years ago, Planned Parenthood Federation of America has sought to end compulsory parenthood by making birth control devices accessible to all who want them. Taking up their cause in local communities and courtrooms throughout the nation, Planned Parenthood has committed itself to making all Americans aware of the problems caused by unrestrained population growth, both here and abroad.

Planned Parenthood's educational goals are equally far-reaching. In the offices of all of its affiliates, basic birth control information is provided through films, group discussions, and individual counseling sessions. In addition, many affiliates offer special discussion groups for young people, where participants can talk about their anxieties, ask their questions, and share their problems in a supportive environment.

All the agency's affiliates also provide educational services within the community. Its trainers prepare teachers, social workers, nurses, and clergy to educate others in matters related to human sexuality and birth control.

Planned Parenthood's activities literally span the globe. The International Planned Parenthood Federation (IPPF) is the world's largest voluntary family planning organization. Dedicated to the formation and support of national family planning associations throughout the world, it assists in developing programs to educate people about the personal, social, and economic benefits of family planning. IPPF also provides technical information to several agencies of the United Nations and gives national associations financial support and technical assistance.

To contact Planned Parenthood, write:

Planned Parenthood Federation of America
810 Seventh Ave.
New York, NY 10019

WHICH CONTRACEPTIVE METHOD IS RIGHT FOR YOU?

If you are sexually active, you need to use the contraceptive method that will work best for you. The process of choosing and using a contraceptive method can be complex and varies greatly from one couple to another. Each individual must consider many variables in deciding which method is most acceptable and appropriate for her or him. Important considerations include:

1. *Individual health risks of each method in terms of personal and family medical history.* IUDs are not recommended for any young women without children, because of an increased risk of pelvic infection and subsequent infertility. Hormonal methods should be used only after a clinical evaluation of one's medical history. Other methods have only minor and local side effects.

2. *Implications of unwanted pregnancy and therefore the importance of effectiveness.* Hormonal methods, when used correctly, offer by far the best protection against pregnancy. Condoms, diaphragms, and cervical caps should be combined with a spermicide and used with every intercourse. Neither FAM nor withdrawal is very effective and should never be relied upon when pregnancy prevention is important. (The box "Improving the Effectiveness of Your Contraceptive Method" gives further details.)

3. *Possible risks of sexually transmissible diseases.* Condom use, preferably with foam, is of critical importance whenever any risk of STD is present. This is especially true when you are not in an exclusive, long-term relationship or when you are taking the pill, because cervical changes occurring during hormone use may lead to increased vulnerability to certain diseases. Abstinence or activities that don't involve intercourse or any other exchange of body fluids can be a satisfactory alternative for some individuals and couples.

4. *Convenience and comfort of the method as viewed by each partner.* The hormonal methods are generally ranked high in this category unless there are negative side effects and health risks or if forgetting to take pills is a problem with OC use. Some users think condom use disrupts spontaneity and lowers penile sensitivity. (Creative approaches to condom use and improved quality can decrease these complaints.) The diaphragm, cap, sponge, and spermicides can be inserted before intercourse begins, but are still considered a significant bother by some.

5. *Type of relationship.* The barrier methods require more motivation and a sense of responsibility from *each* partner than hormonal methods do. When the method depends on the cooperation of one's partner, assertiveness is necessary, no matter how difficult. This is especially true in new relationships, when condom use is most important. When sexual activity is infrequent, a barrier method may make more sense than an IUD or one of the hormonal methods.

6. *Ease and cost of obtaining and maintaining each method.* With OC use, an annual pelvic exam and periodic clinic checks are required and important. In addition,

Combination oral contraceptive	Follow pill-taking instructions carefully and consistently. Use a backup method such as foam or condoms during the first month.
IUD	Frequently check for IUD's position during the first few months. (User should feel thread in cervical opening but not the stem of the IUD.)
	Use a backup method such as foam or condoms during the first three months and, if desired, at midcycle thereafter.
Condom	Use with every act of intercourse.
	Put condom on erect penis before *any* penis-vagina contact.
	Leave space in tip of condom for semen.
	Remove carefully to avoid spillage.
	Avoid damage to condom; handle carefully.
	Avoid heat and Vaseline or any products containing mineral or vegetable oils.
	Do not use after one year.
	Use foam along with condom.
Diaphragm and jelly	Use with every act of intercourse.
	Ask for thorough instruction with initial fitting.
	Have diaphragm and its fit checked every one to two years by an experienced clinician. Replace if necessary. Also have fit checked after a weight change of more than 10 pounds.
	Always use ample amounts of jelly or cream; add as necessary.
	Check position after insertion. Front rim must be behind pubic bone, and dome must cover cervix.
	Inspect regularly for defects or holes.
	Avoid use of Vaseline or any products containing mineral or vegetable oils or perfumed powders, including talcum powder, as they can damage the latex and irritate the vagina.
Vaginal spermicides	Use with every act of intercourse.
	Follow instructions regarding time limits of effectiveness.
	Use ample amounts.
	When using foam, shake vigorously before use.
	Use condoms along with spermicide.
FAM	Combine calendar, temperature, and mucus methods.
Withdrawal	Avoid penis-vagina contact during secretion of preejaculatory lubricating fluid (very difficult to detect).
	Use foam along with coitus interruptus.

Whenever you discontinue one method, immediately replace it with another. Many unplanned pregnancies occur when couples "take a chance" between methods.

If you are sexually active, you need to use the contraceptive method that will work best for you. A number of factors may be involved in your decision. The following questions will help you sort out these factors and choose an appropriate method. Answer yes (Y) or no (N) for each statement as it applies to you and, if appropriate, your partner.

____ **1.** I like sexual spontaneity and don't want to be bothered with contraception at the time of sexual intercourse.

____ **2.** I need a contraceptive immediately.

____ **3.** It is very important that I do not become pregnant now.

____ **4.** I want a contraceptive method that will protect me and my partner against sexually transmissible diseases.

____ **5.** I prefer a contraceptive method that requires the cooperation and involvement of both partners.

____ **6.** I have sexual intercourse frequently.

____ **7.** I have sexual intercourse infrequently.

____ **8.** I am forgetful or have a variable daily routine.

____ **9.** I have more than one sexual partner.

____ **10.** I have heavy periods with cramps.

____ **11.** I prefer a method that requires little or no action or bother on my part.

____ **12.** I am a nursing mother.

____ **13.** I want the option of conceiving immediately after discontinuing contraception.

____ **14.** I want a contraceptive method with few or no side effects.

If you answered "yes" to the statements listed on the left, the method on the right might be a good choice for you.

1, 3, 6, 10, 11	Oral contraceptives
1, 3, 6, 8, 10, 11	Norplant
1, 3, 6, 8, 10, 11, 12	Depo-Provera
1, 3, 6, 8, 11, 12, 13	IUD
2, 4, 5, 7, 8, 9, 12, 13, 14	Condoms (male and female)
5, 7, 12, 13, 14	Diaphragm and spermicide
5, 7, 12, 13, 14	Cervical cap
2, 5, 7, 8, 12, 13, 14	Sponge
2, 5, 7, 8, 12, 13, 14	Vaginal spermicides
5, 7, 13, 14	FAM

Your answers may indicate that more than one method would be appropriate for you. To help narrow your choices, circle the numbers of the statements that are *most* important for you. Before you make a final choice, talk with your partner(s) and your physician. Consider your own lifestyle and preferences as well as characteristics of each method (effectiveness, side effects, costs, and so on). For maximum protection against pregnancy and STDs, you might want to consider combining two methods. It's also a good idea to be prepared for change—the method that seems right for you now may be inappropriate if your circumstances change.

the cost of the pills themselves tends to be higher than barrier supplies for most couples, although insurance plans will sometimes cover pill expense. The initial cost of Norplant may be high, and use of Depo-Provera involves an injection every 12 weeks. Diaphragms and cervical caps also require an initial exam and fitting.

7. *The method's acceptability in terms of religious or other philosophical beliefs.* According to the religious beliefs of some individuals, abstinence is the only acceptable form of sexual behavior in all premarital relationships. Even after marriage, the Catholic Church holds that all artificial birth control is wrong and that FAM is the only permissible contraceptive method.

Whatever your needs, circumstances, or beliefs, do make a choice about contraception—not choosing anything is the one method known *not* to work. (To help make a choice that's right for you, take the quiz "Which Contraceptive Method Is Right for You and Your Partner?") This is an area in which taking charge of your health has immediate and profound implications for your future. The method you choose today won't necessarily be the one you'll want to use your whole life or even next year. But it should be one that works for you right now. Contraception is something you can't afford to leave to chance.

SUMMARY

Principles of Contraception

- Barrier methods of contraception physically prevent the sperm from reaching the egg; hormonal methods are designed to prevent ovulation, fertilization, and/or implantation; and surgical methods permanently block the movement of sperm or eggs to the site of potential conception.

- Choice of contraceptive method depends on effectiveness, convenience, cost, reversibility, side effects and risk factors, and protection against STDs. The concept of effectiveness includes failure rate and continuation rate.

Reversible Contraceptives

- In oral contraceptives (OCs), a combination of estrogen and progestins prevents ovulation, hinders the movement of sperm, and affects the uterine lining so that implantation is inhibited.

- Advantages of OCs include their high degree of effectiveness, simplicity of use, freedom from interruption during foreplay and intercourse, and reversibility. In addition to minor disadvantages, possible serious side effects for some women include blood clots, stroke, and heart attacks.

- The "morning after" pill prevents implantation of the fertilized embryo. No postcoital contraceptives currently have FDA approval.

- Norplant consists of six hormone-filled capsules that are inserted under the skin. They release steady doses of synthetic progesterone that provide effective, reversible contraceptive protection for up to five years.

- Depo-Provera injections contain a long-acting progestin that protects against pregnancy for a period of three months.

- How intrauterine devices work is not clear; they may cause biochemical changes in the uterus, immobilize sperm in the uterus, shorten the travel time of the egg in the oviduct, or interfere with the implantation of the egg in the uterus.

- Advantages of IUDs include reliability, simplicity of use, freedom from interruption during coitus, and—in the absence of complications—reversibility. Pelvic inflammatory disease (PID), a serious complication

possible with IUD use, can lead to infertility if not treated with antibiotics.

- Condoms are the most popular barrier method, and their use has increased dramatically, partly because of their effectiveness against STDs.

- Advantages of condoms include availability and ease of purchase, simplicity of use, immediate reversibility, protection against STDs, and freedom from side effects.

- Female condoms consist of a polyurethane or latex sheath that can be inserted well before intercourse. They may be less reliable than male condoms in preventing pregnancy and the transmission of STDs.

- When used correctly, with spermicidal cream or jelly, the diaphragm covers the cervix and blocks sperm from entering. Diaphragms require a prescription, and a careful fitting is necessary.

- The cervical cap is a rubber or plastic cup that adheres to the cervix through suction. Effectiveness is similar to that of the diaphragm.

- The sponge is a round absorbent device with a concave dimple on one side that helps it fit snugly over the cervix. It is made of polyurethane and saturated with spermicide. Sponges act as barriers, spermicides, and absorbers of seminal fluid.

- Vaginal spermicides come in the form of foams, creams, jellies, and suppositories. They must be inserted less than one-half hour before intercourse.

- Because of religion, culture, poverty, or lack of information, many people use no contraception at all or use "natural" methods. Abstinence may be chosen out of fear of STDs or because of personal needs.

- The Fertility Awareness Method (FAM) is based on avoiding coitus during the fertile phase of a woman's menstrual cycle. A calendar method, a basal body temperature method, and a mucus method may be used to determine the fertile period.

- When withdrawal is used, the male must remove his penis from the vagina just before he ejaculates.

- Combining methods can increase contraceptive effectiveness and help protect against STDs.

Permanent Contraception—Sterilization

- Sterilization is permanent, and no further contraceptive action is needed. Reversibility can never be guaranteed. Male sterilization may be preferable to female sterilization because it's associated with fewer costs, complications, and feelings of regret.

- Vasectomy—male sterilization—involves severing the vasa deferentia. Female sterilization involves severing or blocking the oviducts so that the egg cannot reach the uterus.

New Methods of Contraception

- Contraceptive techniques currently under investigation include biodegradable implants, the vaginal ring, chemical contraceptives for men, injectable microspheres, contraceptive immunization, reversible sterilization, prostaglandins, and luteinizing hormone-releasing hormone.

Issues in Contraception

- Opinions on when to begin having sexual relations are tied to views on sex education and contraception accessibility. Because women today frequently delay childbearing, decisions about sexual activity and contraception are essential for optimal health.

- Although condom use depends on male cooperation, the implications of not using them are greater for women, both in terms of pregnancy and the consequences of STDs.

- Opinion in the United States is divided on the issues of sex education and availability of contraceptives for teenagers; increasing support for such programs is probably due to fear of HIV infection, although the issue of teen pregnancy needs more attention.

Which Contraceptive Method Is Right for You?

- Issues to be considered in choosing a contraceptive include (1) individual health risks of each method, (2) importance of effectiveness in terms of implications of unwanted pregnancy, (3) possible risk of sexually transmissible diseases, (4) convenience and comfort of the method as viewed by each partner, (5) type of relationship, (6) cost and ease of maintaining each method, (7) acceptability in terms of religious or philosophical beliefs.

TAKE ACTION

1. Make an appointment with a physician or other health care provider to review the health risks of different contraceptive methods as they apply to you. For each contraceptive method, determine if any risk factors associated with its use apply to you or your partner.

2. Visit a local drugstore and make a list of the contraceptives they sell and their prices. Next, investigate the costs of prescription contraceptive methods by contacting your physician, medical clinic, and/or pharmacy. Estimate the yearly cost of regular use of each method and rank the methods from most to least expensive.

3. Devise a public service campaign that will encourage men to become more involved in contraception. Your campaign might use techniques such as TV and print advertisements, radio announcements, and posters. Look at other public service campaigns and advertisements for ideas. What sorts of images do you think would be motivational? What sort of tone and message do you think would be most effective?

JOURNAL ENTRY

1. Consider the different methods of contraception described in this chapter. In your health journal, rank the methods according to how they suit your particular lifestyle. Take into account such considerations as how often you have sexual intercourse, convenience, and cost.

2. In your health journal, list the positive behaviors and attitudes that help you adhere to your beliefs about contraception (for example, not drinking alcohol or drinking only in moderation makes it unlikely that you would make an unwise choice because you had had too much to drink). Are there ways you can strengthen these behaviors? Then list behaviors and attitudes that might interfere with your effective use of contraception. Can you do anything to change or improve any of these?

3. *Critical Thinking:* What are your feelings about sex education for children and teens? Write a brief essay that presents the main arguments both for and against sex education for teens and children. Conclude your essay with a description of the sex education you received and a statement of your own opinion on whether sex education is valuable. Are you satisfied with what you were taught? What effect did it have on your sexual behavior? In general, do you think sex education promotes responsibility or promiscuity or neither?

SELECTED BIBLIOGRAPHY

Association for Voluntary Surgical Contraception (AVSC) statements about vasectomy and prostate cancer. 1991. *Advances in Contraception* 7(2–3): 313–15.

Ballagh, S. A., and D. R. Mishell. 1992. Who is a candidate for Norplant? *Western Journal of Medicine* 156(6): 649.

Broome, M., and K. Fotherby. 1990. Clinical experience with the progestogen-only pill (the mini-pill). *Contraception* 42(5): 489–95.

Brown, R. T., and others. 1992. Adolescent sexuality and issues in contraception. *Obstetrics and Gynecology Clinics of North America* 19(1): 177–91.

Cates, W., and K. M. Stone. 1992. Family planning, sexually transmitted diseases and contraceptive choice: A literature update—Part I. *Family Planning Perspectives* 24(2): 75–84.

———. 1992. Family planning, sexually transmitted diseases and contraceptive choice: A literature update—Part II. *Family Planning Perspectives* 24(3): 122–28.

Danielson, R., and others. 1990. Reproductive health counseling for young men: What does it do? *Family Planning Perspectives* 22(3): 115–21.

DeBuono, B. A., and others. 1990. Sexual behavior of college women in 1975, 1986, and 1989. *New England Journal of Medicine* 322(12): 821–25.

Derman, R. J. 1992. An overview of the noncontraceptive benefits and risks of oral contraception. *International Journal of Fertility* 37(1): 19–26.

Duke, R. C., and J. J. Speidel. 1991. Women's reproductive health: A chronic crisis. *Journal of the American Medical Association* 266(13): 1846–47.

Farley, T. M., and others. 1992. Intrauterine devices and pelvic inflammatory disease: An international perspective. *Lancet* 339: 785–88.

Guinan, M. E. 1992. HIV, heterosexual transmission, and women. *Journal of the American Medical Association* 268(4): 520–21.

Hannaford, P. C. 1991. Cervical cancer and methods of contraception. *Advances in Contraception* 7(4): 317–24.

Hatcher, R. A., and others. 1989. *Contraceptive Technology: International Edition,* 1989. Atlanta, Ga.: Printed Matter.

Holden, C., ed. 1992. Making converts for condoms. *Science* 256: 1514–15.

Miller, W. B., and others. 1991. Tubal sterilization or vasectomy: How do married couples make the choice? *Fertility and Sterility* 56(2): 278–84.

Paul, B. K. 1991. Family planning availability and contraceptive use in rural Bangladesh: An examination of the distance decay effect. *Economic Planning Sciences,* July, 269–83.

Petitti, D. B. 1992. Reconsidering the IUD. *Family Planning Perspectives* 24(1): 33–35.

Rosenberg, M. J., and others. 1992. Barrier contraceptives and sexually transmitted diseases in women: A comparison of female-dependent methods and condoms. *American Journal of Public Health* 82(5): 669–74.

Sadik, N. 1991. World population continues to rise. *The Futurist,* March/April, 9–14.

Stepanek, M. 1992. For Japanese, it's abortion instead of pill. *San Francisco Examiner,* 23 June, A2.

Stone, K. M., and H. B. Peterson. 1992. Spermicides, HIV, and the vaginal sponge [editorial]. *Journal of the American Medical Association* 268(4): 521–23.

Strader, M. K., and others. 1992. Effects of communication with important social referents on beliefs and intentions to use condoms. *Journal of Advanced Nursing* 17(6): 699–703.

Toufexis, A. 1989. Too many mouths. *Time.* 2 January, 48–50.

Wilcox, L. S., and others. 1991. Risk factors for regret after tubal sterilization: Five years of follow-up in a prospective study. *Fertility and Sterility* 55(6): 927–33.

Williams-Deane, M., and L. S. Potter. 1992. Current oral contraceptive use instructions: An analysis of patient package inserts. *Family Planning Perspectives* 24(3): 111–15.

RECOMMENDED READINGS

Boston Women's Health Book Collective. 1992. *The New Our Bodies, Ourselves.* New York: Simon and Schuster. *Comprehensive paperback, written from a woman's viewpoint. Broad coverage of many women's health concerns, with an emphasis on psychological, as well as physical factors. A favorite for many years. Periodically updated.*

Family Planning Perspectives (journal published bimonthly). New York: Alan Guttmacher Institute. *An excellent journal focused entirely on family planning issues. A good source for latest research findings. Some articles are quite technical (science-based and statistics-oriented), but all are very readable.*

Hatcher, R. A. and others. 1992. *Safely Sexual.* New York: Irvington. *Detailed coverage of how to plan for a safer sexual lifestyle. Realistic recommendations regarding the prevention of unplanned pregnancy, as well as HIV infection and other sexually transmissible infections.*

Hatcher, R. A., F. J. Guest, F. H. Stewart, G. K. Stewart, J. Trussell, S. Cerel, and W. Cates. 1990. *Contraceptive Technology 1990–92.* New York: Irvington. *A compact, reliable source of up-to-date information on contraception, with a focus on the technological aspects, rather than the psychological. The information is geared toward health care providers, but suitable for all readers. Many references and sources of information are included. Updated every two to three years.*

Stewart, F. H., and others. 1992. *Understanding Your Body.* New York: Bantam Books. *A broad and inclusive guide to women's gynecological health. Discusses common problems and everyday health care, as well as methods of contraception.*

Zilbergeld, B. 1992. *The New Male Sexuality.* New York: Bantam Books. *An update of the popular* Male Sexuality *(1978). A practical discussion of common issues in male sexuality; includes a chapter on sexual behavior and the single man.*

7

Abortion

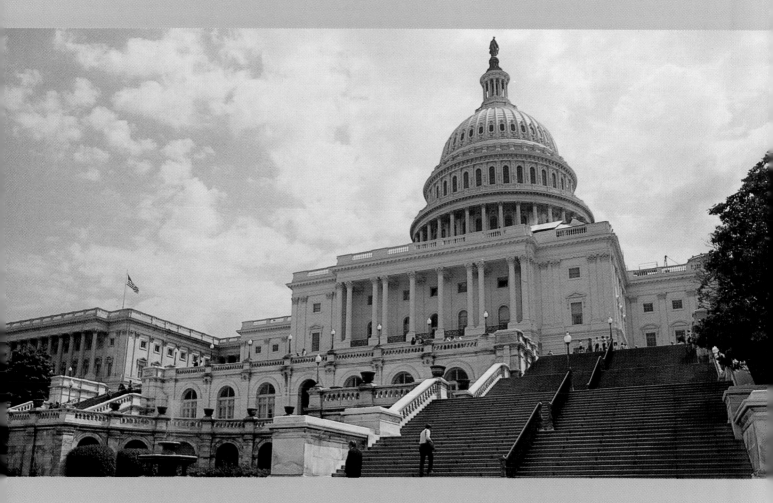

CONTENTS

◗ You and your boyfriend took a chance on having sex without contraception a while ago, and now you've missed your period. You haven't been able to think very clearly about what that might mean or focus on any kind of decisive action. Your boyfriend is pushing you to see a doctor or get a pregnancy test. He says that if you're going to want an abortion, the earlier you have it, the better. You want to wait a little longer and see if you get your next period. Which would be the better course of action?

◗ As the oldest of eight brothers and sisters, you've been around young children and babies your whole life. That's why you don't think you can end your accidental pregnancy with an abortion. It's also why you don't want to have a large family yourself or begin having children at 20. You're leaning toward giving the baby up for adoption, but you're worried that it won't be loved as much as you would love it or have a good home. Are your concerns justified? Is there any way you can ensure your child's well-being? How can you get the information you need to make your decision?

◗ Your roommate had an abortion several months ago. You expected her to be depressed afterwards, but instead she was euphoric. She said she was so relieved that she felt she'd gotten a whole new lease on life. She talked about how blue the spring sky was and how sweet the air smelled. But lately she's been unusually quiet and subdued, avoiding social occasions and spending a lot of time by herself. Could she still be reacting to the abortion? If so, is there anything you can do to help?

◗ You've thought about the abortion issue, but you don't really know where you stand. You recently listened to a discussion about abortion between two of your friends who have opposing opinions. Among the points brought up by your "pro-life" friend is that conception marks the beginning of life and that fetuses are human beings with civil rights. He also says that many abortions are performed on fetuses that could survive outside the womb if given the chance. Your "pro-choice" friend responds that most abortions are performed in the first eight weeks of pregnancy, long before the fetus could survive outside the womb. He also says that a woman has the right to make decisions about her own body. Are some of these claims true and others false? What information do you need to form your own opinion about abortion?

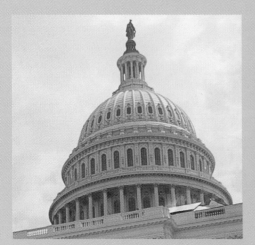

MAKING CONNECTIONS

Whether your connection with the abortion issue is political, social, or personal, it's likely that your life will be touched by this complex and emotional issue in the 1990s. In each of the abortion-related scenarios presented on these pages, individuals have to use information, make a decision, or choose a course of action. How would you act in each of these situations? What response or decision would you make? This chapter provides information about abortion issues and decisions that can be used in situations like these. After finishing the chapter, read the scenarios again. Has what you've learned changed how you would respond?

In the United States today, few issues are as complex and emotion-filled as abortion. While most public attention has focused on legal definitions and restrictions, the most difficult aspects of abortion actually take place at a much more personal level. Because the majority of women having abortions are young, many college students have had some type of direct exposure to these more personal experiences of abortion. This gives them an inside perspective on the dilemma.

On campuses today, as in our society at large, many powerful forces (including the great emphasis on sexuality and on the "good times" that follow alcohol consumption) contribute to the high rate of unintended pregnancy and abortion. At all school levels and in the general public, there is simultaneously great resistance to confronting these related issues openly and honestly—resulting in a lack of programs to deal with the problem at a preventive level.

With their inside vantage point, college students are in a key position to understand and to address the contributing factors as well as the broad effects of unintended pregnancies and abortion. Instead of simply attempting to legislate certain behaviors, they can choose to grapple with the complex human factors that go into the prevention as well as the "treatment" of unintended pregnancy. This chapter will provide basic information on abortion, including the current focuses of controversy. We hope it will act as a springboard for you to form your own views and, more importantly, personal plans for constructive action.

THE ABORTION ISSUE

The following discussion presents various perspectives on abortion. The word **abortion,** by official or strict definition, means the expulsion of a fetus from the uterus before it is sufficiently developed to survive. As commonly used, however, *abortion* refers only to those expulsions that are artificially induced by mechanical means or drugs, and *miscarriage* is the word generally used for a spontaneous abortion, one that occurs naturally with no causal intervention. In this chapter, the word *abortion* will be used as it is commonly, to mean a deliberately induced abortion.

History of Abortion in the United States

For more than two centuries, abortion policy in the United States followed English common law, which made the practice a crime only when performed after "quickening" (fetal movement that begins at about 20 weeks). There was little public objection to this policy until the early 1800s when an anti-abortion movement began, led primarily by physicians who questioned the doctrine of quickening and who objected to the growing practice of abortion by untrained persons (in part because it weakened their control of medical services).

This anti-abortion drive gained minimal attention until the mid-1800s, when newspaper advertisements for abortion preparations became common and concern grew that women were using abortion as a means of birth control (and perhaps to cover up extramarital activity). There was much discussion about the corruption of morality among women in the United States, and by the 1900s, virtually all states had anti-abortion laws. These laws stayed in effect until the 1960s, when courts began to invalidate them on the grounds of constitutional vagueness and violation of right to privacy.

Current Legal Status

In 1973, the abortion issue was thrust to the center of legal debate when the U.S. Supreme Court made abortion legal in the landmark case of *Roe vs. Wade.* To replace the restrictions most states still imposed at that time, the justices devised new standards to govern abortion decisions. They divided pregnancy into three parts, or trimesters, giving a pregnant woman less choice about abortion as she advances toward full term. In the first trimester, the abortion decision must be left to the judgment of the pregnant woman and her physician. During the second trimester, similar rights remain but a state may regulate factors that protect the health of the woman, such as type of facility where an abortion may be performed. In the third trimester, when the fetus is viable (capable of survival outside of the uterus), a state may regulate and even bar all abortions except those considered necessary to preserve the mother's life or health.

Since 1973, campaigns have been waged to overturn the Supreme Court decision and to ban abortions altogether. In addition, attempts have been made to add restrictions at local, state, and national levels. Although the Supreme Court has continued to uphold the *Roe* decision, its support for abortion rights has decreased markedly in recent years, with the presidential appointments of several conservative justices.

In July 1989, another legal milestone was reached, when the Supreme Court handed down its decision in *Webster vs. Reproductive Health Services.* The Court did not overturn *Roe,* but did let stand several key restrictions on abortions enacted by the Missouri legislature in 1986. The two most severe restrictions forbid the use of all public facilities, resources, and employees for abortion services and require costly and time-consuming tests to determine fetal viability whenever the doctor estimates the

Abortion The premature expulsion or removal of an embryo or fetus from the uterus.

TERMS

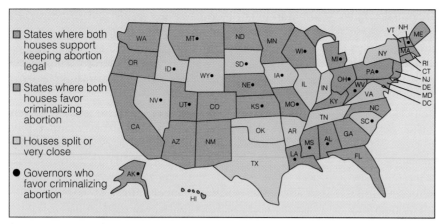

Figure 7-1 *Disparities in attitudes toward legal abortion.*
Source: "Abortion Laws State-by-State." *Time,* 14 May 1992.

fetus to be 20 weeks or older. In June 1992, another major Court decision was handed down in *Planned Parenthood of Southeastern Pennsylvania vs. Casey.* Although this ruling continues to uphold a woman's basic right to abortion, it gives the state further powers to regulate abortion throughout pregnancy, as long as it does not impose an "undue burden" on women seeking the procedure. The Court decided that the following provisions of the Pennsylvania law do not constitute "undue burden" and therefore let these restrictions stand: Women seeking abortion must be told about fetal development and alternatives to ending their pregnancies; they must wait at least 24 hours after receiving that information; minors must get permission from a parent or judge; and physicians are required to keep detailed records, subject to public disclosure. The Court turned down a requirement that married women must notify their husbands of their intention to have an abortion.

Since the Webster and Casey decisions gave few guidelines (other than that further state restrictions will probably be upheld), chaos can be expected at the state levels. Great disparities in the availability of legal abortion are likely to exist from one area of the country to another, causing a checkerboard effect (Figure 7-1). States where abortion laws had been liberalized prior to the 1973 *Roe* decision, mostly in the West, the Northeast, and the Middle Atlantic regions, probably will not change their laws significantly. Other states, mainly those where fundamentalist or Mormon influence is strong, are likely to end up with numerous restrictive measures, but not the outright prohibition many have been seeking. Those states in between will probably add fewer but similar regulations, including those enacted in Missouri and Pennsylvania.

While not banning abortion outright, the addition of these various regulations will seriously restrict accessibility to abortion for many women, especially those with limited resources. For example, the indigent and the young will be most affected by any prohibitions placed on public facilities and funding. These are the same women who will be most affected by legal changes necessitating travel for a legal abortion and laws requiring additional tests in the case of late abortion (since they make up the bulk of those having late abortion). Concerns have been expressed that the new regulations may result in a two-tiered health care system, one for women with means and another for those without.

The complete overturning of *Roe vs. Wade* by the Supreme Court may occur as numerous new test cases are brought for its consideration. Such a reversal would permit, but not require, states to prohibit all abortion. In the absence of federal legislation, differences in availability, cost, and timing of abortion would continue to exist from one state to another, depending on each one's laws and court interpretations. Both pro-choice and pro-life groups will most likely move to the national level, seeking federal legislation, the former to ensure abortion rights (as found in the Freedom of Choice Act) and the latter to make abortion a federal crime (laws pertaining to the health care provider and/or the woman having the abortion).

Attention is also being focused on political campaigns and the backing of candidates with well-defined views on abortion. In the foreseeable future, heated debate is likely to continue.

Personal Insight   Some people believe that teenagers should have their parents' permission before they can have an abortion and married women should have their husband's permission before they can have an abortion. How do you feel about these restrictions?

Moral Considerations

Along with the legal debates have come ongoing arguments between "pro-life" and "pro-choice" groups regard-

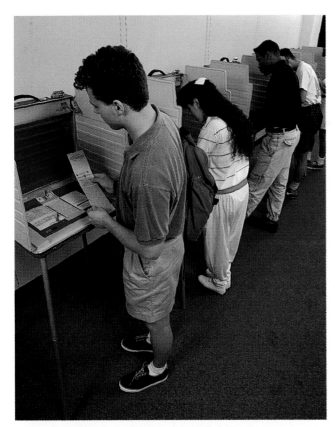

Voting for political candidates with well-defined views on abortion is one way in which individuals can influence the legal status of abortion in the United States.

decision possible must be determined according to each individual situation and that in some cases greater injustice would result if abortion were not an option. If legal abortions were not available, some pro-choice supporters say, "back-alley shops" and do-it-yourself techniques, with their many health risks, as well as the births of unplanned children, would again grow in number. Others argue that discrimination in health care would result, since wealthy women could more easily make the travel arrangements necessary for a legal abortion elsewhere. Still others emphasize that some physicians, because of their strong personal convictions regarding abortion rights, would feel forced into becoming lawbreakers.

Some individuals strongly identify exclusively with either the pro-life or the pro-choice stance, but many people have moral beliefs that are blurred, less defined, and in some cases a mixture of the two. A common assumption is that all religious organizations and individuals adhere to the pro-life position. This notion can be misleading. Although some generalizations can be made, moral positions regarding abortion can vary widely among religious believers just as they can differ markedly among individuals who consider themselves nonreligious.

Personal Insight How do you define life? When do you think it begins? How does your answer affect your position on abortion?

ing the ethics of abortion, what is right and what is wrong in a moral sense (see the box "The Opposing Views"). Central to the pro-life position is the belief that the fertilized egg must be valued as a human being from the moment of conception and that abortion at any time is equivalent to murder. This group holds that any woman who has sexual intercourse knows that pregnancy is a possibility, and should she willingly have intercourse and get pregnant she is morally obligated to carry the pregnancy through. Pro-life followers encourage adoption for women who feel they are unable to raise the child and point out how many couples are seeking babies for adoption. Pro-lifers do not see the availability of legal abortion as essential to women's well-being, but view it instead as having an overall destructive effect on our traditional morals and values.

By contrast, the pro-choice viewpoint holds that distinctions must be made between the stages of fetal development and that preserving the fetus of early gestation is not always the ultimate moral concern. Members of this group maintain that women must have the freedom to decide whether and when to have children; they argue that pregnancy can result from contraceptive failure or other factors out of a woman's control. When pregnancy does occur, pro-choice individuals believe that the most moral

Public Opinion

In general, U.S. public opinion on abortion is somewhat flexible and seems to change depending on the specific situation. Many individuals approve of legal abortion as an option when destructive health or welfare consequences could result from continuing pregnancy, but they do not advocate abortion as a simple way out of an inconvenient situation. Overall, most adults in the United States continue to approve of legal abortion and are opposed to overturning the basic right to abortion established in *Roe vs. Wade* (see the box "Public Opinion on Abortion"). But the amount of public support will vary considerably, depending on the circumstances surrounding the abortion request. Most people see many areas of ambiguity in the abortion issue.

For example, people who feel that abortion should be available in early pregnancy often question at which stage in later pregnancy the fetus's rights should take precedence over the woman's rights. The 1973 U.S. Supreme Court decision considered viability the key criterion in establishing the point beyond which a woman's right to choose abortion becomes markedly restricted. In 1973, viability was generally considered to be about 26 to 28 weeks. Today it is about 24 weeks, with isolated cases of survival at 23 weeks. Although neonatal intensive care *by Kate Michelman*

Let's start with the big lie: Pro-choice is pro-abortion. That single line, that total distortion, is the battle cry of the New Right. It is the banner flying over their crusade to eliminate a woman's freedom to choose.

Pro-choice is not pro-abortion. Pro-choice is pro-freedom, pro-family, and pro-children. Pro-choice is about the lives, health, and security of women, their children, and their families. It's about freedom—freedom of religion, freedom of conscience, freedom of speech, and the right to privacy. It's about the freedom to choose whether or not to bear a child. No other choice has more impact on our community and our nation.

When it comes to taxation or regulation, the New Right demands the right to privacy, the right to dignity, the right to freedom from government intervention. Doesn't a woman facing a crisis pregnancy deserve as much?

Reducing the need for abortion—not increasing the dangers and difficulties—should be our nation's goal. No one wants an abortion. We all wish we could sail through life without difficult, painful choices. But we live in a complex and uncertain world filled with risk, temptation, illusion, and sometimes terror. No matter how strong the outer protection of love, marriage, income, and stability, each pregnancy comes down to a separate judgment, a different choice.

Women should have the freedom to make that choice.

For most women, the choice of abortion is the hardest choice of all. Abortion is not a choice of convenience. It's a choice wrapped in questions of morality, religion, and ethics. Abortion is filled with wrenching ambivalence and deep matters of the heart. Abortion or not, a woman's right to make this decision should be guaranteed.

In 1973 the question before the Supreme Court in *Roe vs. Wade* was, Who should make the deeply personal and profound decision about pregnancy and childbirth?
Answer: The woman.

Roe is a compromise that balances the woman and the unborn. It favors one at first and then the other as term approaches. It chooses the middle ground, the essence of pro-choice. *Roe* is neither libertine nor Draconian. It is neither pro-abortion nor anti-abortion. *Roe* strikes a delicate balance between freedom and a responsibility.

For years women have considered the right to choose an abortion to be a basic freedom no less than freedom of speech or freedom of worship. However, in June 1992 the *Casey* decision imposed restrictions that pushed *Roe* to the very precipice. The Court took the most fundamental American freedom and shattered it into jagged parts.

People once said we shouldn't make choice a political issue. I wish we didn't have to. I wish we could count on the fundamental American right to privacy and dignity. But we've learned the hard way that we can't.

The pro-choice agenda goes beyond the right to choose abortion. It is aimed at creating an America that respects the lives of women, protects the lives of children, and makes whole and happy families.

In a nation with one of the highest rates of unintended pregnancy, we must address the social conditions that force millions of women each year to face the abortion question. Abortion and teen pregnancy are on the rise. Contraception is still hidden behind counters. Expectant mothers still give birth without prenatal care. When it comes to birth control, America is an underdeveloped nation.

America's national policy is fragmented and incoherent. We strongly believe that government has the obligation to pull the pieces together and form a comprehensive reproductive health policy. The central goal of the pro-choice agenda is to reduce abortions. The pro-choice plan seeks to ensure that women who choose to have children can do so in a supportive and healthy environment. We need fundamental and widespread education in human development and sexuality. Our children must understand not just the mechanics of sex and contraception but also the tremendous consequences of pregnancy and birth. It is not enough to counsel abstinence. We've got to foster joint parent/school programs to educate our children in the realities of sex, contraception, and choice. We need to clarify the options and consequences of having children. Not just the joys but the responsibilities. Not just the gifts but the costs.

Between 1980 and 1990 federal grants to nonprofit organizations for family planning services were cut by almost two-thirds. That's got to be reversed. We also urge the federal government to get behind school-linked health clinics. To effectively promote child and teen health, a comprehensive plan must include counseling on pregnancy prevention, drugs, and jobs. Any national reproductive health care plan must guarantee access to prenatal care, treatment for drug-dependent pregnant women, child care, and family and medical leave.

This is not an insurmountable agenda. These are not demands from the political extremes or appeals to break the bank. These are the simple, minimum steps toward a civilized, humane, durable reproductive policy—a policy Americans support.

Kate Michelman is president of the National Abortion Rights Action League.

J. C. Willke, M.D.

In looking at abortion, the first question to ask is, What is this that grows within the woman? Is this human life? Or, when will it be? If it's not human life, then a case can be made to permit abortion. If, however, this being is fully human, sexed, alive, complete, and intact from the first-cell stage, then a second human life exists and we have a collision of the rights of two humans.

So, first, let's ask: Is this human life? The answer lies in books on biology, embryology, and fetology. In these sciences there is no disagreement on the facts of when human life begins. At the union of sperm and ovum there exists a living, single-celled, complete human organism. It is already male or female, is alive and growing, and is human, as the 46 human chromosomes in the cell's nucleus mark this microscopic being as a member of the human family. This is arguably the most complicated cell in the entire world; it contains more information than could be contained in all of NASA's computers. As this single-celled human organism divides and subdivides, each cell in turn contains progressively less information, is more specialized.

At one week of life, this embryonic human attaches to the nutrient lining of the woman's womb and soon sends into her body a hormonal message that stops her period. About four days after the time when the woman's period would have begun, the embryo's heart begins to beat. At 40 days brain waves can be recorded. By 10 weeks the structure of the body is completely formed. By three months all organ systems are functioning. To deny that fully human life begins at fertilization is to deny the known facts of fetal development and biological science.

Some argue that life existed in the sperm and ovum and will exist in the future. True, but we are not asking about generic life, but rather about this one unique individual's human life, which begins at fertilization and ends at death.

Some would measure the beginning of human life with a theologic yardstick, speaking of soul, God, and creation. In a secular state, however, we cannot use a theologic belief to define when human life beings for the purpose of making laws that either protect or allow the destruction of that life.

Others use various philosophic definitions of when the fullness of humanness exists, such as when cognition and self-consciousness are possible, when love is exchanged, when a being is declared to be "humanized" or "socialized," or when certain biologic mileposts are reached. Though these definitions are arrived at by intellectual processes, they cannot be scientifically proven. Open to diametric disagreement among people of good will, these definitions are also beliefs. We should not impose either religious or philosophic beliefs upon others in our culture. If one defines human life from the facts of natural science, human life, complete and intact, begins at fertilization. That is a fact that we must face and work with.

Because this is human life from the very moment of conception, the issues touching that life are civil rights and human rights and the laws protecting those rights.

Now, let us ask a second question: Should there be equal protection under the law for all living humans? Or, should the law discriminate fatally against entire classes of humans, in this case against those still living in the womb?

Interestingly enough, our nation faced a similar situation once before—slavery. In 1857 the Supreme Court ruled in the Dred Scott case that black people were not legal persons before the law. They were the property of the slave owner, who could buy, sell, or even kill them. Abolitionists' protests were countered: "Now look, you find slavery morally offensive? Well, you don't have to own a slave. But don't force your morality on the owner, for he has the constitutional right to choose to own a slave." In 1973 the Court did it again. In *Roe vs. Wade,* also by a 7 to 2 margin, it ruled that unborn people were not legal persons. They were the property of the owner (the mother), who could keep or kill. Pro-lifers objected, to hear the same response. "Look, you find abortion morally offensive. Well, you don't have to have one. But don't force your morality on the owner (the woman) for she now has the constitutional right to choose, to kill."

The Dred Scott decision discriminated by skin color; *Roe vs. Wade* discriminates by place of residence: still living in the womb. Each is a civil rights outrage.

A woman has a right to her own body, but to say that the little passenger residing within her is a part of her body is to utter a biologic absurdity.

But she does not want this child? Since when does anyone's right to live depend upon someone else wanting them? Killing the unwanted is a monstrous evil.

A woman's issue? Did you know that women make up the overwhelming majority in the pro-life movement and that opinion polls consistently show more opposition to abortion from females than from males?

So, should a woman have the right to choose? I have a right to free speech, but not to shout "fire" in a theater. A person's right to anything stops when it injures or kills another living human.

No one should minimize the problems of pregnant women. With adequate counseling, informed consent, involvement of parents, husbands, and friends, we can help solve most of their problems, but sadly, never all of them. The pivotal question is, Should any civilized nation give to one citizen the absolute legal right to kill another to solve that first person's personal problem? I think not. We must give women far more help, both privately and publicly, than is available today. But we simply cannot continue to solve their personal problems by allowing the ghastly violence of killing tiny, innocent humans.

J. C. Willke is president of the Life Issues Institute and The International Right to Life Federation.

A majority of Americans believe that women should retain the right to abortion as established in *Roe vs. Wade* in 1973. But a majority also are in favor of some types of limits on abortion. The graph shown here illustrates how opinion about the legality of abortion has changed since Roe vs. Wade. The public opinion poll shows how Americans currently view the question of the legality of abortion and certain proposed limitations on its availability.

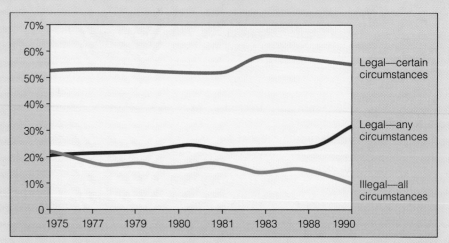

Legal—certain circumstances

Legal—any circumstances

Illegal—all circumstances

Responses to the question, Do you think abortions should be legal under any circumstances, legal only under certain circumstances, or illegal in all circumstances?

Source: Gallup Poll. The results are based on telephone interviews with nearly 2,500 adults conducted in April 1990. The margin of error is ± 3 percentage points

Abortion Views

		Favor	Oppose
1. Do you favor or oppose the U.S. Supreme Court ruling in 1973 that a woman can have an abortion if she wants one at any time during the first three months of pregnancy?		55%	38%

		Yes	No
2. During the first 3 months of pregnancy, do you think abortion should be legal . . .			
. . . when the woman's life is endangered?		87	10
. . . if the family cannot afford to have the child?		39	57
3. Do you think that a pregnant teenager under the age of 18 should be required by law to notify a parent before she could obtain a legal abortion?		80	18
4. Do you think that a pregnant married woman should be required by law to obtain the permission of her husband before she could obtain a legal abortion?		63	33
5. If the Supreme Court changes its view of the law so that each state could make its own laws about abortion, would you want your state to put limits on the availability of abortion?		56	41

Source: Washington Post, 1 July 1992.

Note: Results for first four questions are based on a national random sample by the *Washington Post* interviewd March 27–31. Results in final question are based on CBS-*New York Times* poll conducted June 17-20.

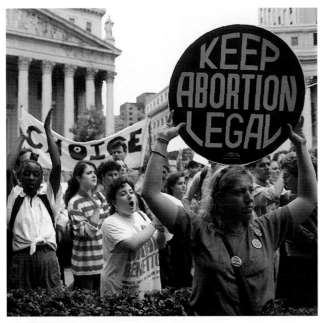

Pro-choice groups believe that the decision to end or continue a pregnancy is a personal matter that should be left up to the individual.

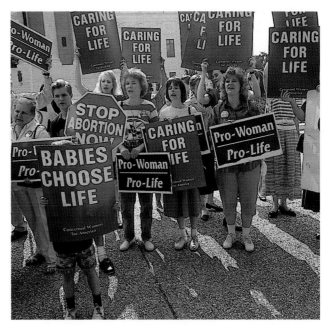

Pro-life groups oppose abortion on the basis of their belief that life begins at the moment of conception.

units continue to advance technologically, most experts feel that viability cannot ever be expected beyond this limit.

Other individuals associate fetal rights not with viability but with earlier developmental characteristics such as onset of heartbeat, brain size, and nervous system maturity. *The Silent Scream,* a widely shown film that used computer-enhanced ultrasound images, purports to depict a 12-week-old fetus "screaming in pain" during an abortion procedure, attributing a fully human response to the fetus. Critics contend that the film was manipulated, with portions of the footage being sped up to project the illusion of a fetus thrashing in terror. Experts in fetal medicine have refuted the film's medical premises, stating that at 12 weeks fetal responses are simply reflex activity and that brain and nervous systems are insufficiently developed to feel pain. In fact, researchers have recently described evidence that minimal nervous system connections necessary for brain function don't develop until after the fifth month of pregnancy.

Still other individuals argue that the embryo becomes a human being at the point of individuation or twinning, which occurs about two weeks after conception. (Before that time, the embryo has not yet differentiated into either a single or an identical twin pregnancy.) Others believe that the moment of conception is the only critical point to consider. For them, all other developmental stages are irrelevant to the abortion debate. As can be seen from such wide variation of opinion, objective measures of humanness and clear-cut guidelines regarding fetal rights are elusive, and decisions ambiguous.

Although opinions vary as to whether, or when, in pregnancy, abortion rights should be tightly regulated by law, most people agree that abortions done later in pregnancy present more difficulties in personal, medical, philosophical, and social terms. Who are the women who have late abortions? Of all abortions done after the twenty-first week of gestation, 44 percent are performed on teenagers. Possible explanations include teenagers' ignorance, denial, fear, and lack of supportive family or friends. Other typical recipients of late abortions include low-income women who may have more difficulty finding suitable facilities as well as necessary funds, and premenopausal women who fail to recognize a delayed period as pregnancy. Another small group of women who may seek late abortion are those who have learned through **amniocentesis** (the withdrawal and analysis of amniotic fluid) that the fetus is suffering from a specific abnormality, such as Down's syndrome. Because the results of this test are usually not available until the sixteenth week of pregnancy, abortion, if chosen, is necessarily delayed. (Chorionic villus sampling, a genetic diagnosis technique that can be performed in the first trimester, is becoming more available. However, this technique does not diagnose neural tube defects and also carries slightly more risk of miscarriage.)

Amniocentesis	Withdrawal of fluid from the amniotic sac.

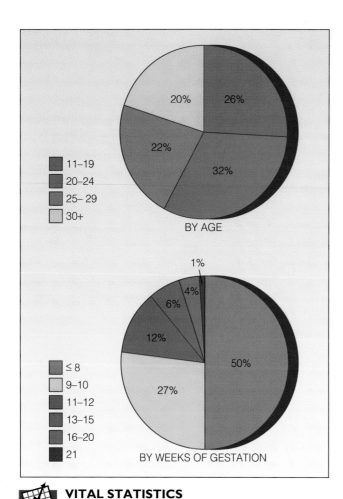

11–19
20–24
25– 29
30+

20%   26%

22%   32%

BY AGE

≤ 8
9–10
11–12
13–15
16–20
21

1%
4%
6%
12%   50%

27%

BY WEEKS OF GESTATION

VITAL STATISTICS

Figure 7-2 *Percentage distribution of all women who had abortions in 1988.*

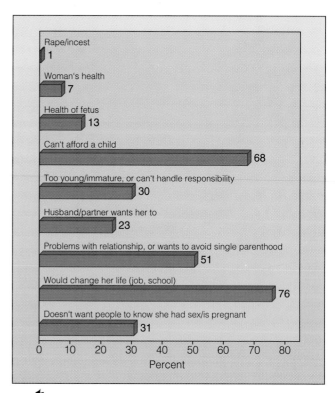

Rape/incest 1
Woman's health 7
Health of fetus 13
Can't afford a child 68
Too young/immature, or can't handle responsibility 30
Husband/partner wants her to 23
Problems with relationship, or wants to avoid single parenthood 51
Would change her life (job, school) 76
Doesn't want people to know she had sex/is pregnant 31

0 10 20 30 40 50 60 70 80
Percent

VITAL STATISTICS

Figure 7-3 *The reasons women choose abortions (respondents could give more than one answer).*

Personal Considerations

For the pregnant woman who is considering abortion, the usual legal and moral arguments may sound meaningless as she attempts to weigh the many short- and long-term ramifications for all lives directly concerned. If she chooses abortion, can she accept that decision in terms of her own religious and moral beliefs? What are her long-range feelings likely to be regarding this decision? What are her partner's feelings regarding abortion, and how will she deal with his responses? Does she have a supportive relative or friend who will help her through this time of emotional adjustment? Which medical facility offering abortions would be most suitable for her? What about transportation and costs? (See Figures 7-2 and 7-3 for information about women who choose abortion.)

For the woman who decides against abortion and chooses instead to continue the pregnancy, there are other questions. If she decides to raise the child herself, will she have the critical resources to do it well? Is a supportive, lasting relationship with her partner likely? If not, how does she feel about being a single parent? Are family members available to help with the many demands of child rearing? If she is young, what will the effects be on her own growth? Will she be able to continue with her educational and other personal goals? What about the ongoing financial responsibilities?

If the pregnant woman considers adoption, she will have to try to predict what her emotional responses will be throughout the full-term pregnancy and the adoption process. What are her long-range feelings likely to be? What is the best setting for her during her pregnancy? How can she best maintain continuity with the rest of her life and her long-term goals? Which adoption facility is likely to make the most suitable arrangements for her and her baby? A public or a private agency? Is anonymity between the adoptive parents and herself desirable or not? Does she have someone she trusts to help her with these difficult decisions? (The box "Adoption: How Viable an Alternative?" addresses some of these questions.)

Personal Insight How would you feel if you discovered that a fetus you were carrying (or your partner was carrying) had a serious genetic defect? Would you be likely to choose abortion? How much would the nature of the defect and its consequences for the baby and you affect your decision?

Adoption: How Viable an Alternative?

Many people encourage women to deal with unwanted pregnancies through adoption rather than through abortion. But adoption is much less commonly chosen than the other alternatives—abortion or keeping the baby—and adoption rates are falling. The proportion of married or once-married women who adopted a child in 1987 was 1.7 percent, down from 2.2 percent in 1982. And according to figures from the National Center for Health Statistics, only 200,000 women sought to adopt a child in 1988, about one-tenth the number expected. Why is adoption not a more attractive alternative to marriage, single parenthood, or abortion, and why are adoption rates falling?

One reason for this change is that many more women are keeping their babies than in the past. Thirty years ago, about 50 percent of single white women under 25 who became pregnant routinely gave up their babies for adoption. Today, partly because of the diminished social stigma attached to unmarried pregnancy, many young women are choosing to be single mothers rather than relinquish their babies.

Another reason is the current prevailing assumption that children are better off with their biological parents under almost any circumstances. Government policies and laws provide financial incentives—in the form of food stamps, food supplements, Aid to Families with Dependent Children, and other assistance—for biological families to stay together. The effect of such policies is to discourage adoption.

These and other factors have worked together to produce a smaller pool of babies placed for adoption each year—at least the babies most in demand, who are healthy, white newborns. Many more babies and children are in need of homes but are less likely to be adopted, including older children, siblings who must be adopted together, children with disabilities, babies born to drug-addicted mothers, babies with HIV infection, and children with physical, mental, emotional, or behavioral problems.

Additionally, cross-racial adoptions are often discouraged, reducing the chances that minority children will be adopted, since many more potential adoptive parents are white than black. Finally, financial factors can be barriers to adoption. In 1990 the average fee for receiving a child, not including some legal costs, was $8,500.

A factor that may change this pattern of falling adoption rates is the trend toward "open" adoptions. In the past, adoptions were usually conducted in secrecy. Mothers unable to care for their children handed them over to adoption agencies and stepped out of the picture, supposedly forever. Records were sealed, preventing any future contact between biological parents and children. But in the 1970s many adults who had been adopted began searching for their biological mothers, and many mothers acknowledged that they were unable to forget the child they had given up. Awareness of these difficulties has contributed to the movement toward open adoptions, in which names, addresses, health records, family histories, and other information are available to all parties involved.

Today, between 60 and 90 percent of all adoptions are open. Couples seeking a baby may put personal ads in newspapers and send letters to lawyers, obstetricians, and clergy across the nation in the hope of finding a pregnant woman willing to relinquish her baby. They usually pay the mother's medical expenses and sometimes her living expenses before and after the baby is born. The biological mother has the opportunity to choose the adoptive family and in many cases to keep in touch with them and her child.

Although open adoption can ease the difficult transition during which the baby passes from biological mother to adoptive parents, adoption is never carefree. Even for women who choose their child's adoptive parents, the transition can be accompanied by intense feelings of loss, grief, and regret. For other women, however, adoption may be the best of all possible solutions.

Adapted from "Abortion and the Adoption Option," *Washington Post Health,* 15 August 1989, p. 607; "Where Have All the Babies Gone?" *Money,* December 1988, pp. 164–76; "The Adoption Option," *American Demographics,* October 1989, p. 11; "Project Provides Help, Hope," *San Francisco Chronicle,* 7 July 1987; "Joys and Fears of Adopting a Child," *San Francisco Chronicle,* 6 March 1990, p. B3–B5; "Quiet Revolution in U.S. Adoption," *San Francisco Chronicle,* 24 September 1992.

Current Trends

Clearly, all responses to unintended pregnancy can be difficult, including abortion and especially late abortion. Fortunately, with the increased accessibility to legalized abortion following the mid-1970s, the rate of late abortions dropped steadily, until fewer than 1 percent of all abortions were performed at more than 20 weeks and fewer than 11 percent at more than 12 weeks by the mid-1980s. Also, the overall abortion *rate,* which rose during most of the 1970s and leveled off around 1980, fell gradually between 1982 and 1988 (Figure 7-4).

The effects of the 1989 *Webster* and 1992 *Casey* decisions and related restrictions are hard to predict. While some foresee a sharp decrease in the number of abortions in the United States, others argue that the overall total will change very little. Women seeking abortions usually do so with very strong motivation and determination and are not likely to be deterred easily. With the current availability of interstate transportation, many women may be able to travel whatever distances are necessary for a legal abortion. Others might well turn to more accessible, but illegal, nonmedical practitioners. Still others may find local

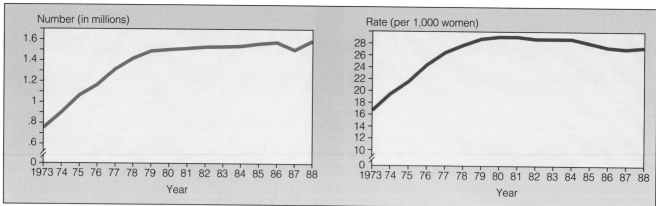

VITAL STATISTICS

Figure 7-4 *Abortion in the United States.*
(a) Number of legal abortions. (b) Rate of abortions per 1,000 women aged 15–44.

physicians who feel strongly about abortion rights and who therefore continue to perform abortions even under illegal circumstances, finding reassurance from those legal scholars who predict that many juries would not be willing to convict either the woman or the doctor of criminal activity. Although even women living in highly restricted areas may continue to obtain abortions, they are likely in most cases to face significant increases in expense and time delays (see the box "Facts About Abortion").

There is also growing speculation regarding the possible impact of the new "abortion pill," RU-486, now approved for use in several countries (see discussion later in this chapter). Although only recently approved for preliminary testing in the United States, this pill may become widely available through illegal channels, according to experts who point to the many other illicit drugs prevalent in our society. Other groups are suggesting that menstrual extraction kits, packaged with use instructions for lay individuals, may offer a self-help option for abortion seekers. Although both of these measures when used without medical supervision could carry serious health risks, they would undoubtedly be sought out by a certain number of women. Of great concern is the fact that "home remedies" may simply damage the fetus instead of causing an abortion.

Unless coupled with attention to the prevention of unwanted pregnancy, especially among the young and single women who make up the majority of those seeking abortions, legal changes alone will probably not reduce the number of abortions dramatically. Refer to the box "Abortion Around the World" for a broader perspective on the abortion issue.

We hope the recent surge of public interest in sexual behavior (largely due to fear of sexually transmissible diseases) will lead to more open discussion regarding sexuality and contraception for individuals who choose to be sexually active. With more communication and broader understanding of personal needs (including needs for intimacy and closeness), individuals and couples could perhaps choose more wisely the social and sexual behavior that would best meet those needs, in both the short and the long run. For those who choose to include sexual intercourse as part of their relationships, birth control should be made readily available and effectively used (see Chapter 6). Other measures that might help to decrease the demand for abortion include the following economic and social reforms: increased options for working women, more dual parenting, maternal/paternal leaves, improved child care facilities, and quality pre- and postnatal care available for all economic levels.

Personal Insight   Some men feel strongly that they should have a say when their partner is considering abortion. Others feel it's up to the woman. How do you feel about men's roles and rights in decisions about abortion?

METHODS OF ABORTION

"Morning after" pills (see Chapter 6) and IUDs inserted immediately after unprotected sexual elations are generally not considered **abortifacients** (agents that produce abortion) from a medical viewpoint, because they act before implantation of the fertilized egg, should one be present. (During this initial period, the female body naturally washes away an estimated 40 percent of fertilized eggs.) Therefore, these topics are not discussed here.

TERMS

Abortifacient   Agent or substance that produces abortion.

Incidence of Abortion

- More than 50 percent of the pregnancies among American women are unintended—one-half of these are terminated by abortion.

- In 1988, there were about 1.6 million abortions in the United States.

- Each year about 3 out of 100 women aged 15–44 have an abortion.

- The abortion rate—the number of abortions per 1,000 women aged 15–44—in 1975 was 22; in 1980, 29; in 1985, 28; and in 1988, 27.

Who Has Abortions?

- The majority of women having abortions are young: 58 percent are under age 25, including about 26 percent who are teenagers (age 11–19); only 20 percent are over 30.

- 18–19-year-old women have the highest abortion rate—64 per 1,000 women.

- The proportion of pregnancies terminated by abortion is higher among unmarried women (56 percent), women aged 40 and older (44 percent), and teenagers (41 percent) than among all women (29 percent).

- Women of low income are about three times more likely than women who are financially better off to have abortions. Nevertheless, 11 percent of abortions are obtained by women whose household incomes are $50,000 or more.

- Women who report no religious affiliation have a higher rate of abortion than do women who report some affiliation. Catholic women are about as likely to obtain an abortion as are all women nationally, and Protestants and Jews are less likely.

- One in six abortion patients in 1987 described herself as a born-again or evangelical Christian; they are half as likely as other women to obtain an abortion.

- 70 percent of women having an abortion say that they intend to have children in the future.

- Most women who have an abortion after 15 weeks of pregnancy have had problems detecting their pregnancy, and almost one-half are delayed because of problems, usually financial, in arranging an abortion.

- Women using contraceptives account for 43 percent of the unintended pregnancies a year, or 1.7 million pregnancies. Fifty-seven percent of unintended pregnancies a year (1.9 million) are among those not using contraceptives.

Abortion and Teenagers

- Among teenagers, 82 percent of pregnancies are unintended.

- Of the 1.6 million abortions obtained by American women in 1988, 406,000 were obtained by teenagers.

- 41 percent of women who become pregnant as teenagers choose abortion, while 59 percent continue their pregnancies to term (excluding those who miscarry).

- Of teenagers having abortions, three-fourths say they cannot afford to have a baby, and two-thirds think they are not mature enough.

- More than one-fourth of unmarried teenagers under age 18 who get abortions have never used birth control. Of those who have, most have often used one of the less effective methods.

- Teenagers are more likely than older women to have abortions during the second three months of pregnancy, when health risks associated with abortion increase significantly.

- 55 percent of teenagers under age 18 who obtain an abortion do so with their parents' knowledge—the younger the teenager, the more likely that her parents know.

Source: Facts in Brief: Abortion in the United States. (New York: The Alan Guttmacher Institute), April 1992.

RU-486

RU-486 (trade name Mifepristone) is commonly known as the abortion pill. This drug, which must be taken by the forty-ninth day following the last menstrual period, blocks uterine absorption of progesterone, thereby causing the uterine lining and any fertilized egg to shed. When RU-486 is given in combination with another drug and under medical supervision, its rate of completed abortion is about 96 percent. Because it does not involve a surgical procedure, it allows for more privacy and involves less cost than do other early abortion options.

Common side effects of the two-drug regimen include nausea, vomiting, diarrhea, and abdominal pain. In addition, a few cases of serious cardiovascular problems have been reported, including one fatal heart attack. Such cardiac complications seem to occur almost exclusively in women with preexisting risk factors, such as women over age 35 who are smokers.

The only other potentially serious side effect known to

In 1979 Chinese leaders, fearing that China would face massive food and housing shortages by the year 2000, undertook a program to cut the nation's soaring birth rate. To limit family size, the government began to promote abortion as a primary means of birth control. Under a policy known as "one family, one child," strict limits were put on childbearing. Today, any family having more than one child may be fined one year's wages unless local authorities authorize a second child. Once a mother has two children, the government requires an abortion if she becomes pregnant again. Estimates of the number of abortions under this policy range from 5 to 20 million a year. Although China is still the most populous nation on earth, its population growth rate was cut in half between 1980 and 1990, to 1.4 percent a year.

As the Chinese example illustrates, attitudes toward abortion around the world can be very different from those in the United States. According to statistics from the Population Crisis Committee, a family planning group in Washington, D.C., 49 countries totally prohibit abortion or allow it only when it will save the mother's life. These countries include most of the nations in Africa, Latin America, and the Middle East, as well as Ireland and Belgium. Another 73 countries allow abortion for a variety of different reasons, ranging from maternal health risk to economic hardship. And 22 countries allow abortion on request, usually limited to the first 20 to 25 weeks of pregnancy, without regard for reason. Even in countries where the practice is illegal, though, women still undergo abortions. Some studies estimate that in many developing countries, the number of deaths from illegal abortions ranges from 100,000 to 200,000 women a year.

How do other nations view abortion? Here is a brief survey of selected nations:

Botswana: Abortion is illegal except to save the mother's life, as it is in most African countries. Pregnancy is common among teenagers, as are illegal abortions.

Brazil: Abortion is illegal except in cases of rape, incest, or maternal health risk, as it is in most Latin American countries. Estimates of illegal abortions performed each year in Brazil range from half a million to 4 million.

Canada: Abortion is legal throughout pregnancy. The cost of abortions performed in hospitals is covered by national health insurance.

Egypt: Abortion is illegal unless the woman's life is in danger. Illegal abortions are quietly available for those who can pay.

France: Abortion is legal for any reason until the tenth week of pregnancy. Cost is covered by national health insurance. Parental consent is required for unmarried minors.

India: Abortion is legal on several grounds, including social or economic hardship, but access to services is difficult in many rural areas. The Indian government is concerned that families are disproportionately aborting female fetuses, after determining their sex through prenatal tests, due to a strong cultural preference for males.

Iran: Abortion is illegal except to save the mother's life. Policies are strongly influenced by Islamic fundamentalism. Pregnancy among teenagers and unmarried women is said to be rare.

Italy: Abortion is legal for any reason up to the twelfth week of pregnancy. Cost is covered by national health insurance. Parental consent is required for minors.

Japan: Abortion is generally legal up to 22 weeks and can be performed after that to protect the mother's life. National health does not pay. Husband or partner's consent is usually required.

Russia/Former Soviet Union: Abortion is legal and used as a primary means of birth control, partly because other forms of contraception are in short supply. The former Soviet Union is believed to have the highest abortion rate in the world. The average woman has 4 abortions in her lifetime; some women have as many as 15. Abortion services are free.

Adapted from "Abortion Around the World." *Time,* 4 May 1992; and Phil Sudo. 1990. "World of Difference." *Scholastic Update,* 20 April.

---

be associated with the use of RU-486 is vaginal bleeding. In most cases, bleeding is more prolonged than with surgical abortion, but total blood loss is similar. In a small number of cases, bleeding is heavy and a follow-up vacuum aspiration is necessary. Although investigations involving several thousand French women have been completed, some medical leaders argue that the RU-486 regimen may have long-term effects as yet unrecognized and that more research is needed before it replaces the well-studied vacuum aspiration.

RU-486 is manufactured by a French company, Roussel-Uclaf, and is currently available or being tested in France, China, England, India, and Sweden. Largely because of the strong anti-abortion lobby in the United States, political forces have blocked its entry into this country. Without FDA approval, the drug cannot be imported or sold.

In recent years, various American groups have been demanding the availability of RU-486 for testing purposes, for abortion as well as for other possible medical

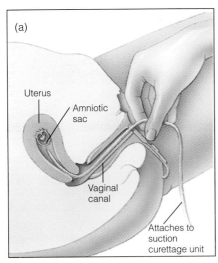

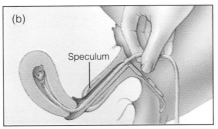

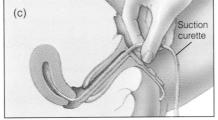

(a)

Uterus

Amniotic sac

Vaginal canal

Attaches to suction curettage unit

(b)

Speculum

(c)

Suction curette

Figure 7-5 Vacuum aspiration takes only five to ten minutes and can be performed up to the twelfth week of pregnancy.

uses, including the treatment of breast cancer, endometriosis, certain brain tumors, and Cushing's syndrome (a disorder of the adrenal gland). Grassroots groups, various health-related organizations, and legislative bodies at all levels have been challenging the FDA's import ban and are working to remove political and legal obstacles. A first step toward making RU-486 available in the United States was taken in 1993 when Roussel-Uclaf agreed to license RU-486 to the U.S. Population Council, a nonprofit organization based in New York City, which will run clinical tests. However, the battle over RU-486 is likely to continue on all fronts.

Menstrual Extraction

Developed in the early 1970s, **menstrual extraction** is the vacuum aspiration of uterine contents shortly after a missed period. It was originally defined as a procedure to be done up to the forty-second day after the last menstrual period and before the absence or presence of a pregnancy was confirmed. Initially, menstrual extraction was seen as safe, cost-effective, and as especially suitable for those women uncomfortable with the notion of abortion. Complication rates, including incomplete evacuation, infection, and continuing pregnancy, were higher than expected, however, and menstrual extraction is now rarely performed in the United States.

With the likelihood of increased restrictions on abortion, however, interest in menstrual extraction has again emerged in certain groups as a possible self-help option. Physicians warn that such procedures can be dangerous; complications include missing the fertilized egg, lacerating the cervix, perforating the uterus, and spreading bacterial infection.

Vacuum Aspiration

First developed in China in 1958, **vacuum aspiration** (also called suction curettage) has rapidly become the

preferred method for abortions up to the twelfth week of pregnancy. It can be done quickly, and the risk of hemorrhage or other complications is small. It is usually done on an outpatient basis.

A sedative may be given, along with a **local anesthetic.** A speculum, a device used to open the vaginal entrance, is inserted into the vagina, and the cervix is cleansed with a surgical solution. The cervix is dilated and a suction curette—a specially designed hollow tube—is then inserted into the uterus. The curette is attached to the rubber tubing of an electric pump, and suction is applied (see Figure 7-5). In about 20 to 30 seconds the uterus is emptied. Moderate cramping is common during evacuation. To ensure that no fragments of tissue are left in the uterus, the doctor usually scrapes the uterine lining with a metal curette, an instrument with a spoonlike tip. The entire vacuum aspiration operation takes only 5 to 10 minutes.

After a few hours in a recovering area, the woman can return home. She is usually instructed not to douche, have coitus, or use tampons for the first week or two after the abortion and to return for a two-week postabortion examination. This examination is important to verify that the abortion was complete and that no signs of infection are present.

Menstrual extraction The vacuum aspiration of uterine contents shortly after a missed period.

Vacuum aspiration Also called *suction curettage*, this procedure involves removal of the embryo or fetus by means of suction.

Local anesthesia (also called regional anesthesia) Use of agents that block the nerves carrying pain signals to the brain; in abortion and childbirth, the nerves running from the pelvic area to the brain are affected while leaving the woman awake and alert.

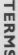

TERMS

Dilation and Curettage

In **dilation and curettage** (commonly called **D & C**) the embryo and placenta are removed by surgical instruments rather than by suction. After the cervix is dilated, a curette is used to scrape the tissues from the wall of the uterus; an ovum forceps, a long grasping instrument, is also used. Because a D & C takes longer, causes a greater loss of blood, and requires a longer recovery period, it has been largely replaced by vacuum aspiration.

Dilation and Excavation

The method most commonly used between 13 and 15 weeks of pregnancy and now preferred by some physicians up to and past 20 weeks is **dilation and evacuation** (often referred to as D & E). This procedure combines and extends both vacuum aspiration and D & C, using greater cervical dilation, larger suction curettes, and heavier forceps as required. Intravenous fluid that includes a medication to increase uterine contractions and thus limit blood loss is often given during or after the procedure. Either local or **general anesthesia** is used. Both the time required for the D & E and the recovery time are slightly longer than for vacuum aspiration.

Medical Methods

After the fifteenth week of pregnancy, one of the following medical methods is used in many centers because suction becomes more difficult. With saline instillation, the oldest of these methods, a local anesthetic is given, and a long needle is inserted through the abdominal and uterine walls into the **amniotic sac**. Amniotic fluid is drained from the sac and replaced with an equal amount of 20 percent salt solution. The injection must be made slowly and with great care to avoid introducing the solution into the woman's circulation. The woman must be fully awake to report pain or other symptoms.

The death of the fetus, which occurs immediately due to the disruption in chemical balances essential to life, is followed by labor and delivery within a day or two. The uterus is scraped to reduce chances of infection or hemorrhage. The recovery period is slightly longer than for suction (vacuum) curettage, and complications are more frequent.

Prostaglandins, a group of naturally occurring chemicals, also bring on abortion, apparently by stimulating contractions of the uterus. They can be injected into the amniotic sac or inserted through the cervical canal into the uterus. Their major shortcoming is their effect on the muscles of the digestive tract, which produces nausea, vomiting, and diarrhea. Synthetic prostaglandins have fewer side effects than natural ones. Another chemical, urea, is often used in combination with prostaglandins to facilitate labor.

Hysterotomy

Abortion by **hysterotomy** is a major surgical procedure (a modified **cesarean section**) usually performed under a general anesthetic, although a spinal anesthetic may be effective. Incisions are made in the walls of the abdomen and the uterus, and the fetus and placenta are removed. Some doctors insist that cesarean section be used for all subsequent deliveries to avoid the risk that the uterus will rupture during labor contractions, but this practice is decreasing. The saline and prostaglandin methods have largely replaced hysterotomy.

ABORTION COMPLICATIONS

Along with questions regarding the actual procedure of abortion, many individuals have concerns regarding possible aftereffects. In recent years, several detailed and long-term studies have focused on both physical and psychological concerns; slowly, more information is being gathered on this important subject.

Possible Physical Effects

The incidence of immediate problems following abortion (infection, bleeding, trauma to the cervix or uterus, and incomplete abortion requiring repeat curettage) varies widely. The overall incidence is significantly reduced with good patient health, early timing of abortion, use of the suction method and local anesthesia, performance by a well-trained clinician, and availability and use of prompt follow-up care.

Problems related specifically to infection can be decreased through pre-abortion testing and treatment of asymptomatic gonorrhea, chlamydia, and other infections. Also, some clinicians routinely give antibiotics after abortion, while others treat only those patients who have a history of or current symptoms of pelvic infection. All patients should thoroughly understand the postabortion

TERMS

Dilation and curettage (D & C) Dilation of the cervix and scraping of the uterus to remove the embryo or fetus or for other medical conditions of the uterus.

Dilation and evacuation (D & E) The method of abortion most commonly used between 13 and 15 weeks of pregnancy. Following dilation of the cervix, both vacuum aspiration and instruments are used as needed.

General anesthesia Use of agents that usually produce unconsciousness to relieve pain.

Amniotic sac/amniotic fluid The bag of watery fluid lining the uterus, which envelops and protects the fetus.

Hysterotomy A modified cesarean section in which the fetus is removed.

Cesarean section A surgical incision through the abdominal wall and uterus; performed when vaginal delivery of a baby is not advisable.

TABLE 7-1 Danger Signs After Abortion

Fever or chills

Tiredness or muscle aches

Abdominal pain, cramping, or backache

Tenderness (to pressure) in the abdomen

Prolonged or heavy bleeding

Foul vaginal discharge

Delay (6 weeks or more) in resuming menstrual periods

Source: R. A. Hatcher and others. 1990. *Contraceptive Technology 1990–1992.* (New York: Irvington), p. 457.

danger signs (Table 7-1) and should not hesitate to report any concerns.

Excessive bleeding during or after abortion is rare with early vacuum aspiration. In later pregnancies, the use of uterus-contracting medications reduces the risk significantly. Again, early reporting and treatment of any heavy bleeding are very important.

Cervical trauma or laceration and uterus perforation are uncommon as well, especially in early abortion with a well-trained clinician. In more advanced pregnancies, slow and careful dilation of the cervix before abortion can diminish these risks.

Incomplete abortion means that some pregnancy tissue has remained in the uterus. With this condition, or when blood clots form in the uterus shortly after abortion, severe cramping and signs of infection often occur and a repeat vacuum aspiration is usually needed. On rare occasions, a pregnancy may continue after incomplete abortion. The recommended two-week postabortion exam is important to establish that the abortion was complete.

Studies on long-term complications (subsequent infertility, spontaneous second abortions, premature delivery, and babies of low birth weight) have not revealed any major risks with the most common abortion methods. The risk of postabortion infertility seems to be very low, especially when any signs of infection are reported and treated promptly.

Also, there is apparently no effect on outcome of future pregnancies when an early vacuum aspiration is performed with minimal cervical dilation; with later abortions and with repeated or multiple abortions, there is only a slight risk, if any. For Rh-negative women, dangerous sensitization (the buildup of antibodies) can be minimized by an injection of Rh-**immune globulin** given within 72 hours of the procedure.

The risk of mortality associated with childbirth is about 11 times as high as that associated with abortion. The risk of death associated with abortion increases with the length of pregnancy, from 1 death for every 500,000 abortions at 8 weeks or less to 1 per 30,000 at 16 to 20 weeks and 1 per 8,000 at 21 or more weeks. The risk of death associated with abortion decreased more than fivefold from 1973 to 1985, with 3.4 deaths per 100,000 legal abortions in 1973 declining to 0.4 in 1985.

Possible Psychological Effects

Psychological side effects of abortion are less clearly defined. Responses vary and depend on the individual woman's psychological makeup, family background, current personal and social relationships, surrounding cultural attitudes, and many other factors. A woman who has specific goals with a somewhat structured life pattern may incorporate her decision to abort as the unequivocally "best" and acceptable decision more easily than may a woman who feels uncertain about her future.

Although many women experience great relief after abortion and virtually no negative feelings, some go through a period of ambivalence. Along with relief, they often feel a mixture of other responses, such as guilt, regret, loss, sadness, and/or anger. When a woman feels she was pressured into sexual intercourse or into the abortion, she may feel bitter. If she has strongly believed abortion to be immoral, she may wonder if she is still a good person. Many of these feelings are strongest immediately after abortion, when hormonal shifts are occurring; such feelings often pass quite rapidly. Others take time and fade only slowly. It is important for a woman to realize that such a mixture of feelings is natural, enabling her to accept all her reactions and to share them with others (see the box "Personal Decisions About Abortion").

For a woman who does experience painful feelings, talking freely with a close friend or family member who is understanding and trustworthy can be very helpful. Supportive people can help her feel positive about herself and her decision. Although a legal and common procedure in the United States, abortion is still treated very secretively in most of our society, so it is easy for a woman to feel unique, isolated, and alone. Some women may specifically seek out other women who have had an abortion. Many clinical centers that offer abortions make such peer counseling available. Other women find they can identify with case histories in books written on abortion, which can help them deal with their own reactions. In a few

Immune globulin A sterile solution of specific proteins that carry many antibodies normally present in human blood; a passive immunizing agent derived from adult human blood. One type of immune globulin carries antibodies to the Rh factor in the blood.

TERMS

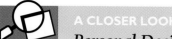

A CLOSER LOOK
Personal Decisions About Abortion

Susan

Susan was a first-year college student and was caught up in her new academic and social activities. Bill (another student) and she had been dating for about three months, when one evening she decided to "take a chance" and not use contraception since she had just finished her menstrual period. When her next period was two weeks overdue, she had a pregnancy test. It was positive.

From the moment she found out, Susan considered only one option—abortion. "I couldn't have raised a child," she said. "And I wouldn't bring a child into the world unless I could take the responsibility for it. I think it would be worse to ruin my future and a baby's life because of a mistake." When Bill first learned of the pregnancy, he became distant, but he did agree to help pay for the abortion. Soon, however, he withdrew completely and had no further contact with Susan.

The hardest time for Susan was before the abortion when she found herself crying frequently. She talked a lot with a close girlfriend, who went with her to the clinic and stayed with her after the abortion. Like all women who have abortions, Susan needed comforting.

After the abortion, Susan felt very strongly that she had made the best decision, but she did occasionally wonder how she would feel in future years. After meeting a new boyfriend with whom she could talk openly, Susan felt more certain than ever that she had made the right choice.

Helen

Helen was attending a junior college and working part time when she found out she was pregnant. She and Mike had met just a couple of months before the pregnancy. They both planned to become parents at some point in their lives, but this was earlier than either of them had expected. They discussed all the options, and they agreed that getting married and keeping their child was the only acceptable solution.

Helen gave up school for the time being, and Mike took on more hours at work to help pay for the additional ex-

pense of a child. Six months after they were married, their daughter was born. Helen and Mike say that it was at this period of their life that they really got to know one another. "Our apartment was so small, we couldn't help but learn everything about each other."

It's now eight years later, and Helen and Mike have two children. Mike works full time but hopes to return to school and complete his degree in the future. Helen works part time and attends evening classes twice a week. They'd like to move to a larger apartment and to travel more, but they can't afford to. "We've given up a lot, and it's still a struggle. But we're a happy family, and we know that we made the right choice for us."

Anna

Anna was shocked when she found out she was pregnant. She was sure she wasn't ready to be a parent herself—she was too young and still hadn't sorted out who she was or what she wanted from life. But Anna also felt that having an abortion would be wrong. So she decided to have the baby and put it up for adoption. "I myself am adopted, so adoption seemed a natural choice, and the best one available to me."

Her boyfriend broke up with her when she told him. But her parents were supportive and helped arrange for her baby's placement in a good home. Anna knew she would have to give her baby up as soon as it was born, but during her pregnancy she developed a powerful bond with her child. Anna delivered her son and left the hospital three days later. "I had to just give the baby to the nurse and walk out. My parents and I cried. I spent nine months preparing for that moment, but it was still so painful."

After a year Anna still hurts, but she doesn't regret her decision. "Keeping him would have changed my life completely, and I knew I wasn't ready to be a mother. I couldn't have given my son the kind of life I want him to have." She's proud that she went through her pregnancy. As an adopted child herself, Anna felt she owed her son the same chance that her biological mother gave her.

---

cases, unresolved emotions may persist, and a woman should seek more professional counseling.

DECISON MAKING AND UNINTENDED PREGNANCY

When faced with an unintended pregnancy, women differ greatly in their approach to decision making. Unprotected sexual intercourse may be followed immediately by a vague sense of anxiety. When symptoms of pregnancy

appear, some women (especially young women) respond with denial, ascribing the delayed menstruation and other signs to other causes. Several days or weeks may elapse before the woman finally has the pregnancy confirmed (a major cause of late abortions). After a positive test, women often feel a mixture of anxiety, depression, guilt, and anger, sometimes tinged with some anticipation and delight. The actual decision making can vary widely. Some women calmly and resolutely make a choice within a very short time, whole others, feeling panic and chaos, wrestle with the decision for several weeks. For some

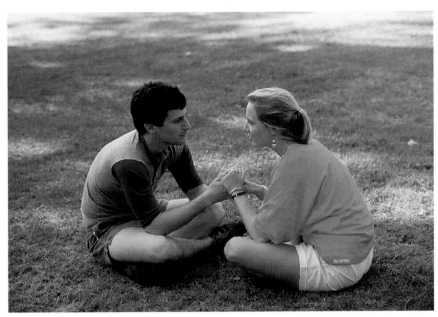

When an unintended pregnancy occurs, both partners can weigh important considerations and help choose an appropriate course of action.

women, it is the first time in their lives that they feel unable to find a "right" answer and instead must settle for a "best" but difficult solution.

The response of a woman's partner can have a significant influence on how she experiences an unintended pregnancy. Men's emotional reactions can vary considerably. Some withdraw and choose to remain completely detached; others simply press for the most expedient solution (usually abortion). Still others feel very emotionally involved and wish to play an active role in decision making. Partners can be very helpful, both in weighing important considerations and in actually helping with the chosen course of action. Some couples find that an abortion experience draws them closer together; for others, it's the last straw in an already unstable relationship. When one or both partners decide the relationship is at a dead end, they have to give it up and move on.

Parents can also be helpful. However, when there are marked disagreements, a stressful situation can become even more difficult. According to most state laws, the woman, who is the one most directly affected by unintended pregnancy, has the final rights in the decision. Pressure is growing, however, to require spousal and/or parental consent in an increasing number of states.

No matter which of the available options to unintended pregnancy is chosen, a series of questions is likely to arise that must be addressed (see the section on personal considerations). Although a prompt decision carries critical advantages, careful consideration is important. If there are strong feelings of uncertainty or ambivalence, hasty action should be avoided.

Having a supportive confidant, such as a male partner, other close friend, or family member, can be very impor-

tant in sorting out complex feelings. Along with listening and offering understanding and perspective, supportive people can help find suitable medical personnel and plan financial arrangements. Once a course of action has been chosen, a sense of moving ahead usually follows and the next step toward resolution can occur.

Personal Insight Women choose abortion for a wide variety of reasons: the pregnancy threatens their health; having a child would interfere with their educational or career plans; the pregnancy resulted from rape or incest; they can't afford to have a child; they don't want to be single parents; prenatal tests reveal fetal abnormalities; and so on. Under what circumstances (if any) do you think abortion is justified?

SUMMARY

- Most people in our society resist confronting the interrelated issues of sexuality, unintended pregnancy, and abortion; as a result, pregnancy-prevention programs are limited in number and scope.

The Abortion Issue

- The common use of the word *abortion* refers only to artificially induced expulsion of the fetus (using drugs or mechanical means).

- Until the mid-1800s abortion in the United States was legal if it took place before the twentieth week; more restrictive laws passed by the various states remained in effect until they began to be invalidated by courts in the 1960s.

- The 1973 *Roe vs. Wade* Supreme Court case devised new standards to govern abortion decisions; it was based on the trimesters of pregnancy and limited a woman's choices as she advanced through pregnancy.

- Although the Supreme court continued to uphold its 1973 decision, challenges were made to it nearly every year; in 1989 in *Webster vs. Reproductive Health Services,* the Court let stand restrictions imposed by Missouri and in 1992 in *Planned Parenthood of Southeastern Pennsylvania vs Casey,* it gave the state further powers to regulate abortion throughout pregnancy, as long as it does not impose an "undue burden" on women seeking the procedure. *Webster* and *Casey* did not overturn Roe and gave few guidelines, leaving room for further restrictions to be enacted by the states.

- Among the results of *Webster* and *Casey* will probably be great differences in laws between the states and perhaps discrimination in health care because wealthier women will be able to travel to get legal abortions.

- The controversy between pro-life and pro-choice movements centers on the issue of when life begins. Pro-life groups believe that a fertilized egg is a human life from the moment of conception and that any abortion is a murder. Pro-choice groups distinguish between stages of fetal development and argue that the woman and not the government regulations should determine the final decision regarding her pregnancy.

- Overall public opinion in the United States supports legal abortion and opposes overturning *Roe vs. Wade.* Opinion changes according to individual situations, and fetal viability outside the uterus is usually the criterion for deciding when the fetus's rights supersede the woman's.

- Most people agree that abortions done late in pregnancy present personal, medical, philosophical, and social problems. Almost half of these are done on teenagers, but other recipients include poor women, women nearing menopause, and women who have waited for the results of amniocentesis.

- The woman considering abortion needs to consider her own religious and moral beliefs, her long-range feelings, support from others, availability, and cost. The woman who decides against abortion needs to make decisions about keeping the child, perhaps being a single parent, or choosing adoption.

- Although the overall abortion *rate* rose during the 1970s, it leveled off around 1980 and fell gradually between 1982 and 1988.

Methods of Abortion

- RU-486, an abortion pill, blocks uterine absorption of progesterone, which causes the uterine lining and any fertilized egg to shed. It is not available in the United States.

- Menstrual extraction is the vacuum aspiration of uterine contents shortly after a missed period; complication rates are high, and it is rarely used in the United States.

- Vacuum aspiration, the preferred method of abortion until the twelfth week of pregnancy, uses an electric pump to remove the uterine contents; the physician also scrapes the uterine lining with a metal curette.

- Dilation and curettage (D & C) uses surgical instruments rather than suction to remove the uterine contents. Dilation and evacuation (D & E) combines and extends vacuum aspiration and D & C and is the most commonly used method between 13 and 15 weeks.

- Saline installation or prostaglandins are used for abortions after the 15th week of pregnancy; the saline solution causes fetal death, and prostaglandins stimulate uterine contractions. Hysterotomy, a major surgical procedure, has generally been replaced by prostaglandins and saline installation.

Abortion Complications

- Physical complications following abortion can be reduced with good patient health, early timing, use of the suction method and local anesthesia, a well-trained physician, and follow-up care. Infections can be reduced through pre-abortion testing and use of antibiotics. A two-week postabortion exam can establish that the abortion was complete.

- The risk of postabortion complications is very low.

- Psychological side effects of abortion vary with the individual. Many women go through a period of ambivalence; the strongest feelings usually occur immediately after the abortion. Having a supportive partner, friend, and family can be helpful.

Decision Making and Unintended Pregnancy

- Women who face unintended pregnancy differ in the way they make decisions; some make their choice calmly and quickly, while others struggle for weeks. It is often a matter of finding the "best," not necessarily the "right" solution.

- The woman's partner can positively influence her experience of an unintended pregnancy—giving support and helping with the decision. On the other hand, unintended pregnancies often mean the end of an unstable or unsatisfactory relationship.

- Parents can be helpful, unless disagreements lead to more stress; in most states today, the woman has the final say in the matter, though new legal changes in several states may change that.

TAKE ACTION

1. Now that you have information about abortion, reevaluate your contraceptive practices. If they aren't adequate to prevent unintended pregnancy, make any changes that you consider necessary to protect yourself.

2. Survey your classmates about their position on the abortion issue. How many people consider themselves pro-choice and how many pro-life? How strong are their opinions? What, if anything, might cause them to change their minds? Do opinions seem to depend on age, gender, or any other factor?

JOURNAL ENTRY

1. *Critical Thinking:* Write a one-page essay presenting your personal opinion on the abortion issue. Include arguments to refute the points typically made by the opposing side. Then write an essay presenting a convincing case for the opposite position. Make sure your arguments are clearly stated and that you can defend them, where appropriate, with facts.

2. Describe in writing the feelings you would have if you were faced with a decision about abortion right now. Decide on a course of action, and then project the consequences of your decision into the future. Describe how your decision might affect the course of your life and how you might feel about it a month from now, a year from now, 10 years from now, and 20 years from now.

SELECTED BIBLIOGRAPHY

Adler, N. E., and others. 1990. Psychological responses after abortion. *Science* 248:41–44.

Casper, L. M. 1990. Does family interaction prevent adolescent pregnancy? *Family Planning Perspectives* 22(3):109–114.

Dagg, P. K. 1991. The psychological sequelae of therapeutic abortion—denied and completed. *American Journal of Psychiatry* 148(5):578–85.

Frank, P. I., and others. 1991. The effect of induced abortion on subsequent pregnancy outcome. *British Journal of Obstetrics and Gynaecology* 98(10):1015–24.

Franz, W., and D. Reardon. 1992. Differential impact of abortion on adolescents and adults. *Adolescence* 27(105):161–72.

Hakim-Elahi, E., and others. 1990. Complications of first-trimester abortion: A report on 170,000 cases. *Obstetrics and Gynecology* 76(1):129–35.

Hardy, J. E. 1990. Abortion in America (plus several other cover stories on abortion). *Scholastic Update,* 20 April, 4–6.

Heikinheimo, O., and others. 1992. Antiprogesterone RU 486—a drug for non-surgical abortion. *Annals of Medicine* 22(2):75–84.

Henshaw, S. 1990. Induced abortion: A world review, 1990. *Family Planning Perspectives* 22(2):76–89.

The high and middle ground [Supreme Court decision on abortion restrictions; American survey]. 1992. *The Economist,* 4 July, 25–26.

Hugins, G. R., and V. E. Cullins. 1990. Fertility after contraception or abortion. *Fertility and Sterility* 54(4):559–73.

Klitsch, M. 1991. Antiprogestins and the abortion controversy: A progress report. *Family Planning Perspectives* 23(6):275–82.

Lacayo, R. 1992. Abortion: The future is already here (plus other cover stories on abortion). *Time,* 4 May, 26–31.

Mandelson, M. T., and others. 1992. Low birth weight in relation to multiple induced abortions. *American Journal of Public Health* 82(3):391–94.

Ralson, J., and others. 1992. The great divide [Pro-life vs. pro-choice]. *Life,* July, 32–42.

Rovner, J. 1992. The Supreme Court's ruling holds to a middle course [Pennsylvania's abortion law, plus several other cover stories on abortion]. *Congressional Quarterly Weekly Report* (50)27:4 July, 1950–60.

Rosenfeld, J. A. 1992. Emotional responses to therapeutic abortion. *American Family Physician* 45(1):137–40.

Salholz, E. 1992. Abortion angst [Supreme Court ruling on Pennsylvania's abortion law]. *Newsweek,* 13 July, 16–20.

Shapiro, J. P. 1992. The teen pregnancy boom. *U.S. News and World Report,* 13 July, 38.

Silvestre, L., and others. 1990. Voluntary interruption of pregnancy with Mifepristone (RU 486) and a prostaglandin analogue: A large-scale French experience. *New England Journal of Medicine* 322(10):645–48.

Supreme Court's 1992 term. (Notes and comment) *The New Yorker,* 13 July, 23–24.

Zolese, G., and C. V. Blacker. 1992. The psychological complications of therapeutic abortion. *British Journal of Psychiatry* 160:742–49.

RECOMMENDED READINGS

Henshaw, S. K., and J. Van Vort, eds. 1992. *Abortion Factbook—1992 Edition: Readings, Trends, and State and Local Data to 1988.* New York: Alan Guttmacher Institute. *A collection of articles and tables that depict abortion in the United States today, including medical services, political phenomena, and related issues.*

Mohr, J. D. 1978. *Abortion in America: The Origins and Evolution of National Policy, 1800–1900.* New York: Oxford University Press. *A historical perspective of views on abortion within American society. Includes a discussion of the powerful role that physicians played in the formation of public opinion and related legal decisions.*

Rosenblatt, Roger. 1992. *Life Itself: Abortion in the American Mind.* New York: Random House. *The author, who is pro-choice, describes the schism in American society over the abortion issue. He argues that Americans can repair the rift by learning to live with conflicting feelings on the issue, as we have done on other issues.*

Stewart, F., and others. 1987. *Understanding Your Body: Every Woman's Guide to Gynecology and Health.* New York: Bantam Books. *A comprehensive guide to women's gynecological health. Describes various treatment options for common problems. Includes up-to-date information on contraception and abortion.*

8

Pregnancy and Childbirth

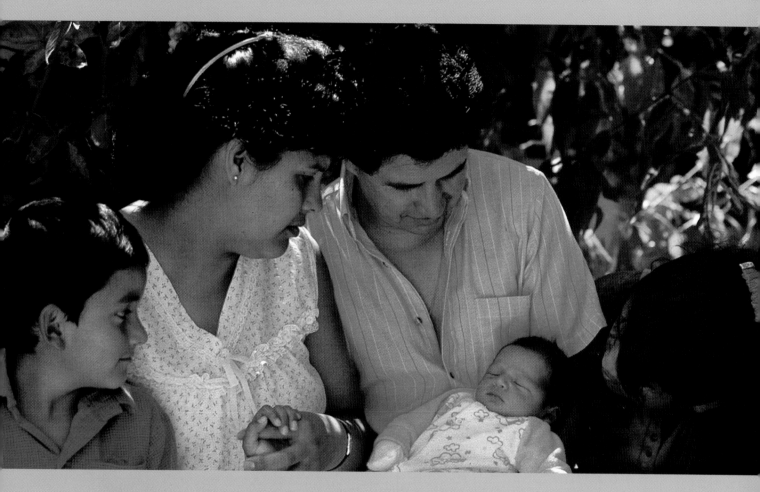

CONTENTS

◗ Your brother and his wife have decided that they're ready to start a family. They're committed to doing everything they can to ensure a healthy pregnancy. Your sister-in-law plans to visit a physician as soon as she knows she's pregnant so she can begin prenatal care right away. But they're wondering if there's anything else they should be doing. What advice can you give them?

◗ You recently found out that you're pregnant, and although you couldn't be more excited, you're giving some thought to two of your daily habits—having a beer with dinner and smoking about half a pack of cigarettes a day. You'd like to give up these habits while you're pregnant, but all the excitement makes it hard to quit. A friend thinks drinking and smoking don't matter until the fourth or fifth month of pregnancy, when the baby really starts to gain weight. Is your friend right? Do you have some time before it makes a difference?

◗ Your sister and her husband have been trying to have a baby for eight months, and she's still not pregnant. She's getting discouraged and is beginning to feel as if there's something wrong with her. She doesn't know what to think or do about her situation. Does she have a fertility problem? How can she find out? What options are open to her if a problem is discovered? What advice can you give her?

◗ You and your partner are taking prepared childbirth classes, and some of the other parents-to-be have some very clear expectations and opinions about childbirth and infant care. They make it sound as if any woman who takes pain-relieving drugs during birth, receives any type of medical monitoring or treatment, has a cesarean delivery, or doesn't breastfeed is a failure, or worse. You're afraid that you'll be setting yourselves up for guilt and disappointment if you adopt the same attitude. Is there only one "right" way to give birth? Are there some circumstances in which medical intervention might be better for the infant and mother than a more "natural" delivery? Will it be harmful to the baby if you decide not to breastfeed?

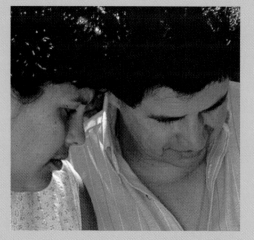

MAKING CONNECTIONS

Some people have a child when they're in their teens or twenties, others wait until they hear their "biological clock" ticking in their mid- or late thirties, and still others never have children at all. Whatever your choice, it's critical for your health and happiness that you take control of your fertility and make the decisions that are right for you. In each of the scenarios relating to pregnancy and childbirth on this page, individuals have to use information, make a decision, or choose a course of action. How would you act in each of these situations? What response or decision would you make? This chapter provides information about pregnancy and childbirth that can be used in situations like these. After finishing the chapter, read the scenarios again. Has what you've learned changed how you would respond?

Deciding whether to become a parent is one of the most important decisions you will ever make. Having a child changes your life forever; deciding not to have children has equally far-reaching implications. Yet many people approach this momentous decision with only the vaguest notion of what is involved in pregnancy and childbirth. An estimated half of the approximately 3.6 million babies born every year in the United States are from unintentional pregnancies.

Today, with changing cultural expectations and increasingly sophisticated contraceptive technology, you have more choice about becoming a parent than people have ever had before. Until recently it was expected that virtually every married couple would have children. Now you can choose whether, when, and how you want to have a child. And you don't have to be part of a couple to have a child; the number of women choosing to have children on their own has risen dramatically.

Pregnancy is a relatively comfortable experience for most women and the outcome predictably happy. Yet for some, problems occur. Some couples who have always planned for children may find that they are unable to conceive; others may face complications during pregnancy. Some problems are impossible to prevent, but you can make choices that minimize the risks and maximize the benefits for yourself, your partner, and your children.

Having a child is one of the most arduous, important, and rewarding enterprises that human beings undertake. The more you know about it—about conception and pregnancy, fetal development and prenatal care, childbirth and parenting—the more capable you will be of making intelligent, informed decisions about it. This chapter presents information that you can use both now and later in your life to make the choices about pregnancy and childbirth that are right for you.

PREPARATION FOR PARENTHOOD

Before you decide whether or when to become a parent, you'll want to consider your suitability and readiness to parent. If you make the decision to become a parent, there are actions you can take before the pregnancy begins to help ensure a healthy outcome for all.

Deciding to Become a Parent

Many factors have to be taken into account when you are considering parenthood. The following are some questions you should ask yourself and some issues you should consider when making this decision. Some issues are relevant to both men and women; others apply only to women.

- Your physical health and your age. Are you in reasonably good health? If not, can you improve your health by changing your lifestyle, perhaps by modifying your diet or giving up cigarettes or drugs? Do you have physical conditions, such as overweight or diabetes, that will require extra care and medical attention during pregnancy? Do you or your partner have a family history of genetic problems that a baby might inherit? Does your age place you or your baby at risk? (Teenagers and women over 35 have a higher incidence of some problems.) Improving your health before pregnancy—discussed in the next section—can help ensure a trouble-free pregnancy and a healthy baby.

- Your financial circumstances. Can you afford a child? Will your health insurance cover the costs of pregnancy, prenatal tests, delivery, and medical attention for mother and baby before and after the birth, including physicians' fees and hospital costs? Supplies for the baby are expensive too—diapers, bedding, cribs, strollers, car seats, clothing, food and medical supplies, and child care. Depending on a variety of factors, including family income and region of residence, the annual cost of raising a child varies from about $4,100 to $9,800. To raise a child to age 17 costs between about $80,000 and $160,000. If one parent has quit his or her job to care for the child or is on parental leave, the family must live on one income.

- Your relationship with your partner. Are you in a stable relationship, and do both of you want a child? Are your views compatible on such issues as child-rearing goals, the distribution of responsibility for the child, and work and housework?

- Your educational, career, and child care plans. Have you completed as much of your education as you want right now? Have you sufficiently established yourself in a career, if that is something you want to do? Have you investigated parental leave and company-sponsored child care? Do you and your partner agree on child care arrangements, and does such child care exist in your community? Some child development experts advise against full-time child care for babies under 1 year of age because it can disrupt their attachment to their parents. The child care issue, which some people consider the most difficult one in parenting, requires a great deal of thought.

- Your emotional readiness for parenthood. Are you prepared to have a helpless being completely dependent on you 24 hours a day? Do you have the emotional reserves to care for and nurture an infant? Are you willing to change your lifestyle to provide the best conditions for a baby's development, both before and after birth?

- Your social support system. Do you have a network of family and friends who will help you with the baby?

Are there community resources that you can call on for additional assistance? A family's social support system is one of the most important factors affecting their ability to adjust to a baby and cope with new responsibilities.

- Your personal qualities, attitudes toward children, and aptitude for parenting. Do you like infants, young children, and adolescents? Do you think time with children is time well spent? Do you feel good enough about yourself to love and respect others? Do you have safe ways of handling anger, frustration, and impatience?

- Your philosophical beliefs. Some people question the value of bringing more people into an already overcrowded world. Many countries have yet to stabilize their populations, the United States among them; worldwide population is expected to soar from 5 billion in 1990 to 9 billion in 2030. Given these figures, some people feel that human beings have already fulfilled the biblical directive to be fruitful and multiply, and they choose not to have children.

Personal Insight Do you want to have children? What is the basis for your feelings and desires? Can you distinguish personal reasons from cultural expectations? What do you think people would think of you if you decided not to have children?

Preconception Care

The birth of a healthy baby depends in part on the mother's general health and well-being *before* conception. The U.S. Public Health Service has recommended that all women receive health care to help them prepare for pregnancy. **Preconception care** should include assessment of health risks, promotion of healthy lifestyle behaviors, and any treatments necessary to reduce risk. The following are some of the questions, tests, and treatments that you and your partner may encounter during preconception care:

- Do you have any preexisting medical conditions, such as diabetes, epilepsy, asthma, high blood pressure, or anemia? There may be things you can do to improve the chances of a trouble-free pregnancy and a positive outcome.

- Are you currently taking any medications? Some medications can harm the **fetus**, so you may need to change or discontinue their use to help ensure a healthy pregnancy.

- Have you had any prior problems with pregnancy and delivery, including miscarriage, preterm birth, ectopic pregnancy, or delivery complications? Some problems are due to physical or hormonal difficulties that can be treated.

- Does your age place you at risk for infertility or health problems during pregnancy, or does it increase the likelihood that your baby may have a genetic or chromosomal disorder? Pregnant teenagers may need special nutritional counseling during pregnancy to supply the needs of their own growing bodies as well as the baby's. Women under 20 and over 35 have babies with a higher incidence of Down's syndrome; genetic testing and counseling may be indicated. Older women may also find it harder to become pregnant.

- Do you smoke, drink, or take other drugs? These habits are dangerous for the baby; and a health care professional can recommend treatment programs.

- Do you currently have any infections or do you need any additional vaccinations? Women at risk for hepatitis B or who are not immunized against rubella (German measles) should be vaccinated. Women not immune to toxoplasmosis (a disease transmitted from animals, especially cats, which can cause birth defects or fetal death) can be counseled about ways to prevent infection during pregnancy. Testing for tuberculosis and certain sexually transmissible diseases (STDs) allows these illnesses to be treated before pregnancy. (See Chapters 17 and 18 for more information about STDs and other infectious diseases.)

- Are you at risk for HIV infection (see Chapter 17)? If so, you should be tested before you or your partner becomes pregnant. About 25 to 30 percent of babies born to HIV-infected mothers become infected; most die before age 2.

- Do you eat a balanced diet? Are you particularly underweight or overweight? Do you suffer from an eating disorder? Do you have special dietary habits such as vegetarianism? Nutritional counseling can help you create a plan for eating that is right for you before and during pregnancy. Your physician may also prescribe multivitamins, particularly folic acid. The U.S. Public Health Service has recommended that all women of childbearing age take extra folic acid

TERMS

Preconception care   Health care to prepare for pregnancy.

Fetus   Developmental stage of a human from the ninth week after conception to the moment of birth.

Conception   The formation of a zygote (fertilized egg), the cell resulting from the fusion of ovum and sperm, and in normal conditions capable of survival and maturation in the uterus.

Ovary   One of the two female reproductive glands that produce ova (eggs) and sex hormones.

Follicles   The thousands of protecting, enclosing spherical bubbles in the ovaries in which ova mature. Each follicle contains a liquid supplied with estrogen.

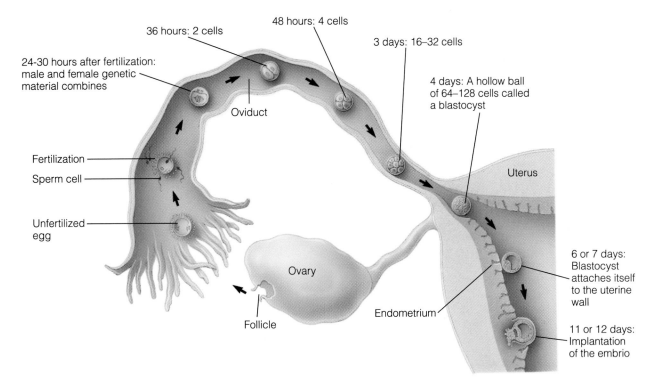

24-30 hours after fertilization: male and female genetic material combines

36 hours: 2 cells

48 hours: 4 cells

3 days: 16–32 cells

4 days: A hollow ball of 64–128 cells called a blastocyst

Oviduct

Fertilization

Sperm cell

Unfertilized egg

Ovary

Follicle

Uterus

Endometrium

6 or 7 days: Blastocyst attaches itself to the uterine wall

11 or 12 days: Implantation of the embrio

Figure 8-1 *Fertilization and early development of the embryo.*
The unfertilized egg is released from an ovarian follicle into the oviduct, where it is fertilized by a sperm cell. As the fertilized egg moves through the oviduct toward the uterus, the genetic material from the male and female germ cells combine, and the egg begins to divide. When the egg reaches the uterus, it is in the form of a hollow ball of cells called a blastocyst, which becomes implanted in the endometrium.

because an adequate intake of folic acid during the first few weeks of pregnancy reduces the risk of neural tube defects such as spina bifida.

- Are you a diethylstilbestrol (DES) baby? Daughters born to women who were given DES during pregnancy to prevent miscarriage—a common practice from the 1940s to early 1970s—are at higher-than-normal risk for a variety of problems with conception and pregnancy. DES daughters may need special monitoring and care to identify and treat problems as soon as they develop.

- Do twins or multiple births run in either your or your partner's family? If so, it may increase the likelihood of a multiple birth.

- Do either you or your partner have a family history of genetic disease? Have you or any family member had a child with a birth defect or mental retardation? Genetic testing and counseling may determine if you are a carrier for a specific disease, what the effects of the disease would be, and whether a baby you conceive can be tested prenatally. Members of certain ethnic groups are at higher risk for genetic disorders that are more prevalent within their groups than in the general population. For more information on

these disorders, refer to the box "Ethnicity and Genetic Diseases."

Additional tests or changes in behavior may be recommended if you have recently traveled outside the United States; if you work with chemicals, radiation, or toxic substances; if you participate in physically demanding or hazardous activities or occupations; or if you face significant psychosocial risks, including homelessness, an unsafe home environment, or mental illness.

UNDERSTANDING FERTILITY

Conceiving is a highly complex process. Although many couples conceive readily, others can testify to the difficulties that can be encountered.

Conception

The process of **conception** involves the fusion of an egg (ovum) from a woman's ovary with a sperm from a man (Figure 8-1). Every month during a woman's fertile years, her body prepares itself for conception and pregnancy. In one of her **ovaries** an egg ripens and is released from its **follicle.** The egg—about the size of a pinpoint, 1/250

The genetic code, formed when egg and sperm combine, is a set of chemical instructions that determines the development of hundreds of individual traits in each human being. Many of these traits are visible—will the baby have blue eyes or brown, be tall or short, be fat or thin? But some important determinants are invisible. One such invisible set of genetic instructions determines whether genetic diseases will be passed from the parents to the child.

Two genes, one from each parent, are involved in determining a given characteristic such as whether the baby will inherit a genetic disease. And each of these genes is either very powerful—*dominant*—or less powerful, or *recessive*. Dominant genes are expressed in the offspring even if the child inherits only one. Diseases that are carried by dominant genes seldom skip a generation; anyone who carries the gene will probably get the disease.

Recessive genes are expressed as traits only if *both* genes in the pair are positive for the trait. Many common diseases caused by recessive genes occur disproportionately in certain ethnic groups. Prospective parents who come from the same ethnic group should be tested for any recessive diseases found in that group to make sure they are not both carriers. If they are, each of their children will have about a one-in-four risk of developing the disease.

Learning all you can about diseases that affect members of your ethnic group can be a lifesaver. Not only can you learn about the risk to your children, but you may also discover that there are things you can do to manage the disease and reduce its impact.

Diseases and Predispositions Related to Ethnicity

Sickle cell anemia affects about 1 out of every 625 African Americans. In this disease, the red blood cells, which carry oxygen to the body's tissues, change shape—the normal doughnut-shaped cells become crescent-shaped, like sickles. These altered cells carry less oxygen and clog small blood vessels.

People who inherit one gene for sickle cell anemia experience only mild symptoms; those with two genes become severely, often fatally, ill. Interestingly, people who inherit one sickle cell gene are far more resistant to malaria than are those without the gene, leading geneticists to conclude that the sickle cell trait might have developed in tropical regions as an adaptation to the presence of malaria, the most widespread tropical disease.

If you are at risk for sickle cell anemia, you can

- Get genetic counseling to help determine your family's genetic pattern and the degree of risk to you and your potential offspring

- Take particular care to reduce stress and respond to minor infections, since red blood cells become sickle-shaped during periods of stress on the body

- Get regular medical checkups

Tay-Sachs disease occurs annually in approximately 1 out of every 1,000 Jews of Eastern European ancestry. People with Tay-Sachs disease are unable to metabolize fat properly; as a result, the brain and other nerve tissues deteriorate. Affected children begin by showing weaknesses in their movements and eventually develop blindness, seizures, and death. This disease is lethal, and death usually occurs by age 3 or 4.

If you are of Eastern European Jewish ancestry and are planning to have children, genetic counseling will help you assess the chances that you and your mate will produce a child with Tay-Sachs disease.

Cystic fibrosis occurs in 1 in every 2,000 Caucasians per year. Because essential enzymes of the pancreas are deficient, thick mucus impairs function in the lungs and intestinal tracts of people with this disease. The disease is often fatal in early childhood, but medical treatments are increasingly effective in reducing symptoms and prolonging life. In some cases, symptoms do not appear until early adulthood.

If there is a history of cystic fibrosis in your family and you plan to have children, genetic counseling can help in assessing the risk to your prospective offspring.

Thalassemia is a blood disease found most often among Italians, Greeks, and, to a lesser extent, African Americans and Asians. When inherited from one parent, this form of anemia is mild; when two genes are present, the disease is severe and can cause fetal death or, after birth, a condition called Cooley's anemia. Children with this condition must

---

inch in diameter—is then drawn into an **oviduct** (or **fallopian tube**) through which it travels to the **uterus.** The journey takes three to four days. The lining of the uterus has already thickened to assist the implantation of a **fertilized egg,** or zygote. If the egg is not fertilized, it lasts about 24 hours and then disintegrates. It is expelled along with the uterine lining during menstruation.

Sperm cells are produced in the man's testes and ejaculated from his penis into the woman's vagina during sexual intercourse (except in cases of artificial insemination or in vitro fertilization; see below). Sperm cells are much smaller than eggs (1/8000 inch in diameter). The typical ejaculate contains millions of sperm, but only a few complete the long journey through the uterus and up the fallopian tube to the egg. Many sperm cells do not survive the acidic environment of the vagina. Once through the cervix and into the uterus, many sperm cells are diverted to the wrong oviduct or get stuck along the way. Of those that reach the egg, only one will be allowed to penetrate the hard outer layer of the egg. As sperm approach the be treated with repeated blood transfusions, and these eventually result in a damaging iron buildup. New medical interventions, such as genetic engineering, bone marrow transplants, and chemicals that bind with excess iron and remove it from the body, offer promise.

If you are at risk of carrying thalassemia, you can

- Get regular checkups and monitor your health for symptoms
- Learn symptom management
- Get genetic counseling to assess the risk to your offspring

Lactose intolerance is a condition found in most Asian people, many African Americans and Native Americans, and a small proportion of people of Northern European ancestry. Although all humans are dependent on milk in the early years, by about age 4 many lose the ability to absorb lactose, the chief nutrient in milk. This lactose intolerance results from an absence of *lactase,* an enzyme that permits the efficient digestion of milk. When lactose-intolerant people ingest milk or dairy products, they suffer from gas pains and diarrhea. Studies show that lactose intolerance is especially high in cultures in which milk is relatively unimportant after weaning, suggesting that evolutionary adaptation has played a role in its development.

If you are lactose intolerant, you can

- Manage your food intake carefully
- Occasionally, to enjoy a dairy food, take commercially available lactase, a nonprescription product

Diabetes is 55 percent more common among African Americans than among white Americans. Native Americans are also at increased risk for adult-onset diabetes. The risk in Mexican Americans is related to their percentage of Native American ancestry. Asians have a predisposition for adult-onset diabetes that surfaces with American diets.

There are many steps you can take if you are at risk for diabetes. They include managing your diet, getting plenty of exercise, and monitoring your blood sugar level. Further details are provided in Chapter 12 in the box "Digestive and Metabolic Disorders."

Osteoporosis is more likely to develop in light-skinned people of Northern European ancestry than in dark-skinned people. This condition is a gradual loss of bone mass that can result in multiple fractures, crippling, deformity, and constant pain. Many factors besides ethnicity increase the risk of osteoporosis—for example, sex, body type, age, diet, reproductive history, hormones, drug intake, and exercise habits.

If you are at risk, you can

- Consult with a physician or nutritionist to devise a diet that enhances bone strength
- Maintain a regular endurance exercise program
- Eliminate smoking and drinking, which contribute to osteoporosis

Alcoholism is the result of many contributing factors, and it is difficult to distinguish psychological, social, and cultural contributors from genetic ones. But studies of twins have revealed that heredity does play a role in alcoholism—when one identical twin suffers from alcoholism, chances are high that the other will be alcoholic too. For a number of years, experts considered this true for men only; today it's known that alcoholism in women is also influenced by heredity.

Rates of alcoholism vary from one group to another. Alcoholism is particularly prevalent among some Native Americans. Many studies have suggested that Native Americans metabolize alcohol more quickly than do whites. However, Native Americans who function successfully in modern cultures while retaining meaningful values from their traditional cultures are the least likely among Native Americans to abuse alcohol. Those lacking social support and good survival skills are most likely to become not only alcoholics but also alcohol-related suicides.

If you are at risk for alcoholism, you can

- Be particularly cautious about alcohol intake
- Acquaint yourself with the signs and symptoms of alcoholism and monitor your own behavior around alcohol carefully
- Familiarize yourself with support services and recovery programs available to alcoholics in your community

---

egg, they release enzymes that soften the outer layer of the egg. Enzymes from hundreds of sperm must be released in order for the egg's outer layers to soften enough to allow a sperm to penetrate. The first sperm cell that bumps into a spot that is soft enough can swim into the cell. It then merges with the nucleus of the egg and **fertilization** occurs. The sperm's tail, its means of locomotion, gets stuck in the outer membrane and drops off, leaving the sperm head inside the egg. The egg then releases a chemical that makes it impregnable by other sperm.

Oviducts (fallopian tubes) The two passages through which ova travel from the ovaries to the uterus; "normal" place for fertilization.

Uterus The hollow, thick-walled, muscular organ in which the egg develops into a child; located directly above the vagina; the source of menstrual flow; the womb.

Fertilized egg The egg after it has been penetrated by a sperm; a zygote.

Sperm cell A mature male germ cell that serves to impregnate the ovum.

TERMS

Creating a Family Health Tree

The genetic inheritance that each of us receives from our parents—and that our children receive from us—contains more than just physical characteristics such as eye and hair color. Heredity also contributes directly to our risk of developing certain diseases and disorders.

For certain uncommon diseases such as hemophilia and sickle cell anemia, heredity is the primary cause; if your parents give you the necessary genes, you'll almost always get the disease. But heredity plays a subtler role in many other diseases, which are caused at least in part by "environmental" influences such as infection, cancer-causing chemicals, or an artery-clogging diet. While your genes alone will not produce those diseases, they can determine how susceptible you are. Researchers have found a genetic influence in many common disorders, including coronary heart disease, diabetes, certain forms of cancer, depression, and alcoholism.

Knowing that a specific disease runs in your family can save your life. It allows you to watch for early warning signs and get screening tests more often than you otherwise would. Changing health habits, too, can be valuable for people with a family history of certain diseases. A smoker with a close relative who had lung cancer, for example, is 14 times more likely to get the disease than other smokers.

In general, the more relatives that had a genetically transmitted disease and the closer they are to you, the greater your risk. However, nongenetic facts such as health habits can also play a role. Signs of strong hereditary influence include early onset of the disease, appearance of the disease largely or exclusively on one side of the family, onset of the same disease at the same age in more than one relative, and disease despite good health habits.

You can put together a simple family tree by compiling a few key facts on your primary relatives: siblings, parents, aunts and uncles, and grandparents. Those facts include the date of birth, major diseases, health-related conditions and habits, and, for deceased relatives, the date and cause of death. (For a free family-medical-history form and guidelines on what to ask, write The March of Dimes Birth Defects Foundation, 1275 Mamaroneck Avenue, White Plains, NY 10605.) Once you've collected the information you want, create a tree using the example here as a guide. Then show your tree to your physician to get a full picture of what the information means for your or your children's health.

A Sample Family Health Tree and What It Means

In this sample family tree, the prostate cancer that killed the man's father means that he should be tested for a prostate tumor at a younger age and more frequently than is generally recommended.

His sisters may need to have earlier, more frequent mammograms because of their mother's breast cancer. If they're overweight, they can reduce their risk by losing weight.

One grandmother and one uncle each died of a heart attack. There are several reasons not to worry too much about that: The two relatives were from different sides of the family; both had the attack at a relatively old age; both had two other major risk factors for coronary heart disease—smoking and either diabetes or obesity; and neither of the man's parents had any apparent heart trouble. He should check to see whether either relative had highly elevated cholesterol levels, a possible sign of familial hypercholesterolemia.

The colon cancer that struck another grandmother and uncle is a different story. Two factors suggest a possible hereditary link: They were mother and son, and they both developed the disease at nearly the same comparatively young age. So the man should be screened early and often.

Finally, alcoholism seems to run in the family. The man should be aware that such a history could indicate a hereditary susceptibility to the problem, though the habit might simply have been passed down by example.

Source: "What's Lurking in Your Family Tree?" *Consumer Reports on Health,* September 1992.

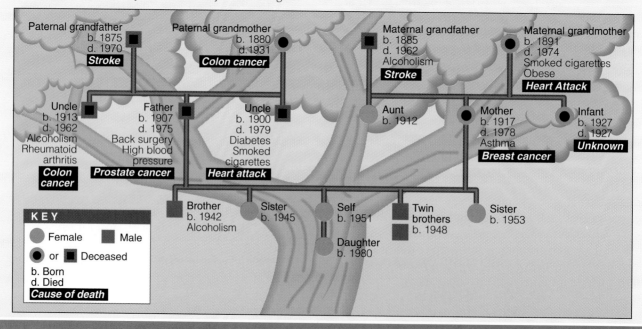

The ovum carries the hereditary characteristics of the mother and her ancestors; sperm cells carry the hereditary characteristics of the father and his ancestors. Together they contain the **genetic code,** a set of instructions for development. Each parent cell—egg or sperm—contains 23 chromosomes, and each of these chromosomes contains many genes, so small that they cannot be seen through a microscope. These genes are packages of chemical instructions for designing every part of a new baby. They specify that the infant will be human; what its sex will be; whether it will tend to be (depending also on its environment) short, tall, thin, fat, healthy, or sickly; and hundreds of other characteristics. Together, they provide the blueprint for a new and unique person (see the box "Creating a Family Health Tree").

As soon as fertilization occurs, the fertilized egg begins to undergo the cell division that allows it to grow. About three or four days after fertilization, the cluster of 16 to 32 cells enters the uterus. About six or seven days after fertilization, the cluster of cells attaches itself to the uterine wall; and four or five days after that, it becomes embedded there.

The usual course of events at conception is that one egg and one sperm unite to produce one fertilized egg and one baby. But if the ovaries release two (or more) eggs during ovulation, and if both eggs are fertilized, two babies will develop. These twins will be no more alike than will be siblings born from different pregnancies, because each came from a different fertilized egg. Twins who develop this way are referred to as **fraternal twins;** they may be the same sex or different sexes. Twins can also develop from the division of a single fertilized egg into two cells that develop separately. Because these babies share all genetic material, they will be **identical twins.**

Infertility

Although the main concern for many women and men, especially if they are young and single, is how *not* to get pregnant, the reverse is true for millions of couples who have difficulty conceiving. **Infertility** is usually defined as the inability to conceive a child after trying for a year or more. About 1 out of 12 or 13 American couples are unable to have the children they want. Over a million couples seek treatment for infertility each year, and about 60 percent of couples with serious infertility problems will eventually achieve a pregnancy.

Female Infertility The leading cause of infertility among women is blocked fallopian tubes. This blockage is usually the result of pelvic inflammatory disease (PID), a serious complication of several different sexually transmitted diseases; most occurrences are associated with untreated cases of chlamydia or gonorrhea. About 1.7 million cases of PID were treated in 1986, but physicians estimate that half may go untreated due to lack of symp-

toms. Other causes of PID include unsterile abortions, abdominal surgery, and certain types of older IUDs. Surgery may restore fertility if the damage is not too severe.

The second leading cause of infertility in women is endometriosis. In this disease, uterine tissue grows outside the uterus, usually in the ovaries, the oviducts (where it may cause blockage), and/or the abdominal cavity. This tissue may bleed each month in response to the hormonal stimulation that controls menstruation. Hormonal therapy and surgery are used to treat endometriosis.

Other causes of infertility among women include benign growths in the uterus and hormonal imbalances that prevent ovulation. Some women develop an allergic response that kills their partner's sperm. Exposure to toxic chemicals or radiation appears to reduce fertility, as does cigarette smoking. Evidence also indicates that the daughters of mothers who were prescribed DES have a significantly higher infertility rate. Beginning around age 30, women's fertility naturally begins to decline, and by age 35, about one out of four women are infertile.

Male Infertility The leading causes of infertility among men are low sperm count, lack of sperm motility (the ability to move spontaneously), or blocked passageways between the testes and the urethra. Some studies indicate that men's sperm counts have dropped by as much as 50 percent over the last 30 years. Evidence suggests that toxic substances, such as lead, chemical pollutants, and radiation, are responsible for this decrease in sperm counts (see the box "The Susceptible Sperm: Men's Role in Genetic Health"). Smoking may produce reduced sperm counts or abnormal sperm. Sons of mothers who took DES may have increased sperm abnormalities and fertility problems. Certain prescription and illegal drugs also affect the number of sperm. Large doses of marijuana, for example, cause lower sperm counts and suppress certain reproductive hormones. Other causes of sperm problems include injury of the testicles, infection (especially from mumps during adulthood), birth defects, or subjecting the testicles to high temperatures, such as those produced by hot baths or tight-fitting underwear. In many cases, fertility increases when the causative factor has been removed.

Fertilization The initiation of biological reproduction, as, for example, when the sperm and ovum unite to form a zygote (fertilized egg).

Genetic code Master blueprint message directing the body's growth and cell differentiation, contained in genetic material.

Fraternal twins Twins who develop from separate fertilized eggs; not genetically identical.

Identical twins Twins who develop from the division of a single zygote; genetically identical.

Infertility The inability to conceive after trying for a year or more.

TERMS

In a perfect union, male and female contribute equal amounts of healthy genetic material to their offspring. But when something goes wrong, scientists have traditionally examined the egg to find out why. The assumption has been that the egg is fragile and susceptible to the damaging effects of radiation, poisons, and the hazards of everyday living. The sperm—seen as a tight little capsule of DNA with a tail—was thought to be impervious to environmental dangers.

In recent years, however, reproductive scientists have found that a substantial number of sperm produced by fertile, apparently healthy men are abnormal. Physically, they may be misshapen, have extra tails or heads, or be poor swimmers. Genetically, they may carry the wrong number of chromosomes or have bits and pieces of genetic material out of place. Although many of these variations seem to occur normally—with 300 million sperm in one ejaculate, a certain number of imperfections are to be expected—researchers are investigating both what may cause them and what their effects may be.

Some evidence indicates that paternal exposure to drugs, alcohol, radiation, and workplace toxins contributes to impaired fertility. Researchers have found, for example, that men who work in dry-cleaning establishments and breathe the solvent perchloroethylene experience changes in sperm mobility. The researchers aren't sure that breathing the fumes lowers fertility, but they do know that the wives of men who had higher exposures took longer to become pregnant. There is also some evidence that firemen, subjected to numerous potential toxins in smoke, may produce an unusually high number of abnormal sperm and be less fertile than other males.

Paternal exposure to environmental hazards may also be implicated in miscarriages, stillbirths, congenital defects, low birth weight, behavioral or learning difficulties in children, and even some types of childhood cancer. Several studies suggest that men exposed to high levels of lead, vinyl chloride, and about a dozen other chemicals have children who are at higher risk for serious medical problems. For example, men who work in the aircraft industry or handle paints or chemical solvents may be at higher risk for producing children with brain tumors. Paternal exposure to paints has been linked with childhood leukemias. And investigators have observed elevated rates of leukemia among children of men who were exposed to low-level radiation while working at a nuclear power facility in England. Although other studies have had contradictory results, studies of animals indicate that paternal exposure to environmental toxins—ranging from recreational drugs to industrial chemicals—apparently contributes to numerous problems in offspring.

Where does this leave prospective parents? Current research indicates that exposure of either the mother or the father to a variety of agents may increase the risk of problems in fertility, pregnancy, or childhood health. Prudence dictates that during the reproductive years, both men and women be judicious about the use of alcohol, tobacco, and other drugs. Until recently, most advice about parental exposure to drugs, chemicals, and pollutants was directed toward women. Now that sperm are recognized as being susceptible to some of the same dangers, men also need to protect themselves—not just for their own sake but also for the sake of their future children.

Adapted from P. Thomas. 1992. "A Father's Role." *Harvard Health Letter*, October; and D. Ansley. 1992. "Sperm Tales." *Discover*, June.

Treating Infertility Some kinds of infertility can be treated; others cannot. About 90 percent of infertile couples receive a physical diagnosis for their condition; for the remaining 10 percent, the cause of the infertility remains unexplained. Surgery can sometimes repair oviducts, clear up endometriosis, and correct anatomical problems in both men and women. Fertility drugs can help a woman ovulate, although they carry the risk of causing multiple births.

If these procedures don't work, more advanced techniques may help (see the box "Different Ways to Start a Family"). Male infertility can sometimes be overcome by collecting and concentrating the man's sperm and introducing it mechanically into the woman's vagina or uterus, a procedure known as **artificial or intrauterine insemination.** The sperm can be provided by the woman's partner or, if there are severe problems with his sperm, by a

donor. Donor sperm is also used in cases where the man carries a serious genetically transmitted disorder and by single women and lesbian couples who wish to conceive using artificial insemination. Intrauterine insemination has a success rate of about 60 percent for infertile couples. On average, women who become pregnant have received two inseminations a month (just prior to ovulation) for two to four months. The American Fertility Society estimates that there are about 30,000 births each year as a result of intrauterine insemination.

Some kinds of female infertility can be bypassed with **in vitro fertilization.** In this procedure, eggs are removed from the woman's ovary and fertilized in a laboratory dish by her partner's sperm. One or more of the resulting embryos is implanted in the woman's uterus. Embryos that aren't used are often frozen and stored for the couple to use later. If one partner is infertile, a donor can supply the

Traditional

1. Couple conceives a child.

2. The child stays with the couple, who are its genetic and legal parents.

Intrauterine Insemination

1. Couple is unable to conceive because male has impaired fertility or is infertile. (This procedure is also sometimes used by single women and lesbian couples.)

2. Sperm from the male or from a donor is concentrated and placed in the woman's vagina using the technique of artificial insemination.

3. The child is genetically linked to both parents unless a donor is used. In cases where a donor provides the sperm, he—the biological father—usually has no legal link to the child.

In Vitro Fertilization

1. Although the male and female produce sperm and eggs, the couple is unable to conceive. (If one or the other partner is infertile, a donor may provide the sperm or egg.)

2. Sperm and egg are combined in a laboratory.

3. The fertilized egg is implanted back into the woman.

4. The child is genetically linked to both parents unless a donor is used. In cases where a donor is used, the donor usually has no legal link to the child.

Surrogate Mother

1. Couple is unable to conceive because the female is infertile or pregnancy would be too risky.

2. A second woman is selected to be inseminated with the father's sperm. She signs a contract agreeing to bear the child and give it up after birth, usually for a sum of money.

3. Shortly after birth, the child is given to the couple. The child is genetically linked to the father but not to the mother. Whether the woman who bore the child—the biological mother—has the right to change her mind and keep the child is still open to question.

Adoptive

1. Couple is unable to conceive or chooses not to. (Single men and women and gay and lesbian couples may also choose to adopt a child.)

2. An adoption agency matches the couple with child to be adopted, or the couple or a lawyer arranges an open adoption with a pregnant woman.

3. Adoption papers are signed. Couple accepts parental responsibilities but has no genetic link to the child.

---

sperm or egg. In vitro fertilization is a costly procedure and usually has to be repeated a number of times before a viable pregnancy results; success rates between 12 and 20 percent are usually reported. In addition, some aspects of in vitro fertilization have sparked intense moral and legal debate. Recent court cases have involved the status of frozen embryos after the parents divorced and the status of frozen embryos as heirs to the estate of their parents, who were both killed in a plane crash before the embryos could be implanted. People are also debating the moral implications of allowing research to be conducted on embryos that have been frozen.

The most controversial of all approaches to infertility is surrogate motherhood. This practice involves a contract between a fertile woman who agrees to carry a fetus and a couple who wishes to have a child but cannot because the woman is infertile. The surrogate mother agrees to be artificially inseminated by the father's sperm, carry the baby to term, and give it to the couple at birth. In return, the couple pays her for her services. Some people question the morality of paying a woman to carry a baby. They see surrogate motherhood as an arrangement essentially to sell a baby, and they worry about the psychological consequences for children who learn that their biological mothers "sold" them. Experience has shown, too, that some surrogate mothers have a very difficult time giving up the baby they have carried and are unwilling to fulfill the contract after the birth, causing emotional trauma for themselves and the couple. There are thought to be several hundred births to surrogate mothers each year in the United States.

All these treatments for infertility are expensive and emotionally draining, and their success is uncertain. Some infertile couples choose not to try to have children, while others turn to adoption, which can also be difficult

Artificial (intrauterine) insemination The introduction of semen into the vagina by artificial means, usually a syringe.

In vitro fertilization Combining ovum and sperm outside the body, usually in a laboratory dish, for the purpose of fertilization.

TERMS

and expensive. One measure that you can take now to avoid infertility is to protect yourself against STDs and to treat promptly and completely any diseases you do contract.

Emotional Responses to Infertility   Couples who seek treatment for infertility have often already confronted the possibility of not being able to become biological parents. Many infertile couples feel they have lost control over a major area of their lives. They may lose perspective on the rest of their lives as they focus more and more on the reasons for their infertility and on treatment. Infertile couples may need to set their own limits on how much treatment they are willing to undergo. Support groups for infertile couples can provide help in this difficult situation, but there are few easy answers to infertility. If treatment is unsuccessful, couples must mourn the loss of the children they will never bear. They must make some kind of decision about their future, whether to pursue plans for adoption or another treatment or to adjust to childlessness and go on with their lives.

> ***Personal Insight***   How do you think you would feel if you discovered that you were infertile? Would you consider extraordinary measures—artificial insemination or in vitro fertilization, for example—in order to become a parent? Would you consider adoption?

PREGNANCY

Pregnancy is usually discussed in terms of **trimesters**—three periods of about three months (or 13 weeks) each. During the first trimester, the mother experiences a few bodily changes and some fairly common symptoms. During the second trimester, often the most peaceful time of pregnancy, the mother gains weight, looks noticeably pregnant, and may experience a general sense of well-being if she is happy about having a child. The third trimester is the hardest for the mother because she must breathe, digest, excrete, and circulate blood for herself and the growing fetus. The weight of the fetus, the pressure of its body on her organs, and its increased demands on her system cause discomfort and fatigue and may make the mother increasingly impatient to give birth.

Pregnancy Tests

The earliest tests for pregnancy are chemical tests designed to detect the presence of **human chorionic gonadotropin (HCG)**, a hormone produced by the implanted fertilized egg. Home pregnancy test kits, which are sold over the counter in drugstores, come equipped with a small sample of red blood cells coated with HCG

antibodies, to which the user can add a small amount of her own urine. If the concentration of HCG is great enough, it will clump together with the HCG antibodies, indicating that the user is pregnant. If the directions are followed carefully, home pregnancy tests are 85–95 percent reliable. Inaccurate results can be caused by unclean conditions, vaginal or urinary infections, taking certain drugs or oral contraceptives, hormonal changes due to menopause, and moving the test while it's working. Blood and urine tests analyzed by a medical laboratory give more accurate results, but no absolute certainty of pregnancy exists until a fetal heartbeat and movements can be detected or an **ultrasound** is performed.

Changes in the Woman's Body

Hormonal changes begin as soon as the egg is fertilized, and for the next nine months the woman's body nourishes the fetus and adjusts to its growth. Let's take a closer look at the changes of early, middle, and late pregnancy (Figure 8-2).

Early Signs and Symptoms   Early recognition of pregnancy is important, especially for women with physical problems and nutritional deficiencies. The following symptoms of pregnancy are not absolute indications of pregnancy, but they are reasons to visit a gynecologist.

- Missed menstrual period. If an egg has been fertilized and implanted in the uterine wall, the uterine lining is retained to nourish the embryo. A woman who misses a period after having unprotected intercourse may be pregnant.

- Slight bleeding. Slight bleeding may follow the implanting of the fertilized egg in the uterine wall. Because this happens about the time a period is expected, the bleeding is sometimes mistaken for menstrual flow. It usually lasts only a few days.

- Nausea. About two-thirds of pregnant women feel nauseated, probably as a reaction to increased levels of progesterone and other hormones. The nausea is often called morning sickness, but some women have it all day long. It frequently disappears by the twelfth week.

- Breast tenderness. Some women experience breast tenderness, swelling, and tingling, usually described as different from the tenderness experienced before menstruation.

- Sleepiness, fatigue, and emotional upset. These symptoms result from hormonal changes.

Chemical tests for pregnancy can be done within weeks of fertilization. The first reliable physical signs of pregnancy can be distinguished about four weeks after a woman misses her menstrual period. (At this point the woman would be considered to be eight weeks pregnant because physicians calculate pregnancy from the time of

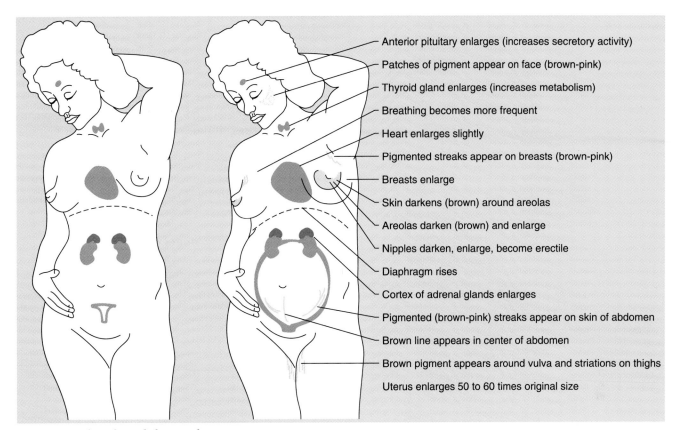

Figure 8-2 *Physiological changes during pregnancy.*
(Left) the female body at the time of conception; (right) development after 30 weeks of pregnancy.

The following labels point to the figure:

- Anterior pituitary enlarges (increases secretory activity)
- Patches of pigment appear on face (brown-pink)
- Thyroid gland enlarges (increases metabolism)
- Breathing becomes more frequent
- Heart enlarges slightly
- Pigmented streaks appear on breasts (brown-pink)
- Breasts enlarge
- Skin darkens (brown) around areolas
- Areolas darken (brown) and enlarge
- Nipples darken, enlarge, become erectile
- Diaphragm rises
- Cortex of adrenal glands enlarges
- Pigmented (brown-pink) streaks appear on skin of abdomen
- Brown line appears in center of abdomen
- Brown pigment appears around vulva and striations on thighs
- Uterus enlarges 50 to 60 times original size

the woman's last menstrual period rather than from the time of actual fertilization, since the latter date is often difficult to determine.) A softening of the uterus just above the cervix, called **Hegar's sign,** and other changes in the cervix and pelvis are apparent during a pelvic examination. The labia minora and the cervix may take on a purple color rather than their usual pink hue.

Continuing Changes in the Woman's Body   The most obvious changes during pregnancy occur in the reproductive organs. During the first three months, the uterus enlarges to about three times its nonpregnant size, but it still cannot be felt in the abdomen. By the fourth month, it is large enough to make the abdomen protrude. By the seventh or eighth month, the uterus pushes up into the rib cage, which makes breathing slightly more difficult. The breasts enlarge and are sensitive by the eighth week and may tingle or throb. The pigmented area around the nipple, the areola, darkens and broadens. After the tenth week, **colostrum,** a thin milky fluid, may be squeezed from the mother's nipples, but actual secretion of milk is prevented by high levels of estrogen and progesterone.

Other changes are going on as well. Early in pregnancy, the muscles and ligaments attached to bones begin to soften and stretch. The joints between the pelvic bones loosen and spread, making it easier to have a baby but

harder to walk. The circulatory system becomes more efficient to accommodate the blood volume, which increases by 50 percent, and the heart pumps it more rapidly. Much of the increased blood flow goes to the uterus and placenta. The mother's lungs also become more efficient, and her rib cage widens to permit her to inhale up to 40 percent more air. Again, much of the oxygen goes to the fetus. The kidneys become highly efficient, removing waste products from fetal circulation and producing large amounts of urine by midpregnancy.

How much weight should a woman gain during pregnancy? Women of normal weight gain an average of 18 to 25 percent of their initial weight: 20 to 28 pounds for a woman weighing 110; 23 to 32 pounds for a woman weighing 128 pounds. Reducing diets during pregnancy

Trimester   One of the three 13-week periods of pregnancy.
Human chorionic gonadatropin (HCG)   A hormone produced by the fertilized egg that can be detected in the urine or blood of the mother within a few weeks of conception.
Hegar's sign   A softening of the uterus just above the cervix that may be an early indication of pregnancy.
Colostrum   The thin, milky fluid secreted by the mammary glands around the time of childbirth until milk comes in, about the third day.

TERMS

duction darkens the skin in 90 percent of pregnant women, especially in places that have stretched.

Sexual activity often changes during pregnancy. Varying hormone levels and increased sensitivity in the genital area cause some women to become more interested in sexual intercourse and others less interested. Both responses are common and are influenced by the woman's and her partner's attitudes toward sexuality during pregnancy. Intercourse is possible throughout pregnancy, but physical awkwardness in later months may interfere with comfort. Open communication between the partners is essential to a satisfying sexual relationship during pregnancy.

Changes of the Later Stages of Pregnancy By the end of the sixth month, the increased needs of the fetus place a burden on the mother's lungs, heart, and kidneys. Her back may ache from the pressure of the baby's weight and from having to throw her shoulders back to keep her balance while standing (Figure 8-3). Her body retains more water, perhaps up to three extra quarts of fluid. Her legs, hands, ankles, or feet may swell, and she may be bothered by leg cramps, heartburn, or constipation. Despite discomfort, both her digestion and her metabolism are working at top efficiency.

The uterus prepares for childbirth throughout pregnancy with preliminary contractions, called **Braxton Hicks contractions.** Unlike true labor contractions, these are usually short, irregular, and painless. The mother may only be aware that at times her abdomen is hard to the touch. These contractions become more frequent and intense as the delivery date approaches.

In the ninth month, the baby settles into the pelvic bones, usually head down, fitting snugly. This process, called **lightening,** allows the uterus to sink down about two inches, producing a visible change in the mother's profile. Pelvic pressure increases and pressure on the diaphragm lightens. Breathing becomes easier; urination becomes more frequent. Sometimes, after a first pregnancy, the baby doesn't settle down into the pelvis until **labor** begins.

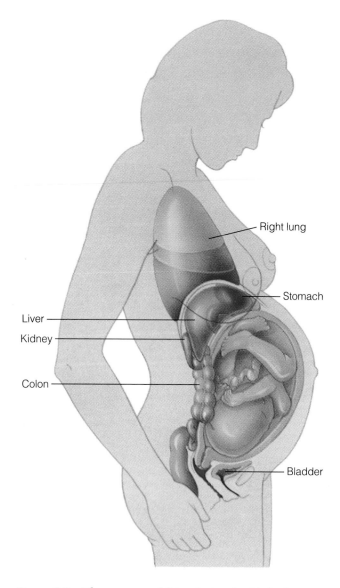

Figure 8-3 *The woman and fetus during the third trimester of pregnancy.*
Pressure from the rapidly growing fetus on the mother's lungs, bladder, stomach, and other organs may cause shortness of breath, heartburn, and the need for frequent urination. The mother's uterus has expanded to 50 or 60 times its original size.

Right lung
Stomach
Liver
Kidney
Colon
Bladder

Personal Insight How do you feel about the changes in a woman's appearance during pregnancy? Do you have an emotional reaction to these changes? Do you think pregnancy makes a woman more or less attractive? Why do you think you feel the way you do?

Emotional Responses to Pregnancy

A woman's feelings during pregnancy will vary dramatically depending on her circumstances—her self-image, how she feels about pregnancy and motherhood, whether the pregnancy was planned, what type of relationship she

can deprive the fetus of needed nutrients, and they are discouraged even among overweight mothers. About 60 percent of weight gained relates directly to the baby—about 7.5 pounds for the baby and 8.5 pounds for the placenta, amniotic fluid, heavier breasts and uterus—and 40 percent accumulates over the mother's entire body as fluid (blood, about 4 pounds) and fat (4 to 8 pounds). But gains in total pregnancy pounds vary strikingly, and similarities in total weight gain appear to conceal large differences in components of gain. As the woman's skin stretches, small breaks may occur in the elastic fibers of the lower layer of skin, producing "stretch marks" on her abdomen, hips, breasts, or thighs. Increased pigment pro-has with her partner, whether she has a secure home situation, and many other factors. A first pregnancy is especially important because it has traditionally symbolized the transition to maturity and is a major developmental milestone in the lives of mothers—and fathers as well.

Pregnancy is likely to change a couple's relationship. Communication is especially important because people may have preconceived ideas about how they and their partners should feel. Both partners may have fears about the approaching birth, their ability to be good parents, and the ways in which the baby will affect their own relationship. These concerns are normal, and sharing them can deepen and strengthen a relationship. For a woman without a partner or whose partner is not supportive, it's important that she find other sources of support, perhaps from friends, family members, or support groups. The relationships that parents-to-be have with their own parents may also undergo changes. Impending parenthood may allow them to assert their independence from their parents but may also allow them to identify with their parents' own experience of pregnancy, childbirth, and parenting.

Rapid changes in hormone levels can cause a pregnant woman to experience unpredictable emotions. A great part of pregnancy is beyond the woman's control—her changing appearance, her energy level, her variable moods—and some women need extra support and reassurance to keep on an even keel. Hormonal changes can also make women feel exhilarated and euphoric, although for some women such moods are temporary.

Like the physical changes that accompany pregnancy, emotional responses also change as the pregnancy develops. During the first trimester, the pregnant woman may fear that she may miscarry or that the child will not be normal. Education about pregnancy and childbirth as well as support from her partner, friends, relatives, and health care professionals are important antidotes to these fears. During the second trimester, the pregnant woman can feel the fetus move within her and worries about miscarriages will probably begin to diminish. The pregnant woman may look and feel radiantly happy and be delighted as her pregnancy begins to show. However, a woman may also worry that her increasing size makes her unattractive. Reassurance from her partner can ease these fears.

The third trimester is the time of greatest physical stress during the pregnancy. A woman may find that her physical abilities are limited by her size. Because they feel physically awkward and sexually unattractive, some women may experience periods of depression. But many also feel a great deal of happy excitement and anticipation. The fetus may already be looked upon as a member of the family, and both parents may begin talking to the fetus and interacting with it by patting the mother's belly. The upcoming birth will probably be a focus for both the woman and her partner.

Fetal Development

Now that we've seen what happens to the mother's body during pregnancy, let's consider the development of the fetus. By the end of the first trimester, the anatomy of the fetus is almost completely formed; further refinements are made during the second trimester; and needed fat and pounds are added during the third trimester (Figure 8-4).

First Trimester   About 30 hours after the egg is fertilized the cell reproduces itself by dividing in half. The process of cell division repeats many times. As the cluster of cells drifts down the oviduct, several different kinds of cells emerge. The entire genetic code is passed to every cell, but each cell follows only a segment of the code; if this were not the case, there would be no different organs or body parts. For example, all cells carry genes for hair color and eye color, but only the cells of the hair follicles and irises respond to that information.

On about the fourth day after fertilization, the cluster, now about 64 to 128 cells and hollow, arrives in the uterus. In this form it is known as a **blastocyst**. On the sixth or seventh day, the blastocyst burrows into the uterine lining, usually along the upper curve. One week after conception the cells number over 100, and the cluster is now considered an **embryo.** It begins to draw nourishment from the **endometrium,** the uterine lining.

Soon, the spherical cluster collapses in on itself, and the inner cells now transform themselves by separating into three layers. One layer composes inner body parts, the digestive and respiratory systems; another layer becomes the skin, hair, and nervous tissue; and the middle layer becomes muscle, bone, marrow, blood, kidneys, and sex glands.

The outermost shell of blastocyst cells becomes the **placenta,** umbilical cord, and **amniotic sac** (Figure 8-5).

Braxton Hicks contractions   Uterine contractions that occur periodically throughout pregnancy.

Lightening   A labor process in which the uterus sinks downward about 2 inches because the baby's head, or other body part, settles far down into the pelvic area.

Labor   The act or process of giving birth to a child, expelling it with the placenta from the mother's body by means of uterine contractions.

Blastocyst   A stage of human development, lasting only from about the sixth to the fourteenth day, during which the cell cluster divides into the embryo and the placenta.

Embryo   The developing cluster of cells from the end of the first week to the end of the eighth week following conception.

Endometrium   The mucous membrane that forms the inner lining of the cavity of the uterus.

Placenta   The organ through which the fetus receives nourishment and empties waste via the mother's circulatory system; after birth, the placenta is expelled from the uterus.

Amniotic sac   Fluid-filled membrane pouch enclosing and protecting the fetus.

TERMS

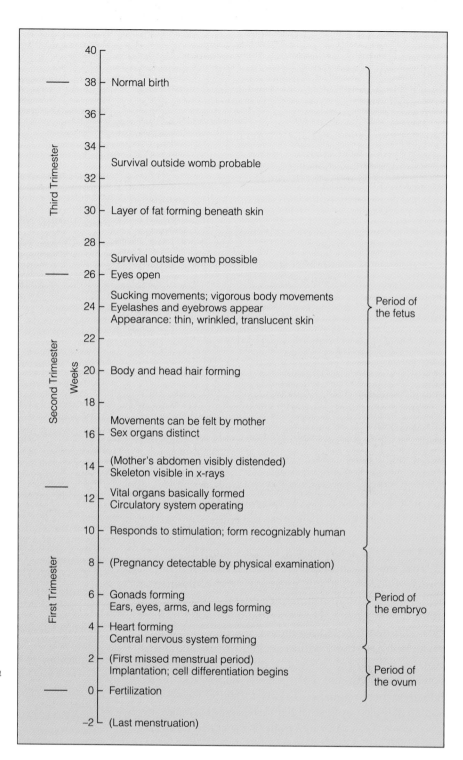

Figure 8-4 *Chronology of milestones in prenatal development.*
Source: Judith Schickedanz, David Schickedanz, Karen Hansen, and Peggy Forsyth. 1993. *Understanding Children.* 2nd ed. (Mountain View, Calif.: Mayfield), p. 86.

A network of roots called **chorionic villi** sprouts from the blastocyst and eventually forms the placenta. The human placenta is a two-way street, allowing the transfer of some materials between the mother and the fetus. The placenta brings oxygen and nutrients to the fetus and transports waste products out. The placenta does not provide a perfect barrier between the fetal circulation and the maternal circulation, however. Some blood cells are exchanged and some substances, such as alcohol, pass freely from the maternal circulation through the placenta to the fetus.

The period between the second and ninth weeks of development is a time of rapid differentiation and change. All the major body structures are formed during this time, including the heart, brain, liver, lungs, and sex organs; the eyes, nose, ears, arms, and legs also appear. Some organs begin to function—the heart begins to beat and the liver starts producing blood cells. Because body structures are forming, the developing organism is vulnerable to damage from environmental influences such as drugs and infections (discussed in detail below).

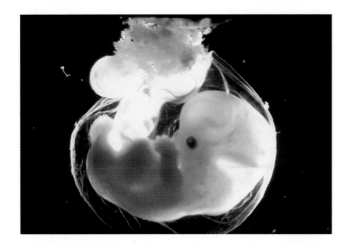

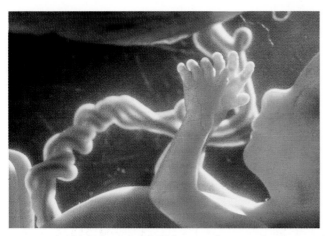

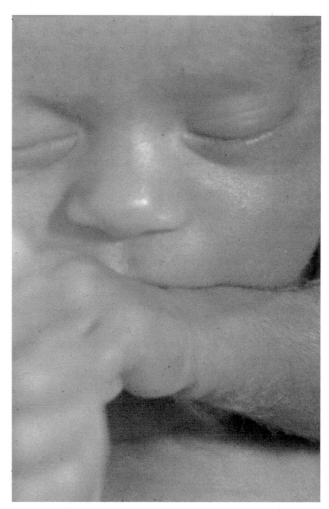

A six-week-old embryo (top left) has simple internal organs, including a beating heart, and is about 1 inch long. By the end of the first trimester, all the major body structures are formed, and some systems are functioning. By the fourth month, the fetus (bottom left) is growing rapidly and is about 10 inches long. Weighing about 6 ounces, it moves vigorously in the uterus and can suck, frown, and turn its head. At seven months, the fetus (right) weighs about 3 pounds and has grown to about 15 inches. Although it can now survive if born prematurely, it needs two more months in the womb to gain weight and acquire a layer of fat.

By the end of the second month, the brain sends out impulses that coordinate the functioning of other organs. The embryo is now considered a fetus, and most further bodily changes will be in the size and refinement of working parts. In the third month the fetus begins to be quite active. By the end of the first trimester, the fetus is about 4 inches long and weighs 1 ounce.

Second Trimester   To achieve its growth during the second trimester—to about 14 inches and 2 pounds—the fetus must have large amounts of food, oxygen, and water, which come from the mother through the placenta. All body systems are operating, and the fetal heartbeat can be heard with a stethoscope. Fetal movements can be felt by the mother beginning in the fourth or fifth month.

Against great odds, a fetus born prematurely at the end of the second trimester might survive.

Third Trimester   The fetus gains most of its birth weight during the last three months. Some of the weight is fatty tissue under the skin that insulates the fetus and supplies food. The fetus must obtain large amounts of calcium, iron, and nitrogen from the food the mother eats. Some

Chorionic villi   Threadlike blood vessels that sprout from the blastocyst into the mother's vessels to draw out blood and nourishment.

TERMS

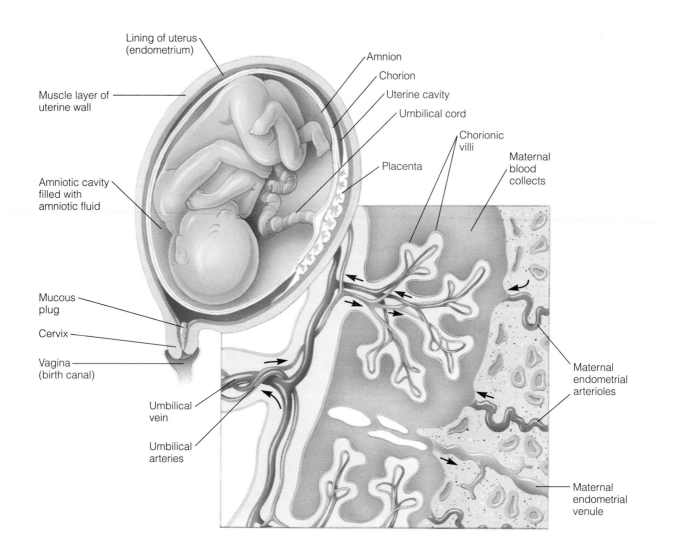

Figure 8-5 *A cross section of the uterus in pregnancy.*

85 percent of the calcium and iron she consumes goes into the fetal bloodstream.

Although the fetus may live if it is born during the seventh month, it needs the fat layer acquired in the eighth month and time for the organs, especially the respiratory and digestive organs, to develop. It also needs the immunities that the mother's blood supplies in the last three months. Her blood protects the fetus against many of the diseases to which she has acquired immunity. These immunities wear off within six months after birth, but they can be replenished by the mother's milk if the baby is breastfed.

Diagnosing Abnormalities of the Fetus Information about the health and sex of a fetus can be obtained before it's born through prenatal testing. The most common tests now used are ultrasound, alpha-fetoprotein (AFP) screening, amniocentesis, and chorionic villus sampling. **Ultrasound** examinations use high-frequency sound waves to create a visual image (**sonogram**) of the fetus in the

uterus. Sonograms show the position of the fetus, its size and gestational age, and the presence of certain anatomical problems, such as cleft palate; sonograms can sometimes be used to determine the sex of the fetus. Studies have not identified problems in humans associated with ultrasound, but high levels of ultrasound have created problems in animal fetuses.

Alpha-fetoprotein (AFP) is a protein produced by the fetus and present in the amniotic fluid and in the mother's blood. **Alpha-fetoprotein (AFP) screening**, usually done between 15 and 20 weeks into the pregnancy, involves analysis of AFP levels in a sample of the mother's blood. Although not foolproof, high levels of AFP may indicate the presence of neural tube defects such as anencephaly (absence of part or all of the brain) and spina bifida. A low level of AFP sometimes indicates a chromosomal defect, such as Down's syndrome. Particularly high or low results may also indicate that the dates of the pregnancy are wrong. If the results of AFP indicate a possible problem, other tests are done to confirm the results.

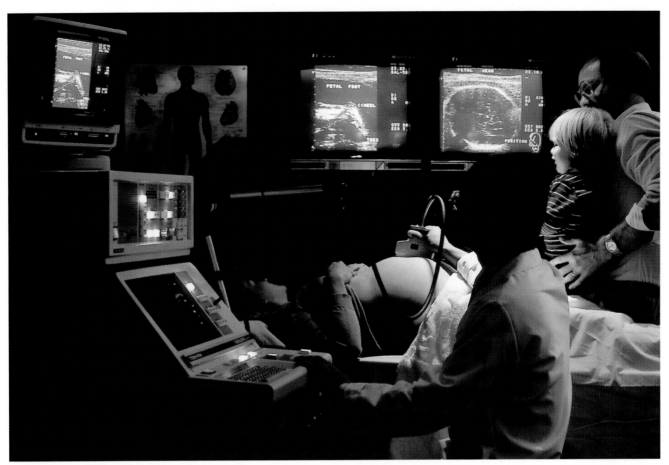

Ultrasound provides information about the position, size, and physical condition of a fetus in the uterus. This couple can see the baby move and perhaps tell its sex by watching it on the screen.

Amniocentesis involves the removal of fluid from the uterus with a long, thin needle inserted through the abdominal wall. It is usually performed at about 16 weeks of gestation. A genetic analysis of the fetal cells contained in the fluid can reveal the presence of possible birth defects such as Down's syndrome, Tay-Sachs disease, spina bifida, and other conditions caused by chromosomal abnormalities. The sex of the fetus can also be determined. Most amniocentesis tests are performed on mothers over the age of 35, who face a greater risk for chromosomal abnormalities, or in cases where the fetus is known to be at risk for a particular chromosomal defect. Amniocentesis carries a slight risk (a 0.5 to 2 percent chance of fetal death).

A newer alternative to amniocentesis is **chorionic villus sampling (CVS)**, which can be performed between the ninth and eleventh weeks of gestation. This procedure involves removal through the cervix (by catheter) or abdomen (by needle) of a tiny piece of the chorionic villi, which contains fetal cells that can be analyzed. CVS also carries a slight risk of fetal death.

Genetic counselors explain the results of the different tests so that parents can understand their implications. If a fetus is found to have a defect, it may be carried to term, aborted, or, in rare instances, surgically treated while still in the uterus. The results of CVS are usually available during the first trimester, allowing for a first-trimester abortion in case of a defect. The results of amniocentesis and AFP screening are usually not available until the second trimester of pregnancy. Consequently, if the pregnancy is terminated through abortion at this stage, it's likely to be physically and emotionally difficult.

TERMS

Ultrasound   High-frequency sound waves used to view the fetus by a method called ultrasonography.

Sonogram   The visual image of the fetus produced through the use of ultrasound.

Alpha-fetoprotein (AFP) screening   Tests of the level of alpha-fetoprotein in a pregnant woman's blood that can reveal the possible presence of fetal abnormalities.

Amniocentesis   A process in which amniotic fluid is removed to detect possible birth defects.

Chorionic villus sampling   Surgical removal of a tiny piece of chorionic villi to be analyzed for genetic defects.

The Importance of Prenatal Care

Adequate prenatal care—appropriate diet, exercise, and rest, avoidance of drugs, and regular medical evaluation—is essential to the health of both mother and baby. The pregnant woman cannot help but be responsible for the condition of the baby she carries. Everything she eats, drinks, and does affects the fetus to one degree or another. The fetus gets its nutrients and oxygen from the mother's bloodstream and has its wastes removed the same way. Many harmful substances can also be passed on to the fetus via the placenta and umbilical cord. For these reasons, taking care of her health during pregnancy is a lifelong investment in her child's health.

Regular Checkups

In the woman's first visit to her obstetrician, she will be asked for a detailed medical history of herself and her family. The physician or midwife will note especially any hereditary conditions that may assume increased significance during pregnancy. The tendency to develop gestational diabetes (diabetes during pregnancy only), for example, can be inherited. Appropriate treatment during pregnancy reduces the risk of serious harm from the condition, if it does develop.

The woman is given a complete physical exam and is informed about appropriate diet. She returns for regular checkups throughout the pregnancy, during which her blood pressure and weight gain are measured and tracked and the size and position of the fetus are monitored. Regular prenatal visits also give the mother a chance to discuss her concerns and to assure herself that everything is proceeding normally. Early advice from physicians, midwives, health educators, and teachers of childbirth classes provides the mother with invaluable information.

Blood Tests

A blood sample is taken during the initial prenatal visit to reveal blood type, anemia, and Rh incompatibilities. The Rh factor is a protein found in the blood. If an Rh-positive father and an Rh-negative mother conceive an Rh-positive baby, the baby's blood will be incompatible with the mother's. If some of the baby's blood enters the mother's bloodstream during delivery, she will develop antibodies to it just as she would toward a virus. If she has subsequent Rh-positive babies, the antibodies in the mother's blood, passing through the placenta, will destroy the fetus's red blood cells, possibly leading to jaundice, anemia, mental retardation, or death. This condition is completely treatable with a serum called Rh-immune globulin, which destroys Rh-positive cells as they enter the mother's body and prevents her from forming antibodies to them. (Blood tests can also reveal the presence of some sexually transmissible diseases, discussed later in the chapter.)

Prenatal Nutrition

An appropriate diet throughout pregnancy is essential for both the fetus and the mother. Not only does the baby get all its nutrients from the mother, but it also competes with her for nutrients not sufficiently available to meet both their needs. When a woman's diet is low in iron or calcium, the fetus receives most of it and the mother may become deficient in it. To meet the increased nutritional demands of her body, a pregnant woman shouldn't just eat more; she should make sure that her diet is adequate in all the basic nutritional categories. In the second and third trimesters, requirements increase for calories and most nutrients, including protein, calcium, the B vitamins, vitamins A, C, D, and E, iodine, iron, magnesium, and zinc. With the possible exception of iron, for which some authorities recommend a supplement, all these nutrients can be obtained from a sensible, varied diet designed for a healthy pregnancy. Table 8-1 provides nutritional guidelines for pregnancy.

Avoiding Drugs and Other Environmental Hazards

In addition to the food the mother eats, the drugs she takes and the chemicals she is exposed to affect the fetus. Some experts believe that everything the mother ingests eventually reaches the fetus in some proportion. Some drugs harm the fetus but not the mother because the fetus is in the process of developing and because the proper dose for the mother represents a massive dose for the fetus.

During the first trimester, when basic body structures are rapidly forming, the fetus is extremely vulnerable to environmental factors such as viral infections, radiation, drugs, and other **teratogens,** any of which can cause **congenital malformations** (birth defects). The most susceptible body parts are those growing most rapidly at the time of exposure. The rubella (German measles) virus, for example, can cause a congenital malformation of a delicate system such as the eyes or ears, leading to blindness or deafness, if exposure occurs during the first trimester, but it does no damage later in the pregnancy. Similarly, the tranquilizer thalidomide taken early in pregnancy prevented the formation of arms and legs in fetuses, but taken later, when limbs were already formed, it caused no damage. Other drugs can cause damage throughout prenatal development.

Currently, there is an alarming increase in the number of babies born who were exposed during the prenatal period to damaging psychoactive drugs, most notably cocaine. Babies exposed to cocaine are likely to be born prematurely and to have malformed hearts and skulls. They tend to be extremely irritable, ultrasensitive to noise and touch, difficult to comfort or console, and unable to re-

TERMS

Teratogen An agent or influence that causes physical defects in a developing embryo.

Congenital malformation A physical defect existing at the time of birth, either inherited or caused during gestation.

TABLE 8-1 Nutritional Guidelines for Pregnancy

Food Group	Nutrients Provided	Daily Requirements	Sources and Equivalents
Milk and milk products	Calcium, protein, vitamins, minerals, calories	4 servings	1 serving = 1 C milk, yogurt, custard, or milk pudding 1½ oz. cheddar-type cheese 1½ C cottage cheese
Meat and other protein sources	Protein, minerals, vitamins, calories	3 servings, 2–3 oz. each	1 3 oz. serving = 1 chicken leg ½ chicken breast 1 lean hamburger 1 medium pork chop 1 small fish fillet ½ serving = 3 T peanut butter 2 oz. cheddar-type cheese ¾ C cooked dried beans, chickpeas, or lentils ¾ C cottage cheese 1 C tofu 4 T sunflower seeds 1½ C yogurt 2 eggs
Fruit and vegetables	Vitamins C and A, other vitamins and minerals, fiber, calories	1 serving vitamin C source every day, 1 serving vitamin A source every other day + 3–7 additional servings (5–9 servings total)	Vitamin C sources: broccoli, brussels sprouts, cabbage, cantaloupe, cauliflower, citrus fruits, bell pepper, spinach, strawberries, potatoes, tomatoes Vitamin A sources: dried apricots, cantaloupe, carrots, squash, sweet potatoes, leafy green vegetables, broccoli, cabbage, pumpkin
Enriched or whole-grain breads and cereals	Protein, iron, B vitamins, other vitamins and minerals, calories	6–11 servings	1 serving = 1 slice bread ½ bagel or English muffin 1 biscuit or dinner roll ½ C cooked cereal ½–¾ C dry cereal 5–7 crackers ½ C cooked macaroni, noodles, or spaghetti 1 tortilla 1 pancake ½ C cooked rice
Fats and sweets	calories	No specific recommendations beyond nonpregnant requirement of 1 T polyunsaturated fat per day	These fat sources all have about 45 calories: 1 t butter or margarine 1 slice bacon 2 T half and half 1½ T sour cream 1 T cream cheese 1 t salad oil 1 t mayonnaise 1 T French dressing ⅛ avocado 6 small nuts

Sources: Ellen Satter. 1986. *Child of Mine* (Palo Alto, Calif.: Bull Publishing); Mike Samuels and Nancy Samuels. 1979. *The Well Baby Book* (New York: Summit Books); Laurel Robertson, Carol Flinders, and Bronwen Godfrey. 1976. *Laurel's Kitchen* (Petaluma, Calif.: Nilgiri Press); U.S. Department of Agriculture. *Food Guide Pyramid.* Home and Garden Bulletin No. 249.

spond normally to the people who care for them. These early problems affect every area of functioning, including social, emotional, language, and intellectual development.

An even more prevalent problem is prenatal exposure to alcohol, another teratogen. A high level of alcohol consumption during pregnancy is associated with miscarriages, stillbirths, and, in live babies, **fetal alcohol syndrome (FAS)**. A baby born with FAS is likely to suffer from mental retardation, low birth weight, abnormal smallness of the head, unusual facial characteristics, congenital heart defects, defective joints, and abnormal behavior patterns. The Centers for Disease Control estimate that more than 8,000 alcohol-affected babies are born every year in the United States. Although occasional or moderate drinking was earlier thought to have no negative effects on the fetus, researchers now doubt that any level of alcohol consumption is safe, and they recommend total abstinence during pregnancy. See Chapter 10 for more information on FAS.

Cigarette smoking is associated with several adverse conditions in newborns, including low birth weight. Researchers have observed that fetal breathing and movement become more rapid and agitated when the level of nicotine in the mother's bloodstream is high. A direct cause-and-effect relationship is difficult to establish between cigarette smoking and problems at birth, but infants whose parents smoke are unusually susceptible to pneumonia and bronchitis during their first year. Since no benefits for either the mother or the fetus come from smoking, many mothers stop smoking during pregnancy.

Some prescription drugs can also harm the fetus, so they should be used only under medical supervision. Accutane, a popular anti-acne drug, is thought to be responsible for over 1,000 cases of severe birth defects in the 1980s. Vitamins, aspirin and other over-the-counter drugs, and large quantities of caffeine-containing foods and beverages should be avoided or used only under a physician's direction. Large doses of vitamin A, for example, can cause birth defects. Chemicals and pollutants can also pose a danger to the fetus. Mercury, from fish contaminated by industrial pollution, is known to cause physical deformities. Continuous exposure to lead, found in some paint products and in water from lead pipes, has been implicated as a cause of a variety of learning disorders. Any product containing chemicals—including chemical fertilizers, solvents, and pesticides—should be avoided or used with extreme caution. Other agents and conditions known to affect prenatal development are shown in Table 8-2.

Infections, including those that are sexually transmitted, are another serious problem for the fetus, if contracted either before or during birth. If a mother contracts rubella during the first trimester, her child may be born with physical or mental disabilities. Immunization against measles must take place before pregnancy, because the immunization is harmful to the fetus. Syphilis can infect and kill a fetus; if the baby is born alive, it will have syphilis. Penicillin given to the mother during pregnancy cures syphilis in both mother and fetus. Gonorrhea can infect the baby during delivery and cause blindness. Because gonorrhea is often asymptomatic, in many states newborns' eyes are routinely treated with silver nitrate or another antibiotic to destroy gonorrheal bacteria. In 1988, the Centers for Disease Control recommended that all pregnant women be tested for hepatitis B, a virus that can be passed from the mother to the infant at birth. If a woman tests positive, her infant can be immunized shortly after birth.

Herpes simplex can damage the baby's eyes and brain and cause death, and no cure has yet been discovered for it. About 2,000 babies die each year from neonatal herpes. Genital herpes can be transmitted to the baby during delivery if the mother's infection is in the active phase. If this is the case, the baby is delivered by cesarean section. An initial outbreak of herpes can be dangerous if it occurs during pregnancy because the virus may pass through the placenta to the fetus. For this reason, testing for genital herpes is recommended for both expectant parents. Once the baby is born, any caregiver who is experiencing a herpes outbreak should wash his or her hands often and not permit contact between hands or contaminated objects and the baby's mucous membranes (inside of eyes, mouth, nose, penis, vagina, vulva, and rectum).

Infection by the human immunodeficiency virus (HIV) is perhaps the most serious infection affecting newborns. The HIV virus, which causes AIDS, can be passed to the fetus by an HIV-infected mother during pregnancy or during labor and delivery. (A small number of cases of transmission through breastfeeding have also been reported.) A woman with HIV infection has about a 25 to 30 percent chance of passing the virus to the fetus. Nationwide, more than 4,000 children have AIDS, and three times that number are estimated to be infected with HIV. The babies most at risk for this fatal disease are those whose mothers are intravenous (IV) drug users or the sexual partners of IV drug users. Physicians now recommend that all women at risk for HIV infection have a blood test before becoming pregnant. And of course, women should also take all the necessary precautions to keep from becoming infected with HIV during and after pregnancy.

Prenatal Activity and Exercise Physical activity during pregnancy contributes to mental and physical well-being. Many women continue working at their jobs until late in their pregnancies, provided the work isn't so phys-

TERMS

Fetal alcohol syndrome A combination of birth defects caused by excessive alcohol consumption by the mother during pregnancy.

TABLE 8-2 *Environmental Factors Associated with Impairments During Prenatal Development*

Agent or Condition	Effects
Rubella (German measles)	Blindness; deafness; heart abnormalities; stillbirth
Cytomegalovirus (CMV)	Microcephaly (smaller than normal head); motor disabilities; hearing loss
Syphilis	Mental retardation; physical deformities; in utero death and miscarriage
HIV infection	Impaired immune response, leading eventually to death
Addictive drugs	Low birth weight; possible addiction of infant to the drug; hypersensitivity to stimuli; higher risk for stroke and respiratory distress
Smoking	Prematurity; low birth weight and length
Alcohol	Mental retardation; growth retardation; increased spontaneous abortion rate; microcephaly; structural abnormalities in the face; lowered IQ
Irradiation	Physical deformities; mental retardation
Inadequate diet	Reduction in brain growth; smaller than average birth weight; decrease in birth length; rickets
Tetracycline	Discoloration of teeth
Streptomycin	Eighth cranial nerve damage (hearing loss)
Quinine	Deafness
Barbiturates	Congenital malformations
DES (diethylstilbestrol)	Increased incidence of vaginal cancer in adolescent female offspring; impaired reproductive performance in male and female offspring
Valium	Cleft lip and palate
Accutane (13-cis-retinoic acid, a drug used to treat acne)	Small or absent ears; small jaws; hydrocephaly; heart defects
Endocrine disorders	Cretinism; microcephaly
Maternal age under 18	Prematurity; stillbirth; increased incidence of Down's syndrome
Maternal age over 35	Increased incidence of Down's syndrome
Malnutrition	Lower birth weight; abnormal reflexes and irritability; altered brain growth
Environmental chemicals (e.g., benzene, formaldehyde, PCBs, etc.)	Chromosome damage; spontaneous abortions; low birth weight

Source: Judith Schickedanz, David Schickedanz, Karen Hansen, and Peggy Forsyth. 1993. *Understanding Children,* 2nd ed. (Mountain View, Calif.: Mayfield), p. 104.

ically demanding that it jeopardizes their health. At the same time, pregnant women need more rest and sleep. They become fatigued more easily because the energy demands on their bodies are so great. They need adequate rest and sleep to maintain their own and the fetus's well-being.

The prospective mother can and should continue all reasonable exercising that she is accustomed to, such as tennis, swimming, low-impact aerobics, or dancing, unless or until her pregnancy inhibits movement. The amniotic sac protects the fetus so that normal activities will not harm it. More strenuous activities that could result in a fall, such as skiing, skating, or horseback riding, are best delayed until after the birth. A pregnant woman who hasn't been exercising and wants to start should first consult with her physician. Additional recommendations for

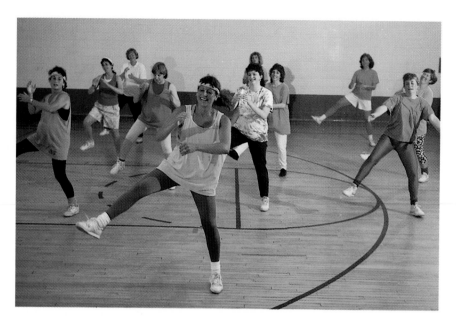

A woman's body changes drastically during pregnancy to accommodate and nourish the growing fetus. Prenatal exercise helps these women stay healthy while their bodies work to sustain two lives.

exercise during pregnancy from the American College of Obstetricians and Gynecologists (ACOG) include the following: Don't exercise strenuously for more than 15 minutes; keep heart rate below 140 beats per minute and body temperature below 100.4° F (38° C); avoid exercising in hot, humid weather or while you have a fever; don't hold your breath; avoid jarring movements or exercises that require deep flexion or extension of joints; and drink plenty of fluids before, during, and after exercise.

Prenatal exercise classes are valuable because they teach exercises that tone the body muscles involved in birth, especially those of the abdomen, back, and legs. Toned-up muscles aid delivery and help the body regain its nonpregnant shape afterward. A program of prenatal exercises is illustrated in the box "Exercises for Pregnancy and Birth."

Preparing for Birth As hospital childbirth practices have been increasingly challenged over the last 20 years, many women have chosen to learn techniques in childbirth preparation classes that help them deal with the discomfort of labor and delivery without pain-relieving drugs. One method of **prepared childbirth** was developed by Dr. Grantly Dick-Read, an English physician. Dick-Read believed that the pain experienced by women during birth results from learned fears that interfere, through tension, with the birth process.

To dispel these fears, childbirth educators teach parents the details of the birth process as well as relaxation techniques to use during labor and birth. Several similar methods of childbirth training are used now, including the Bradley method and the Lamaze method, all designed to ease birth through knowledge, relaxation, and physical conditioning. Most hospitals and childbirth educators tend to instruct parents in a combination of Lamaze and other relaxation techniques.

Childbirth classes are almost a routine part of the prenatal experience for both mothers and fathers these days. The mother learns and practices a variety of techniques so she can choose what works best for her during labor. The father typically acts as a coach, supporting the mother emotionally and helping her with her breathing and relaxing. He remains with the mother throughout labor and delivery, even when a cesarean section is performed. It can be an important and fulfilling time for the parents to be together.

Complications of Pregnancy and Pregnancy Loss

Pregnancy usually proceeds without major complications. Sometimes, however, complications may prevent full-term development of the fetus or affect the health of the infant at birth. As discussed earlier in the chapter, exposure to harmful substances, such as alcohol and cocaine, can harm the fetus. Other complications are caused by physiological problems or genetic abnormalities.

Ectopic Pregnancy In **ectopic pregnancy,** the fertilized egg implants itself and begins to develop outside the uterus, usually in an oviduct. Ectopic pregnancies usually occur because the tube is blocked, most often as a result of pelvic inflammatory disease. The embryo may spontaneously abort or the embryo and placenta may continue to expand until they rupture the oviduct. Sharp pain on one side of the abdomen or in the lower back, usually in about the seventh or eighth week of gestation, may signal an ectopic pregnancy; often there is also irregular bleeding. If bleeding from a rupture is severe, the woman may go into shock, characterized by low blood pressure, high pulse rate, weakness, and fainting. Surgical removal of the embryo and the tube may be necessary to save the mother's life, although microsurgery can sometimes be used to repair the damaged tube. The incidence of ectopic pregnancy has more than quadrupled in the last 20 years, and it is the leading cause of pregnancy-related death in the United States.

Spontaneous Abortion   A **spontaneous abortion** or **miscarriage** is a pregnancy that ends before the twentieth week of gestation. Although the exact frequency of spontaneous abortion is unknown, it is estimated that 10–40 percent of pregnancies end this way, some without the woman's awareness that she was pregnant. Most miscarriages occur between the sixth and eighth weeks of pregnancy, and most—about 60 percent—are due to chromosomal abnormalities in the fetus. Certain occupations that involve exposure to chemicals may increase the likelihood of spontaneous abortions.

Vaginal bleeding ("spotting") is usually the first sign that a pregnant woman may miscarry. She may also develop pelvic cramps and her symptoms of pregnancy may disappear. One miscarriage doesn't mean that later pregnancies will be unsuccessful, and about 70–90 percent of women who miscarry eventually become pregnant again. About 1 percent of women suffer three or more miscarriages, possibly because of anatomic, hormonal, genetic, or immunological factors.

Toxemia   A potentially serious condition that occasionally develops in the later months of pregnancy (usually not before the twentieth week) is **toxemia,** characterized by high blood pressure and fluid retention. The early stages of toxemia, known as **preeclampsia,** can usually be treated through nutritional means. However, if left untreated, blood pressure continues to rise, the face and legs swell, and excess protein appears in the urine. In the later stages, known as **eclampsia,** vision blurs and the head aches continuously, leading eventually to convulsions, coma, and even death. Toxemia is not common and it can be prevented or controlled through diet, rest, and sometimes medication. A woman who notices facial edema (swelling) should see her physician immediately. Changes in blood pressure and the presence of excess protein in the urine are normally noticed and tracked during routine prenatal examinations.

Low Birth Weight   A **low birth weight (LBW)** baby usually weighs less than 5.5 pounds at birth. LBW babies may be premature (born before the thirty-seventh week of pregnancy) or full-term. Babies who are born small even though they're full-term are referred to as small-for-date babies. Most LBW babies will grow normally, but some will experience disabilities. Although they are at greater risk than bigger babies for complications during infancy, small-for-date babies tend to have fewer problems than premature infants.

The most fundamental problem of prematurity is that many of the infant's organs are not sufficiently developed.

Premature infants are subject to respiratory problems and infections. They may have difficulty eating because they may be too small to suck a breast or bottle and their swallowing mechanism may be underdeveloped. As they get older, premature infants may have problems such as low intelligence, learning difficulties, poor hearing and vision, and physical awkwardness.

Low birth weight affects about 7 percent of infants born each year in the United States. About half of all cases of LBW are related to teenage pregnancy, cigarette smoking, poor nutrition, and poor health of the mother. One study found a sixfold increase in the risk of LBW if the mother had financial problems during the pregnancy. Adequate prenatal care is the best means of preventing LBW.

Infant Mortality   The rate of **infant mortality** (the death of a child of less than one year of age) in the United States is at its lowest point ever; however, it remains far higher than that of most of the developed world. The United States ranks twenty-fourth in the world for low infant mortality, with 8.9 deaths for every 1,000 live births in 1991. Many of these deaths are due to poverty and lack of adequate health care; in some inner-city areas in Detroit and parts of Oakland (California), the infant mortality rate approaches that of nonindustrialized countries, with more than 20 deaths per 1,000 births. Poverty-related infant mortality could be reduced by making sure that all pregnant women receive prenatal care and that all infants and young children receive adequate health care and immunizations.

Although many infants die of poverty-related conditions, others die from congenital problems, infectious diseases, injuries, and other causes. About 1 out of every 375

Prepared childbirth   Preparation for birth that includes physical conditioning, instruction in the process of birth and what to expect, and psychological and emotional conditioning so that fear and anxiety are kept to a minimum, making childbirth as pain-free as possible. It can include but does not require labor and delivery without drugs.

Ectopic pregnancy   A pregnancy in which the embryo develops outside the uterus, most typically in the fallopian tube.

Spontaneous abortion (miscarriage)   Termination of pregnancy when the uterine contents are expelled; causes vary, but can include an abnormal uterus, insufficient hormones, and genetic or physical fetal defects.

Toxemia   A condition of pregnancy characterized by high blood pressure and edema; preeclampsia and eclampsia.

Preeclampsia   Early stage of toxemia characterized by increasingly high blood pressure, edema, and protein in the urine.

Eclampsia   Severe form of toxemia characterized by convulsions, coma, and possibly death (in addition to the symptoms of preeclampsia).

Low birth weight (LBW)   Weighing less than 5 pounds at birth, often the result of prematurity.

Infant mortality   Death of a child of less than 1 year of age.

TERMS

The following series of 10 exercises takes about 15 or 20 minutes to perform. You can do them daily, if you wish.

1. **Kegel exercise**
   (to strengthen the muscles of the pelvic floor)
   This exercise can be done in any position. Contract your perineal muscles and hold for about 5 seconds. (To learn the exercise, try stopping and starting the flow of urine while you are urinating; this is the muscle action you want to imitate.) Work up to a series of 5 or 10 repetitions.

2. **Groin stretch**
   (helps make the delivery position more comfortable)

   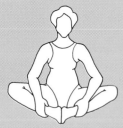

   Start by holding your ankles with the soles of your feet touching each other. Lean forward and press your knees down with your elbows, feeling a gentle stretch in your groin and inner thighs. Hold the position for 10 to 30 seconds. Repeat three times.

3. **Single knee tuck**
   (stretches lower back to help prevent or reduce back pain)

   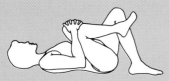

   Start on your back with knees bent and the soles of your feet flat. Bring one knee to your chest feeling a gentle stretch of the lower back. Relax the lower back as you hold for 10 seconds. Switch knees and repeat the entire cycle three times. (The American College of Obstetricians and Gynecologists—ACOG—recommends that women not perform any exercises in the supine position after the fourth month of pregnancy, but recent research has shown that it is safe for short periods of time.)

4. **Hamstring stretch**
   (to stretch the hamstring muscles)

   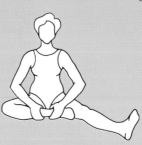

   Start with one leg straight, the other tucked in. Reach for the ankle of the extended leg, feeling the gentle stretch of the muscles in the back of the thigh. Hold the stretch for 10 to 30 seconds. Switch legs and repeat the entire cycle three times.

5. **Pelvic tilting on back**
   (to strengthen the abdominal muscles)

   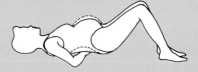

   Start on your back with knees bent. Place one hand in the hollow of your back, the other on the rim of the hip. Slowly tighten the abdominal and buttock muscles by pushing down on your hand with the small of your back. Rock the baby back into the pelvic cradle as you roll your hips back gently. Breathe out as you contract the abdominal muscles. Hold the contraction for 3 to 6 seconds and then relax as you breathe in. Keep your back flat throughout. Repeat three to five times. (ACOG recommends that women not perform any exercises in the supine position after the fourth month of pregnancy, but recent research has shown that it is safe for short periods of time.)

---

infant deaths is due to **sudden infant death syndrome (SIDS),** in which an apparently healthy infant dies suddenly while sleeping.

Coping with Loss Parents form a deep attachment to their children even before birth, and parents who lose an infant before or during birth usually experience a deep grief reaction. Initial feelings of shocked disbelief and numbness may give way to sadness, anger, crying spells, and preoccupation with the loss. Physical sensations such as tightness in the chest or stomach, loss of appetite, and sleeplessness may also occur. For the mother, physical exhaustion and hormone imbalances can compound the emotional and physical stress.

Experiencing the pain of loss is part of the healing process, which can take up to a year or more. Keeping active with work or travel can help renew interest in life. Support groups or professional counseling is also often helpful. Planning the next pregnancy, with a physician's input, can be an important step toward recovery, as long

TERMS

Sudden infant death syndrome (SIDS) Sudden death of an apparently healthy infant during sleep.

6. **Chest push**
(for strength and endurance of the chest muscles)

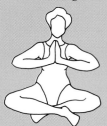

Start with your elbows bent and palms together. Press your palms firmly together so that you can feel the tightening of the pectoral muscles under the breasts. Hold the press for 3 to 6 seconds. Repeat three times.

7. **Sit-back**
(for abdominal strength and endurance)

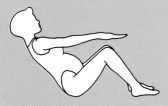

Start in an upright sitting position. Reach forward with your arms and sit back to a 45° angle. Hold the V-like position for 3 to 6 seconds. Repeat three times.

8. **Pelvic tilting on all fours**
(to strengthen abdominal muscles)

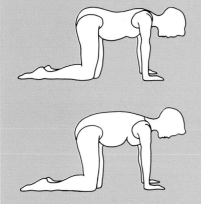

Start in a kneeling position with your arms extended for support. Pull your back and pelvis up into a catlike position. Hold for 3 to 6 seconds and relax to the starting position, but never let your spine sag. Repeat three times.

9. **Squat**
(to strengthen thigh and hip muscles)

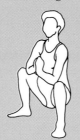

If you have no knee problems, start with your feet flat on the floor, squatting halfway down. Hold for 3 to 6 seconds, then stand up. Eventually go into full squat. If necessary, have a partner hold your hands to assist with balance. Repeat three times. If you have knee problems, limit movement to half squat.

10. **Wall push-away**
(for strength and endurance of the arms and shoulders and for flexibility of the Achilles tendon)

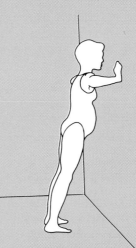

Start supporting yourself with your arms extended against the wall. Bend your arms, allowing your head and upper body to slowly come toward the wall. Hold this position for 10 seconds so that you can feel the stretch of your calves and Achilles tendon. Push away slowly to starting position. Repeat three times.

Source: Ivan Kusinitz and Morton Fine. 1991. *Your Guide to Getting Fit,* 2nd ed. (Mountain View, Calif.: Mayfield), pp. 216–218.

---

as the mind and body are given time to heal. If future pregnancies are ruled out, couples can consider other options, including adoption.

CHILDBIRTH

By the end of the ninth month of pregnancy, most women are tired of being pregnant; both mother and father are impatient to start a new phase of their lives. Most couples find the actual process of birth to be an exciting and positive experience.

Choices in Childbirth

Many couples today can choose the type of practitioner and the environment they want for the birth of their child. A high-risk pregnancy is probably best handled by a specialist physician in a hospital with a nursery, but for low-risk births, a wide variety of options is available.

Parents can choose to have their baby delivered by a physician (an obstetrician or family practitioner) or by a certified nurse-midwife. Certified nurse-midwives are registered nurses with special training in obstetrical techniques, and they are well qualified for prenatal and postnatal care, routine deliveries, and minor medical emergencies. They are usually much less expensive than physicians, and they often are part of a complete medical team that includes a backup physician in case of emergency. Nurse-midwives can usually participate in births in any setting, although this may vary according to hospital policy, state law, and the midwife's preferences. More than 90,000 babies each year are delivered by nurse-midwives.

Most babies in the United States are delivered in hospitals or in freestanding alternative birth centers; only about 2 percent of women choose to have their babies at home. Many hospitals have introduced alternative birth centers in response to criticisms of traditional hospital routines. Alternative birth centers provide a comfortable, emotionally supportive environment in close proximity to up-to-date medical equipment.

The impersonal, routine quality of hospital birth is increasingly being questioned, and many hospitals and physicians offer a variety of options to parents regarding many aspects of childbirth. It's important for parents-to-be to discuss all aspects of labor and delivery with their physician or midwife beforehand, so they can learn what to expect and, where appropriate, can state their preferences.

- Will the father be allowed in the delivery room? What about other family members or another support person? Will young siblings be allowed to visit the mother and new baby? Most hospitals now allow the father to stay in the delivery room. In alternative birth centers, the entire family may be allowed to witness the birth.

- What type of room will the mother be in during labor, delivery, and recovery? How many times will she be moved? Some hospitals and centers allow women to remain in one room during their entire stay.

- What type of tables, beds, or birthing chairs are available? A flat hospital table with stirrups for the woman's feet means the baby is delivered against the force of gravity. In most cultures, a woman gives birth while sitting in a birthing chair, kneeling, or squatting. Some hospitals and centers allow mothers to choose the position most comfortable for them or use birthing chairs that can be raised, lowered, or

TERMS

Electronic fetal monitoring (EFM) The use of an external or internal electronic monitor during labor to measure uterine contractions and fetal heart rate.

Episiotomy Incision in the perineum (from the vagina toward the anus) made to prevent uncontrolled tearing during childbirth.

Cesarean section A surgical incision through the abdominal wall and uterus, performed to extract a fetus.

Rooming-in The practice of allowing the mother and baby to remain together in the hospital or birth center after delivery.

tilted according to the needs of the physician and the mother.

- Will the mother receive any routine preparation, such as an enema, intravenous feeding, or shaving of the pubic area?

- Under what circumstances does the physician or midwife administer drugs to induce or augment labor? The use of these drugs tends to change the course of labor and carries a small risk.

- Does the physician or midwife typically use **electronic fetal monitoring (EFM)** during labor? About three-quarters of all births are electronically monitored, but there is disagreement among medical authorities about the risks and benefits of EFM. Although useful for high-risk pregnancies, studies indicate that routine EFM doesn't produce healthier babies for women with low-risk pregnancies. The American College of Obstetricians and Gynecologists recommends periodic monitoring using a stethoscope rather than EFM for low-risk pregnancies.

- Under what circumstances does the physician or midwife perform an **episiotomy?** Are any steps taken to avoid it? An episiotomy is currently performed in about 85 to 90 percent of births but some medical authorities question the need for routine episiotomies.

- Under what circumstances does the physician or midwife use forceps or vacuum extraction? In some cases of fetal distress, the use of forceps or vacuum extraction may be necessary to save the infant's life. These techniques are sometimes also used in cases in which delivery is proceeding slowly, but some authorities believe that if the fetus is not in distress, delivery can safely proceed naturally. Currently, about 10 percent of hospital deliveries include the use of forceps or vacuum extraction.

- What types of medications are typically used? Some form of anesthetic is usually administered during most hospital deliveries, as are hormones that intensify the contractions and shrink the uterus after delivery. The administration of anesthesia must balance the need for pain relief for the mother and the need to prevent exposing the fetus to drugs. The anesthetics most often used are short-acting narcotics, which ease the pain of labor somewhat and allow the mother to relax more between contractions, and regional nerve blocks, which numb the nerves from the uterus and the vagina. A local anesthetic may also be used to numb the tissue in the vaginal canal as the baby's head emerges or when an episiotomy is performed. A general anesthetic is usually used only when the baby is delivered by **cesarean section.**

- Under what circumstances does the physician perform a cesarean section? What is his or her rate of cesarean section? Some medical authorities feel that

The number of cesarean deliveries performed in the United States has risen dramatically in the past 30 years, causing concern among both parents and medical personnel. In 1970, 5.5 percent of American babies were delivered by cesarean section; today, nearly one out of every four babies—close to 25 percent—is delivered by cesarean. Yet according to national health statistics, there is no clear evidence that maternal and child health has improved as a result of this increase. Why are babies delivered by cesarean section, and why is the number of such operations increasing? What can be done to lower the rate of cesarean deliveries in the United States?

Cesarean sections are necessary when a baby can't be delivered vaginally. If the baby's head is bigger than the pelvic girdle of the mother, the baby may need to be delivered by cesarean. If the baby is in an unusual position—feet down, buttocks down, or lying sideways across the uterus—instead of in the usual head-down position, vaginal birth is more difficult. If the mother has a serious health condition such as kidney or heart disease, diabetes, high blood pressure, or toxemia, she may need to have a cesarean to avoid the stress of a long labor and a vaginal delivery. Sometimes a woman is unable to sustain labor, and a physician may perform a cesarean to reduce the risk of infection to the newborn. Other reasons for cesarean delivery include abnormal or difficult labor and fetal distress.

A substantial part of the increase in cesarean births is due to repeat cesarean deliveries. In the United States, fewer than about 10 percent of women who have had a cesarean in the past deliver subsequent babies vaginally; in other countries, the rate of vaginal birth after cesarean section is closer to 50 percent. The American College of Obstetricians and Gynecologists now recommends that low-risk women who have had one previous cesarean birth be encouraged to attempt labor and vaginal delivery in their current pregnancy.

Cesarean sections are major surgery and carry some risk themselves, although much less than in the past. Improved medical care—including better antibiotics and better use of anesthesia—make the procedure relatively safe. A local anesthetic may be used so the woman remains conscious during the operation. The father may be present in the delivery room during a cesarean. Advocates of increased reliance on cesareans claim that the procedure makes birth safer for mothers and babies in some situations. They point to reduced rates of maternal and neonatal mortality and the better health of newborns.

Critics of increased reliance on cesarean deliveries, including many physicians, believe that cesareans are often performed unnecessarily. They claim that American medical personnel don't manage labor very well and cannot always interpret signs of fetal distress or abnormal labor accurately. They suggest that cesareans are often performed more for the convenience of the physician than out of consideration for the mother's or baby's health. They point to studies that indicate that cesareans carry a risk of maternal death 2 to 26 times higher than that of vaginal delivery. And they note that other countries with rates of maternal and infant death as low as those in the United States have much lower rates of cesarean section.

The U.S. Department of Health and Human Services has set a goal for reducing the rate of cesarean delivery to no more than 15 percent by the year 2000. Several strategies have been suggested to help lower this rate.

- *Addressing malpractice concerns.* Physicians may perform cesareans because they are afraid of being sued if something goes wrong.

- *Eliminating financial incentives for physicians and hospitals.* Cesareans are more lucrative than vaginal deliveries. Statistics indicate that for-profit hospitals have higher rates of cesarean section than nonprofit hospitals. In addition, a woman with private insurance is more likely to have a cesarean than is a woman who is without insurance or covered by Medicaid. Reimbursing vaginal and cesarean deliveries equally would eliminate any financial incentive.

- *Publishing cesarean delivery rates of individual physicians and hospitals.* Increasing public awareness would alert people to differences in practice and allow them to make informed choices about practitioners.

- *Increasing training in normal labor and vaginal deliveries.* Current training tends to emphasize high-risk care and the reliance on advanced technological devices to assess and manage labor. Older, more experienced physicians perform significantly fewer cesarean sections for difficult labor and unusual fetal position. The use of secondary tests to confirm a diagnosis of fetal distress based on electronic fetal monitoring has also been shown to lower rates of cesarean delivery.

many of the cesarean sections performed in the United States each year are unnecessary. About 24 percent of all babies are now born by cesarean section, an increase of more than 400 percent over the past 20 years. See the box "Cesarean Births" for more information.

- How often will the baby be brought to the mother while they remain in the hospital or birthing center? Can the baby stay in the mother's room rather than in the nursery (a practice known as **rooming-in**)?

A variety of birth situations can have positive physical and psychological outcomes, and parents should choose

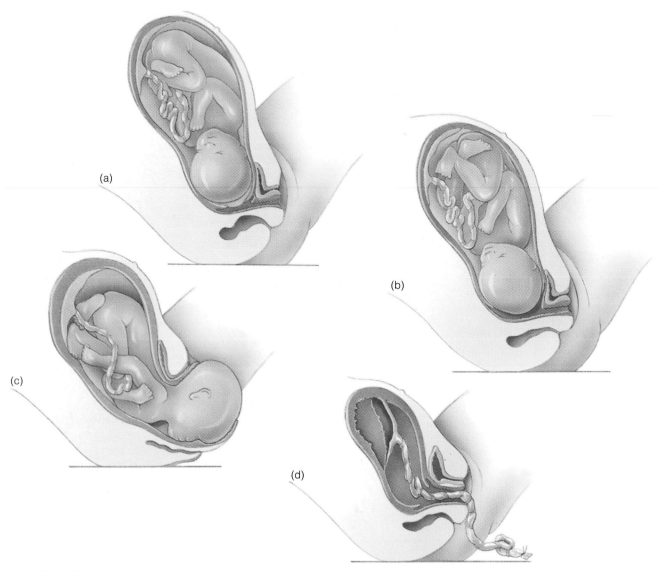

Figure 8-6   *The birth process.*
(a) early stages of labor; cervix begins to dilate; (b) second stage of labor; cervix completely dilated; (c) late stage of labor; baby's head is completely turned; head begins to emerge; (d) final stage of labor; delivery of the placenta.

what is appropriate for their medical circumstances and what feels most comfortable to them. The important thing is that people give sufficient thought to the issues so that they can make the choices that are right for them.

> ***Personal Insight***   If you are a woman and want to have a child, what kind of birth experience do you want to have? If you are a man, do you want to participate and have a role in your partner's birth experience, or would you rather just leave it to her? Where do you think your ideas come from?

Labor and Delivery

The birth process occurs in three stages (Figure 8-6). Labor starts when hormonal changes in both the mother and the baby cause strong, rhythmic uterine **contractions** to begin. These contractions exert pressure on the cervix and cause the lengthwise muscles of the uterus to pull on the circular muscles around the cervix, causing effacement (thinning) and dilation (opening) of the cervix. The contractions also pressure the baby to descend into the mother's pelvis, if it hasn't already. The entire process of labor and delivery usually takes from 2 to 36 hours, depending on the size of the baby, the baby's position in the uterus, the size of the mother's pelvis, and other factors. The length of labor is generally shorter for second and

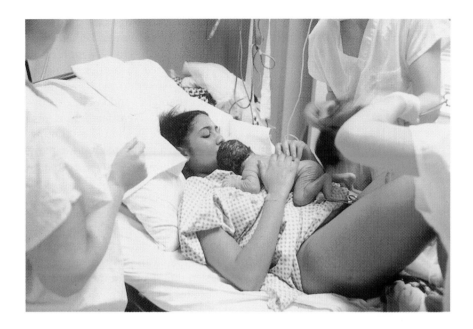

The second stage of labor ends with the birth of the baby. Attachment between mother and her new child begins immediately after birth as the baby is placed on the mother's body.

subsequent births.

The first stage of labor averages about 13 hours for a first birth, although there is a wide variation among women. Contractions usually last about 30 seconds and come every 15 to 20 minutes at first, more often later. The prepared mother relaxes as much as possible during these contractions to allow labor to proceed without being blocked by tension. Early in the first stage, a small amount of bleeding may occur as a plug of slightly bloody mucus that blocked the opening of the cervix during pregnancy is expelled. In some women, the amniotic sac ruptures and the fluid rushes out—sometimes referred to as "breaking of the waters."

The end of the first stage of labor, called **transition,** is characterized by strong and frequent contractions, much more intense than in the early stages of labor. Contractions may last 60 to 90 seconds and occur every 1 to 3 minutes. It is during transition that the cervix opens completely, to a diameter of about 10 centimeters. Since the head of the fetus usually measures between 9 and 10 centimeters, once the cervix has dilated completely, the head can pass through. Many women report that transition, which normally lasts about 30 minutes to an hour, is the most difficult part of labor. The mother may become angry or fearful and will need the support of her helpers.

The second stage of labor begins when the baby's head moves into the birth canal and ends when the baby is born. The baby is slowly pushed down, through the bones of the pelvic ring, past the cervix, and into the vagina, which it stretches open. The mother bears down with the contractions to help push the baby down and out. Some women find this the most difficult part of labor, while others find that the contractions and bearing down bring a sense of euphoria. The baby's back bends, the head turns to fit through the narrowest parts of the

passageway, and the soft bones of the baby's skull move together and overlap as it is squeezed through the pelvis. When the top of the head appears at the vaginal opening, the baby is said to be crowning.

As the head of the baby emerges, the physician or midwife will remove any mucus from the mouth and nose, wipe the baby's face, and check to ensure that the umbilical cord is not around the neck. With a few more contractions, the baby's shoulders and body emerge. As the baby is squeezed through the pelvis, cervix, and vagina, the fluid in the lungs is forced out by the pressure on the baby's chest. Once this pressure is released as the baby emerges from the vagina, the chest expands and the lungs fill with air for the first time. The baby will still be connected to the mother via the umbilical cord, which is not cut until it stops pulsating. The baby will appear wet and often is covered with a milky substance. The baby's head may be oddly shaped at first, due to the molding of the soft plates of bone during birth, but it usually takes on a normal appearance within 24 hours.

In the third stage of labor, the uterus continues to contract until the placenta is delivered. This stage usually takes 5 to 20 minutes. If the placenta does not come out on its own, the physician or midwife may exert gentle pressure on the abdomen to help with its delivery. It is important that the entire placenta be expelled; if part re-

Contraction (uterine) Shortening of the muscles in the uterine wall, which causes effacement and dilation of the cervix and assists in expelling the fetus.

Transition The final phase of the first stage of labor during which the cervix becomes fully dilated, characterized by intense and frequent contractions.

TERMS

mains in the uterus, it may cause infection or bleeding. Breastfeeding soon after delivery helps control uterine bleeding because it stimulates the secretion of a hormone that makes the uterus contract; massaging the abdomen may also help.

In the meantime, the physical condition of the baby will be assessed: Heart rate, respiration, color, reflexes, and muscle tone are individually rated with a score of 0 to 2. The total, called an **Apgar score,** will be at least 7 if the child is healthy. The baby is then usually wrapped tightly in a blanket and returned to the mother, who may begin to nurse the baby right away.

> *Personal Insight* When you think about having a baby, what do you imagine the birth will be like? Do you consider the possibility of having a cesarean delivery? How do you think you would react to having a cesarean?

The Postpartum Period

The three or so months following childbirth are considered the **postpartum period,** a time of critical family adjustments. Parenthood—a job that goes on around the clock without relief—begins literally overnight, and the transition can cause considerable physical and emotional stress.

Following a vaginal delivery, mothers usually leave the hospital within one to three days; after a cesarean section, they usually stay three to five days. Uterine contractions will occur from time to time for several days after the birth as the uterus begins to return to its prebirth size. It usually takes six or eight weeks for a woman's reproductive organs to return to their prebirth condition. She will have a bloody discharge called **lochia** for several weeks after the birth.

Currently, just over 50 percent of mothers breastfeed their infants, up from about 10 percent in 1970 but down from over 60 percent in the early 1980s. **Lactation**—the production of milk—begins about three days after childbirth. Prior to that time (sometimes as early as the second trimester), a yellowish liquid called colostrum is secreted by the nipples. Colostrum contains antibodies that help protect the newborn from infectious diseases and is also high in protein. The American Academy of Pediatricians recommends breastfeeding for a baby's first six months. In general, breastfeeding is preferred to bottlefeeding because human milk is perfectly suited to the baby's nutritional needs and digestive capabilities and because it supplies the baby with antibodies. Breastfeeding is also beneficial to the mother, because it stimulates contractions that help the uterus return to normal more rapidly. It may also contribute to weight loss after pregnancy. Nursing also provides a sense of closeness and emotional well-being for mother and child. For women who want to breastfeed but who have problems, help is available from support groups, books, or a lactation consultant.

For some women, physical problems such as tenderness or infection of the nipples can make breastfeeding difficult. If a woman has an illness or requires drug treatment, she may have to bottlefeed her baby because drugs and infectious agents may show up in breast milk. Some parents choose bottlefeeding because breastfeeding can be restrictive—mothers may not be able to leave the baby for more than a few hours at a time. Companies rarely provide part-time employment or nursing breaks for their female employees, so bottlefeeding or the use of a breast pump (to express milk for use while the mother is away from her infant) may be the only practical alternatives. Bottlefeeding makes it easier to tell how much milk an infant is taking in and bottlefed infants tend to sleep longer. Bottlefeeding also allows the father or other caregiver to share in the nurturing process. Both breastfeeding and bottlefeeding can be part of loving, secure parent-child relationships.

When a mother doesn't nurse, menstruation usually begins within about ten weeks. Breastfeeding can prevent the return of menstruation for as long as six months because the hormone prolactin, which aids milk production, suppresses hormones vital to the development of mature eggs. However, ovulation—and pregnancy—can occur before menstruation returns, so breastfeeding is not a contraceptive method. If a woman wishes to avoid pregnancy, she should use a reliable method of contraception. If the mother becomes pregnant while still nursing, she should stop nursing to ensure good nutrition for the unborn child.

Many women experience fluctuating emotions during the postpartum period as hormone levels change. The physical stress of labor, as well as dehydration, blood loss, and other physical factors, contribute to lowering the woman's stamina. About 50–80 percent of new mothers experience "baby blues," characterized by episodes of sadness, weeping, anxiety, headache, sleep disorders, or irritability. She may feel lonely and anxious about caring for her infant. About 10 percent of new mothers experience **postpartum depression,** a more disabling syndrome characterized by despondency, mood swings, guilt, and occasional hostility. Rest, sharing feelings and

TERMS

Apgar score A number that reflects the general condition of the newborn soon after birth.

Postpartum period The period of about three months after the birth.

Lochia Bloody discharge from the uterus and vagina that continues for several weeks after childbirth.

Lactation The production of milk.

Postpartum depression An emotional low experienced by the mother following childbirth; infrequently intensifies until medical attention is necessary.

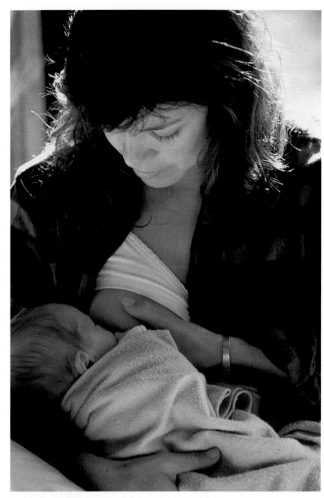

Breastfeeding is an ideal method of feeding an infant because the mother's milk contains antibodies against disease and is perfectly suited to the baby's nutritional needs. But women who choose bottlefeeding can still experience the physical contact and emotional closeness that are such an important part of the parent-child relationship.

concerns with others, and relying on supportive relatives and friends for assistance are usually helpful in dealing with mild cases of the baby blues or postpartum depression, which generally lasts only a few weeks. If the depression is serious, professional treatment may be needed. Some men also seem to get a form of postpartum depression, characterized by anxiety about their changing roles and feelings of inadequacy. Both mothers and fathers need time to adjust to their new roles as parents.

Another feature of the postpartum period is the development of attachment—the strong emotional tie that grows between the baby and the adult who cares for the baby. Parents can foster secure attachment relationships in the early weeks and months by responding sensitively to the baby's true needs. Parents who respond appropriately to the baby's signals of gazing, looking away, smiling, and crying establish feelings of trust and effectiveness in

their child. They feed the baby when it's hungry, for example; respond when it cries; interact with it when it gazes, smiles, or babbles; and stop stimulating it when it frowns or looks away. A secure attachment relationship helps the child to develop and function well socially, emotionally, and intellectually.

For most people, the arrival of a child is one of life's most important events, providing a deep sense of joy and accomplishment. However, adjusting to parenthood requires effort and energy. Talking with friends and relatives about their experiences during the first few weeks or months with a baby can help prepare new parents for the period when the baby's needs may require all the energy that both parents have to expend. But the pleasures of nurturing a new baby are substantial, and many parents look back on this time as one of the most significant and joyful of their lives.

SUMMARY

- Today it's possible to choose whether, when, and how to have a child.

Preparation for Parenthood

- Factors to consider when deciding if and when to have a child include (1) physical health and age, (2) financial circumstances, (3) relationship with partner, (4) educational, career, and child care plans, (5) emotional readiness for parenthood, (6) social support system, (7) personal qualities, attitudes toward children, and aptitude for parenting, and (8) philosophical beliefs.
- Health care before pregnancy can reduce risks for both mother and child. Preconception care examines factors such as preexisting medical conditions, current medications, past history of pregnancy, age of the mother, lifestyle behaviors, infections, nutritional status, and family history of genetic disease.

Understanding Fertility

- Fertilization is a complex process culminating when a sperm penetrates the membrane of the egg released from the woman's ovary.
- Infertility affects about 1 out of every 12 or 13 American couples. Among women, the leading causes of infertility include blocked oviducts and endometriosis. Among men, exposure to toxic substances, use of certain drugs, injury of the testicles, and infection can all cause infertility.
- Surgery and drugs can cure some problems; more advanced techniques include in vitro fertilization and artificial insemination.

- One way to avoid some forms of infertility is to protect oneself against STDs and to get treatment for any disease contracted.

Pregnancy

- Pregnancy is usually divided into trimesters based on fetal development.

- Early pregnancy tests detect the presence of human chorionic gonadotropin in the urine or blood of the mother.

- Early signs and symptoms include a missed menstrual period; slight bleeding; nausea; breast tenderness; sleepiness, fatigue, and emotional upset; and a softening of the uterus just above the cervix.

- During pregnancy, the uterus enlarges until it pushes up into the rib cage; the breasts enlarge and may secrete colostrum; the muscles and ligaments soften and stretch; and the circulatory system, lungs, and kidneys become more efficient.

- Pregnancy may lead to either increased or decreased interest in sexual activity. Mood changes are common throughout pregnancy.

- The fetal anatomy is almost completely formed in the first trimester and is refined in the second; needed fats and pounds are added during the third trimester.

- As the fertilized egg divides, its outer cells develop into the placenta, umbilical cord, and amniotic sac.

- Information about the health and sex of a fetus can be obtained through prenatal tests such as ultrasound, alpha-fetoprotein screening, amniocentesis, and chorionic villus sampling.

- Health care during pregnancy includes a complete history and physical at the beginning and regular checkups for blood pressure, weight gain, and size and position of the fetus. Blood tests reveal blood type, anemia, STDs, and Rh incompatibilities.

- Important elements of prenatal care include good nutrition; avoiding drugs, alcohol, tobacco, infections, and other harmful agents or conditions; regular physical activity; and childbirth classes.

- Pregnancy usually proceeds without major complications. Problems that can occur include ectopic pregnancy, spontaneous abortion, toxemia, and low birth weight. The loss of a fetus or infant will cause a deep grief reaction in the parents.

Childbirth

- Couples preparing for childbirth may have many options to choose from. These include type of practitioner; type of facility, room, and bed or chair for labor and delivery; and under what circumstances some medical procedures will be carried out.

- The first stage of labor begins with contractions that exert pressure on the cervix, causing effacement and dilation. The period of transition is characterized by frequent and intense contractions.

- The second stage of labor begins when the cervix is dilated to about 10 centimeters. The baby is pushed down into the vagina, and the mother bears down until the baby emerges.

- The third stage of labor is delivery of the placenta. The umbilical cord is cut and the baby takes its first breath.

- During the postpartum period, the mother's body begins to return to its prepregnancy state, and she may begin to breastfeed. Both mother and father must adjust to their new roles as parents as they develop a strong emotional tie to their baby.

TAKE ACTION

1. Interview your parents to find out what your birth was like. What were the cultural conditions like at the time, and what were their personal preferences? Find out as much as you can about hospital procedure, use of anesthesia, length of hospital stay, and so on. Did your father have a role in your birth? If possible, interview your grandparents or someone of their generation. How was their experience different from your parents'?

2. Investigate the childbirth facilities in your community. If possible, visit the maternity wing of a hospital and an alternative birth center. What do you like about them, and what do you not like? What types of child-birth preparation classes do they offer? Which of these do you feel most comfortable with and why?

JOURNAL ENTRY

1. Would you take advantage of a prenatal diagnostic tool like amniocentesis to find out ahead of time if your child had a genetic abnormality? If such an abnormality was discovered, would you choose to terminate the pregnancy? Write an essay describing what you would do and why. What criteria would you use to make your decision?

2. *Critical Thinking:* There have been many legal cases involving the status of sperm or embryos frozen as part of an infertility treatment such as artificial insemination or in vitro fertilization. Research one or more of these cases and write an essay outlining some of the moral and legal implications of this technology. What guidelines would you suggest for regulating the

use and status of frozen sperm and embryos? What evidence can you give to support your position?

3. Do you think you are ready to become a parent? Make a list of the qualities you possess that you think would make you a good parent. Then list those qualities that might be a hindrance to good parenting. Do you think your partner (if you have one) is ready to become a parent? Create the same type of lists based on his or her personal qualities.

SELECTED BIBLIOGRAPHY

American College of Obstetricians and Gynecologists. 1985. *Exercise During Pregnancy and the Postnatal Period (ACOG Home Exercise Programs)*. Washington, D.C.: ACOG.

Carroll, J. 1990. Tracing the causes of infertility. *San Francisco Chronicle,* 5 March.

Centers for Disease Control. 1992. *HIV/AIDS Surveillance Report,* October.

Department of Health and Human Services. 1991. *Healthy People 2000: National Health Promotion and Disease Prevention Objectives.* Washington, D.C.: U.S. Government Printing Office, Pub. No. (PHS)91-50212.

Diabetes: Living successfully with a lifelong challenge. 1992. Medical Essay, Supplement to *Mayo Clinic Health Letter,* June.

Downes, N. J. 1991. *Ethnic Americans—for the Health Professional.* 2nd ed. Available from author at San Jose State University.

Fackelmann, K. A. 1991. HIV poses hazards for breast feeding. *Science News* 140:135.

Faludi, S. 1991. *Backlash: The Undeclared War Against American Women.* New York: Crown.

Golombok, S. 1992. Psychological functioning of infertility patients. *Human Reproduction* 7(2): 208–212.

Gray, M. J., and others. 1991. *The Woman's Guide to Good Health.* Yonkers, N.Y.: Consumers Union.

Gross, D. 1992. *Discovering Anthropology.* Mountain View, Calif.: Mayfield.

Hilts, P. 1990. Growing concern over pelvic infection in women. *New York Times,* 11 October.

Jack, B. W., and L. Culpepper. 1990. Preconception care: Risk reduction and health promotion in preparation for pregnancy. *Journal of the American Medical Association* 264(9): 1147–49.

Laurent, S. L., and others. 1992. An epidemiologic study of smoking and primary infertility in women. *Fertility and Sterility* 57(3): 565–72.

Lino, M. 1990. Expenditures on a child by husband-wife families. *Family Economics Review* 3(3): 2–12.

Morales, K., and C. B. Inlander. 1991. *Take This Book to the Obstetrician with You: A Consumer's Guide to Pregnancy and Childbirth.* Reading, Mass.: Addison-Wesley.

Mueller, B. A., and others. 1992. Risk factors for tubal infertility: Influence of history of prior pelvic inflammatory disease. *Sexually Transmitted Diseases* 19(1): 28–34.

Myers, S. A., and N. Gleicher. 1988. A successful program to

lower cesarean-section rates. *New England Journal of Medicine* 319(23): 1511–16.

Nesler, C. L., and others. 1988. Effects of supine exercise on fetal heart rate in the second and third trimesters. *American Journal of Perinatology* 5:159–63.

Notzon, F. C. 1990. International differences in the use of obstetric interventions. *Journal of the American Medical Association* 263(24): 3286–91.

Olshansky, E. F. 1992. Redefining the concepts of success and failure in infertility treatment. *Naacogs Clinical Issues in Perinatal and Women's Health Nursing* 3(2): 343–46.

Pear, R. 1992. The U.S. reports rise in low-weight births. *The New York Times,* 22 April.

Petit, C. 1990. New study to ask why so many infants die. *San Francisco Chronicle,* 9 May.

Schickedanz, J., and others. 1993. *Understanding Children.* 2nd ed. Mountain View, Calif.: Mayfield.

Scott, S. G., and others. 1990. Therapeutic donor insemination with frozen semen. *Canadian Medical Association Journal* 143(4): 273–78.

Study calls for limiting use of episiotomy in childbirth. 1992. *Los Angeles Times,* 2 July, A1.

Stafford, R. S. 1991. The impact of nonclinical factors on repeat cesarean section. *Journal of the American Medical Association* 265(1): 59–63.

Weiss, P. 1992. The bond of mother's milk. *San Jose Mercury News,* 18 August, 1–2E.

Ziporyn, T. 1992. Postpartum depression: True blue? *Harvard Health Letter,* February.

Zylke, J. W. 1991. Another consequence of uncontrolled spread of HIV among adults: Vertical transmission. *Journal of the American Medical Association* 265(14): 1798–99.

RECOMMENDED READINGS

Armstrong, P., and S. Feldman. 1990. *A Wise Birth.* New York: William Morrow. *A thought-provoking exploration of the effects of medical technology and technological thinking on modern childbirth.*

Dunham, C. (The Body Shop Staff). 1992. *Mamototo: A Celebration of Birth.* New York: Viking Penguin. *An exploration of childbirth in many cultures using text and photos.*

Eisenberg, A., and others. 1991. *What to Expect While You're Expecting.* Rev. 2nd ed. New York: Workman. *A highly readable guide to pregnancy, childbirth, and the postpartum period.*

Kitzinger, S. 1989. *The Complete Book of Pregnancy and Childbirth.* New York: Alfred A. Knopf. *A comprehensive and easy-to-read manual for those who are contemplating pregnancy or those who want to know more about its physiological and psychological aspects.*

Menning, B. E. 1988. *Infertility: A Guide for the Childless Couple.* 2nd ed. Englewood Cliffs, N.J.: Prentice-Hall. *A useful guide for couples facing infertility.*

Nilsson, L., and L. Hamberger. 1990. *A Child Is Born.* New York: Delacorte/Seymour Lawrence. *The story of birth, beginning with fertilization, told in stunning photographs with additional text.*

Panuthos, C., and C. Romeo. 1984. *Ended Beginnings: Healing*

Childbearing Losses. New York: Warner Books. *A sensitive guide to dealing with the grief involved in miscarriages, stillbirths, and infant deaths.*

Strong, B., and C. Devault. 1994. *Human Sexuality: The Intimate Environment.* Mountain View, Calif.: Mayfield. *A comprehensive introduction to human sexuality based on current research; includes coverage of pregnancy and reproductive issues.*

9

Toward a Tobacco-free Society

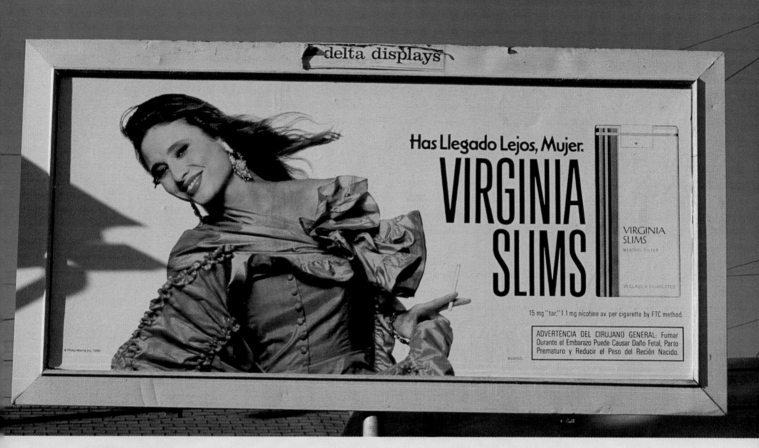

CONTENTS

▶ You've been smoking cigarettes for the last two years, and you promised yourself you'd quit right after high school. Then you gave yourself until college started in September. Well, September has come and gone. You still plan to quit, though . . . just as soon as you get through finals. A friend recently commented that this pattern of postponing your quit date is evidence you're hooked. Your first reaction to his comment was anger, but now you're reconsidering. Could your friend be right? If you really can quit anytime you want, as you've always maintained, then why haven't you?

▶ While you're waiting for a bus in a crowded terminal, the person sitting next to you lights up a cigarette. You ask her if she would mind not smoking, since you don't want to breathe the smoke. She replies that she *would* mind and suggests that you find another seat. "You nonsmoking fanatics are always talking about your right to breathe clean air," she says. "What about *my* rights? I've got a right to smoke if I want to." Does she have a point? What should you do?

▶ It seems as though at least half the guys on the intramural baseball team dip snuff, and you can't help but find the habit attractive. When a friend offers you some, saying it will give you a pleasant lift, you're tempted to try it. You reason that it can't be as bad for you as cigarettes are because you don't inhale any smoke. You've also noticed that lots of professional athletes use chewing tobacco and endorse it in ads—things they wouldn't do if it were dangerous. How valid are these arguments? Should you give it a try?

▶ On a visit home from school you discover that your 15-year-old sister has started smoking cigarettes. She says she and some of her friends are smoking because they heard it was a good way to keep their weight under control. You point out that smoking is a health hazard, but she says that you have to smoke for years before it has any negative effects. She's just going to enjoy it while she's young and stop smoking before it affects her health. Besides, she tells you, she can quit any time she wants. How much of what she says is true? What advice can you give her?

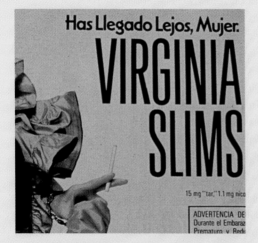

MAKING CONNECTIONS

Smoking is hazardous to everyone's health, smoker and nonsmoker alike. This is part of the reason that the tobacco issue is likely to remain a battleground for conflicting rights and opposing interests throughout the 1990s. In each of the tobacco-related scenarios presented on these pages, individuals have to use information, make a decision, or choose a course of action. How would you act in each of these situations? What response or decision would you make? This chapter provides information about tobacco use, health hazards associated with tobacco, and how to beat the nicotine habit that can be used in situations like these. After finishing the chapter, read the scenarios again. Has what you've learned changed how you would respond?

Once considered a glamorous and sophisticated habit, smoking is now viewed with increasing disapproval. The recognition of the health risks of smoking is a primary cause of this change in public opinion, and it has led to significant changes in the behavior of many Americans. Over the past four decades, the proportion of cigarette smokers among adults in the United States has dropped 30 percent, and the prevalence of pipe and cigar smoking among men has plummeted by 80 percent. Private businesses and all levels of government also have jumped on the nonsmoking bandwagon: Almost every state now restricts smoking in public places, and more than a third of states restrict it in private-sector workplaces as well.

Despite such progress, **tobacco** use remains widespread and is the single most preventable cause of death in this country. Nearly one in three American adults smokes. Every day about 700 people die from tobacco-related heart and lung diseases, and another 375 die from cancer caused by tobacco use. Nonsmokers subjected to the smoke of others also suffer: Exposure to **environmental tobacco smoke (ETS)** kills an estimated 53,000 Americans each year. In addition, smoking by pregnant women results in an estimated 4,600 infant deaths each year in the United States. Smokeless tobacco has enjoyed a troubling resurgence. Production of smokeless tobacco products has jumped 40 percent since 1970, and nearly 20 percent of male high school students now use this potentially deadly form of tobacco.

Given the overwhelming evidence against tobacco, why would anyone today begin using it? How does it exercise its hold over users? What can smokers and nonsmokers do to help achieve a tobacco-free society? In this chapter we explore answers to these and other questions.

WHY PEOPLE USE TOBACCO

If the United States is to become a tobacco-free society, the problem of tobacco use needs to be addressed not just in terms of cure but also in terms of prevention. This section examines the personal and societal forces that induce people to start smoking, as well as the forces that encourage them to continue.

Nicotine Addiction

The primary reason people continue to use tobacco despite the health risks is that they have become addicted to a powerful **psychoactive drug—nicotine.** Nicotine reaches the brain via the bloodstream seconds after it is inhaled or, in the case of smokeless tobacco, absorbed through membranes of the mouth or nose. Like other psychoactive drugs such as cocaine and heroin, nicotine acts by triggering the release of powerful chemical messengers in the brain, including epinephrine, norepinephrine, and dopamine. But unlike street drugs, most of which are used to achieve a "high," nicotine's primary attraction seems to lie in its ability to modulate everyday emotions.

At low doses, nicotine appears to act as a stimulant: It increases heart rate and blood pressure and can enhance alertness, concentration, rapid information processing, memory, and learning. People type faster on nicotine, for instance. At high doses, on the other hand, nicotine appears to act as a sedative—it can reduce aggression and alleviate the stress response. Tobacco users may be able to fine-tune nicotine's effects and regulate their moods by increasing or decreasing their intake of the drug. Studies have shown that smokers experience milder mood variation than nonsmokers while performing long, boring tasks or while watching emotional movies, for example.

All tobacco products contain nicotine, and use of any of them can lead to addiction (see the box "Nicotine Dependence: Are You Hooked?"). Physicians define an addictive drug as one that produces loss of control; pharmacological tolerance, in which progressively higher doses of a drug are needed in order to produce the same effect; and, when its use is abruptly stopped, a withdrawal syndrome.

Loss of Control Three out of four smokers want to quit but find they cannot. Of the 60 to 80 percent of people who kick cigarettes at stop-smoking clinics, 75 percent start smoking again within a year—a relapse rate similar to rates for alcoholics and heroin addicts. Some evidence suggests quitting is even harder for smokeless users: In one study, only 1 of 14 smokeless tobacco users who participated in a tobacco-cessation clinic was able to stop for more than four hours.

Regular tobacco users live according to a rigid cycle of need and gratification. On average, they can go no more than 40 minutes between doses of nicotine; otherwise, they begin feeling edgy and irritable and have trouble concentrating. If ignored, nicotine cravings build until getting a cigarette or some smokeless tobacco becomes a paramount concern, crowding out other thoughts. Tobacco users become adept, therefore, at keeping a steady amount of nicotine circulating in the blood and going to the brain. In one experiment, smokers were given cigarettes that looked and tasted alike but varied in nicotine content. The subjects automatically adjusted their rate

Tobacco The leaves of cultivated tobacco plants (genus *Nicotiana*) prepared for smoking, chewing, or use as snuff.

Environmental tobacco smoke Smoke that enters the atmosphere from the burning end of a cigarette, cigar, or pipe, as well as smoke that is exhaled by smokers.

Psychoactive drug A drug that affects the brain or nervous system.

Nicotine A poisonous, addictive substance found in tobacco and responsible for many of the effects of tobacco.

TERMS

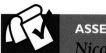
Nicotine Dependence: Are You Hooked?

Answer each question in the list below, giving yourself the appropriate points.

	0 points	1 point	2 points
____ 1. How soon after you wake up do you smoke your first cigarette?	After 30 minutes	Within 30 minutes	—
____ 2. Do you find it difficult to refrain from smoking in places where it is forbidden, such as the library, theater, doctor's office?	No	Yes	—
____ 3. Which of all the cigarettes you smoke in a day is the most satisfying?	Any other than the first one in the morning	The first one in the morning	—
____ 4. How many cigarettes a day do you smoke?	1–15	16–25	26+
____ 5. Do you smoke more during the morning than during the rest of the day?	No	Yes	—
____ 6. Do you smoke when you are so ill that you are in bed most of the day?	No	Yes	—
____ 7. Does the brand you smoke have a low, medium, or high nicotine content?	Low	Medium	High
____ 8. How often do you inhale the smoke?	Never	Sometimes	Always
____ Total			

Scoring

More than 6 points—very dependent

Less than 6 points—low to moderate dependence.

Source: American Lung Association: Fagerstom Test.

and depth of inhalation so that they absorbed their usual amount of nicotine. In other studies, heavy smokers were given nicotine without knowing it—and they cut down on their smoking without a conscious effort. Smokeless tobacco users maintain bloodstream nicotine levels as high as those of cigarette smokers.

Tolerance and Withdrawal Syndrome Tobacco use also produces **tolerance.** Where one cigarette may make a beginning smoker nauseated and dizzy, a long-term smoker may have to chain-smoke a pack or more to experience the same effects. For most regular tobacco users, sudden abstinence from nicotine produces a predictable **withdrawal syndrome** as well. Symptoms, which come on several hours after the last dose of nicotine, include severe cravings, insomnia, confusion, tremors, difficulty concentrating, fatigue, muscle pains, headache, nausea, irritability, anger, and depression. Sufferers undergo measurable changes in brain waves, heart rate, and blood pressure, and they perform poorly on tasks requiring sustained attention. While most of these symptoms pass in two to three days, many ex-smokers report intermittent, intense urges to smoke for years after quitting. In his 1991 book, *Smoking: The Artificial Passion,* David Krogh describes how smokers went to unusual lengths to ward off withdrawal symptoms during wartime tobacco shortages. Even starving smokers traded food for cigarettes, preferring hunger to nicotine cravings. Others, disregarding dignity, decorum, and hygiene, smoked cigarette butts they picked up off the streets.

Social and Psychological Factors

Why do tobacco users have such a hard time quitting even when they want to? Social and psychological forces combine with physiological addiction to maintain the tobacco habit (see the box "For Smokers Only: Why Do You Smoke?"). Many people, for example, have established habits of smoking while doing something else—while talking, working, drinking, and so on. The smokeless tobacco habit is also associated with certain situations—studying, drinking coffee, or playing sports. It's difficult

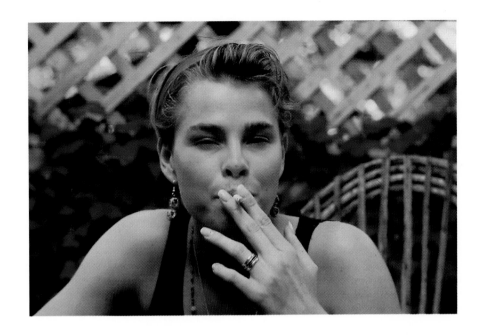

Most adults who smoke begin as teenagers. Like this young woman, they imagine that smoking will give them an air of worldly sophistication and help them lose weight—just as the tobacco companies would have them believe.

for these people to break their habits because the activities they associate with tobacco use continue to trigger their urge. Psychologists call such activities **secondary reinforcers**; they act together with the physiological addiction to keep the user dependent on tobacco.

Why Start in the First Place?

A junior high school girl takes up smoking in an attempt to appear older. A high school boy uses smokeless tobacco in the bullpen, emulating the major league ball players he admires. An overweight first-year college student turns to cigarettes in hopes they will curb her appetite. Although smoking rates among American youth have declined by about one-third since the late 1970s, children and teenagers still constitute 90 percent of all new smokers in this country: Every day, an estimated 3,000 adolescents become regular cigarette smokers, while hundreds of others take up snuff or chewing tobacco. The average age for starting smokers? Thirteen. For smokeless tobacco users? Ten. Meanwhile, children—especially girls—are beginning to experiment with tobacco at ever-younger ages. For example, a 1991 study of more than 1,000 first-graders in the United States found that 36 percent of the boys and 27 percent of the girls had already tried a cigarette; 10 percent of the first-grade boys and 5 percent of the girls had tried two or more. The trends are particularly worrisome because the earlier people begin smoking, the more likely they are to become heavy smokers—and to die of tobacco-related disease. For more statistics on tobacco use and its consequences, see the box "Facts About Smoking."

Swayed by seductive advertising or older role models like siblings or sports stars, these young people have decided that the touted benefits of tobacco—sexual attrac-

tiveness, slenderness, confidence, and popularity, to name a few—outweigh the risks. Making such a decision requires minimizing or denying both the health risks of tobacco use and the tremendous pain, disability, emotional trauma, family stress, and financial expense involved in tobacco-related diseases such as cancer and emphysema. A sense of invincibility, characteristic of many adolescents and young adults, also contributes to the decision to use tobacco. These young people may persuade themselves they are too intelligent, too lucky, or too robustly healthy to be vulnerable to tobacco's dangers. "I'm not dumb enough to get hooked," they may argue. "I'll be able to quit before I do myself any real harm." Other typical rationalizations: "My grandmother smoked and she lived to be 80" and "You can get killed just by crossing the street."

Personal Insight   Did people in your family smoke when you were growing up? Do you think it has affected your feelings and attitudes about smoking today? If so, how?

TERMS

Tolerance   A phenomenon in which increased doses of a drug or medication are required to achieve the same effect.

Withdrawal syndrome   A set of physical and psychological symptoms that occur when a person suddenly stops taking a drug to which he or she has been addicted.

Secondary reinforcers   Stimuli that are not necessarily pleasurable in themselves, but have been associated with other stimuli that are pleasurable.

What kind of smoker are you? What do you get out of smoking? This test is designed to provide you with a score on each of six factors that describe many people's smoking. Your scores will help you identify what you use smoking for and what kind of satisfactions it gives you. Circle one number for each statement. Be sure you answer every question.

	Always	Frequently	Occasionally	Seldom	Never
A. I smoke cigarettes in order to keep myself from slowing down.	5	4	3	2	1
B. Handling a cigarette is part of the enjoyment of smoking it.	5	4	3	2	1
C. Smoking cigarettes is pleasant and relaxing.	5	4	3	2	1
D. I light up a cigarette when I feel angry about something.	5	4	3	2	1
E. When I have run out of cigarettes, I find it almost unbearable until I can get them.	5	4	3	2	1
F. I smoke cigarettes automatically without even being aware of it.	5	4	3	2	1
G. I smoke cigarettes to stimulate me, to perk myself up.	5	4	3	2	1
H. Part of the enjoyment of smoking a cigarette comes from the steps I take to light up.	5	4	3	2	1
I. I find cigarettes pleasurable.	5	4	3	2	1
J. When I feel uncomfortable or upset about something, I light up a cigarette.	5	4	3	2	1
K. I am very much aware of the fact when I am not smoking a cigarette.	5	4	3	2	1
L. I light up a cigarette without realizing I still have one burning in the ashtray.	5	4	3	2	1
M. I smoke cigarettes to give me a "lift."	5	4	3	2	1
N. I enjoy watching the smoke as I exhale it.	5	4	3	2	1
O. I want a cigarette most when I am comfortable and relaxed.	5	4	3	2	1
P. When I feel "blue" or want to take my mind off cares and worries, I smoke cigarettes.	5	4	3	2	1
Q. I get a real gnawing hunger for a cigarette when I haven't smoked for a while.	5	4	3	2	1
R. I've found a cigarette in my mouth and didn't remember putting it there.	5	4	3	2	1

How to Score

1. Enter the numbers you have circled to the smoking questions in the scoring chart, putting the number you have circled to question A over line A, to question B over line B, and so on.

2. Total the 3 scores on each line to get your totals. For example, the sum of your scores over lines A, G, and M gives you your score on *Stimulation*—lines B, H, and N give the score on *Handling*, etc.

Scoring Chart

TOTALS

____ A	+ ____ G	+ ____ M	= ____	STIMULATION
____ B	+ ____ H	+ ____ N	= ____	HANDLING
____ C	+ ____ I	+ ____ O	= ____	PLEASURABLE RELAXATION
____ D	+ ____ J	+ ____ P	= ____	CRUTCH: TENSION REDUCTION
____ E	+ ____ K	+ ____ Q	= ____	CRAVING: STRONG PHYSIOLOGICAL OR PSYCHOLOGICAL ADDICTION
____ F	+ ____ L	+ ____ R	= ____	HABIT

ASSESS YOURSELF

For Smokers Only: Why Do You Smoke? (continued)

What Your Scores Mean

Scores can vary from 3 to 15. Any score 11 and above is *high*; any score 7 and below is *low*. The higher your score, the more important a particular factor is in your smoking and the more useful the discussion of that factor can be in your attempt to quit.

Stimulation   If you score high on this factor, it means that you are stimulated by cigarettes—you feel that they help wake you up, organize your energies, and keep you going. Try substituting a brisk walk or moderate exercise whenever you feel the urge to smoke.

Handling   A high score suggests you gain satisfaction from handling a cigarette. Try doodling or toying with a pen, pencil, or other small object.

Accentuation of Pleasure—Pleasurable Relaxation   A high score on this factor suggests that you receive pleasure from smoking. Try substituting other pleasant situations or events such as social or physical activities.

Reduction of Negative Feelings, or "Crutch"   A high score on this factor means you use cigarettes as a kind of crutch in moments of stress or discomfort. Physical exertion or social activity may serve as useful substitutes for cigarettes. Refer back to Chapter 2 for other strategies for dealing with stress.

Craving or Strong Addiction   A high score on this factor indicates that you have a strong psychological craving for cigarettes. "Cold turkey" is probably your best approach to quitting. It may be helpful for you to smoke more than usual for a day or two, so that your taste for cigarettes is spoiled, and then isolate yourself completely from cigarettes until the craving is gone.

Habit   A high score on this factor indicates that you smoke out of habit, not because smoking gives you satisfaction. Being aware of every cigarette you smoke and cutting down gradually may be effective quitting strategies for you.

Summary

Quitting smoking isn't easy. It usually means giving up something pleasurable that has a definite place in your life. In the end, of course, it's worth it. Now that you have some ideas about why you smoke, read the Behavior Change Strategy at the end of the chapter for a plan that will help you quit.

Adapted from "Why Do You Smoke?" Washington, D.C.: NIH Publication No. 90-1822, reprinted March 1990.

Who Uses Tobacco?

Not all young people are equally vulnerable to the lure of tobacco. Research suggests that the more of the following characteristics that apply to a child or adolescent, the more likely he or she is to use tobacco:

- A parent uses tobacco.
- A sibling uses tobacco.
- Peers use tobacco.
- The child comes from a blue-collar family.
- The child comes from a low-income home.
- The family is headed by a single parent.
- The child performs poorly in school.
- The child drops out of school. (Dropouts are more than three times as likely to smoke as are students who remain in school.)
- The child has positive attitudes about tobacco use.
- The child is white. (Compared to other ethnic groups, whites begin smoking at younger ages.)

In 1990, about 28 percent of men and 23 percent of women smoked cigarettes (Table 9-1). Rates of smoking varied, based on gender, age, racial or ethnic group, and education level. Adults with less than a twelfth-grade education are more than twice as likely to smoke as are those with college degrees.

An estimated 20 percent of male high school students used smokeless tobacco in 1990. Rates of use were highest among white students, with male Latino teens in second place. Studies of college students indicate one-fourth to one-half of male varsity and intramural athletes use smokeless tobacco; among major league baseball players, about 34 percent report regular use of smokeless tobacco.

Drug addicts are another major group of tobacco users. Some studies have found that over 90 percent of heroin addicts and 80 percent of alcoholics are heavy cigarette smokers. Other recent studies suggest that smokers are more likely than nonsmokers to have suffered from depression. Such findings lead some researchers to suggest that underlying psychological or physiological traits may predispose people to drug use, including tobacco.

Personal Insight   How do you think you would feel if you found your 12-year-old child smoking? Would your feelings depend on whether you yourself were a smoker or a nonsmoker?

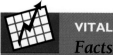

- In 1915, most tobacco was used for pipes, cigars, and chewing tobacco, and cigarette smoking was uncommon. Lung cancer was virtually unknown.

- In 1964—the year of the first Surgeon General's Report linking smoking with heart disease—42 percent of adult Americans smoked.

- Today, about 30 percent of the adult population smoke cigarettes, and 400,000 people in the United States die of lung cancer and other tobacco-related diseases every year.

- Nearly 20 percent of high school boys use smokeless tobacco. The average age for starting is 10.

- Nearly 70 percent of smokers under age 50 say they would like to quit.

- Half of all smokers began to smoke regularly before the age of 18; every day, 3,000 American teenagers take up cigarettes.

- 1,200 people quit smoking every day—by dying. That is equivalent to two fully loaded jumbo jets crashing every day, with no survivors.

- Smoking by pregnant women causes 4,600 infant deaths in the United States each year. Twenty to 25 percent of pregnant American women continue to smoke throughout pregnancy.

- Environmental tobacco smoke kills 53,000 involuntary smokers in this country each year.

- Tobacco smoke contains over 4,000 chemical compounds, including at least 43 that are carcinogenic (cancer-causing).

- High prices, health concerns, and declining social acceptance of smoking have led to decreased per capita consumption of cigarettes in the United States. However, domestic cigarette output increases about 7 percent a year, in part due to aggressive overseas marketing by American tobacco companies. U.S. cigarette exports have jumped by 180 percent since 1985.

- It costs the American economy approximately $52 billion a year to cover cigarette-related health care costs and loss of worker productivity.

- According to recent polls, 30 percent of the American public are unaware that smoking causes heart disease. Nearly 50 percent of women polled did not know that smoking during pregnancy increases the risk of stillbirth and miscarriage.

Sources: American Cancer Society, *Cancer Facts and Figures 1993*; Centers for Disease Control; Coalition of Smoking on Health.

HEALTH HAZARDS

Tobacco adversely affects nearly every part of the body including brain, stomach, mouth, and reproductive organs.

Tobacco Smoke: A Poisonous Mix

Tobacco smoke contains hundreds of damaging chemical substances. Smoke from a typical unfiltered cigarette contains about 5 billion particles per cubic millimeter—50,000 times as many as are found in an equal volume of smoggy urban air. These particles, when condensed, form the brown, sticky mass called **cigarette tar.**

Some chemicals in tobacco tar are linked to the development of cancer. Some, such as benzopyrene and vinyl chloride, are **carcinogens;** that is, they directly cause cancer. Other chemicals, such as formaldehyde and phenol, are **cocarcinogens;** they do not themselves cause cancer but combine with other chemicals to stimulate the growth of certain cancers, at least in laboratory animals. Other substances in tobacco cause health problems because they damage the lining of the respiratory tract or decrease the lungs' ability to fight off infection (Table 9-2).

Tobacco also contains poisonous substances, including arsenic. In addition to being an addictive psychoactive drug, nicotine is also a poison and can be fatal in high doses. Many cases of nicotine poisoning occur each year in toddlers and infants who eat tobacco.

Cigarette smoke contains carbon monoxide, the deadly gas in automobile exhaust, in concentrations 400 times greater than is considered safe in industrial workplaces. Not surprisingly, smokers often complain of breathlessness when they require a burst of energy to run across campus for their next class. Carbon monoxide displaces oxygen in red blood cells, depleting the body's supply of life-giving oxygen for extra work. Carbon monoxide also impairs visual acuity, especially at night.

All smokers absorb some gases, tars, and nicotine from cigarette smoke, but smokers who inhale bring most of

TERMS

Cigarette tar Brown sticky mass created when the chemical particles in tobacco smoke condense.

Carcinogen A substance that causes cancer.

Cocarcinogen A substance that works with a carcinogen to produce cancer.

Cerebral cortex The outer layer of the brain, which controls the complex behavior and mental activity of human beings.

TABLE 9-1 Who Smokes? Percentage of Adults Who Smoke Cigarettes by Gender, Age, Race, and Education—United States, 1990

	Men	Women	Total
Age (yrs)			
14–17	33	31	32
18–24	27	23	25
25–44	33	27	30
45–64	29	25	27
65–74	18	16	17
>74	8	6	7
Race/ethnic group			
White	28	24	26
Black	33	21	26
Asian/Pacific Islander	25	6	16
American Indian/ Alaskan Native	40	36	38
Hispanic Origin			
Hispanic	31	16	23
Non-Hispanic	28	23	26
Education (yrs)			
<12	37	27	32
12	34	27	30
13–15	26	20	23
>15	15	12	14
Total	28	23	26

TABLE 9-2 Hazards of Selected Substances in Cigarettes

Substance	Hazard
Arsenic	Poisonous, carcinogenic
Benzopyrene	Carcinogenic
Carbon monoxide	Reduces the oxygen-carrying capacity of blood
Formaldehyde	Cocarcinogen
Hydrogen cyanide	Reduces the cilia function of lungs
Nicotine	Poisonous, addictive
Nitrogen dioxide	Irritates respiratory tract
Nitrous oxide	Reduces the number of white blood cells that help protect the lungs from infectious agents
Phenol	Cocarcinogen
Vinyl chloride	Carcinogen

Some smokers switch to low-tar, low-nicotine, or filtered cigarettes because they believe them to be healthier alternatives that expose the smoker to fewer harmful chemicals. But researchers warn that there is no such thing as a "safe" cigarette. Low-tar or low-nicotine cigarettes may reduce some health risks. However, some smokers who switch to low-tar or low-nicotine cigarettes change their smoking habits to compensate for their change in brands. They smoke more cigarettes and inhale more deeply to meet their craving for nicotine. Some filtered brands of cigarettes have been found to deliver even more carbon monoxide than unfiltered brands. And smokers sometimes offset the effects of the filters by partially blocking them.

Immediate Effects of Smoking

The beginning smoker often has symptoms of mild *nicotine poisoning*: dizziness; faintness; rapid pulse; cold, clammy skin; and sometimes nausea, vomiting, and diarrhea. The seasoned smoker occasionally suffers these effects of nicotine poisoning, particularly after quitting and returning to a previous level of consumption. The effects of nicotine on smokers vary, depending greatly on the size of the nicotine dose and how much tolerance previous smoking has built up. Nicotine can either excite or tranquilize the nervous system, depending on dosage.

Nicotine has many other immediate effects. It stimulates the part of the brain called the **cerebral cortex.** It

these substances into their bodies and keep them there. In one year, a typical one-pack-per-day smoker takes in 50,000 to 70,000 puffs. Smoke from a cigarette, pipe, or cigar directly assaults mouth, throat, and respiratory tract; the nose—which normally filters about 75 percent of foreign matter in the air we breathe—is completely bypassed.

In a cigarette, the unburned tobacco itself acts as a filter. As a cigarette burns down, there is less and less filter. Thus, more chemicals are absorbed into the body during the last third of a cigarette than during the first. A smoker can cut down on absorption of harmful chemicals by not smoking cigarettes down to short butts. Any gains, of course, will be offset by smoking more cigarettes, inhaling deeper, or puffing more frequently.

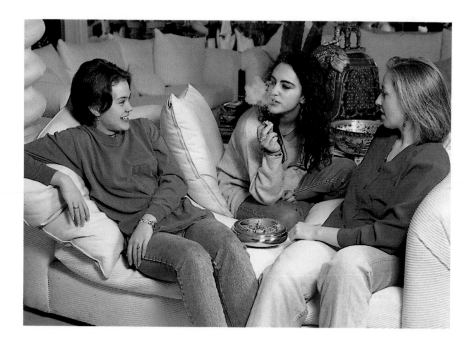

Cigarette smoke contains many toxic and carcinogenic chemicals that affect both the person smoking and the people breathing the environmental tobacco smoke. A growing body of evidence links ETS with lung cancer and respiratory and cardiovascular diseases.

also stimulates the adrenal glands to discharge adrenalin. And it inhibits the formation of urine, constricts the blood vessels, especially in the skin, increases the heart rate, and elevates blood pressure. Higher blood pressure, faster heart rate, and constricted blood vessels require the heart to pump more blood. In healthy people, the heart can usually meet this demand, but in people whose coronary arteries are damaged enough to interfere with the flow of blood, the heart muscle may be strained.

People who smoke often do not feel as hungry as people who do not. Smoking depresses hunger contractions and causes the liver to release glycogen, which slightly raises the level of sugar in the blood. Smoking also dulls taste buds so that food does not taste as good. People who quit smoking usually notice how much better food tastes. Figure 9-1 summarizes these immediate effects.

Long-Term Effects of Smoking

Smoking is a dangerous habit linked to many deadly and disabling diseases (Table 9-3). Research indicates that the total amount of tobacco smoke inhaled is a key factor contributing to disease. People who smoke more cigarettes per day, inhale deeply, puff frequently, smoke cigarettes down to the butts, or begin smoking at an early age run a greater risk of disease than do those who behave more moderately or who do not smoke at all. Many diseases have already been linked to smoking; and as more research is done, even more diseases associated with smoking are being uncovered. The most costly ones, to society as well as to the individual, are cardiovascular diseases, respiratory diseases such as emphysema and lung cancer, and other cancers. Although cancer tends to receive the most publicity, one form of cardiovascular dis-

ease, **coronary heart disease (CHD),** is actually the most widespread single cause of death for cigarette smokers.

Cardiovascular Disease   Cigarette smoking is strongly related to various cardiovascular disorders that involve the heart and blood vessels. CHD is one type and often results from a disease called **atherosclerosis,** in which fatty deposits called **plaques** form on the inner walls of heart arteries, causing them to narrow and stiffen. The crushing chest pain of **angina pectoris,** a primary symptom of CHD, results when the heart muscle or **myocardium** does not get enough oxygen. Sometimes a plaque forms at a narrow point in a main coronary artery. If the plaque completely blocks the flow of blood to a portion of the heart, that portion may die. This type of heart attack is called a **myocardial infarction.** CHD can also interfere with the normal electrical activity of the heart, resulting in disturbances of the normal heartbeat rhythm. Sudden and unexpected death is a common result of CHD, particularly among smokers. (See Chapter 15 for a more extensive discussion of cardiovascular disease.) Smokers have a 70 percent higher death rate from CHD than non-smokers. Deaths from CHD associated with cigarette smoking are most common in people 40 to 50 years old. (By contrast, deaths from lung cancer caused by smoking are most likely to occur in 60- to 70-year-olds.) Cigar and pipe smokers run a lower risk than do cigarette smokers.

We do not completely understand how cigarette smoking increases the risk of CHD. Researchers, however, are beginning to shed light on the process. Smoking reduces the amount of **HDL** cholesterol (**high-density lipoprotein,** the "good" cholesterol) and thus promotes plaque formation and speeds blood clotting. Smoking may also increase tension in the heart muscle walls, speed up the

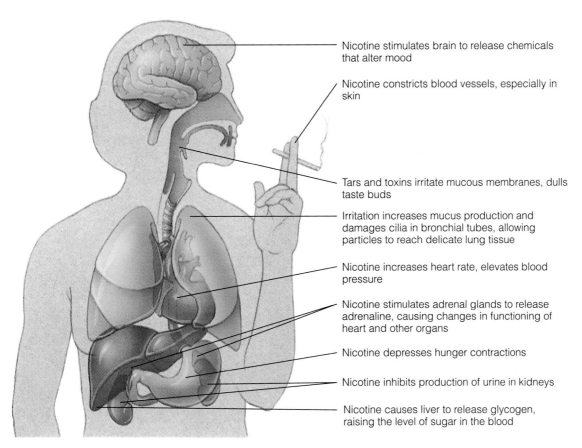

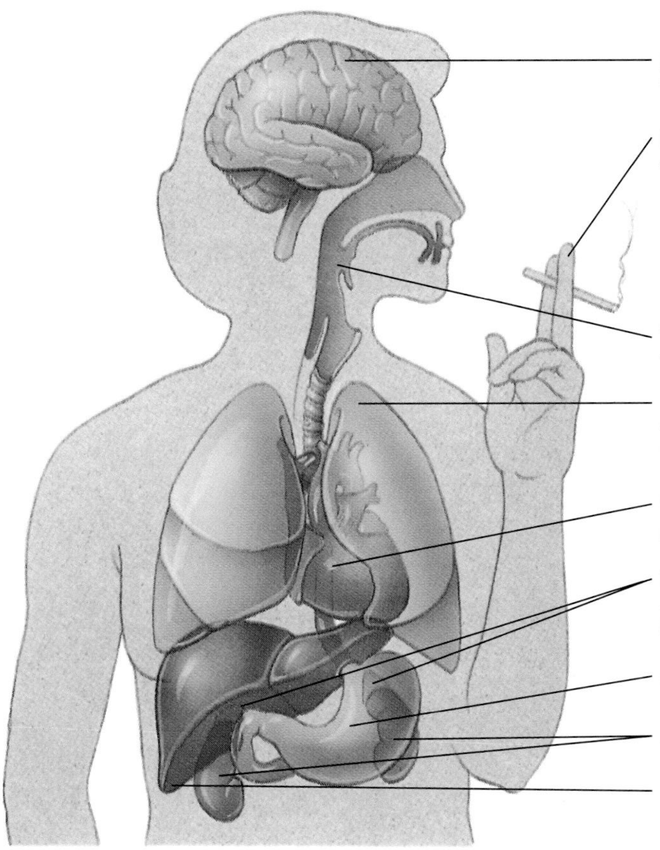
Nicotine stimulates brain to release chemicals that alter mood
Nicotine constricts blood vessels, especially in skin
Tars and toxins irritate mucous membranes, dulls taste buds
Irritation increases mucus production and damages cilia in bronchial tubes, allowing particles to reach delicate lung tissue
Nicotine increases heart rate, elevates blood pressure
Nicotine stimulates adrenal glands to release adrenaline, causing changes in functioning of heart and other organs
Nicotine depresses hunger contractions
Nicotine inhibits production of urine in kidneys
Nicotine causes liver to release glycogen, raising the level of sugar in the blood

Figure 9-1 *How does smoking a cigarette affect your body?*

rate of muscular contraction, and increase the heart rate. The workload of the heart thus increases, as does its need for oxygen and other nutrients. Carbon monoxide produced by cigarette smoking combines with hemoglobin in the red blood cells, displacing oxygen and thus providing less oxygen to the heart.

As suggested earlier, the risks of CHD decrease rapidly when the person stops smoking, particularly for younger smokers whose coronary arteries haven't yet been extensively damaged. Cigarette smoking has also been linked to other cardiovascular diseases, including:

- Stroke, a sudden interference with the circulation of blood in a part of the brain, resulting in the destruction of brain cells
- Aortic aneurysm, a bulge in the aorta caused by weakening in its walls
- Pulmonary heart disease, a disorder of the right side of the heart, caused by changes in the blood vessels of the lungs

Lung and Other Cancers Cigarette smoking is the primary cause of lung cancer. Smokers are 12 (women) to 22 (men) times more likely to die from it than are nonsmokers. The dramatic rise in lung cancer among women clearly parallels the increase of smoking in this group; lung cancer now exceeds breast cancer as the leading cause of cancer deaths among women. The risk of developing lung cancer increases with the number of cigarettes smoked each day, the number of years smoking, and the age at which the person started smoking.

While cigar and pipe smokers run a higher risk for lung cancer than nonsmokers do, the risk is lower than for cigarette smokers. Smoking filter-tipped cigarettes slightly reduces health hazards, unless the smoker compensates by smoking more, as is often the case.

TERMS

Coronary heart disease (CHD) Heart disease caused by hardening of the arteries that supply oxygen to the heart muscle.

Atherosclerosis Cardiovascular disease caused by the deposit of fatty substances in the walls of the arteries.

Plaque A deposit on the inner wall of blood vessels. Blood can coagulate around plaque and form a clot.

Angina pectoris Chest pain due to coronary heart disease.

Myocardium The muscle of the heart.

Myocardial infarction Heart attack caused by complete blockage of a main coronary artery.

High-density lipoprotein (HDL) Blood fats that help keep cholesterol in a watery state and thus protect against cardiovascular diseases.

TABLE 9-3 Adverse Effects of Cigarette Smoking

Disease and death risks	Maternal/fetal risks	Other health and cosmetic concerns
Cardiovascular disease • Coronary heart disease • Atherosclerosis • Heart attack • Stroke • High blood pressure • High cholesterol Lung disease • Emphysema • Chronic bronchitis • Hoarseness Cancer • Lung • Trachea • Larynx • Esophagus • Liver • Colon • Pancreas • Kidney • Bladder • Cervix Dental disease • Tooth decay • Gum disease • Periodontal disease • Halitosis (bad breath) Other diseases • Peptic and duodenal ulcers • Osteoporosis • Diabetes	Delayed conception or infertility Increased fetal death • Miscarriage • Ectopic pregnancy Preterm birth Stillbirth Low birth weight **Childhood complications** Sudden infant death syndrome Slow growth rate Learning delays **Effects of environmental tobacco smoke on healthy nonsmokers** In adults • Increased risk of cardiovascular disease, lung cancer, and other diseases In children • Increased frequency of respiratory infection and respiratory symptoms such as coughing and wheezing • Increased risk of hospitalization for bronchitis and pneumonia	Circulatory problems Complications from diabetes Acceleration of multiple sclerosis Menstrual disorders Infertility in men and women Early menopause Shortness of breath Decreased sense of taste and smell Decreased energy level Increased susceptibility to colds Increased hair loss Increased facial wrinkling Stained teeth Discolored fingers Increased risk of fire Increased risk of auto accidents **Economic costs** Average of $1.25 per pack of cigarettes, or $460 per year for a pack-a-day habit Increased health and home insurance premiums More frequent dry cleaning of clothes More frequent cleaning of teeth More frequent cleaning of house and office Burnt clothing, upholstery, and carpeting

Adapted from "Smoking Cessation." *Postgraduate Medicine*, vol. 90, no. 1, July 1991.

The evidence suggests that after a year without smoking the risk of lung cancer decreases substantially. After 10 years, the incidence of lung cancer among ex-smokers approaches the incidence of those who never smoked. If smoking is stopped before cancer has started, lung tissue tends to repair itself, even if cellular changes that can lead to cancer are already present.

Research has also linked smoking to cancers of the trachea, mouth, pharynx, esophagus, larynx, pancreas, bladder, kidney, cervix, stomach, liver, and colon.

Chronic Obstructive Lung Disease   The lungs of a smoker are constantly exposed to dangerous chemicals and irritants, and they must work harder to function adequately. The stresses placed on the lungs by smoking can permanently damage lung function and lead to chronic obstructive lung disease (COLD), also known as chronic obstructive pulmonary disease (COPD). This progressive

and disabling disorder consists of several different but related diseases; emphysema and chronic bronchitis are two of the most common.

Cigarette smokers are up to 18 times more likely to die from emphysema and chronic bronchitis than are nonsmokers. (Pipe and cigarette smokers are more likely to die from COLD than are nonsmokers, but they have a smaller risk than do cigarette smokers.) The risk of developing COLD rises with the number of cigarettes smoked and falls when smoking ceases. For most people in the United States, cigarette smoking is a more important cause of COLD than air pollution. But exposure to both air pollution and cigarette smoking is more dangerous than exposure to either by itself.

Emphysema   Smoking is the primary cause of **emphysema,** a particularly disabling condition in which the walls of the air sacs in the lungs lose their elasticity and

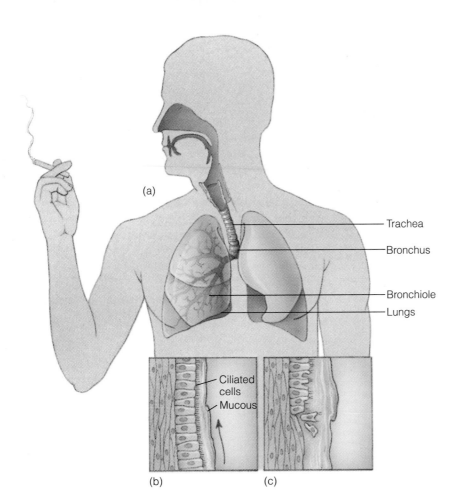

Figure 9-2 *Damage to the lungs caused by smoking.*

(a) The respiratory system. (b) View of the inside of a bronchiole of a nonsmoker. Foreign particles are collected by a thin layer of sticky mucus and transported out of the lungs, up toward the mouth, by the action of cilia. (c) View of the inside of a bronchiole of a smoker. Smoking irritates the lung tissue and causes increased mucus production, which can overwhelm the action of the cilia. A smoker develops a chronic cough as the lungs try to rid themselves of foreign particles and excess mucus. Eventually the cilia are destroyed, leaving the delicate lung tissue exposed to injury from foreign substances.

(a)

Trachea

Bronchus

Bronchiole

Lungs

Ciliated cells

Mucous

(b)   (c)

are gradually destroyed. The lungs' ability to obtain oxygen and remove carbon dioxide is impaired. A person with emphysema is breathless, is constantly gasping for air, and has the feeling of drowning. The heart must pump harder and may become enlarged. People with emphysema often die from a damaged heart. There is no known way to reverse this disease. In its advanced stage, the victim is bedridden and severely disabled.

Chronic Bronchitis   Chronic bronchitis is persistent, recurrent inflammation of the bronchial tubes. When the cell lining of the bronchial tubes is irritated, it secretes excess mucus. Bronchial congestion is followed by a chronic cough, which makes breathing more and more difficult. If smokers have chronic bronchitis, they face a greater risk of lung cancer, no matter how old they are or how many (or few) cigarettes they smoke. Chronic bronchitis seems to be a shortcut to lung cancer.

Other Respiratory Damage   Even when the smoker shows no signs of lung impairment or disease, cigarette smoking damages the respiratory system. Normally the cells lining the bronchial tubes secrete mucus, a sticky fluid that collects particles of soot, dust, and other substances in inhaled air. Mucus is carried up to the mouth by the continuous motion of the cilia, hairlike structures

that protrude from the inner surface of the bronchial tubes (Figure 9-2). If the cilia are destroyed or don't work or if the pollution of inhaled air is more than the system can remove, the protection provided by cilia is lost.

Cigarette smoke first slows, then stops the action of the cilia. Eventually it destroys them, leaving delicate membranes exposed to injury from substances inhaled in cigarette smoke or from the polluted air in which the person lives or works. Special cells of the body, the **macrophages** (literally "big eaters"), also work to remove foreign particles from the respiratory tract by engulfing them. Smoking appears to make macrophages work less efficiently. This interference with the functioning of the respiratory system often leads rapidly to the conditions called smoker's throat and smoker's cough, as well as to shortness of breath. Even smokers of high school age show impaired respiratory function, compared with nonsmokers of the same age.

Emphysema   Loss of lung tissue elasticity and breakup of the many small air sacs in the lungs so that fewer, larger, and less elastic air sacs are formed. The progressive accumulation of air causes difficulty in breathing.

Macrophages   Large cells in the body that absorb dead tissue and dead cells.

TERMS

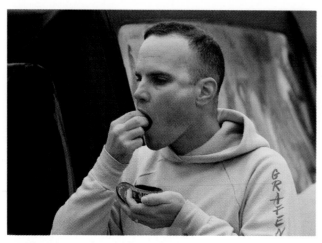

Nearly one out of every five male high school students uses smokeless tobacco, a habit linked to oral cancer, dental problems, dulling of the senses of taste and smell, and possibly cardiovascular problems.

Although cigarette smoking can cause many respiratory disorders and diseases, the damage is not always permanent. Once a person stops smoking, steady improvement in overall lung function usually takes place. Chronic coughing subsides, phlegm (mucus) production returns to normal, and breathing becomes easier. The likelihood of lung disease drops sharply. People of all ages, even those who have been smoking for decades, improve after they stop smoking. If given a chance, the human body has remarkable powers to restore itself.

Additional Health Hazards Besides respiratory problems, common physical complaints of smoking include loss of appetite, diarrhea, fatigue, hoarseness, weight loss, stomach pains, and insomnia. These conditions usually disappear in people who stop smoking. People who smoke cigarettes are more likely to develop peptic ulcers than nonsmokers and are more likely to die from them, especially from ulcers of the stomach. People with ulcers should stop smoking immediately because smoking impairs the ability of the ulcer to heal. Many of the hazards associated with tobacco use have only recently been discovered, so we are not sure if they are causally related or if they merely exist together. Premature skin wrinkling, premature baldness, gum disorders, tooth decay, and allergies have all been associated with cigarette smoking. Recent research also suggests that smoking may harm the immune system. Further research may link tobacco use to still other disorders.

Cumulative Effects The cumulative effects of tobacco use fall into two general categories. The first category is reduced life expectancy. A male who takes up smoking before age 15 and continues to smoke is only half as likely to live to age 75 as is a male who never smokes. If he in-

hales deeply, he risks losing one minute of life for every minute of smoking. Females who have similar smoking habits also have a reduced life expectancy.

The second category involves quality of life. A national health survey begun in 1964 shows that smokers spend one-third more time away from their jobs because of illness than do nonsmokers. Female smokers spend 17 percent more days sick in bed than do female nonsmokers. Lost work days associated with cigarette smoking number in the millions.

Both men and women smokers show a greater rate of acute and chronic disease than do those who have never smoked. The U.S. Public Health Service estimates that if all people had the same rate of disease as those who never smoked, there would be 1 million fewer cases of chronic bronchitis, 1.8 million fewer cases of sinusitis, and 1 million fewer cases of peptic ulcers in the country every year.

Other Forms of Tobacco Use

Many smokers have switched from cigarettes to other forms of tobacco, such as cigars, pipes, clove cigarettes, and smokeless tobacco. However, each of these alternatives is far from safe.

Smokeless Tobacco In the United States in recent years there has been a disturbing resurgence in the use of all forms of smokeless tobacco, especially among teenage boys and young adult males. The U.S. Centers for Disease Control reported in 1990 that 19 percent of male high school students used smokeless tobacco. There are two main categories of smokeless tobacco products—chewing tobacco and snuff. In chewing tobacco, the tobacco leaf may be shredded ("leaf"), pressed into bricks or cakes ("plugs"), or dried and twisted into ropelike strands ("twists"). Chewing tobacco is usually treated with molasses and other flavorings. The user places a wad of tobacco (often referred to as a "quid") in his or her mouth and then chews or sucks it to release the nicotine. In snuff, the leaf is processed into a coarse, moist powder. "Dipping" snuff involves placing a pinch of tobacco between the cheek and gum. All types of smokeless tobacco cause an increase in saliva production, and the resulting tobacco juice is spit out or swallowed.

The nicotine in smokeless tobacco—along with a number of flavorings, additives, and carcinogenic chemicals—is absorbed through the gums and lining of the mouth. The dose of nicotine that the user of smokeless tobacco products receives is comparable to that provided by cigarettes. Because of its nicotine content, smokeless tobacco is highly addictive. Some users keep it in their mouth even while sleeping.

Although not as dangerous as cigarettes, the use of smokeless tobacco carries many health risks. Changes can occur in the mouth after only a few weeks of use: Gums and lips become dried and irritated and may bleed, and precancerous white or red patches may appear inside the mouth. Oral cancers occur several times more frequently among snuff users than among those who don't use tobacco at all. Long-term snuff use may increase the risk of cancer of the cheek and gum by as much as 50 times. Smokeless tobacco use also can cause bad breath, tooth decay, and gingivitis (inflammation) and recession of the gums, especially where the tobacco is usually placed. The senses of taste and smell are usually dulled. Data on the incidence of heart disease in smokeless tobacco users have not yet been collected. But it is known that chewing and dipping produce blood levels of nicotine similar to those in cigarette smokers that have dangerous effects on the cardiovascular system, including elevation of blood pressure, heart rate, and blood levels of certain fats. Other chemicals in smokeless tobacco are believed to pose risks to developing fetuses in female users who are pregnant.

Cigars and Pipes Cigar and pipe smoking has declined in recent years, but many people, mostly men, still use one of these dangerous forms of tobacco. Cigars are made from rolled whole tobacco leaves. Pipe tobacco is made from shredded leaves; it is often flavored. Users of cigars and pipes absorb nicotine through the gums and lining of the mouth.

Some cigar and pipe users don't inhale; others do. Those who don't inhale have lower risks for cardiovascular and respiratory diseases than do cigarette smokers; however, their risks are higher than those of nonsmokers. Cigar and pipe smoke is more irritating to the lungs than cigarette smoke, so people who do inhale have even higher rates of respiratory and cardiovascular disease than cigarette smokers. All cigar and pipe smokers face an increased risk for cancers of the lip, mouth, throat, and esophagus.

Clove Cigarettes Called "kreteks" or "chicartas" and imported primarily from Indonesia, clove cigarettes are made of tobacco mixed with chopped cloves. Despite the addition of cloves, tests show that clove cigarettes deliver more tar, nicotine, and carbon monoxide than ordinary tobacco cigarettes. Clove cigarettes thus offer all the known hazards of tobacco cigarettes plus the unknown hazards of the chemical constituents of cloves. One of the most suspicious of these compounds is eugenol, an anesthetic that may damage the respiratory system's ability to detect and defend against foreign particles. Some individuals may also have severe allergic reactions to eugenol.

Since the early 1980s, when clove cigarettes first became a fad in the United States, there have been two confirmed reports of deaths from these "natural" cigarettes. Clove cigarettes have also been blamed for eight other cases of serious respiratory system injuries, including pneumonia and lung abscesses, among young adults. Publicity over the deaths and injuries has caused imports of clove cigarettes into the United States to fall in recent years; however, they are still available. Health officials stress that clove cigarettes are not a safe or healthy alternative to tobacco cigarettes.

THE EFFECTS OF SMOKING ON THE NONSMOKER

The movement to protect people from environmental tobacco smoke (ETS) is gaining strength. Nonsmokers are insisting on the right to breathe clean air. Federal Aviation Administration regulations now prohibit smoking on all flights in the continental limits of the United States of six hours or less, which effectively prohibits smoking on all domestic flights. Most states and hundreds of cities have enacted laws restricting smoking in public places like museums and theaters and in public-sector workplaces like courthouses and other government offices. Every year, laws restricting smoking in private-sector workplaces are enacted.

Environmental Tobacco Smoke

Environmental tobacco smoke consists of mainstream smoke and sidestream smoke. Smoke exhaled by smokers is referred to as **mainstream smoke. Sidestream smoke,** also called secondhand smoke, enters the atmosphere from the burning end of the cigarette, cigar, or pipe. Undiluted sidestream smoke, because it isn't filtered through either a cigarette filter or a smoker's lungs, has significantly higher concentrations of the toxic and carcinogenic compounds found in mainstream smoke. For example, compared to mainstream smoke, sidestream smoke has (1) twice as much tar and nicotine, (2) three times as much benzopyrene, a cancer-causing agent, (3) almost three times as much carbon monoxide, which displaces oxygen from red blood cells and forms **carboxyhemoglobin,** a dangerous compound that seriously limits the body's ability to use oxygen, and (4) three times as much ammonia. Nearly 85 percent of the smoke in a room where someone is smoking comes from sidestream smoke. Of course, sidestream smoke is diffused through the air, so nonsmokers don't inhale the same concentrations of toxic chemicals that the smoker does. Still, the concentrations can be considerable. In rooms where people are smoking, levels of carbon monoxide, for instance,

Mainstream smoke   Smoke that is inhaled by a smoker and then exhaled into the atmosphere.
Sidestream smoke   "Secondhand smoke" that comes from the burning end of a cigarette, cigar, or pipe.
Carboxyhemoglobin   A compound formed when carbon monoxide displaces oxygen from red blood cells; it seriously limits the body's ability to use oxygen.

TERMS

Everyone knows that smoking is dangerous to your health. It shortens life expectancy and increases the risk of cancer, lung disease, and heart disease. But did you know that smoking carries special risks for women? Many of these risks are associated with reproduction and the reproductive organs. The risk of cervical cancer, for example, is higher in women who smoke than in women who don't. For women trying to become pregnant, smoking may impair fertility. For pregnant women, smoking increases the risk of ectopic (tubal) pregnancy, miscarriage, and stillbirth.

Babies born to women who smoke during pregnancy may suffer from growth retardation in the womb and are typically lower in birth weight than are babies born to non-smoking women. As a group, they also perform worse on tests in both infancy and childhood. Babies whose mothers smoked during pregnancy are at higher risk for sudden infant death syndrome (SIDS) than are babies of nonsmokers.

Smoking interacts with oral contraceptives in dangerous ways; women who smoke and take birth control pills have a higher risk of developing potentially fatal blood clots than do other women. They are also at greater risk for fatal heart attacks and hemorrhagic strokes.

Smoking increases women's chances of developing osteoporosis, a disease in which bones become thinner and more brittle. Estrogen is often prescribed to prevent this bone loss after menopause, but estrogen works less well in preventing osteoporosis when a woman smokes. Older women who smoke are thus more likely to suffer hip fractures from falls.

Right now, for the first time in U.S. history, teenage girls are taking up smoking in greater numbers than teenage boys. If the trend continues, female smokers will outnumber male smokers in the adult population by the year 2000. We can expect to see a corresponding increase in tobacco-related diseases among women. Already, lung cancer has surpassed breast cancer as the most common form of cancer in American women. Unfortunately, we can also expect to see more of these debilitating and life-threatening tobacco-related diseases that are unique to women.

can exceed those permitted by Federal Air Quality Standards for outside air.

Effects of ETS

Studies show that up to 25 percent of nonsmokers subjected to ETS develop coughs, 30 percent develop headaches and nasal discomfort, and 70 percent suffer eye irritation. Other symptoms range from breathlessness to sinus problems. People with allergies tend to suffer the worst symptoms. Tobacco odor—which clings to skin and clothes—is another unpleasant effect of ETS.

But ETS causes more than just annoyance and discomfort. In early 1993 the U.S. Environmental Protection Agency classified ETS as a Class A carcinogen—an agent known to cause cancer in humans. This classification puts ETS in the same category as arsenic and asbestos and will make it easier for nonsmokers to demand protection from it. The EPA's indictment stems from studies in eight different countries, all showing that nonsmoking wives of smoking husbands suffer significantly more than their share of lung cancer. Based on these and other studies, the EPA estimates that people who live or work among smokers face a 20 to 30 percent increase in lung-cancer risk and that 3,000 Americans die from lung cancer caused by ETS each year. ETS also contributes to heart disease. According to the American Cancer Society, about 36,000 deaths from heart disease can be attributed to ETS each year. ETS also aggravates asthma, itself an increasing cause of sudden death in otherwise healthy adults. Ominously, scientists have been able to measure changes capable of contributing to lung tissue damage and potential tumor promotion in the bloodstreams of healthy young test subjects who spend just three hours in a smoke-filled room. And nonsmokers can still be affected by the harmful effects of ETS hours after they have left a smoky environment. Carbon monoxide, for example, lingers in the bloodstream five hours later.

Children and ETS

The U.S. Environmental Protection Agency estimates that environmental tobacco smoke triggers up to 300,000 cases of bronchitis, pneumonia, and other respiratory infections in babies every year, resulting in as many as 15,000 hospitalizations. Older children suffer, too: The EPA blames ETS for as many as 26,000 new cases of asthma in previously unaffected children every year and says it exacerbates asthma symptoms in up to 1 million children who already have the condition. The EPA also links ETS to reduced lung function in children and labels it a known cause of middle-ear infections, a leading reason for childhood surgery.

Why are infants and children so vulnerable? Because they breathe faster than adults, they inhale more air—and more of the pollutants in the air. Because they also weigh less, they inhale three times more pollutants per unit of body weight than do adults. And because their young lungs are still growing, this intake can impair optimal development. The problem is widespread. The American

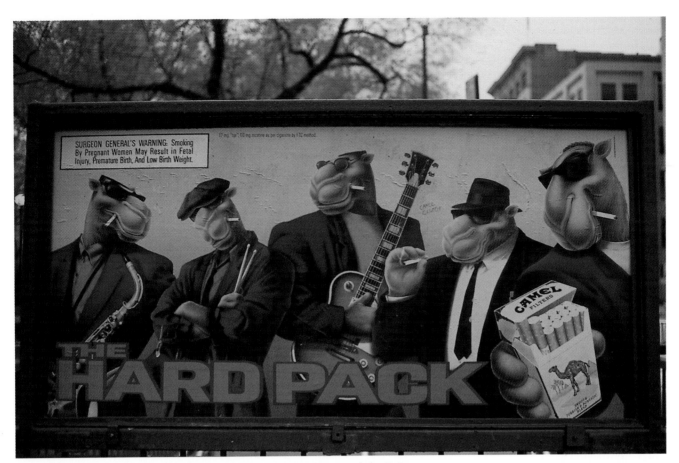

The Surgeon General and the American Medical Association pressured the R. J. Reynolds Tobacco Company to withdraw its "Old Joe" cartoon camel cigarette ads because the character is so appealing to children. One study found that more than half of children aged 3 to 6 recognized "Old Joe" as a cigarette ad.

Academy of Pediatrics estimates some 9 million American children are exposed to ETS, usually in the home. A mother's smoking has the most impact on a child's health, no doubt because mothers continue to provide more child care than fathers, even when both parents work.

Smoking and Pregnancy

Smoking almost doubles a pregnant woman's chance of suffering a miscarriage, and women who smoke also face an increased risk of ectopic pregnancy (see the box "Special Risks for Women Who Smoke"). Maternal smoking causes an estimated 4,600 infant deaths in the United States each year, primarily due to premature delivery and smoking-related problems with the placenta, the organ that delivers blood, oxygen, and nutrients to the fetus. Infants whose mothers smoked during pregnancy are also more likely to die from sudden infant death syndrome (SIDS). Maternal smoking causes fetal growth retardation, too. It is a major factor in low birth weight, which puts newborns at high risk for infections and other potentially fatal problems. Babies born to mothers who smoke more

than two packs per day perform poorly on developmental tests in the first hours after birth when compared with babies of nonsmoking mothers. Later in life, hyperactivity, short attention span, and lower scores on spelling and reading tests all occur more frequently in children whose mothers smoked throughout pregnancy than in those born to nonsmoking mothers. If these problems weren't enough, animal research suggests certain cancers are more common in animals that were exposed to cigarette smoke as fetuses. Nevertheless, 20 to 25 percent of pregnant Americans continue to smoke throughout pregnancy.

Personal Insight How do you feel when someone near you lights up a cigarette? What knowledge or experience influences your feelings? If it bothers you, but you have difficulty asserting yourself, what feelings are making you uncomfortable? Can you think of ways to deal with them?

Early in 1967, John F. Banzhaf III, outraged by a television commercial that equated smoking with masculinity, fired off a petition to the Federal Communications Commission. In it, Banzhaf, then 26 and fresh out of law school, demanded that foes of cigarettes be given a chance to air their side. On June 2, 1967, the FCC issued a watershed decision agreeing with him. The agency ordered broadcasters to provide "significant" free air time for anti-cigarette announcements. Four years later, Congress banned all cigarette advertising from TV and radio.

Two decades later, Eric D. Blom, fed up with seeing the ubiquitous Marlboro cigarette logo at the Indianapolis 500, rounded up a loose coalition of fellow auto racing fans concerned that the Indy was lending tobacco an image of glamour and daring. With his backers, Blom, an Indianapolis speech pathologist, gathered $50,000 in contributions and sponsored a car they christened "Tobacco Free America." On May 24, 1992, "Tobacco Free America" crossed the finish line at the Indy 500—ahead of two red-and-white Marlboro entries.

In both cases, individuals acted on their own to combat tobacco use, arguably the deadliest plague of our time. Every hour, 50 Americans die from preventable smoking-related diseases. Today there are more avenues than ever before for individual and group action against this major public health threat.

Action at the Local Level

Health activists now view local laws and ordinances as among the most effective anti-tobacco weapons. Here's why: While the mighty tobacco industry might be able to defeat or cripple anti-smoking laws in Congress and the 50 states, it can't hope to fight anti-tobacco statutes and rules in hundreds of school boards, town councils, city halls, and county boards of supervisors across the country. Among recent local actions: West Virginia University banned smoking at its baseball park effective in 1993. In 1992 the Houston City Council banned smoking in the Astrodome and other sports facilities, as well as in theaters, airports, and all city-owned buildings.

Action at the State and Federal Levels

By 1990, all but six states had laws restricting smoking in public places. All but a dozen had laws restricting smoking in public-sector workplaces. Seventeen had laws restricting smoking in private-sector job sites. Recent state measures include a 1992 Kentucky law that raised the age limit for buying tobacco products from 16 to 18 and a 1991 Florida regulation banning smoking in the state's 14,825 beauty parlors.

Federal action has ranged from a campaign by the U.S. Surgeon General aimed at pressuring the R. J. Reynolds

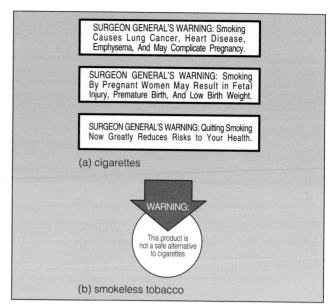

Figure 9-3 *Selected tobacco warning labels.*

Tobacco Company into dropping "Old Joe," the Camel cigarette logo that appeals to kids, to a 1992 Congressional measure calling for enforcement of laws prohibiting tobacco sales to youth. As the decade opened, federal health officials unveiled their "Healthy People 2000" objectives. A major goal is to reduce the proportion of Americans who smoke to 15 percent by decade's end. Federal courts and agencies have bolstered nonsmokers' rights by holding that people who are sensitive to ETS are "handicapped persons" and can take legal action to require employers to provide a "reasonable accommodation" to the handicap. The smoking ban on domestic airline flights ranks as one of Congress's hardest-fought anti-tobacco battles. The Comprehensive Smokeless Tobacco Health Education Act, passed by Congress in 1986, requires manufacturers of chewing tobacco and snuff to include health warning labels on packages (Figure 9-3). The law also bans radio and television advertising of the products and requires manufacturers to reveal to the U.S. Department of Health and Human Services what additives and flavorings they contain.

Such local, state, and national efforts represent progress, but more needs to be done. Of the 41 states that had enacted smoking restrictions by 1989, for example, just 22 had laws limiting smoking in restaurants. Action especially needs to be taken in smaller cities and in tobacco-producing states.

Individual Action

When a smoker violates a nonsmoking designation, complain. If your favorite restaurant or shop doesn't have a nonsmoking policy, ask the manager to adopt one. If you see children using cigarette vending machines or buying tobacco in stores, report this illegal activity to the facility manager or the police. Learn more about addiction and tobacco cessation so you can better support the tobacco users you know (see the box "How You Can Help a Tobacco User Quit.") Follow local, state, and national politics. Vote for politicians who support anti-tobacco measures. Write to elected officials to let them know your views. Cancel your subscriptions to magazines that carry tobacco advertising; include a note to the publisher or editor explaining your decision. Volunteer with the American Lung Association, the American Cancer Society, or the American Heart Association. These are just some of the many ways individuals can help support tobacco prevention and cessation efforts. Nonsmokers not only have the right to breathe clean air, but they also have the right to take action to help solve one of society's most serious public health threats (Figure 9-4 is a Nonsmoker's Bill of Rights).

Checking Tobacco Interests

With their immensely profitable industry shrinking, tobacco companies are concentrating on appealing to narrower and narrower market segments with an ever-increasing array of brands and styles—over 350 in all. As tobacco use has declined among better-educated, wealthier segments of the American population, tobacco companies have redirected their marketing efforts toward minorities, the poor, and young women, populations among whom smoking rates are still high. This practice of targeting specific segments of the market has become controversial, especially when the segment has unusually high risk for fatal diseases caused by tobacco use.

The rise in popularity of smokeless tobacco is one example of targeted marketing. Advertisements for smokeless tobacco associate chewing and dipping with a "macho" image and athletic prowess. Ads for smokeless tobacco have appeared mainly in male-oriented outdoor publications such as *Field and Stream, Outdoor Life,* and *Sporting News.* U.S. Tobacco Company's Skoal has been a major sponsor of Atlanta Braves baseball telecasts. The company has also promoted its products through scholarship offers to rodeo riders. A. J. Foyt, four-time winner of the Indianapolis 500, has raced automobiles bearing bold logos for Copenhagen snuff. Prominent baseball and football players have appeared in testimonial ads as well.

Pressure placed on tobacco companies in response to such targeted marketing campaigns has had an effect, however. The R. J. Reynolds Tobacco Company recently canceled its plans to market Uptown, a brand of cigarettes designed to appeal to African Americans, after the U.S. Secretary of Health and Human Services accused the company of "promoting a culture of cancer." The American Cancer Society saw the Uptown campaign as an escalation in the exploitation of African Americans, who, despite a significant drop in smoking rates in recent years, suffer a disproportionate number of health problems from smoking. In 1992, R. J. Reynolds pulled its new Dakota cigarettes off the test market. The cigarettes had been targeted to 18- to 20-year-old women, the only group of Americans whose rate of smoking continues to increase. Cigarette companies continue their efforts to appeal specifically to women, however, usually by connecting smoking with thinness (the dominant women's brand is Virginia Slims). In addition, tobacco companies have be-

Figure 9-4 *Nonsmoker's Bill of Rights.*

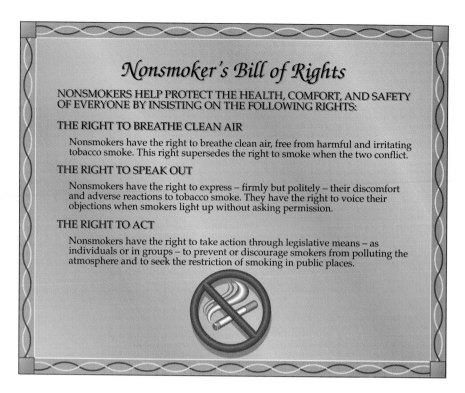

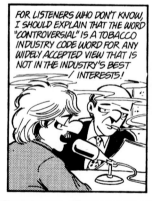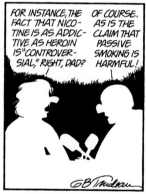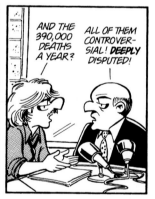

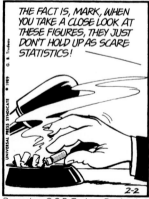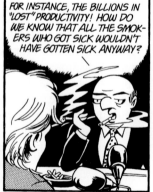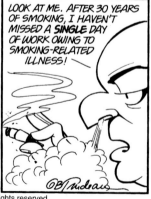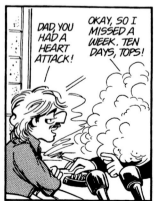

The Tobacco Trade: Exporting the Nicotine Habit

In 1989 the World Health Organization calculated how many people now living will be killed by tobacco-related diseases if current smoking patterns persist. The figure: 500 million people, one-tenth of the world's population. Another estimate suggests that by 2020 about 70 percent of the world's tobacco-related deaths will occur in the poorest nations of the globe.

Since the U.S. Surgeon General confirmed the dangers of smoking in 1964, tobacco consumption in the United States has steadily declined. Thirty-eight million American adults, or nearly half of all those who ever smoked, have quit smoking. To compensate for the loss in revenues, the U.S. tobacco industry, the world's number one tobacco exporter, has stepped up its efforts to sell to foreign markets, especially those in developing nations. Historically, poor countries have put fewer, if any, restrictions on tobacco advertising. Exported cigarettes usually have no health warnings on them, despite the fact that they contain more tar and nicotine than those sold in the United States.

The tobacco industry's aggressive advertising, lavish sponsorship of sports events, liberal distribution of free cig-arette samples, and relentless pursuit of new smokers—including very young smokers—have all succeeded in developing markets for U.S. tobacco products abroad. Even more effective has been the industry's recent success in enlisting the support of the federal government. In the past few years, the U.S. Trade Office has been threatening sanctions against countries that restrict the sale of American tobacco products. The federal government has pressured several countries into allowing advertising of American cigarettes, causing sharp increases in smoking among teenagers in countries like Japan, Korea, and Taiwan. In Japan, tobacco ads on television appear even during children's shows.

Health advocates are lobbying fiercely against the growing presence of Western tobacco firms in developing countries. They cite anemic local health policies, lax advertising regulations, and the American government's role in encouraging tobacco-marketing campaigns abroad that it would never tolerate at home. Nevertheless, smoking continues to increase globally. About 5.5 trillion cigarettes were consumed by the world's smokers in 1991, 2 percent more than in 1990.

---

gun focusing on increasing the export of cigarettes, particularly to developing nations (see box "The Tobacco Trade: Exporting the Nicotine Habit"). As companies compete for customers in the years ahead, the need to exercise public pressure to keep the powerful tobacco interests in check will persist.

HOW CAN A TOBACCO USER QUIT?

Giving up tobacco is a long-term, intricate process. Heavy smokers who say they've just stopped "cold turkey" aren't revealing the thinking and struggling and other mental processes that contributed to their final conquest over this powerful addiction. Research shows tobacco users move through predictable stages from being uninterested in stopping, to thinking about change, to making a concerted effort to stop, to finally maintaining abstinence. But most attempt to quit several times before they finally succeed. Relapse is a normal part of the process.

Quitting on Your Own

Some 85 to 95 percent of smokers who quit do so on their own. The National Cancer Institute, the American Cancer Society, and the American Lung Association publish information for would-be quitters on going it alone. But one recent study of solo quitters found that those who used such materials were no more successful than those who didn't. Some factors did seem to increase the chances of success, however. Smokers who quit cold turkey stood a slightly better chance of remaining tobacco-free for seven months than did those who tapered off gradually or switched brands before quitting. Successful quitters were also more likely to have support from others and to exercise. On the other hand, focusing on the negative effects of tobacco use has not proved to be a strategy associated with success. And another study showed that the more alcohol an individual drank, the less likely he or she was to succeed in quitting. The Behavior Change Strategy at the end of the chapter outlines a plan for quitting.

Group Programs

Formal programs are particularly recommended for people who have tried repeatedly to quit on their own without success. The American Cancer Society, the American Lung Association, and the Seventh-day Adventist Church all offer well-respected smoking cessation programs. Your college health center or community hospital may also do so. Some programs now are geared specifically to smokeless tobacco users. Studies show 15 to 30 percent of the people who enroll in formal quit-smoking programs remain tobacco-free a year later. When quitters enrolled in quit-smoking clinics also use nicotine gum, the success rate climbs as high as 47 percent.

Nicotine replacement therapy—in which a tobacco user is supplied with nicotine from a source other than standard tobacco products—can help break a tobacco habit by dividing the process of quitting into several steps. Nicotine replacement therapy allows a tobacco user to overcome the psychological and behavioral aspects of the tobacco habit without having to simultaneously endure the physical symptoms of nicotine withdrawal. Nicotine replacements can be taken in the form of chewing gum or through the use of the newly introduced skin patches; both types of products require a prescription. Each piece of gum delivers about as much nicotine as one cigarette; each patch delivers a timed dose of nicotine equal to as much as three-quarters of a pack of cigarettes over a 24-hour period. After a few weeks or months of using either nicotine gum or the nicotine patch, the reforming tobacco user begins to gradually taper off use of the replacement, avoiding withdrawal symptoms.

Nicotine replacements can be effective in helping people quit. Of those who try to quit without using this therapy, only about 5 or 10 percent avoid relapse for a year. Nicotine replacement therapy increases the success rate to about 15 percent; if combined with counseling and behavioral therapy to help break psychological dependence, the success rate climbs to about 30 percent.

There are drawbacks to nicotine replacement therapy, however. Many people find it difficult to manage the dosage of nicotine while using nicotine gum. Possible side effects of the gum include burning sensations in the mouth and throat, nausea, and vomiting. Certain foods and drinks can interfere with the absorption of nicotine from the gum. About 20 percent of people who use nicotine gum get hooked on the cure. These gum abusers confess they stockpile chewed gum wads for emergencies and, in a pinch, will chew even a dusty, stale, and lint-covered wad. Because the gum is available only by prescription, chewers may visit numerous physicians in different cities or even states to maintain their supply. A serious gum habit can cost more than $80 per week.

Skin patches avoid some of the problems of nicotine gum, mainly because they deliver a steady dose of nicotine. However, patches are associated with skin inflammation in about 7 percent of people who try them. Some users suffer from insomnia or nightmares. Patches cost up to $25 or $30 per week.

The most serious problem that may be associated with nicotine replacement therapy involves misuse of the nicotine replacement products. Some people use nicotine replacements *and* smoke, a practice that the products' packaging specifically warns against. Nicotine is a dangerous drug that narrows the blood vessels leading to the heart and increases the propensity of the blood to form clots. These effects can contribute to heart attacks. In 1992, federal health authorities began investigating a number of deaths by heart attack in people who wore nicotine patches while continuing to smoke.

But despite the potential for problems, specialists in addiction medications have welcomed nicotine replacement therapy as an effective pharmacological aid for tobacco users who want to quit. And using nicotine alone is still safer than smoking cigarettes, which deliver carbon monoxide, more than 30 carcinogens, and thousands of toxins on top of nicotine.

Adapted from "Nicotine Patches: A Better Way to Quit Smoking?" *Consumer Reports on Health*, September 1992.

Prescription Help

Physicians can now prescribe nicotine in gum or skin-patch form to help ease quitters' withdrawal symptoms (see the box "Nicotine Replacement Therapy: A New Hope?"). Clonidine, a drug used to help heroin addicts during withdrawal, is also prescribed to help some smokers quit. Meanwhile, researchers are investigating the usefulness of antidepressants and antianxiety drugs in smoking cessation and are experimenting with nicotine nose drops and sprays.

Benefits of Quitting

Giving up tobacco provides immediate health benefits to men and women of all ages. People who quit smoking find food tastes better. Their sense of smell increases. Circulation improves, heart rate and blood pressure drop, and lung function and heart efficiency increase. People have more "wind," and their capacity for exercise improves. Many ex-smokers report feeling more energetic and alert. They experience fewer headaches. Even their complexions may improve. Quitting also has a positive effect on long-term disease risk. From the first day without tobacco, quitters begin to decrease their risks of cancer of the lung, larynx, esophagus, mouth, pancreas, bladder, cervix, and other sites. Risks of heart attack, stroke, and other cardiovascular diseases drop quickly, too.

The younger people are when they stop smoking, the more pronounced the health improvements. And these improvements gradually but invariably increase as the period of nonsmoking increases (Table 9-4). It's never too late to quit, though. According to a 1990 U.S. Surgeon General's report, people who quit smoking, regardless of age, live longer than people who continue to smoke. Even smokers who have already developed chronic bronchitis or emphysema show some improvement when they quit.

TABLE 9-4 Benefits of Quitting Smoking

Disease or Consequence	Effect of Quitting on Risk
Chronic obstructive pulmonary disease	Within 1 year of quitting, risk is reduced to half that of continuing smokers. After 15 years, risk is the same as for people who have never smoked.
Lung cancer	Risk is as much as halved compared to continuing smokers 10 years after quitting.
Stroke	Risk is reduced to that of people who have never smoked 5 to 15 years after quitting.
Cancers of the mouth, throat, and esophagus	Risk is halved compared to continuing smokers 5 years after quitting.
Cancer of the larynx, ulcers	Risk is reduced compared to continuing smokers after quitting.
Pancreatic cancer	Risk is reduced compared to continuing smokers 10 years after quitting.
Cancers of the bladder and cervix	Risk is reduced compared to continuing smokers a few years after quitting.
Low-birth-weight baby	Risk is reduced to that of nonsmokers for women who quit before pregnancy or during their first trimester.

Adapted from *The Health Benefits of Smoking Cessation: A Report of The Surgeon General, 1990, At a Glance.* Atlanta: Centers for Disease Control, Office on Smoking and Health.

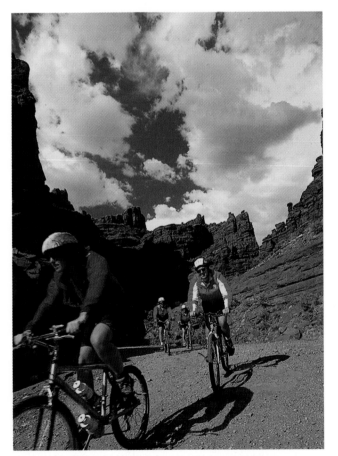

Quitting smoking improves quality of life. In addition to reducing their long-term disease risks, these ex-smokers have more energy and an improved capacity for exercise.

SUMMARY

- Smoking is the largest preventable cause of ill health and death in the United States. Nevertheless, millions of Americans continue to use tobacco.

Why People Use Tobacco

- Regular tobacco use causes physical dependence on nicotine, characterized by loss of control, tolerance, and the appearance of a withdrawal syndrome when tobacco use ceases. Habits can become associated with tobacco use and trigger the urge for a cigarette or other tobacco product.
- People who begin smoking are usually imitating others or responding to seductive advertising. They often deny or minimize the risks of smoking.
- Tobacco use is associated with low education level and the use of other drugs. Although cigarette, pipe, and cigar smoking have been decreasing, use of smokeless tobacco is increasing.

Health Hazards

- Tobacco smoke is made up of particles of several hundred different chemicals, including some that are carcinogenic or poisonous or that damage or irritate the respiratory system. Carbon monoxide in cigarette smoke displaces oxygen in red blood cells, depleting the body's supply of oxygen.

- Depending on dosage, nicotine acts on the nervous system as a stimulant or a tranquilizer. Nicotine can cause blood pressure and heart rate to increase, straining the heart.
- Cardiovascular disease is the most widespread cause of death for cigarette smokers. Smoking's reduction of high-density lipoproteins probably promotes the formation of deposits in the arteries and speeds blood clotting. Cigarette smoking has also been linked to stroke, aortic aneurysm, and pulmonary heart disease.
- Cigarette smoking is the primary cause of lung cancer and is linked to many other cancers as well.
- Smoking can permanently damage lung function and lead to chronic obstructive lung disease (COLD). In emphysema, the walls of the air sacs in the lungs lose their elasticity and are gradually destroyed, causing severe disability and death. Chronic bronchitis, characterized by congestion and a chronic cough, is linked to a high risk of lung cancer.
- Cigarette smoking decreases lung function, damages the cilia in the bronchial tubes, and hinders the work of macrophages.
- Damage from smoking may not always be permanent, and lung function usually improves when a person quits.
- Cigarette smokers are more likely to develop peptic ulcers and to die from them than are nonsmokers. Also associated with smoking are gum disorders, premature skin wrinkling and baldness, and allergies. Tobacco use leads to lower life expectancy and to a diminished quality of life.
- The use of chewing tobacco or snuff leads to nicotine addiction and is linked to oral cancers.
- Cigars, pipes, and clove cigarettes are not safe alternatives to cigarettes.

The Effects of Smoking on the Nonsmoker

- Environmental tobacco smoke (ETS) contains high concentrations of toxic chemicals and can cause headaches, eye and nasal irritation, and sinus problems. Long-term exposure to ETS can cause lung cancer and heart disease.
- Babies and young children inhale more air than adults do and so take in more pollutants; children whose parents smoke are especially susceptible to respiratory diseases.
- Smoking during pregnancy increases the risk of spontaneous abortion, stillbirth, congenital abnormalities, premature birth, and low birth weight. Crib death and long-term impairments in physical and intellectual development are also risks.

What Can Be Done?

- There are many avenues individuals and groups can take to act against tobacco use. Nonsmokers can use social pressure and legislative channels to discourage smokers from polluting the air and assert their rights to breathe clean air.
- Congress has placed warnings on cigarette packages and restricted smoking on airplanes and in public-sector workplaces.
- Recently tobacco companies have aimed marketing programs at narrower segments of the population in which smoking is still popular.

How Can a Tobacco User Quit?

- Giving up smoking is a difficult and long-term process. Although most ex-smokers quit on their own, some smokers benefit from stop-smoking programs. Prescription medications can ease withdrawal symptoms, and support groups or counseling can help deal with psychological factors.

TAKE ACTION

1. Interview one or two ex-tobacco users about their experiences with tobacco and the methods they used to quit. Why did they start using tobacco and how long did their habit continue? What made them decide to quit? How did they go about quitting? What could a current tobacco user learn from their experience of quitting?

2. Make a tour of the public facilities in your community and on your campus, such as movie theaters, auditoriums, business and school offices, and classrooms. What kinds of restrictions on smoking do these places have? In your opinion, are they appropriate? If you feel more or different restrictions are in order, write a letter to the editor of your school or local newspaper making your case. Support it with convincing arguments and appropriate facts.

3. Plan what you will say or do the next time you want to ask a smoker to stop smoking around you. Draw up a list of statements you might make to a smoker in various situations. You'll increase the effectiveness of your statements if they are courteous and don't threaten the person's dignity. Practice saying these statements in a way that is assertive rather than aggressive or passive. The next time you're in an appropriate situation, use one of your statements. If it doesn't have the desired effect, think about why and modify it for the next time.

1. *Critical Thinking:* Examine the ads for cigarettes and smokeless tobacco on billboards and in some popular magazines. What markets are they targeting? How do they try to appeal to their audience? How do the advertisers deal with the Surgeon General's warning? Write a short essay describing your findings.

2. *Critical Thinking:* Restrictions on smoking are increasing in our society. Do you think they're fair? Do they infringe on people's rights? Do they go too far or not far enough? Write a brief essay stating your position on smoking restrictions. Be sure to explain your reasoning. What are the most important factors in your decision? Why do you think you hold the opinion you do?

3. *Critical Thinking:* Research the roles the U.S. government plays in tobacco use and sales. Describe these roles and their effects. Do you think the government is acting appropriately? In your opinion, what role should the government have regarding tobacco use and sales?

BEHAVIOR CHANGE STRATEGY

KICKING THE TOBACCO HABIT

You can look forward to a longer and healthier life if you join the 39 million Americans who have quit using tobacco. The steps for quitting described below are discussed in terms of the most popular tobacco product in the United States—cigarettes—but they can be adapted for all forms of tobacco use. Begin by taking the quiz in the box "For Smokers Only: Why Do You Smoke?" Clues and information about the reasons you smoke, the ways you respond to nicotine addiction, and other aspects of your behavior will be helpful as you plan a strategy for quitting.

Gather Information

Collect personal smoking information in a detailed journal about your smoking behavior. Use your journal to collect two major types of information—cigarettes smoked and smoking urges. Part of the job is to identify patterns of smoking that are connected with routine situations (for example, the coffee break smoke, the after-dinner cigarette, the tension-reduction cigarette, and so on). Use this information in combination with your self-assessment scores to discover the behavior chains involved in your smoking habit.

Set a Target Quitting Date

Choose a date in the near future when you expect to be relatively stress-free and can give quitting the energy and attention it will require. Don't choose a date right before or during finals week, for instance. Consider making quitting a gift: Choose your birthday as your quit date, for example, or make quitting a Father's Day or Mother's Day present. You might also want to coordinate your quit date with a buddy—a fellow tobacco user who wants to quit or a nonsmoker who wants to give up another bad habit or begin an exercise program. Tell your friends and family when you plan to quit. Ask them to offer encouragement and help hold you to your goal.

Prepare to Quit

One of the most important things you can do to prepare to quit is to develop and practice nonsmoking relaxation methods. Many smokers find that they use cigarettes to help them unwind in tense situations or to relax at other times. If this is true for you, you'll need to find and develop effective substitutes. It takes time to become proficient at relaxation techniques, so begin practicing before your quit date. Refer to the detailed discussion of relaxation techniques found in Chapter 2.

Other things you can do to help prepare for quitting include the following:

- Make an appointment to see your physician. Ask about some of the new prescription aids for tobacco cessation and whether one might be appropriate for you.
- Make a dentist's appointment to have your teeth cleaned the day after your target quit date.
- Start an easy exercise program if you're not exercising regularly already. Get in the habit of going to bed and getting up at the same time. Don't let yourself become overworked or fall behind at school or on the job.
- Buy some sugarless gum. Stock your kitchen with low-calorie snacks.
- Throw away all your cigarette-related paraphernalia (ashtrays, lighters, and so on).

Quitting

Complete a personal contract for quitting that specifies the day and time when you will stop smoking as well as possible rewards for quitting (see sample contract below). When drawing up your contract, you may be torn between quitting abruptly ("cold turkey") and quitting gradually. Research favors the abrupt approach but with enough time set aside to learn and practice effective quitting skills.

Your first few days without cigarettes will probably be the most difficult. It's hard to give up such a strongly ingrained habit, but remember that 39 million Americans

Cues and High-Risk Situations	Suggested Strategies
Awakening in morning	Brush your teeth as soon as you wake up. Stay busy and try not to think about smoking.
Drinking coffee	Do something else with your hands. Drink tea or another beverage instead.
Eating meals	Eat in a different location. Sit in nonsmoking sections at restaurants. Get up from the table right away after eating and start another activity. Brush your teeth right after eating.
Driving a car	Have the car cleaned when you quit smoking. Chew sugarless gum or eat a low-calorie snack. Take public transportation or ride your bike.
Socializing with friends who smoke	Suggest nonsmoking events (movies, theatre, shopping). Tell them you've quit and ask them not to smoke around you, offer you cigarettes, or give you cigarettes if you ask for them.
Drinking at a bar, restaurant, or party	Try to take a nonsmoker with you or associate with nonsmokers. Let friends know you've just quit. Moderate your intake of alcohol (it can weaken your resolve).
Encountering stressful situations	Practice relaxation techniques. Get out of your room or house. Go somewhere that doesn't allow smoking. Take a shower, chew gum, call a friend, or exercise.

Adapted from *Postgraduate Medicine,* vol. 90, no. 1, July 1991.

have done it—and you can too. Plan and rehearse the steps you will take when you experience a powerful craving. For example, try drinking a glass of water, chewing gum, taking a walk or a shower, going swimming, or practicing a relaxation technique. Avoid or control situations that you know from your journal are powerfully associated with your smoking (see table below). If your hands feel empty without a cigarette, try holding or fiddling with a small object such as a paper clip or pencil.

Social support can also be a big help. Arrange with a buddy to help you with your weak moments—call him or her whenever you feel overwhelmed by an urge to smoke. Tell people you've just quit. You may discover many inspiring former smokers who can encourage you and reassure you that it's possible to quit and lead a happier, healthier life.

Maintaining Nonsmoking

Maintaining nonsmoking over time is the ultimate goal of any stop-smoking program. The lingering smoking urges that remain once you've quit should be carefully tracked and controlled because they can cause relapses if left unattended. Keep track of these urges in your smoking journal to help you deal with them. If certain situations still trigger the urge for a cigarette, change something about the situation to break past associations. If stress or boredom causes strong smoking urges, use a relaxation technique, take a brisk walk, have a stick of gum, or substitute some other activity for smoking.

Don't set yourself up for a relapse. If you allow yourself to get overwhelmed at school or work or to gain weight, it will be easier to convince yourself that now isn't the right time to quit. This *is* the right time. Continue to practice time management and relaxation techniques. Exercise regularly, eat sensibly, and get enough sleep. These habits will not only ensure your success at remaining tobacco-free, but they will also serve you well in stressful times throughout your life.

Watch out for patterns of thinking that can make nonsmoking more difficult. Testing yourself ("I'll put the pack out in front of me to prove my strength") or remembering

My Personal Contract for Quitting

I agree to stop all smoking on ___Nov 1st___ at ___7:00 a.m.___.
I understand that it is important for me to make a strong personal effort at this particular time so that I can become a permanent ex-smoker. I will reward myself for reaching each of the following goals:

	Reward
1 day without a cigarette	movie
3 days without a cigarette	new CD
1 week without a cigarette	tickets to basketball game
2 weeks without a cigarette	hike
1 month without a cigarette	concert tickets
3 months without a cigarette	camping trip

I will keep a smoking diary to track my urges for cigarettes. I will combat my smoking urges with the following strategies: __brush my teeth first thing in the morning; drink tea or juice instead of coffee; go for a walk right after dinner__

I sign this contract as an indication of my personal commitment to stop smoking.

___Vipul Singh___   10/19

A personal contract for quitting cigarettes.

cigarettes as long-lost friends or part of a better time in your life ("the good old days") can erode your sense of resolve and your skills in resisting smoking urges. Focus on the positive aspects of not smoking and give yourself lots of praise—you deserve it.

Keep track of the emerging benefits that come from having quit. Items that might appear on your list include improved stamina, an increased sense of pride at having kicked a strong addiction, improved sense of taste and smell, no more smoker's cough, and so on. Keep track of the money you're saving by not smoking and spend it on things you really enjoy. And if you do lapse, be gentle with yourself. Lapses are a normal part of quitting. Forgive yourself and pick up where you left off.

SELECTED BIBLIOGRAPHY

Barry, M. 1991. The influence of the U.S. tobacco industry on the health, economy, and environment of developing countries. *The New England Journal of Medicine* 324(13): 917–19.

Benowitz, N. L. 1991. Nicotine replacement therapy during pregnancy. *Journal of the American Medical Association* 266(22): 3174–75.

Bircher, A. J., and others. 1991. Adverse skin reactions to nicotine in a transdermal therapeutic system. *Contact Dermatitis* 25:230–36.

Blum, A. 1991. The Marlboro Grand Prix: Circumvention of the television ban on tobacco advertising. *New England Journal of Medicine* 324(13): 913–17.

Botvin, G. J., and others. 1992. Correlates and predictors of smoking among black adolescents. *Addictive Behaviors* 17:97–103.

Bowen, D. J., and K. Dahl. 1991. Descriptions of early triers. *Addictive Behaviors* 16:95–101.

Burros, M. 1988. The smoking law revisited. *New York Times,* 12 October.

Cancer Facts and Figures. 1993. New York: American Cancer Society.

Centers for Disease Control. 1989. Cigarette smoking among reproductive-aged women: Behavioral risk factor surveillance system. *Morbidity and Mortality Weekly Report* 40(42).

———. 1991. Cigarette smoking among youth—United States, 1989. *Morbidity and Mortality Weekly Report* 40(41).

———. 1991. Current tobacco, alcohol, marijuana, and cocaine use among high school students—United States, 1990. *Morbidity and Mortality Weekly Report* 40(38).

———. 1991. Differences in the age of smoking initiation between blacks and whites—United States. *Morbidity and Mortality Weekly Report* 40(44).

———. 1991. State tobacco prevention, control activities: Results of 1989–1990 Association of State, Territorial Health Officials survey—final report. *Morbidity and Mortality Weekly Report* 40(40).

———. 1991. Tobacco use among high school students—United States, 1990. *Morbidity and Mortality Weekly Report* 40(36).

———. 1992. Cigarette smoking among adults—United States, 1990. *Morbidity and Mortality Weekly Report* 41(20).

———. 1992. Cigarette smoking among Chinese, Vietnamese, and Hispanics—California, 1989–1991. *Morbidity and Mortality Weekly Report* 41(20).

Clearman, D. R., and D. R. Jacobs, Jr. 1991. Relationships between weight and caloric intake of men who stop smoking: The multiple risk factor intervention trial. *Addictive Behaviors* 16:401–410.

Committee on Substance Abuse. 1991. Hazards of clove cigarettes. *Pediatrics* 88(2): 395–96.

Coreil, J., and others. 1991. Predictors of smoking among Mexican-Americans: Findings from the Hispanic HANES. *Preventive Medicine* 20:508–517.

DiFranza, J. P., and others. 1991. RJR Nabisco's cartoon camel promotes Camel cigarettes to children. *Journal of the American Medical Association* 266(22): 3149–53.

DuNah, R., Jr., and others. 1991. Demographics and cigarette smoking among women. *Preventive Medicine* 20:262–70.

Eriksen, M. P., C. A. LeMaistre, and G. R. Newell. 1988. The health hazards of passive smoking. *Annual Review of Public Health* 9:47–70.

Feighery, E., and others. 1991. The effects of combining education and enforcement to reduce tobacco sales to minors. *Journal of the American Medical Association* 266(22): 3168–71.

Fischer, P. M., and others. 1991. Brand logo recognition by children aged 3 to 6 years. *Journal of the American Medical Association* 266(22): 3145–48.

Gerace, T. A., and others. 1991. Smoking cessation and change in diastolic blood pressure, body weight, and plasma lipids. *Preventive Medicine* 20:602–620.

Gingiss, P. L., and N. H. Gottlieb. 1991. A comparison of smokeless tobacco and smoking practices of university varsity and intramural baseball players. *Addictive Behaviors* 16:335–40.

Glynn, T., and others. 1991. Tobacco-use reduction among high-risk youth: Recommendations of a National Cancer Institute expert advisory panel. *Preventive Medicine* 20:279–91.

Gostin, L. O., and others. 1991. Tobacco liability and public health policy. *Journal of the American Medical Association* 266(22): 3178–82.

Guidotti, T. L., and others. 1989. Clove cigarettes: The basis for concern regarding health effects. *Western Journal of Medicine* 151:220–28.

Heart Facts. 1992. New York: American Heart Association.

Hymowitz, N., and others. 1991. Baseline factors associated with smoking cessation and relapse. *Preventive Medicine* 20:590–601.

Jason, L. A., and others. 1991. Active enforcement of cigarette control laws in the prevention of cigarette sales to minors. *Journal of the American Medical Association* 266(22): 3159–61.

Lando, H. A., and others. 1991. A comparison of self-help approaches to smoking cessation. *Addictive Behaviors* 16:183–93.

Manley, M., and others. 1991. Clinical interventions in tobacco control. *Journal of the American Medical Association* 266(22): 3172–73.

McGovern, P. G., and H. A. Lando. 1991. Reduced nicotine exposure and abstinence outcome in two nicotine fading methods. *Addictive Behaviors* 16:11–20.

———. 1992. An assessment of nicotine gum as an adjunct to freedom from smoking cessation clinics. *Addictive Behaviors* 17:137–47.

McMaster, C., and C. Lee. 1991. Cognitive dissonance in tobacco smokers. *Addictive Behaviors* 16:349–53.

Mintz, J., and others. 1991. Combined use of alcohol and nicotine gum. *Addictive Behaviors* 16:1–10.

Mintz, M. 1991. Tobacco roads. *The Progressive,* May, 24–29.

Patel, C. H., and R. M. Davis. 1989. Trends in cigarette smoking in the U.S.—The changing influence of gender and race. *Journal of the American Medical Association* 261:2843.

Pierce, J. P., and others. 1991. Does tobacco advertising target young people to start smoking? Evidence from California. *Journal of the American Medical Association* 266(22): 3154–58.

Rigotti, N. A., and C. L. Pashos. 1991. No-smoking laws in the United States. *Journal of the American Medical Association* 266(22): 3162–67.

Schinke, S., and others. 1992. Substance use among Hispanic and non-Hispanic adolescents. *Addictive Behaviors* 17:117–24.

The tobacco trade: The search for El Dorado. 1991. *The Economist,* 16 May, 21–24.

Transdermal Nicotine Study Group. 1991. Transdermal nicotine for smoking cessation. *Journal of the American Medical Association* 266(22): 3133–38.

U.S. Surgeon General. 1989. *Reducing the Health Consequences of Smoking.* Bethesda, Md.: U.S. Department of Health and Human Services.

RECOMMENDED READINGS

Boyd, G., and C. M. Darbey, eds. 1990. *Smokeless Tobacco Use in the United States.* NCI Monograph, National Cancer Institute. *A comprehensive examination of the role of smokeless tobacco in causing cancer.*

Cahalan, D. 1991. *An Ounce of Prevention: Strategies for Solving Tobacco, Alcohol, and Drug Problems.* San Francisco: Jossey-Bass. *A cogent analysis of proposed solutions to the problem of tobacco and other drug addictions.*

Journal of the American Medical Association, 6 January 1989. *This issue of JAMA is devoted mostly to smoking and includes the following articles: Trends in cigarette smoking in the United States, the cost-effectiveness of counseling smokers to quit, and many others.*

Krogh, D. 1992. *Smoking: The Artificial Passion.* New York: W. H. Freeman. *Probes the roots of smoking.*

Leventhal, H., K. Glynn, and R. Fleming. 1987. Is the smoking decision an "informed choice"? Effect of smoking risk factors on smoking beliefs. *Journal of the American Medical Association* 257(24):3373–76. *A cogent exploration of the kinds of apparent psychological options people have and their willingness to engage in detrimental behaviors.*

A Lifetime of Freedom from Smoking. 1989. New York: American Lung Association. *Useful for anyone who wants to quit, or wants anyone else to quit.*

Schelling, T. C. 1986. Economics and cigarettes. *Preventive Medicine* 15(5):549–60. *A discussion of how politics and the marketplace drive the consumption of cigarettes.*

———. 1992. Addictive drugs: The cigarette experience. *Science* 255:430–33. *A fascinating look at addiction and tobacco.*

10

The Responsible Use of Alcohol

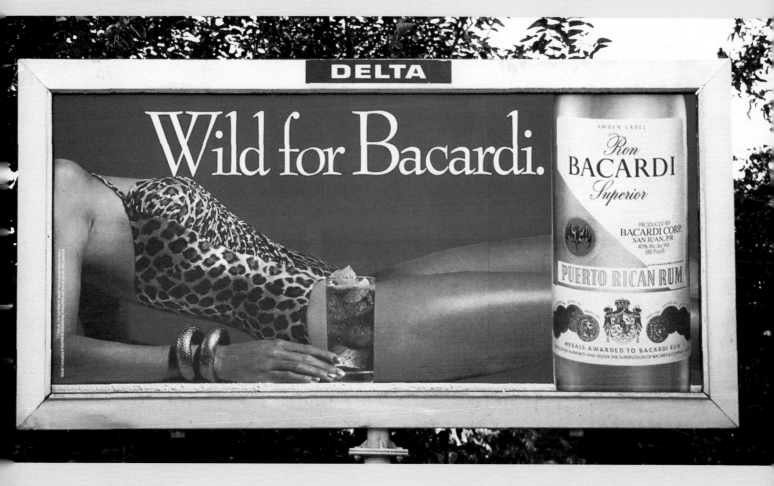

CONTENTS

● You didn't realize it was getting so late and find that you're still feeling slightly drunk when it's time to drive your moped home from a Friday night gathering at a local pub. A friend orders you a cup of strong coffee and urges you to eat a lot of potato chips to speed absorption of the alcohol in your stomach. She says if you take several deep breaths and do a few jumping jacks when you get outside, you'll be just fine. Is she right that these are good activities to help you sober up?

● You wanted everyone to have a good time at a party you gave in your apartment, so you made sure there was plenty of beer and wine. But now, as your guests are leaving, you realize that one person who is quite drunk has to drive himself and his date home. Other guests are expressing concern about them to you and urging that you insist that they stay overnight. They even say you should take the man's car keys. You're not sure you have the right to do that. After all, he's an adult and freely made the choice to drink as much as he did. What are your responsibilities in this situation? Should you intercede, or should you let them go?

● You like your Uncle Joe a lot when he's not drinking, but he's hard to take when he's under the influence. He's spoiled innumerable Thanksgivings, Christmases, and other family celebrations with his drunken behavior, which is sometimes angry, sometimes weepy, and always loud. You're going home for the holidays and really feel compelled to say or do something about it, for the sake of both your family and your Uncle Joe. Your mother has always said that he takes after their father and that there's nothing you can do about it. Is it true that you can't influence him? Should you say something to him and, if so, what?

● Your fraternity is doing its usual planning for the Homecoming weekend party, which includes huge quantities of beer, wine, and hard liquor. During past Homecomings, some outrageous things have been done at your house. This year, you've been asked by your college administration to take measures to control your guests. They've specifically asked you to limit the consumption of alcohol. What kinds of things can you do to comply with this request and yet ensure that people have a good time?

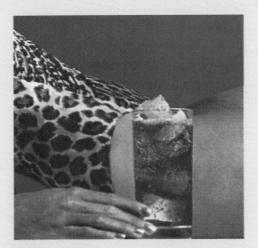

MAKING CONNECTIONS

The use of alcohol pervades our culture. Although personal and social expectations vary, the reality is that virtually everyone, at some point, is faced with a decision about whether, what, or how much to drink. Knowing your options is the best guarantee that you will make the right choice. In each of the alcohol-related scenarios on this page, individuals have to use information, make a decision, or choose a course of action. How would you act in each of these situations? What response or decision would you make? This chapter provides information about alcohol that can be used in situations like these. After finishing the chapter, read the scenarios again. Has what you've learned changed how you would respond?

People long ago recognized the power of alcoholic beverages: The "spirit" changed feelings and behavior. Ever since, **alcohol** has had a somewhat contradictory role in human life. It is associated with good times, cheerfulness, and conviviality, but it is also associated with escape, slow suicide, and self-destructiveness. Many of our slang expressions for **intoxication** reflect its less positive aspects; we say we're "smashed," "bombed," "wasted."

Alcohol is probably the oldest drug in the world. There is evidence that beer and berry wine were used by 6400 B.C., and probably even earlier. Once the **distillation** process was developed (about A.D. 800), the spirit could be concentrated in a purer and more potent form. It was called *al-kuhl,* an Arabic word meaning "finely divided spirit."

Alcohol has been used in religious ceremonies, in feasts and celebrations, and as a medicine for thousands of years. Throughout history, alcohol has been more popular than any other drug in the Western world, despite numerous prohibitions against it. In fact, forbidding the use of alcohol seems only to make it more popular. Even the newer **psychoactive drugs** have not diminished its popularity.

Most of us think of alcohol the way it's portrayed in advertisements, on television, and in movies—as part of good times at the beach, social occasions, and elegant gatherings. Used in moderation, alcohol can enhance social occasions by loosening inhibitions and creating a pleasant feeling of relaxation. For some people, alcohol is an integral part of celebrations and special events. But the use of alcohol can also be an unhealthy adaptation. Like other drugs, alcohol has definite physiological effects on the body that can impair functioning in the short term and cause devastating damage in the long term. For some, alcohol becomes an addiction, leading to a lifetime of recovery or, for a few, to debilitation and death.

Two-thirds of Americans over the age of 15 drink alcohol in some form. If the total amount of alcohol consumed in the United States in a year were evenly divided among drinkers, each would consume the equivalent of 10 gallons of whiskey, 30 gallons of wine, or 90 gallons of beer. But heavy drinkers, who constitute about 10 percent of the American drinking population, account for over half of all the alcohol consumed, as well as a disproportionate amount of the social, economic, and medical costs of alcohol abuse (estimated at $120 billion per year). And through automobile and other accidents, alcohol is the leading cause of death among people between the ages of 15 and 24.

The use of alcohol is a complex issue, one that demands conscious thought and informed decisions. In our society, some people choose to drink in moderation, some choose not to drink at all, and others realize too late that they've made an unwise choice—when they become dependent on alcohol, are involved in an alcohol-related auto crash, or simply wake up to discover they've done something they regret. This chapter discusses the complexities of alcohol use and provides information that will help you make the choice that's right for you.

> *Personal Insight*   How was alcohol used in your family when you were growing up, and what are your associations with it? Was it used for family celebrations? Was there alcohol abuse in your family? If so, how did you react at the time? How do you feel about it now?

THE NATURE OF ALCOHOL

How does alcohol affect people? Does it affect some people differently than others? Can some people "handle" alcohol? Is it possible to drink a safe amount of alcohol? Many of the misconceptions about the effects of alcohol can be cleared up by examining the chemistry of alcohol and how it is absorbed and metabolized by the body.

The Chemistry of Alcohol

Ethyl alcohol is the common psychoactive ingredient in all alcoholic beverages. Beer, a mild intoxicant brewed from a mixture of grains, usually contains between 3 and 6 percent alcohol by volume. Wines are made by **fermenting** the juices of grapes or other fruits. The concentration of alcohol in table wines is about 9 to 14 percent. *Fortified wines*—so named because distilled alcohol has been added to them—contain about 20 percent alcohol; these include sherry, port, and Madeira. Stronger alcoholic beverages, called *hard liquors,* are made by distilling brewed or fermented grains or other products. These beverages, including gin, whiskey, brandy, rum, and liqueurs, usually contain from 35 to 50 percent alcohol.

The concentration of alcohol in a beverage is indicated by the **proof value,** which is two times the percentage

Alcohol   The intoxicating ingredient in fermented liquors. A colorless, pungent liquid.

Intoxication   The state of being mentally affected by a chemical (literally, a state of being poisoned).

Distillation   The process of heating a mixture and recondensing the vapor. This process changes the proportions of the mixture, for example, increasing the percentage of alcohol in the condensed vapor. Distillation is used in manufacturing whiskey and brandy.

Psychoactive drugs   Drugs that affect the brain or nervous system.

Fermented   Describes a substance in which complex molecules have been broken down by the action of yeast or bacteria. Fermentation of certain substances produces alcohol.

Proof value   Two times the percentage of alcohol by volume. A beverage that is 50 percent alcohol by volume is 100 proof.

TERMS

Do you notice that you react differently to alcohol than some of your friends do? If so, you may be noticing genetic differences in alcohol metabolism that are associated with gender or ethnicity. Alcohol is metabolized mainly in the liver, but some alcohol is broken down in the stomach before it can be sent into the bloodstream and on to the liver. Once it's circulating in the bloodstream, alcohol produces the well-known feelings of intoxication. Studies have shown that women metabolize less alcohol in the stomach than men do, so they release more unmetabolized alcohol into the bloodstream. Although the biochemical explanation for this phenomenon is still unknown, the practical implication is that women feel the effect of alcohol sooner and to a greater degree than men do. The same amount of alcohol will have more effect on a woman than on a man.

Other differences in alcohol metabolism are associated with ethnicity. Alcohol is broken down in the liver by an enzyme called alcohol dehydrogenase, producing a by-product called acetaldehyde (see figure). Acetaldehyde is responsible for many of the unpleasant effects of alcohol abuse. Another enzyme, acetaldehyde dehydrogenase, breaks this product down further. Some people, including many of Asian descent, have genetic information that causes them to produce somewhat different forms of the two enzymes that metabolize alcohol. The result is high concentrations of acetaldehyde in the brain and other tissues, producing a host of unpleasant symptoms. When people with these enzymes drink alcohol, they experience a physiological reaction referred to as "flushing syndrome." Their skin feels hot, their heart and respiration rates increase, and they may get a headache, vomit, or break out in hives. Drinking makes them so uncomfortable that it's unlikely they could ever become addicted to alcohol. The body's response to acetaldehyde is the basis for treating alcohol abuse with the drug disulfiram (Antabuse), which inhibits the action of acetaldehyde dehydrogenase. When a person taking disulfiram ingests alcohol, acetaldehyde levels increase rapidly, and he or she develops an intense flushing reaction along with weakness, nausea, vomiting, and other disagreeable symptoms.

How people behave in relation to alcohol is influenced in complex ways by many factors, including social and cultural ones. But in these two cases at least, individual choices and behavior are strongly influenced by a specific genetic/biological characteristic.

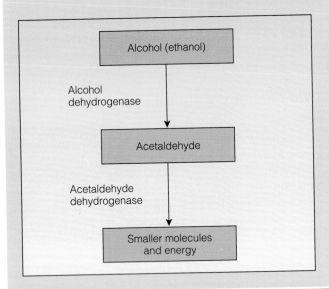

concentration. For example, if a beverage is 100 proof, it contains 50 percent alcohol. Two ounces of 100-proof whiskey contain one ounce of pure alcohol. The proof value of hard liquors can usually be found on the bottle labels. When alcohol consumption is discussed, "one drink" refers to the typical 12-ounce bottle of beer, or to a 5-ounce glass of table wine, or to a cocktail with 1½ ounces of liquor. Each of these different drinks contain approximately the same amount of alcohol—about 0.6 ounces.

There are a number of different kinds of alcohol. In this chapter, the term *alcohol* refers to ethyl alcohol, which is the only kind of alcohol that can be consumed. Other kinds of alcohol such as methanol (wood alcohol) and isopropyl alcohol (rubbing alcohol) are also intoxicating, but they can cause blindness and other serious problems when consumed even in low doses.

Absorption

When a person ingests alcohol, about 20 percent is rapidly absorbed from the stomach into the bloodstream. About 75 percent is absorbed through the upper part of the small intestine. Any remaining alcohol enters the bloodstream further down the gastrointestinal tract. The rate of absorption is affected by a variety of factors. For example, the carbonation in a beverage like champagne increases the rate of alcohol absorption. Food in the stomach slows the rate of absorption, as does the drinking of highly concentrated alcoholic beverages such as hard liquor. Remember, though, *all* alcohol consumed is eventually absorbed.

Metabolism and Excretion

Alcohol is quickly transported throughout the body by

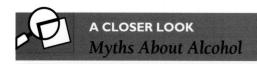

A CLOSER LOOK
Myths About Alcohol

Myth You can speed up the metabolism of alcohol by exercising, drinking coffee or taking other central nervous system stimulants, or by breathing fresh air.

Fact Once alcohol is absorbed, there are no ways of appreciably accelerating its breakdown.

Myth Alcoholics can "handle their alcohol" better than nonalcoholics.

Fact In the early stages of alcoholism, this is sometimes true. However, in later stages of alcoholism, tolerance to alcohol often decreases. In some severe alcoholics, tolerance fluctuates from day to day: on one day a liter of wine has little behavioral effect; on another day, one glass of wine causes intoxication.

Myth When you are under the influence of alcohol, you are so relaxed you are less likely to get hurt in an accident.

Fact Alcohol slows protective reflexes and impairs coordination. People under the influence of alcohol are at much greater risk of injury (and death) from accidents.

Myth Most alcoholics are consciously aware of drinking too much.

Fact Denial—the unconscious psychological process that blocks awareness of reality—is an almost universal charac-

teristic of alcoholics and other drug abusers. There is a clinical adage: "the two hallmarks of alcoholism are drinking too much and denying that you drink too much."

Myth An alcoholic must want help before he or she will respond to it.

Fact Many alcoholics respond to coercive intervention—to save their relationships, their careers, or their driver's licenses—even though they continue to deny their drinking problems.

Myth Only an alcoholic can understand and help another.

Fact Recovering alcoholics do have something unique to offer—a positive, encouraging example. But most of us have experienced and can empathize with the feelings associated with excessive drinking—anxiety, depression, loneliness, remorse.

Myth An alcoholic must "hit bottom" before he or she is ready to stop drinking.

Fact Alcoholics do not have to lose all before they are motivated to stop. People vary markedly in what induces them to change their behavior. For some, the first blackout or alcohol-related automobile crash fosters abstinence.

the blood. Because alcohol easily moves through most biological membranes, it is rapidly distributed throughout most body tissues. The main site of alcohol **metabolism** is the liver, though a small amount of alcohol is metabolized in the stomach. (See the box "Metabolizing Alcohol: Our Bodies Work Differently" for more information.)

About 2 to 10 percent of ingested alcohol is not metabolized in the liver or other tissues, but is excreted unchanged by the lungs, kidneys, and sweat glands. Excreted alcohol causes the telltale smell on a drinker's breath and is the basis of breath and urine analyses for alcohol levels. Such analyses do not give precise measurements of alcohol concentrations in the blood (the measure of intoxication), but they do provide a reasonable approximation if done correctly.

Alcohol Intake and Blood Alcohol Concentration

Blood alcohol concentration (BAC) is determined by the amount of alcohol consumed and by individual factors such as body weight and amount of body fat. In most cases, a smaller person develops a higher BAC than a larger person after drinking the same amount of alcohol. This is because a smaller person has less overall body tissue into which alcohol can be distributed. A person with a higher percentage of body fat will usually develop a

higher BAC than a more muscular person who weighs the same. This is because alcohol does not concentrate as much in fatty tissue as in muscle and most other tissues, in part because fat has fewer blood vessels. Since women generally have a higher percentage of fat at any given weight than men do, they usually have higher BACs after consuming the same amount of alcohol.

BAC also depends on the balance between the rate of alcohol absorption and the rate of alcohol metabolism. A man who weighs 154 pounds and has normal liver function metabolizes about 0.3 to 0.5 ounces of alcohol per hour—the equivalent of slightly less than a 12-ounce bottle of beer or a 5-ounce glass of wine. The rate of alcohol metabolism varies among individuals and is largely determined by genetics. Contrary to popular myths, this metabolic rate cannot be influenced by exercise, breathing deeply, eating, drinking coffee, or taking other drugs. The rate of alcohol metabolism is the same whether a person is asleep or awake (see the box "Myths About Alcohol").

Metabolism The chemical transformation of food and other substances in the body into energy and wastes.

Blood alcohol concentration (BAC) The amount of alcohol in the blood in terms of weight per unit volume.

TERMS

TABLE 10-1 Effects of Alcohol

Blood Alcohol Concentrations (Percent)	Common Behavioral Effects	Hours Required for Alcohol to Be Metabolized
0.00–0.05	Slight change in feelings—usually relaxation and euphoria. Decreased alertness.	2–3
0.05–0.10	Emotional liability with exaggerated feelings and behavior. Reduced social inhibitions. Impairment of reaction time and fine motor coordination. Increasingly impaired during driving. Legally drunk at 0.08 in many states and 0.10 in others.	4–6
0.10–0.15	Unsteadiness in standing and walking. Loss of peripheral vision. Driving is extremely dangerous. Legally drunk at 0.15 in all states.	6–10
0.15–0.30	Staggering gait. Slurred speech. Pain and other sensory perceptions greatly impaired.	10–24
More than 0.30	Stupor or unconsciousness. Anesthesia. Death possible at 0.35 and above.	More than 24

If a person absorbs slightly less alcohol each hour than he or she can metabolize in an hour, the BAC remains low. People can drink large amounts of alcohol this way over a long period of time without becoming noticeably intoxicated; however, they do run the risk of significant long-term health hazards, as described later in this chapter. If a person is absorbing alcohol more quickly than it can be metabolized, the BAC will steadily increase, and he or she will become more and more drunk (Table 10-1).

ALCOHOL AND HEALTH

The effects of alcohol consumption on health depend on the individual, the circumstances, and the amount of alcohol consumed. What are the effects of alcohol on your body? Can drinking be part of a lifestyle devoted to wellness?

Immediate Effects of Alcohol

The BAC is a primary factor determining the effects of alcohol (see Table 10-1). At low concentrations, alcohol tends to make people feel relaxed and jovial, but at higher concentrations people are more likely to feel angry, **sedated,** or sleepy. Alcohol is a **central nervous system (CNS) depressant,** and its effects vary because body systems are affected to different degrees at different BACs.

The effects of alcohol can first be felt at a BAC of about 0.03 to 0.05 percent. These effects may include light-headedness, relaxation, and release of inhibitions. Most drinkers experience mild euphoria and become more sociable. When people drink in social settings, alcohol often seems to act as a **stimulant,** enhancing conviviality or as-

sertiveness. This apparent stimulation occurs because alcohol depresses inhibitory centers in the brain.

At higher concentrations, these pleasant effects tend to be replaced by more negative ones—interference with motor coordination, verbal performance, and intellectual functions. The drinker often becomes irritable and may be easily angered or given to crying. When the BAC reaches 0.1 percent, most sensory and motor functioning is reduced, and many people become sedated, or sleepy. Vision, smell, taste, and hearing become less acute. At 0.2 percent, most drinkers are completely unable to function, either physically or psychologically, because of the pronounced depression of the central nervous system, muscles, and other body systems. Coma usually occurs at a BAC of 0.35 percent, and any higher level can be fatal.

At any given BAC, the effects of alcohol are more pronounced when the BAC is rapidly increasing compared to when the BAC is slowly increasing, level, or decreasing. The effects of alcohol are more pronounced if a person drinks on an empty stomach because alcohol is absorbed more quickly and the BAC rises more quickly. If alcohol is taken with other drugs that depress the central nervous system, the drugs can interact to produce a dangerous degree of central nervous system depression. Antihistamines and sleeping pills are examples of other central nervous system depressants.

Statistics show that being drunk is hazardous to your health. The combination of impaired judgment, weakened sensory perception, reduced inhibitions, impaired motor coordination, and, often, increased aggressiveness and hostility that characterizes alcohol intoxication can be dangerous or even deadly. See the box "The Dangers of Drinking" for some statistics on the increased risks associated with alcohol use.

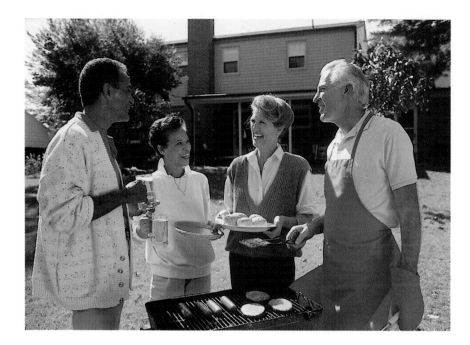

Alcoholic beverages like beer and wine are an integral part of social occasions for many people. A central nervous system depressant, alcohol acts to loosen inhibitions; when used in moderation, it tends to make people feel more relaxed and sociable.

Shakespeare accurately described the effects of alcohol on sexual functioning. He said (in *Macbeth*) that "it stirs up desire, but it takes away the performance." Small doses may improve sexual functioning for individuals who are especially anxious or self-conscious, but higher doses usually have a negative effect. Excessive alcohol use on either an acute or chronic basis can result in reduced erection response and reduced vaginal lubrication.

Alcohol causes blood vessels near the skin to dilate, so drinkers often feel warm; their skin flushes, and they may sweat more. Flushing and sweating contribute to loss of heat, and so the internal body temperature falls. High doses of alcohol may impair the body's ability to regulate temperature, causing it to drop sharply, especially if the surrounding temperature is low. Drinking alcoholic beverages to keep warm in cold weather does not work, and it can even be dangerous.

Alcohol, particularly in large amounts, definitely changes sleep patterns. Alcohol may facilitate falling asleep more quickly, but the sleep is often light, punctuated with awakenings, and unrefreshing. Even after the habitual drinker stops drinking, his or her sleep may be altered for weeks or months. Users of alcohol frequently awaken with a "hangover"—headache, nausea, stomach distress, and generalized discomfort.

Personal Insight Have you ever said or done anything while under the influence of alcohol that you regretted later? If so, how did you deal with the consequences? Did you change your behavior so it didn't happen again?

Drinking and Driving

Drunk driving continues to be one of the most serious public health and safety problems in the United States. Every year, about 500,000 people are injured in alcohol-related automobile crashes—an average of one person injured every minute. Over half of the more than 40,000 traffic crash fatalities each year are alcohol-related.

Figure 10-1 illustrates the results of a study of the relationship between drinking and driving. There is a **dose-response relationship** between the amount of alcohol consumed and the risk of auto accidents—higher doses of alcohol are associated with a much greater probability of accidents. The estimated number of drinks is shown on the bottom axis of Figure 10-1, and the approximate BAC associated with that number of drinks is shown on the top axis. For the purposes of the graph, the drinker is assumed to be a man of about 150 pounds, and the drinking takes place in one hour. (As explained earlier, it takes more drinks to achieve a given BAC if a person weighs more, if he or she has eaten recently, or if the drinking is done more slowly; it takes less time for a woman to achieve a given BAC.) The vertical axis represents how

Sedate To calm by the use of a drug that quiets the activity of the nerves.

Central nervous system depressant Any chemical that affects the brain or spinal cord and decreases nervous or muscular activity.

Stimulant Something that increases nervous or muscular activity.

Dose-response relationship The relationship between the amount of a drug taken and the intensity or type of drug effect.

TERMS

- Drunk drivers as a group are eight times more likely to be involved in a fatal crash than are sober drivers.

- Alcohol use more than triples the chances of fatal accidents during leisure activities such as swimming or boating.

- 69 percent of drowning deaths are alcohol-related.

- Alcohol is involved in up to 50 percent of all fatal falls.

- 35 percent of suicide victims between the ages of 15 and 34 have been drinking.

- Alcohol is related to increased risk of death in a fire.

- Over 50 percent of the perpetrators of murder, assault, and rape were drinking before the crime.

- Alcohol is especially common in "victim-precipitated homicides," in which the eventual victim strikes the first blow.

- Through homicide, automobile crashes, and other incidents, alcohol is the fourth leading killer in the United States. For people aged 15 to 24, it is the leading cause of death.

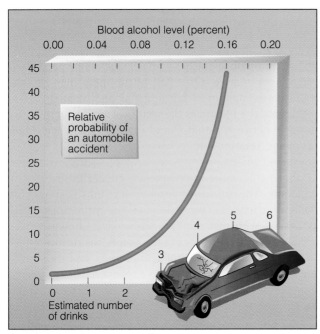

VITAL STATISTICS
Figure 10-1 *The dose-response relationship of alcohol levels and automobile crashes.*

In addition to increased risk of injury and death, driving while intoxicated can have serious legal consequences. Drunk driving is against the law. The legal limit for BAC is 0.10 percent or lower in nearly all states. There are stiff penalties for driving while drunk, and many cities have set up checkpoints where drivers are stopped and checked for intoxication.

Even low doses of alcohol increase the risk of an automobile crash somewhat, especially in crowded conditions; but as the dose increases, the risk increases at a spectacular rate. The number of drinks it takes the average person to reach the legal BAC limit is shown in Figure 10-2. Remember that these amounts are approximate, since BACs vary depending on many factors, including gender. While you can do something about your own drinking, it's harder to protect yourself against someone else; the box "Protecting Yourself on the Road" gives some hints.

Effects of Chronic Use

Because alcohol is distributed throughout most of the body, it can affect many different organs and tissues (Figure 10-3). Problems associated with chronic use of alcohol include diseases of the digestive and cardiovascular systems and some cancers. Drinking during pregnancy risks the health of both the woman and the developing fetus.

Digestive System Even in relatively small amounts, alcohol can alter liver function. With continued use of al-

likely the drinker is to have an automobile accident compared to a sober driver. In other words, a man driving with a BAC of 0.10 percent is about 10 times more likely to be involved in an accident than someone with no alcohol in his or her blood.

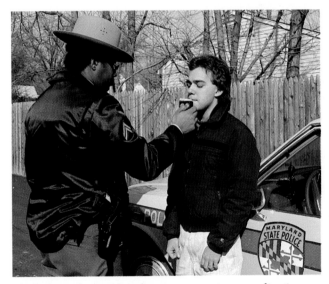

BAC Zones:	90–109 lbs.	110–129 lbs.	130–149 lbs.	150–169 lbs.	170–189 lbs.	190–209 lbs.	210 lbs. & Up
TIME FROM 1st DRINK	TOTAL DRINKS 1 2 3 4 5 6 7 8	TOTAL DRINKS 1 2 3 4 5 6 7 8	TOTAL DRINKS 1 2 3 4 5 6 7 8	TOTAL DRINKS 1 2 3 4 5 6 7 8	TOTAL DRINKS 1 2 3 4 5 6 7 8	TOTAL DRINKS 1 2 3 4 5 6 7 8	TOTAL DRINKS 1 2 3 4 5 6 7 8
1 hr							
2 hrs							
3 hrs							
4 hrs							

■ (0.01%–0.04%) Sometimes impaired   ■ (0.05%–0.07%) Usually impaired   ■ (0.08% and up) Always impaired

Figure 10-2 *Approximate blood alcohol concentration and body weight.*
A BAC of 0.08 is considered legally drunk in some states and a BAC of 0.10 is considered legally drunk in most others. However, alcohol impairs the user at much lower BACs. This chart illustrates the BAC an average person of a given weight would reach after drinking the specified number of drinks in the time given.
Source: California Department of Motor Vehicles.

cohol, liver cells are damaged and then progressively destroyed. The destroyed cells are often replaced by fibrous scar tissue, a condition known as **cirrhosis of the liver.** As cirrhosis develops, a drinker may gradually lose his or her capacity to tolerate alcohol, because there are fewer and fewer healthy cells remaining in the liver to metabolize it. Alcohol-precipitated cirrhosis is a major cause of death in the United States.

As with most health hazards, the risk of cirrhosis depends on an individual's susceptibility—largely determined by genetics—as well as the amount of alcohol consumed over time. Some people show signs of cirrhosis after a few years of consuming three or four drinks per day. Early signs of cirrhosis include jaundice—a yellowing of the skin and white part of the eyes—and the accumulation of fluid in the abdomen and lower extremities. Treatment for cirrhosis includes a balanced diet and complete abstinence from alcohol.

Alcohol can also inflame the pancreas, causing nausea, vomiting, abnormal digestion, and severe abdominal pain. Irritation of the stomach lining by alcohol can cause bleeding and contribute to the formation of ulcers.

Cardiovascular System The effects of alcohol on the cardiovascular system depend on the amount of alcohol consumed. Moderate doses of alcohol—one or two drinks a day—may reduce slightly the chances of heart attack in some people. The reasons for this finding are poorly understood, but it may be that moderate amounts of alcohol increase blood levels of **high-density lipoproteins (HDLs).** Red wines may also include a chemical that inhibits blood clotting.

Alcohol interferes with judgment, perception, coordination, and other areas of mental and physical functioning and is a factor in a majority of all fatal automobile crashes. This driver is lucky that he was stopped by a suspicious police officer before a crash occurred. He is being given a breathalyzer test to determine his blood alcohol concentration.

Cirrhosis of the liver A disease caused by excessive and chronic drinking in which liver cells are destroyed and replaced by fibrous scar tissue.
High-density lipoprotein (HDL) Waxy substance in the blood thought to protect against heart disease.

TERMS

Social drinkers and alcoholics alike are a menace behind the wheel. One-half of all traffic fatalities are associated with alcohol use, and one-third of all alcohol-related traffic accidents involve drivers between the ages of 16 and 24. People who drink and drive are unable to drive responsibly because their judgment is impaired, their reaction time is slower, and their coordination is reduced. No one can drive skillfully and safely when under the influence of alcohol.

What can you do to protect yourself from alcohol-related accidents on the road? If you are out of your home and drinking, follow the practice of having a "designated driver," an individual who refrains from drinking in order to provide safe transportation home for others in the group. The responsibility is rotated, so different people take the role of designated drivers on different occasions. In Sweden and the United Kingdom, where the practice originated, designated drivers place their car keys in their empty beverage glasses so they are not served. In the United States, designated drivers sometimes wear a special button to indicate their role for that evening.

Of course, even if you follow safe practices, you may encounter a drunk driver on the road. To reduce your chances of being involved in a crash caused by someone else, learn to be alert to the erratic driving that signals an impaired driver. Warning signs include the following:

- Unusually wide turns
- Straddling the center line or lane marker
- Driving with one's head out of the window or with the window down in cold weather
- Nearly striking an object or another vehicle
- Weaving or swerving
- Driving on other than the designated roadway

- Stopping with no apparent cause
- Following too closely
- Responding slowly to traffic signals
- Abrupt or illegal turns
- Rapid acceleration or deceleration
- Driving with headlights off at night

If you see any of these warning signs, what should you do?

- If the driver is ahead of you, maintain a safe following distance. Do not try to pass, because the driver may swerve into your car.
- If the driver is behind you, turn right at the nearest intersection. Let the driver pass and then return to your route.
- If the driver is approaching your car, move to the shoulder and stop. Avoid a head-on collision by sounding your horn or flashing your lights.
- When approaching an intersection, slow down and expect the unexpected.
- Make sure your seat belt is fastened, children are in approved safety seats, and keep your doors locked.
- Report suspected impaired drivers to the nearest law enforcement agency by phone. Give a description of the vehicle, license number, location, and direction the vehicle is headed.

Don't become a statistic. Be alert, don't drink and drive, and use a designated driver to make sure you come home alive and safe.

Adapted from "The Designated Driver: Being a Friend." *Healthline,* December 1986.

Higher doses of alcohol have harmful effects. In some people, more than two drinks a day will elevate blood pressure, making strokes and heart attacks more likely. Some alcoholics show weakening of the heart muscle, a condition known as **cardiac myopathy.** Cardiac myopathy can be caused by the direct toxic effects of alcohol, or indirectly by the malnutrition and vitamin deficiencies that many alcoholics experience from their poor diets and gastrointestinal disturbances. Although the relationships between alcohol and cardiovascular disease are multiple and complex, it is clear that excessive drinking increases the risk of disease. These health risks progressively increase as the amount of excessive drinking increases.

Mortality An ancient proverb states "Those who worship Bacchus [the god of wine] die young." Modern research supports that statement. In addition to increasing the risk of injury and death as detailed in the box "The Dangers of Drinking," alcohol is associated with early death from cancer. Alcoholics have a cancer rate that is about 10 times higher than would be expected in the general population. They are particularly vulnerable to cancers of the throat, larynx, esophagus, upper stomach, liver, and pancreas. Women who abuse alcohol are at increased risk for breast cancer. Altogether, alcoholics have life spans that are 10 to 12 years shorter than those of nonalcoholics.

Fetal Alcohol Syndrome Studies of animals and humans indicate that alcohol ingested during pregnancy can harm the fetus. Alcohol and its metabolic product acetaldehyde quickly cross the placenta. As with many drug

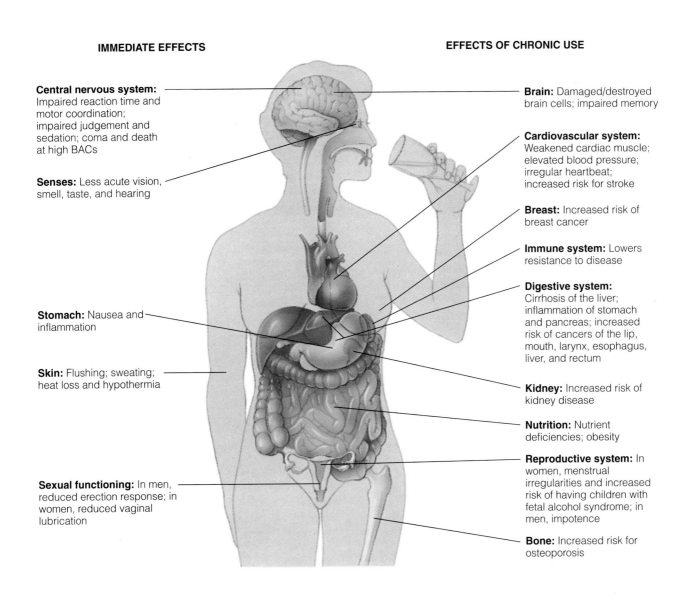

IMMEDIATE EFFECTS

Central nervous system: Impaired reaction time and motor coordination; impaired judgement and sedation; coma and death at high BACs

Senses: Less acute vision, smell, taste, and hearing

Stomach: Nausea and inflammation

Skin: Flushing; sweating; heat loss and hypothermia

Sexual functioning: In men, reduced erection response; in women, reduced vaginal lubrication

EFFECTS OF CHRONIC USE

Brain: Damaged/destroyed brain cells; impaired memory

Cardiovascular system: Weakened cardiac muscle; elevated blood pressure; irregular heartbeat; increased risk for stroke

Breast: Increased risk of breast cancer

Immune system: Lowers resistance to disease

Digestive system: Cirrhosis of the liver; inflammation of stomach and pancreas; increased risk of cancers of the lip, mouth, larynx, esophagus, liver, and rectum

Kidney: Increased risk of kidney disease

Nutrition: Nutrient deficiencies; obesity

Reproductive system: In women, menstrual irregularities and increased risk of having children with fetal alcohol syndrome; in men, impotence

Bone: Increased risk for osteoporosis

Figure 10-3 *Immediate and long-term effects of alcohol use.*

hazards, the effects of alcohol on the fetus are dose-related. Below-normal birth weights occur when pregnant mothers consume as few as two alcoholic drinks a day. With heavier drinking, a collection of birth defects known as the **fetal alcohol syndrome** becomes increasingly likely. These children have a characteristic mixture of deformities that include small teeth with faulty enamel; irregular ear lobes; small, wide-set eyes and other facial deformities. They are usually small and may have heart defects. Even with the best of care, their physical and mental growth rate is slower than normal during childhood. In adolescence they sometimes catch up with their age mates in terms of physical size, but not usually in mental abilities. Most remain mentally retarded with IQs in the 40 to 80 range (normal is 90–110). Fetal alcohol ef-

fects also include more subtle changes in fine motor coordination and learning problems.

Although researchers initially thought that fetal alcohol syndrome was caused by poor nutrition associated with the alcoholism of the mother, subsequent research indicates that it results directly from excessive alcohol intake. There is no precise blood alcohol threshold level

Cardiac myopathy Weakening of the heart muscle through disease.

Fetal alcohol syndrome A characteristic group of birth defects caused by excessive alcohol consumption by the mother, including facial deformities, heart defects, and physical and mental impairments.

TERMS

above which damage occurs and below which there is no danger. Instead, the frequency and severity of defects progressively increase as the amount of drinking increases. Exposing the fetus to alcohol or other drugs during the first 12 or 13 weeks of pregnancy is particularly hazardous because, during this time, the critical formation of the central nervous system, heart, and other organs occurs. As discussed in Chapter 8, the safest course of action is abstinence. Occasionally, newly born babies of alcoholic mothers show withdrawal reactions. These withdrawal problems are similar to those experienced by older individuals.

Any alcohol consumed by a nursing mother quickly enters the breast milk. What impact this has on the child or the mother's milk production is a matter of controversy. Dosage may again be the key issue. Some pediatricians argue that very small amounts of alcohol—half a glass of wine—may provide some useful relaxation to mother and child, but that large amounts are too sedating and may interfere with subsequent child development.

Medical Uses and Possible Health Benefits of Alcohol

Alcohol can be effective for some medical purposes. Alcohol sponges are commonly used to reduce fever because alcohol cools the skin by evaporation. In concentrations of 70 percent by weight, alcohol kills bacteria. It is used as an astringent and skin cleanser in treating skin disorders. The type of alcohol used for these medicinal purposes, however, is not ethyl alcohol—the kind in beverages—but isopropyl alcohol or another form of denatured alcohol. Contrary to popular myth, no kind of alcohol is a good antiseptic for open wounds. All kinds of alcohol injure exposed tissue and may form a coagulant that protects rather than destroys bacteria. The best course of action is just to cleanse the wound with water and soap and try to keep it clean while seeking medical attention.

People who associate alcohol with dining pleasure may feel hungrier and digest their food better if they take a small amount of alcohol—a glass of beer or wine—with their meals. Drinking alcohol has been thought by some to be useful in treating angina pectoris, a painful disorder in which the heart is unable to get enough oxygen. Most physicians feel that there are much more effective drugs for this condition, and any beneficial effect of alcohol is due to sedation rather than improvement in blood circulation.

Relationships between alcohol use and mortality rates are complex. As one would predict, both abstainers and moderate drinkers live longer than heavy drinkers. Some recent studies also suggest that people who regularly drink moderate amounts of alcohol—fewer than three drinks per day—live longer than those who abstain completely. As noted earlier, one or two drinks a day—but not more—may reduce the risks of heart attack somewhat.

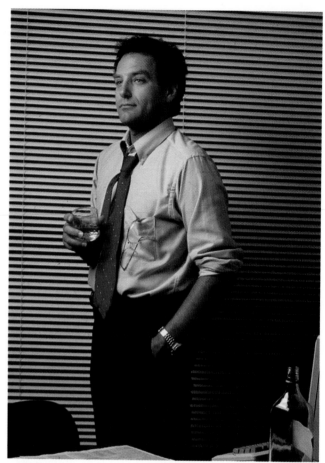

Drinking alone during the day is a sign of alcohol abuse. Although alcohol may seem to provide temporary relief from uncomfortable feelings, it offers no actual solutions to personal problems.

MISUSE OF ALCOHOL

Addiction to alcohol—like addiction to tobacco and other psychoactive drugs—affects more than just the user. Alcoholics can wreak havoc within a family, and children are often those most severely affected. But alcohol can be abused even when there's no true addiction; even though the rate is falling, too many victims of car crashes are actually victims of weekend drinkers.

Alcohol Abuse

Recent definitions make a distinction between alcohol abuse and alcohol dependence, or alcoholism. According to the third edition (revised) of the *Diagnostic and Statistical Manual of Mental Disorders* (1987) of the American Psychiatric Association, **alcohol abuse** involves either (1) continued use of alcohol despite knowledge of having a persistent or recurrent social, occupational, psychological, or physical problem that is caused by or exacerbated by use of alcohol, or (2) recurrent use of alcohol in situations when use is physically hazardous (such as driving

When You're the Guest

- Let your waistline be your incentive. For the same 215 calories in two 7-ounce gin and tonics, you can have a nutritious snack.

- At a restaurant, order the food first, not a drink. Then if you want a drink you'll probably have time for only one before the meal is served.

- Avoid drinks made with carbonated mixers, especially if you're thirsty. You'll gulp them down.

- Remember that the pressure to have a drink may often be in your imagination. It is becoming more and more acceptable to say "no thanks" to alcohol.

When You're the Host

- Have plenty of nonalcoholic beverages on hand and make sure they are as accessible and as attractive as the alcoholic drinks.

- If it's a dinner party, try to serve dinner on schedule, before there's time for a second drink.

- Experiment with various juices and beverages until you come up with an alcohol-free concoction all your own. Or stick to traditional punches and blends, but leave out the alcohol.

Adapted from *University of California at Berkeley Wellness Letter,* April 1987.

---

while intoxicated). The term **alcohol dependence,** which is also called **alcoholism,** refers to more extensive problems with alcohol use, usually involving tolerance or withdrawal.

Other authorities use different definitions to describe problems associated with drinking. The important point is that one does not have to be an alcoholic to have problems with alcohol. The person who drinks only once a month, perhaps after an exam, but then drives while intoxicated is an alcohol abuser.

How can you tell if you are beginning to abuse alcohol or if someone you know is doing so? Look for the following warning signs:

1. Drinking alone or secretively.

2. Using alcohol deliberately and repeatedly to perform or get through difficult situations.

3. Feeling uncomfortable on certain occasions when alcohol is not available.

4. Escalating alcohol consumption beyond an already established drinking pattern.

5. Consuming alcohol heavily in risky situations; for example, before driving.

6. Getting drunk regularly or more frequently than in the past.

7. Drinking in the morning or at other unusual times.

The box "Keeping Social Drinking Social" gives some hints to help cut back on drinking.

Alcoholism

Alcoholism, or alcohol dependency, is similar to nicotine dependency (described in Chapter 9) in its being usually characterized by tolerance to alcohol and withdrawal. Everyone who drinks—even nonalcoholics—develops tolerance to alcohol after repeated use. **Tolerance** means that a drinker needs more alcohol to achieve intoxication or the desired effect, that the effects of continued use of the same amount of alcohol are diminished, or that the drinker can function adequately at doses or blood levels of alcohol that would produce significant impairment in a casual user. Heavy users of alcohol may need to consume about 50 percent more than they originally needed to experience the same degree of intoxication. In addition to these examples of *acquired* tolerance, people vary considerably in their *inborn* tolerance, the amount of alcohol they can tolerate independent of their drinking experience. Inborn tolerance depends both on people's individual abilities to metabolize alcohol and on inherent differences in the sensitivity of their tissues to alcohol.

Withdrawal from alcohol occurs when someone who has been using alcohol heavily for several days or more suddenly stops drinking or markedly reduces intake of alcohol. Symptoms of withdrawal can include trembling hands, sweating, and weakness.

Alcohol abuse   The use of alcohol to a degree that causes physical damage, impairs functioning, or results in behavior harmful to others.

Alcohol dependence   Either pathological use of alcohol or impairment in functioning due to alcohol and tolerance or withdrawal; alcoholism.

Alcoholism   Chronic psychological and nutritional disorder from excessive and compulsive drinking; alcohol dependence.

Tolerance   Lower sensitivity to a drug so that a given dose no longer exerts the usual effect and larger doses are needed.

Withdrawal   Unpleasant physical and mental sensations experienced when abstaining from a drug to which one is addicted.

TERMS

Alcohol abusers come from all socioeconomic classes and cultural groups, but there are notable differences in patterns of drinking among various racial and ethnic groups.

African Americans

Alcohol abuse is a serious problem for African Americans. Blacks face disproportionately high levels of alcohol-related birth defects, cirrhosis, cancer, hypertension, and other medical problems. In addition, blacks are more likely than members of other ethnic groups to be victims of alcohol-related homicides, criminal assaults, and accidents. Black women are more likely to abstain from alcohol use than are white women; but among black women who drink, there is a higher percentage of heavy drinkers. Urban black males commonly start drinking excessively and develop serious neurological illnesses at an earlier age than do urban white males. They also have a higher rate of alcoholism-related suicide.

AA groups comprising predominantly African Americans have been shown to provide effective treatment, perhaps because essential elements of AA—sharing common experiences, mutual acceptance of one another as human beings, and trusting a higher power—are already a part of African American culture. Treatment efforts that utilize the extended family and include occupational training are also especially effective.

Hispanic Americans

Hispanic American men have rates of alcohol abuse higher than the national average. Deaths and injuries from drunk driving and cirrhosis are particular problems. Hispanic women are more likely to abstain from alcohol than are white or black women, but those who do drink are at special risk for problems. Treating the entire family as a unit is an important part of treatment because family pride, solidarity, and support are important aspects of Latino culture. Some Hispanics do better during treatment if treatment efforts are integrated with the techniques of curanderos (folk healers) and espiritistas (spiritists).

Asian Americans

As a group, Asian Americans and Pacific Islanders have lower-than-average rates of alcohol abuse. However, acculturation may weaken somewhat the generally strong Asian taboos and community sanctions against alcohol use. For many Asian Americans, though, the genetically based physiologic aversion to alcohol remains a deterrent to abuse. For those needing treatment, ethnic agencies, health professionals, and ministers seem to be the most effective sources.

Native Americans and Alaskan Natives

Alcohol abuse is one of the most widespread and severe health problems among Native Americans and Alaskan Natives, especially for adolescents and young adults. Excessive drinking varies from tribe to tribe but is generally high among both men and women. The rate of alcoholism among Native Americans is twice that of the general population, and the death rate from alcohol-related causes is about eight times higher. Treatment efforts should reflect the value the Native American culture places on noninterference in the lives of others, which runs contrary to the Anglo-American tendency to bring aid in the form of counseling and advice to those with problems. Treatment efforts that emphasize maintaining sobriety so that the individual can contribute to family, community, and tribe are generally more effective than confrontational techniques or AA-type methods that stress public disclosure of alcohol problems.

Patterns and Prevalence Alcoholism is found among people of all races, ethnic groups, and socioeconomic classes (see the box "Alcohol Abuse and Treatment: Variations Among Different Populations"). The stereotype of the alcoholic skid row bum actually accounts for less than 5 percent of all alcohol-dependent people—and usually represents the final stage of a drinking career that began years earlier. There are different patterns of alcohol dependence, including these four common ones:

1. *Regular daily intake of large amounts.* This continuous pattern is the most common adult pattern of excessive consumption in most countries.

2. *Regular heavy drinking limited to weekends.* This continuous pattern is often followed by teenagers and college students.

3. *Long periods of sobriety interspersed with binges of daily heavy drinking lasting for weeks or months.* This episodic or "bender" pattern is common in the United States but quite uncommon in France, although the per capita consumption of alcohol is higher in France.

4. *Heavy drinking limited to periods of stress.* This "reactive" pattern is associated with periods of anxiety or depression; for example, at times of test or other performance fears, interpersonal problems, school or work pressures.

Among white American men, excessive drinking often begins in the teens or twenties and progresses gradually through the thirties until the individual is clearly identifiable as an alcoholic by the time he is in his late thirties or early forties. Other men remain controlled drinkers until later in life, sometimes becoming alcoholic in association with retirement, the inevitable losses of aging, boredom, illness, or psychiatric disturbances.

The progression of alcoholism in women is usually different. Women tend to become alcoholic at a later age and with fewer years of heavy drinking. It is not unusual for women in their forties or fifties to become alcoholic after years of controlled drinking. Women alcoholics develop cirrhosis and other medical complications somewhat more often than men. Some authorities feel that women alcoholics suffer more medical problems because they are less likely to seek early treatment, in part because of the strong stigma placed on women who abuse alcohol. In addition, there may be an inherently greater biological risk for women who drink because, as discussed earlier, they have a smaller tissue mass in which alcohol is distributed and they metabolize alcohol more slowly than men.

Primary alcoholism, which accounts for about 80 percent of all alcoholism and is the focus of this chapter, develops in people who show no prior evidence of major psychiatric problems such as schizophrenia and depression. About 20 percent of alcoholics do not show signs of alcoholism until after they develop psychiatric symptoms. Their excessive use of alcohol may represent an attempt at self-medication for anxiety, hallucinations, or other psychiatric symptoms.

Once established, primary alcoholism often exhibits a pattern of exacerbations and remissions. The alcoholic may stop drinking and abstain from alcohol for days or months after a frightening problem develops. After a period of abstinence, an alcoholic often attempts controlled drinking, which almost inevitably leads to an escalation in drinking and more problems. Alcoholism is not hopeless, however; many alcoholics do achieve permanent abstinence.

Estimating the prevalence of alcoholism in the United States is complicated by disagreements about definition and other methodological problems. In 1992 the National Council on Alcoholism reported that 13 million Americans were alcoholics. Studies of smaller geographic areas such as counties or states suggest that the lifetime risk for primary alcoholism in the United States is about 10 percent for men and about 3 percent for women. The risk for women has been increasing in recent years as women's roles in our society have expanded.

Causes of Alcoholism   The precise causes of alcoholism are unknown, but a variety of factors is probably involved. Recent studies of twins and adopted children clearly demonstrate the importance of genetics. If one of a pair of fraternal twins is alcoholic, then the other has about twice the chance of the general population of becoming alcoholic. For the identical twin of an alcoholic, the risk of alcoholism is about four times that of the general population. These risks persist even when the twins

have little contact with each other or their biological parents. Similarly, adoption studies show an increased risk for children of alcoholics even if they were adopted away at birth into nondrinking families and raised without knowing about the problems of their biological parents. Alcoholism in adoptive parents, on the other hand, does not make individuals either more or less likely to become alcoholics. Some studies suggest that as much as 50 percent of a person's risk for alcoholism is determined by genetic factors.

Not all children of alcoholics become alcoholic, however, and it is clear that other factors are involved. A person's risk of developing alcoholism may be increased by certain personality disorders, having been subjected as a child to destructive child-rearing practices, and imitating the alcohol abuse of peers and other role models. People who begin drinking excessively in their teens are especially prone to alcoholism later in life. Common psychological features of individuals who abuse alcohol are denial ("I don't have a problem") and rationalization ("I drink because I need to socialize with my customers"). Certain social factors have also been linked with alcoholism, including urbanization, disappearance of the extended family, general loosening of kinship ties, increased mobility, and changing religious and philosophical values.

Health Effects of Alcoholism   The main characteristics of alcoholism—tolerance and withdrawal—can have a severe impact on health. An alcoholic requires greater and greater amounts to produce the same psychological effect, and these larger doses increase the chances of adverse physical effects. When alcoholics stop drinking or sharply decrease their intake, they have withdrawal symptoms. The jitters, or "shakes," are the most common withdrawal symptom and may continue for as long as two weeks. Seizures, or "rum fits," are less common, but are more serious. Still less common is the severe withdrawal reaction known as the **DTs (delirium tremens)**, a medical emergency characterized by disorientation, confusion, and vivid **hallucinations**, often of vermin and small animals. The mortality rate from DTs may be as high as 15 percent.

Because alcohol is distributed throughout the body's organs and tissues, alcoholism takes a heavy physical and psychological toll. Alcoholics face all the physical health risks associated with intoxication and chronic drinking that were described earlier in the chapter. Some of the

DTs (delirium tremens)   A state of confusion brought on by reduction of alcohol intake in a person addicted to alcohol. Other symptoms are sweating, trembling, anxiety, and hallucinations.

Hallucinations   False perceptions that do not correspond to external reality. A person who hears voices that are not there or who sees visions is having hallucinations.

TERMS

One out of eight Americans—about 30 million people—grow up in alcoholic households, according to the Children of Alcoholics Foundation. For these children, life is a struggle to deal with constant stress, anxiety, and embarrassment. Family life centers on the drinking parent, and children's needs are often ignored.

Children in alcoholic households often adapt to their situation by learning patterns of interaction and methods of coping that help them survive childhood but that don't support their own healthy development. They may be victims of violence, abuse, neglect, or incest in the home, all of which contribute to long-lasting emotional scars. When they grow up, children of alcoholics are more likely to become alcoholic and to marry an alcoholic than is the general population. They are also more likely to abuse other drugs and develop an eating disorder.

Until recently, children of alcoholics were considered no different from other children with family difficulties and were largely ignored by treatment programs, which tended to focus on the alcoholic parent. But today, professionals recognize the special problems and needs of children of alcoholics, and family-oriented therapy has become a major focus of alcoholism rehabilitation.

If you are the child of an alcoholic, be aware, first, that you are not alone. Millions of people across the country have been through the same problem and have dreamed of having a happy family life in which drinking is not an issue. Realize, too, that other people can understand what you have been through and can help. Find a person you can trust—perhaps a teacher, a friend, a member of the clergy—and confide in him or her. It may seem safer to keep your feelings secret, but talking about the problem is the first step toward a healthy readjustment. Finally, acknowledge that your parent's alcoholism is not your fault. Many children of alcoholics carry a burden of guilt from early childhood, when they could not understand that they weren't the cause of their parent's behavior. This unexamined assumption causes part of the emotional pain experienced by children of alcoholics.

Several support groups exist for children of alcoholics. To get help for yourself or someone you know, call one of the local Al-Anon or AlaTeen agencies listed in your telephone book. You can also write the Children of Alcoholics Foundation at 540 Madison Avenue, New York, NY 10022.

---

damage is worsened by nutritional deficiencies that often accompany alcoholism. Some people develop alcoholic **paranoia**, characterized by delusions, jealousy, suspicion, and mistrust. Other psychiatric problems associated with alcoholism include profound memory gaps (amnesia), which are sometimes filled by conscious or unconscious lying (confabulation).

The specific health effects of alcoholism tend to vary from person to person. One individual may suffer primarily from problems with memory and defects of the central nervous system while having no liver or gastrointestinal problems. Another alcoholic with a similar drinking and nutritional history may have advanced liver disease but no memory defects.

Social and Psychological Effects Alcohol use causes more serious social and psychological problems than all other forms of drug abuse combined. For every person who is an alcoholic, another three or four people are directly affected. In a 1989 Gallup poll, 20 percent of Americans said that drinking had been a cause of trouble in their family (see the box "Children of Alcoholics: The Struggle to Recover").

An estimated 4 million 14- to 17-year-olds show signs of potential alcohol dependency. These numbers are far greater than those associated with cocaine, heroin, or marijuana use. The social and psychological consequences of excessive drinking in young people are more difficult to measure than the risks to physical health. One of the consequences is that excessive drinking interferes with learning the interpersonal and work skills that are required for adult life. Excessive drinkers sometimes narrow their circle of friends to other heavy drinkers and thus limit the range of people they can learn from. Perhaps most important is that people who were excessive drinkers in college are more likely to have social, occupational, and health problems 20 years later. (For more information about college drinking, refer to the box "Facts About Drinking Among College Students.") Despite media attention to cocaine and other chemicals, alcohol remains our society's number one drug problem.

Treatment Some alcoholics recover without professional help. How often this occurs is unknown, but perhaps as many as 25 percent of alcoholics stop drinking on their own or reduce their drinking enough to eliminate problems. Often these spontaneous recoveries are linked

TERMS

Paranoia A mental disorder characterized by persistent delusions—fixed, false beliefs that would not be accepted by the individual's culture. Hallucinations, if any, are not prominent and intelligence is not impaired.

Facts About Drinking Among College Students

The Scope of College Drinking

- Approximately 9 out of 10 college students drink alcohol. About three-quarters of all college students consume alcohol every month. Four percent drink every day.

- College students drink less on a daily basis than their noncollege peers, but they are more likely to "binge" drink. About 40 percent of American college students engage in a bout of heavy drinking (five or more drinks in a row) at least once every two weeks. This pattern indicates that students are more likely to confine their drinking to weekends, but then to drink heavily.

- More than twice as many male students as female students drink daily. On average, fraternity members drink greater quantities than do other college students, drink more frequently, and drink more heavily.

- The average yearly consumption of alcoholic beverages per student is over 34 gallons. Beer is the most commonly consumed beverage; as a group, American college students consume almost 4 billion cans of beer each year.

- Different studies indicate that between 53 and 84 percent of students get drunk at least once a year; between 26 and 48 percent get drunk each month.

- In the last decade, there has been a small but significant downward trend in the prevalence of alcohol use.

The Consequences of College Drinking

- A 1991 survey indicated that approximately 40 percent of students' academic problems and 28 percent of dropouts were related to alcohol use. Over 7 percent of first-year students drop out of college for alcohol-related reasons.

- Students with high academic standing drink less in almost all contexts than do their peers with low academic standing. There is a negative relationship between college grades and the amount of alcohol consumed.

- Surveys indicate that alcohol is involved in about 68 percent of the violent behavior and 52 percent of the physical injuries that occur on campuses. College students are particularly vulnerable to other risks that alcohol exacerbates, such as suicide, automobile crashes, and falls.

- Drinking alcohol increases the risk that a college student will commit a crime and also makes it more likely that he or she will be a crime victim.

- Surveys indicate that one-half to two-thirds of undergraduates have driven while intoxicated or have been a passenger in a car when the driver was intoxicated.

- Of the college students currently enrolled in the United States, approximately the same number will eventually die from alcohol-related causes as will get master's degrees and doctorates combined.

Adapted from L. D. Eigen. 1991. *Alcohol Practices, Policies, and Potentials of American Colleges and Universities: An Office for Substance Abuse Prevention White Paper.* Washington, D.C.: U.S. Department of Health and Human Services, September.

---

to an alcohol-related crisis, such as a health problem or the threat of being fired.

Most alcoholics, however, require a treatment program of some kind in order to stop drinking. Many different kinds of programs exist. No one treatment works for everyone, so a person may have to try different programs before finding the right one. Over 1 million Americans enter treatment for alcoholism every year.

Although not all alcoholics can be successfully treated, considerable optimism has replaced the older view that nothing could be done. One encouraging note is that many alcoholics have patterns of drinking that fluctuate widely over time. These fluctuations indicate that their alcohol abuse is a response to environmental factors, such as life stressors or social pressures, and therefore may be influenced by treatment.

One of the oldest and best-known recovery programs is Alcoholics Anonymous. AA consists of self-help groups that meet weekly in most communities and follow a "twelve step" program. Important steps for people in these programs include recognizing that they are "powerless over alcohol" and must seek help from a "higher power" in order to regain control of their lives. By verbalizing these steps, the alcoholic directly addresses the denial that is often prominent in alcoholism and other addictions. Many AA members have a "sponsor" of their choosing who is available by phone 24 hours a day for individual support and crisis intervention. AA convincingly shows the alcoholic that abstinence can be achieved and also provides a sober peer group of people who share the same identity—that of "recovering alcoholics."

A companion program to AA is Al-Anon, which consists of groups for families and friends of alcoholics. In Al-Anon spouses and others explore how they "enabled" the alcoholic to drink by denying, rationalizing, or covering up his or her drinking and how they can change this "codependent" behavior. Other self-help programs exist as well. Some of them, like Rational Recovery, Secular Organizations for Sobriety, and Women for Sobriety, deliberately avoid any emphasis on higher spiritual powers.

Employee assistance programs and school-based programs represent another approach to alcoholism treatment that works for some people. One of the advantages of these programs is that they can deal directly with work and campus issues—often important sources of stress for the alcohol abuser. In these programs there might be an emphasis on distinguishing internal and external sources of distress. If the person is stressed by self-imposed performance standards, the focus might be on learning relaxation of self-reinforcement skills. If environmental stressors are more problematic, the focus might be on learning assertiveness skills or other coping responses. Individuals might also benefit from learning new cognitive concepts, such as a self-identity that doesn't involve drinking.

Inpatient hospital rehabilitation is useful for some alcoholics, especially if they have serious medical or psychiatric problems or if life stressors threaten to overwhelm them. When the person returns to the community, however, it is critical that there be some form of active, continuing, long-term treatment. Patients who return to a spouse or family often require ongoing treatment on issues involving those significant others, such as establishing new routines and planning shared recreational activities that don't involve drinking. As time goes by, family, friends, and work become more important influences on subsequent drinking behavior than is the treatment program.

There are also some chemical treatments for alcoholism. One involves the use of disulfiram (trade name, Antabuse), which inhibits the metabolic breakdown of alcohol into acetaldehyde (see the box "Metabolizing Alcohol: Our Bodies Work Differently"). Disulfiram causes patients to become violently ill when they drink and thus prevents impulse drinking. However, it is dangerous and must be coupled with ongoing therapy to be useful over time. Sometimes drugs are prescribed to replace alcohol, such as diazepam (Valium) or chlordiazepoxide (Librium). Most therapists feel that such chemical substitutes are useful for only a week or so and that ongoing work on the underlying problems is essential.

> **Personal Insight** What is your attitude about alcoholism? Do you think of it as a disease, a weakness, an affliction, a choice? What is the basis for your attitude?

Helping Someone with an Alcohol Problem

Helping a friend or relative with an alcohol problem requires skill and tact. One of the first steps is making sure you are not an "enabler" or "codependent"—someone who, perhaps unknowingly, allows another to continue excessive use of alcohol. Enabling takes many forms. One of the most common is making excuses or covering up for the alcohol abuser—saying "he has the flu" when it is really a hangover. Whenever you find yourself minimizing or lying about someone's drinking behavior, a warning bell should sound (see the box "Codependency" in Chapter 11). Often another important step is open, honest labeling—"I think you have a problem with alcohol." Such explicit statements usually elicit emotional rebuttals and may endanger a relationship. In the long run, however, you are seldom most helpful to your friends when you allow them to deny their problems with alcohol or other drugs. Even when problems are acknowledged, there is commonly reluctance to obtain help. Your best role might be to obtain information about the available resources and persistently encourage their use.

DRINKING BEHAVIOR AND RESPONSIBILITY

The responsible use of alcohol means drinking in such a way as to keep your BAC low so that your behavior is always under your control. Sometimes people lose control when they misjudge how much they can drink; other times they set out deliberately to get drunk. When you want to drink responsibly, it's helpful to know, first of all, why you drink. The following are the 10 most common reasons given by college students for drinking alcohol:

1. "It increases my feelings of sociability."
2. "It relieves anxiety or tension."
3. "It makes me feel elated or euphoric."
4. "It makes me less inhibited in thinking, saying, or doing certain things."
5. "It enables me to go along with my friends."
6. "It enables me to experience a different state of consciousness."
7. "It makes me less inhibited sexually."
8. "It enables me to stop worrying."
9. "It alleviates depression."
10. "It makes me less self-conscious."

If you drink, what are your reasons for doing so? Are you attempting to meet underlying needs that could best be addressed by other means? Or is your drinking moderate and responsible? To assess your drinking habits, take the quiz in the box "Do You Have a Problem with Alcohol?" Here are some tips for keeping your drinking under control:

- *Drink slowly.* Learn to sip your drinks rather than gulp them. It helps to develop the habit of deliberately tasting and smelling the nuances of alcoholic beverages so that you can determine their similarities and differences. Learn to compare and contrast the

To determine if you have a problem with alcohol, answer yes (Y) or no (N) to the following questions about your drinking behavior. Refer to the scale at the end of the quiz for evaluation of your answers.

____ 1. Do you occasionally drink heavily after a disappointment or a quarrel or when your parents or boss gives you a hard time?

____ 2. When you have trouble or feel pressured at school or at work, do you always drink more heavily than usual?

____ 3. Have you noticed that you are able to handle more liquor than you did when you were first drinking?

____ 4. Did you ever wake up the "morning after" and discover that you could not remember part of the evening before, even though your friends tell you that you did not pass out?

____ 5. When drinking with other people, do you try to have a few extra drinks that others don't notice?

____ 6. Are there certain occasions when you feel uncomfortable if alcohol is not available?

____ 7. Have you recently noticed that when you begin drinking you are in more of a hurry to get the first drink than you used to be?

____ 8. Do you sometimes feel a little guilty about your drinking?

____ 9. Are you secretly irritated when your family or friends discuss your drinking?

____ 10. Have you recently noticed an increase in the frequency of your memory blackouts?

____ 11. Do you often find that you wish to continue drinking after your friends say they have had enough?

____ 12. Do you usually have a reason for the occasions when you drink heavily?

____ 13. When you are sober, do you often regret things you did or said while drinking?

____ 14. Have you tried switching brands or following different plans for controlling your drinking?

____ 15. Have you often failed to keep the promises you've made to yourself about controlling or cutting down on your drinking?

____ 16. Have you ever tried to control your drinking by changing jobs or moving to a new location?

____ 17. Do you try to avoid family or close friends while you are drinking?

____ 18. Are you having an increasing number of financial and academic problems?

____ 19. Do more people seem to be treating you unfairly without good reason?

____ 20. Do you eat very little or irregularly when you are drinking?

____ 21. Do you sometimes have the shakes in the morning and find that it helps to have a drink?

____ 22. Have you recently noticed that you cannot drink as much as you once did?

____ 23. Do you sometimes stay drunk for several days at a time?

____ 24. Do you sometimes feel very depressed and wonder whether life is worth living?

____ 25. Sometimes after a period of drinking, do you see or hear things that aren't there?

____ 26. Do you get terribly frightened after you have been drinking heavily?

If you answer yes to two or three of these questions, you may wish to evaluate your drinking in these areas. Yes answers to *several* of these questions may indicate one of the following stages of alcoholism:

Questions 1–8 (early stage): Drinking is a regular part of your life.

Questions 9–21 (middle stage): You are having trouble controlling when, where, and how much you drink.

Questions 22–26 (beginning of the final stage): You no longer can control your desire to drink.

Source: National Council on Alcoholism.

different kinds of wines and beers. Don't drink alcoholic beverages to quench your thirst.

• *Space your drinks.* Learn to drink nonalcoholic drinks at parties—juices or tonic water without the alcohol, for example—or intersperse these with alcoholic drinks. Learn to refuse a round: "I've had enough for right now." Parties are easier for some people if they hold a glass of anything nonalcoholic that has ice and

a twist of lime floating in it so that it looks as if they are drinking alcohol. Other people are comfortable in openly requesting "mocktails"—drinks that have all the ingredients of the cocktail except the alcoholic beverage. Such requests provide a healthy model for others.

• *Eat before and while drinking.* Avoid drinking on an empty stomach. Food in your stomach will not

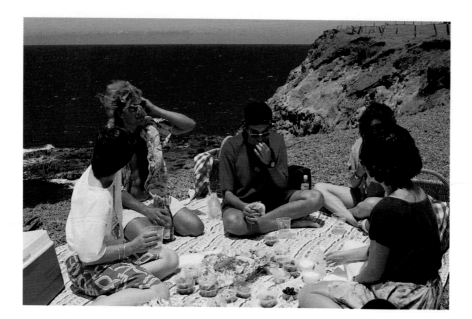

People who choose to drink should do so responsibly, which means keeping BAC low and behavior under control. These picnickers are using several good strategies for keeping their drinking moderate and responsible, including eating while drinking and having a designated driver who abstains from alcohol.

prevent the alcohol from eventually being absorbed, but it will slow down the rate somewhat, and thus the peak blood alcohol level will usually be lower.

- *Know your limits and your drinks.* Learn how different blood alcohol concentrations affect you. In a safe setting such as your home, with your roommate or a friend, see how a set amount—say, two drinks an hour—affects you. A good test is walking heel to toe in a straight line with your eyes closed or standing with your feet crossed and trying to touch your finger to your nose with your eyes closed.

  However, be aware that in different settings your performance, and especially your ability to judge your behavior, may change. At a given blood alcohol concentration, you will perform less well when surrounded by activity and boisterous companions than you will in a quiet test setting with just one or two other people. This impairment results partially because alcohol reduces your ability to perform when your brain is bombarded by multiple stimuli. It is useful to discover the rate at which you can drink without increasing your BAC. Be able to calculate the approximate amount a given drink increases your BAC.

- *Cultivate and model responsible attitudes toward alcohol.* Our society teaches us attitudes toward drinking that increase the chances for alcohol-related problems, if not for ourselves, then for others. Many of us have difficulty expressing disapproval to someone who has drunk too much. We are amused by the antics of the "funny" drunk. We tend to accept the alcohol industry's linkage of drinking with virility or sexuality. And we treat abstainers as odd. These attitudes are not healthy. We need to demonstrate that in driving, operating complicated machinery, and other hazardous situations, abstinence is the appropriate

choice (see the box "Young People Take Action: Students Against Driving Drunk").

- *Learn to be a responsible host or hostess regarding alcohol.* In medieval England an important legal precedent, called the dramskeeper's principle, was established. This principle put the responsibility for alcohol-related injuries or untoward results of the guest's drunken behavior on the innkeeper or tavern owner. Although the legal force of this principle has been muted over the centuries, it is a useful guide for our obligations to our guests. Acquire the habit of serving nonalcoholic beverages as well as alcohol. Popular nonalcoholic drinks include soft drinks, sparkling water and fruit juice in a variety of flavors (sales of these beverages have increased 600 percent in the last decade), drinks made from mixers without the alcohol, and alcohol-free wine and beer. Always serve food along with alcohol, and stop serving alcohol an hour or more before people will leave. Eliminate one drink more—for the road. Be able to insist that a guest who had too much take a taxi, ride with someone else, or stay at your house rather than drive.

- *Hold the drinker responsible.* When any alcohol is consumed, the individual must take full responsibility for his or her behavior. Pardoning unacceptable behavior fosters the attitude that the behavior is due to the drug. The drinker is thereby excused from responsibility and learns to expect minimal adverse consequences for his or her behavior. Research indicates the opposite approach—holding the individual fully accountable for his or her behavior—is a more effective policy. For example, alcohol-impaired drivers who receive legal penalties have fewer subsequent accidents and rearrests than do those who receive only mandatory treatment.

Students Against Driving Drunk (SADD) was established in 1981 to improve young people's knowledge and attitudes about alcohol and drugs to help save their lives—and the lives of others. The program has three major components.

First, it provides a series of lesson plans to present the facts about drinking and driving, permitting students to make informed decisions.

Second, it mobilizes students to help one another through peer pressure to face up to the potential dangers of mixing driving with alcohol or drugs.

And third, it promotes a frank dialogue between teenagers and their parents through the SADD "Contract." Under this agreement both students and their parents pledge to contact each other should they ever find themselves in a potential DWI (driving while intoxicated) situation.

- *Learn about alcohol abuse prevention programs at your school.* What alternatives are being developed to "keg parties" and other events where heavy drinking is fostered? Are programs available for students who are at high risk for alcohol abuse—such as students whose parents abused alcohol? Are counseling or self-help programs like Alcoholics Anonymous available for students who are having problems with alcohol?

- *Refer to the Behavior Change Strategy at the end of this chapter* for more suggestions on developing responsible drinking habits.

Personal Insight   How do you perceive a nondrinker in a social situation where others are drinking? Does it seem like an acceptable choice to you? What is the basis for your attitude?

SUMMARY

- Although alcohol has long been a part of human celebrations, it is a drug capable of causing addiction and harmful physiological effects.

The Nature of Alcohol

- Ethyl alcohol is the psychoactive ingredient in alcoholic beverages. The proof value of an alcoholic beverage is two times the percentage concentration.

- How long it takes for alcohol to be absorbed into the bloodstream depends on the amount, type, and proof of the beverage, the time taken to drink it, and whether there is food in the stomach.

- After alcohol is absorbed, it is distributed throughout the body via the bloodstream. The liver metabolizes alcohol as the blood circulates through it. A small amount of alcohol is excreted via the lungs and kidneys.

- If people drink less alcohol each hour than the amount they can metabolize in an hour, the blood alcohol content remains low. The BAC increases when people drink more than they can metabolize. The rate of alcohol metabolism depends on a variety of individual factors, including gender, body weight, and percentage body fat.

Alcohol and Health

- Alcohol helps people relax; in social settings it often acts as a stimulant, probably because it helps people lose their inhibitions. At higher doses, alcohol interferes with motor coordination, intellectual functions, and verbal performance. At very high doses, coma and even death are possible.

- Alcohol affects internal body temperature, changes sleep patterns, and has an adverse effect on sexual functioning. Driving under the influence of alcohol, even with BAC below the limit, increases the chances of being involved in an automobile crash.

- Continued alcohol use causes cirrhosis, in which damaged and destroyed liver cells are replaced by fibrous scar tissue.

- Although moderate doses of alcohol may reduce the chances of heart attack, higher doses are associated with cardiovascular problems, including cardiac myopathy.

- Alcohol has also been related to certain cancers and abusers have shorter life spans than the average.

- Women who drink while pregnant risk giving birth to children with fetal alcohol syndrome, a characteristic group of birth defects including physical abnormalities and mental retardation. There is no safe level of drinking during pregnancy.

Misuse of Alcohol

- Alcohol abuse involves either (1) continued use of alcohol despite knowledge that it causes recurrent social, occupational, physical, and psychological problems, or (2) recurrent use of alcohol in situations where use is physically hazardous.

- Alcohol dependence, or alcoholism, involves more extensive problems with alcohol abuse, usually involving tolerance or withdrawal.

- Alcohol abuse follows different patterns, such as daily intake of large amounts, heavy weekend drinking, long periods of sobriety interspersed with binges of heavy drinking, or heavy drinking limited to periods of stress.

- Warning signs of alcohol abuse include drinking alone, using alcohol to get through difficult situations, feeling uncomfortable when alcohol is not available, escalating alcohol consumption, heavy use in risky situations, getting drunk regularly, and drinking at unusual times.

- Alcoholism affects people from all social and economic classes; excessive drinking often begins in the teens and twenties for men, though later for women.

- There is a genetic contribution to alcoholism, but other factors are involved, including personality disorders, destructive child-rearing practices, and the desire to imitate others. Social factors include urbanization, disappearance of the extended family, increased mobility, and changing values.

- When tolerance develops after continued use, the chances of adverse psychological and physical effects increase. When alcohol has been used so long and so excessively that liver damage occurs, tolerance begins to decrease.

- Withdrawal symptoms occur when alcoholics stop drinking or drastically reduce their intake. These vary from unpleasant sensations to life-threatening disorders.

- Psychiatric problems involved with alcohol abuse include paranoia and memory loss.

- Alcoholism causes many social problems; it especially affects the children in a family. Furthermore, millions of teenagers show signs of potential alcohol dependency; they risk not only their physical health but also their occupational and social lives.

- Some alcoholics recover without professional help; most require some treatment. A variety of approaches to treatment exists, including self-help support groups like AA, work- and school-based programs, inpatient hospital programs, and chemical treatments.

- Helping someone who abuses alcohol means avoiding being an enabler. Open, honest labeling is important; the best way to help might be to obtain information about available resources and persistently encourage their use.

Drinking Behavior and Responsibility

- The responsible use of alcohol means keeping the BAC low and behavior always under control. Ways to do so include drinking slowly and spacing drinks, eating before and while drinking, being a responsible host or hostess, holding a drinker responsible, and learning about alcohol abuse prevention programs.

TAKE ACTION

1. Interview some of your fellow students about their drinking habits. How much do they drink and how often? Are they more likely to drink on certain days or in certain circumstances? Are there any habits that seem to be common to most students? How do your own drinking habits compare to those of people you interviewed?

2. Some Alcoholics Anonymous groups encourage visitors. If your local chapter does so, attend a meeting to see how the organization functions. What behavioral techniques are used to help people stop drinking? How effective do these techniques seem to be? If there is a local "codependent" or Al-Anon group, attend one of their meetings. What themes are emphasized? Do any themes apply to your relationships?

3. Plan an alcohol-free party. What would you serve to eat and drink? What would you tell people about the party when you invite them?

JOURNAL ENTRY

1. In your health journal, list the positive behaviors that help you drink responsibly. Consider how you can strengthen these behaviors. Then list the behaviors that interfere with responsible drinking for you. Which ones can you change?

2. *Critical Thinking:* Look at advertisements for alcoholic beverages in magazines and on billboards. Analyze several of these ads. What psychological techniques are used to sell the products? What are the hidden messages? Write an essay outlining your opinion of alcohol advertising and marketing. Do you think it's ethical to sell a potentially dangerous substance by appealing to people's desires and vulnerabilities? Do you think liquor manufacturers ought to be held responsible for the damage alcohol inflicts on some people? Explain your reasoning.

3. Make a list of statements you might make to a person you care about who you think is developing a

drinking problem; statements you might make to a person planning to drive under the influence of alcohol, both with and without you in the car; and questions you might ask a friend about your own behavior when you drink. Consider using some of these statements when an appropriate situation arises.

BEHAVIOR CHANGE STRATEGY

DEVELOPING RESPONSIBLE DRINKING HABITS

How much do you drink? Is it the right amount for you? You may know the answer to this question already, or you may not have given it much thought. Many people learn through a single unpleasant experience how alcohol affects their bodies or minds. Others suffer ill effects but choose to ignore or deny them.

To make responsible, informed choices about alcohol, consider, first, whether there is any history of alcohol abuse in your family. Since there seems to be a genetic component to the problem, this information is important to your decisions about alcohol. If someone in your family is dependent on alcohol, you may have a higher-than-average likelihood of becoming dependent too.

Second, consider whether you are dependent on other substances. Do you smoke, drink strong coffee every day, use other drugs regularly? Does some habit control your life (going out for a pack of cigarettes in the middle of the night, taking risks to get drugs)? Some people have more of a tendency to become addicted than others, and a person with one addiction is often likely to have other addictions as well. If this is the case for you, again, you may need to be more cautious with alcohol.

Keep a Record

Once you have answered these questions, find out more about your alcohol-related behavior by keeping track of your drinking for two weeks in your health journal. Keep a daily alcohol behavior record like the one illustrated in Chapter 1 for eating behavior. For every drink, include

- The time of day
- What the drink was
- How fast you drank it
- Where you were
- What else you were doing
- How others influenced you
- What made you want to drink
- Your feelings at the time
- Your thoughts and concerns at the time
- Changes in your feelings while you were drinking and afterwards

- Changes in your behavior after drinking, such as silliness, assertiveness, aggression, or depression
- Any further consequences of having the drink

Analyze Your Record

Next, analyze your record to detect patterns of feelings and environmental cues. Do you always drink when you're at a certain place or with certain people? Do you sometimes drink just to be sociable, when you don't really want a drink and would be satisfied with a nonalcoholic beverage? Do you drink alcohol when you're thirsty? Refer to the list in this chapter of reasons given by college students for drinking to see if any of your reasons are the same. Also refer to the list of warning signs of alcohol abuse given in the text. Are any of them true for you? For example, do you feel uncomfortable in a social situation if alcohol is *not* available?

Set Goals

Now that you've analyzed your record, think about whether you want to change any of your behaviors. This might be the case if you tend to drink too much, even without driving, because alcohol damages your body. It should definitely be the case if you drink and drive or if you're becoming dependent on alcohol. Decide on goals that will give you the best health and safety returns, such as a beer or a glass of wine with dinner, one drink per hour at a party, or no alcohol at all.

Devise a Plan

Refer back to your health journal to see what kinds of patterns your drinking falls into and where you can intervene to break the behavior chain. You may be able to change the antecedents of your behavior, such as by stocking your refrigerator with alternative beverages like juices or sparkling water. If you feel self-conscious about ordering a nonalcoholic drink when you're out with a group, try recruiting a friend to do the same. If it's impossible to avoid drinking in some situations, such as at a bar or a beer party, you may decide to avoid those situations for a period of time.

Instead of drinking, you can try other activities that produce the same effect. For example, if you drink to relieve anxiety or tension, try adding 20 or 30 minutes of exercise to your schedule to help you manage stress. Or try doing a relaxation exercise or going for a brisk walk to help reduce anxiety before a party or date. If you drink to relieve depression or to stop worrying, consider finding a trustworthy person (perhaps a professional counselor) to talk to about the problem that's bothering you. If you drink to feel more comfortable sexually, consider ways to improve communication with your partner so you can deal with sexual issues more openly. When these activities are successful, they will reinforce your responsible drinking decisions and make it more likely that you'll make the same decisions again in the future.

For other ways to monitor and control your drinking behavior, see the suggestions given in the box "Keeping Social Drinking Social" and in the section "Drinking Behavior and Responsibility."

Reward Yourself and Monitor Your Progress

If changing your drinking behavior turns out to be difficult, it may be a clue that drinking was becoming a problem for you—all the more reason to get it under control now. Be sure to reward yourself as you learn to drink responsibly (or not at all), using the personal rewards you listed in your health journal at the beginning of this course. You may lose weight, look better, feel better, and have higher self-esteem as a result of limiting your drinking. Keep track of your progress in your health journal and revise your strategy if you start to revert to unhealthy or out-of-control patterns. Stay with your program by recruiting support, using a buddy, looking to a role model, and managing stress with healthy coping techniques. Remember, when you establish sensible drinking habits, you're planning not just for this week or month but for your whole life.

SELECTED BIBLIOGRAPHY

American Psychiatric Association. 1987. *Diagnostic and Statistical Manual of Mental Disorders* (DSM-III-R). 3rd ed. revised. Washington, D.C.: American Psychiatric Association.

Baer, J. S., A. Stacy, and M. Larimer. 1991. Biases in the perception of drinking norms among college students. *Journal of Studies on Alcohol* 52(6): 580–6.

Blot, W. J. 1992. Alcohol and cancer. *Cancer Research* 52(7 suppl): 2119s–23s.

Cermak, T. L. 1991. Co-addiction as a disease. *Psychiatric Annals* 21:266–72.

Geller, S. E., M. J. Kalsher, and S. W. Clarke. 1991. Beer versus mixed-drink consumption at fraternity parties: A time and place for low-alcohol alternatives. *Journal of Studies on Alcohol* 52(3): 197–204.

Goldstein, A., and H. Kalant. 1990. Drug policy: Striking the right balance. *Science* 249:1513–22.

Hansen, W. B., A. E. Raynor, and B. H. Wolkenstein. 1991. Perceived personal immunity to the consequences of drinking alcohol: The relationship between behavior and perception. *Journal of Studies on Alcohol* 14(3): 205–24.

Holden, C. 1991. Probing the complex genetics of alcoholism. *Science* 251:163–64.

Kendler, K. S., A. C. Heath, M. C. Neale, R. C. Kessler, and L. J. Eaves. 1992. A population-based twin study of alcoholism in women. *Journal of the American Medical Association* 268(14): 1877–82.

Lund, A. K., and A. C. Wolfe, 1991. Changes in the incidence of alcohol-impaired driving in the United States, 1973–1986. *Journal of Studies on Alcohol* 52(4): 293–301.

Martin, M. J., and M. E. Pritchard. 1991. Factors associated with alcohol use in later adolescence. *Journal of Studies on Alcohol* 52(1): 5–9.

Menella, J. A., and G. K. Beauchamp. 1991. The transfer of alcohol to human milk: Effects on flavor and the infant's behavior. *New England Journal of Medicine* 325(14): 981–85.

Miller, N. S. 1991. *Comprehensive Handbook of Drug and Alcohol Addiction*. New York: Marcel Dekker.

Moos, R. H., J. W. Finney, and R. C. Cronkite. 1990. *Alcoholism Treatment: Context, Process, and Outcome*. New York: Oxford University Press.

Neff, J. A., T. J. Prihoda, and S. K. Hoppe. 1991. "Machismo," self-esteem, education and high maximum drinking among Anglo, black and Mexican-American male drinkers. *Journal of Studies on Alcohol* 52(5): 458–63.

Roeleveld, N., and others. 1992. Mental retardation associated with parental smoking and alcohol consumption before, during, and after pregnancy. *Preventive Medicine* 21(1): 110–19.

Schuckit, M. A. 1991. Keeping current with the DSMs and substance use disorders. In *Current Psychiatric Therapy*. Ed. D. Dunner. Philadelphia: W. B. Saunders.

Smart, R. G., and R. E. Mann. 1991. Factors in recent reductions in liver cirrhosis deaths. *Journal of Studies on Alcohol* 52(3): 232–40.

U.S. Public Health Service. 1990. *Seventh Special Report to the U.S. Congress on Alcohol and Health*. Rockville, Md.: National Institute of Alcohol Abuse and Alcoholism.

RECOMMENDED READINGS

Alcoholics Anonymous, 3rd ed. 1976. New York: Alcoholics Anonymous World Services. *This is the "Big Book," the basic text for AA. It includes the founding tenets of AA and vivid histories of recovering alcoholics.*

Dorris, M. 1992. *The Broken Cord*. New York: HarperCollins. *A personal story and a current source of information on fetal alcohol syndrome.*

Ray, O., and C. Ksir. 1991. *Drugs, Society, and Human Behavior*, 5th ed. St. Louis: Mosby-Yearbook. *An entertaining, popular college text that skillfully underscores societal factors that influence alcohol use.*

Vaillant, G. E. 1983. *The Natural History of Alcoholism*. Cambridge: Harvard University Press. *A well-written description of an important longitudinal study of alcoholism.*

Vogel-Sprott, M. 1992. *Alcohol Tolerance and Social Drinking: Learning the Consequences*. New York: Guilford Press. *An interesting book on recent research into behavioral aspects of alcohol use.*

11

The Use and Abuse of Psychoactive Drugs

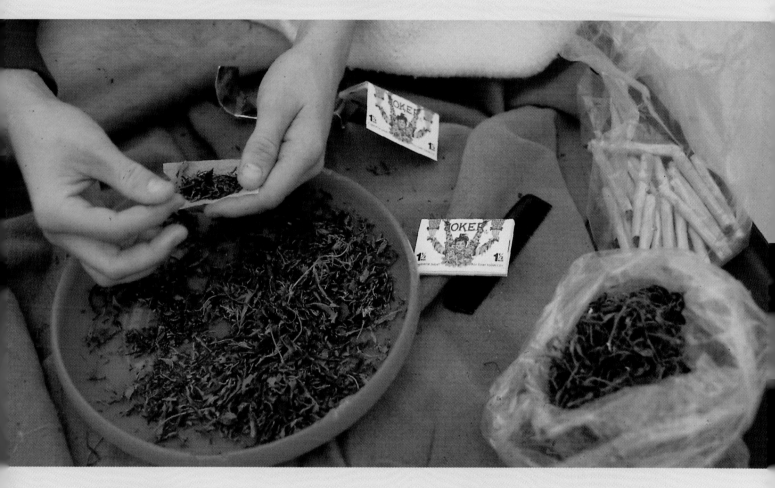

CONTENTS

◗ Last summer, while working in an office and living at home with your parents, you got into the habit of drinking quite a lot of coffee. You had coffee at home in the morning, coffee all day long at work, and more coffee after dinner. You didn't think too much about it until you returned to school in the fall. During your first few days back you developed a terrible headache, had trouble focusing your thoughts, and had absolutely no energy. To try to wake up for afternoon classes one day, you got a double cappuccino at the student union. It helped—a lot. Not only did you have more energy, but your headache also disappeared and you felt alert and clear-headed for the first time in days. You're surprised that coffee—and lack of it—could have such an effect on you. Is it possible that caffeine is that potent? Can a person be addicted to it? Is there a way to cut back without feeling so bad?

◗ One of your housemates smokes marijuana every evening and before every social occasion. She's a good friend and sometimes you worry about her. Last week you asked her why she smokes every night, and she said it makes things more fun. You pointed out that it can't be good for her health, and she responded that a single joint can't do any harm. "Look at all the people who smoke 10 or 20 cigarettes a day," she said. "Now, *that's* a bad habit! Marijuana isn't bad for you, and it isn't addictive." Is it true that marijuana is harmless? Can you be addicted to it? Are there any long-term effects?

◗ A friend of yours has been using cocaine occasionally for the last few months. Recently he's been jumpy, harried, and distracted a lot of the time. He says he's too smart and too careful to get hooked, but you're starting to wonder just how much he's taking. He's borrowed money from you and hasn't paid you back, and you've caught him in a number of minor lies. Now he wants to borrow money again. He's a good friend and you'd like to lend it to him, but you're worried that you might just be helping him get into more trouble. Is it likely that your friend has a drug problem? Should you lend him the money? Should you confront him with your concerns? What's the best thing to do in this situation?

◗ You've been feeling pretty bad ever since you and your boyfriend broke up three weeks ago. You're not sleeping well, you can't concentrate on school, and most of the time you feel either depressed or anxious. A woman in your dorm says she has a prescription for Valium and will give you some. She says it will help you relax and feel better. Would this be a good way to deal with your current situation? Are there any risks involved?

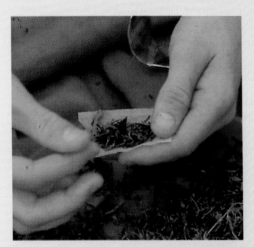

MAKING CONNECTIONS

Some drugs improve people's lives; others destroy them. Drugs are everywhere in our society, and knowing how to handle situations involving them is crucial to maintaining control of your life. In each of the scenarios presented on this page, all related to drug use, individuals have to use information, make a decision, or choose a course of action. What would you do in each situation? What response or decision would you make? This chapter provides information about drug use and abuse of psychoactive drugs that can be used in situations like these. After finishing the chapter, read the scenarios again. Has what you've learned changed how you would respond?

We live in a drug society. The use of drugs for both medical and social purposes is common and widespread. Too many Americans believe that all problems, large and small, have chemical solutions. They turn to caffeine when they're tired, sedatives when they can't sleep, and alcohol or other recreational drugs when they're anxious, tense, or bored. Advertisements, social pressures, medical research, and our own desires for quick fixes to life's difficult problems all contribute to the prevailing attitude that drugs can ease even the mildest physical and emotional complaints.

Drugs are defined as chemicals other than food intended to affect the structure or function of the body. They include prescription medicines, such as antibiotics or tranquilizers; over-the-counter remedies, such as alcohol, tobacco, and caffeine products; and illegal substances, such as cocaine, marijuana, and heroin. This chapter focuses primarily on **psychoactive drugs**, chemicals that can alter a person's experiences or consciousness. Two of the most widely used psychoactive drugs—nicotine and alcohol—were discussed in earlier chapters.

THE DRUG TRADITION

Using drugs to alter consciousness is an ancient and universal pursuit. As described in Chapter 10, people have used alcohol to celebrate and intoxicate for thousands of years. Native populations in all parts of the world discovered the psychoactive properties of various local plants, such as the coca plant in South America and the opium poppy in the Middle East and Far East.

In the nineteenth century, chemists were successful in extracting the active elements from medicinal plants, such as morphine from the opium poppy and atropine, a muscle spasm reliever, from belladonna. This was the beginning of *pharmacy,* the art of compounding drugs, and of *pharmacology,* the science and study of drugs. From this point on, a variety of drugs began to be produced, including morphine, cocaine, heroin, and codeine (Figure 11-1).

Before their potential for abuse became apparent, these drugs weren't regulated. Many could be purchased without a prescription; even Coca-Cola originally contained a small amount of cocaine, which accounted for the "lift" it provided. Thanks to easy availability, by 1900, many people in Europe and the United States were addicted to drugs. This situation prompted enactment of drug legislation to protect consumers. Over the course of the next 50 years, drug use and addiction dropped sharply.

In the 1960s, there was a surge in the recreational use of drugs such as marijuana, cocaine, amphetamines, LSD, and other psychoactive drugs synthesized in laboratories. Use continued to rise until the late 1970s, when it stabilized and began to decline slightly, at least for many drugs. The exceptions are "crack" cocaine and methamphetamine, or "ice," whose use and abuse continue to grow in some populations. Today, the drug scene in the United States is dominated by a multibillion-dollar criminal drug industry that thrives on the dependencies and recreational habits of large segments of the population.

Personal Insight What was your family's attitude about drugs when you were growing up? Did your parents discuss drugs with you? Did they set rules or offer advice about how to deal with situations involving drugs? How did their attitudes affect your current values? Do you share your parents' attitudes about drugs or have you adopted a different position?

USE, ABUSE, AND DEPENDENCE

People use drugs for a variety of reasons and in a variety of ways. For some, drug use can lead to the serious problems of abuse and physical and psychological dependence.

Who Uses Drugs?

Use and abuse of drugs occurs at all income and education levels, among all races and ethnic groups, and at all ages. Unborn babies can become involuntary drug users if their mothers use drugs during pregnancy; great-grandmothers can become unintentional abusers of prescription drugs.

But some people are at higher-than-average risk for trying illicit drugs. Risk factors include being male, being an adolescent or young adult, and having frequent exposure to drugs through family members or peers. Risk is also higher for people who come from a single-parent family, for those whose mothers failed to complete high school, for those who are uninterested in school and earn poor grades, and for those who feel lonely or isolated. A risk-taking personality is another factor. People who drive too fast or who don't wear seat belts may have this personality type, which is characterized by a sense of invincibility. Believing themselves invulnerable, such people find it easy to dismiss warnings of danger, whether about drugs or seat belts—"That only happens to other people; it could never happen to me."

These risk factors predict drug use irrespective of race or ethnicity. Hispanic adolescents, for example, aren't any more likely to have substance abuse problems than are

Drugs Chemicals other than food intended to affect the structure or function of the body.

Psychoactive drug Any chemical other than food that, when taken into the body, can alter the user's consciousness.

TERMS

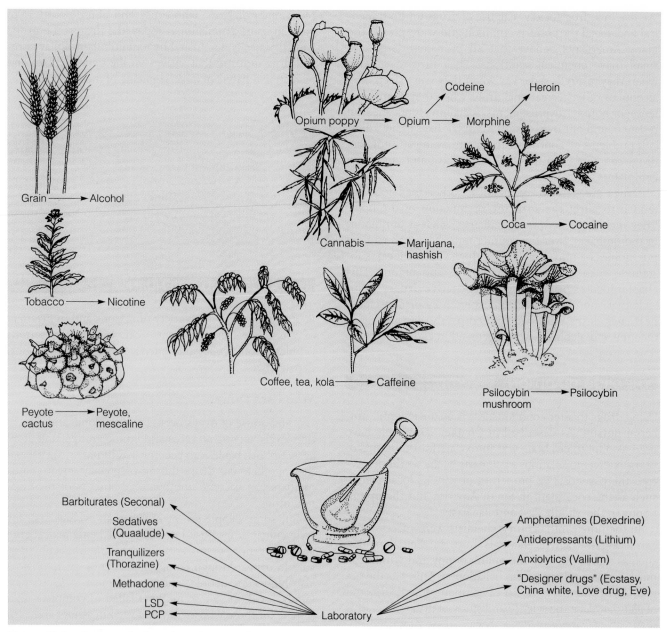

Grain ──→ Alcohol

Opium poppy ──→ Opium ──→ Morphine
Morphine ──→ Codeine
Morphine ──→ Heroin

Cannabis ──→ Marijuana, hashish

Coca ──→ Cocaine

Tobacco ──→ Nicotine

Coffee, tea, kola ──→ Caffeine

Psilocybin mushroom ──→ Psilocybin

Peyote cactus ──→ Peyote, mescaline

Barbiturates (Seconal)
Sedatives (Quaalude)
Tranquilizers (Thorazine)
Methadone
LSD
PCP

Laboratory

Amphetamines (Dexedrine)
Antidepressants (Lithium)
Anxiolytics (Vallium)
"Designer drugs" (Ecstasy, China white, Love drug, Eve)

Figure 11-1 *Sources of selected psychoactive drugs.*

non-Hispanic white adolescents with the same social and family characteristics. This may seem obvious, but researchers had to undertake careful studies over the past decade to document that our nation's drug crisis is driven by socioeconomic problems, not by inherent racial or ethnic characteristics.

What about people who *don't* use drugs? As a group, non-users also share some characteristics. Drug use is less common among young people who attend school regularly, get good grades, have strong personal identities, are religious, have a good relationship with their parents, and are independent thinkers whose actions aren't controlled by peer pressure. Coming from a strong family, one that

has a clear policy on drug use and where crises and conflicts are dealt with constructively, is another factor associated with people who don't use drugs. Identifying the personality characteristics and skills that help people resist pressure to use drugs is an important focus of research today (see the box "Students' Reasons for Avoiding Drugs").

Why Do People Use Drugs?

The answer to this question depends on both the user and the drug. Young people, especially those from middle-class backgrounds, are frequently drawn to drugs by the

Much has been made of young people's reasons for using and abusing drugs. What about their reasons for *not* using drugs or for stopping once they start? Here are the five most common reasons students give for abstaining from drug use:

1. Concern about health risks, including developing dependency.

2. Peers don't approve of drug use.

3. Role models (parents, older friends) don't use drugs.

4. Fear of getting caught and shaming others.

5. Individual doesn't view self as drug user.

Adapted from R. A. Selan, *Stanford Report,* 1990, and D. F. Duncan, *Journal of Drug Education,* 1988.

And here are the four most common reasons students give for discontinuing marijuana use:

1. Health reasons.

2. Disliked the effects.

3. Mental or emotional problems.

4. Athletic training or lifestyle changes.

The majority of students don't use drugs. Their reasons show a healthy respect for the risks and growing sense of self-responsibility.

allure of the exciting and illicit. They may be curious, rebellious, or vulnerable to peer pressure. They may want to appear to be daring and to be part of the group. They may want to imitate adult models in their lives or in the movies. Most people who have taken illicit drugs have done so on an experimental basis, typically trying the drug one or more times but not continuing beyond that. The main factors in the initial choice of a drug are whether it is available and whether other people around are already using it.

Although some people use drugs because they have a desire to alter their mood or are seeking a spiritual experience, others are motivated primarily by a desire to escape boredom, anxiety, depression, feelings of worthlessness, or other distressing symptoms of psychological problems. They use drugs as a way to cope with the difficulties they are experiencing in life. The common practice in our society of seeking a drug solution to every problem is a factor in the widespread reliance on both illicit drugs and prescription drugs like Valium.

For people living in poverty in the inner cities, many of these reasons for using drugs are magnified. The problems are more devastating, the need for escape more compelling. The buying and selling of drugs reflect issues of discrimination, prejudice, class, and economics.

Drug Abuse

What exactly is **drug abuse?** This is a tough question to answer because it's difficult to separate drug use from drug abuse and drug abuse from drug dependence. Many addiction experts describe drug abuse as a maladaptive pattern of use of any substance that persists despite adverse social, psychological, or medical consequences. As described in Chapter 10 for alcohol, the pattern of abuse may be constant or intermittent, and **physical depen-**

dence may or may not be present. For example, a person who drinks excessively once a month and then drives is abusing alcohol, even if he or she is not physically dependent. People who continue to smoke marijuana on the weekends even though it makes them feel sluggish and forgetful (and consumes money they should be saving) are abusing the drug.

Personal Insight   Have you ever misused or abused a drug, even coffee or an over-the-counter remedy? If so, what were your reasons and motivations? Was it hard to stop? How did the experience affect your current attitudes and behavior?

Drug Dependence

Drug abuse can become drug **dependence,** also known as addiction. A person is dependent on a drug if he or she takes it compulsively, neglects constructive activities because of it, and experiences adverse social effects resulting

TERMS

Drug abuse   A maladaptive pattern of use of any substance that persists despite adverse social, psychological, or medical consequences. The pattern may be intermittent, with or without tolerance and physical dependence.

Physical dependence   The result of physiological adaptations that occur in response to the frequent presence of a drug; interruption of drug use is followed by withdrawal syndrome. Also known as physical addiction.

Dependence (dependency)   The compulsive use of a drug that results in neglect of constructive activities and adverse social consequences. Tolerance and physical dependence are often present. Also known as *addiction.*

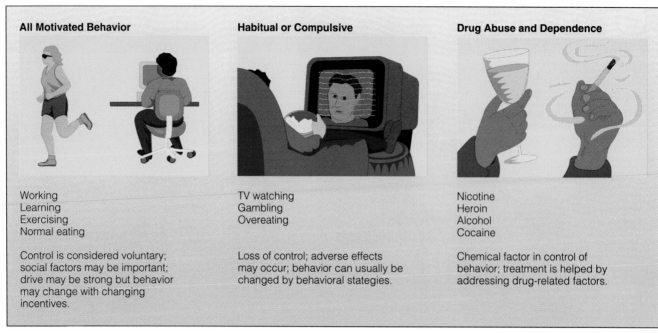

All Motivated Behavior	Habitual or Compulsive	Drug Abuse and Dependence
Working Learning Exercising Normal eating	TV watching Gambling Overeating	Nicotine Heroin Alcohol Cocaine
Control is considered voluntary; social factors may be important; drive may be strong but behavior may change with changing incentives.	Loss of control; adverse effects may occur; behavior can usually be changed by behavioral stategies.	Chemical factor in control of behavior; treatment is helped by addressing drug-related factors.

Figure 11-2 *Behavior control.*
A progression from normal to dependent behavior occurs in some areas of life for some people. The key feature of this progression is loss of control.

from its use. Drug dependence can be physical and/or psychological.

Physical Dependence As described in the chapters on nicotine and alcohol, the hallmarks of physical dependence on a drug are **tolerance** and withdrawal. Tolerance occurs when the body adapts to the repeated effects of a drug so that higher doses are required to achieve the same effect. Tolerance increases with daily doses and can lead to levels of drug use that produce physical dependence. The usual starting dose of heroin, for example, is about 3 milligrams, but after several months of continual use, a dose of 1,000 milligrams may be required to produce the same effects.

Physical addiction has occurred if a **withdrawal syndrome** follows interruption of the use of the drug. Withdrawal occurs because the user's body has gradually become accustomed to high levels of the drug, and when the drug is withdrawn, the body must rapidly adjust to the sudden drop in the concentration of the drug. Withdrawal symptoms begin as soon as blood levels of the drug begin to fall and may last several days or longer. Symptoms can be mild or potentially fatal, depending on the type of drug and on the degree of physical dependence. The specific symptoms of withdrawal tend to be the opposite of the effects of the drug. For example, symptoms of withdrawal from sedatives include restlessness, sleep disturbances, anxiety, shaking, and occasionally life-threatening seizures. Withdrawal from stimulants, on the other hand, tends to produce intense fatigue and deep depression.

Psychological Dependence Some experts in addiction also consider psychological aspects of dependence. **Psychological dependence** involves an intense repetitive need, or craving, for the changes in feelings and mood that a particular drug provides. Physical changes contribute to these cravings, so psychological dependence has a physical component, but it can develop independently of physical dependence. Psychological dependence can develop more rapidly than physical dependence, particularly for drugs that have strong, immediate effects.

Psychological dependence is strongly affected by social factors. Particular situations, times of day, or people may trigger the compulsive craving for a drug. Personality traits can also play a role in whether a person develops a psychological dependence on a particular drug. In some ways, people can become psychologically dependent on things other than drugs, too, such as gambling, overeating, or sexual activity (Figure 11-2).

Risk Factors for Dependence Some people are able to use psychoactive drugs without falling into a pattern of abuse or becoming dependent. Others aren't as lucky. Why do some people become dependent? The answer seems to be in a combination of physical, psychological, and social factors. Some research indicates that some people may be born with certain characteristics of brain chemistry or metabolism that make them more vulnerable to drug dependence. Other research suggests that people who were exposed to drugs while still in the womb may have an increased risk of abusing drugs themselves later in life. One possible explanation for this is that prenatal exposure may "imprint" a desire for a drug on a developing fetus. People who suffer chronic pain, such as those with back injuries, are also at risk of developing a dependence on the drugs they take to control pain.

Psychological risk factors for drug dependence include difficulty in controlling impulses and having a strong need for excitement, stimulation, and immediate gratification. Feelings of rejection, hostility, aggression, anxiety, or depression are also associated with drug dependence. People may turn to drugs to blot out their emotional pain. People with psychiatric illnesses have a very high risk for drug dependence.

Social factors that involve risk for drug dependence include growing up in a family in which a parent or sibling abused drugs, belonging to a peer group that emphasizes and encourages drug abuse, and poverty. Because they have easy access to drugs, health professionals also face an increased risk for drug dependence.

To determine if you may have a problem with drug abuse or dependence, take the quiz in the box "Do You Have a Problem with Drugs?"

HOW DRUGS AFFECT THE BODY

Like alcohol and tobacco, the psychoactive drugs discussed in this chapter have complex and variable effects. The same drug may affect different users differently or the same user in different ways under different circumstances. The effects of a drug depend on three general categories of factors: (1) drug factors—the properties of the drug itself and differences in how it's used, (2) user factors—the physical and psychological characteristics of the user, and (3) social factors.

Drug Factors

When different drugs or dosages produce different effects, the differences are usually caused by one or more of five different drug factors:

- The **pharmacological properties** of the drug are its overall effects on a person's body chemistry, behavior, and psychology. Of all the millions of chemicals known, only a few have pharmacological properties that lead humans to use and abuse them. These self-administered chemicals are alcohol, nicotine, and the drug groups discussed in this chapter—opiates; barbiturates and other sedative-hypnotics; tranquilizers; caffeine, cocaine, and amphetamine-like stimulants; psychedelics; certain deliriants; and marijuana.

- The **dose-response function** is the relationship between the amount of drug taken and the intensity or type of drug effect. This relationship is not necessarily a direct one in which increasing the dose simply increases or intensifies the effect. Rather, the effect can change with a higher dosage. A familiar example is the person who becomes friendly after one cocktail but belligerent and hostile after four. With some drugs there is a plateau in the dose-response function in which a larger dose has no effect on the response. With LSD, for example, the greatest changes in perception occur at a certain dose, and no further changes in perception take place if higher doses are taken.

- The **time-action function** is the relationship between the time elapsed since a drug was taken and the intensity of its effect. The effects of a drug are greatest when concentrations of the drug in the tissues are changing the fastest, especially if they are increasing. For example, with alcohol, immediately after a person takes a drink, the alcohol begins to be absorbed in the digestive tract and the level of alcohol in the blood begins to rise rapidly. As the alcohol is metabolized, the blood alcohol level gradually falls, as explained in Chapter 10. Intoxication is usually greater when the level is rising than when it is falling, even though there may actually be somewhat less alcohol in the blood when it is rising.

- The *cumulative effects* of psychoactive drugs may be different from the effects of a single dose, because over time the drugs produce physiological alterations in the body that change their effects. A given amount of alcohol, for example, will generally affect a habitual drinker less than an occasional drinker. Tolerance to some drugs, such as LSD, builds rapidly. To experience the same effect, a user has to abstain from the drug for a period of time before that dosage will again exert its original effects.

- The *method of use* has a direct effect on how strong a response a drug produces. Methods of use include

---

TERMS

Tolerance   Lower sensitivity to a drug so that a given dose no longer exerts the usual effect and larger doses are needed.

Withdrawal syndrome   The cluster of physical and psychological symptoms that follow interruption of use of a drug on which a user is physically dependent; symptoms may be mild or life-threatening.

Psychological dependence   A strong repetitive need, or craving, for the change in feelings and mood that a particular drug provides.

Pharmacological properties   The overall effects of a drug on the individual's behavior, psychology, and chemistry. This term also refers to the amount of the drug required to exert various effects, the time course of these effects, and other characteristics of the drug, such as its chemical composition.

Dose-response function   The relationship between the amount of a drug taken and the intensity or type of drug effect.

Time-action function   The relationship between the time elapsed since a drug was taken and the intensity of a drug effect.

If you wonder whether *you* are becoming dependent on a drug, ask yourself the following questions. Answer yes (Y) or no (N).

1. Do you take the drug on a regular basis? _____

2. Have you been taking the drug for a long time? _____

3. Do you always take the drug in certain situations or when you're with certain people? _____

4. Do you find it difficult to stop using the drug? Do you feel powerless to quit? _____

5. Have you tried repeatedly to cut down or control your use of the drug? _____

6. Do you need to take a larger dose of the drug in order to get the same high you're used to? _____

7. Do you feel specific symptoms if you cut back or stop using the drug? _____

8. Do you frequently take another psychoactive substance to relieve withdrawal symptoms? _____

9. Do you take the drug to feel "normal"? _____

10. Do you go to extreme lengths or put yourself in dangerous situations to get the drug? _____

11. Do you hide your drug use from others? Have you ever lied about what you're using or how much you use? _____

12. Do people close to you ask you about your drug use? _____

13. Are you spending more and more time with people who use the drug you use? _____

14. Do you think about the drug when you're not high, figuring out ways to get it? _____

15. If you stop taking the drug, do you feel bad until you can take it again? _____

16. Does the drug interfere with your ability to study, work, or socialize? _____

17. Do you skip important school, occupational, social, or recreational activities in order to obtain or use the drug? _____

18. Do you continue to use the drug despite a physical or mental disorder or despite a significant problem that you know is worsened by drug use? _____

19. Have you developed a mental or physical condition or disorder because of prolonged drug use? _____

20. Have you done something dangerous or that you regret while under the influence of the drug? _____

The more times you answer yes, the more likely it is that you are developing a physical or psychological dependency on the drug. If your answers suggest dependency, talk to someone at your school health clinic or to your physician about taking care of the problem before it gets worse.

ingestion, inhalation, injection, and absorption through the skin or tissue linings. Drugs are usually injected one of three ways: intravenously (IV, or mainlining), intramuscularly (IM), or subcutaneously (SQ, or "skin popping").

If a drug is taken by a method that allows the drug to enter the bloodstream and reach the brain rapidly, the effects are usually stronger and the potential for dependence is greater than when the method involves slower absorption. For example, injecting a drug generally produces stronger effects than swallowing the same drug.

Different methods of drug use are associated with different "costs," or risks. For example, injecting drugs often involves the sharing of needles, which may be contaminated with disease agents from another user's blood. For this reason, intravenous drug users are at high risk for hepatitis B and HIV

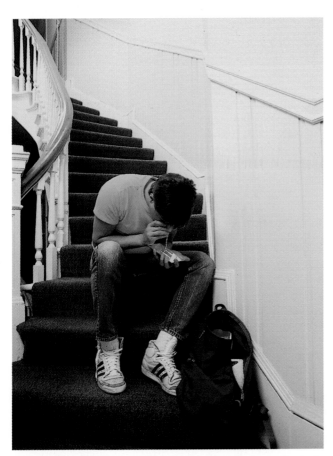

Most middle-class users sniff, or "snort," cocaine, a method of use that produces effects in two to three minutes. With other methods, such as injecting it intravenously, inhaling vapors, or smoking crack, the effects of cocaine are felt within seconds. Method of use is just one variable in the overall effect of a drug on the body.

infection (see the box "Drugs and HIV Infection/AIDS"). The surest way to prevent transmission of disease is never to share needles. Sterilizing needles using bleach may kill the HIV virus, but sterilization has to be done carefully because viruses can be transmitted in very small amounts of blood. (See Chapter 17 for more information about preventing HIV infection and hepatitis B.) Other dangers associated with injecting drugs include tetanus, collapse of veins, and scarring and abscesses at the site of injection.

User Factors

The second category of factors that determine how a person will respond to a particular drug involves the person's physical characteristics. Body mass is one variable. The effects of certain drugs on a 100-pound person will be twice as great as the effect of the same amount of the drug on a 200-pound person. Other variables include general health and various subtle **biochemical** states, including

genetic factors. For example, some people have an inherited ability to rapidly metabolize a cough suppressant called dextromethorphan, which also has psychoactive properties. These people must take a higher-than-normal dose to get a given cough-suppressant effect.

If a person's biochemical state is already altered by another drug, this too can make a difference. Some drugs intensify the effects of other drugs, as is the case with alcohol and barbiturates. Some drugs block the effects of other drugs, such as when a **tranquilizer** is used to relieve anxiety caused by cocaine. Interactions between drugs, including many prescription and over-the-counter drugs, can be unpredictable and dangerous.

One physical condition that requires special precautions is pregnancy. It can be risky for a woman to use any drugs at all during pregnancy, including alcohol and common over-the-counter drugs like cough medicine. The risks are greatest during the first trimester of pregnancy when the fetus's body is rapidly forming and even small chemical alterations in the mother's body can have a devastating effect on development. Even later, the fetus is more susceptible than the mother to the adverse effects of any drugs she takes. The fetus may even become physically dependent on a drug being taken by the mother and suffer withdrawal symptoms after birth.

Sometimes response to a drug is affected strongly by the user's expectations about how he or she will respond to the drug. With large doses, the chemical properties of the drug do seem to have the strongest influence on the user's response. But with small doses, psychological (and social) factors are often more important. The **set** is the user's expectations about how he or she is going to respond to the drug. When people strongly believe that a given drug will affect them a certain way, they are likely to experience those effects regardless of the drug's pharmacological properties. The **placebo** effect—when an individual receives an inert substance and yet responds as if it were an active drug—is a well-documented example of set.

Social Factors

The **setting** is the physical and social environment surrounding the drug use. If a person uses marijuana at home with trusted friends and pleasant music, the effects

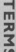

Biochemical Describes the branch of chemistry that deals with the life processes of plants and animals.

Tranquilizers Central nervous system depressants that reduce tension and anxiety.

Set A person's expectations or preconceptions in a given situation.

Placebo An inert or innocuous medication that is given in place of an active drug; it is often called a sugar pill.

Setting The environment in which something is done.

The first wave of HIV infection in the United States struck primarily gay and bisexual men. The second wave, spread by the sharing of contaminated hypodermic needles, affected intravenous (IV) drug users. The third wave of infection is affecting women and children—the sexual partners and children of IV drug users.

By early 1993, 25,000 women and 4,000 children with AIDS had been reported to the Centers for Disease Control; many more are infected with HIV but have not yet developed AIDS. Nearly three-quarters of these women became infected through IV drug use or through sex with an HIV-infected IV drug user. And over 90 percent of children with AIDS acquired the infection from their mothers, either in the womb, at birth, or from breast milk. By 1992, HIV infection/AIDS was the leading cause of death in New York state among Hispanic children between the ages of 1 and 4 and the second leading cause of death among African American preschoolers. Over 50,000 cases of AIDS among men can be attributed to IV drug use or sexual contact with IV drug users.

No easy solutions are in sight. Education and prevention campaigns, which have succeeded in slowing the spread of HIV through the gay community, are far less effective at changing behavior among IV drug users. Most IV drug users are removed from the social and medical mainstream and lack access to the standard sources of education about health issues. For those dependent on drugs, the physical and psychological cravings for drugs are powerful motivators of behavior; thoughts of safety alone aren't strong enough to change behavior.

Heroin and other injectable opiates are responsible for much of the spread of HIV infection among IV drug users. Crack cocaine, even though it is smoked rather than injected, has also played a major role in the spread of HIV among young heterosexuals. Crack fosters transmission of HIV in two ways. First, many crack users also engage in IV drug use; "speedballs," injected cocaine-heroin mixes, enjoyed an alarming increase in popularity in the late 1980s and early 1990s. Second, crack use frequently leads to increased sexual activity. Many users trade sex for drugs or sex for money to buy drugs. Rates of syphilis and other sexually transmissible diseases (STDs) have skyrocketed among crack users, also contributing to the spread of HIV. (The presence of genital sores related to STDs greatly increases the likelihood that a person will contract HIV from an infected sexual partner.)

Some public health experts believe free public needle-exchange programs—in which IV drug users turn in a used syringe and get a new, clean one back—could help stem the spread of HIV. A handful of experimental needle exchange programs have been introduced, and supporters are working to expand them. But opponents argue that supplying addicts with syringes gives them the message that illegal drug use is acceptable and could exacerbate the nation's drug problem.

Concerned people on both sides of the needle-exchange debate agree that getting people off drugs is the best solution. But government resources have been inadequate for the task. In 1991, for example, 60 percent of New York City's estimated 200,000 injecting drug users were infected with HIV. The city had resources to provide drug treatment for only 40,000 addicts at a time. Clearly, the spread of HIV among drug users in the United States constitutes a medical and social emergency, one that we will face for years to come.

Adapted from D. W. Wara, "Perinatal AIDS and HIV: Diagnosis and Treatment Update," presented at the 1992 meeting of the American Academy of Pediatrics in San Francisco; and C. Morain, "Necessary But Illegal." *American Medical News,* 12 August 1991.

---

are likely to be different from the effects if the same dose is taken in an austere experimental laboratory with an impassive research technician. Similarly, the dose of alcohol that produces mild euphoria and stimulation at a noisy, active cocktail party might induce sleepiness and slight depression when taken at home while alone.

Experiments have been conducted in which some subjects smoked small quantities of marijuana while others (unknowingly) smoked a substance that smelled and tasted like marijuana but was not. The intensity of the **"high"** the subjects experienced was not related to whether they had actually smoked marijuana. In other studies, subjects who smoked low doses of real marijuana that they believed to be a placebo experienced no effects from the drug. Clearly, the setting and the set had greater effects on the smokers than the drug itself.

REPRESENTATIVE PSYCHOACTIVE DRUGS

What are the major psychoactive drugs, and how do they produce their effects? We discuss six different representative groups in this chapter: (1) opiates, (2) **central nervous system (CNS)** depressants, (3) CNS stimulants, (4) psychedelics, (5) marijuana and other cannabis products, and (6) deliriants. Some of these drugs are classified according to how they affect the body; others—the opiates and the cannabis products—are classified according to their chemical makeup. See Figure 11-1 for sources of selected psychoactive drugs.

Opiates

The opiates, also called narcotics, are natural or synthetic

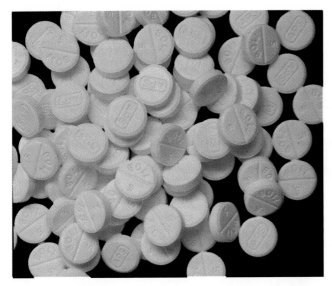

Drugs that relieve anxiety have a place in medical treatment, but they are easily abused. Valium, pictured here, can produce dependency even when taken exactly as directed.

(laboratory-made) drugs that relieve pain, cause drowsiness, and induce **euphoria.** Opium, morphine, heroin, methadone, codeine, meperidine, and fentanyl are examples of drugs in this class. The opiates tend to reduce anxiety and to produce lethargy, apathy, and an inability to concentrate. Opiate users become less active and less responsive to frustration, hunger, and sexual stimulation. These effects are more pronounced in novice users; with repeated use, many effects diminish.

Although the euphoria associated with opiates is an important factor in their abuse, many individuals experience a feeling of vague uneasiness when they first use these drugs. They may feel nauseated, vomit, or have other unpleasant sensations. Opiates are often dependency-producing.

The various opiates have similar effects, but they do differ in dose-response and time-action characteristics. They are sometimes injected under the skin, into the muscles, or directly into the veins. They may also be taken into the body by **absorption** from the stomach and intestine, the nasal membranes, or the lungs. As mentioned earlier, how the drug is taken determines how quickly it enters body tissue. If it is injected intravenously or smoked, the tissue level will change rapidly, and more immediate behavioral changes will result.

Media reports in the early 1990s indicate a resurgence in heroin use. This may primarily be the result of heroin use by crack cocaine users.

Central Nervous System Depressants

Central nervous system **depressants,** or **sedative-hypnotics,** slow down the overall activity of the nervous system. The result can range from mild **sedation** to death,

depending on the various factors involved—which drug is used, how it's taken, how tolerant the user is, and so on. CNS depressants include alcohol (discussed in Chapter 10), **barbiturates,** antianxiety agents, and various other drugs with similar effects.

Effects CNS depressants reduce anxiety and produce mood changes, muscular incoordination, slurring of speech, and drowsiness or sleep. Mental and motor functioning are also affected, but the degree varies from person to person and also depends on the kind of task the person is trying to do. Most people become drowsy with small doses, although a few become more active. When people take these drugs deliberately to alter their awareness or for social reasons, they can overcome most of the sedative effects and remain awake even with large doses, particularly if they have developed tolerance or if the environment is exciting. However, even though users may remain awake, their mental and motor functioning is affected.

Types A variety of barbiturates is available. They are similar in chemical composition and action, but they do differ in how quickly they act and how long their action lasts. Drug users call barbiturates "downers" or "downs" and refer to specific brands by names that describe the color and design of the capsules: "reds" or "red devils" for Seconal, "yellows" or "yellow jackets" for Nembutal, "blue heavens" for Amytal, and "trees" for Tuinal (a combination of secobarbital and amobarbital). People usually take barbiturates in capsules, but injecting them is also common.

Antianxiety agents, also termed tranquilizers, include the benzodiazepines such as Valium and Librium. Other CNS depressants include methaqualone (Quaalude is the trade name of a common methaqualone compound), ethchlorvynol (Placidyl), and chloral hydrate.

Medical Uses Barbiturates, antianxiety agents, and other sedative-hypnotics are widely used to treat insom-

"High" The subjectively pleasing effects of a drug, usually felt quite soon after the drug is taken.

Central nervous system The brain and spinal cord.

Euphoria An exaggerated feeling of well-being.

Absorption The passage of substances through the skin, lungs, or gastrointestinal tract into the blood.

Depressant Something that decreases nervous or muscular activity.

Sedative-hypnotics Another term for central nervous system depressants. These drugs cause drowsiness or sleep.

Sedation The induction of a calm, relaxed, often sleepy state.

Barbiturate A common sedative-hypnotic drug.

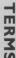

TERMS

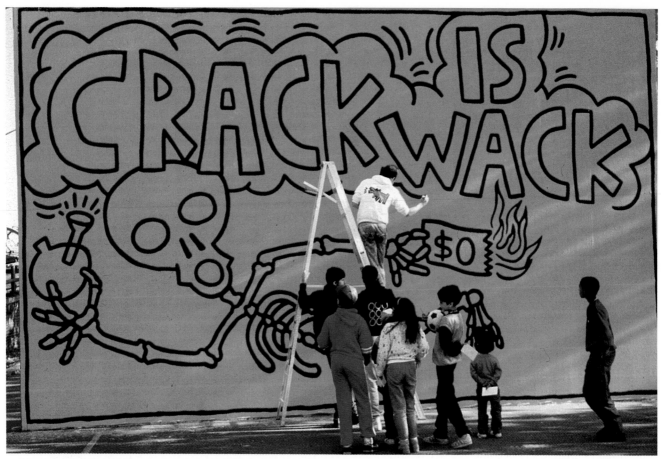

With the introduction of crack cocaine in the 1980s, the use of drugs and the incidence of associated crime rose dramatically in the United States, especially in the cities. This playground backboard, painted by the late Keith Haring, attempts to raise awareness among young people about the consequences of crack use.

nia and anxiety disorders and to control seizures. They are also used to modify the effects of other drugs (for example, to reduce the excessive physical activity that often accompanies the use of CNS stimulants). Some CNS depressants are used for their calming properties in combination with **anesthetic agents** before operations and other medical or dental procedures.

From Use to Abuse   People are usually introduced to CNS depressants either through a medical prescription or through drug-using peers. Abuse of CNS depressants for the medical patient may begin with repeated use for insomnia and progress to dependency through bigger and bigger doses at night coupled with a few capsules at stressful times during the day. The abuse of tranquilizers such as Valium often involves increasingly frequent doses during the day. If a person tries to reduce or stop the medication, feelings of anxiety may occur; the anxiety is "treated" with another dose.

Most CNS depressants, including alcohol and the barbiturates, can lead to classical physical dependence. Tolerance, sometimes for up to 15 times the usual dose, can develop during a year or two of repeated use. Tranquilizers have been shown to produce physical dependence even at ordinary prescribed doses. Withdrawal symptoms can be as severe as those accompanying opiate dependence and are similar to the DTs of alcoholism. They may begin as anxiety, shaking, and weakness but may turn into convulsions and possible cardiovascular collapse, which may result in death.

While intoxicated, people on depressants cannot function very well. They are mentally confused and are frequently obstinate, irritable, and abusive. After long-term use, depressants like alcohol can lead to generally poor health and brain damage, with impaired ability to reason and make judgments. The lack of judgment and physical coordination caused by these drugs often results in injuries and accidents.

Barbiturate dependents, like alcoholics and opiate addicts, often become preoccupied with having enough of the drug and sometimes resort to criminal activities to make sure they do. Violent behavior has also been linked with barbiturate dependence and with the use of methaqualone.

TABLE 11-1 Why Crack Cocaine Poses Particular Problems

Crack Cocaine	Comparison Drugs
Rapid onset of effects.	Drugs ingested or sniffed have much slower onset.
Initial effect usually intense euphoria.	Other drugs less intense.
More "brain rewarding" than any other drug.	Preferred over all other drugs in animal self-administration studies.
Short duration of effects with abrupt termination of pleasurable effects.	Almost all other drugs have more gradual termination of their effects. "Let-down" less intense.
Often no obvious side effects.	Alcohol and other CNS depressants often cause slurring of speech, etc. Opiates often cause drowsiness.
No odor.	Marijuana and alcohol have distinctive odors.
Can be smoked.	"Regular" cocaine does not vaporize and thus is usually sniffed or injected.
Sold in smaller, less expensive doses.	"Regular" cocaine is too expensive for many people to use.

Overdosing with CNS Depressants   Barbiturates and other sedative-hypnotics are common agents of self-destruction. Barbiturate overdose is one of the most frequent methods of suicide among American women and accounts for over 3,000 known deaths each year in the United States. Accidental overdose can occur because the margin between a dose that produces the effects the user wants and a dose that is lethal narrows as tolerance develops. Accidental deaths can also result when people use two or more CNS depressants together, such as barbiturates and alcohol. Even if a single dose of either would not have been fatal, the combined depressant effects of both can halt breathing.

Central Nervous System Stimulants

CNS **stimulants** speed up the activity of the nervous system. Under their influence, heart rate accelerates, blood pressure rises, blood vessels constrict, the pupils of the eyes and the bronchial tubes dilate, and gastric and adrenal secretions increase. There is greater muscular tension and sometimes an increase in motor activity. Small

doses usually make people feel more awake and alert, less fatigued and bored. The most common CNS stimulants are cocaine, amphetamine, nicotine (discussed in Chapter 9), and caffeine.

Cocaine   Usually derived from the leaves of coca shrubs that grow high in the Andes Mountains, cocaine is a potent CNS stimulant. For centuries natives of the Andes have chewed coca leaves both for pleasure and to increase their endurance. For a short time in the nineteenth century, some physicians were enthusiastic about the use of cocaine to cure alcoholism and addiction to morphine, which was used as a painkiller. As is so often the case with new drug treatments, enthusiasm waned after the adverse side effects became apparent.

Cocaine—also known as "coke" or "snow"—quickly produces a feeling of euphoria, which makes it a popular recreational drug. Cocaine—snorted, or inhaled—enjoyed a rapid surge in popularity during the early 1980s, when the drug's high price made it a "status" drug. Since 1985, cocaine use among casual drug users appears to have leveled off, but the drug remains one of this country's leading public health problems. As its price has dropped, it has entered virtually all social and economic groups in this country. The last 10 years have seen a dramatic increase in the popularity of injecting it with another drug such as heroin and of smoking it. Cocaine-related deaths and emergency room visits have increased over the same period.

Methods of Use   Cocaine is usually snorted or injected intravenously, since those methods of administration provide more rapid increases of the drug's concentration in the blood and hence more intense effects. Another method of use involves heating the cocaine with ether or other chemicals and then inhaling its vapors. In "free-basing," as this practice is called, the user risks burns from sudden combustion.

A chemically similar method of processing cocaine involves baking soda and water. This yields a ready-to-smoke form of free-base cocaine, often called crack. Crack is typically available as small beads or pellets smokable in glass pipes or sprinkled on tobacco or marijuana. The tiny but potent beads can be handled more easily than cocaine powder and marketed in smaller, less expensive doses. Thus, processing cocaine into crack has increased cocaine availability to young people and others who couldn't afford to buy more expensive preparations (Table 11-1). The crack epidemic, meanwhile, now plays

Anesthetic agents   Drugs that produce loss of sensation with or without loss of consciousness.

Stimulant   Something that increases nervous or muscular activity.

TERMS

a major role in the spread of HIV infection. Crack use often involves the exchange of sex for drugs or sex for money to buy drugs.

Effects   The effects of cocaine are usually intense but short-lived. The euphoria lasts from 5 to 20 minutes and ends abruptly, to be replaced by irritability, anxiety, or slight depression. When cocaine is absorbed via the lungs, either by smoking or inhalation, it reaches the brain in 10 seconds or so, and the effects are particularly intense. This is part of the appeal of both free-basing and smoking crack. The effects from intravenous injections occur almost as quickly—20 seconds. Since the mucous membranes in the nose briefly slow absorption, the onset of effects from snorting takes 2 or 3 minutes. Heavy users who want to maintain the effects inject cocaine intravenously every 10 to 20 minutes.

The larger the dose of cocaine and the more rapidly it is absorbed into the bloodstream, the greater the immediate—and sometimes lethal—effects. Sudden death from cocaine is most commonly the result of excessive CNS stimulation that causes convulsions and respiratory collapse, cardiac arrhythmias (irregularities in heartbeat), excessive constriction of the arteries to the heart causing ischemia (lack of oxygen to heart muscle), and possibly heart attacks or strokes. Although rare, fatalities can occur in young, athletic people who have no underlying health problems.

Cocaine users sometimes try to alter or control their experience by using "speedball" mixtures, which combine cocaine with a depressant. However, the rapid changes thus imposed on the CNS are sometimes fatal. Comedian John Belushi died from a combination of intravenous cocaine and heroin.

Cocaine constricts the blood vessels and it acts as a local anesthetic. It is still used for minor nose surgery where bleeding is a problem. However, in the chronic cocaine snorter, repeated **vasoconstriction** produces inflammation of the nasal mucosa, which can lead to persistent bleeding and ulceration of the septum between the nostrils. Cocaine users may also become paranoid or violent.

Abuse and Dependence   When steady cocaine users stop taking the drug, they experience a sudden "crash," characterized by depression, agitation, and fatigue, followed by a period of withdrawal. Their depression can be temporarily relieved by taking more cocaine, so its continued use is reinforced. Cocaine use follows different patterns among different individuals. A binge cocaine user may go for weeks or months without using any co-

caine and then take large amounts repeatedly. Although not physically dependent, a binge cocaine user who misses work or school and risks serious health consequences is clearly abusing the drug.

Cocaine Use During Pregnancy   An alarming number of babies are being exposed to cocaine before birth. A survey by the U.S. Department of Health and Human Services reported that nearly 9,000 "crack babies" were born in eight major cities in 1989. Cocaine rapidly crosses the placenta and has many serious effects on the fetus. A woman who uses cocaine during pregnancy is at higher risk for premature labor and stillbirth. Her infant is at increased risk for limb and heart defects, hearing problems, stroke, heart rhythm irregularities, intestinal problems, and death from sudden infant death syndrome; the type of problem depends on a variety of factors, including when during pregnancy the cocaine was used.

Infants whose mothers use cocaine may also be born dependent on the drug. These infants often experience withdrawal after birth. They are typically irritable, jittery, and do not eat or sleep properly. They don't respond to people in the way healthy babies do, and they are difficult to comfort or console. These characteristics affect their social and emotional development because it's difficult for adults to interact with them.

Cocaine-affected children are at increased risk for developmental delays and learning and behavior problems in their first year of life. Recent research suggests that some of these problems can disappear later in childhood if the drug-exposed infants receive adequate nutrition and skilled parenting. But children who grow up in cocaine-abusing families are at high risk for continuing problems, including accidental drug poisoning. Infants and children can also become intoxicated from the environmental smoke of free-base or crack cocaine. Cocaine passes into breast milk, as well, where it can intoxicate a breastfeeding infant.

It's estimated that the cost of caring for cocaine-affected babies could total $500 million for hospital and foster care through age 5 and an additional 1.5 billion for preparing them for school. Clearly, this is one of the major problems our society faces in the coming years.

Amphetamines   Amphetamines are a group of synthetic chemicals that are potent CNS stimulants. Some common amphetamines are dextroamphetamine (Dexedrine), *d-1*-amphetamine (Benzedrine), and methamphetamine (Methedrine). Popular names for these drugs change often and are different in different parts of the country. Some of the more common names are "speed," "crank," "crystal," and "meth."

"Ice," a smokeable, high-potency form of methamphetamine, has grown rapidly in popularity in recent years, especially on the West Coast and in Hawaii. Easy to manufacture, ice is cheaper than crack and produces a eu-

TERMS

Vasoconstriction   A constriction of the blood vessels.
State dependency   Situation where information learned in a drug-induced state is difficult to recall when the effects of the drugs wear off.

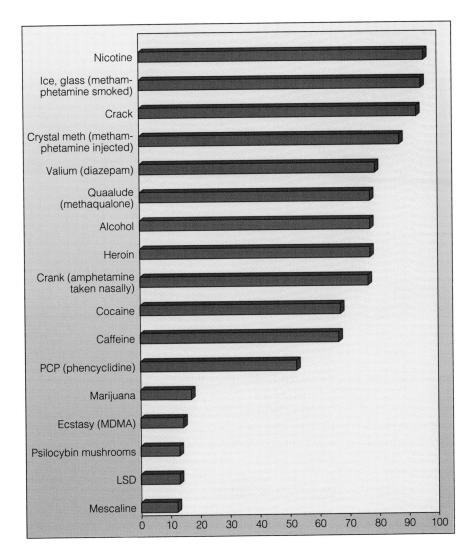

Figure 11-3 *How easy is it to get hooked on drugs?*
The numbers at the bottom of the chart are relative rankings. *Source:* L. Davis. 1990. "Why Do People Take Drugs?" *In Health,* November/December.

phoria similar to that produced by cocaine but lasting much longer. Use of ice can quickly lead to dependence (Figure 11-3). In Hawaii, law enforcement officials reported in 1990 that ice had surpassed crack as that state's number one drug problem. As the decade opened, many emergency rooms on the West Coast were treating more ice users than cocaine users for drug-related problems.

Effects Small doses of amphetamines usually make people feel better, more alert and wide-awake, and less fatigued or bored. Small doses can produce some improvement in activities—like certain athletic contests or military maneuvers—that require extreme physical effort or endurance. Amphetamines generally increase motor activity but do not measurably alter a normal, rested person's ability to perform tasks calling for complex motor skills or high-level thinking. When amphetamines do improve performance, it's primarily by counteracting fatigue and boredom. Amphetamines in small doses also increase the heart rate and blood pressure and change sleep patterns.

Amphetamines are sometimes used to curb appetite, but after a few weeks the user develops tolerance, and higher doses are necessary. When people stop taking the drug, their appetites usually rebound, and they gain back the weight they lost unless they have made permanent changes in eating behavior. Amphetamines have other medical uses, but many physicians doubt their usefulness and consider other approaches more worthwhile and not as risky.

From Use to Abuse Much amphetamine abuse begins as an attempt to cope with a passing situation. A student cramming for exams or an exhausted long-haul truck driver can go a little longer by "popping a benny," but the results can be disastrous. The likelihood of making bad judgments significantly increases. An additional danger is that the stimulating effects may wear off suddenly, and the user may precipitously feel exhausted or fall asleep ("crash").

Another problem is **state dependency,** the phenomenon whereby information learned in a certain drug-induced state is difficult to recall when the person is not in that same physiological state. Test performance may dete-

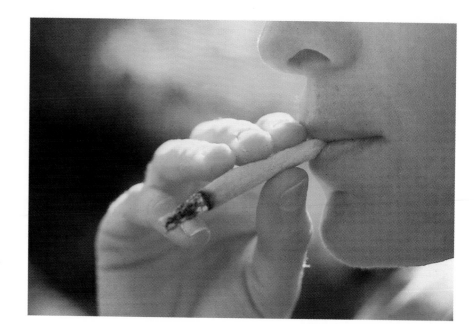

Marijuana is the most widely used illicit drug in the United States. At low doses, marijuana users typically experience euphoria and a relaxed attitude. Further research is needed to determine its precise physiological and psychological effects, particularly for chronic use.

riorate when students use drugs to study and then take tests in their normal, nondrug state.

Dependence   Repeated use of amphetamines, even in moderate doses, often leads to tolerance and the need for larger and larger doses. The result can be severe disturbances in behavior, including paranoid **psychosis** with illusions, hostility, delusions of persecution, and unprovoked violence. It is just like a nondrug psychosis except that it ends if the person stops taking the drug.

If injected in large doses, amphetamines produce a feeling of intense pleasure, followed by sensations of vigor and euphoria that last for several hours. As these feelings wear off, they are replaced by feelings of irritability and vague uneasiness. Long-term use of ice at high doses can cause paranoia, hallucinations, delusions, and incoherence. Withdrawal symptoms may include muscle aches and tremors, along with profound fatigue, deep depression, despair, and apathy. Chronic high-dose amphetamine use is often associated with pronounced psychological dependence. Chronic abusers frequently spend much of their time obsessively seeking drugs.

Women who use amphetamines during pregnancy risk premature birth, stillbirth, and early infant death. Babies born to amphetamine-using mothers have a higher incidence of cleft palate, cleft lip, and missing or deformed limbs. They may also be born dependent on amphetamines.

Other hazards of amphetamine use include malnutrition, weight loss, damage to blood vessels, strokes, and other changes in the heart and blood vessels. The use of the injection method brings an added danger, the risk of HIV infection and other blood-borne diseases from contaminated needles.

Caffeine   Caffeine is probably the most popular psychoactive drug and also one of the most ancient. It is found in coffee, tea, cocoa, soft drinks, headache remedies, and over-the-counter drugs like No-Doz. In ordinary doses caffeine produces greater alertness and a sense of well-being. It also cuts down on feelings of fatigue or boredom, and using caffeine may enable a person to keep at physically exhausting or repetitive tasks longer. Such use is usually followed, however, by a sudden letdown. Caffeine does not noticeably influence a person's ability to perform complex intellectual tasks unless fatigue, boredom, alcohol, or other factors have already affected normal performance.

Caffeine mildly stimulates the heart and respiratory system, it increases muscular tremor, and it enhances gastric secretion. Higher doses may cause nervousness, anxiety, irritability, headache, disturbed sleep, and gastric irritation or peptic ulcers. In women, excessive caffeine consumption may aggravate the symptoms associated with premenstrual syndrome. Some people, especially children, are quite vulnerable to the adverse effects of caffeine. They become "wired"—hyperactive and exquisitely sensitive to any stimulation in their environment. In rare instances, the disturbance is so severe that there is misperception of their surroundings—a toxic psychosis.

TERMS

Psychosis   A severe mental disorder in which there is a distortion of reality. Symptoms might include delusions or hallucinations.

Depersonalization   A state in which a person loses the sense of his or her own reality or perceives his or her own body as unreal.

TABLE 11-2 The Daily Dose

This chart will help you calculate your daily caffeine intake. But remember, caffeine content varies widely, depending on the product you use and how it's prepared.

Beverages	Serving Size	Caffeine (mg)
Coffee, drip	7.5 oz	115–175
Coffee, perk	7.5 oz	80–135
Coffee, instant	7.5 oz	65–100
Coffee, decaffeinated	7.5 oz	3–4
Tea, 1 minute steep	5 oz	20
Tea, 3-minute steep	5 oz	35
Tea, iced	12 oz	70
Coca-Cola	12 oz	45
Mountain Dew	12 oz	54
Dr. Pepper	12 oz	40
Pepsi Cola	12 oz	38
7 Up	12 oz	0

Foods	Serving Size	Caffeine (mg)
Milk chocolate	1 oz	1–15
Bittersweet chocolate	1 oz	5–35
Chocolate cake	1 slice	20–30

Over-the-Counter Drugs	Dose	Caffeine (mg)
Anacin, Empirin, or Midol	2	64
Excedrin	2	130
NoDoz	2	200
Aqua-Ban (diuretic)	2	200
Dexatrim (weight control aid)	1	200

Sources: Tony Chou. 1992. "Wake Up and Smell the Coffee." *Western Journal of Medicine* 157:544–53; "Caffeine Update: The News Is Mostly Good." *University of California at Berkeley Wellness Letter,* July 1988.

Drinks containing caffeine are rarely harmful for most individuals, but some tolerance develops and withdrawal symptoms of irritability, headaches, and even mild depression do occur. Thus, although we don't usually think of caffeine as a dependency-producing drug, it is. People can usually avoid problems by simply decreasing their daily intake of caffeine (Table 11-2).

Marijuana and Other Cannabis Products

Marijuana is the most widely used illicit drug in the United States (cocaine is second), although use is not as high as it was in the late 1970s. The National Institute on Drug Abuse reports that nearly 62 million Americans over the age of 12—about one in three—have tried marijuana at least once. In 1991, an estimated 26 percent of high school students had tried marijuana and 11 percent were current users.

Marijuana is a crude preparation of various parts of the Indian hemp plant, *Cannabis sativa,* which grows in most parts of the world. THC (tetrahydrocannabinol) is the main active ingredient in marijuana. Hashish is a potent cannabis preparation derived mainly from the thick resinous materials of the flowering tops and upper leaves of the plant. THC can be synthesized, but it is an expensive process. Because of the cost, pure THC is virtually never available on the illicit market. Drugs sold as THC are almost always something else, such as methamphetamine.

Marijuana is usually smoked, but can also be ingested. Although it is usually thought of as a psychedelic, the classification of marijuana is a matter of some debate. For this reason, it is treated separately here.

Short-Term Effects and Uses As is true with most psychoactive drugs, the effects of a low dose of marijuana are strongly influenced by what the user expects and what his or her previous experience with the drug has been. At low doses, marijuana users typically experience euphoria, heightening of subjective sensory experiences, slowing down of the time sense, and a relaxed, "laid-back" attitude. These pleasant effects are the reason why this drug is so widely used. With moderate doses, these effects become stronger, and the user can also expect to have impaired memory function, disturbed thought patterns, lapses of attention, and feelings of **depersonalization,** in which the mind seems to be separated from the body. Decreased driving and workplace safety can also be expected.

The effects of marijuana with higher doses are determined mostly by the drug itself rather than by set and setting. Very high doses produce feelings of depersonalization as well as marked sensory distortion and changes in body image (such as a feeling that the body is very light). People who have not had much experience with marijuana sometimes think these sensations mean that they are going crazy and become anxious or even panicky. Such reactions resemble a bad trip on LSD, but they happen much less often, are less severe, and do not last as long.

Physiologically, marijuana chiefly acts to cause increases in heart rate and dilation of certain blood vessels in the eyes, which creates the characteristic bloodshot eyes. The user also feels less inclination for physical exertion.

Cannabis preparations were once medically prescribed for a variety of human illnesses, including insomnia, migraine, depression, and epilepsy. Now, however, none of these uses can be supported. Its medical use for sedative or euphoric effects is limited because of the perceptual and cognitive changes it brings about and also because individual reactions cannot be predicted. Somewhat more promising are current investigations into the use of THC to reduce nausea and improve appetite during cancer chemotherapy. In this situation, adverse side effects are less critical. THC and related compounds are also being studied for possible use in certain forms of glaucoma, an eye disease that causes blindness.

Long-Term Effects Marijuana remains a complex, poorly understood drug; further research is needed to determine its precise physiological and psychological effects. Chronic bronchial irritation is one of the few widely agreed upon long-term effects of chronic marijuana use. Other potential adverse effects include impairment of long-term memory; gum disease; increased risk of cancers of the mouth, jaw, tongue, and lung; and impairment of the immune system. Some studies suggest that long-term marijuana use may result in decreased testosterone levels, decreased sperm counts, and increased sperm abnormalities in male users. Heavy marijuana use during pregnancy may cause impaired fetal growth and development. Some studies also indicate that children whose mothers smoked marijuana just before or during pregnancy may be at increased risk for a rare form of leukemia.

When we consider the long-term effects of marijuana (and of any other drugs), we should keep in mind the time-lag factor. A period of time must pass before long-term effects of a drug can be recognized. Tobacco, for example, was long thought to be a "harmless" drug. Widespread marijuana use has been common for only about 20 years, and some effects may take longer than that to appear.

Dependence Regular users of marijuana can develop a marked tolerance to the drug, but physical dependence characterized by significant withdrawal symptoms has not been well established for marijuana use in either human or animal studies. However, as with all drugs that relieve "bad" feelings and produce "good" feelings, marijuana can become the focus of the user's life to the exclusion of other activities. The chronic marijuana user will not necessarily limit his or her drug use to cannabis. Drug uses appear to be related, and the chronic marijuana user is more likely to be a heavy user of tobacco, alcohol, and other dangerous drugs. The person who buys marijuana is in touch with the illicit drug market, and that contact may be the key to the association between marijuana use and the increased rate of subsequent use of cocaine and heroin.

Psychedelics

The term *psychedelics* refers to a group of drugs whose predominant pharmacological effect is to alter perception, feelings, and thoughts in the user. These drugs are also called hallucinogens, although at low doses hallucinations are not one of their major effects. The psychedelics include LSD (lysergic acid diethylamide), mescaline, psilocybin, STP (dimethoxy-methyl-amphetamine), DMT (dimethyl-tryptamine), and many others. These drugs are most commonly ingested or smoked. LSD ("acid") is the most widely known of the psychedelics, and we discuss it in detail here as an example of the entire group.

LSD LSD is one of the most powerful psychoactive drugs. Tiny doses will produce noticeable effects in most people. These effects include an altered sense of time, disorders of vision, an improved sense of hearing, changes in mood, and distortions in how people perceive their bodies. There is almost always dilation of the pupils, and there may also be slight dizziness, weakness, and nausea. With larger doses, users may experience a phenomenon known as **synesthesia,** feelings of depersonalization, and other alterations in the perceived relationship between self and external reality.

Many psychedelics induce biological tolerance so quickly that after a few days' use their effects are reduced greatly. The user must then stop taking the drug for several days before his or her system can be receptive to it again. These drugs cause little drug-seeking behavior and no physical dependence or withdrawal symptoms.

The immediate effects of low doses of psychedelics are largely determined by set and setting. Many effects of psychedelics are hard to describe because they involve subjective and unusual dimensions of awareness—the **altered states of consciousness** for which psychedelics are famous. For this reason, psychedelics have acquired a certain aura not associated with other drugs. Some people have taken LSD in search of a religious or mystical experience, or in the hope of exploring new worlds, or as therapy, in an attempt to solve their problems.

A severe panic reaction, which can be terrifying in the extreme, can occur at any dose of LSD. It is impossible to predict when a panic reaction will occur. Some LSD users report having hundreds of pleasurable and ecstatic experiences before an inexplicable "bad trip," or "bummer." If the user is already in a serene mood and feels no anger or hostility and if he or she is in secure surroundings with trusted companions, a bad trip may be less likely, but a tranquil experience is not guaranteed.

Even after the drug's chemical effects have worn off, spontaneous flashbacks and other psychological disturbances can occur. Flashbacks are perceptual distortions and bizarre thoughts that occur after the drug has been entirely eliminated from the body. Flashbacks are relatively rare phenomena, but they can be extremely distressing. They are often triggered by specific psychological cues associated with the drug-taking experience, such as certain mood states or even types of music.

Researchers in the 1970s claimed that LSD damages

chromosomes. Evidence so far indicates that LSD in moderate doses, at least the pure LSD produced in the laboratory, does not damage chromosomes, cause detectable genetic damage, or produce birth defects.

A federal Drug Enforcement Administration survey released in 1991 suggests that LSD may be enjoying a revival among high school students. The survey found nearly 19 percent of white males in some affluent suburban high schools had tried LSD or another hallucinogen. Overall, 6 percent of the high school seniors surveyed had tried LSD or another hallucinogen during the previous year, more than the 4 percent who reported using cocaine during the preceding 12 months. Among college students surveyed, almost 10 percent reported having tried LSD at least once.

Other Psychedelics   Most other psychedelics have the same general effects that LSD has, but there are some variations. As in LSD use, the effects of small doses depend largely on psychological and social factors, the set, and the setting. A DMT high does not last as long as an LSD high. An STP trip, in contrast, lasts longer than an LSD trip. Ditran and related compounds cause greater intellectual impairment and confusion than do other psychedelics.

Mescaline (peyote), the ceremonial drug of the Native North American Church, supposedly produces a trip different from that caused by LSD. Obtaining mescaline costs far more than making LSD, however, so most street mescaline is LSD that has been highly diluted. Psychedelic effects can be obtained from certain mushrooms (*Psilocybe mexicana,* or "magic mushrooms"), certain morning glory seeds, nutmeg, jimsonweed, and other botanical products, but unpleasant side effects, such as dizziness, have limited the popularity of these products.

Deliriants

Many drugs, and other substances not usually thought of as drugs, can bring on a form of abnormal behavior called **delirium,** or toxic psychosis. Delirium results from a temporary impairment of brain function. Different chemicals act on the brain in different ways, but the results are generally similar. They consist of changing levels of awareness to surrounding events, decreased ability to maintain attention to a task, and variable amounts of mental confusion. The user may also experience hallucinations, especially visual ones.

PCP   Phencyclidine, also known as "angel dust," "PCP," "hog," and "peace pill," is a widely used synthetic drug that can be considered a deliriant. PCP reduces and distorts sensory input, especially **proprioception** (awareness of the position of arms and legs, joints, and so forth), and creates a state of sensory deprivation. This drug was initially used as a human anesthetic, but was unsatisfactory because of the postoperative agitation, confusion, and delirium its use caused. Since the ingredients of PCP are readily obtainable and it can be easily made, it is often available on the illicit market and is sometimes used as a cheap adulterant for other psychoactive agents.

Following the faddish pattern of use of most psychedelics, PCP was extensively used in the mid-1960s. It declined in popularity when that generation became aware of the prevalence of adverse side effects, including convulsions, memory impairments, coma, and occasionally death. In the mid-1970s PCP again became widely used and now in the 1990s is again a major drug problem.

Inhalants   Delirium can be produced by inhaling certain chemicals, such as some glues, gases in aerosols, kerosene, gasoline, butyl nitrite, and anesthetic agents like laughing gas (nitrous oxide). Most inhaled chemicals interfere directly with brain function, but some do so indirectly by interfering with oxygen exchange in the lungs. Inhalants can be very dangerous to health; high concentrations of these substances in the blood can cause brain, liver, and kidney damage or even asphyxiation.

Designer Drugs

A relatively recent addition to the group of psychoactive chemicals, **"designer drugs"** are new compounds produced in clandestine laboratories. They are created by modifying existing drugs to produce **analogues.** An analogue has effects similar to those of the drug it is designed to mimic, but its origins and chemical structure are different. Use of designer drugs is increasing.

Two types of synthetic opiates have become popular designer drugs because of their heroin-like effects (Table 11-3). Analogues of the drug meperidine (Demerol), marketed as "new heroin" or "synthetic heroin," first came to the attention of physicians because some people devel-

---

TERMS

Synesthesia   A condition in which a stimulus evokes not only the sensation appropriate to it but also another sensation of a different character. An example is when a color evokes a specific smell.

Altered states of consciousness   Profound changes in mood, thinking, and perception.

Chromosome   Microscopic bodies in the cell nucleus. The chromosomes carry the genes that convey hereditary characteristics.

Delirium   A reversible state of mental confusion sometimes marked by emotional excitement.

Proprioception   The sensory processes that identify the position and movement of muscles, tendons, and joints.

Designer drugs   Drugs created by altering the chemical structure of existing compounds to produce analogues with similar effects.

Analogue   A drug similar in function to the drug from which it is derived, but with a different origin.

TABLE 11-3 Common "Designer" Drugs

Fentanyl derivatives
  alpha-methyl-fentanyl ("China white")
  3-methyl-fentanyl

Meperidine derivatives
  MPPP
  MPTP

Mescaline-methamphetamine derivatives
  MDMA ("Ecstasy," "XTC," "Adam," "M & M," "Hug drug")
  MDA ("Love drug")
  MDEA ("Eve")

Phencyclidine (PCP) derivatives
  PCPy
  PCE
  TCP

Adapted from G. L. Sternback and J. Varon. 1991. "Designer Drugs: Recognizing and Managing Their Toxic Effects." *Postgraduate Medicine* 91(8).

another designer drug category. MDA, known on the street as the "love drug," became a popular drug of abuse in the late 1960s. This amphetamine analogue produces a mild euphoria. Those who take it experience a desire to be with and talk to people. Like amphetamine, which it mimics, MDA can be fatal.

MDMA, known as "ecstasy" or "Adam" on the street, is chemically similar to both methamphetamine and mescaline. The drug stimulates the central nervous system and causes hallucinogenic effects. MDMA can elevate users' moods and increase feelings of intimacy with others. But it also may cause panic, anxiety, paranoid thinking, rapid heart rate, jaw clenching, involuntary eye twitching, and shaking. An overdose can cause life-threatening disturbances in heart rhythm, high blood pressure, and seizures. After a number of deaths were linked to its use during the 1980s, the United States Drug Enforcement Administration (DEA) designated MDMA a controlled substance. Designer drug manufacturers responded to the DEA action by synthesizing a similar analogue, known on the street as "Eve." Eve is not yet regulated, but is capable of producing adverse effects similar to those produced by amphetamine and other amphetamine analogues.

oped irreversible **parkinsonism** after taking the drug. Sufferers of this neurological condition experience loss of facial expression, drooling, a shuffling gait, and tremor of the hands, arms, and legs. An occasional by-product of designer heroin production caused the parkinsonism. Analogues of the drug fentanyl (Sublimaze) make up a second type of designer opiate. The best known is sold on the street as "China white." Initially touted as a safe alternative to heroin, the drug turned out to be a thousand times more potent than heroin. Numerous cases of fatal overdoses of China white have been reported since its introduction in 1979.

Methamphetamine and mescaline analogues constitute

DRUG USE: THE DECADES AHEAD

Drug research will undoubtedly provide new information, new treatments, and new chemical combinations in the decades ahead. New psychoactive drugs may present unexpected possibilities for therapy, social use, and abuse. Making honest and unbiased information about drugs available to everyone, however, may cut down on their abuse. Lies about the dangers of drugs—"scare tactics"—can lead some people to disbelieve any reports of drug dangers, no matter how soundly based and well documented they are.

Although the use of some drugs, both legal and illegal,

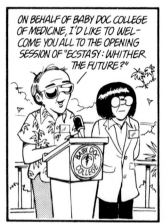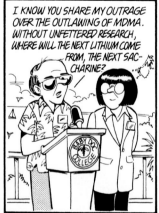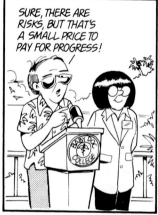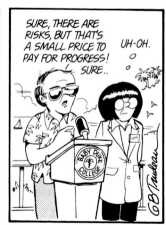

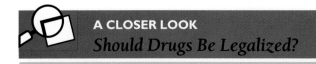

In a reversal of their usual political stances, some liberals are calling for increased drug-law enforcement and some conservatives are calling for controlled legalization of drugs. The conservative position reflects a growing sense of pessimism over the effectiveness of the nation's drug programs, as well as doubt that the present system of seizure, punishment, and treatment will ever eliminate the drug problem.

Ethan A. Nadelman, assistant professor of politics and public affairs at Princeton University, writes that drug traffickers—from the notorious foreign drug cartels to the local dealers—are the greatest beneficiaries of present anti-drug laws. He draws a tight connection between illicit drugs and crime, pointing out that crimes by drug users usually are committed to buy drugs that cost relatively more than alcohol and tobacco because they are produced illegally.

Contradicting popular wisdom, Nadelman believes that the drugs themselves are not the problem. He claims that most users of cocaine don't get into trouble with the drug itself. The nation's leaders should look at illicit drugs the same way they look at alcohol and tobacco, according to Nadelman. Some people drink and smoke to excess and require some forms of treatment, but many don't. Legalization of both tobacco and liquor have eliminated crimes associated with their sale.

Opponents of legalization respond that alcohol and tobacco are major causes of disease and death in our society and that they shouldn't be used as a model for other practices. They feel that regardless of practical issues, decriminalization would give drugs an approval that they don't now have. This factor would be particularly important in how children and teenagers regard drugs. Many opponents of legalization believe that government, as the agent of society, is responsible for helping to instill certain values and virtues in people, such as decency, dignity, self-control, duty, and responsibility. Drug-dependent people, they claim, are unlikely to make productive workers, good parents, reliable neighbors, or safe drivers—qualities considered desirable by most people.

Opponents of legalization also believe that more people would use drugs if they were legal, especially since they would be less expensive and easier to get, and that this would lead to a greater number of drug-degraded people in our society. There would still be tremendous costs associated with drugs for regulation and enforcement of controls. Opponents of legalization believe that the best ways to stop drugs are intensified prosecution and enforcement, widespread testing, community cooperation with police to reassert public control over streets and parks, and improved drug education programs in the schools.

What do you think?

Adapted from R. G. Fichenberg. 1989. "Schultz Backs Legalized Drugs." *San Francisco Examiner,* 31 October; and J. Q. Wilson and J. J. Dilulio, Jr. 1989. "Crackdown." *The New Republic,* 10 July.

---

has declined dramatically since the 1970s, the use of others has held steady, or increased. Mounting public concern has led to great debate and a wide range of opinions about what should be done. Efforts to combat the problem include workplace drug testing; tougher law enforcement and prosecution; and treatment and education. The legalization of drugs has also been proposed as a strategy to help control our nation's drug problem (see the box "Should Drugs Be Legalized?"). With drugs entering the country on a massive scale from South America, Southeast Asia, and elsewhere and distributed through tightly controlled drug-smuggling organizations and street gangs, it remains to be seen how effective any program will be.

Drug Testing

One of the more controversial issues in American politics is drug testing in the workplace. It has been estimated that many workers, perhaps 1 in 10, use psychoactive drugs on the job. For some occupations, such as air traffic controllers, truck drivers, and train conductors, drug use can create significant dangers, sometimes involving hundreds of people. Some people believe that the dangers are so great that all workers should be tested and that anyone found to have traces of drugs in the blood or urine should be fired or treated. Others insist that this would violate people's right to privacy and to the freedom from unreasonable search guaranteed by the Fourth Amendment. Proponents then ask whether companies who don't test for drugs should be liable for damages if their employees cause harm to others.

Many employers now test their employees, and the U.S. armed forces test military personnel on a regular basis. However, drug testing is expensive, with costs running as high as $100 per individual test; and questions about accuracy and reliability complicate the issue. Another factor to be considered is that most jobs don't involve hazards, so employees who are on drugs aren't any

Parkinsonism A syndrome characterized by a masklike expression, shuffling gait, drooling, and tremor; can be drug-induced.

TERMS

A Traditional Approach to a Modern Problem

At Four Cedars Medicine Lodge in northern Washington state, several young Native Americans cluster inside a heated sweat lodge. Crouched there in the small, dark space, they burn sage, sweet grass, and other wild herbs in a purifying ceremony. They perform a ritual using stones, feathers, and other symbolic objects that are believed to help release and absorb feelings. And as they pass around the circle a pebble that signals their turn to talk, they describe their struggles with alcohol and drugs and the support they get from their own cultural traditions.

Four Cedars Medicine Lodge is just one of hundreds of substance-abuse programs across the country funded by the U.S. Public Health Service and run by Native American health professionals. Many of these programs incorporate elements from Native American belief systems—ceremonies, rituals, prayers, chants—to prevent and treat alcohol and drug abuse. "You get strength to carry you through your lifetime from your culture," says Norma Joseph, director of Four Cedars and a member of the Sauk tribe with a master's degree in anthropology from UCLA. Dan Flavin, medical director for the National Council on Alcohol and Drug Abuse, agrees that "the development of a cultural identity is very important" in preventing alcohol and drug dependence.

Four Cedars is operated by seven tribes located in northern Washington. In addition to canvas teepees and sweat houses, there are dormitories, a library, a gym, and classrooms with computers. The youths in the program are considered at risk for alcohol abuse and have been referred by schools, social service agencies, and courts. They spend from 2 to 10 weeks at the lodge, taking classes, receiving counseling, and learning traditional ways from tribal elders. Participants discover that their native culture offers resources to help them resist alcohol and drugs—family and community support; the opportunity to talk, listen, and share with peers and elders; pride in themselves and their cultural heritage; and practical alternatives for real-life situations.

These treatment and prevention programs aren't aimed at just adolescents and young adults. In Seattle, an after-school, neighborhood-based program called the Children of the Circle provides both a gathering place and a sense of community for the 1,400 Native American children enrolled in city elementary schools. Children beat drums with elders, sing in their native languages, and practice traditional arts and crafts. They also learn about the dangers of drug and alcohol abuse and the healthy alternatives offered by their own culture.

Currently the Indian Health Service, a division of the U.S. Public Health Service, provides substance-abuse treatment for over 20,000 Native Americans through 340 community-based programs from Florida to Alaska. Nearly all the programs have a cultural component. In contrast to earlier programs, which were often perceived as imposed by outside agencies, these programs arise from within the community and make sense in the context of Native American traditions.

How effective are the programs? Success is difficult to assess, but many believe the alcoholism problem among Native Americans is improving because of traditional approaches. To measure the impact of alcoholism, the Indian Health Service uses alcohol-related mortality rates. When these programs were just getting started, in 1969, the mortality rate from alcoholism was 56.6 per 100,000 population. In 1988 it was 33.9 per 100,000. Officials in the Indian Health Service say the treatment programs account for this decrease: "Communities have now taken responsibility for their own wellness. That's having a big impact." In addition to community responsibility, these successes can be attributed to the nature of the programs themselves, with their focus on social support, feelings of pride and belonging, and practical alternatives to alcohol and drugs.

Adapted from: K. D. Rauch. 1992. "How Indian Youths Defeat Addictions." *Washington Post Health,* 10 March.

---

more dangerous than employees who aren't on drugs. All these legal and practical issues mean that drug testing is likely to remain controversial in the 1990s.

Treatment for Drug Dependence

A variety of programs is available to help people break their drug habits. Professional treatment programs usually take the form of drug substitution programs or programs operated by rehabilitation centers. Nonprofessional self-help groups and peer counseling are also available. There is no single best method of treatment, and the relapse rate is high for all types of treatment (Figure 11-4). To be successful, a treatment program must deal with the reasons behind people's drug abuse and

help them develop behaviors, attitudes, and a social support system that will help them remain drug-free (see the box "A Traditional Approach to a Modern Problem").

Drug Substitution Programs   Sometimes a less debilitating drug can be substituted for one with many damaging effects, thus reducing the "costs," or risks, of the drug use. Methadone is a synthetic drug used as a substitute for heroin. When methadone is used, addicts can stop taking heroin without experiencing severe withdrawal reactions. Methadone is addictive too, but it decreases the craving for heroin and allows the individual to function normally in personal, social, and vocational activities. It also blocks the action of narcotics, so addicts don't get high even if they take heroin. Methadone maintenance treatment al-

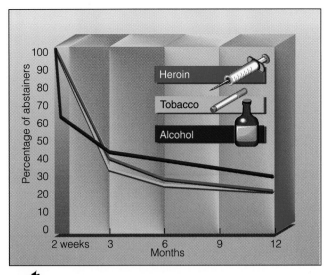

Figure 11-4 *Percentage of people who continue to abstain over time after giving up heroin, tobacco, and alcohol.*

lows many former heroin abusers to live more useful lives.

One disadvantage of methadone is that it is metabolized fairly rapidly (although not as rapidly as heroin) and thus must be taken on a daily basis. Newer heroin substitutes, such as LAAM, are metabolized more slowly still and need to be taken only two to three times a week. Preliminary tests of another new drug, buprenorphine, indicate that it is less addicting and causes fewer withdrawal symptoms than methadone; buprenorphine may become another important treatment for opiate addiction.

Because they are relatively inexpensive to administer, drug substitute programs are a popular form of treatment. However, there is a significant relapse rate from methadone and LAAM treatment programs, as is the case with all drug dependency treatment efforts. This rate is reduced when psychological and social services are also provided, underscoring the importance of psychological factors in drug dependency.

Treatment Centers   The 1980s saw a boom in drug rehabilitation centers. Some national chains built or bought hospitals devoted solely to treating chemical dependency, and many general hospitals opened drug rehabilitation or chemical dependency units. But as the 1990s opened, skyrocketing health care costs caused the closure of many of these centers. Health insurance policies that once covered 30-day stays at drug rehabilitation centers now cover only limited outpatient visits or have no coverage for drug treatment at all. Many people with drug problems may find themselves in an impossible situation: Their employers demand a drug-free workforce but no longer offer insurance that pays for treatment for drug dependence.

Public drug treatment facilities, especially those in urban areas, usually have long waiting lists, sometimes of a year or more. The challenge for the years ahead will be for chemical dependency centers to prove—and improve—their effectiveness and for private employers and public agencies to develop cost-effective ways to meet the needs of people in our society with drug problems.

Most treatment centers offer a variety of short- and long-term services, including hospitalization, detoxification, counseling, and other psychiatric services. A specific type of center is the therapeutic community, a residential program run in a completely drug-free atmosphere. Administered by ex-addicts, these programs use confrontation, strict discipline, and unrelenting peer pressure to attempt to resocialize the addict with a different set of values. "Halfway houses," transition settings between a 24-hour-a-day program and independent living, are an important phase of treatment for some people.

Treatment centers often also offer counseling for those close to drug abusers. Drug abuse takes a toll on friends and family members, and counseling can help people work through painful feelings of guilt and powerlessness. Sometimes people close to a drug abuser develop patterns of behavior that help or enable the person to remain drug-dependent (see the box "Codependency"). Counseling can help people adopt realistic ideas about their role in their loved one's dependence and recovery and identify and change any problematic patterns of behavior.

For help in locating a treatment program in your area, call the National Drug Information and Treatment Hotline at 1-800-662-HELP (Spanish-speaking callers can phone 1-800-66-AYUDA).

Self-Help Groups and Peer Counseling   Groups such as Alcoholics Anonymous (AA) and Narcotics Anonymous (NA) have helped many people. People treated in drug substitution programs or chemical dependency treatment centers are often urged or required to join a self-help group as part of their recovery. As described in Chapter 10, these groups follow a "twelve-step" program. The first step for people in the program is to acknowledge that they have a problem over which they have no control. Peer support is a critical ingredient of these programs. Members usually meet at least once a week. They are paired with buddies they can call for advice and support if a craving or temptation to relapse becomes overwhelming. With such support, thousands of drug-dependent people have been able to recover, remain abstinent, and reclaim their lives. Chapters of AA and NA meet on some college campuses; community-based chapters are listed in the phone book.

Many colleges also have peer counseling programs, in which students are trained to help other students who have drug problems. Students are often drawn to peer counseling work because of a personal or family experience with drug dependency. Depending on the particular

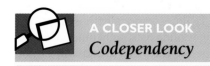

Codependency became a trendy term in the late 1980s, and popular authors attributed a long list of personal and social problems to what they termed "codependent behavior." However, the concept is a useful one for looking at the relationships between drug abusers (and people with other types of self-destructive habits) and those close to them. A codependent is a person who is in a continuing relationship with a drug-abusing person and whose actions help or enable that person to remain dependent. Codependency, also called enabling, removes or softens the effects of the drug use on the user. People often become enablers spontaneously and naturally. When someone they love becomes dependent on a drug, they want to help, and they assume that their good intentions will persuade the drug user to stop. Unfortunately, alcoholics and drug-dependent people have a system of denial that is strengthened rather than diminished by well-meaning attempts to help.

The habit of enabling hinders a drug-dependent person's recovery because the person never has to experience the consequences of his or her behavior. Frequently, the enabler is dependent too—on the pattern of interaction in the relationship. People who need to take care of people often marry people who need to be taken care of. Children in these families often develop the same pattern of behavior as one of their parents, either by becoming helpless or by becoming a caregiver. This is why treatment programs for drug dependency, such as Alcoholics Anonymous, Narcotics Anonymous, and Cocaine Anonymous, involve the whole family.

Have you ever been an enabler in a relationship? You may have if you have ever done any of the following:

- Given someone one more chance to stop abusing drugs, then another, and another . . .

- Made excuses or lied for someone to his or her friends, teachers, or employer

- Joined someone in drug use and blamed others for your behavior

- Lent money to someone to continue drug use

- Stayed up late waiting or gone out searching for someone who uses drugs

- Felt embarrassed or angry about the actions of someone who uses drugs

- Ignored the drug use because the person got defensive when you brought it up

- Not confronted a friend or relative who was obviously intoxicated or high on a drug

There are a number of books available in bookstores on codependency. If you come from a codependent family or see yourself developing relationships like this, consider acting now to make changes in your patterns of interaction.

If you notice changes in behavior and mood in someone you know, they may signal a growing dependence on drugs. Signs that a person's life is beginning to center on drugs include the following:

- Sudden withdrawal or emotional distance

- Rebellious or unusually irritable behavior

- Loss of interest in usual activities or hobbies

- Decline in school performance

- Sudden change in group of friends

- Changes in sleeping or eating habits

- Frequent borrowing of money or stealing

- Secretive behavior about personal possessions, such as a backpack or the contents of a drawer

- Deterioration of physical appearance

If you believe a family member or friend has a drug problem, obtain information about resources for drug treatment available on your campus or in your community. Communicate your concern, provide him or her with information about treatment options, and offer your support during treatment. If the individual continues to deny having a problem, you may want to talk with an experienced counselor about setting up an "intervention"—a formal, structured confrontation designed to end denial by having family, friends, and other caring individuals present their concerns to the drug user. Participants in an intervention may stress the ways in which the individual is hurting others as well as himself or herself. If your friend or family member agrees to treatment, encourage him or her to attend a support group such as Narcotics Anonymous or Alcoholics Anonymous. And finally, examine your relationship with the abuser for signs of codependency. If necessary, get help for yourself; friends and family of drug users often can benefit from counseling.

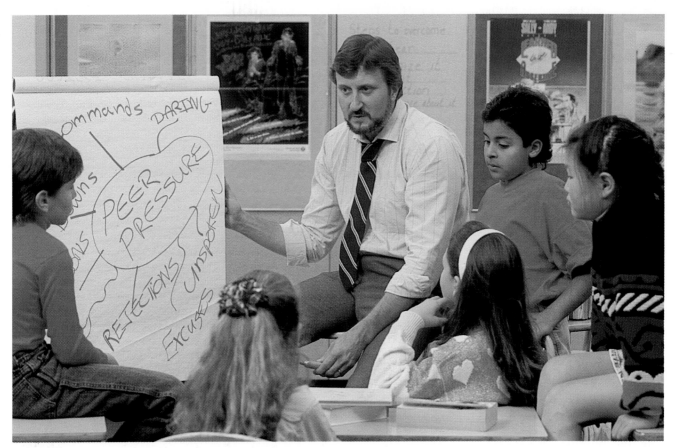

Giving young people information about the adverse effects of drugs and teaching them strategies for resisting peer pressure to use drugs may help prevent future drug abuse. Young children may respond to education programs involving a respected or well-known adult.

program and college, a peer counselor's role may be as limited as referring a student to a professional with expertise in chemical dependency for an evaluation or as involved as helping to arrange a leave of absence from school to allow participation in a drug treatment program. Most peer counseling programs are founded on principles of strict confidentiality. Peer counselors may also be able to assist students who are concerned about a classmate or loved one with an apparent drug problem (see the box "If Someone You Know Has a Drug Problem . . ."). Information about peer counseling programs is usually available from the student health center.

Prevention of Drug Abuse

Clearly, the best solution to drug abuse is prevention. Government attempts at controlling the drug problem tend to focus on stopping the production, importation, and distribution of illicit drugs. Creative effort also has to be put into stopping the demand for drugs. Developing persuasive antidrug educational programs offers the best hope for solving the drug problem in the future. Indirect approaches to prevention involve building young people's

Personal Insight   What is your attitude toward drug dependency? Do you view it more as a moral violation, a criminal act, or an illness? Where do you think your ideas come from?

self-esteem, improving their academic skills, and increasing their recreational opportunities. Direct approaches involve giving information about the adverse effects of drugs and teaching tactics that help students resist peer pressure to use drugs in various situations. Developing strategies for resisting peer pressure is one of the more effective techniques.

Prevention in the 1990s will probably focus on the different motivations individuals have for using and abusing specific drugs at different ages. For example, grade school children seem receptive to programs that involve their parents or well-known adults like professional athletes. Adolescents in junior or senior high school are often more responsive to peer counselors. Many young adults tend to be influenced by efforts focusing on health education. For all ages, it is important to provide nondrug alternatives

- Bored? Go for a walk or a run; stimulate your senses at a museum or a movie; challenge your mind with a new game or book; introduce yourself to someone new.

- Stressed? Practice relaxation or visualization; try to slow down and open your senses to the natural world; get some exercise.

- Shy, lonely? Talk to a counselor; enroll in a shyness clinic; learn and practice communication techniques.

- Feeling low on self-esteem? Focus on the areas in which you are competent; give yourself credit for the things you do well. A program of regular exercise can also enhance self-esteem.

- Depressed, anxious? Talk to a friend, parent, or counselor.

- Apathetic, lethargic? Force yourself to get up and get some exercise to energize yourself; assume responsibility for someone or something outside yourself; volunteer.

- Searching for meaning? Try yoga or meditation; explore spiritual experiences through religious groups, church, prayer, or reading.

- Afraid to say no? Take a course in assertiveness training; get support from others who don't want to use drugs; remind yourself that you have the right and the responsibility to make your own decisions.

- Still feeling peer pressure? Begin to look for new friends or roommates. Take a class or join an organization that attracts other health-conscious people.

that speak to that individual's or group's specific reasons for using drugs, such as recreational facilities, counseling, greater opportunities for leisure activities, or places to socialize (see the box "What to Do Instead of Drugs").

The Role of Drugs in Your Life

Where do you fit into this complex picture of drug use and abuse? Chances are good that you've had experience with over-the-counter and prescription drugs, and you may or may not have had experience with one or more of the drugs described in this chapter. You probably know someone who has used or abused a psychoactive drug. Whatever your experience up to now, it's likely that you will encounter drugs at some point in your life. To make sure you'll have the inner resources to resist peer pressure and make your own decision, cultivate a variety of activities you enjoy doing, realize that you are entitled to have your own opinion, and don't neglect your self-esteem. Like other aspects of health behavior, making responsible decisions about drug use depends on information, knowledge, and insight into yourself. Many choices are possible; making the ones that are right for you is what counts.

SUMMARY

The Drug Tradition

- Naturally occurring drugs have been used throughout history for religious, medicinal, and personal reasons. Although drug use dropped after 1900, it surged again in the 1960s; it has been declining overall since the late 1970s, although certain drugs are enjoying a revival in certain populations.

Use, Abuse, and Dependence

- People of all incomes, education levels, and ethnic backgrounds use drugs. Risk factors for drug use include being male, being young, having frequent exposure to drugs, and having a risk-taking personality.

- Reasons for using drugs include the lure of the illicit; curiosity; rebellion; peer pressure; and the desire to alter one's mood or escape boredom, anxiety, depression, or other psychological problems.

- Drug abuse is a maladaptive pattern of drug use that persists despite adverse social, psychological, or medical consequences.

- Drug dependence involves taking a drug compulsively, neglecting constructive activities because of it, and experiencing adverse social effects resulting from its use. Tolerance, physical dependence, and a withdrawal syndrome are usually present.

- Psychological dependence involves a craving for the mood changes that a drug provides; it is strongly affected by social factors.

How Drugs Affect the Body

- The effects of a drug depend on drug factors, user factors, and social factors.

- Drug factors include pharmacological properties, dose-response function, time-action function, cumulative effects, and method of use.

- User factors include a person's physical and psychological characteristics, such as body mass, general health, and other drugs being taken.
- The psychological set and social setting are sometimes more important in determining effects than the drug itself, if low doses are involved.

Representative Psychoactive Drugs

- Opiates relieve pain, cause drowsiness, and induce euphoria; they reduce anxiety and produce lethargy, apathy, and an inability to concentrate.
- Central nervous system depressants slow down the overall activity of the nerves; they reduce anxiety and produce mood changes, muscular incoordination, slurring of speech, and drowsiness or sleep. Physical dependency is possible with most CNS drugs, and withdrawal symptoms can be severe.
- Central nervous system stimulants speed up the activity of the nerves, causing acceleration of heart rate, rise in blood pressure, dilation of pupils and bronchial tubes, and an increase in gastric and adrenal secretions. Tolerance and physical and psychological dependence are associated with the use of CNS stimulants.
- Cocaine produces an intense euphoria; it is usually sniffed, snorted, or injected intravenously. Crack is a less expensive, ready-to-smoke version of cocaine.
- Amphetamines make people feel more alert and less fatigued or bored. Paranoid psychoses, including delusions and unprovoked violence, can result from abuse. Other dangers include damage to blood vessels, strokes, and other changes in heart and blood vessels.
- Caffeine mildly stimulates the heart and respiratory system, increases muscular tremor, and enhances gastric secretion. Tolerance can develop and withdrawal symptoms can appear.
- Marijuana usually causes euphoria and a relaxed attitude at low doses; very high doses produce feelings of depersonalization and sensory distortion. Marijuana use increases heart rate and dilation of blood vessels in the eyes. Possible effects of long-term use include bronchial irritation, changes in brain function, and fertility problems. Tolerance to marijuana can develop.
- Psychedelics alter perception, feelings, and thought. LSD is the most widely known; its effects include an altered sense of time, disorders of vision, and changes in mood. Large doses may lead to synesthesia and depersonalization. Tolerance to psychedelics occurs, but there are no withdrawal symptoms. Panic reactions and flashbacks are among the adverse effects of LSD use.

- Deliriants cause temporary impairment of brain function—changing levels of awareness to surrounding events, decreased ability to maintain attention to a task, confusion, and perhaps hallucinations. PCP is a widely used deliriant with dangerous side effects.
- Inhalants, such as glue, kerosene, butyl nitrite, and nitrous oxide, can produce delirium; their use can lead to brain, liver, and kidney damage.
- Designer drugs are created by modifying existing drugs to produce compounds that have similar effects.

Drug Use: The Decades Ahead

- Honest and unbiased information about drugs may help cut down on their abuse; scare tactics and exaggerations are ineffective.
- Drug testing, a controversial issue in American politics, involves a basic conflict between public safety and the individual's right to privacy and freedom from unreasonable search.
- Drug substitution programs using methadone and other drugs attempt to reduce the costs, or risks, of drug abuse.
- Features of drug treatment centers include hospitalization, detoxification, counseling, and other psychiatric services. Therapeutic communities use confrontation, strict discipline, and peer pressure to resocialize addicts. Halfway houses provide a bridge to independent living. Counseling for friends and relatives of drug abusers is also often available.
- Self-help groups and peer counseling are helpful forms of treatment for some drug abusers.
- Government attempts to control the drug problem focus on production, importation, and distribution. Persuasive antidrug educational programs are necessary; especially important is helping students develop strategies for resisting peer pressure. Providing nondrug alternatives that address an individual's or group's specific reasons for using drugs is essential.

TAKE ACTION

1. Find out what type of services are available on your campus or in your community to handle drug dependence. If there are none, what services are needed? Locate the school official and public health agency responsible for your campus and community and ask why these needs aren't being met.
2. Survey three older adults and three young students about their attitudes toward legalizing marijuana. Are

there any differences? If so, what accounts for these differences? What kinds of reasons do they give for their positions?

3. Look at a recent film or television program, paying special attention to how drug use is portrayed. What messages are being conveyed? If possible, compare a recent movie with a movie made 10 or 15 years ago. Has the presentation of drug use changed? If so, how?

JOURNAL ENTRY

1. Keep track of your own drug use for a week, noting in your health journal the name of the drug, the approximate dosage, the time of day, and what you think your reasons were for taking each dose. Don't forget to include coffee, soft drinks, and over-the-counter medications. What types of drugs are you taking? Are there any patterns? Are there any signs of abuse or dependence? If you'd like to cut down, begin by making a list of alternative behaviors you could substitute for drug use.

2. *Critical Thinking:* Does a woman have an obligation to avoid alcohol and other drugs during pregnancy? What about smoking cigarettes and eating junk food? If she doesn't follow her physician's advice, should she be held legally responsible for the effects on her child? What rights do the mother and child have in this situation? In your health journal, write an essay stating your opinion; be sure to defend your position.

3. *Critical Thinking:* Do you think there is such a thing as responsible use of illegal psychoactive drugs? Are they a legitimate recreational activity? Would you change any of the current laws governing drugs? If so, how would you draw the line between legitimate and illegitimate use? Write an essay describing your position.

BEHAVIOR CHANGE STRATEGY

CHANGING YOUR DRUG HABITS

We have chosen to devote this behavior change strategy to one of the most commonly used drugs—caffeine. If there is another drug you want to cut down on or stop using, you can devise your own plan based on this one and on the steps outlined in Chapter 1.

Because caffeine supports certain behaviors that are characteristic of our culture, such as sedentary, stressful work, you may find yourself relying on coffee (or tea, chocolate, or colas) to get through a busy schedule. Such habits often begin in college. Fortunately, it's easier to

break a habit before it becomes entrenched as a lifelong dependency.

Caffeine overdose can have some harmful effects on you, and knowing what they are can help motivate you to reduce your intake. You may feel increased anxiety and irritability; some people may be especially sensitive to caffeine and may find such exaggerated states hard to manage.

When you are studying for exams, the forced physical inactivity and the need to concentrate even when fatigued may lead you to overuse caffeine. But caffeine doesn't "help" unless you are already sleepy. And it does not relieve any underlying condition (you are just more tired when it wears off). So how can you change this pattern?

Self-Monitoring

Keep a log of how much caffeine you eat or drink. Use a measuring cup to measure coffee or tea. Using Table 11-2, convert the amounts you eat or drink into an estimate expressed in milligrams of caffeine. Be sure to include all forms, such as chocolate bars and over-the-counter medications, as well as caffeine candy, colas, cocoa or hot chocolate, chocolate cake, tea, and coffee.

Self-Assessment

At the end of the week, add up your daily totals and divide by 7 to get your daily average in milligrams. How much is too much? At more than 250 mg per day, you may well be experiencing some adverse symptoms. Are you experiencing at least five of the following? If so, you may want to cut down.

- Restlessness
- Nervousness
- Excitement
- Insomnia
- Flushed face
- Excessive sweating
- Gastrointestinal problems
- Muscle twitching
- Rambling flow of thought and speech
- Irregularities in rhythm of heartbeats
- Periods of inexhaustibility
- Excessive pacing or need to constantly move around

Set Limits

Can you restrict your caffeine intake to a daily total, and stick to this contract? If so, set a cutoff point, such as one cup of coffee. Pegging it to a specific time of day can be helpful, because then you don't confront a decision at any other point (and possibly fail). If you find you cannot stick to your limit, you may want to cut out caffeine altogether; abstinence can be easier than moderation for some people. If you experience caffeine withdrawal symptoms (headache, fatigue) when you decrease your caffeine consumption, you may want to cut your intake more gradually.

Find Other Ways to Keep Your Energy Up

If you are fatigued, it makes sense to get enough sleep or to exercise more rather than drowning the problem in coffee. Different individuals need different amounts of sleep; you may also need more sleep at different times, such as during a personal crisis or an illness. Also, exercise raises your metabolic rate for hours afterward—a handy fact to exploit when you want to feel more awake and want to avoid an irritable coffee jag. And if you've been compounding your fatigue by not eating properly, try filling up on complex carbohydrates such as whole-grain bread or potatoes instead of candy bars.

Some Tips on Cutting Out Caffeine   Here are some more ways to decrease your consumption of caffeine:

1. Keep some noncaffeine drink on hand, perhaps decaffeinated coffee, herbal teas, hot water, or bouillon.
2. Alternate between hot and very cold liquids.
3. Fill your coffee cup only halfway.
4. Avoid the office or school lunchroom or cafeteria and the chocolate area of the grocery store. (Often people drink coffee or tea and eat chocolate simply because it's there.)

SELECTED BIBLIOGRAPHY

American Psychiatric Association. 1987. *Diagnostic and Statistical Manual of Mental Disorders,* 3rd ed., revised (DSM-III-R). Washington, D.C.: American Psychiatric Association Press.

Blaine, J. D., and W. Ling. 1992. Psychopharmacologic treatment of cocaine dependence. *Psychopharmacology Bulletin* 28(1): 11–14.

Boodman, S. G. 1989. Up against it. *Washington Post Health,* 5 September.

Brook, J. S., and others. 1992. Childhood precursors of adolescent drug use: A longitudinal analysis. *Genetic, Social and General Psychology Monographs* 118(2): 195–213.

Chavez, E. L., and R. C. Swaim. 1992. An epidemiological comparison of Mexican-American and white non-Hispanic eighth and twelfth grade students' substance abuse. *American Journal of Public Health* 82(3): 445–47.

Cohen, S. 1985. *The Substance Abuse Problems.* Vol. 2, *New Issues for the 80s.* New York: Haworth Press.

Compton, D. R., and others. 1990. Cannabis dependence and tolerance production. *Advances in Alcoholism and Substance Abuse* 9(1–2): 129–47.

Craig, R. J., and R. Olson. 1992. MMPI subtypes for cocaine abusers. *American Journal of Drug and Alcohol Abuse* 18(2): 197–205.

Cregler, L. L., and H. Mark. 1986. Cardiovascular dangers of cocaine abuse. *American Journal of Cardiology* 57:1185.

Darling, M. R., and T. M. Arendorf. 1992. Review of the effects of cannabis smoking on oral health. *International Dental Journal* 42(1): 19–22.

Day, N. L., and G. A. Richardson. 1991. Prenatal marijuana use: epidemiology, methodologic issues and infant outcome. *Clinics in Perinatology* 18(1): 77–91.

Derlet, R. W., and B. Heischober. 1990. Methamphetamine: Stimulant of the '90s? *Western Journal of Medicine* 153(6): 625–28.

Duncan, D. F., and R. S. Gold. 1982. *Drugs and the Whole Person.* New York: John Wiley.

Ecstasy-fueled 'Rave' parties become dances of death for English youths. 1992. *Journal of the American Medical Association* 268(12): 1505–6.

Fisher, S., A. Raskin, and E. H. Uhlenhuth, eds. 1987. *Cocaine: Clinical and Biobehavioral Aspects.* New York: Oxford University Press.

Hawkins, J. D., and others. 1992. Risk and protective factors for alcohol and other drug problems in adolescence and early adolescence: Importance for substance use prevention. *Psychological Bulletin* 112(1): 64–105.

Hecht, M. L., and others. 1992. Resistance to drug offers among college students. *International Journal of the Addictions* 27(8): 995–1017.

Imperato, P. J. 1992. Syphilis, AIDS and crack cocaine. *Journal of Community Health* 17(2): 69–71.

Inciardi, J. A., and others. 1992. A heroin revival in Miami: Notes from a street survey. *Journal of Psychoactive Drugs* 24(1): 57–62.

Kaplan, C. D., and others. 1992. Are there 'casual users' of cocaine? *CIBA Foundation Symposium* 166:57–73; 73–80.

Klonger, R. A., and others. 1992. The effects of acute and chronic cocaine use on the heart. *Circulation* 85(2): 407–19.

Moss, P. D., and P. D. Werner. 1992. An MMPI typology of cocaine abusers. *Journal of Personality Assessment* 58(2): 269–76.

Nahas, G., and C. Latour. 1992. The human toxicity of marijuana. *Medical Journal of Australia* 156(7): 495–97.

Sternbach, G. L., and J. Varon. 1992. 'Designer drugs': Recognizing and managing their toxic effects. *Postgraduate Medicine* 91(8): 169–171; 175–176.

Strunin, L., and Hingson, R. 1992. Alcohol, drugs, and adolescent sexual behavior. *International Journal of the Addictions* 27(2): 129–46.

Tobler, N. S. 1992. Drug prevention programs can work: Research findings. *Journal of Addictive Diseases* 11(3): 1–28.

U.S. Centers for Disease Control. 1992. Tobacco, alcohol and other drug use among high school students—United States. 41(37): 698–703.

U.S. Public Health Service. 1987. *Prevention Research: Deterring Drug Abuse Among Children and Adolescents.* Washington, D.C.: U.S. Department of Health and Human Services.

U.S. Public Health Service. 1988. *Mechanisms of Tolerance and Dependence.* Washington, D.C.: U.S. Department of Health and Human Services.

U.S. Public Health Service. 1988. *Progress in the Development of Cost-Effective Treatment for Drug Abusers.* Washington, D.C.: U.S. Department of Health and Human Services.

Westermeyer, J. 1992. Substance abuse disorders: Predictions for the 1990s. *American Journal of Drug and Alcohol Abuse* 18(1): 1–11.

Young, S. L., and others. 1992. Cocaine: Its effects on maternal and child health. *Pharmacotherapy* 12(1): 2–17.

Zimmerman, S., and A. M. Zimmerman. 1990–91. Genetic effects of marijuana. *International Journal of the Addictions* 25(1A): 19–33.

RECOMMENDED READINGS

Beattie, M. 1990. *Codependents' Guide to the Twelve Steps.* New York: HarperCollins. *A useful book for friends and loved ones of substance abusers by the writer who first popularized the now-trendy term "codependent."*

Kaplan, J. 1970. *Marijuana—The New Prohibition.* New York: World Publishing. *The classic book on the politics of marijuana control in the United States.*

Kaplan, J. 1983. *The Hardest Drug: Heroin and Public Policy.* Chicago: University of Chicago Press. *An excellent description of the scientific and political issues involving heroin.*

Keller-Phelps, J., and A. E. Nourse. 1992. *The Hidden Addiction.* Boston: Little, Brown. *Written by two physicians, this book gives straightforward information about a range of addicting substances, from caffeine to cocaine, along with advice for avoiding or overcoming dependency problems.*

Mooney, A. J. 1992. *The Recovery Book.* New York: Workman. *Written by a physician, this helpful guide covers family relationships, support groups, work, money, and other issues involved in chemical dependency.*

Nadelman, E. A. 1988. U.S. drug policy: A bad export. *Foreign Policy* 70:83–107, Spring. *Nadelman is a vocal advocate of the controlled legalization of currently illicit drugs.*

Schuckit, M. A. 1989. *Drug and Alcohol Abuse: A Clinical Guide to Diagnosis and Treatment.* 3rd ed. New York: Plenum Press. *A balanced, informative text that focuses on the clinical aspects of drug use.*

Siegel, R. 1989. *Intoxication: Life in Pursuit of Artificial Paradise.* New York: E. P. Dutton. *A thoughtful, historical look at the causes and effects of substance abuse.*

U.S. Journal, Inc. 1992. *The Treatment Directory: National Directory of Alcohol, Drug Addiction and Other Addiction Treatment Programs.* Deerfield Beach, Fla.: U.S. Journal, Inc. *A helpful reference for people seeking information about treatment options for themselves or loved ones.*

12

Nutrition Facts and Fallacies

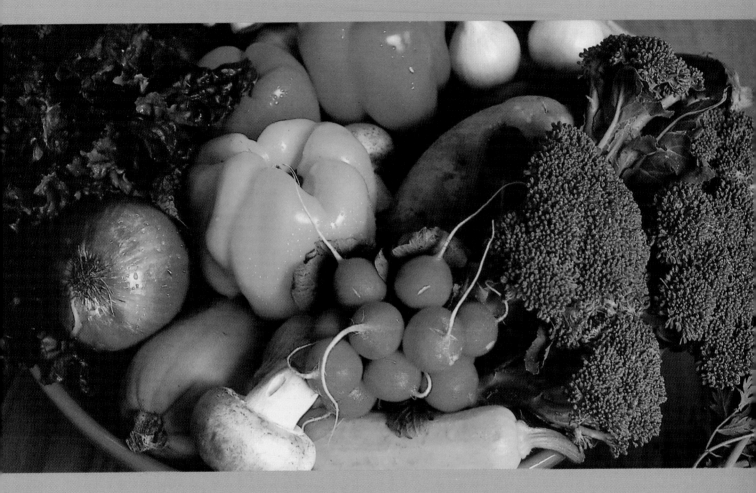

CONTENTS

Nutritional Requirements: Components of a Healthy Diet
Proteins—The Basis of Body Structure
Fats—Essential in Small Amounts
Carbohydrates—An Ideal Source of Energy
Dietary Fiber—A Closer Look
Vitamins—Organic Micronutrients
Water—Vital but Often Ignored
Minerals—Inorganic Micronutrients

Nutritional Guidelines: Planning Your Diet
Recommended Dietary Allowances
Food Guide Pyramid
Dietary Guidelines for Americans
The Vegetarian Alternative

A Personal Plan: Making Intelligent Choices About Food
Reading Food Labels to Learn More About What You Eat
Who Should Take Vitamin or Mineral Supplements?
Getting Reliable Nutritional Advice
The Food Supply: Is It Safe?
Additives in Food: Are They Dangerous?

Appendix: The Facts About Fast Food

BOXES
How to Calculate Your Fat Intake
Digestive and Metabolic Disorders
Keeping the Nutrient Value in Your Food
Osteoporosis: Reducing Your Risk
Reducing the Fat in Your Diet
Nutrition Checklist
Ethnic Diets and Cuisines
Food Safety

▶ You and your date go out to dinner one night at a popular restaurant that has a reputation for fresh, healthy foods. You order spaghetti with marinara sauce, and she decides on salad. She returns from the salad bar with a mix of lettuce, marinated mushrooms, chopped green pepper, tomato, bacon bits, croutons, hard-boiled eggs, shredded cheese, avocado, and sunflower seeds, topped with creamy Italian dressing. She says, "I'm glad I'm eating a healthy, nonfattening meal for a change. Why don't you try salad next time? It's better for you." Is she right?

▶ Your grandmother has suffered from osteoporosis for many years and is now stooped over and considerably shorter than she used to be. Your mother recently started taking hormones to protect herself from bone loss. You're a healthy 23-year-old woman of average weight (although you do smoke). How great is your risk of developing osteoporosis? Is there anything you can do now to protect yourself?

▶ You want to improve your diet, so instead of buying cookies at the store for a snack, you bought some all-natural granola bars. While you're eating one, you glance at the list of ingredients on the side of the box and notice that it's unusually long. Reading it, you notice seven different sweeteners—sugar, honey, molasses, corn syrup, brown sugar, dextrose, and malt syrup—and three different kinds of hydrogenated oil. Also listed are ingredients like sorbitol, citric acid, sulfiting agents, and BHA. It doesn't seem much like a health food. What are all these ingredients for? Are these granola bars a healthy snack?

▶ When you were growing up, your family had beef, pork, or lamb for dinner almost every night, and the refrigerator was always stocked with cold cuts and cheese for sandwiches at lunch. Breakfast was usually bacon and eggs. The freezer always had ice cream; the cupboards held cookies and chips. Yet you and your sister aren't overweight, and you rarely get sick. Now you're sharing a house with three people who rarely eat red meat, and when they do, eat only very small amounts. Three or four nights a week, they eat no meat at all—just pasta, or beans and rice, with a salad or steamed vegetables. Breakfast is usually cereal and skim milk, and snacks and desserts are fruit and nonfat yogurt. This strikes you as a very experimental way to eat. The foods your family ate, in contrast, have a long track record. Can your family's diet really be all that bad? Aren't your roommates risking protein deprivation?

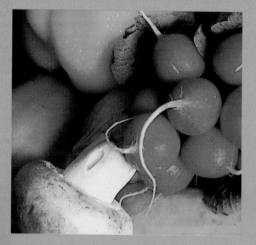

MAKING CONNECTIONS

Of all your daily behaviors and habits, choosing a nutritious diet is probably the single most important action you can take to influence your health in a positive way. Some kinds of diets are linked with vitality, energy, and well-being; others are linked with a host of diseases, including cancer and heart disease. In each of the nutrition-related scenarios presented on these pages, individuals have to use information, make a decision, or choose a course of action. How would you act in each of these situations? What response or decision would you make? This chapter provides information about nutrition that can be used in situations like these. After finishing the chapter, read the scenarios again. Has what you've learned changed how you would respond?

In your lifetime, you'll spend about six years eating—about 70,000 meals and 60 tons of food. What you choose to eat can have profound effects on your health and well-being. Poor nutrient intake can make you more susceptible to diseases like osteoporosis and iron-deficiency anemia, while overzealous use of vitamin and mineral supplements can lead to toxicity. Your nutritional habits also affect your risk for the major chronic "killer" diseases, including heart disease, cancer, stroke, and diabetes. Choosing foods that provide adequate amounts of the nutrients you need while avoiding the substances linked to disease should be an important part of your daily life. The food choices you make will significantly influence your health both now and later in your life.

If you're confused about the right diet for you, this chapter can offer some help. Although the science of **nutrition** is relatively young, we know what nutrients are needed for an adequate diet and what foods provide them. Understanding just the basics of a healthy diet—variety, balance, and moderation—can help you eat sensibly and protect yourself against many nutrition-related problems. For most Americans, the most likely dietary problems are overeating and an imbalance in the nutrients consumed. The *Healthy People 2000* report highlights some of the most important dietary changes that Americans can make to safeguard their health and well-being; these include reducing consumption of fat and sodium, increasing consumption of complex carbohydrates and dietary fiber, and consuming adequate amounts of iron and calcium. Reading this chapter will help you understand the reasons behind these recommendations and provide you with the tools to incorporate them into your own diet.

NUTRITIONAL REQUIREMENTS: COMPONENTS OF A HEALTHY DIET

When you think about your diet you probably do so in terms of the foods you like to eat—a turkey sandwich and a glass of milk or a steak and a baked potato. What's important for your health, though, is the nutrients contained in those foods. Your body requires carbohydrates, proteins, fats, vitamins, minerals, and water—about 45 **essential nutrients.** The word *essential* in this context means that you must get these substances from food because your body is unable to manufacture them at all, or at least not fast enough to meet body needs. Plants use light from the sun to convert chemicals from the air, water, and soil into all the complex chemicals they need. Animals, including humans, must eat foods to obtain the nutrients necessary to keep their bodies growing and functioning properly. Your body obtains these nutrients when the foods you eat are broken down (digested) into compounds that your gastrointestinal tract can absorb and your body can use. A diet containing adequate amounts of all essential nutrients is vital because nutrients provide energy, help build and maintain body tissues, and help regulate body functions.

The energy in foods is expressed as **kilocalories.** One kilocalorie represents the amount of heat it takes to raise the temperature of 1 liter of water 1° C. A person needs about 2,000 kilocalories per day to meet his or her energy needs. In common usage, people often refer to kilocalories as *calories* (a calorie is actually a very small energy unit; a kilocalorie contains 1,000 calories). We'll use the more popular term *calorie* in this chapter to stand for the larger energy unit.

Three classes of nutrients supply energy—protein, carbohydrates, and fats. Alcohol, though it's not an essential nutrient and has no nutritional value, also supplies energy. Fats provide the most energy at 9 calories per gram; protein and carbohydrates each provide 4 calories per gram. The high caloric content of fat is one reason experts continually advise against high fat consumption—most of us don't need the extra calories. Alcohol provides 7 calories per gram. And although alcohol has no general nutritional role, alcoholic beverages are the third leading calorie contributor (6 percent of the total) to the American diet, after white bread, rolls, and crackers (10 percent) and doughnuts, cookies, and cakes (6 percent).

Just meeting energy needs is not enough; our bodies require adequate amounts of all the essential nutrients to grow and function properly. Many of the diet patterns followed around the world can supply these essential nutrients. Water is the major component in both foods and the human body—we are about 60 percent water—and we can live only a few days without it. Our needs for proteins, fats, carbohydrates, **vitamins,** and **minerals,** in terms of weight, are much less, but still vital. Practically all foods contain mixtures of nutrients, although foods are commonly classified according to the predominant nutrient; for example, spaghetti is thought of as a "carbohydrate" food. Let's take a closer look at the function and sources of each class of nutrients.

Nutrition   The science of food and how the body uses it in health and disease.

Essential nutrients   Substances your body must get from foods because (with minor exceptions) the body cannot manufacture them at all or fast enough to meet body needs. These nutrients include vitamins, minerals, some amino acids, linoleic acid, and water.

Kilocalorie   Unit of fuel potential in a diet; 1 calorie represents the amount of heat needed to raise the temperature of 1 liter of water 1° C.

Vitamins   Carbon-containing substances needed in small amounts to help promote and regulate chemical reactions and processes in the body.

Minerals   Inorganic compounds needed in relatively small amounts for regulation, growth, and maintenance of body tissues and functions.

TERMS

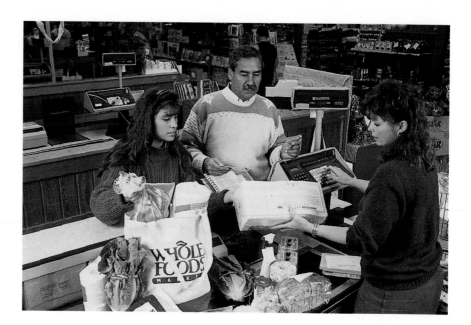

Our bodies require adequate amounts of all essential nutrients—water, proteins, carbohydrates, fats, vitamins, and minerals—in order to grow and function properly. Choosing foods to fulfill these nutritional requirements is an important part of a healthy lifestyle.

Proteins—The Basis of Body Structure

Proteins form important parts of the body's main structural components—muscles and bones. Proteins also form important parts of blood, enzymes, some hormones, and cell membranes. As mentioned above, proteins can provide energy for the body (4 calories per gram).

The building blocks of proteins are called **amino acids.** Twenty common amino acids are found in food; nine of these are essential parts of an adult diet: histidine, isoleucine, leucine, lysine, methionine, phenylalanine, threonine, tryptophan, and valine. The other 11 amino acids can be produced by the body, given the presence of the needed building blocks supplied by foods.

Individual protein sources are considered "complete" or "high quality" if they supply all the essential amino acids in adequate amounts and "incomplete" or "low quality" if they do not. Meat, fish, poultry, eggs, milk, cheese, and other foods from animal sources provide complete proteins. Incomplete proteins, which come from plant sources such as beans, peas, and nuts, are good sources of most essential amino acids, but are usually low in one or two.

Your concern with amino acids and complete protein in your diet should focus on what a meal supplies, rather than on what each individual food supplies. Combining two vegetable proteins, such as wheat and peanuts in a peanut butter and jelly sandwich, allows each vegetable protein to make up for the amino acids missing in the other protein. The combination yields a complete protein for the meal. By having plant proteins complement each other so that all essential amino acids are consumed in a meal, vegetarians can get the amino acids they need to synthesize the proteins their bodies require. (Healthy vegetarian diets are discussed in detail later in this chapter.)

The leading sources of protein in the American diet are (1) beef, steaks, and roasts, (2) hamburger and meatloaf, (3) white bread, rolls, and crackers, (4) milk, and (5) pork. About two-thirds of the protein in the American diet comes from animal sources; hence, the American diet is rich in amino acids. Most Americans consume nearly twice the amount of protein they need each day. Protein consumed beyond protein needs is synthesized into fat for energy storage or burned for energy needs. For most of us, this extra protein in our diet is not harmful; it simply reflects the high standard of living and the dietary habits that we enjoy. Nutritionists have recommended, however, that our protein intake not exceed twice our needs on a daily basis. The amount of protein you eat should represent about 10–15 percent of your total calorie intake (Figure 12-1).

Fats—Essential in Small Amounts

Fats, also known as lipids, are the most concentrated source of energy at 9 calories per gram. The fats stored in your body represent usable energy and help insulate your body and support and cushion your organs. Fats in the diet help your body absorb fat-soluble vitamins, as well as add important flavor and texture to foods. Fats are the major fuel for the body during rest and light activity: Carbohydrates fuel the nervous system, brain, and red blood cells, while fats fuel most of the rest of the body's organ systems. Two fats—linoleic acid and alpha-linolenic acid—are essential components of the diet. They are key to the regulation of body functions, such as the maintenance of blood pressure and the progress of a healthy pregnancy.

Most of the fats in food are in the form of triglycerides, which are composed of a glycerol molecule (an alcohol) plus three fatty acids. Fatty acids differ in the length of their carbon atom chains and in their degree of saturation

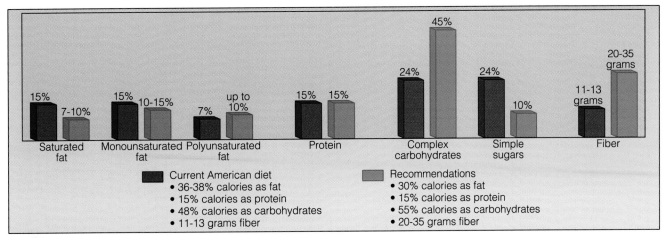

 VITAL STATISTICS

Figure 12-1 *The current American diet versus the recommended American diet.*

(the number of double bonds contained between the carbon atoms). If no double bonds exist between the carbon atoms, the fatty acid is called **saturated.** Fatty acids with one double bond are called **monounsaturated,** and fatty acids with two or more double bonds are called **polyunsaturated.**

Food fats are often composed of both saturated and unsaturated fatty acids; the dominant type of fatty acid determines the fat's characteristics. Food fats containing large amounts of saturated fatty acids are usually solid at room temperature (these are called "fats"); they are generally found in animal products. The leading sources of saturated fat in the American diet are unprocessed animal flesh (hamburger, steak, roasts), whole milk, cheese, and hot dogs/lunch meats; other significant sources include poultry skin, ice cream, and many baked products. Food fats containing large amounts of monounsaturated and polyunsaturated fatty acids are usually from plant sources and are liquid at room temperature (these are called "oils"). Olive, canola, and peanut oils contain mostly monounsaturated fatty acids. Sunflower, corn, and safflower oils contain mostly polyunsaturated fatty acids.

Notable exceptions to these generalizations are palm oil and coconut oil, often used in processed foods; though derived from plants, these oils are highly saturated. Hydrogenated vegetable oils are also highly saturated. The process of **hydrogenation** turns many of the double bonds in unsaturated fatty acids into single bonds and produces a more solid fat from a liquid oil. Food manufacturers use this process to extend the shelf life of fats; the more double bonds a fat contains, the more likely it is to break down and turn rancid. The more solid fats that result from hydrogenation also have the texture needed to make better pastry and cake products. Hydrogenation prevents oil from separating out in peanut butter.

You need only about 1 tablespoon of vegetable oil per day incorporated into your diet to supply the essential fats. The average American diet supplies much more than this amount; in fact, fats make up about 36 to 38 percent of our calorie intake. Health experts recommend that we reduce our fat intake to 30 percent or less of total calories, with no more than 7 to 10 percent coming from saturated fat (see Figure 12-1). The fat content of many common foods is given in Table 12-1; the box "How to Calculate Your Fat Intake" explains how to determine the percentage of calories from fat in foods.

Controlling the amount of saturated fat in your diet is the most important diet-related action you can take to control your **serum (blood) cholesterol** level. An elevated serum cholesterol level is associated with an increased risk for premature heart disease (see Chapter 15). All adults, especially those who have high blood cholesterol levels (over 200 milligrams of cholesterol per 100 milliliters of blood serum), should minimize their saturated fat intake. Consuming hydrogenated and partially hydrogenated vegetable oils, including margarine and shortening, may also pose a risk to health because the process of hydrogenation produces some **trans fatty acids,** which may increase serum cholesterol levels.

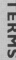

TABLE 12-1 Foods and Their Fat

Percentage Fat	Food
95–100	Butter, margarine, mayonnaise, salad oil, olives, Italian dressing, heavy cream
90–95	Pecans, macadamia nuts, baking chocolate
85–90	Walnuts, egg yolk, avocado, sour cream
80–85	Almonds, cream cheese, frankfurter, pork spareribs
75–80	Peanut butter, sunflower seeds, salami, bacon, half and half
70–75	Cheddar cheese, lamb chop
65–70	American cheese, mozzarella cheese, tuna fish in oil, ground chuck
60–65	Sweet chocolate, coconut, eggs, potato chips, rich ice cream
55–60	Veal chop, milk chocolate, pie crust
50–55	Roast beef, pork chop, roast chicken with skin
45–50	Regular ice cream, whole milk, club steak, salmon
40–45	Granola, banana bread, buttered popcorn, french fries, chili, Ritz crackers
35–40	Lasagna, hamburger on a bun, chocolate chip cookies
30–35	Chicken (skinless dark meat), 2% milk
25–30	Pizza, ground round, sea bass
20–25	Chicken (skinless white meat), liver, turkey, chicken noodle soup, chocolate pudding
15–20	Halibut, oatmeal
10–15	Plain popcorn, pretzels, bread, fig bar, low-fat cottage cheese
5-10	Tortilla, brown rice, sherbet, haddock, honeydew melon, raisins
0–5	Skim milk, white rice, egg white, spaghetti, potatoes, most fruits and vegetables, beer, wine, most cereals, clear soups

Certain forms of polyunsaturated fatty acids—those found in fish—may have a positive effect on cardiovascular health. If the double bonds of a polyunsaturated fat begin after the third carbon on the fatty acid chain, an **omega-3** form is produced. If the double bonds start after the sixth carbon atom, an omega-6 form is produced. Most of the polyunsaturated fats currently consumed by Americans are omega-6 forms, primarily from corn oil and soybean oil. However, consumption of omega-3 fatty acids found in fish has been shown to reduce the tendency of blood to clot and to decrease inflammatory responses in the body; it even appears to lower the risk of heart disease. Because of these benefits, nutritionists now recommend that Americans increase the proportion of omega-3 polyunsaturated fats in their diet by increasing their consumption of fish. Mackerel, whitefish, herring, salmon, oysters, and lake trout are all good sources of omega-3 fatty acids.

Personal Insight Do you have emotional attachments to particular kinds of foods or meals, such as those you eat on holidays or at family gatherings? If so, do your attachments make it hard for you to evaluate those foods objectively and admit that some of them may not be good for you?

Carbohydrates—An Ideal Source of Energy

Carbohydrates are needed in the diet primarily to supply energy for body cells. Some cells, such as those found in the brain and other parts of the nervous system and in blood, use only carbohydrates for fuel. During high-intensity exercise, muscles also use primarily carbohydrates for fuel. When we don't eat enough carbohydrates to satisfy the needs of the brain and red blood cells, our bodies synthesize carbohydrates from proteins. This synthesis is expensive in terms of both the **metabolism** needed (see Chapters 13 and 14) and the original cost of protein foods (compare the cost of a 1-pound loaf of whole wheat bread to that of three-quarters of a pound of lean beef, which both yield about 1,100 calories). In situations of extreme deprivation, when the diet lacks a sufficient amount of both carbohydrates and proteins, the body turns to its own proteins, causing severe muscle wasting. The average American would have to struggle to consume a diet so low in carbohydrates that it would force the body to synthesize carbohydrates from dietary or body proteins—consuming just three or four slices of bread supplies the body's daily need for carbohydrates, sparing protein for more essential functions. Crash diets and medically supervised very low carbohydrate diets used in weight reduction are the only common situations in which this would take place.

Carbohydrates can be divided into two groups: simple

To calculate how much fat a food contains, you first need to know the total number of calories and grams of fat it contains. Nutrition labels often provide this information. Multiply the grams of fat by 9 (because there are 9 calories in a gram of fat). Then divide that number by the total calories. For example, a tablespoon of peanut butter has 8 grams of fat and 95 calories. So $8 \times 9 = 72$, divided by the number of calories (95) equals 0.76, or about 76 percent calories from fat.

To monitor the fat percentage in your diet, multiply the grams of fat in any individual food by 9. If the result is more than a third of the total calories, the food is relatively high in fat. You can still eat it, but make sure you limit the amount you eat—especially if it's also high in saturated fat. And make sure that you balance it with low-fat foods.

Your goal is to end up with fewer than 30 percent of your total daily calories from fat. This can be accomplished by set-ting a goal for fat consumption and then keeping track of the amount of fat you consume during the day. To set a goal for your daily fat consumption, first determine approximately how many calories you consume per day. Depending on your activity level, daily caloric needs range from about 2,200 to 3,500 calories for men and from about 1,700 to 2,500 for women. Multiply your chosen daily calorie intake by 30 percent (0.3) to get the maximum fat calories allowed per day. Divide this figure by 9 to get the maximum number of grams of fat you can consume per day and still stay within the 30 percent guideline at your level of caloric intake. For example, if you consume about 1,800 calories per day, your maximum fat intake would be $1,800 \times 0.3 = 540$ calories from fat, or 60 grams of fat. By checking nutrition labels you can keep a running total of the grams of fat you consume and make food choices that keep you within the limit you've set for yourself.

and complex. Table sugar, honey, fructose, glucose, and corn syrup are simple carbohydrates and contain only one or two sugar units in each molecule. Simple carbohydrates provide much of the sweetness in foods. Starches and most types of dietary fiber are complex carbohydrates; they consist of chains of many sugar units. During **digestion** in the mouth and small intestine, your body breaks down starches and double sugars into single sugar molecules, such as **glucose,** for absorption (Figure 12-2). Once glucose is in the bloodstream, cells take it up and use it for energy. The liver and muscles also take up glucose to provide carbohydrate storage in the form of the animal starch called **glycogen.** Our bodies cannot break down the links between the sugar molecules in dietary fiber, so fiber is not a source of carbohydrates. However, consumption of dietary fiber *is* necessary for good health, for reasons discussed in the next section. Some people have problems metabolizing glucose, a disorder called **diabetes mellitus;** refer to the box "Digestive and Metabolic Disorders" for more information on diabetes.

Carbohydrates consumed beyond body needs for carbohydrate and energy are synthesized into fat and stored as such once glycogen stores are full. Any type of diet where calorie intake exceeds calorie needs can lead to fat storage and weight gain. This is true whether these excess calories come from carbohydrate, protein, fat, or alcohol.

Carbohydrates are found primarily in plant foods, especially grains, vegetables, and fruits; milk is the only significant animal source. On average, Americans consume over 200 grams of carbohydrates per day (about 48 percent of total calorie intake), well above the minimum of 50 to 100 grams of essential carbohydrate required by the body. However, health experts recommend that Americans increase their consumption of carbohydrates—particularly complex carbohydrates—to 55 percent of total calories. This increase in carbohydrate consumption should take place at the expense of fat intake. Potatoes, rice, pasta, bread, vegetables, and beans are all good sources of complex carbohydrates.

Athletes in training can especially benefit from high-carbohydrate diets, which enhance the amount of carbohydrates stored in their muscles (as glycogen) and therefore provide more carbohydrate fuel for use during endurance events or long workouts. In addition, carbohydrates consumed during prolonged athletic events can help fuel muscles and extend the availability of the glycogen stored in muscles. A discussion of "carbohydrate loading" is included in Chapter 14.

Omega-3 fatty acid A polyunsaturated fatty acid in which the double bonds occur after the third carbon atom on the chain.

Metabolism The sum of the biochemical activities within your body. Substances changed by chemical reactions within your body are said to be *metabolized.*

Digestion Process of breaking down foods in the gastrointestinal tract into compounds your body can absorb.

Glucose A simple sugar that is your body's basic fuel.

Glycogen An animal starch stored in the liver and muscles.

Diabetes mellitus A disorder characterized by high blood sugar levels and the inability of the body to take up and use glucose; it is caused by an insufficient supply of the hormone insulin.

TERMS

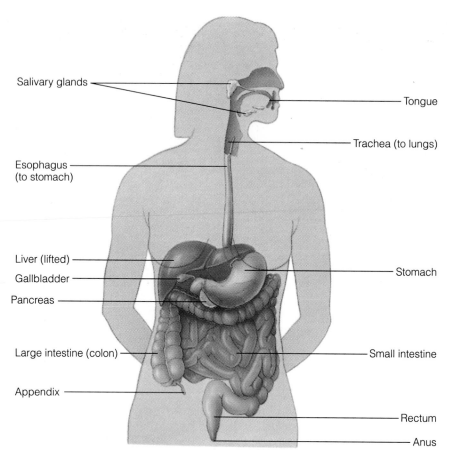

Salivary glands

Tongue

Trachea (to lungs)

Esophagus
(to stomach)

Liver (lifted)

Gallbladder

Pancreas

Stomach

Large intestine (colon)

Small intestine

Appendix

Rectum

Anus

Figure 12-2 *The digestive tract.*
Digestion of carbohydrates begins in the
mouth, but most digestion takes place in
the small intestine and stomach.

Dietary Fiber—A Closer Look

Dietary fiber (also known as "bulk" or "roughage") includes plant substances that are difficult or impossible for humans to digest. Fiber passes through your intestinal tract and provides bulk for feces (stool) in the large intestine; this facilitates elimination. Some types of fiber are metabolized by bacteria in the large intestine into products such as acids and gases; too much fiber intake can therefore lead to intestinal gas.

Nutritionists classify fibers as soluble or insoluble; each group has important physiological effects on your body. **Soluble fiber** binds cholesterol-containing compounds in the intestine, thereby lowering your blood cholesterol level. Soluble fiber also slows your body's absorption of glucose. Therefore, under medical supervision, a diet high in soluble fiber has a place in the treatment of diabetes and high serum cholesterol levels. Chapter 15 will discuss the latest research findings on the effect of fiber on blood cholesterol in more detail.

Insoluble fiber primarily binds water, making feces bulkier and softer so they pass more quickly and easily through the intestines. A diet high in insoluble fiber can help prevent a variety of health problems, including constipation, hemorrhoids, and diverticulitis (a painful condition in which abnormal pouches in the wall of the large intestine are produced and then become inflamed). Stud-

ies have linked high levels of insoluble fiber in the diet with lower incidences of colon cancer; conversely, a low-fiber diet can increase the risk for colon cancer. There is even some evidence that high levels of insoluble fiber can suppress and reverse precancerous changes that can lead to colon and rectal cancer.

All plant foods contain some dietary fiber. Fruits, **legumes,** oats (especially oat bran), barley, and psyllium (found in some laxatives) are rich in soluble fiber. Wheat (especially wheat bran), cereals, grains, and vegetables are good sources of insoluble fiber. Processing can remove fiber from foods, so fresh fruits and vegetables and foods made from whole grains are the richest sources of dietary fiber.

Although it's not yet clear exactly how much and what types of fiber would be ideal to consume, most experts feel that the average American would benefit from an increase in daily fiber intake. We currently consume about 11–13 grams a day; a better goal would be 20–35 grams a day. Emphasizing fruits, vegetables, cereals, legumes, and whole grains in the diet makes this fiber goal easy to obtain and gives a nice mixture of both soluble and insoluble fibers. Eating a fiber-rich cereal for breakfast is one way to get a good start on this goal each day. Follow that with a sandwich made of whole wheat bread for lunch and a piece of fruit. Finally, have one or more servings of vegetables with dinner.

TABLE 12-2 Vitamins: Their Functions and Food Sources

Vitamin	Function	Food Sources
Thiamin	Conversion of carbohydrates into usable forms of energy	Yeast, mushrooms, whole-grain and enriched breads and cereals, liver, pork, lean meats, poultry, eggs, fish, beans, nuts
Riboflavin	Energy release; maintenance of skin, mucous membranes, and nervous structures	Dairy products, liver, whole-grain and enriched breads and cereals, lean meats, poultry, leafy vegetables
Niacin	Conversion of carbohydrates, fats, and protein into usable forms of energy; essential for growth, synthesis of hormones	Eggs, chicken, turkey, fish, milk, grains, nuts, enriched breads and cereals, lean meats
B-6 (pyridoxine, pyridoxal, pyridoxamine)	More than 60 enzyme reactions, mostly involving proteins	Liver, lean meats, fish, poultry, whole grains, legumes
B-12	Synthesis of red and white blood cells; other metabolic reactions	Liver, meat, eggs, milk
Folate	Blood cell production, maintenance of nervous system	Liver, leafy vegetables, oranges, whole grains
Biotin	Metabolism of fats, carbohydrates, and proteins	Cauliflower, egg yolks, nuts, cheese
Pantothenic acid	Metabolism of carbohydrates, fats, and proteins	Widely distributed in all foods.
A (retinol)	Maintenance of eyes, vision, skin, linings of the nose, mouth, digestive and urinary tracts, immune function	Liver, milk, butter, cheese, fortified margarine, carrots, spinach, most other vegetables and fruits that are dark green, yellow, or orange
C (ascorbic acid)	Maintenance and repair of connective tissue, bones, teeth, cartilage; promotes wound healing	Peppers, broccoli, brussel sprouts, citrus fruits, tomatoes, potatoes, cabbage
D (cholecalciferol)	Aids in calcium and phosphorus metabolism; promotion of calcium absorption; development and maintenance of bones and teeth	Fortified milk, fish liver oils; sunlight on skin produces vitamin D
E (tocopherol)	Protection and maintenance of cellular membranes	Vegetable oils, whole grains, leafy vegetables, asparagus, peaches; smaller amounts widespread in foods
K	Production of prothrombin and other factors essential for blood clotting	Green leafy vegetables, other vegetables, liver, milk; widespread in other foods

Too much fiber—about 40 to 60 or more grams per day—can cause health problems, such as producing stools that are too large or binding important minerals and preventing their absorption. Thus, moderation in fiber intake, as with other nutrients, is an important dietary prescription. And stick to foods—use supplements only when directed by a physician.

Vitamins—Organic Micronutrients

Vitamins are organic (carbon-containing) substances required in very small amounts to promote specific chemical reactions within living cells (Table 12-2). Humans need 13 vitamins. Four are fat-soluble (A, D, E, and K), while nine are water-soluble (C, and the eight "B-complex" vitamins: thiamin, riboflavin, niacin, vitamin B-6, folate, vitamin B-12, biotin, and pantothenic acid). Be-

Soluble fiber Fiber that dissolves in water or is broken down by bacteria in the large intestine.

Insoluble fiber Fiber that does not dissolve in water and is not broken down by bacteria in the large intestine.

Legumes Vegetables such as peas and beans that are high in fiber and are also important sources of protein in a vegetarian diet.

TERMS

Digestion is the complex process by which nutrients—such as carbohydrates, proteins, and fats—are taken in by the body and broken down into simpler forms—such as glucose—for use by various cells. It involves the digestive tract, including the stomach and intestines, as well as the digestive organs and glands—the liver, gallbladder, and pancreas. From the process of digestion, the body gains the energy it needs for metabolism.

Usually the digestive process runs smoothly—but not always. Digestive problems afflict virtually everyone at one time or another. Most problems are minor or of short duration; examples include heartburn, nausea, and diarrhea. These problems can usually be self-treated (refer to the self-care appendix following Chapter 21). Other digestive and metabolic problems are more serious and require the attention or advice of a physician. These include diabetes mellitus, ulcers, gallbladder disease, and irritable bowel syndrome.

Diabetes Mellitus

Diabetes mellitus is a disease of the pancreas that causes a disruption of normal metabolism. The pancreas, a long, thin organ located behind the stomach, normally secretes the hormone insulin, which stimulates cells to take up glucose. In a person with diabetes, the pancreas either produces too little insulin or stops producing it completely. The result is low absorption of glucose by cells, which need it for energy, and by the liver, which normally stores it for future use. There is a corresponding buildup of glucose in the blood.

Approximately 14 million Americans have one of the two forms of diabetes. The most common is Type 2, also known as adult-onset or non-insulin-dependent diabetes; it usually affects people over 40, especially people who are overweight. In this type of diabetes, the pancreas produces some insulin but not enough to regulate blood sugar levels; the insulin that is produced may also be less effective.

About 10 percent of all people with diabetes have the more serious form, Type 1, also known as juvenile-onset or insulin-dependent diabetes. In this type of diabetes, the pancreas produces almost no insulin, so daily doses of insulin are required. Type 1 usually strikes before age 30.

If left untreated, diabetes can be fatal; it is currently the seventh leading cause of death in the United States. Without insulin, a person with Type 1 diabetes can lapse into a coma. Over the long term, diabetes is associated with kidney failure, circulation problems, blindness, and increased rates of heart attack, stroke, and hypertension.

The major factors involved in the development of diabetes are age, obesity, a family history of diabetes, and lifestyle. Ethnic background also plays a role. African Americans and people of Hispanic background are 55 percent more likely than non-Hispanic whites to develop Type 2 diabetes. Native Americans also have a higher-than-average incidence of diabetes.

Although there is no cure for diabetes, both types can be successfully managed. The first step is to recognize the symptoms: frequent urination, increased thirst, extreme hunger or fatigue, unexplained weight loss, or blurred vision. A person with Type 2 may also experience tingling or numbness in the feet and frequent vaginal or skin infections.

Treatment for diabetes involves keeping blood sugar within safe limits through diet, exercise, and, if necessary, medication. Blood sugar levels can be monitored using a home test. About 80 percent of Type 2 diabetes patients are overweight when they're diagnosed, and the first step in diabetes treatment is usually to lose weight. People with diabetes should eat regular meals, avoid alcohol, and eat foods that are high in complex carbohydrates and low in sugar and fat. Regular exercise, together with a healthy diet, is often sufficient to control Type 2 diabetes. By adding exercise to their lives, some people are able to reduce or eliminate their diabetes medication. Recent studies have shown that exercise actually prevents the development of Type 2 diabetes, a benefit especially important in individuals with one or more risk factors for the disease. People with Type 1 diabetes have to exercise and manage their diet as well as take insulin on a daily basis.

cause patients can survive for many years without becoming ill on intravenous feeding formulated with just these substances and the other essential nutrients, it appears that no vitamins remain to be discovered.

Many vitamins act with catalysts to initiate or speed up chemical reactions. Vitamins provide no energy to the body directly but instead are used to unleash the energy stored in carbohydrates, proteins, and fats. Some vitamins form substances that act as **antioxidants.** These are compounds that can decrease the breakdown of foodstuffs, such as when the vitamin C in orange juice is used to stop sliced bananas from turning brown. Antioxidants also aid in the preservation of healthy cells in the body. When the body uses oxygen or breaks down certain fats, it gives rise to substances called "free radicals." In their search for electrons, free radicals react with fats, proteins, and DNA, damaging cell membranes and mutating genes. Antioxidants react with free radicals and donate electrons, rendering them harmless. Key vitamin antioxidants in our diet are vitamin E, vitamin C, and the vitamin A derivative beta-carotene. Obtaining a regular intake of these nutrients is vital for maintaining the health of the body.

If your diet lacks a particular vitamin, or if you don't consume enough of it, characteristic symptoms of defi-

Peptic Ulcers

A peptic ulcer is a raw area, usually about ½ to 1 inch wide, in the lining of the stomach or duodenum (the tube that leads from the stomach to the small intestine). Ulcers are caused by the erosion of the mucous lining of the stomach or duodenum by acid and digestive enzymes. About 1 in 5 men and 1 in 10 women develop an ulcer at some time. Stomach ulcers are more common among women and the elderly; duodenal ulcers occur more often in young people.

Stress may be a factor in the development of an ulcer, since acid secretions in the stomach increase during the alarm phase of the stress response. Elderly people are at higher risk for ulcers, as are people who smoke or drink heavily, take painkillers containing aspirin, or have hurried or irregular meals. Recent evidence suggests that infection with the bacteria *Helicobacter pylori* may set the stage for the development of an ulcer.

The main symptom of an ulcer is abdominal pain that occurs several hours after a meal, caused by the continuing action of stomach acids on tissue after the food has left the stomach. The primary risk of ulcers is perforation of the stomach or intestinal wall. If this happens, the contents spill into the abdomen, causing massive infection. An ulcer may also erode a blood vessel, leading to serious blood loss.

In the past, the treatment for ulcers was usually surgery to remove the eroded area. Today, ulcers are commonly treated with antacids, coating agents, antibiotics, and substances that reduce acid secretions. Lifestyle changes are also important in treating ulcers. A person with an ulcer should shun tobacco and alcohol; eat small, frequent meals; avoid aspirin; and take steps to manage stress effectively.

Gallbladder Disease

The gallbladder is a small, muscular sac that stores bile, a fluid secreted by the liver and used to digest fats. About 10 percent of the U.S. population—an estimated 25 million Americans—develop gallstones. These small, hard masses, made up primarily of cholesterol, form in the gallbladder and bile duct (which carries bile to the duodenum). In many cases, gallstones cause no symptoms, but if a gallstone blocks the bile duct, it can cause intense pain. Treatment usually involves surgical removal of the gallstones and gallbladder.

The cause of gallstones is unknown. Risk factors include obesity, certain gastrointestinal disorders, and some drugs. There is also a genetic factor. Women are about twice as likely as men to have gallstones; the incidence among Native Americans can be as high as 65 percent.

Irritable Bowel Syndrome

Irritable bowel syndrome—also known as irritable or spastic colon—is a common condition that primarily affects women, usually in early adulthood. It is characterized by a disruption of the normal pattern of muscular contractions that move waste through the intestines. The result is either diarrhea or constipation or alternating bouts of both. Other symptoms include abdominal pain or swelling, feelings of excessive fullness, gas, painful bowel movements, indigestion, heartburn, and nausea. Since these symptoms can occur with other disorders, diagnosis by a physician is crucial.

The cause of irritable bowel syndrome is unknown, and there is no cure, but symptoms can be controlled. Anxiety is commonly associated with attacks, so stress reduction and management are an important part of treatment. People with irritable bowel syndrome should avoid tobacco, gradually add fiber to their diet (though a bland, low-fiber diet seems to be best during an attack), and, if recommended by their physician, use a bulk laxative to add volume to their stool. A physician may also prescribe medications that relieve pain and control muscle spasms.

---

ciency develop. Vitamin A deficiency can cause blindness, niacin deficiency can lead to mental illness, vitamin B-6 deficiency can cause seizures, vitamin B-12 deficiency can cause a severe type of anemia, and vitamin D deficiency can cause growth retardation. The best known deficiency disease is probably **scurvy,** caused by vitamin C deficiency; it killed many sailors on long ocean voyages until people realized in the eighteenth century that eating oranges and lemons could prevent it. Even today people develop scurvy; its presence suggests a very poor intake of fruits and vegetables, which are often rich sources of vitamin C.

Vitamin deficiency diseases are most often seen in developing countries. They are rare in the United States because vitamins are readily available from our food supply. People suffering from alcoholism currently run the great-

Antioxidants Substances that can lessen the breakdown of foodstuffs or body constituents. Their actions include binding oxygen and electrons (free radicals) and preventing the activity of certain enzymes.

Scurvy A disease caused by lack of vitamin C in which the gums bleed and teeth are loosened.

TERMS

1. Consume or process vegetables immediately after purchasing (or harvesting).

   The longer vegetables are kept before they are eaten or processed, the more vitamins are lost, especially vitamin C and folate.

2. Store vegetables and fruits properly.

   If you can't eat fruits and vegetables immediately after purchasing (or harvesting) but plan to do so within a few days, keep them in the refrigerator. Place them in covered containers or plastic bags to lessen moisture loss.

   The best method for longer-term preservation is to freeze fruits and vegetables when possible. Canning fruits and vegetables preserves them, but it's a lot of work and causes a greater nutrient loss.

3. Reduce preparation and cooking of vegetables and other foods.

   The more preparation and cooking of foods that is done before eating, the greater the nutrient loss. To reduce the losses:

- Avoid soaking vegetables in water.
- When possible, cook vegetables, like potatoes, in their skins.
- Don't soak and rinse rice before cooking; you'll wash off the B vitamins.
- Cook in as little water as possible.
- Bake, steam, or broil vegetables. Microwave cooking retains vitamins. If you stew meats, consume the broth too.
- When boiling, use tight-fitting lids to diminish evaporation of water.
- Cook vegetables in as short a time as possible. Develop a taste for a more crunchy texture.
- Don't thaw frozen vegetables before cooking.
- Prepare lettuce salads right before eating.

---

est risk of vitamin deficiencies, especially from the water-soluble vitamins thiamin, vitamin B-6, and folate. Vitamins are abundant in fruits, vegetables, and grains. In addition, many foods, such as flour and breakfast cereals, are enriched with certain vitamins. A few vitamins can also be made by your body: Vitamin D is made in your skin when it is exposed to sunlight, and biotin and vitamin K are made by intestinal bacteria. Vitamins (and minerals) can be lost or destroyed when foods are prepared, stored, and cooked. To retain the maximum nutritional value, follow the tips listed in the box "Keeping the Nutrient Value in Your Food."

Extra vitamins in the diet can be harmful, especially when taken as supplements. High doses of vitamin A are toxic to the person taking them and, if taken during pregnancy, also to the fetus. Many aspects of cell growth and maintenance are hampered, resulting in hair loss, bone disorders, and liver damage. Vitamin D toxicity causes calcium deposits in vital organs. Cases of irreversible nerve damage have recently been seen in women consuming large amounts of vitamin B-6 in an attempt to alleviate the symptoms of premenstrual syndrome. High doses of niacin are sometimes used to lower elevated serum cholesterol levels. This therapy is effective, but may cause side effects such as flushing of the skin and liver disorders. Later in this chapter we will discuss when a vitamin supplement might be advisable. For now, keep in mind that some vitamins can produce toxic results when regularly consumed in high quantities; as always, the dose determines the effect—health or ill health.

Water—Vital but Often Ignored

Water is the major component in both foods and the human body—you are about 60 percent water. Your need for other nutrients, in terms of weight, is much less than your need for water. You can live up to 50 days without food, but only a few days without water.

Water is distributed all over the body—among lean and other tissues and in urine and other body fluids. Water is used in the digestion and absorption of food and is the medium in which most of the chemical reactions take place within the body. Some water-based fluids like blood transport substances around the body, while other fluids serve as lubricants or cushions (for example, the synovial fluid within joints). Water also helps regulate body temperature.

Water is contained in almost all foods, particularly in liquids, fruits, and vegetables. The foods and fluids you consume provide 80 to 90 percent of your daily water intake; the remainder is generated through the metabolism of energy nutrients. You lose water each day in urine, feces, and sweat and through evaporation in your lungs. To maintain a balance between water consumed and water lost, you need to take in about 1 milliliter of water for each calorie you burn—that's about 2 liters or 8 cups of

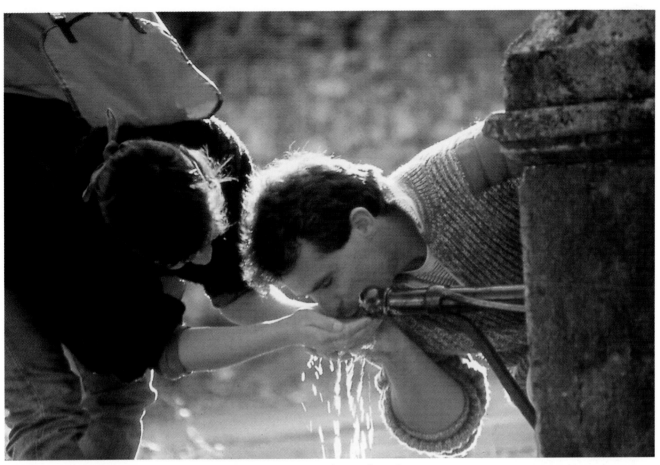

Often overlooked but absolutely crucial to life, water is an essential part of our diet.

fluid per day—more if you live in a hot climate or engage in vigorous exercise.

Thirst is the body's first sign of dehydration, a signal that it needs more water. If this thirst mechanism is faulty, as it may be during illness or vigorous exercise, hormonal mechanisms can help conserve water by reducing the output of urine. Severe dehydration causes weakness and can lead to death.

Minerals—Inorganic Micronutrients

Minerals are inorganic (non-carbon-containing) compounds you need in relatively small amounts to help regulate body functions, aid in growth and maintenance of body tissues, and act as catalysts in the release of energy (Table 12-3). There are about 17 essential minerals. The major minerals—those that the body needs in amounts exceeding 100 milligrams—include calcium, phosphorus, magnesium, sodium, potassium, and chloride. The essential trace minerals—those that you need in minute amounts—include copper, fluoride, iodide, iron, selenium, and zinc.

Characteristic symptoms develop if an essential mineral is consumed in a quantity too small or too large for good health. The minerals most commonly lacking in our diets are iron and calcium—and possibly zinc and magnesium. We should focus on good food choices for these nutrients. Lean meats are rich in iron and zinc, while low-fat or skim milk is an excellent choice for calcium. Plant foods are good sources of magnesium. Iron-deficiency **anemia** is a problem in many age groups and researchers fear poor calcium intakes are sowing the seeds for future **osteoporosis,** especially in women. See the box "Osteoporosis: Reducing Your Risk" to learn more.

NUTRITIONAL GUIDELINES: PLANNING YOUR DIET

Various scientific and governmental groups have established sets of nutrition guidelines to help you plan a

Anemia   A deficiency in the oxygen-carrying material in the red blood cells.

Osteoporosis   A condition, mostly affecting women, in which the bones become extremely thin and brittle.

Osteoporosis is a condition in which the bones become dangerously thin and fragile over time. As the disease progresses, losses in bone density lead first to poor bone strength and then to an increased risk of fractures, back pain, height loss, and a curving of the spine. Osteoporosis develops gradually over the years, although everyone develops it. After the age of 35, we all lose more bone mass than our bodies replace, but most of us retain enough throughout our lives to avoid serious problems.

Who Is at Risk?

Osteoporosis afflicts four times as many women as men. Women are more susceptible because they generally have less bone mass to begin with. More importantly, women commonly experience rapid bone loss in the first few years following menopause. There is also an important genetic factor—Caucasian and Asian women get osteoporosis more often than do black women, and the risk is even greater for small-boned women and those with a family history of osteoporosis.

Other factors can increase the likelihood of osteoporosis: abnormal menstrual periods, early menopause or surgical removal of the ovaries, a history of anorexia nervosa, the use of certain drugs, smoking, and the habitual consumption of alcohol.

What Can You Do?

Childhood, adolescence, and the first years of adulthood are the times to build bones strong enough to cover bone loss in later years. However, lifestyle factors at any point during the lifespan can decrease the loss of bone density over time.

Exercise can help prevent osteoporosis by strengthening the bones that are most likely to be affected. Many experts recommend a regular routine of weight-bearing exercise, such as walking, running, or aerobic dancing. But any benefit derived from exercise may be lost within a year after the exercising stops. Therefore, exercising is just as important for a woman in her forties and fifties who is trying to prevent bone loss as it is for a younger woman who is trying to increase her bone mass.

Exercise alone is not a sufficient defense against the kind of bone loss that can lead to osteoporosis. Sufficient calcium and adequate vitamin D are both important in preventing the condition. Calcium is necessary for healthy bones, especially during childhood and adolescence, when bones are growing. The recommended dietary allowance of calcium for people between 19 and 24 is 1,200 milligrams per day, approximately as much as in a quart of milk. After age 25, the recommended amount drops down to 800 milligrams daily, although pregnant and nursing women need more.

Getting enough calcium in the diet takes some careful planning, especially since foods traditionally recognized as high in calcium are also high in fat. One 8-ounce glass of milk contains about 300 mg of calcium; and other dairy products, such as cheese and ice cream, are also excellent sources. But so are low-fat and nonfat dairy products such as skim milk and nonfat yogurt. Tofu, canned salmon, and sardines eaten with the bones are also calcium-rich foods. Other good sources are dark-green vegetables such as collard or turnip greens, bok choy, kale, and broccoli.

Vitamin D is necessary for the body to absorb calcium. The body makes its own vitamin D when it is exposed to the sun, and the vitamin is also available in such foods as milk and egg yolk.

The Menopause Connection

Menopause is a natural accelerator of bone loss. The presence of estrogen inhibits bone loss, but after menopause a woman's body stops producing estrogen, and bone loss increases rapidly. Whether the loss of bone mass will lead to osteoporosis is determined by the specific constellation of interacting factors such as heredity, diet, and the individual's particular bone-mass density.

Estrogen replacement at menopause seems to virtually stop further bone loss, but there is a question about whether its long-term use increases cancer risk. It is therefore recommended that estrogen-replacement therapy be considered on an individual basis by women and their physicians.

---

healthy diet. The **Recommended Dietary Allowances (RDAs),** Estimated Safe and Adequate Daily Dietary Intakes (ESADDIs), and Estimated Minimum Requirements are standards for nutrient intake designed to prevent nutrient deficiencies. The **Food Guide Pyramid** then translates these nutrient recommendations into a food-group plan that, when followed, ensures a balanced intake of the essential nutrients. To provide further guidance in choosing foods, **Dietary Guidelines for Americans** have been established to address the prevention of certain diet-related chronic diseases.

Personal Insight How have your eating habits changed since you've entered college? Do you feel more comfortable with your current habits or less? Why?

Recommended Dietary Allowances (RDAs)

The Food and Nutrition Board of the National Academy of Sciences meets approximately every five years to set RDAs and related guidelines; the most recent version was

TABLE 12-3 Selected Minerals: Their Functions and Food Sources

Mineral	Function	Food Sources
Calcium	Maintenance of bones and teeth; blood clotting; maintenance of cell membranes; control of nerve impulses	Milk and milk products, tofu, fortified orange juice, sardines, leafy vegetables
Phosphorus	Bone growth and maintenance (teams with calcium); energy transfer in cells	Present in nearly all foods, especially milk, cheese, bakery products, and meats
Magnesium	Transmission of nerve impulses; energy transfer; composition of many enzyme systems	Widespread in foods and water (except soft water) and especially found in wheat bran, milk products, beans, nuts, and leafy vegetables
Iron	Component of hemoglobin (carries oxygen to tissues) and myoglobin (in muscle fibers) and enzymes	Liver, lean meats, legumes, enriched flour; absorption enhanced by presence of vitamin C
Iodide	Essential part of thyroid hormones; regulation of body metabolism	Iodized salt, seafood
Zinc	More than 70 enzyme reactions including synthesis of proteins, RNA, and DNA	Meat, eggs, liver, and seafood (especially oysters), milk, whole grains
Copper	Iron metabolism and red blood cell formation	Liver, shellfish, nuts, dried beans

published in 1989 (Table 12-4). The RDA for a vitamin or mineral is set by estimating the range for normal human needs, selecting the number at the high end of the range, and then adding amounts to account for needed body storage and losses during food preparation. To cover the range of individual variation, these recommendations are generally higher than most people need.

Intake recommendations are set for individual nutrients in one of three categories: (1) Recommended Dietary Allowances (RDAs) themselves, which give specific recommended intakes of nutrients that are well-known and well-researched—calories, protein, 11 vitamins, and seven minerals; (2) Estimated Safe and Adequate Daily Dietary Intakes (ESADDIs), which provide a range of values for nutrients (two vitamins and five minerals) about which our knowledge is still sketchy; and (3) Estimated Minimum Requirements, which provide minimum values for three minerals—sodium, potassium, and chloride.

The aim of the RDAs is to guide you in meeting your nutrition needs with food, rather than with vitamin and mineral supplements. This aim is important because recommendations have not yet been set for some essential nutrients; not enough is known about these nutrients for the Food and Nutrition Board to actually set a recommended level of intake. Because many supplements contain only nutrients with established RDAs, using them to meet nutrient needs can leave you deficient in other nutrients. Meeting these recommendations with food ensures a balanced intake of all essential nutrients.

No nutrient is absolutely needed daily. You can survive for a few days on a diet without water and about one year on a diet without vitamin A. But diets meeting only half the recommended intake levels are likely to be insufficient to replace daily losses of nutrients and thus over the long run can lead to a deficiency. Signs and symptoms of nutritional deficiency may be subtle and develop slowly. Decreased effectiveness of the immune system, reduced organ function, decreased ability to carry oxygen in the bloodstream, and general ongoing cell damage may not be apparent for a long period of time. You may become ill more often and not really know why. Though your diet may be inadequate, you still may show no telltale signs. So it's best to eat a diet that meets your projected nutrient needs on a daily basis.

A variant of the RDA is the **U.S. Recommended Daily Allowances** (U.S. RDAs). These are usually the largest values for each age and gender category of the RDA values set in 1968. Percentages of the U.S. RDAs are listed on

Recommended Dietary Allowances (RDAs) Amounts of certain nutrients considered adequate to meet the needs of most healthy people.

Food Guide Pyramid Food-group plan that provides practical advice to ensure balanced intake of the essential nutrients.

Dietary Guidelines for Americans Seven general principles of good nutrition intended to help prevent certain diet-related diseases.

U.S. Recommended Daily Allowances A simplified version of the RDAs used in food-product labels.

TERMS

TABLE 12-4 Recommended Dietary Allowances, Revised 1989[a,b,c]

		Weight[d]		Height[d]		Protein (g)	Fat-Soluble Vitamins			
Category	Age (years) or Condition	(kg)	(lb)	(cm)	(in)		Vita-min A (µg RE)	Vita-min D (µg)	Vita-min E (mg α-TE)	Vita-min K (µg)
Infants	0.0–0.5	6	13	60	24	13	375	7.5	3	5
	0.5–1.0	9	20	71	28	14	375	10	4	10
Children	1–3	13	29	90	35	16	400	10	6	15
	4–6	20	44	112	44	24	500	10	7	20
	7–10	28	62	132	52	28	700	10	7	30
Males	11–14	45	99	157	62	45	1,000	10	10	45
	15–18	66	145	176	69	59	1,000	10	10	65
	19–24	72	160	177	70	58	1,000	10	10	70
	25–50	79	174	176	70	63	1,000	5	10	80
	51 +	77	170	173	68	63	1,000	5	10	80
Females	11–14	46	101	157	62	46	800	10	8	45
	15–18	55	120	163	64	44	800	10	8	55
	19–24	58	128	164	65	46	800	10	8	60
	25–50	63	138	163	64	50	800	5	8	65
	51 +	65	143	160	63	50	800	5	8	65
Pregnant						60	800	10	10	65
Lactating	1st 6 Months					65	1,300	10	12	65
	2nd 6 Months					62	1,200	10	11	65

[a]The allowances, expressed as average daily intakes over time, are intended to provide for individual variations among most normal people as they live in the United States under usual environmental stresses. Diets should be based on a variety of common foods in order to provide other nutrients for which human requirements have been less well defined.
[b]Estimated Safe and Adequate Daily Dietary Intakes (ESADDIs) for adults: 30–100 µg biotin; 4.0–7.0 mg pantothenic acid; 1.5–3.0 mg copper; 2.0–5.0 mg manganese; 1.0–4.0 mg fluoride; 50–200 µg chromium; 75–250 mg molybdenum. (See *Recommended Dietary Allowances*, 10th edition, for information on other age groups.)
[c]Estimated Minimum Requirements of healthy adults: 500 mg sodium; 750 mg chloride; 2,000 mg potassium. (See *Recommended Dietary Allowances*, 10th edition, for information on other age groups.)
[d]Weights and heights of reference adults are actual medians for the U.S. population of the designated age. The use of these figures does not imply that the height-to-weight ratios are ideal.

nutrition labels, such as those seen on cereal boxes. These are soon to be updated using the 1989 RDAs, but there is ongoing debate over the timing of the update; their new name will be listed under Daily Values (DVs).

Many countries publish their own nutrient guides, as does the World Health Organization (WHO). These guidelines differ slightly from one another because there is disagreement among scientists about requirements and because different diets can lead to slightly different vitamin and mineral needs.

Food Guide Pyramid

Most of us learned about food groups in grade school. We learned that by choosing foods from each group, we could have a healthy diet. The fundamental principles of this food guide are moderation, variety, and balance—a theme echoed throughout this chapter. A diet is balanced if it contains appropriate amounts of each nutrient; choosing foods from each of the food groups helps insure that. The latest version of the food-group plan is the U.S. Department of Agriculture's Food Guide Pyramid (Figure 12-3). It is based on a recommended number of servings from six food groups: (1) a milk, yogurt, and cheese group; (2) a meat, poultry, fish, dry beans, eggs, and nut group; (3) a fruit group; (4) a vegetables group; (5) a breads, cereals, rice, and pasta group; and (6) a fats, oils, and sweets group. Caution is advised when choosing from the last group, although foods within that group can supply the essential fats for your diet (Table 12-5).

If you're worried about maintaining a healthy weight or want to lose weight, the Food Guide Pyramid can help you create food plans that contain as few as 1,600 calories and meet the adult RDAs of all essential nutrients. To

TABLE 12-4 Recommended Dietary Allowances, Revised 1989 (continued)

Water-Soluble Vitamins							Minerals						
Vita-min C (mg)	Thia-min (mg)	Ribo-flavin (mg)	Niacin (mg)	Vita-min B-6 (mg)	Fo-late (μg)	Vita-min B-12 (μg)	Cal-cium (mg)	Phos-phorus (mg)	Mag-nesium (mg)	Iron (mg)	Zinc (mg)	Iodine (μg)	Sele-nium (μg)
30	0.3	0.4	5	0.3	25	0.3	400	300	40	6	5	40	10
35	0.4	0.5	6	0.6	35	0.5	600	500	60	10	5	50	15
40	0.7	0.8	9	1.0	50	0.7	800	800	80	10	10	70	20
45	0.9	1.1	12	1.1	75	1.0	800	800	120	10	10	90	20
45	1.0	1.2	13	1.4	100	1.4	800	800	170	10	10	120	30
50	1.3	1.5	17	1.7	150	2.0	1,200	1,200	270	12	15	150	40
60	1.5	1.8	20	2.0	200	2.0	1,200	1,200	400	12	15	150	50
60	1.5	1.7	19	2.0	200	2.0	1,200	1,200	350	10	15	150	70
60	1.5	1.7	19	2.0	200	2.0	800	800	350	10	15	150	70
60	1.2	1.4	15	2.0	200	2.0	800	800	350	10	15	150	70
50	1.1	1.3	15	1.4	150	2.0	1,200	1,200	280	15	12	150	45
60	1.1	1.3	15	1.5	180	2.0	1,200	1,200	300	15	12	150	50
60	1.1	1.3	15	1.6	180	2.0	1,200	1,200	280	15	12	150	55
60	1.1	1.3	15	1.6	180	2.0	800	800	280	15	12	150	55
60	1.0	1.2	13	1.6	180	2.0	800	800	280	10	12	150	55
70	1.5	1.6	17	2.2	400	2.2	1,200	1,200	320	30	15	175	65
95	1.6	1.8	20	2.1	280	2.6	1,200	1,200	355	15	19	200	75
90	1.6	1.7	20	2.1	260	2.6	1,200	1,200	340	15	16	200	75

maximize the nutrient value of the plan, choose a serving of plant proteins (grains, legumes, and nuts) as part of your servings from the group containing meat, poultry, eggs, and fish. For fruits, include a vitamin C source. For vegetables, include a dark-green or orange vegetable each day. For breads, cereals, rice, and pasta, most of your servings should be whole-grained. Finally, include a tablespoon of vegetable oil (if not already present in other food products). A diet like this, using low-fat food choices, contains only about 1,600 calories but meets known nutritional needs, except possibly for iron in some women who have heavy menstrual flow. For those women, foods fortified in iron, such as breakfast cereals, can supply the deficit.

If 1,600 calories is too many calories for you, first try to become more active; it's hard to design an adequate diet for young adults that supplies fewer than 1,600 calories. If you can't increase your energy output, you can include some nutrient-fortified foods. If your diet doesn't include meat or other animal products, see the recommendations made in the discussion of vegetarianism.

Dietary Guidelines for Americans

To provide further guidance for choosing a healthy diet, the U.S. Department of Agriculture and the Department of Health and Human Services have issued Dietary Guidelines for Americans, most recently in 1990. What follows is a summary of the advice provided by the Dietary Guidelines, with additional comments from various health-related organizations, including the Surgeon General, the American Heart Association, the National Cancer Institute, and the National Academy of Sciences.

1. *Eat a variety of foods.* Focus on the Food Guide Pyramid we just discussed, choosing an appropriate number of servings from each group. Choose a variety of foods from within each group to take advantage of the fact that certain foods are better sources of some nutrients than other foods are. Everyone, especially adolescent girls and women, should take special care to meet their RDA for calcium and iron. Limit your protein intake to no more than twice the RDA and don't take a nutrient supplement in quantities greater than the U.S. RDA in any one day.

2. *Maintain healthy weight.* Emphasize balancing food intake with regular physical activity to avoid creeping overweight and eventual obesity. Excess body fat increases the risk for diabetes, heart disease, cancer,

Chapter 12   Nutrition Facts and Fallacies   319

TABLE 12-5 *Food Guide Pyramid*

This guide lets you easily turn the RDA into food choices. You can get all essential nutrients by eating a balanced variety of foods each day from the food groups listed here. Eat a variety of foods in each food group and adjust serving sizes appropriately to reach and maintain a desirable weight. This pattern will yield only about 1,600 calories.

Choosing some plant proteins and following the other suggestions listed should provide a diet adequate in all nutrients, except possibly iron for women who experience a heavy menstrual flow.

Food Group	Serving	Major Contributions	Foods and Serving Sizes*
Milk, yogurt, and cheese	2 (adult‖) 3 (children, teens, young adults, and pregnant or lactating women)	Calcium Riboflavin Protein Potassium Zinc	1 cup milk 1½ oz cheese 2 oz processed cheese 1 cup yogurt 2 cups cottage cheese 1 cup custard/pudding 1½ cups ice cream
Meat, poultry, fish, dry beans, eggs, and nuts	2–3	Protein Niacin Iron Vitamin B-6 Zinc Thiamin Vitamin B-12†	2–3 oz cooked meat, poultry, fish 1–1½ cups cooked dry beans 4 T peanut butter 2 eggs ½–1 cup nuts
Fruits	2–4	Vitamin C Carbohydrates Fiber	¼ cup dried fruit ½ cup cooked fruit ¾ cup juice 1 whole piece of fruit 1 melon wedge
Vegetables	3–5	Vitamin A Vitamin C Folate Magnesium Carbohydrates Fiber	½ cup raw or cooked vegetables 1 cup raw leafy vegetables
Bread, cereals, rice, and pasta	6–11	Starch Thiamin Riboflavin§ Iron Niacin Folate Magnesium‡ Carbohydrates Fiber‡ Zinc‡	1 slice of bread 1 oz ready-to-eat cereal ½–¾ cup cooked cereal, rice, or pasta
Fats, oils, and sweets			Foods from this group should not replace any from the other groups. Amounts consumed should be determined by individual energy needs.

*May be reduced for child servings
†Only in animal food choices
‡Whole grains especially
§If enriched
‖25 years of age or older

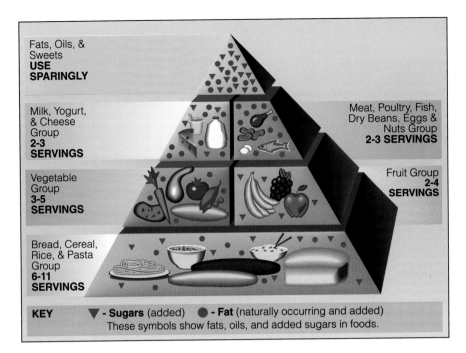

Figure 12-3 *The Food Guide Pyramid: a guide to daily food choices.* The Pyramid is an outline of what to eat each day. It's not a rigid prescription, but a general guide that lets you choose a healthful diet that's right for you. The Pyramid calls for eating a variety of foods to get the nutrients you need and at the same time the right amount of calories to maintain a healthy weight. The Pyramid also focuses on fat because many Americans eat too much fat, especially saturated fat. *Source:* U.S. Department of Agriculture, Human Nutrition Information Service. 1992. *Food Guide Pyramid.* Home and Garden Bulletin No. 249.

and other diseases. Those who are overweight shouldn't try to lose more than ½ to 1 pound per week. Weight loss should be accomplished by increasing physical activity and eating low-calorie, nutrient-rich foods—grains, vegetables, and fruits—not fat and fatty foods, sugar and sweets, and alcoholic beverages. Diets with fewer than 800–1,000 calories per day can be hazardous and should be followed only under medical supervision.

3. *Choose a diet low in fat, saturated fat, and cholesterol.* Limit your fat intake to 30 percent or less of total calories. Limit your intake of saturated fat to one-third of your total fat intake (10 percent of total calories) and dietary cholesterol to 300 milligrams per day. The average American consumes 15 percent of total calories as saturated fat and about 300–500 milligrams of dietary cholesterol per day. Experts recommend choosing lean meat, fish, poultry, and dry beans and peas as protein sources; using nonfat or low-fat milk and milk products; limiting your intake of fat-rich foods and oils high in saturated fat; trimming fat off meats; broiling, baking, or boiling instead of frying; and moderate use of fat-containing foods such as breaded or deep-fried foods. Refer to the box "Reducing the Fat in Your Diet" for more suggestions.

How many times a week do you eat at your favorite fast-food restaurant? The Appendix at the end of this chapter lists nutrition information for many of the fast foods we grab when we're on the run. If you look at the last column, you'll see that very few of them have a percentage of calories as fat that is less than 40 percent. If you eat a meal at a fast-food

restaurant, you'll need to choose low-fat foods during the rest of the day to stay within recommended levels of fat intake.

4. *Choose a diet with plenty of vegetables, fruits, and grain products.* Emphasize complex, rather than simple carbohydrates. Five or more servings of vegetables or fruits daily and six or more servings of breads, cereals, and legumes daily is a good goal and will help you reach a daily dietary fiber consumption of 20–35 grams.

5. *Use sugars only in moderation.* Some authorities recommend that no more than 10 percent of your total calories come from sugar. This would amount to about 40 pounds per person per year, as opposed to our current consumption of about 145 pounds per person per year.

6. *Use salt and sodium only in moderation.* Sodium is an essential nutrient, but you need only about 500 milligrams per day—that translates into only about ¼ teaspoon of salt. Most Americans consume 8 to 12 times this amount. It's recommended that you limit your sodium intake to no more than 2.4 to 3 grams per day, or about 1¼ to 1½ teaspoons of salt. A restriction of this magnitude does require a change in food habits for many people, such as eliminating processed (lunch) meats, salted snack foods, most canned and prepared soups, regular cheese, and many tomato-based products. You can begin to make this change by learning to enjoy the flavors of unsalted foods, adding little or no salt during cooking or at the table, and flavoring foods with herbs, spices, or lemon juice.

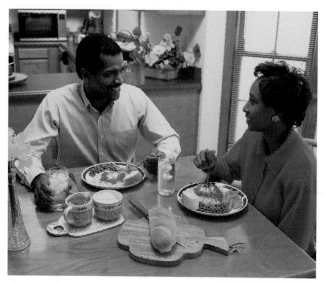

This couple's dinner of spaghetti with marinara sauce, carrots, peas, and bread is high in complex carbohydrates, vitamin A, vitamin C, folate, and dietary fiber.

TACTICS AND TIPS
Reducing the Fat in Your Diet

- Steam, boil, or bake vegetables, or stir fry them in a small amount of vegetable oil.

- Season vegetables with herbs and spices rather than with sauces, butter, or margarine.

- Try lemon juice on salad or use a yogurt-based salad dressing instead of mayonnaise or sour cream dressings.

- Use vegetable oil instead of butter or margarine when possible. Use tub margarine instead of stick margarine in baked products.

- Replace whole milk with skim or low-fat milk in puddings, soups, and baked products. Substitute plain low-fat yogurt, blender-whipped cottage cheese, or buttermilk in recipes that call for sour cream.

- Choose lean cuts of meat, and trim any visible fat from meat before and after cooking. Remove skin from poultry before or after cooking.

- Roast, bake, or broil meat, poultry, or fish so that fat drains away as the food cooks.

- Use a nonstick pan for cooking so added fat will be unnecessary; use a vegetable spray for frying.

- Chill broths from meat or poultry until the fat becomes solid. Spoon off the fat before using the broth.

- Eat a low-fat vegetarian main dish at least once a week.

7. *If you drink alcoholic beverages, do so in moderation.* Men should consume no more than two drinks daily. Women should drink no more than one drink daily, and alcohol should not be consumed during pregnancy. One drink is the equivalent of 5 ounces of wine, 12 ounces of beer, or 1½ ounces of distilled spirits. Remember, alcoholic beverages are high in calories and low in nutrients.

One further recommendation geared specifically for cancer prevention is to use moderation when consuming salt-cured, smoked, and nitrate-cured foods (such as bacon and sausage) because these may increase the risk of colon and other gastrointestinal cancers.

These guidelines do not apply equally to everyone. We vary in our susceptibility to developing high serum cholesterol levels, high blood pressure, obesity, cancer, and the other health problems these guidelines seek to counteract. You should consider your own health status and apply these guidelines appropriately to address current or potential health problems.

How does the average American diet measure up against these guidelines? Despite reported trends in the American diet away from saturated fats (whole milk and cream being replaced by low-fat and nonfat milk, for instance), not all the recent dietary news is good. In fact, whole milk and whole-milk beverages continue to be one of the five major contributors of calories to the American diet. The other four are white bread, rolls, and crackers; doughnuts, cakes, and cookies; alcoholic beverages; and hamburgers, cheeseburgers, and meatloaf. Some of these foods have some nutritional value, but were the American diet truly moving toward the ideas we've just discussed— a decrease in alcohol, sugar, and saturated fats, along with an increase in dietary fiber—we wouldn't expect to find these foods at the top of the list. We feel that low-fat and nonfat milk, whole-wheat bread and whole-grain cereals, lean meat, tuna, beans, and other vegetable proteins should replace these as contributors of calories and that oranges, romaine lettuce, carrots, and broccoli should also be major sources of nutrients. What would your list look like? You can further evaluate your current eating and food preparation habits by completing the nearby "Nutrition Checklist."

> *Personal Insight* Do you feel good after you eat a healthy meal? Are your good feelings physical or emotional or both?

The Vegetarian Alternative

Some people choose a diet with one essential difference from the diets we've already described—foods of animal origin (meat, poultry, fish, eggs, milk) are eliminated or restricted. Today, several million Americans follow a veg-

The Food Guide Pyramid provides a general basis for good nutrition. Your choice of foods within each group and methods of food preparation are also important. Evaluate some of your dietary habits by answering the following questions with yes (Y) or no (N). A "no" answer indicates a behavior you might want to change.

_____ 1. I rarely add salt to my food when cooking or eating.

_____ 2. I take time to read food labels when shopping.

_____ 3. I choose foods that are fresh and unprocessed whenever possible.

_____ 4. I eat a wide variety of foods.

_____ 5. I remove fat and skin before cooking meat, poultry, or fish.

_____ 6. I sometimes have meatless days, substituting healthy alternatives to meat.

_____ 7. I broil, boil, or bake rather than fry meat, fish, and poultry.

_____ 8. I choose nonfat or low-fat milk and milk products.

_____ 9. I eat sherbet or frozen yogurt rather than ice cream.

_____ 10. I use vegetable oil instead of butter or margarine.

_____ 11. I choose whole-grain breads rather than white.

_____ 12. I choose cereals that are high in fiber.

_____ 13. I choose cereals, crackers, bread, and other foods that are low in added sugar and low in fat.

_____ 14. I have at least one serving of a citrus fruit each day.

_____ 15. I have at least one serving of a dark green or orange vegetable every day.

_____ 16. I eat fresh or frozen fruits and vegetables rather than canned whenever possible.

_____ 17. When I cook vegetables, I generally steam them.

_____ 18. I avoid frequent consumption of salt-cured, smoked, or nitrate-cured foods.

_____ 19. I consume alcohol in moderation.

_____ 20. I use nonstick pans or sprays when cooking to avoid adding extra fat to my food.

---

etarian diet. Most do so because they think foods of plant origin are a more natural way to nourish the body. Some do so for religious, health, ethical, or philosophical reasons. If you choose to be a vegetarian, you can be confident you can meet your nutritional needs by following a few basic rules. (Vegetarian diets for children and pregnant women warrant individual professional guidance.)

There is a variety of vegetarian styles; the wider the variety of the diet eaten, the easier it is to meet nutritional needs. **Vegans** eat only plant foods. **Lacto-vegetarians** eat plant foods and dairy products. **Lacto-ovo-vegetarians** eat plant foods, dairy products, and eggs. Finally, **partial** or **semivegetarians** eat plant foods, dairy products, eggs, and usually a small selection of poultry, fish, and other seafood. Including some animal protein in a diet makes planning much easier.

A food-group plan has been developed for lacto-vegetarians; it includes six servings from a protein group that contains grains, legumes, nuts, and seeds. Three or more servings from a vegetable group, one to four servings from a fruit group, and two or more servings from the milk and/or eggs group complete the plan. By following this plan, the lacto-vegetarian should have no problem obtaining an adequate diet. Consuming fruits with most meals is especially helpful, because any vitamin C present will improve iron absorption (the iron in plants is more difficult to absorb than is that in animal sources).

In contrast to those who eat dairy products, the vegan has to do much more special diet planning to obtain all essential nutrients. A vegan must take special care to consume adequate amounts of protein, riboflavin, vitamin D, vitamin B-12, calcium, iron, and zinc; good strategies for obtaining these nutrients include the following:

• Eat proteins from a wide variety of sources and include a couple of protein sources at each meal. A good rule of thumb is that 60 percent of the protein should be from grains; 35 percent from legumes, which include black-eyed peas, peanuts, split peas,

Vegans Vegetarians who eat no animal products at all.

Lacto-vegetarians Vegetarians who include milk and cheese products in their diet.

Partial or semivegetarians Vegetarians who include eggs, dairy products, and small amounts of poultry and seafood in their diet.

Lacto-ovo-vegetarians Vegetarians who eat no meat, poultry, or fish, but do eat eggs and milk products.

TERMS

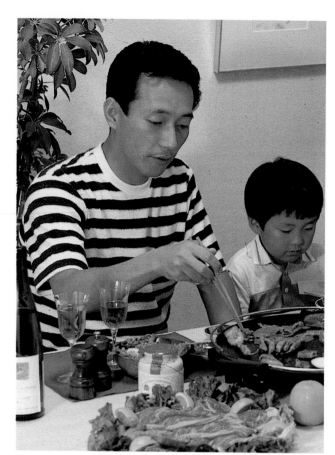

Many different cultural dietary patterns provide adequate nutrients and encompass the dietary practices recommended by nutrition experts. The adult eating habits of this boy will be powerfully influenced—both positively and negatively—by the foods he eats as he's growing up.

garbanzos, **tofu** (soybean curd), lentils, and many other types of beans and peas; and 5 percent from dark-green leafy vegetables.

- Eat green leafy vegetables, whole grains, yeast, and legumes to obtain riboflavin.

- Obtain vitamin D by spending at least one-half hour a day out in the sun or—if that is not possible on a regular basis—by taking a supplement of 200 I.U. or 5 micrograms.

- Obtain vitamin B-12 (found only in animal foods) from a supplement or by consuming foods fortified with vitamin B-12, such as special yeast products, soy milks, and breakfast cereals. (Vitamin B-12 deficiency takes a long time to develop, but it can cause irreversible nerve damage.)

TERMS

Tofu A custardlike food made from soybeans.

- Consume fortified tofu, green leafy vegetables, nuts, and fortified orange juice and soy milk to obtain calcium. Supplements may be necessary.

- Consume whole grains, dried fruits, nuts, and legumes to obtain iron.

- Obtain zinc from whole grains and legumes.

It takes a little planning and common sense to put together a good vegetarian diet. If you are a vegetarian or are considering becoming one, devote some extra time and thought to your diet. It's especially important that you eat as wide a variety of foods as possible to ensure that all of your nutritional needs are filled.

A PERSONAL PLAN: MAKING INTELLIGENT CHOICES ABOUT FOOD

Now that you understand the basis of good nutrition and a healthy diet, you can put together a diet that works for you. There probably is an ideal diet for you based on your particular nutrition and health status, but there is no single type of diet that provides optimal health for everyone. Many cultural dietary patterns encompass the practices recommended by nutrition experts: eating a variety of foods, maintaining a healthy body weight, and maintaining a physically active lifestyle (refer to the box "Ethnic Diets and Cuisines" for more information). For you, the key now is to focus on the likely causes of health problems in your life and to make specific dietary changes to address those. Beyond this, there are some specific areas that may be of concern to you, such as deciphering food labels, deciding whether to use a vitamin supplement, choosing an expert to help you plan a diet, avoiding foodborne illness, and understanding food additives. We turn to these and other issues next.

Reading Food Labels to Learn More About What You Eat

To make intelligent choices about food, you should learn to read and understand food labels. In December 1992, the federal government enacted new and dramatically different guidelines for food labels. All food packages are required to have the new labels in place no later than May 1994, though some will begin using them earlier.

Under the old regulations, food labels giving nutritional content were required only if the manufacturer made a nutritional claim about the food or if nutrients were added to the food. These labels list the number of calories; the amount (by weight) of protein, carbohydrate, fat, and sodium; and the percentage of U.S. RDA of protein and various vitamins and minerals.

The new labels are designed to help consumers make food choices based on the nutrients of most concern to health. Under the new regulations, all food packages will

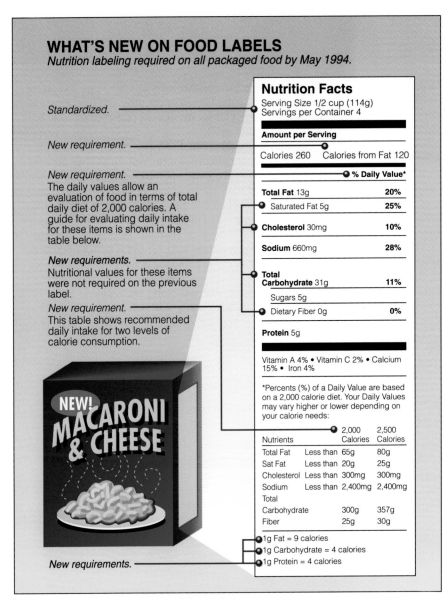

WHAT'S NEW ON FOOD LABELS
Nutrition labeling required on all packaged food by May 1994.

Standardized.

New requirement.

New requirement.
The daily values allow an evaluation of food in terms of total daily diet of 2,000 calories. A guide for evaluating daily intake for these items is shown in the table below.

New requirements.
Nutritional values for these items were not required on the previous label.

New requirement.
This table shows recommended daily intake for two levels of calorie consumption.

New requirements.

Nutrition Facts
Serving Size 1/2 cup (114g)
Servings per Container 4

Amount per Serving

Calories 260   Calories from Fat 120

	% Daily Value*
Total Fat 13g	20%
Saturated Fat 5g	25%
Cholesterol 30mg	10%
Sodium 660mg	28%
Total Carbohydrate 31g	11%
Sugars 5g	
Dietary Fiber 0g	0%

Protein 5g

Vitamin A 4% • Vitamin C 2% • Calcium 15% • Iron 4%

*Percents (%) of a Daily Value are based on a 2,000 calorie diet. Your Daily Values may vary higher or lower depending on your calorie needs:

Nutrients		2,000 Calories	2,500 Calories
Total Fat	Less than	65g	80g
Sat Fat	Less than	20g	25g
Cholesterol	Less than	300mg	300mg
Sodium	Less than	2,400mg	2,400mg
Total Carbohydrate		300g	357g
Fiber		25g	30g

1g Fat = 9 calories
1g Carbohydrate = 4 calories
1g Protein = 4 calories

Figure 12-4   *The new, improved food label.*
A sample label for macaroni and cheese is shown here.

have to show how much fat, saturated fat, cholesterol, protein, dietary fiber, and sodium they contain. In addition to listing nutrient content by weight, the new labels put the information in the context of a daily diet of 2,000 calories that includes no more than 65 grams of fat (approximately 30 percent of total calories). For example, if a serving of a particular product has 260 calories and 13 grams of fat, the label will tell you that that amount of fat is 20 percent of the total amount of fat recommended for a daily diet of 2,000 calories.

The new labels require uniform serving sizes. This means that consumers looking at different brands of salad dressing, for example, can compare calories and fat content based on the same serving amount. The new regula-

tions also require that foods meet strict definitions if their packaging includes the terms "light," "low-fat," or "high-fiber." A footnote on the label gives suggested intakes of fat, saturated fat, cholesterol, sodium, carbohydrate, and fiber for both a 2,000-calorie diet and a 2,500-calorie diet. A sample label is shown in Figure 12-4.

Who Should Take Vitamin or Mineral Supplements?

You may wonder whether or not to take vitamin or mineral supplements. To answer this question, first look closely at your diet. Does it follow the Food Guide Pyramid, especially emphasizing whole grains, low-fat and

Every cultural group has its own eating practices—its own habitually eaten foods (its diet) and its own manner of preparing foods (its cuisine). These culture-based eating practices are influenced by many factors, including availability of food items, cultural and religious beliefs and values about what people can and can't eat, and even the symbolic meaning of various foods.

In the United States, where so many different groups have mingled, eating practices are a blend of many traditions. The diets of the native peoples of the Western Hemisphere included corn, beans, squash, tomatoes, chili peppers, fish, game, wild nuts, wild fruits, and wild greens. The earliest immigrants, most of them from England and other northern European countries, brought with them a meat-heavy diet and cuisine that reflected the cultural importance of hunting. Dinners consisted of large portions of meat, side dishes of cabbage or carrots, and fruit pie for dessert. For breakfast, these European Americans ate eggs, bacon or other cuts of meat, and bread or biscuits. Also from England came the concept of three meals a day, the evening meal being the most substantial.

To the extent they could, African Americans also preserved their food traditions. From West Africa they brought such food as peanuts, okra, and black-eyed peas, and they combined them with native American foods such as greens, sweet potatoes, and wild fish and game. French immigrants, far fewer in number than the English, preserved their French country-cooking heritage in southern Louisiana. A gradual blending of their practices with African American practices produced Cajun cuisine, reflecting both French and African influences. This cuisine includes spicy, thick soups (gumbo, jambalaya), sausage, rice, red beans, and seafood.

Other food traditions came with later immigrants—Chinese, Japanese, Mexican, Southern European, Caribbean,

TABLE 1 *Characteristics of Selected American Ethnic Diets*

	Hispanic Diet	African American Diet (Southern)	Chinese American Diet
Meats and other proteins	Legumes (pinto beans, black beans), chicken, pork, eggs, cheese, seafood, tripe, sausages	Legumes (white beans, black-eyed peas), pork, chicken, fish, pickled meats, pecans, peanuts	Pork, beef, chicken, duck, fish, shellfish, eggs, tofu, soy milk, nuts
Vegetables and fruits	Corn, potatoes, red and green chilis, tomatoes, onions, cactus, jicama, squash, bananas, plantains, melons, avocados, oranges, mangoes, guavas, papayas	Corn, potatoes, onions, sweet potatoes, tomatoes, okra, swiss chard, collard greens, cabbage, squash, melons, peaches, bananas, limes, oranges	Carrots, onions, bok choy and other cabbage, broccoli, celery, mushrooms, green beans, squash, bean sprouts, bamboo shoots, pea pods, citrus fruits, kumquats, melons, grapes, apples, bananas
Grains	Corn and wheat tortillas, macaroni, rice, bread, baked and fried pastries of refined flour	Biscuits, fried breads, cornbread, hominy grits, rice, baked desserts of refined flour	Rice, wheat-flour dumplings and steamed breads, fried noodles
Fats used in cooking	Lard, salt pork, bacon fat, margarine	Lard, palm oil, butter, margarine	Peanut oil, soybean oil, sesame oil, lard
Strengths of the diet	A variety of fruits and vegetables are available to the diet. Beans, corn, and rice provide high-quality, complementary protein.	Leafy green vegetables such as collard greens are an excellent source of vitamins, minerals, and fiber. Sweet potatoes, used in a variety of dishes, are high in vitamins and minerals.	A wide range of vegetables is available, including many anticarcinogenic vegetables. This diet is rich in vitamins, minerals, and fiber and low in saturated fat and sugar. Most foods are stir-fried, using little cooking oil. Desserts usually consist of fresh fruit.
Weaknesses of the diet	Many foods are fried or contain high amounts of animal fats. The diet lacks leafy green vegetables, calcium-rich foods, and fiber.	Many foods are fried or contain high amounts of animal fats. The diet tends to depend on meat as a main dish and tends not to include fresh fruit daily. Although good sources of protein, peanuts and pecans are high in saturated fat. The diet tends to be high in salt.	There are few options in the grains category; steamed rice is the predominant grain. Condiments such as MSG (monosodium glutamate) and soy sauce are high in sodium. The diet tends to be low in calcium.

Middle Eastern, and Southeast Asian, to name just a few. Many of their recipes changed over the years, adapting to the absence or availability of ingredients and to changing tastes. At the same time, elements from all these diets and cuisines were assimilated into existing American food patterns.

Although the American diet is a rich hybrid, some foods are thought of as "typically American," including hamburgers, hot dogs, pizza, fried chicken, turkey, steak, potatoes, sweet potatoes, corn, lobster, pies, layer cakes, ice cream, and many prepared foods. Probably the most distinctive feature of the American diet is the central position given to meat, a legacy of our northern European roots. Diets and cuisines that maintain their distinctiveness within American culture, usually associated with more recent immigrant groups, are often referred to as ethnic diets and ethnic cuisines. Many items from these cuisines, such as nachos, bean burritos, Chinese chicken salad, fettucine alfredo, and falafel, are commonly available in restaurants all over the country. Other items are available in "ethnic" restaurants.

Is there one diet that clearly surpasses all the others in providing people with healthful foods? The answer is no; the diet of every culture has evolved as a means of meeting people's nutritional requirements within the limits of available resources. However, every diet has its advantages and disadvantages, so within each cuisine, some foods are better choices. It is in this area of personal choice that individuals can make a difference in their own health, whether they follow a traditional ethnic diet exclusively or just like to eat out at an Indian or Chinese restaurant on Saturday night.

Table 1 lists some of the foods that make up the typical diet of selected American ethnic groups, along with the advantages and disadvantages of each. Table 2 lists the more and less healthful choices individuals can make when they eat out at various ethnic restaurants.

	Japanese American Diet	Diet of Middle-Eastern Americans	Diet of Southeast-Asian Americans
Meats and other proteins	Fresh, smoked, canned, dried, and raw fish; tofu; soy milk; eggs; chicken; pork; beef; red beans; seafood such as squid and eel	Lamb, chicken, beef, seafood, chick peas, lentils, cheese, yogurt, tahini (ground sesame seeds)	Fresh, dried, and salted fish; fish sauces; pork; beef; chicken; eggs; peanuts; tofu; sweetened, condensed milk
Vegetables and fruits	Sea vegetables, mushrooms, onions, cabbage, bamboo shoots, carrots, celery, daikon (white radish), spinach, eggplant, persimmons, pears, apples, bananas, oranges, grapes, melons, pickled fruits such as plums	Eggplants, tomatoes, onions, peppers, garlic, leeks, artichokes, zucchini, fava beans, olives, melons, pomegranates, lemons, oranges, dates, figs, apricots	Cauliflower, leafy greens, squash, mushrooms, bamboo shoots, bok choy and other cabbage, carrots, sweet potatoes, cucumbers, lemon grass, mint, bananas, mangoes, papayas, pineapple, melons, coconut, oranges, tamarind
Grains	Rice, rice noodles, buckwheat noodles, bread, baked and steamed sweet rolls sometimes filled with sweet red bean paste	Rice, tabouli (cracked wheat), couscous (ground wheat), bread, millet, barley, pastries of refined flour	Rice, bread, noodles
Fats used in cooking	Soybean oil, rice oil, suet	Olive oil	Lard, vegetable oil, coconut oil, peanut oil, sesame oil, butter
Strengths of the diet	This diet is low in saturated fat. A wide range of vegetables and fruits is available. Sea vegetables are excellent sources of vitamins and minerals and are versatile foods.	Whole grains are eaten with nearly every meal, providing complex carbohydrates and fiber. The main cooking oil, olive oil, reduces cholesterol. Fresh and dried fruit are consumed regularly.	Most foods are stir-fried or broiled, so the diet can be relatively low in fat. The diet can contain excellent sources of calcium—small fish bones and vinegar in which animal bones have soaked. A variety of fruit and vegetables is available.
Weaknesses of the diet	Sea vegetables are high in salt. Raw fish, an important food in the diet, can carry intestinal parasites.	This diet emphasizes protein, especially from animal sources. It lacks leafy green vegetables and is low in calcium.	Heavy use of MSG and foods preserved by pickling or salting results in a high-salt diet. Coconut oil and coconut milk, commonly used in sauces, are high in fat. French bread made from refined flour (eaten regularly by Vietnamese Americans) is low in fiber and nutritional value.

(continued)

TABLE 2 When You're Dining Out . . .

	Choose Often	Choose Less Often
Chinese	Chinese greens	Crispy duck
	Rice, brown or white	Egg rolls
	Steamed beef with pea pods	Fried rice
	Stir-fry dishes	Kung pao (fried chicken)
	Wonton soup	Pork spare ribs
Japanese	Chiri nabe (fish stew)	Age tofu (fried tofu)
	Sushi, sashimi (raw fish)	Tonkatsu (fried pork)
	Yakitori (grilled chicken)	Tempura (fried chicken, shrimp, or vegetables)
Thai	Forest salad	Fried fish, duck, or chicken
	Larb (minty chicken salad)	Curries with coconut milk
	Po tak (seafood soup)	Yum koon chaing (sausage with peppers)
	Yum neua (broiled beef with onions)	
Italian	Cioppino (seafood stew)	Antipasto
	Minestrone soup (vegetarian)	Cannelloni, ravioli
	Pasta with marinara sauce	Fettucini alfredo
	Pasta primavera (pasta with vegetables)	Garlic bread
		White clam sauce
Mexican	Beans and rice	Chiles rellenos
	Black bean/vegetable soup	Chimichangas
	Burritos, bean	Enchiladas, beef or cheese
	Enchiladas, bean	Flautas
	Gazpacho	Guacamole
	Tortillas, steamed	Nachos or fried tortillas
	Tostadas, bean or chicken	Quesadillas
Indian	Chapati (tortilla-like bread)	Bhatura (fried bread)
	Dal (lentils)	Coconut milk
	Karni (chick-pea soup)	Ghee (clarified butter)
	Khur (milk/rice dessert)	Korma (rich meat dish)
	Tandoori, chicken or fish	Samosa (fried meat and vegetables in dough)

Source: Runner's World, January 1990, p. 25.

nonfat dairy products, leafy and dark-green vegetables, foods containing vitamin C, and a serving of vegetable oils? If so, men are probably meeting their nutrient needs; some women (those with heavy menstrual flows) may still need more iron to compensate for that lost. Secondly, do you regularly consume a fortified breakfast cereal? Most breakfast cereals have extra vitamins and minerals added, some even matching the adult U.S. RDA.

Nutrition scientists generally agree that most people can obtain needed vitamins and minerals from a healthy diet. Improve your diet where needed. After that, consider whether you need a supplement. Talk to a registered dietitian and your physician as well, because there is some risk in consuming even standard multivitamin and mineral supplements, not necessarily megadoses. These risks include iron toxicity in individuals genetically prone to a certain liver disease (hemochromatosis) and birth defects during the early months of pregnancy.

Recently a panel of nutrition scientists suggested certain cases when vitamin and mineral supplements should be considered.

• Women with excessive bleeding during menses may need iron.

• Women who are pregnant or breastfeeding may need extra iron, folate, and calcium.

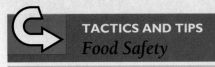

- Thoroughly wash hands with hot soapy water before and after handling food, especially raw meat, fish, poultry, or eggs, which may contain *Salmonella* bacteria.

- Don't let groceries sit in a warm car; bacteria will grow in warm temperatures. Get them home to the refrigerator or freezer promptly.

- Don't buy food in containers that leak, bulge, or are severely dented—the deadly botulism toxin may be present.

- Make sure counters, cutting boards, dishes, and other equipment are thoroughly cleaned before and after use, especially if they have come in contact with raw meat, fish, poultry, or eggs.

- Thoroughly rinse and scrub fruits and vegetables, with a brush, if possible. Peel them, if appropriate, even though you'll peel away some of the nutrients. Remove outer leaves of leafy vegetables, such as lettuce and cabbage.

- If possible, use separate cutting boards for meat and for foods that will be eaten raw, such as fruits or vegetables. Recent research indicates that wood cutting boards may be more sanitary than plastic ones for cutting up raw meat and poultry.

- Cook foods thoroughly, especially beef, poultry, fish, pork, and eggs. Cooking kills most microbes. Don't eat raw animal products.

- Trim fat from meat, poultry, and fish and remove skin (which contains most of the fat) from poultry and fish. Discard fats and oils found in broths and pan drippings. (Pesticide residues concentrate in the animals' fat.)

- Cook stuffing separately from poultry; or wash poultry thoroughly, stuff immediately before cooking, and then transfer the stuffing to a clean bowl immediately after cooking.

- Store foods below 40° or above 140° F. Do not leave cooked or refrigerated foods, such as meats or salads, at room temperature for more than two hours.

- Avoid coughing or sneezing over foods, even when you are healthy, and cover any cuts on your hands.

- Use only pasteurized milk.

- Throw back the big fish—the little ones have less time to take up and concentrate pesticides and other harmful residues.

Adapted from Food and Drug Administration. 1988. "Safety First: Protecting America's Food Supply." *FDA Consumer*, November, p. 26.

---

rather to change manufacturing practices to reduce cancer risk.

Compounds such as BHA and BHT prevent changes in color, flavor, or texture that occur when foods are exposed to air. While some studies show that BHT prevents certain forms of cancer in animals, other studies link BHT to some other forms of cancer. The FDA is reviewing use of BHT and BHA, but any risk to the diet from these agents is low. Some companies have stopped using BHA and BHT and substituted other preservatives, such as vitamin C, citric acid, or vitamin E.

Sulfites protect vegetables from turning brown. Their use has been severely limited by the FDA in the last few years because some people develop allergic reactions after eating foods treated with them. These reactions include difficulty in breathing, wheezing, hives, diarrhea, vomiting, abdominal pain, and dizziness after exposure. The FDA currently requires manufacturers to declare the presence of sulfites on labels of packaged foods containing at least 10 parts per million of sulfites. Labels on wine bottles must also have a sulfite warning.

The process of **food irradiation** causes "ionizing" radiation by creating free radicals. The gamma radiation used does not make the food radioactive; however, the energy is strong enough to break chemical bonds. By altering DNA, enzymes, and a variety of proteins, irradiation can prevent the growth of microorganisms, parasites, and insects without creating much heat in the food product. The process is sometimes referred to as "cold sterilization." Since irradiation alters food, it is regulated like food additives.

Food irradiation is a safe and effective way to extend the shelf life of foods, destroy microorganisms, slow the rapid ripening of harvested produce, and reduce the need for pesticides. Extensive studies indicate that foods exposed to low doses of irradiation are safe to eat and do not undergo significant changes in nutrient composition. Irradiation is also used to prepare special foods for astronauts, military personnel, and cancer patients with impaired immunity. The FDA has approved irradiation of spices, dried herbs, pork, fresh fruits, and poultry. So far, however, food companies have been reluctant to market irradiated foods.

Food irradiation A sterilizing process used to preserve food by means of ionizing radiation.

TERMS

Additives That Aid in Processing and Preparation

Some additives help give body and texture to foods, help blend food components, improve baking qualities, control acidity or alkalinity, help retain moisture, and prevent caking or lumping. For example, emulsifiers suspend fat in water, in turn giving a uniform consistency to cakes. Thickeners create smoothness and prevent ice crystals from forming in frozen foods like ice cream. Leavening agents, such as yeast and baking powder, make baked goods rise by releasing carbon dioxide during the cooking process.

Additives That Alter Taste and Appearance

Various products are added to foods to alter their taste and appearance, including coloring agents, natural and artificial flavors, and flavor enhancers such as monosodium glutamate (MSG) and sweeteners. One coloring agent (Yellow No. 5) can cause hives, itching, runny nose, and asthma in some people; it must be listed separately on food labels. Some artificial flavors are chemically identical to their "natural" counterparts, while others are not. Saccharin and aspartame—common alternate sweeteners—fall into the latter category. Some people experience episodes of high blood pressure and sweating after consuming the common flavor enhancer MSG. If you're sensitive to MSG, check food labels when you're shopping and ask to have it left out of dishes you order at restaurants.

Limits for the Use of Additives

The amount of an additive that can be used in food processing must be kept to the lowest amount needed to do the job and is also limited to 0.01 to 0.001 of the dose that is found safe to administer to animals. If the additive is known to cause cancer in animals, then it generally cannot be intentionally used in foods at all. Thus, although additives such as sulfites, MSG, and the yellow dye tartrazine do cause reactions in sensitive individuals, food additives pose no significant health hazard to most people because the levels used are well below any that could produce toxic effects. Check food labels if you think you are sensitive to MSG or tartrazine. Foods containing these products can always be replaced by others free of the additives. If you consume a variety of foods in moderation, the chance of suffering negative health consequences from food additives is minimal.

Overall, the American food supply is outstandingly safe, whether you're concerned with additives, pesticides, or bacteria. With reasonable precautions in preparing food and avoiding substances to which you seem to be sensitive, you can be confident that the food supply is not causing you harm. By far the greatest dietary risks to your long term health come from overconsumption of calories, fat, and sodium.

SUMMARY

- Choosing foods that provide needed nutrients is an important part of daily life. Food choices made in youth can significantly affect health in later years.

Nutritional Requirements: Components of a Healthy Diet

- The fuel potential in our diet is expressed in calories.

- To function at its best, the human body requires about 45 essential nutrients in specific proportions. People get the nutrients needed to fuel their bodies and maintain tissues and organ systems through foods; the body cannot synthesize most of them.

- Proteins, made up of amino acids, form muscles and bones and help make up blood, enzymes, hormones, and cell membranes. Foods from animal sources provide complete proteins; plants provide incomplete proteins, but combinations of plant proteins yield complete proteins. The American diet is generally rich in protein.

- Fats, a concentrated source of energy, also help insulate the body and cushion the organs; 1 tablespoon of vegetable oil per day supplies the essential fats. Dietary fat intake should be limited to 30 percent of total calories. Americans need to reduce consumption of saturated fats especially, replacing them mostly with complex carbohydrates.

- Carbohydrates supply energy to the brain and other parts of the nervous system as well as to red blood cells. The body needs 50–100 grams of carbohydrates a day; much more is usually consumed. During digestion, carbohydrates are broken down into glucose and other simple sugars for energy; some is stored as glycogen.

- Dietary fiber includes plant substances difficult or impossible for humans to digest. Insoluble fibers like wheat bran hold water and increase bulk in the stool; they may prevent or lessen various bowel disorders. Soluble fibers like oat bran bind cholesterol-containing compounds in the intestine and slow glucose absorption; they may help lower elevated cholesterol and glucose levels.

- The 13 vitamins needed in the diet are organic substances that promote specific chemical and cell processes within living tissue. Deficiencies can cause serious illnesses and even death.

- Water is used to digest and absorb food, to transport substances around the body, to lubricate joints and organs, and to regulate body temperature. Lack of water can cause death within a few days.

- The approximately 17 minerals needed in the diet are inorganic substances that regulate body functions, aid in growth and maintenance of body tissues, and help in the release of energy from foods. The minerals most commonly lacking in the diet are iron and calcium.

Nutritional Guidelines: Planning Your Diet

- Various scientific and governmental groups have established nutrition guidelines for preventing nutrient deficiencies, for providing balanced nutrient intake, and for combating specific diseases.

- Recommended Dietary Allowances (RDAs) are recommended intakes for essential nutrients that meet the needs of healthy persons. They are a guide to foods, not to supplements, and are averages for groups.

- The Food Guide Pyramid contains six food groups; choosing foods from each every day helps insure appropriate amounts of necessary nutrients. The fundamental principles of the Food Guide Pyramid are moderation, variety, and balance.

- The Dietary Guidelines for Americans address prevention of diet-related diseases like cardiovascular disease, cancer, and diabetes. The guidelines advise: (1) eat a variety of foods, (2) maintain a healthy weight, (3) choose a diet low in fat, (4) choose a diet with plenty of fruits, vegetables, and grain products, (5) use sugars only in moderation, (6) use sodium only in moderation, and (7) drink alcohol in moderation, if at all.

- A vegetarian diet can meet human nutritional needs. Although including dairy products makes diet planning easier, a vegan can meet all needs through careful planning and a wide variety of foods.

A Personal Plan: Making Intelligent Choices About Food

- No single diet provides wellness for everyone; people should focus on the likely causes of health problems in their lives and make dietary changes to address them.

- New regulations for food labels require all food packages to show how much fat, cholesterol, protein, fiber, and sodium they contain. Serving sizes have been standardized, and health claims are carefully regulated.

- Most people don't need vitamin and mineral supplements. Those who do include pregnant and breastfeeding women, vegetarians, and people who are ill or taking certain medications.

- Reliable nutritional advice can be obtained from registered dietitians; some people will also need consultation with a physician.

- Food-borne illness is a greater threat to health than are additives and environmental contaminants; many cases of "flu" are probably actually food poisoning. Specific precautions in handling and preparing food can help prevent food-borne illness.

- Food additives maintain or improve nutritional quality, maintain freshness, help in processing, and alter taste or appearance. They make up less than 1 percent of our food; the chance of suffering negative health consequences is minimal.

TAKE ACTION

1. Read the list of ingredients on three or four canned or packaged foods that you enjoy eating. If any ingredients are unfamiliar to you, find out what they are and why they have been used. A nutrition textbook from the library may be a helpful resource.

2. Investigate the nutritional and dietary guidelines that are used to prepare the food served in your school. Are they consistent with what you've learned in this chapter? If not, try to find out more about the guidelines that have been used and why they were chosen.

3. Prepare a flavorful low-fat vegetarian and/or ethnic meal. (Use the suggestions in the chapter and check your local library for appropriate cookbooks.) How do the foods included in the meal and the preparation methods differ from what you're used to?

JOURNAL ENTRY

1. In your health journal, keep track of everything you eat and drink for three or four days. Calculate the average number of servings of each food group you consume per day. Then see how well your average daily intake meets the guidelines in the Food Guide Pyramid.

2. Put together three sample daily menus that follow the Food Guide Pyramid. Keep the dietary guidelines in mind as you make your food selections from each group. Also be sure to base your menus around foods you enjoy eating.

3. *Critical Thinking:* Analyze patterns of food advertising on television by recording the number and types of ads that appear each hour. If possible, compare the number and types of products advertised during an hour of cartoons or other children's programs, an hour of daytime programs, and an hour of prime-time programs. What patterns do you see? What types of information do the ads present? Are they geared toward different segments of the population? Do they encourage healthy eating?

IMPROVING YOUR DIET

If you want to alter your diet, some of the major health behavior change strategies we have already examined can help you. Here are some suggestions for behavior management that you can use to lower your fat consumption, raise your fiber intake, or make other changes in your diet.

Establishing a Baseline

Let's say that you want to do two things to your diet: (1) Cut out all candy while walking between classes or while on errands in town and (2) eat more fresh fruits and raw vegetables.

Begin by keeping track of your candy consumption. In a journal jot down the time of day and what occurred before and after you ate the candy. On a chart such as the one shown here, keep track of the number of times each day you eat candy. Because you also want to add more fruits and vegetables to your diet, also keep notes on the kinds of foods you have been eating at meals. You can include this information on the same chart or you can keep two graphs.

Intervention

Once you have established your baseline levels, begin to make some changes in those routines that seem to precede your eating candy. For example, you might find that you have been eating candy from a vending machine that you walk by every day after class. If this is the case, try another route that allows you to avoid the machine. If you find that you usually are hungry at one particular time of day and that you rarely have lunch or a healthful snack with you, try to keep a healthful snack on hand so that

you won't be caught off guard and be pushed toward eating candy (which always seems to be available). Putting fresh or dried fruit in a backpack or pocket every morning can help. You can use the same sort of strategy to increase the number of fruits and vegetables in your diet: Specifically, you will need to shop for these food items *in advance* and prepare them *ahead of time* so that they are readily available.

Revision (If Needed)

You may discover that your initial plan works perfectly or that it works well for three weeks but then loses its effectiveness. Watch out for programs that become stale and lose their strength, and, of course, revise an ineffective program entirely once you have given it a real try. The critical data from your journal can help you to decide how to revise your program. Plotting the data on a prominently displayed chart can encourage you to continue.

Social Eating Events

Avoiding an attractive candy vending machine may be a lot easier than cutting back on late-night pizza binges; the former involves only you while the latter involves you and your friends. It's harder to make adjustments in social eating patterns, but there are some strategies that you can try. First, tell your friends that you would prefer to try something new to eat instead of pizza, such as popcorn. Being assertive in such matters can be very helpful; you may discover some allies who share your views about the type of food you want to eat. Second, try to cut down on these group activities without eliminating them entirely. Of course, you can try to change or limit the kinds of food you eat at these times, but it's generally very difficult to refrain from joining in once you're actually in the social situation.

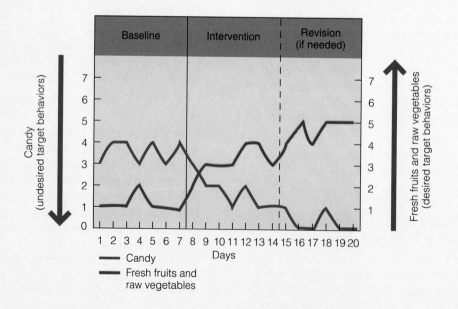

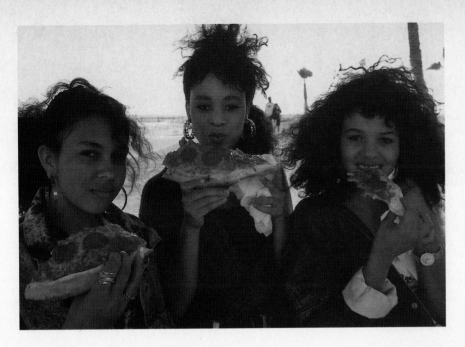

Pizza makes a convenient lunch, but it's not always a good choice. Pizza with lots of cheese and pepperoni can be very high in fat, and the white flour crust may be filling without providing needed nutrients. These young women could improve their meal by adding a salad or a piece of fresh fruit.

Systematic Changes in Other Habits

Many people begin an exercise program or begin to increase their routine activity levels (walks after meals, and so on) at the same time that they try to adjust their diet. While it isn't a good idea to try to make too many significant changes at one time, you may want to experiment with other changes while you're making adjustments in your diet.

SELECTED BIBLIOGRAPHY

Alcorn, J. M. 1992. Colorectal cancer prevention: A primary care approach. *Geriatrics* 47(2): 24.

Alvarado, D. 1992. Bones of contention. *San Jose Mercury News,* 6 May.

Anderson, J. W., and others. 1991. Lipid responses of hypercholesterolemic men to oat-bran and wheat-bran intakes. *American Journal of Clinical Nutrition* 54:678.

Bouchard, C. 1991. Current understanding of the etiology of obesity: Genetic and nongenetic factors. *American Journal of Clinical Nutrition* 53:1561S.

Bray, G. A. 1992. Pathophysiology of obesity. *American Journal of Clinical Nutrition* 55:488S.

Clark, N. 1991. How to pack a meatless diet full of nutrients. *The Physician and Sports Medicine* 19:31.

Cutler, R. G. 1991. Antioxidants and aging. *American Journal of Clinical Nutrition* 53:373S.

Diabetes: Living successfully with a lifelong challenge. 1992. Medical Essay, Supplement to *Mayo Clinic Health Letter,* June.

Diet, nutrition and the prevention of chronic diseases—A report of the WHO study group on diet, nutrition and prevention of noncommunicable diseases. 1991. *Nutrition Reviews* 49:291.

Dinsmoor, R. S. 1992. Exercise and adult-onset diabetes. *Harvard Health Letter,* November.

Donatelle, E. P. 1990. Constipation: Pathophysiology and treatment. *American Family Physician* 42(5): 1335.

Dwyer, J. T. 1991. Dietary change: Convergence of prevention and treatment measures. *Topics of Clinical Nutrition* 6:42.

———. 1991. Nutritional consequences of vegetarianism. *Annual Reviews of Nutrition* 11:61.

Filer, L. J. 1991. Recommended dietary allowances: How did we get where we are? *Nutrition Today,* September/October.

Food and Nutrition Board. 1989. *Recommended Dietary Allowances.* Revised. Washington D.C.: National Academy of Sciences—National Research Council.

Garn, S. M., and W. R. Leonard. 1989. What did our ancestors eat? *Nutrition Reviews* 47:337.

Harper, A. E. 1991. The 1990 Atwater lecture: The science and the practice of nutrition—Reflections and directions. *American Journal of Clinical Nutrition* 53:413.

Hecht, A. 1991. Preventing food-borne illness. *FDA Consumer,* January/February, 18.

Kim, W. W., and others. 1984. Evaluation of long-term dietary intakes of adults consuming self-selected diets. *American Journal of Clinical Nutrition* 40:1327.

Nielsen, F. H. 1991. Nutritional requirements for boron, silicon, vanadium, nickel, and arsenic: Current knowledge and speculation. *FASEB Journal* 5:2661.

Papazian, R. 1991. Osteoporosis treatment advances. *FDA Consumer,* April, 29–32.

Perkin, B. B. 1990. Dietary guidelines for Americans, 1990 edition. *Journal of the American Dietetic Association* 90:1725.

Saling, J. 1992. Staying ahead of osteoporosis. *Take Care,* Winter, 8–10.

Slavin, J. L. 1990. Dietary fiber: Mechanism or magic on disease prevention. *Nutrition Today,* November/December, 6.

Soll, A. H. 1990. Pathogenesis of peptic ulcer and implications for therapy. *New England Journal of Medicine* 322:909.

Spencer, H., and others. 1988. Do protein and phosphorus cause calcium loss? *Journal of Nutrition* 118:657.

Surgeon General's report on nutrition and health. 1988. *Nutrition Today,* September/October, 22.

Webb, L. 1990. Changing dietary habits of consumers. *Topics in Clinical Nutrition* 5:34.

Willard, M. D. 1991. Obesity: Types and treatments. *American Family Physician* 43(6): 2009.

Woteki, C. E., and P. R. Thomas. 1991. *Improving America's Diet and Health.* Washington, D.C.: National Academy Press.

RECOMMENDED READINGS

Committee on Diet and Health, National Research Council, 1989. *Diet and Health.* Washington, D.C.: National Academy Press. *A well-referenced review of nutrition and its relationship to chronic diseases, such as heart disease and cancer.*

Robertson, L., C. Flinders, and B. Godfrey. 1986. *The New Laurel's Kitchen.* Berkeley, Calif.: Ten Speed Press. *The updated classic on vegetarian cooking and nutrition, with solid nutritional information and innovative recipes.*

U.S. Department of Health and Human Services—Public Health Service. 1988. *The Surgeon General's Report on Nutrition and Health.* Washington, D.C.: U.S. Government Printing Office. *A comprehensive guide to the role of nutrition in disease prevention.*

Wardlaw, G. M., and P. M. Insel. 1993. *Perspectives in Nutrition.* 2nd ed. St. Louis: Mosby-Yearbook. *An easy-to-understand review of major concepts in nutrition—from infancy to elderly years.*

Woteki, C. E., and P. R. Thomas. 1992. *Eat for Life.* Washington, D.C.: National Academy Press. *A summary of* Improving America's Diet and Health *(listed above) designed for the lay public. This volume is packed with up-to-date and useful information on the relationship between diet and health status.*

APPENDIX

The Facts About Fast Food

Burger King

	Serving size (gm)	Calories	Protein (gm)	Carbohydrates (gm)	Fat: Total (gm)	Polyunsaturated fat (gm)	Monounsaturated fat (gm)	Saturated fat (gm)	Cholesterol (mg)	Sodium (mg)	Potassium (mg)	Phosphorus	Vitamin A	Vitamin C	Thiamine	Riboflavin	Niacin	Calcium	Iron	Zinc	% cal from fat
														% U.S. RDA							
Whopper	270	614	27	45	36	13	11	12	91	865	N/A	N/A	11	20	24	24	34	8	27	N/A	53
Whopper with cheese	294	706	32	47	44	13	13	16	116	1177	N/A	N/A	19	20	24	28	34	22	27	N/A	56
Hamburger	108	272	15	28	11	1	5	4	37	505	N/A	N/A	3	5	15	15	19	4	15	N/A	36
Bacon double cheeseburger	160	507	33	26	30	2	13	14	108	809	N/A	N/A	8	*	23	29	36	18	21	N/A	53
Burger buddies (pair)	129	349	18	31	17	1	8	7	52	717	N/A	N/A	9	8	32	24	23	11	19	N/A	44
BK Broiler chicken sandwich	154	267	22	28	8	3	3	2	45	728	N/A	N/A	4	6	45	45	60	4	15	N/A	27
Ocean Catch fish fillet sandwich	165	479	16	31	33	12	13	8	45	736	N/A	N/A	*	*	48	25	48	5	13	N/A	62
Chicken tenders (6 piece)	90	236	16	14	13	2	8	3	38	541	N/A	N/A	2	*	7	5	40	*	2	N/A	50
Chunky chicken salad	258	142	20	8	4	1	1	1	49	443	N/A	N/A	92	34	10	10	47	4	7	N/A	25
Garden salad	223	95	6	8	5	0	1	3	15	125	N/A	N/A	100	58	5	6	4	15	6	N/A	47
French fries (medium, salted)	116	372	5	43	20	2	12	5	0	238	N/A	N/A	*	5	5	*	12	*	7	N/A	48
Onion rings	97	339	5	38	19	2	12	5	0	628	N/A	N/A	15	*	10	6	12	11	3	N/A	50
Chocolate shake	284	326	9	49	10	0	4	6	31	198	N/A	N/A	7	4	6	28	*	31	4	N/A	28
Croissan'wich w/bacon, egg, & cheese	118	353	16	19	23	2	12	8	230	780	N/A	N/A	10	*	23	27	15	14	10	N/A	59
Breakfast Buddy	84	255	11	15	16	8	6	16	127	492	N/A	N/A	5	*	19	17	13	8	10	N/A	56

* Contains less than 2% of the U.S. RDA of these nutrients.
N/A—not available

Domino's Pizza

(1 serving = 2 slices)

	Serving size	Calories	Protein	Carbohydrates	Fat: Total	Polyunsaturated fat	Monounsaturated fat	Saturated fat	Cholesterol	Sodium	Potassium	Phosphorus	Vitamin A	Vitamin C	Thiamine	Riboflavin	Niacin	Calcium	Iron	Zinc	% cal from fat
	gm		gm	gm	gm	gm	gm	gm	mg	mg	mg					% U.S. RDA					
Cheese (2 slices)		376	22	56	10	1	3	6	19	483	N/A	N/A	7	<4	33	25	17	17	13	N/A	24
Pepperoni (2 slices)		460	24	56	18	2	7	9	28	825	N/A	N/A	7	<4	37	24	28	19	15	N/A	35
Sausage/mushroom (2 slices)		430	24	55	16	2	6	8	28	552	N/A	N/A	8	<4	40	30	30	20	17	N/A	33
Veggie (2 slices)		498	31	60	19	2	7	10	36	1035	N/A	N/A	10	<6	39	52	25	39	26	N/A	34
Deluxe (2 slices)		498	27	59	20	2	9	9	40	954	N/A	N/A	9	<5	35	23	35	23	23	N/A	36
Ham (2 slices)		417	23	58	11	1	4	6	26	805	N/A	N/A	4	<4	37	19	28	19	19	N/A	24

N/A—not available

KFC

(Kentucky Fried Chicken)

	Serving size	Calories	Protein	Carbohydrates	Fat: Total	Polyunsaturated fat	Monounsaturated fat	Saturated fat	Cholesterol	Sodium	Potassium	Phosphorus	Vitamin A	Vitamin C	Thiamine	Riboflavin	Niacin	Calcium	Iron	Zinc	% cal from fat
	gm		gm	gm	gm	gm	gm	gm	mg	mg	mg					% U.S. RDA					
Original Recipe—wing	53	172	12	5	11	2	6	3	59	383	N/A	N/A	*	*	2	4	15	3	3	N/A	58
center breast	103	260	25	8	14	2	8	4	92	609	N/A	N/A	*	*	5	8	49	3	4	N/A	48
drumstick	57	152	14	3	9	2	5	2	75	269	N/A	N/A	*	*	3	7	13	*	4	N/A	53
Extra Tasty Crispy—wing	57	231	11	8	17	2	10	4	63	319	N/A	N/A	*	*	2	4	15	2	3	N/A	66
center breast	110	344	23	15	21	2	12	5	80	636	N/A	N/A	*	*	5	8	47	2	5	N/A	55
drumstick	68	205	14	7	14	2	8	3	72	292	N/A	N/A	*	*	4	8	17	*	6	N/A	61
Hot & Spicy—wing	62	244	12	9	18	2	10	4	65	459	N/A	N/A	*	*	2	4	16	2	6	N/A	66
center breast	122	382	24	16	25	3	14	6	84	905	N/A	N/A	*	*	7	8	46	2	6	N/A	59
drumstick	70	207	11	10	14	1	8	3	75	406	N/A	N/A	*	*	4	9	16	*	46	N/A	61
Lite 'N Crispy—center breast	86	220	N/A	N/A	12	N/A	N/A	3	57	416	N/A	N/A	N/A	N/A	N/A	N/A	N/A	N/A	N/A	N/A	49
drumstick	47	121	N/A	N/A	7	N/A	N/A	2	51	196	N/A	N/A	N/A	N/A	N/A	N/A	N/A	N/A	N/A	N/A	52
Kentucky nuggets (6)	95	284	16	15	18	2	10	4	66	865	N/A	N/A	*	*	6	7	28	2	4	N/A	57
Buttermilk biscuit (1)	65	235	5	28	12	2	5	3	1	655	N/A	N/A	*	*	16	11	13	10	9	N/A	46
Mashed potatoes & gravy	98	71	2	12	2	—	1	—	<1	339	N/A	N/A	*	*	2	6	2	2	2	N/A	25
Corn-on-the-cob	73	90	3	16	2	1	0	1	<1	11	N/A	N/A	3	2	5	4	5	*	2	N/A	20
Coleslaw	90	114	1	13	6	3	2	1	4	177	N/A	N/A	*	47	2	2	*	3	2	N/A	47

* Contains less than 2% U.S. RDA of these nutrients.
N/A—not available

Jack in the Box

Item	Serving size (gm)	Calories	Protein (gm)	Carbohydrates (gm)	Fat. Total (gm)	Polyunsaturated fat (gm)	Monounsaturated fat (gm)	Saturated fat (gm)	Cholesterol (mg)	Sodium (mg)	Potassium (mg)	Phosphorus	Vitamin A	Vitamin C	Thiamine	Riboflavin	Niacin	Calcium	Iron	Zinc	% cal from fat
														% U.S. RDA							
Breakfast Jack	126	307	18	30	13	2.5	5	5.2	203	871	N/A	N/A	9	*	31	24	15	17	17	N/A	38
Supreme crescent	146	547	20	27	40	7.8	18.9	13.2	178	1053	N/A	N/A	11	*	43	32	21	15	15	N/A	66
Hamburger	96	267	13	28	11	2.0	4.9	4.1	26	556	N/A	N/A	*	*	10	15	10	15	10	N/A	37
Double cheeseburger	149	467	21	33	27	3.1	11.6	12.3	72	842	N/A	N/A	8	*	10	20	30	40	17	N/A	52
Jumbo Jack	222	584	26	42	34	8	13	11	73	733	N/A	N/A	*	*	24	17	9	14	17	N/A	52
Bacon bacon cheeseburger	242	705	35	41	45	8.7	15.7	14.9	113	1240	N/A	N/A	7	13	16	28	44	25	28	N/A	57
Chicken Fajita Pita (1)	189	292	24	29	8	1.4	3.6	2.9	34	703	N/A	N/A	10	*	50	10	30	25	15	N/A	25
Chicken supreme	245	641	27	47	39	11.4	14.8	10	85	1470	N/A	N/A	8	10	26	19	55	24	16	N/A	55
Fish supreme	218	510	24	44	27	7.7	11.4	6.1	55	1040	N/A	N/A	*	9	26	14	21	16	15	N/A	48
Taco salad	402	503	34	28	31	1.6	11.9	13.4	92	1600	N/A	N/A	27	15	19	31	29	41	21	N/A	55
Egg rolls—3 piece	165	437	3	54	24	2.6	12.5	6.8	29	957	N/A	N/A	*	6	39	19	30	8	20	N/A	49
Chicken strips—4 piece	112	285	25	18	13	.7	7.9	3.1	52	695	N/A	N/A	*	*	7	7	56	*	4	N/A	41
Taquitos—5 piece	134	362	15	42	15	1.8	8.4	3.3	24	462	N/A	N/A	*	3	6	7	11	15	15	N/A	37
Seasoned curly fries	109	358	5	3	20	.5	13.3	4.7	0	1030	N/A	N/A	*	9	11	6	15	3	9	N/A	50
Onion rings	103	380	5	38	23	.9	15.2	5.5	0	451	N/A	N/A	*	5	19	10	13	3	12	N/A	54
Chocolate milkshake	322	330	11	55	7	<1	2.1	4.3	25	270	N/A	N/A	*	*	10	35	2	35	4	N/A	19

* Contains less than 2% of the U.S. RDA of these nutrients.
N/A—not available

McDonald's

Item	Serving size (gm)	Calories	Protein (gm)	Carbohydrates (gm)	Fat. Total (gm)	Polyunsaturated fat (gm)	Monounsaturated fat (gm)	Saturated fat (gm)	Cholesterol (mg)	Sodium (mg)	Potassium (mg)	Phosphorus	Vitamin A	Vitamin C	Thiamine	Riboflavin	Niacin	Calcium	Iron	Zinc	% cal from fat
														% U.S. RDA							
Cheeseburger	116	305	15	30	13	1	7	5	50	725	N/A	N/A	8	4	20	15	20	20	15	N/A	38
QuarterPounder®	166	410	23	34	20	1	11	8	85	645	N/A	N/A	4	6	25	15	35	15	20	N/A	44
McLean Deluxe™	206	320	22	35	10	1	5	4	60	670	N/A	N/A	10	10	25	20	35	15	20	N/A	28
Big Mac®	215	500	25	42	26	1	16	9	100	890	N/A	N/A	6	2	30	25	35	25	20	N/A	47
Filet-O-Fish®	141	370	14	38	18	6	8	4	50	730	N/A	N/A	2	*	20	8	45	15	10	N/A	44
McChicken®	187	415	19	39	20	7	9	4	50	830	N/A	N/A	2	4	60	10	45	15	15	N/A	43
Chicken fajitas	82	185	11	20	8	3	3	2	35	310	N/A	N/A	2	8	10	10	20	8	4	N/A	39
Medium french fries	97	320	4	36	17	1.5	12	3.5	0	150	N/A	N/A	*	20	15	*	15	*	4	N/A	48
Chicken McNuggets® 6 pce		270	20	17	15	1.5	10	3.5	55	580	N/A	N/A	*	*	8	8	40	*	6	N/A	50
Chef salad	265	170	17	8	9	1	4	4	111	400	N/A	N/A	100	35	20	15	20	15	15	N/A	48
Chunky chicken salad	255	150	25	7	4	1	2	1	78	230	N/A	N/A	170	45	15	10	45	4	15	N/A	24
Egg McMuffin	135	280	18	28	11	1	6	4	235	710	N/A	N/A	10	*	30	20	20	25	15	N/A	35
Bacon, egg & cheese biscuit	153	440	15	33	26	2	16	8	240	1215	N/A	N/A	10	*	25	20	10	20	15	N/A	53
Breakfast burrito	105	280	12	21	17	7	6	4	135	580	N/A	N/A	10	10	20	15	10	10	8	N/A	55
Chocolate lowfat milkshake	323	320	11	66	1.7	0.1	0.9	0.7	10	240	N/A	N/A	6	*	8	30	2	35	*	N/A	5

* Contains less than 2% of the U.S. RDA of these nutrients.
N/A—not available

Taco Bell

	Serving size	Calories	Protein	Carbohydrates	Fat: Total	Polyunsaturated fat	Monounsaturated fat	Saturated fat	Cholesterol	Sodium	Potassium	Phosphorus	Vitamin A	Vitamin C	Thiamine	Riboflavin	Niacin	Calcium	Iron	Zinc	% cal from fat
	gm		gm	gm	gm	gm	gm	gm	mg	mg	mg	% U.S. RDA									
Taco	78	183	10	11	11	1	N/A	5	32	276	159	N/A	7	2	3	8	6	8	6	N/A	54
Soft taco	92	225	12	18	12	1	N/A	5	32	554	196	N/A	4	2	26	13	14	12	13	N/A	48
Tostada w/red sauce	156	243	9	27	11	1	N/A	4	16	596	401	N/A	13	75	4	10	3	18	9	N/A	41
Chicken soft taco	107	213	14	19	10	2	N/A	4	52	615	233	N/A	4	4	13	13	17	8	35	N/A	42
Taco supreme	92	230	11	12	15	1	N/A	8	32	276	205	N/A	11	5	4	10	6	11	6	N/A	59
Bean burrito w/red sauce	206	357	15	63	14	2	N/A	4	9	1148	495	N/A	7	88	27	117	14	19	21	N/A	35
Burrito supreme w/red sauce	255	503	20	55	22	2	N/A	8	33	1181	501	N/A	18	43	29	123	18	19	22	N/A	39
Fiesta bean burrito	114	226	8	29	9	1	N/A	3	9	652	307	N/A	5	57	12	13	11	15	15	N/A	35
Nachos Bell Grande	287	649	22	61	35	3	N/A	12	36	997	674	N/A	23	96	7	20	11	30	19	N/A	48
Chicken MexiMelt	107	257	14	19	15	2	N/A	7	48	779	150	N/A	10	4	12	14	7	22	20	N/A	53
Mexican pizza	223	575	21	40	37	10	N/A	11	52	1031	408	N/A	20	51	21	19	15	26	21	N/A	58
Taco salad	575	905	34	55	61	12	N/A	19	80	910	673	N/A	33	125	33	33	24	32	33	N/A	61

N/A—not available

Wendy's

	Serving size	Calories	Protein	Carbohydrates	Fat: Total	Polyunsaturated fat	Monounsaturated fat	Saturated fat	Cholesterol	Sodium	Potassium	Phosphorus	Vitamin A	Vitamin C	Thiamine	Riboflavin	Niacin	Calcium	Iron	Zinc	% cal from fat
	gm		gm	gm	gm	gm	gm	gm	mg	mg	mg	% U.S. RDA									
Single with everything	210	420	25	35	21	2.1	7.3	5.5	70	890	430	N/A	5	15	25	10	35	10	30	N/A	45
Wendy's Big Classic	260	570	27	47	33	2.5	7.4	5.6	80	1085	525	N/A	10	20	30	15	35	15	35	N/A	52
Jr. hamburger	111	260	15	33	9.0	1.9	4.0	3.0	35	570	215	N/A	2	4	25	10	20	10	20	N/A	31
Jr. bacon cheeseburger	155	430	22	33	25	2.7	6.9	5.2	50	840	290	N/A	2	15	30	50	25	10	20	N/A	52
Grilled chicken sandwich	175	320	24	37	9	6.9	3.0	2.2	60	815	340	N/A	2	8	30	15	50	10	20	N/A	25
Fish fillet sandwich	170	460	18	42	25	10	9.6	4.7	50	780	320	N/A	2	2	40	25	25	10	15	N/A	49
Country fried steak sandwich	145	440	14	45	25	4.3	7.6	5.7	35	870	215	N/A	2	2	30	15	25	10	20	N/A	51
French fries (small)	91	240	3	33	12	.77	7.98	2.5	0	145	510	N/A	*	10	10	2	10	*	4	N/A	45
Crispy chicken nuggets (6)	93	280	14	12	20	3.8	9.6	4.5	50	600	200	N/A	*	*	6	6	30	4	4	N/A	64
Chili and cheese	403	500	15	71	18	3.3	3.30	4.0	25	630	1270	N/A	15	60	20	100	25	8	28	N/A	32
Salad Dressing Blue Cheese (2oz. packet)	54	324	<1	<1	36	22.14	N/A	6.84	36	378	36	N/A	*	*	*	*	*	*	*	N/A	100
Garden salad	231	70	4	9	2	.23	0	0	0	60	500	N/A	110	70	10	10	6	10	8	N/A	26
Taco salad	490	530	27	55	23	.27	.03	.07	35	825	800	N/A	30	40	20	35	15	40	30	N/A	39
Frosty dairy dessert (small)	243	340	9	57	10	.39	2.58	5	40	200	625	N/A	8	*	8	50	2	30	6	N/A	26

* Contains less than 2% of the U.S. RDA of these nutrients.
N/A—not available.

13

Weight Management

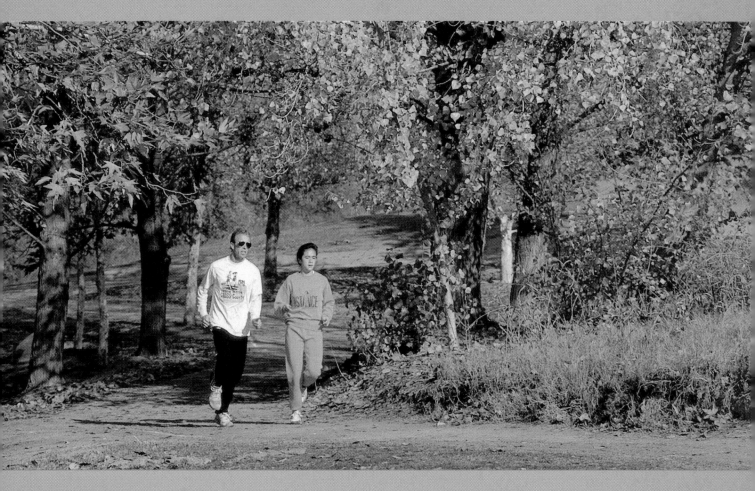

CONTENTS

You and one of your new housemates are about the same size and shape—about ten pounds heavier than you think you should be. You've been on a variety of diets in the past few years, repeatedly losing the weight and then gaining it back. You decide to try to enlist your similarly shaped housemate in your latest diet plan. You're surprised to discover that he's not really interested in losing weight. He says that he focuses on eating a healthy diet and exercising regularly; he figures that whatever he weighs after that is right for him. You've never thought about your weight this way. Is he on to something? Should you try adopting his attitude?

You and a friend have both gained a little weight and have decided to watch your diets. When you go to the cafeteria, she thinks you should get the Vegetarian Fiesta Delight—pinto beans, corn tortilla, spicy rice, salsa, and lettuce. You think that's too starchy. You vote for broiled pork chops with gravy and a salad, because it's high in protein and low in carbohydrates. Which would be the better choice?

Your roommate is driving you crazy—she seems to eat whatever she wants and never gains any weight, while you watch every bite and are just barely able to maintain the weight you want. She says her secret is walking and riding her bike everywhere she goes. You're skeptical that it could make that much difference. She suggests you stop taking the bus for a month and see what happens. Was she just born to be thin or does her activity level have something to do with it? Should you give her idea a try?

Your brother has been dating a woman who talks about her weight and her diet all the time, even though she doesn't appear to you to be overweight. You rarely see her eat anything, and when she does have food in front of her she just plays with it. She also seems to exercise a great deal. Your brother tells you that he's noticed that her apartment is sometimes stocked with large amounts of junk food. He's begun to wonder if she has some kind of eating problem, but he doesn't know what it is or what he should do. He asked if you had any ideas. What information and advice can you give your brother?

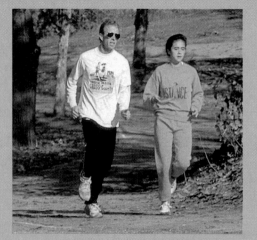

MAKING CONNECTIONS

If you're like most people, you'll probably gain weight as you get older, and that weight will be a burden on your health as the years go by. Maintaining a reasonable body weight requires conscious effort and informed, sensible lifestyle choices. In the scenarios presented on these pages, each related to weight control, individuals have to use information, make a decision, or choose a course of action. How would you act in each of these situations? What response or decision would you make? This chapter provides information about lifestyle and weight management that can be used in situations like these. After finishing the chapter, read the scenarios again. Has what you've learned changed how you would respond?

There is a "secret" to weight management: Maintain a moderate level of total calories, minimize fat calories, and get lots of exercise. Unfortunately, this simple formula is not as exciting as the latest fad diet or the "scientific breakthrough" that promises slimness without effort. If only calories didn't count, or exercising just a few minutes a day could produce a beautifully proportioned body, then the continuing stream of diet books, special programs, dietary supplements, and medical procedures for weight loss that assault the American public year after year might disappear. **Obesity** would not be the public health problem or the personal agony that it is for so many. Fad diets and promises of being able to get something for nothing are the fool's gold of weight control.

Yet more and more Americans are going on diets. At any given time, more than one-third of the American public is engaged in dieting behavior. Research shows that many girls start dieting during adolescence and that the rate of dieting reaches 60 percent or more during the college years. Males too are getting caught up in the dieting craze. Furthermore, this bad habit is taking hold at younger and younger ages; many have started dieting in high school or even grade school. Twenty-two percent of tenth-grade girls reported frequent dieting, and another 10 percent engaged in fasts. There have even been reports of failure to thrive—a syndrome involving undernourishment and retarded growth—in infants whose affluent parents put their babies on a diet, mistakenly thinking this would reduce their child's risk of later obesity! Yet, despite all the concern about body weight, the prevalence of obesity is increasing.

LIFESTYLE AND WEIGHT

At the turn of the century, Americans consumed a diet very different from that of the 1990s, and they got much more exercise. Americans today actually eat somewhat fewer calories overall (down about 3 percent), but they eat more fat and more refined sugars and fewer complex carbohydrates. Since 1910, the percentage of calories consumed from fat increased from 32 percent to 38 percent, while that from complex carbohydrates—vegetables, grains, rice, legumes, and pasta—declined from 38 percent to 24 percent. Eating foods high in fat and refined sugar, usually in the form of candy, ice cream, cookies, and pastries, is a favorite modern way of coping with stress. Fats and simple sugars make up over 60 percent of all calories consumed in the 1990s. In large part, these changes reflect the trend toward more processed foods and away from fresh, unprocessed foods and complex carbohydrates.

Despite the increased interest in fitness during recent years, Americans today get far less exercise than did their great-grandparents. In earlier times, people walked or rode bicycles more often than they drove. Most worked on farms or did manual labor. They were able to eat more and weigh less because they didn't have the dubious benefits of labor-saving devices. Daily energy expenditure has decreased over the past 200 years as our nation has changed from an agricultural, to an industrial, and now to an information economy. Fewer and fewer people have jobs that require strenuous physical labor. From 1965 to 1977 alone, daily energy expenditure was thought to have dropped by 200 calories a day—due largely to automobiles, remote control devices for television and garage doors, and a host of electrical appliances that do our work for us.

People from other countries often deplore the prevalence of obesity in this country. Financially, most Americans can afford to eat more meat than can people in the rest of the world, who still consume mostly complex carbohydrates. Gasoline here is cheap in comparison to its cost elsewhere, and most Americans view automobiles as a necessity. American cities are not particularly safe for walking or riding bicycles, which are still the primary means of transportation for most people in the world. The typical American lifestyle does not naturally promote healthy eating or adequate exercise. And the results of our lifestyle are clear from recent national surveys, which indicate that about 34 million American adults are overweight. More women than men are affected. Overweight is also more common among people of certain racial or ethnic groups, people having low incomes, and people of low educational attainment. The percentage of the American population that is overweight continues to rise. It's no wonder that dieting has practically become an American institution.

More children and adolescents are developing weight problems than ever before. Even so, most young people arrive at early adulthood with the advantage of having a "normal" body weight (that is, neither too fat nor too lean). In fact, many young adults get away with terrible eating and exercise habits and don't develop a weight problem. But as the rapid growth period of adolescence slows, it becomes necessary to adopt a healthy lifestyle in order to maintain normal weight without undue effort. As family and career obligations increase and less time and perhaps motivation are available for other things, living a healthy lifestyle becomes a greater and greater challenge. A good time to develop such a lifestyle is early in adulthood, when healthy habits and behavior patterns have a better chance of taking a firm hold.

Obesity   A complex, health-impairing disorder characterized by excessive accumulation of body fat; also referred to as "overweight."

TERMS

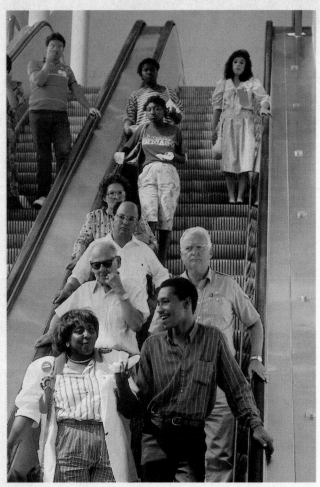

The typical American lifestyle does not lead naturally to healthy weight management. Labor-saving devices such as escalators help reinforce our sedentary habits.

ADOPTING A HEALTHY LIFESTYLE

Four factors are crucial to the kind of lifestyle that will naturally yield a healthy body weight: what goes into your mouth, what you do with your body, what goes on in your head, and how you cope with life. In other words, nutrition, physical activity, thinking and emotions, and habits and behavior patterns are the keys to successful maintenance of normal weight. These four factors are discussed in detail in this section.

Nutrition

Too often nutrition is a topic studied in a class on health, and too seldom does it become personally relevant to most people's lives. Knowing about nutrients and a balanced diet may help, but actually making healthy food choices day to day is what really counts. What goes into your mouth directly affects health and body weight. In particular, too much dietary fat and refined sugar can undermine good health in the long run, whereas eating more complex carbohydrates and keeping total calories at a moderate level produces a healthy body weight with little effort.

Fat   Most experts agree that the real problem in the American diet is overconsumption of dietary fats. Although no more than 30 percent of total calories (and preferably less) should come from fat, Americans get 36 to 38 percent of their calories from fat sources. (See Chapter 12 for the correct method of calculating the percentage of calories from fat.) Oils, margarine, butter, cream, and lard are almost pure fat. Meat and processed foods such as pastries contain a great deal of "hidden" fat, while nuts, seeds, and avocados are plant sources of fat. Most fat in the American diet comes from fatty red meats, dairy products, and processed foods, including snack foods like potato and corn chips. You can substantially decrease your fat consumption by moving closer to a vegetarian (complex carbohydrate) diet: Eating more fruits, vegetables, grains, and legumes and decreasing overall meat consumption. Learn to substitute leaner choices (fish or poultry without the skin) for high-fat choices such as bacon, sausage, and ribs. Refer to the box "Eating Smart—Little Things Add Up" for more suggestions on how to cut your fat intake.

Sugar   Some people equate sugar with fatness, even though there is no evidence that fat people consume more sugar than thin people. Sugar is a health problem primarily because it causes tooth decay. Still, for some who are trying to maintain a reasonable body weight, sugar can be a problem. Sugar is a major component of many favorite foods in the American diet, which are often also high in fat. Ice cream, for example, is 63 percent sugar, 27 percent fat, and only 10 percent protein. An ounce of milk chocolate is 59 percent sugar, 33 percent fat, and 8 percent protein. Under such names as corn syrup, corn sweetener, honey, molasses, fructose, sucrose, and dextrose, sugar is added to processed foods such as breads, crackers, cereals, sauces, salad dressings, fruit-flavored yogurt, soft drinks, pastries and baked goods, and bacon and cured meats.

Protein   Americans worry far too much about the protein content of their diet. The typical American eats an average of 70–100 grams of protein every day. An adult male needs only 60 grams of protein a day and an adult female only 45 grams. Special dietary supplements that provide extra protein are totally unnecessary for most people; and, in fact, protein not needed by the body for growth and tissue repair will be stored as body fat. Foods high in protein are often also high in fat.

Complex Carbohydrates   People concerned about their weight often eliminate bread, pasta, and potatoes—the starches or "carbs" in the diet—in the mistaken belief

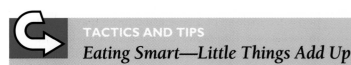

It's easier to incorporate small switches and substitutions in your eating habits than to initiate radical changes. These simple suggestions for a more healthful diet can reduce your fat and calorie intake considerably while still satisfying your appetite. To put these numbers in perspective, if you consume 2,000 calories a day, you should eat no more than about 66 grams of fat—that way fat will contribute less than 30% of your daily calories.

Instead of Eating	Substitute	To Save*
1 croissant	1 plain bagel	35 calories, 10 grams fat
1 whole egg	1 egg white	65 calories, 6 grams fat
1 oz. cheddar cheese	1 oz. part-skim mozzarella	35 calories, 4 grams fat
1 oz. cream cheese	1 oz. cottage cheese (1% fat)	74 calories, 9 grams fat
1 T whipping cream	1 T evaporated skim milk, whipped	32 calories, 5 grams fat
3.5 oz. lamb chop, untrimmed, broiled	3.5 oz. lean leg of lamb, trimmed, broiled	219 calories, 28 grams fat
3.5 oz. pork spare ribs, cooked	3.5 oz. lean-pork loin, trimmed, broiled	157 calories, 17 grams fat
1 oz. regular bacon, cooked	1 oz. Canadian bacon, cooked	111 calories, 12 grams fat
1 oz. hard salami	1 oz. extra-lean roasted ham	75 calories, 8 grams fat
1 beef frankfurter	1 chicken frankfurter	67 calories, 8 grams fat
3 oz. oil-packed tuna, light	3 oz. water-packed tuna, light	60 calories, 6 grams fat
1 regular-size serving fast-food French fries	1 medium-sized baked potato	125 calories, 11 grams fat
1 oz. potato chips	1 oz. thin pretzels	40 calories, 9 grams fat
1 oz. corn chips	1 oz. plain air-popped popcorn	125 calories, 9 grams fat
1 T sour-cream dip	1 T bottled salsa	20 calories, 3 grams fat
1 glazed doughnut	1 slice angel-food cake	110 calories, 13 grams fat
3 chocolate sandwich cookies	3 fig bar cookies	4 grams fat
1 cup ice cream (premium)	1 cup sorbet	320 calories, 34 grams fat

Reprinted permission of *University of California at Berkeley Wellness Letter*, P.O. Box 10922, Des Moines, IA 50340.
*The values listed are the most significant savings; smaller differences are not shown. Weights given for meats are edible portions.

that cutting these calories will help control weight. In fact, complex carbohydrates from these sources as well as from fresh vegetables, legumes, and whole grains help maintain proper weight. In contrast to fat calories, which the body can easily convert to body fat, calories from complex carbohydrates actually cost the body calories to digest. Furthermore, eating a large amount of complex carbohydrates makes you feel full. In fact, eating a high-carbohydrate/low-fat diet can even result in weight loss without conscious restriction of calories and without exercise! The real problem in terms of obesity is not eating too many complex carbohydrates, but adding high-fat sauces and toppings to them. Changing the composition of your diet in favor of a higher carbohydrate-to-fat ratio

may require retraining your taste buds so that you get used to bread without butter, potatoes without sour cream, and pasta with a vegetable sauce instead of a cream sauce or cheese.

Hunger and Satiety What you put in your mouth also affects your experience of hunger and satiety. One theory says that the brain senses hunger when the blood sugar gets too low and that this sensation triggers eating. The resulting increase in blood sugar presumably produces **satiety**—feelings of fullness. However, blood sugar level varies under normal conditions, and it's not clear exactly how variations in blood sugar affect hunger. Another theory says that low levels of **serotonin** (a neurotransmitter) in the brain are associated with feelings of hunger and high levels with satiety. People who eat a diet high in fat and low in complex carbohydrates tend to have lower than normal levels of serotonin in their brains. Theoretically, eating a diet low in fat and high in complex carbohydrates should help us avoid feelings of hunger.

Most people infer that they're hungry when their stomach growls or when they get the "shakes" from not eating. However, research suggests that many people are unable to recognize stomach contractions as a signal of their hunger. They might confuse anxiety or physiological arousal with feeling hungry. Telling such people to "eat only when hungry" is poor advice. It's better to say, "stop eating when full," since people are much better at knowing when they feel full than when they feel hungry. Unfortunately, many people who know they're full keep eating because the food tastes good. We all need to mentally monitor feelings of fullness and be guided by adequate portion control in order to maintain normal weight.

Eating Habits Equally important to weight control is eating small, frequent meals—three a day or more, plus planned, appropriate snacks if desired. Some people—especially young people on the go—skip breakfast and even lunch, thinking they're saving calories. When they do finally eat, they're often so hungry they can't stop eating for the rest of the night. Gradually their eating pattern gets shifted to later and later in the day, until finally they "can't" eat breakfast in the morning. They're still full from the night before! In addition, waiting to eat until late in the day often results in shopping for a meal on an empty stomach and feeling stressed and fatigued from a day without sufficient body fuel. Insufficient energy contributes to poor performance. Failure to do a job well then leads to feelings of stress. This stress can result in making poor food choices, overeating, and possibly drinking too much alcohol. Eating eventually seems to be an effective means of self-soothing and distraction from problems. This cyclical pattern sets the stage for future problems with food.

A healthier approach is to develop a *structure* to guide eating. This structure involves having a more-or-less regular time for meals. (Weekends and vacations may differ from weekdays.) It also means establishing a set of *decision rules* that guide food choices. These rules indicate what choices are "allowed" for breakfast, lunch, and din-

ner, when high-fat or high-sugar choices may be indulged in, what are the preferred substitutions for the less healthy choices, and so forth. For example, the rule governing breakfast choices might be, "Choose a sugar-free, high-fiber cereal with nonfat milk most of the time. Once in a while (no more than once a week) a poached or soft-boiled egg is okay. Save pancakes and waffles for special occasions." The decision rule governing dinner entrees might be, "Choose chicken or fish most of the time. Avoid cream sauces. Once in a while if a steak is desired, make it a small fillet or flank steak."

Decreeing some food "off limits" is generally not a good idea. Doing so sets up a struggle to be vigilant and resist the urge to eat that food, but almost everyone eventually succumbs to the forbidden food rather than feel deprived. The guiding principle should be "everything in moderation." If a particular food becomes troublesome, it could be placed off limits temporarily until control over it is regained.

Exercise and Physical Activity

Regular exercise is a source of many benefits. As described in Chapter 14 and other chapters, regular endurance exercise strengthens the heart and cardiovascular system, creates greater endurance and energy, provides a means of managing stress, and helps prevent osteoporosis. Exercise also burns calories and keeps the **metabolism** geared to using food for energy instead of storing calories. And perhaps most importantly, exercise builds lean body mass, which in turn can increase metabolism. People with low metabolic rates are more likely to become overweight than are those with normal or elevated metabolic rates. The greater the amount of fat-free body mass—muscle—the higher the metabolism. Your body burns more calories when your metabolism is more active, meaning you can eat more without necessarily gaining weight.

Research has established that obese people are clearly less physically active than their nonobese peers, and there is universal agreement that increased physical activity plays a critical role in long-term weight management success. Those who say that exercise isn't worthwhile for weight loss because "you have to play volleyball for 32 hours to burn enough calories to lose just one pound of fat" overlook the metabolic boost that results from exercise—and that lasts even beyond the period of exercise. Calculating the number of calories burned for any given activity is complex—heavy people burn more calories than do lighter ones and the level of a person's physical fitness affects calorie use—but it's possible to estimate the number of calories burned for a given activity (Table 13-1).

A well-rounded exercise program that includes endurance exercise, weight training, and activities to promote flexibility, relaxation, and enjoyment is best for well-

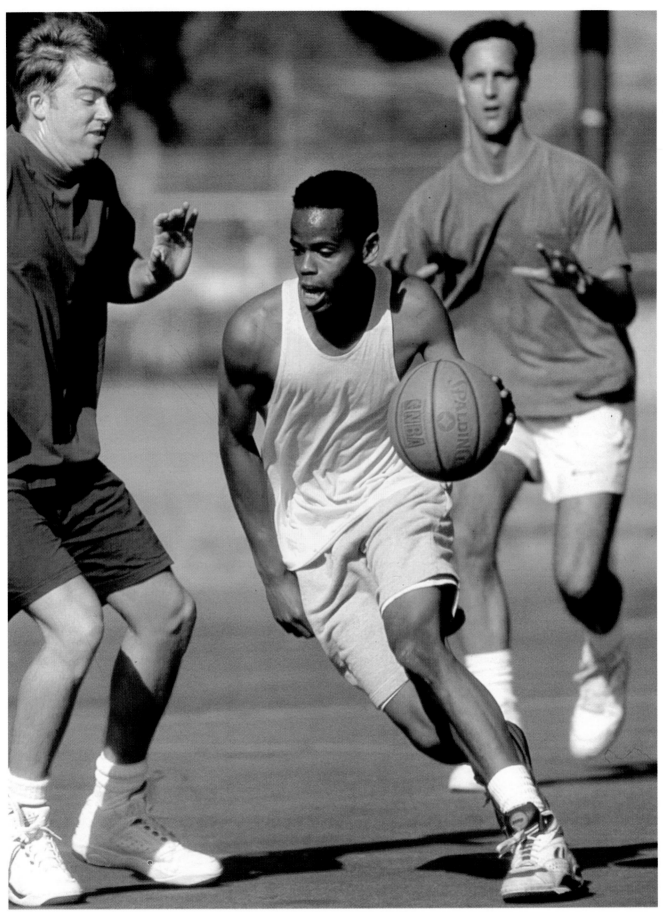

Physical activity is an essential component of any effective weight management plan.
Playing basketball is just one of innumerable activities that can help you keep in shape.

TABLE 13-1 Energy Costs of Selected Physical Activities*

To determine how many calories you burn when you engage in a particular activity, multiply the calorie multiplier given below by your body weight and then by the number of minutes you exercise.

Activity	Cal./lb./min.	× Body weight	× Min.	= Activity cal.
Cycling (13 mph)	.071	_____	____	_____
Digging	.062	_____	____	_____
Driving a car	.020	_____	____	_____
Housework	.029	_____	____	_____
Painting a house	.034	_____	____	_____
Shoveling snow	.052	_____	____	_____
Sitting quietly	.009	_____	____	_____
Sleeping and resting	.008	_____	____	_____
Standing quietly	.012	_____	____	_____
Typing or writing	.013	_____	____	_____
Walking briskly (4.5 mph)	.048	_____	____	_____

Adapted from I. Kusinitz and M. Fine. 1991. *Your Guide to Getting Fit.* 2nd ed. (Mountain View, Calif.: Mayfield).
*See Chapter 14 for energy costs of fitness activities.

ness and weight management. Moderate endurance exercise, sustained for 45 minutes to an hour, can help you lose body fat and keep it off. The longer the duration of a session of endurance exercise, the more fat you'll burn as fuel. Weight training helps increase or maintain lean body mass during diet-induced weight loss. Because of the important role of lean body mass in metabolism, its maintenance means you'll burn more calories even when you're not exercising. (Women need not fear that weight training will result in weight gain and bulky muscles because females lack the necessary hormones to add muscle bulk easily.) Chapter 14 provides information about how to put together a complete exercise program tailored specifically to your needs and preferences.

Living a healthy lifestyle also means taking advantage of routine opportunities to get exercise. Try taking the stairs instead of the elevator, walking or biking instead of driving, and so forth. In the long term, even a small increase in activity level can result in weight loss.

The message about exercise is that regular exercise, maintained throughout life, makes weight management easier. The sooner you establish good habits, the better. The key to success is to make exercise an integral part of the lifestyle you can enjoy now and will enjoy in the future. Chapter 14 contains many suggestions for becoming a more active, physically fit person.

Thinking and Emotions

What goes on in your head is the third component of a healthy lifestyle and successful weight management. The way you think about yourself and your world influences—and is influenced by—how you feel and how you act. Certain kinds of thinking produce negative emotions, which can undermine a healthy lifestyle.

Research on people who have a weight problem indicates that low self-esteem and the negative emotions that accompany it are significant problems. This low self-esteem often results in part from mentally comparing the actual self to an internally held picture of the "ideal self." The greater the discrepancy, the larger the impact on self-esteem and the more likely the presence of negative emotions.

Often our internalized "ideal self" is the result of having adopted perfectionistic goals and beliefs about how we and others "should" be. Examples of such beliefs include, "If I don't do things perfectly, I'm a failure" and "It's terrible if I'm not thin." These irrational beliefs may actually cause stress and emotional disturbance. The remedy is to challenge such beliefs and replace them with more realistic ones.

The beliefs and attitudes you hold give rise to self-talk, an internal dialogue you carry on with yourself about

You need to adopt a weight management plan that will last a lifetime. Look through the following list of strategies and adopt those that will be most useful for you.

- When shopping for food, make a list and stick to it. Don't shop when you're hungry. Avoid aisles that contain problem foods.

- When serving food, use a small food scale to measure out portions before putting them on your plate. Serve meals on small plates and in small bowls to help you eat smaller portions without feeling deprived.

- Eat three meals a day; replace impulse snacking with planned, healthy snacks. Drink plenty of water to help fill you up.

- Eat only in specifically designated spots. Remove food from other areas of your house or apartment. When you eat, just eat—don't do anything else, such as read or watch TV.

- Eat more slowly. Pay attention to every bite and enjoy your food. Try putting your fork or spoon down between bites.

- For problem foods, try eating small amounts under controlled conditions. Go out for a scoop of ice cream, for example, rather than buying half a gallon for your freezer.

- If you cook a large meal for friends, send leftovers home with your guests.

- When you eat out, choose a restaurant where you can make healthy food choices. Ask the waiter or waitress not to put bread and butter on the table before the meal; request that sauces and salad dressings be served on the side.

- If you're eating at a friend's, eat a little and leave the rest. Don't eat to be polite; if someone offers you food you don't want, thank the person and decline firmly. To turn down dessert or second helpings, try "No thank you, I've had enough" or "It's delicious, but I'm full."

- Develop strategies for handling stress—go for a walk or use a relaxation technique. Practice positive self-talk.

- Incorporate more physical activity into your life. Begin a fitness program that includes endurance exercise and resistance weight training, ride your bike or walk instead of driving, take the stairs instead of the elevator, and so on.

- Tell family and friends that you're making some changes in your eating and exercise habits. Ask them to be supportive.

Adapted from J. D. Nash. 1986. *Maximize Your Body Potential.* (Menlo Park, Calif.: Bull Publishing).

events that happen to and around you. Positive self-talk includes leading yourself through the steps of a job and then praising yourself when it's successfully completed. Negative self-talk takes the form of self-deprecating remarks, self-blame, and angry and guilt-producing comments. Negative self-talk can undermine efforts at self-control and lead to feelings of anxiety and depression (see Chapter 3).

Your beliefs and self-talk influence how you interpret what happens to you and what you can expect in the future, as well as how you feel and react. A healthy lifestyle is supported by having realistic beliefs and goals and by engaging in positive self-talk and problem-solving efforts.

Coping Strategies

The fourth component of a healthy lifestyle is adequate and appropriate coping strategies for dealing with the stresses and challenges of life. One strategy that some people adopt for coping is eating. (Others use drugs, alcohol, smoking, spending, gambling, and so on, to cope.)

So, when boredom presents itself, eating can provide entertainment. Food may be used to alleviate loneliness or as a pickup for fatigue. Eating provides distraction from difficult problems and is a means of punishing the self or others for real or imagined transgressions.

People who lead healthy lifestyles have learned more effective ways to get their needs met. They have learned to communicate assertively and to manage interpersonal conflict effectively and don't shrink from problems or overreact. The person with a healthy lifestyle knows how to create and maintain relationships with others and has a solid network of friends and loved ones. Food is used appropriately—to fuel life's activities and growth and for personal satisfaction, not to manage stress.

The healthy lifestyle that naturally and easily results in a reasonable body weight is one characterized by good nutrition, adequate exercise, positive thinking and emotions, and effective coping strategies and behavior patterns. You can make positive changes in your lifestyle to promote permanent weight control; refer to the box "Strategies for Managing Your Weight" for ideas.

Personal Insight Do you sometimes overeat? If so, are you more likely to overeat in certain situations, at certain times of the day, or with particular people? Do you overeat when you're in a particular frame of mind?

A CLOSER LOOK AT BODY WEIGHT

How many times have you or one of your friends said "I'm overweight"? Probably quite a few. But how do you decide whether you or someone else is overweight? At what point does being overweight affect your health? And how much should you weigh?

The answers to these questions are complex. Total body weight—expressed in pounds or kilograms—is the most commonly used measure of overweight. Total body weight can be an indicator of health risks, but a more important measure of the health effects of body weight is the composition of this weight. The human body is composed of lean body mass (bones and teeth, water, muscles, connective and organ tissues) and body fat. The percentage body fat is of primary concern because too much or too little body fat can have negative effects on health. The location of stored body fat also has health implications.

These three factors—body weight, body composition, and the distribution of body fat—can be measured and evaluated by a variety of means. The results of these assessments can help determine whether people face any increased risks due to their weight or percentage of body fat. Although in common usage we tend to use the terms *overweight* and *obese* very loosely, they actually refer to specific ranges of body weight or body fatness, as measured by various techniques. People who meet the criteria for severe overweight or obesity face additional health risks.

In this section, we review some of the techniques for assessing weight and body composition and then look at the health implications of obesity.

Assessing Your Weight and Body Composition

Several different approaches can be used to assess body weight, body composition, and body fat distribution. Each has advantages and disadvantages that need to be considered.

Height-Weight Tables The most common way to assess total body weight is to refer to a height-weight table. These tables are usually based on mortality statistics from life insurance companies. They give ranges of "ideal," "recommended," or "desirable" weights, adjusted for sex, height, and sometimes frame size.

Most experts agree that these tables have inherent problems. First, the ranges of weights recommended in height-weight tables as "healthy" (that is, associated with

TABLE 13-2 Guidelines for "Healthy" Weights*

Height (ft-in)	Suggested Weight (Without Clothes or Shoes)	
	19 to 34 Years	35 Years and Over
5-0	97–128	108–138
5-1	101–132	111–143
5-2	104–137	115–148
5-3	107–141	119–152
5-4	111–146	122–157
5-5	114–150	126–162
5-6	118–155	130–167
5-7	121–160	134–172
5-8	125–164	138–178
5-9	129–169	142–183
5-10	132–174	146–188
5-11	136–179	151–194
6-0	140–184	155–199
6-1	144–189	159–205
6-2	148–195	164–210
6-3	152–200	168–216
6-4	156–205	173–222

*Both sexes are combined in one table; the higher weights generally apply to men, the lower to women.

Source: U.S. Department of Health and Human Services. 1990. *Nutrition and Your Health: Dietary Guidelines for Americans* (Washington, D.C.: U.S. Government Printing Office, Home and Garden Bulletin 232).

minimum mortality) are too narrow. Although there are significant health risks associated with extreme overweight or underweight, a large "gray area" lies between any of the currently recommended ranges of weight and these extremes. Second, these tables rarely take age into account. Age is an important factor because the weights associated with minimum mortality rise with age, so that overweight in a younger person is riskier than overweight in someone older. Third, assessment of frame size is difficult and inaccurate, and frame size categories are arbitrary.

Even if these problems were correctable, however, the present height-weight table recommendations are based on unrepresentative data that may be inaccurate. Minorities and women are underrepresented in the database, and the self-reported weights on which the tables are

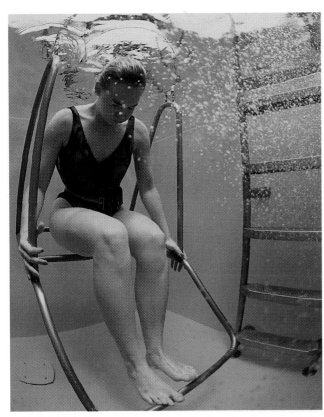

This young woman is being submerged as part of a hydrostatic weighing procedure, one of several methods for measuring the percentage of body weight that is fat. A very high or very low percentage of body fat is associated with health problems.

The range of "normal," healthy values for body fat content in young adults is about 10 to 18 percent for men and 18 to 25 percent for women. The values for women are higher because women need more body fat for certain reproductive functions, including regular menstruation. Individuals who engage in vigorous, regular exercise may have much less body fat. However, too little body fat—less than 8 percent for women or 5 percent for men—can cause health problems, including muscle wasting and fatigue. For women, a very low percentage of body fat is also associated with **amenorrhea** and loss of bone mass.

Skinfold Measurements A more convenient method for determining percentage of body fat is the skinfold thickness technique, which measures the thickness of fat under the skin. A technician grasps a fold of skin at a predetermined location and measures it using an instrument called a caliper. Repeated measurements are taken from several areas of the body, and the results are computed from formulas that predict body fatness from skinfold thickness.

This technique has been criticized because the distribution of body fat is nonuniform and taking the measurements can be difficult. Pinching muscle along with skin can cause measurement errors, as can badly adjusted calipers. Most importantly, there are age, sex, and ethnic differences in skinfolds, and appropriate standards are not always used to take these differences into account.

Electrical Impedance Analysis Body fat can also be assessed by the newly popular technique of electrical impedance analysis. Electrodes are attached to the body in several areas, and a harmless electrical current is transmitted from electrode to electrode. The electrical conduction through the body favors the path of the lean tissues over the fat tissues. A computer can calculate fat percentage from these current measurements.

Like the other methods, electrical impedance analysis is subject to error. Electrical impedance equipment is calibrated with the same equations used in underwater weighing, making it subject to the same criticisms about standards. Furthermore, the margin of error with this equipment may be even greater than with skinfold or hydrostatic techniques. If the person being analyzed does anything that affects water retention or the electrolyte balance of the body—such as using diuretic medications or doing vigorous exercise—additional error can be introduced. For an accurate measurement, the person being

based may be lower than people's true weights in some cases. Despite these limitations, the U.S. Food and Drug Administration and the Health and Human Services Department have recently published a new height-weight table (Table 13-2). The table gives a range of suggested weights based on height and age. Both sexes are included in one table; the higher weights in each range generally apply to men, the lower to women.

Underwater Weighing One of the most accurate methods for assessing body composition is *hydrostatic weighing*, or weighing under water. Since the density of fat is different from that of lean tissue, these masses can be estimated by either measuring the amount of water displaced or by comparing the difference between the underwater and the dry weighings. This method is not without problems, however. It can be an intimidating procedure, especially for those who have a fear of water. Underwater weighing is neither convenient nor a widely available procedure. And it is not without error—measurements can be affected by eating foods that create internal gas or engaging in activities that affect fluid retention or cause dehydration. Furthermore, the standards used for assessing the outcome were developed by testing middle-aged sedentary males, so they may be inaccurate for many people.

Amenorrhea   Absence of menstruation.

TERMS

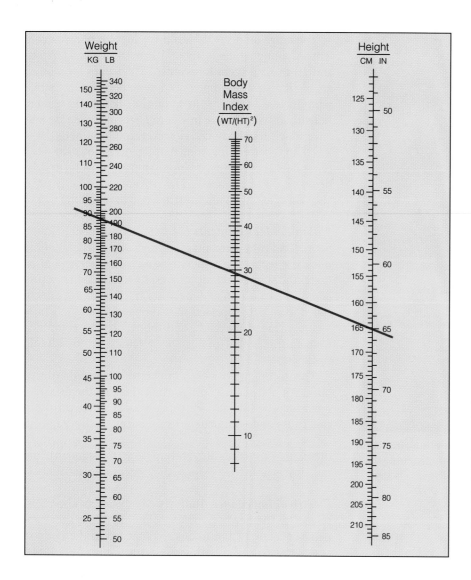

Figure 13-1 *Body mass index (BMI).* To determine your BMI, place a ruler or other straight edge so that it intersects your body weight under the weight column on the left and your height in the height column on the right. Read your BMI where the ruler intersects the center column. For example, the red line shows that a person who weighs 190 pounds and is 65 inches tall has a BMI of 29.5.

measured needs to avoid consuming alcohol for 48 hours and avoid eating for at least 3 hours before the test.

Body Mass Index Another approach to determining whether a person is overweight is **body mass index (BMI),** defined as body weight (in kilograms) divided by the square of height (in meters) or BMI = kg/m² (Figure 13-1). BMI correlates highly with direct measures of body fat.

The National Academy of Sciences (NAS) recommends that people between the ages of 19 and 24 maintain a BMI between 19 and 24 kg/m², with an increase of 1 kg/m² for each succeeding decade. These lower suggested values for young people reflect the fact that even a small degree of overweight at younger ages is associated with serious health problems and lower life expectancy. For all ages and sexes, a BMI below 19 is considered underweight and unhealthy.

Waist-to-Hip Ratio Another approach to assessing overweight and its associated health risks focuses on the distribution of body fat. Fat located in the waist and abdomen is more metabolically active and associated with greater risk of disease and premature death than is fat in the thighs, hips, and buttocks. The higher the ratio of waist to hip measurement, the greater the risk. To determine your ratio, simply measure your waist and hips and then divide the waist measurement by the hip measurement. Ratios of more than 1.0 for men or 0.8 for women suggest elevated risk.

Defining Overweight and Obesity The term **overweight** is usually used in reference to total body weight or body mass index. In terms of height-weight tables—the least accurate approach to body weight assessment—anyone with a body weight above the "healthy" range is considered overweight. In terms of BMI, anyone with a BMI between 27 and 30 is considered overweight, and anyone with a BMI over 30 is considered severely overweight. About 10 percent of Americans have BMI over 30.

Using the body composition approach, researchers have defined obesity as a body-fat content greater than 25

To select a body weight goal for yourself that is reasonable, consider the following criteria. A reasonable weight for you is . . .

- The weight that results from a lifestyle that includes a healthy diet and regular exercise.
- The lowest weight you have maintained as an adult for at least one year (this is a good indicator of your lower limit of reasonable weight).
- Likely to be higher than for others if you have a family history of obesity. (That is, if one or both of your parents were significantly overweight, expect that a reasonable weight for you may be higher than that for others.)

percent of total body weight for males and greater than 30 percent for females. This condition is also termed **overfat.** Using height-weight tables, researchers define obesity as being 20 percent or more above a person's upper limit for weight, adjusted for sex and height (some researchers use 30 percent).

Anyone who meets the criteria for overweight or obesity or who has an elevated waist-to-hip ratio faces increased health risks.

A Radical Answer　For most of us, our body weight and percentage of body fat fall somewhere under the levels associated with significant health risks. For us, these assessment tests don't really answer the question, "How much should I weigh?" Height-weight tables, body composition analyses, and BMI and waist-to-hip ratio measurements can best serve as general guides or estimates for body weight. They can't account for individual genetic, racial, or ethnic differences that cause variations from "average" population weights but that may still be healthy. Perhaps it's time for a radical idea: To answer the question of what you "should" weigh, let your lifestyle be your guide. Don't focus on a particular weight as your goal. Focus on living a lifestyle that includes eating moderate amounts of healthful foods, getting plenty of exercise, thinking positively, and learning to cope with stress. Then let the pounds fall where they may. For most people, the result will be close to the recommended weight ranges discussed earlier. For some, their weight will be somewhat higher than societal standards—but right for them (see box "What Is a Reasonable Weight for You?"). By letting a healthy lifestyle determine your weight, you can avoid the dieting hysteria and fixation on body weight that grips this country.

Health Implications of Obesity

In general, the health risks of obesity increase with its severity, reaching significance when BMI exceeds 27. These risks include higher rates of cardiovascular disease, hypertension, gallbladder disease, and diabetes. Obesity may be associated with a more dangerous blood lipid profile: high levels of triglycerides, total cholesterol, and low-density lipoproteins and low levels of high-density lipoproteins. Obesity is also associated with certain types of cancer, including cancer of the colon, prostate, gallbladder, ovary, endometrium, breast, and cervix. Women who are obese are more likely to suffer from menstrual abnormalities and complications during pregnancy. With more severe obesity, respiratory problems and degenerative joint disease are common.

How dangerous obesity is depends to some extent on where excess fat is located in the body. As mentioned earlier, people who carry their body fat in their trunk and abdomen are at greater risk for health problems than are people who carry fat in their hips, thighs, and buttocks. The risks associated with body fat stored primarily in the midsection include higher rates of heart disease, hypertension, stroke, and diabetes. Men are more likely than women to store excess fat in the midsection and to develop a "beer belly," whether or not they drink alcohol. Women typically store fat in the lower body, but women who exhibit the male pattern of fat distribution face the increased health risks associated with it.

Obesity and body fat distribution are clearly associated with health risks. However, there is controversy over whether obesity adversely affects health *independently* of other risk factors, such as smoking and diabetes. There is also disagreement over the point on the weight spectrum at which this increased risk begins.

TERMS

Body mass index (BMI)　A measure of relative body weight nearly independent of height and correlating highly with more direct measures of body fat. It is calculated by dividing total body weight in kilograms by the square of body height in meters.

Overweight　Body weight or body mass index that falls above the range associated with minimum mortality.

Overfat　A condition in which a person has more body fat than is considered to be healthy. The amount differs according to gender (females naturally have more body fat than males), race, and ethnicity.

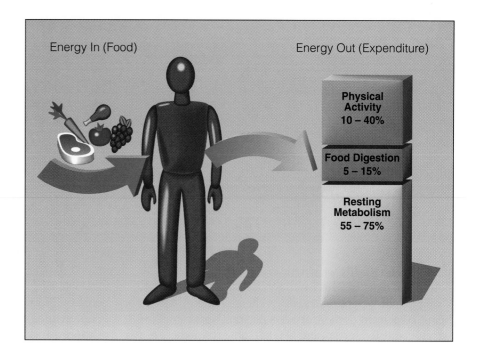

Figure 13-2 *Energy balance equation.*
Total energy expenditure in humans is
composed of physical activity, digestion,
and resting metabolism.

Energy In (Food)

Energy Out (Expenditure)

Physical
Activity
10 – 40%

Food Digestion
5 – 15%

Resting
Metabolism
55 – 75%

OVERCOMING A WEIGHT PROBLEM

Why do some people become obese and others remain thin? A variety of factors work together to determine body weight and body fatness, including genetics, metabolism, and lifestyle. But for whatever reasons it occurs, obesity is a problem that requires action.

What Contributes to a Weight Problem?

Although the picture is far from complete, we know that physical factors, as well as psychological, cultural, and social factors, play a significant role in determining body weight. In particular, heredity and metabolism have been linked to a tendency toward obesity.

Genetic Factors   Obesity can be produced in animals through selective breeding. That is, animals can be bred for higher or lower fat content, and the same principles may hold true for humans. A study comparing 540 adult Danish adoptees and their biological parents concluded that genetic influences played an important role in determining fatness in adults. The best predictor of a woman's weight was her own mother's weight. Furthermore, if both parents are overweight, 73 percent of their offspring are likely to be overweight. If only one parent is overweight, 41 percent of the offspring are likely to be overweight. If neither parent is overweight, only 9 percent tend to be overweight.

Genes influence body type, body size, body weight, and obesity, and the occurrence of obesity in families has long been reported. Even the pattern of fat distribution on the body (that is, whether it tends to accumulate on the hips, at the waist, in the abdomen, etc.) is a function of heredity. Heredity may also be the culprit in certain types of glandular, chromosomal, neurological, or metabolic dysfunctions that produce some kinds of obesity. Nevertheless, probably no more than 5 percent of all obesity problems are attributable to such causes.

Remember that genes are not destiny. With increased exercise and decreased food consumption, even those with a genetic tendency toward obesity can maintain a healthy body weight.

Set Point Theory   Set point theory holds that body weight, or, more precisely, body fat, is automatically regulated at a relatively constant level, in much the same manner as body temperature, blood pressure, and blood glucose levels. The body "defends" this set point and defeats attempts to change levels of body fat with a variety of compensatory responses, such as increasing or decreasing metabolic rate or feelings of hunger. Proponents of this theory claim that the only way to lower set point is through increased exercise. So far, the operation of a set point has been demonstrated conclusively only in animals. Recent research suggests that if a set point for humans exists, it is probably a range rather than a specific point, and it is probably greatly affected by diet and exercise.

Fat Cell Theory   According to fat cell theory, the quantity of fat stored in the body is the result of the number of fat cells that a person has and their size. People with an above-average number of fat cells may have been born with them or may have developed them at certain critical times because of overfeeding. Childhood-onset obesity, or hyperplasia, is thought to be the result of developing too many fat cells. Adult-onset obesity, or hypertrophy, is the result of developing bigger, rather than more, fat cells. Some very obese people are thought to have a combination of both too many fat cells and extraordinarily large fat cells. As the theory goes, having extra fat cells creates a biological pressure to keep these fat cells full. New fat cells are most likely to develop in response to prolonged overeating when existing fat cells reach the limit of their fat storage capacity. Similarly, it seems that the number of fat cells can be decreased if weight is kept off for an extended period. More research is needed to determine the actual relevance of fat cell theory to the development and maintenance of obesity in humans.

Metabolism and Energy Balance   Metabolism is the sum of all the vital processes in which energy and nutrients from foods are made available to and utilized by the body. The largest component of metabolism, measured as **resting metabolic rate (RMR),** is the energy required to maintain vital bodily functions, including respiration, temperature regulation, and blood pressure, while the body is at rest. As shown in Figure 13-2, this component of metabolism accounts for 55 to 75 percent of energy used. The energy required to digest food accounts for an additional 5 to 15 percent of daily energy expenditure. The remaining 10 to 40 percent of energy is expended during physical activity; this represents the biggest variable in energy use among people.

Metabolic rate differs from person to person, depending on a variety of genetic and behavioral factors. A higher percentage of body fat is associated with a lower metabolic rate. Thus, obese people have relatively lower metabolic rates than thin people, partly because thin people dissipate more calories through heat loss. And women, with their larger percentage of body fat, have lower metabolic rates than men.

Recurrent cycles of dieting may lower metabolic rates, according to recent research. When people repeatedly lose weight and then gain it back, their bodies may increase metabolic efficiency by reducing the number of calories required to maintain body functions. This means they lose weight more slowly and gain it back more quickly each time they diet.

Exercise affects metabolic rate in several ways. When people exercise, they increase their RMR (the number of calories their bodies burn at rest), and they also increase their lean body mass, which is associated with a higher metabolic rate. The exercise itself also burns calories, raising total energy expenditure. The higher a person's energy expenditure, the more the person can eat without gaining weight.

Two factors in the energy balance equation illustrated in Figure 13-2 are under individual control—the amount of energy taken in as food and the number of calories expended through physical activity. Exercise is thus an im-

portant part of weight management. Studies have shown that obese adults are less physically active than their average-weight peers. However, this doesn't prove that inactivity causes obesity; it may be that obesity causes inactivity. There is universal agreement, however, that increased physical activity is a critical component of long-term success in weight management.

Overeating   Although "common sense" suggests that overeating is involved in weight gain, most research has not been able to prove that all or even many obese people eat more than normal people. In fact, 12 out of 13 studies of eating behavior found that obese people reported consuming no more calories per day than did their nonobese counterparts, and in some instances reported eating less. However, more recent research using a sophisticated technique to measure energy expenditure has raised serious questions about the accuracy of self-reported caloric intake, and in turn about whether obese people indeed consume no more calories than the nonobese. Both the obese and nonobese have been found to underestimate their caloric intake as recorded in daily diet journals, but obese subjects typically underreport their intakes by 30 to 35 percent—much more than the nonobese.

Even if the obese do not generally overeat, approximately 25 to 45 percent of obese dieters engage in episodes of binge eating, during which they may consume large amounts of food. (The extent of binge eating in the obese who are not involved in a diet program is unknown.) Binge eating may cause some people to become obese.

Psychological Problems   At one time most health professionals believed that obesity was the result of psychological problems. Yet research has shown that overweight people are no more neurotic than are people of normal weight and do not suffer more psychiatric disturbance. No particular personality characteristics are consistently linked with obesity, although some obese people tend to be more dependent and passive than average. Although the obese may be more emotional in certain circumstances, by and large negative emotions are the result of concern about weight and failed efforts to reduce. Dieting per se can cause emotional disturbances—the most common complaints being anxiety, irritability, depression, and a preoccupation with food.

Obese Eating Style   Few consistent differences in eating style have been found between the obese and others.

Resting metabolic rate (RMR)   The energy required to maintain vital bodily functions, including respiration, heart rate, and blood pressure.

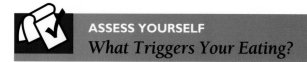

Hunger isn't the only reason people eat. Efforts to maintain a healthy body weight can be sabotaged by eating related to other factors, including emotions, environment, and patterns of thinking. This test is designed to provide you with a score for five factors that describe many people's eating. This information will put you in a better position to manage your eating behavior and control your weight. Circle the number that indicates to what degree each situation is likely to make you start eating.

Social

	Very Unlikely							Very Likely		
1. Arguing or having conflict with someone	1	2	3	4	5	6	7	8	9	10
2. Being with others when they are eating	1	2	3	4	5	6	7	8	9	10
3. Being urged to eat by someone else	1	2	3	4	5	6	7	8	9	10
4. Feeling inadequate around others	1	2	3	4	5	6	7	8	9	10

Emotional

5. Feeling bad, such as being anxious or depressed	1	2	3	4	5	6	7	8	9	10
6. Feeling good, happy, or relaxed	1	2	3	4	5	6	7	8	9	10
7. Feeling bored or having time on my hands	1	2	3	4	5	6	7	8	9	10
8. Feeling stressed or excited	1	2	3	4	5	6	7	8	9	10

Situational

9. Seeing an advertisement for food or eating	1	2	3	4	5	6	7	8	9	10
10. Passing by a bakery, cookie shop, or other enticement to eat	1	2	3	4	5	6	7	8	9	10
11. Being involved in a party, celebration, or special occasion	1	2	3	4	5	6	7	8	9	10
12. Eating out	1	2	3	4	5	6	7	8	9	10

Thinking

13. Making excuses to myself about why it's okay to eat	1	2	3	4	5	6	7	8	9	10
14. Berating myself for being so fat or unable to control my eating	1	2	3	4	5	6	7	8	9	10
15. Worrying about others, or about difficulties I am having	1	2	3	4	5	6	7	8	9	10
16. Thinking about how things should or shouldn't be	1	2	3	4	5	6	7	8	9	10

Physiological

17. Experiencing pain or physical discomfort	1	2	3	4	5	6	7	8	9	10
18. Experiencing trembling, headache, or light-headedness associated with no eating or too much caffeine	1	2	3	4	5	6	7	8	9	10
19. Experiencing fatigue or feeling overtired	1	2	3	4	5	6	7	8	9	10
20. Experiencing hunger pangs or urges to eat, even though I've eaten recently	1	2	3	4	5	6	7	8	9	10

Scoring

Total your scores for each area and enter them below. Then rank the scores by marking the highest score "1," next highest score "2," and so on. Focus on the highest ranked areas first, but any score above 24 is *high* and indicates that you need to work on that area.

Area	Total Score	Rank Order
Social (Items 1–4)	_____	_____
Emotional (Items 5–8)	_____	_____
Situational (Items 9–12)	_____	_____
Thinking (Items 13–16)	_____	_____
Physiological (Items 17–20)	_____	_____

What Your Score Means

Social   A high score on this factor means you are very susceptible to the influence of others. Work on better ways to communicate more assertively, handle conflict, and manage anger. Challenge your beliefs about the need to be polite and the obligations you feel you must fulfill.

Emotional   A high score here means you need to develop effective ways to cope with emotions. Work on developing skills in stress management, time management, and communication. Practicing positive self-talk can help you handle small daily upsets.

Situational   A high score here means you are especially susceptible to external influences. Try to avoid external cues to eat and to respond differently to those you cannot avoid. Control your environment by changing the way you buy, store, cook, and serve food. Anticipate potential problems and have a plan for handling them.

Thinking   A high score here means that the way you think—how you talk to yourself, the beliefs you hold, your memories, and your expectations—have a powerful influence on your eating habits. Try to be less self-critical, less of a perfectionist, and more flexible in your ideas about the way things ought to be. Recognize when you're making excuses or rationalizations that allow you to eat.

Physiological   A high score here means that the way you eat, what you eat, or medications you are taking may be affecting your eating behavior. You may be eating to reduce physical arousal or deal with physical discomfort. Try eating three meals a day, supplemented with regular snacks if needed. Avoid too much caffeine. If any medication you're taking produces adverse physical reactions, switch to an alternative if possible. If your medications may be affecting your hormones, discuss possible alternatives with your physician.

From J. D. Nash. 1986. *Maximize Your Body Potential.* Shortened version. (Menlo Park, Calif.: Bull Publishing).

Both lean and fat people report eating in the absence of hunger, eating rapidly, and having frequent snacks. Only one thing seems to differentiate the obese—good-tasting food keeps them eating longer.

Externality Theory   Externality theory proposes that the obese might be more sensitive to external cues to eat. Researchers looked for evidence that time of day, elapsed time between eating episodes, sight of food, and association of eating with particular cues might account for differences between lean and obese people. Environmental cues *are* intimately linked to eating behavior, but this was found to be true for people in every weight category. Overweight people on the average are more responsive than lean people to food cues in the environment, but many people of normal weight are too. To determine if you're sensitive to environmental or other types of cues, take the quiz in the box "What Triggers Your Eating?"

Lifestyle and Weight   Most weight problems are in fact lifestyle problems. Researchers have found a strong relationship between socioeconomic status (SES) and obesity, with the prevalence of obesity going down as SES level goes up. One major study found that the rate of obesity in women was 30 percent for the lower SES group, 16 percent for the middle group, and only 5 percent for the higher group. More women are obese at lower SES levels than are men, but men are somewhat more obese at the higher SES levels than are women. These differences may reflect the greater sensitivity and concern for a slim physical appearance among upper SES women. It may also reflect the greater acceptance of obesity among low-income and certain ethnic groups, as well as different cultural values related to food choices.

In addition to poor nutrition and lack of adequate exercise, an unhealthy lifestyle is characterized by too many obligations and too few rewards. Sometimes the seeds of an unhealthy lifestyle are planted early, in the family of origin. When a family advocates setting high goals for accomplishment, being a perfectionist, putting work first, and not balancing obligations with personal rewards, it establishes the basis for a lifestyle that may support a weight problem.

Social and cultural influences further complicate the picture. Food is used to show friendship and caring; it is part of the social fabric and is involved in celebrations and social gatherings. In our society, eating well and sharing food with friends are highly valued activities. Food is a symbol of love and caring.

> ***Personal Insight*** What do you recall about your family's eating habits as you were growing up? Were certain foods given as a reward or withheld as a punishment? Were you encouraged to always "clean your plate"? How have these family eating habits affected your attitudes toward food and your current eating behavior?

Hazards and Rewards in the Search for the "Perfect" Body

The American focus on attaining a perfect body has prompted a flood of weight loss programs, fad diets, health clubs, exercise equipment, appetite-reducing medicines, and books on diet, nutrition, and fitness. Presumably, with the right combination of programs, exercise, and eating plans, one can attain the promised rewards of a healthier, slimmer, fitter, more aesthetically appealing body.

Dieting has become part of the American way of life. In one recent survey, nearly one-quarter of all adult men and half of all adult women reported being on diets. The rates are even higher among young people. A 1988 national survey found that 61 percent of adolescent girls and 28 percent of adolescent boys had dieted during the previous year. Another study found that up to 15 percent of girls and 3 percent of boys were "chronic dieters"—that is, they reported that they always dieted or had been on a diet more than 10 times in the past year. Chronic dieting among teenagers can lead to retardation of physical growth, menstrual irregularities, and the development of **eating disorders.** As discussed earlier, chronic dieting may also lower metabolic rate, making weight management more difficult.

During adolescence, both boys and girls become sensitive about their size and physical appearance. Studies have consistently shown a high prevalence of dissatisfaction with body weight or shape among male and female adolescents. The cultural pressure to be thin, especially for female adolescents, coupled with the social stigma of obesity, may well predispose weight-conscious youth to dieting, abnormal eating patterns, and eating disorders.

Setting large weight loss goals in response to cultural ideals of attractiveness can set people up for failure and psychological distress. Dieters may suffer from depression, persistent irritability, inability to concentrate, sleep difficulties, and preoccupation with food and weight. When they fail to attain their goal of thinness, they may feel they're weak or suffer from a character flaw. Such ideas can undermine their chances of developing a truly healthy lifestyle, one that will allow them to maintain a reasonable body weight easily and naturally.

Smaller weight loss goals are much more realistic and can have very beneficial effects. For an obese person, losing as little as 10 pounds can reduce blood pressure as much as antihypertensive medication. People participating in behavioral weight loss programs tend to experience improvement in mood, sometimes after losing as little as 10 pounds.

Obesity *is* a serious health risk, but weight management needs to take place in a positive and realistic atmosphere. The hazards of excessive dieting and overconcern about body weight need to be countered by a change in attitude about what constitutes the perfect body and a reasonable body weight. The current ideals of ultra-thin and ultra-fit need to change. A reasonable body weight must take into account an individual's weight history, social circumstances, metabolic profile, and psychological well-being.

> ***Personal Insight*** How do you feel about your body weight, shape, and size? Do you have strong feelings about what an ideal male and female body should look like? Where do you think you've learned these ideals?

Resources for Getting Help

What should you do if you are overweight? Several approaches are possible.

Doing It Yourself Research indicates that people are far more successful than was previously thought at losing weight and keeping it off. One study found that about 64 percent of the people achieved long-term success without

TERMS

Eating disorder Any of a number of disorders characterized by gross disturbances in eating or eating-related behaviors.

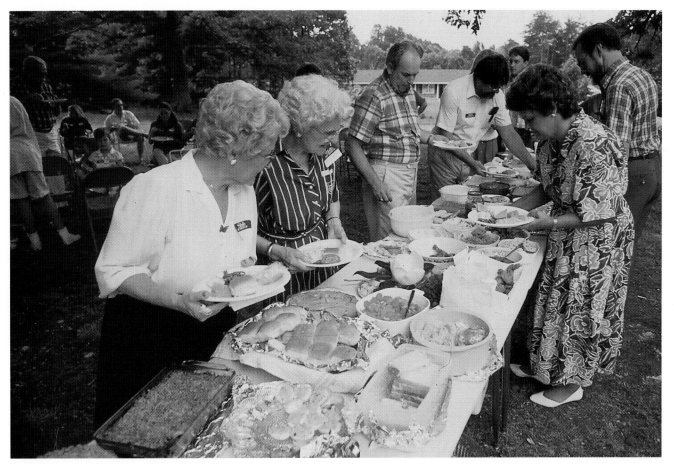

Eating is so intimately bound up with the social fabric of life that people trying to change their diets often meet unexpected obstacles and difficulties. High-fat foods are an integral part of this family reunion, not easily avoided even by those very concerned with their fat intake.

joining a formal program or getting special help. Supporting these findings, a Public Health Service survey indicated that about 50 percent of the general public succeed with long-term weight management.

Other researchers investigated the characteristics that distinguished those who lost at least 20 percent of body weight and maintained this loss for two years or more. Although some had used diet alone to lose weight, some had used exercise alone, and others had used a combination of diet and exercise, virtually all maintained their success by making exercise a permanent part of their lifestyle. They also kept tabs on their weight and habits. In addition, they learned to develop their own diet, exercise, and maintenance plans, and they became more involved in and excited by activities other than eating— such as careers, projects, and special interests.

If you need to lose weight, focus on adopting the healthy lifestyle we've described. The "right" weight for you will naturally evolve, and you won't have to diet. However, if you must diet, do so in combination with exercise, and avoid very-low-calorie diets. Realize that most low-calorie diets cause a rapid loss of body water at first.

When this phase passes, weight loss declines. As a result, dieters are often misled into believing that their efforts are not working. They then give up, not realizing that smaller losses later in the diet are actually better than the initial big losses, because later loss is mostly fat loss, whereas initial loss was primarily fluid (Figure 13-3). For more tips on how to lose weight on your own, refer to the box "Getting Started on a Sensible Weight Loss Program."

Diet Books Many people who try to lose weight by themselves fall prey to one or more of the dozens of diet books on the market. Although a very few of these do contain useful advice and tips for motivation, most make promises they can't fulfill. Some guidelines for evaluating and choosing a diet book can be offered:

1. Reject books that advocate an unbalanced way of eating. These include books advocating a high-carbohydrate-only diet, such as *The Endocrine Control Diet* or *Bloomingdale's Eat Healthy Diet,* or those advocating low-carbohydrate/high-protein diets, such as *The Complete Scarsdale Medical Diet* and *Dr. Atkins' Diet Revolution.*

2. Reject books that claim to be based on a "scientific breakthrough" or to have the "secret" to success. Examples include *The T-Factor Diet, The La Costa Book of Nutrition,* and *The Princeton Plan.*

3. Reject books that use gimmicks, like combining foods in special ways to achieve weight loss, rotating levels of calories, or purporting that a weight problem is due to food allergies, food sensitivities, or yeast infections. Examples include *The Beverly Hills Diet, Fit for Life, The Rotation Diet, The Two-Day Diet,* and *The Diet-Type Weight-Loss Program.*

4. Reject books that promise quick weight loss or limit the selection of foods. An example is *The Paris Diet.*

5. Accept books that advocate a balanced approach to diet plus exercise and sound nutrition advice. Some books to consider include *The I-Don't-Eat (But-I-Can't-Lose) Weight Loss Program,* by Steven Jonas and Virginia Aronson, *Maximize Your Body Potential,* by Joyce D. Nash, and *The Weighting Game,* by Lawrence E. Lamb.

Dangerous Do-It-Yourself Options: Dietary Supplements Using commercially available supplements for modified fasting can be a dangerous option, especially if they are the sole source of nutrition, because there is no medical monitoring by a physician. Such approaches include powders used to make shakes that substitute for some or all of the daily food intake, as well as food bars. Many provide fewer than 800 calories a day. Although the products available today are much improved over the liquid-protein supplements that contributed to many dieters' deaths in the 1970s, only careful medical evaluation and monitoring can significantly reduce the risk of such an approach. Furthermore, dietary supplements teach reliance on patented products, not on sound, lifelong eating habits. And although weight loss can be rapid, muscle tends to be lost too, and weight is often regained.

Over-the-Counter Diet Pills and Diet Aids A large number of over-the-counter diet aids are available to those seeking a magic pill to do away with extra pounds. Many of these tout gimmicks, such as exotic-sounding herbs, grapefruit juice extract, and amino acids (L-glutamine, L-arginine), none of which has been proven to affect appetite or weight loss.

The most common ingredient, in diet aids sold in drug stores is *phenyl propanolamine hydrochloride (PPA).* The Food and Drug Administration (FDA) has declared that PPA is a safe and effective appetite suppressant for weight loss. Though less potent, PPA is similar to amphetamines, a class of drugs available legally only by prescription. It acts as a mild stimulant and suppresses the desire to eat.

Studies on the effectiveness of PPA are contradictory. A recent study found that while PPA was effective in suppressing appetite, the average weight loss of people taking

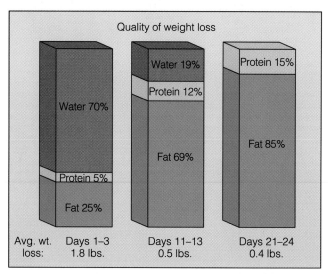

Figure 13-3 *Quality of weight loss.*
In the early stages of dieting, most of the weight lost is fluid. After about three weeks, however, mostly fat is being lost, even though the absolute number of pounds per day decreases. *Source:* F. Grande. 1961. "Nutrition and Energy Balance in Body Composition Studies." In *Techniques for Measuring Body Composition.* (Washington, D.C.: National Academy of Sciences—National Research Council).

it over a six-week period was only two pounds greater than for those receiving a placebo. Without a conscious effort to reduce calorie intake, increase activity, and change eating behavior, such weight loss is unlikely to be maintained. Furthermore, there is concern over the safety of PPA. Some reports suggest it can cause dizziness, headaches, rapid pulse, palpitations, sleeplessness, and hypertension. Use of PPA is not approved by the FDA for periods longer than 12 weeks.

The second most common ingredient of diet aids sold in drug stores is *fiber.* Oat bran, guar gum, hemicellulose, cellulose, corn bran, pectin, psyllium seed, apple fiber, and lignin are all promoted as weight-loss aids. Manufacturers claim these work by "swelling in the stomach and absorbing liquids" to provide a feeling of fullness. In fact, dietary fiber acts as a bulking agent in the large intestine, not in the stomach. The FDA has found no data to warrant classifying any type of fiber as an aid in weight control or as an appetite suppressant. Furthermore, most of these products provide a mere 1 to 3 grams of fiber per day, which doesn't contribute much toward the recommended daily intake of 20 to 35 grams. In 1992, the FDA banned guargum and 110 other ingredients from use in nonprescription diet aids because they had not been proven safe and effective.

The bottom line on over-the-counter diet aids is *caveat emptor*—buyer beware. There is no quick and easy way to lose weight. The most effective answer is to develop healthy diet and exercise habits and to make these part of your lifestyle.

Would you like to lose weight on your own? Here are some tips for getting started on a program of weight management that will last a lifetime.

Motivation and Commitment

Make sure you are motivated and committed before you begin. Failure at weight loss is a frustrating experience that can make it physically and psychologically more difficult to lose weight in the future. Think about the reasons you want to lose weight. Self-focused reasons, such as to feel good about yourself or to have a greater sense of well-being, are often associated with success. Trying to lose weight for others or out of concern for how others view you is a poor foundation for a weight loss program. Make a list of your reasons for wanting to lose weight and post it in a prominent place.

Creating a Negative Energy Balance

When your weight is constant, you are burning approximately the same number of calories as you are taking in. To tip the energy balance toward weight loss, you must either consume fewer calories or burn more calories through physical activity, or both. One pound of body fat represents 3,500 calories. To lose weight at the recommended rate of one-half to one pound per week, you must create a negative energy balance of 1,750 to 3,500 calories per week or 250 to 500 calories per day. To generate your negative energy balance, it's usually best to begin by increasing your activity level rather than decreasing your calorie consumption.

Increasing Your Level of Physical Activity

Exercise is a crucial component of weight management. You can increase your activity level both by beginning a program of regular exercise and by incorporating more physical activity into your daily routine. Just 30 minutes of moderate walking or cycling can provide a significant contribution— 150 calories—toward your daily negative calorie balance; an hour of cycling or slow jogging burns about 500 calories. Chapter 14 has more information about putting together a successful program of regular exercise.

Don't try to use exercise to "spot reduce." Leg lifts, for example, contribute to fat loss only to the extent that they burn calories; they don't burn fat just from your legs. You can make parts of your body appear more fit by exercising them, but the only way you can reduce fat in any specific part of your body is to create an overall negative energy balance.

Making Changes in Your Diet and Eating Habits

If you can't generate a large enough negative calorie balance solely by increasing physical activity, you may want to supplement exercise with small cuts in your calorie intake. Don't think of this as "going on a diet"—your goal is to make small changes in your diet that you can maintain for a lifetime. Focus on cutting your fat intake (refer back to the box on "Eating Smart") and on eating a variety of nutritious foods in moderation. Don't try skipping meals, fasting, or very-low-calorie diets. These strategies seldom work, and they can have negative effects on your ability to manage your weight and on your overall health.

Making changes in eating habits is another important strategy for weight management. If your program centers on conscious restriction of certain food items, you're likely to spend all your time thinking about the forbidden foods. Focus on *how* to eat rather than *what* to eat. Try adopting some of the behaviors listed in the box "Strategies for Managing Your Weight"—you may find that your new eating habits make it much easier for you to achieve and maintain a healthy weight.

Commercial, Group, and Medical Programs A variety of options is available if you want help, support, or advice for your weight management program. Different types of programs may work for different individuals, but a little research can help you locate a program that suits your needs and preferences. Many commercial weight loss programs include counseling sessions, nutrition education, exercise planning, and behavior modification training; they can be expensive, though, and some require purchase of special foods or supplements. If you consider trying a commercial weight loss program, use the suggestions in the box "How to Evaluate Commercial Weight Loss Programs."

Self-help groups that focus on weight management can offer support and encouragement. Your physician or a registered dietitian can also help you put together a successful weight management program. Many registered dietitians can be found in private practice or conducting weight management programs through hospitals or clinics. For cases of severe obesity, a physician's advice is probably indicated.

Getting Psychological Help Although some people do seek individual psychotherapy for treatment of obesity, it is not clear whether psychotherapy alone can help. Often people choose this potential solution when they feel they have tried everything else and failed or when the emotional disturbance from failed dieting efforts becomes unbearable. Although no empirical evidence supports the notion, some clinicians feel that some obesity is associated with early child abuse, particularly sexual abuse. Together with a program specifically focused on managing obesity, individual psychotherapy may be beneficial for some people.

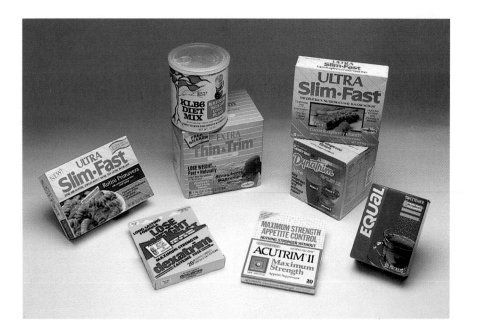

Over-the-counter diet aids such as those shown here can be helpful in controlling hunger and weight in the short term, but they are not a miracle cure. Long-term weight management requires lifelong healthy diet and exercise habits.

Selecting a Weight Reduction Approach

No single approach to weight reduction is appropriate for all individuals, and no one type of program stands above all others. After eliminating those approaches that are dangerous or fraudulent, you will have a number of options. The challenge is to find the one that's best for you.

The first step is to decide how serious your weight problem is. If you are less than 20 percent overweight, you might consider a self-directed approach—cutting back on fat calories and increasing exercise on your own—or reconsidering whether in fact you need to lose weight. Be sure you are pursuing a reasonable weight, given your family history and lifestyle.

If you are 20 to 40 percent overweight, you might consider joining a self-help group, one of the commercial weight loss programs, a behavioral program led by a health professional, or a work site program. More serious degrees of overweight, 40 to 100 percent, may require a more aggressive approach. Consider getting private counseling, joining a hospital-based program, participating in a medically supervised very-low-calorie diet (VLCD) with a maintenance program, or going to a residential program such as Pritikin.

If you are 100 percent or more overweight, or have 100 pounds or more to lose, a medically supervised VLCD should be your first choice. With appropriate pretreatment assessment, open-ended treatment that includes a maintenance program, and the help of a professional staff that includes dietitians, physicians, and psychologists, such an approach has been found to be quite effective for about 65 percent of those who participate. Should this approach fail, the most drastic (but often successful) treatment is surgery. Discuss this alternative with your physician.

Once you narrow your options, take into consideration your own needs and preferences. You may prefer a group program to individual care. You may need supervised exercise, while others may be able to exercise on their own. Choosing a program that fits your lifestyle will increase your chances of success.

EATING DISORDERS

Problems with body weight and weight control are not limited to excessive body fat. A growing number of people, especially adolescent girls and young women, experience what are called "eating disorders," characterized by severe disturbances in eating and eating-related behaviors. The major eating disorders are **anorexia nervosa, bulimia nervosa,** and **binge eating disorder.** Each disorder can be characterized by its primary behavioral manifestation: For anorexia, it is starvation; for bulimia, binging and purging; and for binge eating disorder, compulsive overeating. All eating disorders are associated with increased illness and, in some cases, increased risk of premature death.

Western society's emphasis on extreme thinness as the ideal for females places many young women in conflict about their weight. Although the typical woman under the age of 30 has become heavier by 5 or 6 pounds since the 1960s, the "ideal" body—as reflected by winners of the Miss America Pageant and models—has become thinner. This widening gap between reality and ideal for most young women is reflected in their high rates of body dissatisfaction.

Eating disorders are far more prevalent in industrialized countries than in developing ones. In the United States, eating disorders affect more women than men,

The National Council Against Health Fraud advises against commercial weight loss programs that:

1. Promise or imply dramatic, rapid weight loss (substantially more than 1 percent of total body weight per week).

2. Promote diets that are extremely low in calories (below 800 calories per day; 1,200-calorie diets are preferred) unless under the supervision of competent medical experts.

3. Attempt to make clients dependent upon special products rather than teaching how to make good choices from the conventional food supply. (This does not condemn the marketing of low-calorie convenience foods that may be chosen by consumers.)

4. Do not encourage permanent, realistic lifestyle changes, including regular exercise, and do not address the behavioral aspects of eating, wherein food may be used as a coping device. (Programs should focus upon changing the causes of overweight rather than simply the effect, which is the overweight itself.)

5. Misrepresent salespeople as "counselors," supposedly qualified to give guidance in nutrition and/or general health. Even if adequately trained, such "counselors" would still be objectionable because of the obvious conflict-of-interest that exists when providers profit directly from products they recommend and sell.

6. Require large sums of money at the start or require that clients sign contracts for expensive, long-term programs. Such practices too often have been abused as salespeople focus attention upon signing up new people rather than delivering continuing, satisfactory service to consumers. Programs should be on a pay-as-you-go basis.

7. Fail to inform clients about the risks associated with weight loss in general or the specific program being promoted.

8. Promote unproven or spurious weight loss aids such as human chorionic gonadotropin hormone (HCG), starch blockers, diuretics, sauna belts, body wraps, passive exercise, ear stapling, acupuncture, electric muscle stimulating (EMS) devices, spirulina, amino acid supplements, and so forth.

9. Claim that use of an appetite suppressant or a "bulking agent" enables a person to lose body fat without restricting caloric intake.

10. Claim that a weight loss product contains a unique ingredient or component unless it is unavailable in other weight loss products.

Source: "How to Evaluate Commercial Weight Loss Programs." *Nutrition Forum*, March 1988, vol. 5, no. 3.

---

more whites than nonwhites, and more younger people (under age 30) than older people. Some studies suggest that eating disorders are more prevalent among people of middle and upper-middle socioeconomic status. Certain occupations also appear to be associated with a higher prevalence of eating disorders; these include modeling, ballet, and some sports, in which professional advancement requires maintenance of very low body weight.

Factors in the Development of Eating Disorders

Many factors are probably involved in the development of an eating disorder. Although many widely different explanations have been proposed, they share one central feature—dissatisfaction with body image and body weight. Such dissatisfaction is created by distortions in thinking, including perfectionistic beliefs, unreasonable demands for self-control, and excessive self-criticism.

Dissatisfaction with body weight leads to dysfunctional attitudes about eating, such as fear of fat and preoccupation with food, and problematic eating behaviors, including excessive dieting, constant calorie counting, and frequent weighing. If a significant family dysfunc-

tion—such as a rigid or overprotective parent or a family in which there is hostility, substance abuse, or lack of cohesion—is added to body dissatisfaction, an eating disorder is a likely outcome.

The issue of control is also important in the development of eating disorders. It has been hypothesized that a "fat phobia" is central to anorexia nervosa and that anorexics try to control their lives and avoid having to

Anorexia nervosa An eating disorder characterized by a refusal to eat enough food to maintain normal, healthy body weight and/or the use of measures to produce severe weight loss. Anorexics do experience hunger and appetite but resist the impulse to eat.

Bulimia nervosa An eating disorder characterized by alternating binging and purging by means of vomiting, laxatives or diuretics, or excessive exercise. Bulimics can be normal weight or overweight.

Binge eating disorder An eating disorder characterized by uncontrollable urges to eat. People suffering from binge eating disorder are often overweight.

TERMS

Anorexia Nervosa

A person suffering from anorexia nervosa doesn't eat enough food to maintain a reasonable body weight. Anorexics have an intense fear of gaining weight or becoming fat. Their body image is distorted, so that even when they're emaciated they think they're fat. When confronted about being dangerously thin, anorexics often respond with disbelief. Their entire sense of self-worth is tied up in their evaluation of their body shape and weight.

Anorexics may engage in compulsive behaviors or rituals that help keep them from eating, though some anorexics also binge eat. They commonly use vigorous and prolonged physical activity to reduce body weight as well. Anorexics are often introverted, emotionally reserved, and socially insecure. They tend to favor health foods, be obsessive about health issues, and prepare meals for others without eating them themselves.

Anorexia affects between 1 and 3 million Americans, mostly women. It's been estimated that 1 percent of precollege girls have some form of anorexia nervosa.

Health Risks of Anorexia Nervosa Because of extreme weight loss, the anorexic is likely to stop menstruating, become intolerant of cold, and develop low blood pressure and heart rate. Anorexics develop dry skin that is often covered by fine, neonatal-like body hair called lanugo. Their hands and feet may swell and take on a blue color.

Anorexia nervosa has been linked to a variety of medical complications, including dental problems and disorders of the cardiovascular, gastrointestinal, and endocrine systems. When body fat is virtually gone and muscles are severely wasted, the body turns to its own organs in a desperate search for protein. Death can occur from heart failure caused by electrolyte imbalances. As many as 18 percent of patients with anorexia nervosa die of complications related to the disorder. Depression is also a serious risk, and about half the fatalities due to anorexia are from suicide.

Treatment of Anorexia Nervosa Both the physical and psychological aspects of anorexia must be addressed in treatment. The crucial first step is to restore body weight as much as possible. This usually has to be done in a specialized inpatient setting because anorexics tend to cling to their unrealistic beliefs and resist treatment. Although controversial, drugs may be included as part of the treatment.

Psychotherapy for anorexia includes education, behavior modification, and changing maladaptive patterns of thinking. Anorexics need to learn about the physical risks of self-starvation and the importance of healthy eating habits. They have to adopt habits that will allow them to regain and sustain a healthy weight. They have to change their irrational thinking, learn to tolerate imperfection in

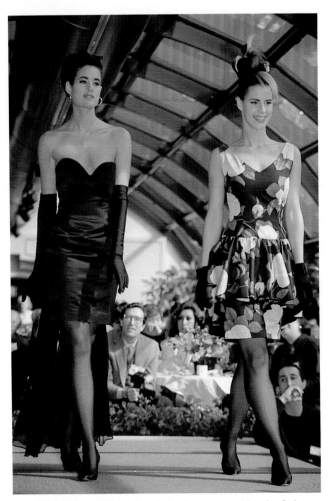

The image of the "ideal" female body promoted by the fashion and fitness industries doesn't reflect the wide range of body shapes and sizes that are associated with good health. Overconcern with body image can contribute to low self-esteem and the development of dangerous eating disorders.

grow up and deal with their emerging sexuality by obliterating secondary sexual characteristics through extreme weight loss. People with anorexia over-control their behavior; bulimics periodically lose control and then regain it. Binge eating disorder is characterized by loss of control.

Eating disorders can also be described as an obsession with weight and an addiction to abnormal eating behavior. A person with an eating disorder experiences obsessive, anxiety-producing thinking, revolving around the fear of gaining weight. The abnormal eating behavior—whether it's starvation, purging, or binging—reduces anxiety by producing numbness and alleviating emotional pain. Thus, an eating disorder is a means of coping with stress and relieving tension. A person who has an eating disorder often lacks an adequate repertoire of skills for dealing with stress.

themselves, and gain some perspective on the arbitrary cultural standard of thinness.

Bulimia Nervosa

Bulimia nervosa is characterized by recurring episodes of binge eating (consuming a huge amount of food in a discrete period of time) followed by purging. During a binge, bulimics feel that they can't stop eating or control what or how much they eat. To compensate for the binge, bulimics induce vomiting and/or use laxatives or diuretics. They may also use strict dieting, fasting, or vigorous exercise to maintain normal weight. Bulimics may binge up to 20 to 30 times per day, consuming over 6,000 calories in 24 hours. Bulimia can be difficult to recognize because bulimics conceal their eating habits and usually maintain normal weight.

Like anorexics, bulimics have a morbid fear of becoming fat, and they base their sense of self-worth on their body shape and weight. Bulimics are typically more socially outgoing than anorexics—and more socially deviant. Bulimics are more likely to smoke and to abuse alcohol and other drugs. They tend to prefer junk food to health food. Bulimics also tend to have fluctuating moods that vary from persistent fatigue and depression to feelings of agitation accompanied by impulsive behaviors. They often have a strong need for social approval. Bulimics place high demands on themselves but have few strategies for coping with stress.

Restrictive eating and purging are attempts made by bulimics to control their bodies and, by extension, their surroundings. Many bulimics have been in relationships (family and interpersonal) that were unpredictable, where they didn't feel safe. The binge-purge cycle has the quality of a ritual: Bulimics are able to plan, follow through, and predict how they will feel during and after the bulimic episode. The sense of security and control the binging and purging brings is what reinforces and perpetuates the behavior.

Among college women, the incidence of bulimia has variously been reported to range from 2 to 19 percent. In a sample of 18- to 30-year-olds in the general population, 3 to 4 percent of women were reported to have bulimia. The number of women who occasionally engage in bulimic behaviors, but don't develop the disorder, may be as high as 14 percent.

Health Risks of Bulimia Nervosa   The binge-purge cycle of bulimia places a tremendous strain on the body and can have serious health effects. Contact with vomited stomach acids erodes tooth enamel. Bulimics often develop dental caries because they binge on foods that contain large amounts of simple sugars. Repeated vomiting or the use of laxatives, in combination with deficient calorie intake, can damage the liver and kidneys and cause cardiac arrhythmia. Chronic hoarseness and esophageal tearing with bleeding may also result from vomiting. More rarely, binge eating can lead to rupture of the stomach. Although many bulimics maintain normal weight, even small amounts of weight loss to a lower-than-normal weight can cause menstrual problems. And although less often associated with suicide or premature death than is anorexia nervosa, bulimia is associated with increased depression, excessive preoccupation with food and body image, and sometimes disturbances in intellectual functioning.

Treatment of Bulimia Nervosa   The symptom that usually brings bulimics into treatment is vomiting, which they often find shameful and distressing. The treatment for bulimia is similar to that of anorexia. Bulimics need to learn about nutrition, the physiology of body weight, and the dangers of their method of weight control. They need to adopt a regular pattern of eating meals and snacks and learn to use moderation rather than restriction in choosing foods. Cognitive techniques for combating bulimia include substituting coping thoughts for anxiety-producing ones and challenging dysfunctional attitudes about food and weight. Antidepressant drugs can be used in cases of depression.

Binge Eating Disorder

Binge eating disorder is a newly recognized eating disorder. The symptoms of this disorder are the same as those of bulimia nervosa, except that the purging behavior does not occur. In addition, loss of control is indicated by the presence of at least three of the following symptoms:

- Eating more rapidly than normal
- Eating until feeling uncomfortably full
- Eating large amounts of food when not feeling physically hungry
- Eating large amounts of food throughout the day with no planned mealtimes
- Eating alone because of being embarrassed by how much one is eating
- Feeling disgusted with oneself, depressed, or very guilty after overeating

A person with binge eating disorder is often overweight; dieters seem to be most susceptible to the disorder. There is evidence that between 25 and 45 percent of obese dieters, most of whom are women, may have binge eating disorder. Whether overweight or normal weight, bingers report more negative moods and emotional disturbances than nonbingers. The binge eater is likely to engage in obsessive thinking and frequently experience anxiety, self-doubt, and guilt.

Health Risks of Binge Eating Disorder   The health risks of compulsive binge eating without purging are not as well documented as those associated with anorexia or

In Quest of the Perfect Body

Human bodies come in a tremendous range of sizes and shapes, and people don't have to fit any particular standard to be healthy. Unfortunately, over the last few decades our society has tended to embrace a single ideal, especially for women—slim but fit. The media expose us to this single "right" look relentlessly, and the beauty and fitness industries promise to help us attain it.

As a result, Americans have become preoccupied with their appearance and ever more dissatisfied with their bodies. In 1972, 15 percent of men and 25 percent of women surveyed said that they were dissatisfied with their bodies. In 1987, 34 percent of men and 38 percent of women surveyed expressed dissatisfaction. The higher levels of dissatisfaction among women reflect the cultural belief that women's value is largely a function of their physical appearance and that they should strive to be beautiful, slim, and fit. Men are also concerned about appearance, but they are taught that their success doesn't depend solely on their looks.

Research indicates that such detailed attention to physical appearance has a negative effect on self-esteem. We become increasingly critical of ourselves for not attaining the right weight and look. Some people (usually women) who are dissatisfied with their appearance also develop a distorted body image. They look in the mirror and see only "flaws"—areas in which they fail to match the culture's physical ideal. They focus critically on these perceived flaws and then generalize from them to their whole body. They may conclude that their bodies are totally unacceptable and even disgusting, when the truth is that they simply don't conform to the cultural ideal.

These distorted ideas about the body may extend to ideas about the self in general. Our bodies shape our sense of identity because they represent how we appear to the rest of the world. When our body image is distorted, it interferes with a healthy sense of self-worth and can lead to feelings of anxiety and depression, as well as to chronic dieting. It also puts people at risk for developing eating disorders.

Research has shown that people can turn dissatisfaction into satisfaction by learning to perceive their bodies differently. One study attempted to correct body image distortions among young women who were of appropriate weight for their height but thought they were overweight. These women tended to think "globally," applying negative thoughts to their entire body. As part of a six-week therapy program, they learned to view themselves more realistically, replacing negative thoughts with positive ones while looking in the mirror. They also learned to put their supposed flaws in perspective. By the end of the program they had become more confident and comfortable with themselves.

Perhaps a more sensible approach in the long run is to change our attitudes about our bodies, replacing faultfinding with respect. What our bodies need is moderate exercise, healthy foods, adequate sleep, and opportunities for relaxation. When we treat our bodies better, we feel better about ourselves. Another thing we can do is add interests to our lives besides counting calories and watching the scale. By broadening our roles and activities, we make it clear to ourselves and others that how we look is not the sum of what we are.

How accurate is your own body image? Do you like your body the way it is, or are you caught up in a quest for "the perfect body"? To assess the health of your attitudes toward your body, answer the questions on the questionnaire that follows. If your score indicates that you have a negative body image, you can take steps to change it. Look in the mirror and notice the features you like. "Forgive" those features you're worried about, and view them realistically as only a part of your entire body. When you see idealized standards presented by the beauty and fitness industries, realize that one of their goals is to increase your dissatisfaction with yourself. Most of all, put your concerns about your physical appearance in perspective. Remember, your worth as a human being is not a function of how you look.

bulimia. Since most people with the disorder are obese, they face all the health risks associated with obesity. In addition, obese bingers are more likely than nonbingers to experience negative moods and emotional distress, especially depression.

Treatment of Binge Eating Disorder

Treatment of Binge Eating Disorder Treatments are just beginning to be developed for binge eating disorders. Obese bingers are more likely to drop out of any kind of obesity treatment than are nonbinging dieters. Thus a primary objective for successful treatment is to find ways to keep bingers in treatment. Bingers need to develop more effective ways to cope with their emotions and to recover from relapses in their weight management programs. An-

other useful strategy is to develop patterns of positive self-talk directed at reaching goals.

When You or Someone You Know Needs Help . . .

How can you tell if you or someone you know needs help? Begin by taking the self-test in the box "In Quest of the Perfect Body." A score of 14 or above indicates that you have a level of body dissatisfaction that may place you at risk for an eating disorder. If you think you may have an eating disorder or be at risk for developing one, contact a psychologist or other licensed therapist who specializes in this kind of problem. For further information, contact one of the resource organizations listed in

In Quest of the Perfect Body (continued)

Assessing Your Body Image	Never	Some-times	Often	Always
1. I dislike seeing myself in mirrors.	0	1	2	3
2. When I shop for clothing, I am more aware of my weight problem, and consequently I find shopping for clothes somewhat unpleasant.	0	1	2	3
3. I'm ashamed to be seen in public.	0	1	2	3
4. I prefer to avoid engaging in sports or public exercise because of my appearance.	0	1	2	3
5. I feel somewhat embarrassed about my body in the presence of someone of the opposite sex.	0	1	2	3
6. I think my body is ugly.	0	1	2	3
7. I feel that other people must think my body is unattractive.	0	1	2	3
8. I feel that my family or friends may be embarrassed to be seen with me.	0	1	2	3
9. I find myself comparing myself with other people to see if they are heavier than I am.	0	1	2	3
10. I find it difficult to enjoy activities because I am self-conscious about my physical appearance.	0	1	2	3
11. Feeling guilty about my weight problem preoccupies most of my thinking.	0	1	2	3
12. My thoughts about my body and physical appearance are negative and self-critical.	0	1	2	3

Now, add up the number of points you have circled in each column: _____   0 + _____ + _____ + _____

Score Interpretation

The lowest possible score is 0, and this indicates a positive body image. The highest possible score is 36, and this indicates an unhealthy body image. A score higher than 14 suggests a need to develop a healthier body image.

Questionnaire used with permission. J. D. Nash. 1986. *Maximize Your Body Potential.* (Palo Alto, Calif.: Bull Publishing).

the self-care appendix that follows Chapter 21. You can help others by learning to recognize the symptoms that suggest the existence of an eating disorder:

- Looking underweight or always wearing baggy clothes
- Not eating in front of others or toying with food
- Disappearing for a while after eating
- Smelling like he or she has vomited
- Exhibiting hyperactivity with no apparent fatigue
- Showing agitated behavior or disorganized thinking
- Complaining of abdominal discomfort
- Complaining of feeling fat but looking normal or even underweight

If more than a few of these signs are present, try talking to your friend about your concerns. Remember that anorexics tend to deny their symptoms and refuse treatment. Bulimics are often more cooperative. Suggest that your friend seek professional help immediately. If she refuses and you feel sure that she is anorexic, you may need to take stronger measures, such as contacting her family or letting a teacher or counselor at school know. Whatever you do, be sure to let your friend know that you care and want to help. It will not be easy for you or your friend to talk about this kind of problem. Admitting to having an eating disorder can be quite painful, and your friend may find it very difficult to accept your help. Reaching out for help is an act of courage.

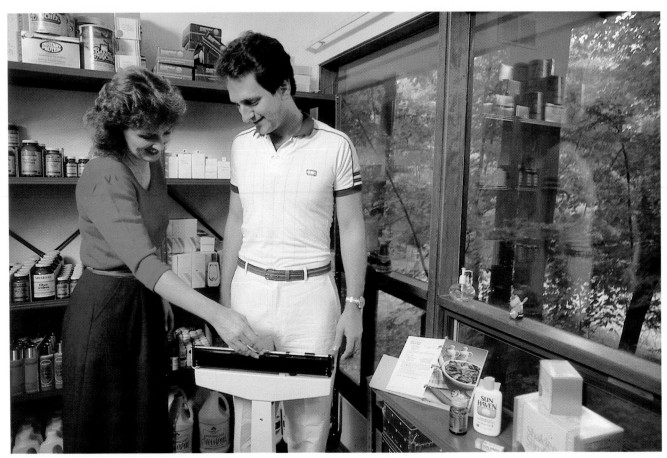

Achieving a specific body weight should not be a goal, since weight alone does not indicate that a person is in good health. An active and healthy lifestyle leads naturally to an appropriate body weight.

Today's Challenge

Eating disorders can be seen as the logical extension of the concern with weight that pervades American society. Most people don't succumb to irrational or distorted ideas about their bodies, but many do become obsessed with dieting. The challenge facing Americans today is achieving a healthy body weight without excessive dieting—by adopting and maintaining sensible eating habits, an active lifestyle, realistic and positive attitudes and emotions, and creative ways to handle stress.

SUMMARY

Lifestyle and Weight Control

- The overweight problem that plagues American society can be traced to a sedentary, high-stress lifestyle and a diet based on overly refined and processed foods.

Adopting a Healthy Lifestyle

- The four key factors in maintaining normal weight are nutrition, physical activity, thinking and emotions, and coping strategies.

- Although sugar causes tooth decay and may be addictive for some people, the real problem in the American diet is too much fat.

- Protein is amply supplied in the typical American diet. Excess dietary protein is stored as body fat.

- Eating more complex carbohydrates is a key component in maintaining a healthy body weight. The body has to expend energy to digest complex carbohydrates, and eating starchy foods makes you feel full.

- Eating small, frequent meals and having a structure to guide eating and decision rules to guide food choices are helpful weight management strategies.

- Physical activity is an important part of weight

management because it burns calories, increases lean body mass, and keeps the metabolism geared up to active levels.

- Many people have an internalized "idealized self," based on perfectionistic irrational beliefs, with which they frequently compare themselves. Such comparisons can lead to low self-esteem and other emotional problems and to negative "self-talk."

- Maintaining a healthy body weight also depends on having a repertoire of appropriate techniques for coping with stress and other emotional and physical challenges.

A Closer Look at Body Weight

- Height-weight tables are a popular, though often inaccurate, means of assessing body weight. Body mass index measures body weight but correlates highly with direct measures of body fat. Techniques for analyzing body composition include hydrostatic weighing, skinfold measurements, and electrical impedance analysis.

- The ratio of waist and hip measurements can be used to assess the health risks of body fat distribution.

- Rather than concerning themselves with elaborate measurements, individuals should focus on the four factors that go into maintaining normal weight.

- Obesity increases a person's risk for a variety of health problems, including cardiovascular disease, gallbladder disease, diabetes, and certain types of cancer. People who tend to carry their body fat in their trunk and abdomen are at greater risk than people who carry body fat in their hips, thighs, and buttocks.

Overcoming a Weight Problem

- Genetic factors influence many physical characteristics, but people can control whether they actually become obese by modifying their behavior and adopting a healthy lifestyle.

- Set point theory suggests that the body has a certain natural weight and resists moving away from it by very much. It's believed that only increased exercise can lower set point.

- Fat cell theory suggests that obese people were born with more or larger fat cells than normal-weight people or developed them during childhood. Now it is thought that the number of fat cells can be increased at any time during life by overeating and decreased by keeping weight off.

- Resting metabolism is the single largest determinant of energy expenditure. Physical activity is the only component of energy expenditure over which we have much control.

- It is not clear whether, in general, obese people eat more than do people of normal weight. Binge eating is a serious problem for many dieters.

- Obese people do not have a distinctive eating style. However, they tend to be more vulnerable to highly palatable, good-tasting food.

- No particular personality characteristics are consistently found among the obese, nor do they have a higher rate of psychological problems.

- There is a strong association between weight problems and socioeconomic status, overweight being more common among people of lower SES.

- The high rate of dieting in the United States is due in part to unrealistic cultural ideals of thinness. Modest weight loss can benefit health.

- People can be successful at losing weight and maintaining a healthy body weight on their own, usually through a combination of diet and exercise.

- Diet books should be carefully evaluated because many advocate useless or dangerous steps. Some over-the-counter diet aids can be helpful, but none is effective without individual effort. Supplements for modified fasting can be dangerous if used without medical monitoring.

- Different approaches to weight reduction are appropriate for different individuals. The best choice depends on how severely overweight a person is and his or her lifestyle and preferences.

Eating Disorders

- Dissatisfaction with body weight and shape are common to all eating disorders. Serious physical and psychological health risks are associated with eating disorders.

- Anorexia nervosa is characterized by self-starvation, increased physical activity, distorted body image, intense fear of gaining weight, and amenorrhea. It is potentially fatal. Treatment involves restoring body weight, addressing underlying psychological problems, and changing eating habits.

- Bulimia nervosa is characterized by intense concern with body weight, recurrent episodes of uncontrolled binge eating, and frequent purging, either by self-induced vomiting or the use of laxatives or diuretics. Treatment usually involves behavior modification and cognitive therapy.

- Binge eating disorder involves binging without compensatory purging. It is most common among obese dieters.

- Although eating disorders are extreme conditions, many Americans are obsessed with dieting. The challenge is to maintain normal body weight by balancing diet and exercise.

1. Interview some people who have successfully lost weight and kept it off. What were their strategies and techniques? Do you think their approach would work for others?

2. Find out what percentage of your body weight is fat by taking one of the tests described in this chapter at your campus health clinic, sports medicine clinic, or health club. If you have too high a proportion of body fat, consider taking steps to reduce it.

JOURNAL ENTRY

1. Monitor your diet for a week to see exactly how much fat and sugar you consume. If these amounts are excessive, make a list of specific steps you can take to reduce them, such as those suggested in the boxes in this chapter.

2. Make a list of at least five things you could do each day to become more physically active. Your list might include things such as riding your bike to class instead of driving and walking up stairs instead of taking the elevator. For each item on your list, describe the lifestyle adjustments you'd need to make—for example, leaving for class five minutes earlier to allow for cycling time.

3. *Critical Thinking:* Evaluate some of the weight loss resources in your community. First, investigate a commercial weight management program that operates in your community. Write an evaluation of it in terms of the 11 criteria listed in the box in this chapter. How does the program measure up? Next, look at the frozen diet dinners in your supermarket, such as Weight Watchers and Lean Cuisine. How do they compare in terms of calories, fat content, and nutritional value?

BEHAVIOR CHANGE STRATEGY

A WEIGHT MANAGEMENT PLAN

The behavior management plan described in Chapter 1 provides an excellent framework for a weight management program. Following are some suggestions about specific ways you can adapt that general plan to controlling your weight.

Goal-setting

Choose a reasonable weight you think you would like to reach over the long term, and be willing to renegotiate it as you get further along. Break your long-term goal into a series of short-term goals. Focus on reaching each short-term goal until you get close to your long-term goal. Likewise, when setting behavioral goals, break them down into small, reasonable steps—big enough to be a challenge but not so big that you can't accomplish each step. Don't try to convert to a new behavior pattern all at once. Shape yourself into a new way of behaving by designing small, manageable steps that will get you to where you want to go.

Self-monitoring

Keep a chart, journal, or record of your weight and behavior change progress. Try keeping a record of everything you eat. Write down what you plan to eat, the quantity, and the caloric content as well. Do this *before* you eat it. You'll find that just having to record something that is "not okay" to eat is likely to stop you from eating it. If you also note what seems to be triggering your urges to eat (for example, you feel bored, it's lunchtime, someone offered you something, it was there so you ate it), you'll become more aware of your weak spots and be better able to take corrective action.

Stimulus Control

Figure out what makes you want to eat. Then engineer your environment so that these cues are eliminated (or avoid them if you can't get rid of them). Go through your pantry and refrigerator and throw out or give away "trouble" food—ice cream, candy, cookies, etc. Avoid driving past the doughnut shop that always beckons you to stop. Ask your friends or fellow students not to offer you snack food. Anticipate problem situations and plan ways to handle them more effectively.

Exercise

Evaluate your energy expenditure. Keep a daily log of both routine daily activity and planned exercise. Consider how you can find ways to increase your energy output simply by increasing routine physical activity, such as walking or taking the stairs. If you are not already involved in a regular exercise routine aimed at increasing endurance and building or maintaining lean body mass, seek help from someone who is competent to help you plan and start an appropriate exercise routine. If you are already doing regular physical exercise, evaluate your program according to the guidelines in Chapter 14.

Social Support

Get others to help. Get someone to join your efforts to adopt a healthy lifestyle. Make an appointment with someone to exercise together. Talk to friends and family about what they can do to support your efforts. Give them lots of praise for helping.

Reward Yourself Appropriately

Use lots of self-praise; avoid self-criticism, even when you slip. Plan special nonfood treats for yourself—a walk, a movie, an afternoon's reprieve from studying—when you accomplish a small step or short-term goal. Don't wait for the long-term goal to reward yourself. Reward yourself often and for anything that counts toward success.

Cognitive Strategies

Give yourself credit for even the smallest successes. Don't discount anything you can possibly count as progress. Tell yourself what you need to do next to stay on track. Think about your accomplishments and achievements. Congratulate yourself. Avoid demanding too much of yourself. Don't be a perfectionist; let yourself be human. Above all, don't criticize yourself!

Learn to Recover from Slips

When you have a slip (and you will, because you are human), learn from it. Decide what you might do to reduce the risk of its happening again. Identify the "high-risk" situations that set you up to backslide. Figure out how you can avoid such situations or change your response so that you win.

SELECTED BIBLIOGRAPHY

Aluli, N. E. 1991. Prevalence of obesity in a native Hawaiian population. *American Journal of Clinical Nutrition* 53: 1556S–60S.

Body-weight perceptions and selected weight-management goals and practices of high school students—United States, 1990. 1991. *Journal of the American Medical Association* 266(20).

Bray, G. A. 1989. Obesity: Basic aspects and clinical applications. *The Medical Clinics of North America* 78(1).

Broussard, B. A., A. Johnson, J. H. Himes, and others. 1991. Prevalence of obesity in American Indians and Alaska natives. *American Journal of Clinical Nutrition* 53:1535S–42S.

Brownell, K. D. 1991. Dieting and the search for the perfect body: Where physiology and culture collide. *Behavior Therapy* 22:1–12.

Brownell, K. D., and T. A. Wadden. 1991. The heterogeneity of obesity: Fitting treatments to individuals. *Behavior Therapy* 22:153–77.

———. 1992. Etiology and treatment of obesity: Understanding a serious, prevalent, and refractory disorder. *Journal of Consulting and Clinical Psychology* 60:505–17.

Curb, J. E., and E. B. Marcus. 1991. Body fat and obesity in Japanese Americans. *American Journal of Clinical Nutrition* 53:1552S–55S.

Dolan, B. 1991. Cross-cultural aspects of anorexia nervosa and bulimia: A review. *International Journal of Eating Disorders* 10:67–78.

Flood, M. 1989. Addictive eating disorders. *Nursing Clinics of North America* 24:45–53.

Gortmaker, S. L., W. H. Dietz, Jr., L. W. Y. Cheung. 1990. Inactivity, diet, and the fattening of America. *Journal of the American Dietetic Association* 90:1247–52.

Jeffery, R. W., R. R. Wing, and S. A. French. 1992. Weight cycling and cardiovascular risk factors in obese men and women. *American Journal of Clinical Nutrition* 55:641–44.

Kuczmarski, R. J. 1992. Prevalence of overweight and weight gain in the United States. *American Journal of Clinical Nutrition* 55:495S–502S.

Marcus, M. D., and R. R. Wing. 1987. Binge eating among the obese. *Annals of Behavioral Medicine* 9:23–27.

Peterkin, B. B. 1990. Dietary guidelines for Americans, 1990 edition. *Journal of the American Dietetic Association* 90: 1725–27.

Pi-Sunyer, F. X. 1991. Health implications of obesity. *American Journal of Clinical Nutrition* 53:1595S–1603S.

Rand, C. S. W., and J. M. Kuldau. 1992. Epidemiology of bulimia and symptoms in a general population: Sex, age, race, and socioeconomic status. *International Journal of Eating Disorders* 11:37–44.

Rodin, J. 1992. Body mania. *Psychology Today,* January/February.

Sacra, C. 1990. Mirror images. *Health,* March.

Sichieri, R., J. E. Everhart, and V. S. Hubbard. 1992. Relative weight classifications in the assessment of underweight and overweight in the United States. *International Journal of Obesity* 16:303–12.

Stallone, D. D., and A. J. Stunkard. 1991. The regulation of body weight: Evidence and clinical implications. *Annals of Behavioral Medicine* 13:220–30.

Steiger, H., F. Y. K. Leung, G. Puentes-Neuman, and N. Gottheil. 1992. *International Journal of Eating Disorders* 11:121–31.

Story, M., K. Rosenwinkel, J. H. Himes, M. Resnick, L. J. Harris, and R. W. Blum. 1991. Demographic and risk factors associated with chronic dieting in adolescents. *American Journal of Diseases in Children* 145:994–98.

Wilson, G. T., and B. T. Walsh. 1991. Eating disorders in the DSM-IV. *Journal of Abnormal Psychology* 100:362–65.

Wooley, S. C., and D. M. Garner. 1991. Obesity treatment: The high cost of false hope. *Journal of the American Dietetic Association* 91:1248–51.

RECOMMENDED READINGS

Finn, S., and L. S. Kass. 1992. *The Real Life Nutrition Book.* New York: Penguin Books. *The philosophy behind this book, which covers the nutrition basics, is that your lifestyle should dictate your nutrition and fitness regimen.*

Goldberg, L. 1991. *The New Controlled ChEATing Weight-Loss and Fitness Program.* Kansas City: Andrews and McMeel. *Entertaining and motivating, this diet book tells how to eat your favorite foods without guilt. Even so, it gives responsible diet advice and advocates that exercise accompany dieting.*

Minirth, F., P. Meier, R. Hemflet, and S. Sneed. 1990. *Love Hunger: Recovery from Food Addiction.* Nashville: Thomas Nelson. *This volume addresses the serious problem of food addiction that affects both uncontrollable binge eaters and bulimics. Reflecting the approaches of Overeaters Anonymous and Alco-*

holics Anonymous, *the book offers valuable advice for those who accept its spiritual orientation.*

Nash, J. D. 1986. *Maximize Your Body Potential.* Palo Alto, Calif.: Bull Publishing. *Called "the most helpful book on lifetime weight management" by the* Journal of Nutrition Education, *this comprehensive book on nutrition, exercise, behavior, and the psychological aspects of weight management helps the reader assess her situation and plan effective action.*

————. 1992. *Now That You've Lost It: How to Maintain Your Best Weight.* Palo Alto, Calif.: Bull Publishing. *Keeping the weight off once one gets to goal weight is often the toughest part of a weight management effort, and this book addresses the psychological and motivational factors that can produce long-lasting success.*

14

Exercise for Health and Fitness

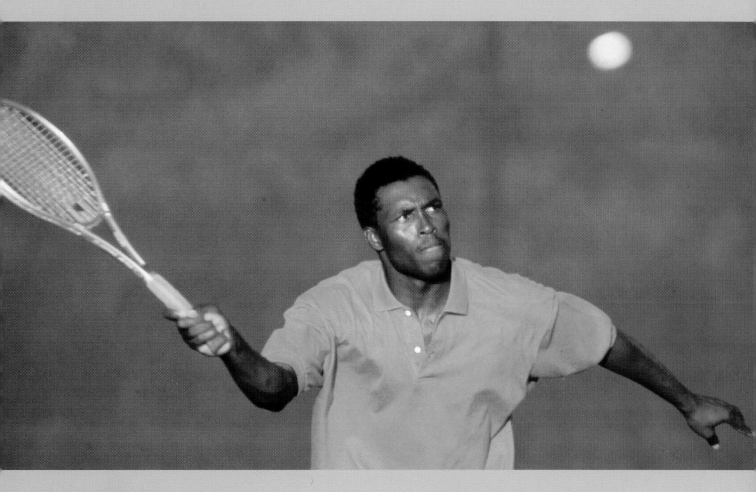

CONTENTS

▶ Your roommate wanted to work some exercise into her crowded schedule, so she decided on swimming during the morning lap swim hours, from six to eight o'clock. At first she loved it and swam for 45 minutes every day. But it's become harder for her as the mornings have grown darker and colder. Last week it was raining every morning when she woke up, and she just couldn't face it. She's been down on herself about losing her motivation, and you'd like to help her out with some support or advice. What can you tell her about getting her fitness program back on track?

▶ You and some friends are planning a cross-country ski vacation and have been looking at the trail maps from the ski resort. You all do resistance weight training at the gym and consider yourselves in excellent shape. One friend wants to tackle the longest and most arduous of the trails, but you're wondering if you should start out with something easier until your muscles get accustomed to the movements involved in cross-country skiing. Your friend says that because you're young and lift weights, you ought to be able to ski the toughest trail. Is he right? What should you plan for your trip?

▶ A friend of yours was a star football player in high school and is going out for the college team. He told you he started taking steroids last summer because he's under pressure from back home to make the team. He's offered to get you some steroids to help you out with your body-building program. You heard they were dangerous, but he says the health risks aren't significant in the short term. He hasn't experienced any ill effects and feels more competitive than ever. Should you give them a try?

▶ Your sister decided she wanted to get in shape, so you suggested she join a health club in her community and take their low-impact aerobics classes. She investigated one club but was intimidated by the whole scene. She said the manager wanted her to sign a three-year contract without taking it home to discuss with anyone else. She thought the instructors were more interested in looking at themselves in the mirror than in helping the students learn the exercises and dance routines. Your sister is discouraged about clubs now but doesn't know what else to do. Are all health clubs like that? What advice can you give her?

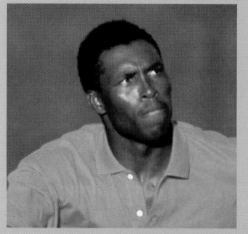

MAKING CONNECTIONS

Exercise has nearly limitless benefits. It helps you control your weight, manage stress, boost your immune system, and protect yourself against heart disease, cancer, and perhaps even premature death. But knowing how and when to exercise can make a big difference in your benefits and enjoyment. In each of the fitness-related scenarios presented on these pages, individuals have to use information, make a decision, or choose a course of action. How would you act in each of these situations? What response or decision would you make? This chapter provides information about exercise and physical fitness that can be used in situations like these. After finishing the chapter, read the scenarios again. Has what you've learned changed how you would respond?

Exercise is part of the lives of millions of Americans. People are walking, jogging, and working out in gyms and fitness centers. They're talking about weight training, aerobic exercise, cardiorespiratory capacity, and body composition. Colleges are stressing regular exercise programs, and businesses are providing recreational and fitness facilities for their employees.

But the "fitness boom" is not without its casualties. Some people start an exercise program without enough thought and drop it a few months later because it's too time-consuming, inconvenient, or boring. Some rush into sports or activities without proper training or knowledge, only to get benched with a sprained ankle or sore knee a week or two later. Many "weekend warriors" suffer overuse injuries from trying to squeeze all their activities into a 48-hour period.

Most of these difficulties arise because people don't have the basic knowledge and understanding they need to exercise properly and get the most from it. Many choose inappropriate activities or do too much too soon. When their program doesn't work out, they become frustrated and discouraged about exercise in general. At the same time, some people remain on the sidelines because they simply don't know where to begin. If you have ever been confused about the best way to get in shape and stay in shape, this chapter will help you understand the basics of exercise so you can put together a physical fitness plan that will work for you. If approached correctly, exercise and sports can contribute immeasurably to health and well-being, add fun and joy to life, and provide the foundation for a lifetime of fitness.

WHAT IS PHYSICAL FITNESS AND WHY IS IT IMPORTANT?

Physical fitness is the ability to adapt to the demands and stresses of physical effort. It has many components, some related to general health and others related more specifically to particular sports or activities. The components most important for health include the following:

- Cardiorespiratory endurance
- Flexibility
- Muscular strength, power, and endurance
- Body composition (proportion of fat to lean body mass)

In addition to some or all of these, physical fitness for a particular sport or activity might include the following:

- Coordination
- Speed
- Agility
- Balance
- Skill

Although some components may overlap, each is largely independent and requires specific types of exercise to develop it. Your body has the ability to adapt to physical stress and improve its function; that is, through specific physical activities, you can increase your heart and lung capacity, develop stronger muscles, become more flexible, improve your performance in particular sports, and so on. In general, your level of physical fitness is directly related to the amount and intensity of your physical activity.

Why is physical fitness so important? Part of the answer to this question lies in your genetic inheritance. Your body is a wonderful moving machine, designed to be active. Your bones, joints, and ligaments provide a support system for movement; your muscles perform the motions of work and play; your heart and lungs nourish your cells as you move through your daily life. Millions of years of evolution have made your body a precision tool capable of astonishing feats of speed, strength, endurance, and skill, all in the service of survival. But your body is made to work best when it is active. Left unchallenged, bones lose their density, joints stiffen, muscles become weak, and cellular energy systems begin to degenerate. To be truly well, you must be active.

Unfortunately, modern life for most Americans provides few built-in occasions for vigorous activity—people don't have to hunt, fight, or work strenuously all day for their dinner, as human beings did in the past. Technological advances have made our lives increasingly inactive and sedentary; we drive cars, ride escalators, watch television, and push papers around at school or work. Growing evidence points to lack of physical activity as a prime contributing factor to the array of perplexing degenerative diseases we now see in our society—heart disease, cancer, stroke, obesity, diabetes, and hypertension, among others. For example, a study of almost 17,000 male Harvard alumni revealed that the death rate from heart disease, respiratory disease, cancers, suicide, and all causes of death combined was significantly higher in sedentary men than in active men. The relationship between exercise and health in women is less clear. Studies suggest that regular exercise reduces the risk of coronary heart disease, hypertension (high blood pressure), cancers of the reproductive system, and bone loss. It also helps control weight and prevent depression. Overall, sedentary people have been found to have up to 50 percent more health problems than people with active lifestyles.

A major physical fitness study that followed 13,000

Physical fitness The extent to which the body can respond to the demands of physical effort.

TERMS

TABLE 14-1 Health Benefits of Exercise

Exercise Tends to Increase or Improve	Exercise Tends to Decrease
Feeling of well-being	Work of the heart (decreased heart rate and increased pumping volume)
Emotional outlook	Electrical irritability of the heart
Oxygen supply to the heart	Glucose intolerance
Function and efficiency of the heart	Progression of coronary heart disease
Electrical stability of the heart	Blood levels of triglycerides, cholesterol, and low-density lipoproteins
Size and strength of blood vessels	Platelet stickiness (overadhesiveness in this type of blood cell has been implicated in the development of CHD)
Blood-flow regulation	
Blood volume	Arterial blood pressure
Number of red cells	Obesity and body fat
Blood-sugar regulation	Muscle loss during dieting
Energy regulation and efficiency in cells	Bone loss
Growth hormone (increases fat use)	"Stress" hormone secretion
Lean body weight	Psychological depression
Efficiency of the thyroid gland	Harmful effects of psychic stress
Tolerance to stress	
Muscle strength in trunk and legs (may decrease back pain)	
Joint range of motion	
Bone mass	
HDL cholesterol	

men and women for eight years found that inactive men were almost 3½ times more likely to die over the course of the eight years than active men, and inactive women were over 4½ times more likely to die than active women. Being sedentary was found to be as risky as having hypertension, high cholesterol, high blood-sugar levels, or obesity. An encouraging finding is that even mild exercise, such as a brisk walk for 30 to 60 minutes a day, every other day, was enough to make a substantial difference in an individual's risk of death. The conclusion is obvious: Exercise and physical activity are good for your health.

There is another basic reason to be physically fit, of course: It's fun and it feels good. Some people are active not because they're thinking about health benefits but simply because they enjoy it, whether they're skiing, swimming, hiking, playing basketball, or engaging in any of innumerable other activities. Sports provide the opportunity to be active, to develop strength and skills, to improve and excel, to challenge yourself or an opponent, to share victory and defeat with fellow team members, to compete. Many people who play sports feel that physical performance is an integral part of an active and exciting lifestyle.

As one of the most important—and most controllable—factors in a person's general health, exercise is mentioned in many other contexts in this book. It can help you to manage stress, to maintain your emotional well-being, to control your weight, to boost your immune system, and to protect yourself against serious diseases later in life. It does all this by improving the overall functioning of your body in ways detailed more fully in the rest of this chapter.

WHY IS EXERCISE SO GOOD FOR YOU?

The health benefits of exercise can be divided into five general categories—improved cardiorespiratory effi-

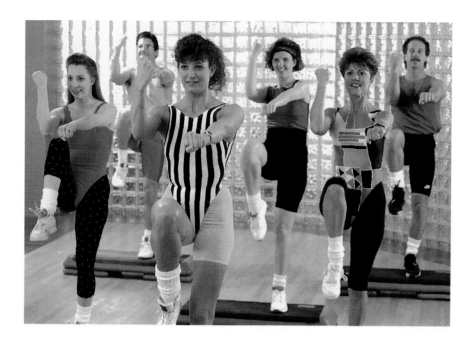

Endurance exercise conditions the heart, improves the function of the entire cardiorespiratory system, and has many other health benefits as well. An effective personal fitness program should be built around an activity like running, walking, biking, swimming, or aerobic dance.

ciency and health, more efficient metabolism and better control of body fat, improved psychological and emotional well-being, improved muscular strength and flexibility, and improved health over the whole life span.

Improved Cardiorespiratory Efficiency

The most important kind of exercise is **cardiorespiratory endurance** (or **aerobic**) **exercise.** It improves heart and lung functioning. As fitness pioneer Kenneth Cooper remarked, "You can live without big muscles or a nice figure, but you can't live without a healthy heart." This type of exercise helps your body become a more efficient machine, better equipped to cope with physical challenges. The many specific effects of moderate to vigorous aerobic exercise on the cardiorespiratory system are outlined in Table 14-1. *Aerobic* means "requiring oxygen." In very-high-intensity exercise, such as sprinting, the body relies on an energy system that doesn't require much oxygen, but that can operate only for short periods of time. For these reasons, very-high-intensity exercise doesn't develop the cardiorespiratory system to the same extent as does aerobic exercise.

The primary effect of endurance exercise is to improve the ability of the heart, lungs, and circulatory system to carry oxygen to the body's tissues. The heart pumps more blood per beat, resting heart rate slows down, the number of red blood cells increases, blood supply to the tissues improves, and resting blood pressure decreases. A fit cardiorespiratory system doesn't have to work as hard at rest and at low levels of exercise, because it functions more efficiently. A healthy heart can better withstand the stresses and strains of daily life and meet the occasional emergencies that make extraordinary demands on the body's cardiorespiratory resources.

Endurance exercise also has a positive effect on the balance of lipids, or fatlike substances such as cholesterol and triglycerides, that are circulating in the blood. As explained in Chapter 15, lipids are involved in the formation of plaques, or fatty deposits, on the inner lining of the coronary arteries. Cholesterol is carried in the blood by **lipoproteins,** which are classified according to size and density. Cholesterol carried by low-density lipoproteins (LDLs) tends to stick to the walls of coronary arteries, and high-density lipoproteins (HDLs) tend to pick up excess cholesterol in the bloodstream and carry it back to the liver for excretion from the body. The total amount of HDL and the relative amounts of HDLs and LDLs in the blood are very important factors involved in the development of coronary heart disease. Recent studies have shown that people with low levels of HDL have an increased risk of coronary heart disease even if their total cholesterol is low. The good news is that one excellent way to increase your HDLs and lower your LDLs is to exercise.

Endurance exercise also protects the cardiorespiratory system from the effects of stress. Many studies have shown that excessive stress and anxiety are associated with poor cardiorespiratory health. Psychological stress

Cardiorespiratory endurance exercise (or aerobic) Rhythmical, large-muscle exercise for a prolonged period of time. Partially dependent on the ability of the cardiovascular system to deliver oxygen to tissues.

Lipoproteins *(low-density lipoproteins, LDL; high-density lipoproteins, HDL)* Substances in blood, classified according to size, density, and chemical composition, that transport fats.

TERMS

If you've ever gone for a long, brisk walk after a hard day's work, you know how refreshing exercise can be. Exercise can improve mood, stimulate creativity, clarify thinking, relieve anxiety, and provide an outlet for anger or aggression. But why does exercise make you feel good? Does it simply take your mind off your problems, or does it cause a physical reaction that affects your mental state?

Until recently, scientists were unable to learn whether the mood-altering effects of physical activity were based on some sort of physical or chemical reaction or whether these effects were merely "in the mind." Current research indicates that exercise triggers many physical changes in the body that can alter mood. Scientists are now trying to explain how and why exercise affects the mind.

Some researchers are looking at the physical structure of the brain. They think the effect of exercise on the mind may be due to the close proximity of two specific areas of the brain—the motor cortex, which is responsible for the movement of muscles in the body, and a nearby area that is responsible for thought and emotion. As muscles work more vigorously, nerve cells transmit signals with much greater frequency, stimulating the motor cortex. This increased brain activity may also stimulate the nearby areas of the brain.

Other researchers suggest that exercise stimulates the release of endorphins, substances that can suppress fatigue, produce euphoria, and decrease pain. Endorphins affect the human body much as the opium-based drug morphine does. The pituitary gland, located in the base of the brain, produces greater amounts of endorphins during vigorous exercise. If you are a long-distance runner, you have probably experienced a sense of euphoria, called a "runner's high," after running several miles. This euphoria, which contributes to an athlete's endurance, is attributed to increased production of endorphins.

In theory, endorphins flow through the bloodstream and find their way into the area of the brain that controls mood. So far, no evidence has been found indicating that they actually reach this part of the brain. The theory remains promising, but further research is needed to determine the exact role of endorphins in our sense of well-being.

A third area of research focuses on changes in brain activity during and after exercise. Currently, researchers recognize that two changes occur. The first is an increase in alpha wave activity. Alpha brain waves indicate a highly relaxed state; meditation also induces alpha wave activity. The increase in alpha waves starts some time after exercise is begun and continues well beyond the end of the exercise period.

The second change is an alteration in the levels of the **neurotransmitters** norepinephrine, dopamine, and serotonin—chemicals that increase alertness and reduce stress. Higher levels of norepinephrine can also improve state of mind in people who suffer from depression. Not only does exercise trigger a change in these neurotransmitters, but some effects of exercise, such as an increase in body temperature, also further alter their levels.

You might wonder how much exercise is needed to improve your overall mood. Some studies have compared a sedentary lifestyle with a lifestyle that included walking a few times a week. After several weeks, the inactive individuals showed no change in before-and-after tests of psychological well-being, but the moderately active individuals showed significant improvement. So no matter what the exact explanation for this mind-body connection turns out to be, it makes sense to take advantage of it today.

Adapted from D. C. Nieman. 1989. "Exercise and the Mind." *Women's Sports and Fitness* 11(17): 54–57; "Fitness Update." *Consumer Reports on Health,* August 1992.

prompts increased secretion of **epinephrine** and **norepinephrine,** the so-called fight-or-flight hormones, which are thought to speed the development of atherosclerosis, or hardening of the arteries. Excessive hostility has also been found to be associated with an increased risk of heart disease. Exercise decreases the secretion of hormones triggered by emotional stress, and it can diffuse hostility by providing an emotional outlet for pent-up anger.

More Efficient Metabolism and Better Control of Body Fat

A second major effect of endurance exercise is to improve the efficiency of the body's metabolism, the complicated process by which the body converts chemical or food energy into mechanical or work energy. This process involves hormones, oxygen, fuels, and enzymes. A physically fit person is better able to generate useful energy, to use fats for energy, and to regulate hormones. One theory holds that the bodies of physically active people process food faster and get rid of cancer-causing agents before they can create a problem. This may explain the lower rates of colon cancer among fit people.

A related effect of endurance exercise, of course, is simply to expend calories and thus help regulate energy balance and body weight. Without exercise, it is extremely difficult to eat a nutritious diet and maintain an ideal body weight. Sedentary people may gain weight on a good diet simply because they are taking in more calories than they are using. Weight training can also help with weight control by increasing or maintaining muscle mass.

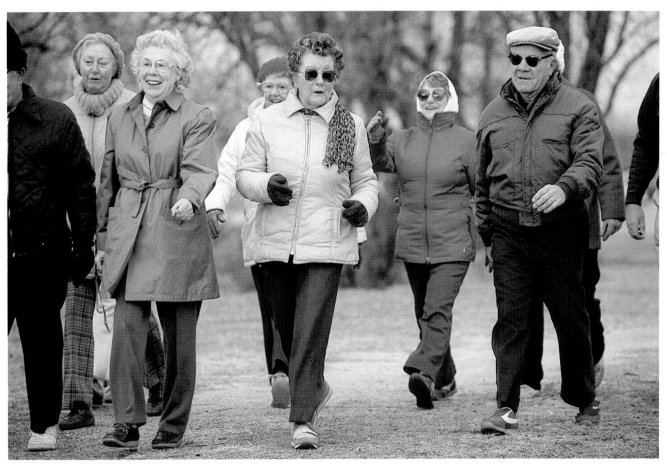

It makes sense to choose activities that will add enjoyment to your life for years to come. In this group of older people we can see the rewards of a lifetime of fitness and smart exercise habits.

Improved Psychological and Emotional Well-Being

Most people who participate in sports or vigorous exercise have noted a number of social, psychological, and emotional benefits of being active. The joy of a well-hit cross-court backhand, the euphoria of a run through the park, or the rush of a downhill schuss through deep snow powder provides pleasure that transcends health benefits alone. Competent performance of a physical activity serves as proof that you can master skills and control your efforts, which in turn enhances your self-image. Exercise improves the appearance of your body, which also tends to make you feel better about yourself. Exercise can offer an arena for harmonious interaction with other people as well as opportunities to strive and excel. Since physically fit people develop greater physical efficiency, they have plenty of energy and lead lives that are full and varied.

Beyond these personal and interpersonal benefits, positive feelings associated with exercise have a physiological basis in hormones and body chemicals. Exercise decreases the secretion of stress-related hormones, as noted earlier, and it alleviates depression and anxiety by providing an emotional outlet. Additionally, researchers are

studying the effect of **endorphins** and other hormonelike substances whose production increases during vigorous exercise. For further discussion of the connection between exercise and emotional well-being, see the box "The Power of Exercise: How It Affects the Mind."

Improved Strength and Flexibility

Most of the benefits already discussed are benefits of cardiorespiratory endurance exercise, but exercises designed to improve muscular strength and endurance, joint flexibility, and posture are also crucial to your physical well-

Epinephrine A hormone secreted principally by the adrenal medulla with a wide variety of functions, such as stimulating the heart, making carbohydrates available in the liver and muscles, and releasing fat from fat cells.

Norepinephrine A hormone released from the adrenal medulla and nerve endings of the autonomic nervous system. Has many of the same effects as epinephrine.

Endorphins Substances resembling opium that are secreted by the brain. They seem to be involved in modulating pain.

Neurotransmitters Substances that transmit nerve impulses.

Among the most dramatic events in the 1992 Summer Olympics in Barcelona were the fiercely competitive wheelchair races, at 800 meters for women and 1,500 meters for men. The elite athletes who participated in these exhibition events made it obvious that people with disabilities can be active, healthy, and extraordinarily fit.

Wheelchair racing is a demonstration sport in the Olympics, but it's just one of many regular competitions in the Paralympics, the premier event for elite athletes with disabilities. Held in the same year and city as the Olympics, the Paralympics has grown dramatically since it was begun in Rome in 1960. In that year, 400 athletes participated, representing 23 countries. In 1992, over 3,100 competitors from 96 countries marched or wheeled into the Barcelona Olympic Stadium for the September opening ceremonies. Competing in 15 sports for over 10 days, they included people with cerebral palsy, people with visual impairments, paraplegics, quadriplegics, and others.

Most of the Paralympic competitions are the same as those in the Olympics, although some are modified, such as wheelchair basketball and tandem cycling, in which a blind cyclist pedals with a sighted athlete. As more people with disabilities become involved in athletics, competition at the Paralympics grows more intense. Some performances approach those seen at events for the able-bodied. In 1981, for example, a Canadian athlete whose right leg was amputated above the knee after a childhood farming accident set a world high-jump record in his class at 2.04 meters—not that far from the 2.44-meter able-bodied record.

Paralympians point out that able-bodied athletes and athletes with disabilities have two important things in common—both are striving for excellence, and both can serve as role models. One athlete commented, "I'd like to let kids who have a disability know there is a sports option. The possibilities are endless. A lot of people still think otherwise, but attitudes have changed a lot."

Currently, between 34 and 43 million Americans are estimated to have chronic, significant disabilities. Some disabilities are the result of injury, such as spinal cord injuries

sustained in car crashes. Other disabilities result from illness, such as the blindness that sometimes occurs as a complication of diabetes or the joint stiffness that accompanies arthritis. And some disabilities are present at birth, as in the case of congenital limb deformities or cerebral palsy. No matter what the cause, disabilities are defined in terms of limited ability to function, either physically or mentally.

Exercise and physical activity are as important for people with disabilities as for able-bodied individuals—if not *more* important. Being active helps prevent secondary conditions that may result from prolonged inactivity, such as circulatory or muscular problems. It also provides an emotional boost that helps support a positive attitude.

People with disabilities don't have to be Olympians to participate in sports and lead an active life. Depending on the nature of the disability, numerous options exist, including tennis, basketball, cycling, swimming, and running. Some fitness centers offer modified aerobics, mild exercise in warm water, and other exercises adapted for people with disabilities.

For those who prefer to get their exercise at home, special aerobic workout videos are available. Most of these videos are produced by hospitals and health associations and are geared to specific disabilities. For example, the Arthritis Foundation produces two videos, at different levels, called "People with Arthritis Can Exercise." There are also workout videos designed especially for individuals with multiple sclerosis; for those with hearing impairments (instructors both speak and sign); for women who have had breast surgery and need to strengthen arm, shoulder, and back muscles; for people with Parkinson's disease; and for people confined to wheelchairs. Some tapes are designed so that both able-bodied people and people with disabilities can participate.

If you want to try one of these videos or participate in some form of adapted physical activity, check with your physician about what's appropriate for you. Remember that no matter what your level of ability or disability, it's possible to make exercise an integral part of your life.

Sources: P. Bodo. 1990. "Hell on Wheels." *Tennis.* July; Mary Nemeth. 1992. "Willing and Able." *Maclean's.* September 7; Marc Silver. 1990. "All the Right Moves." *U.S. News and World Report.* November 12; U.S. Department of Health and Human Services. 1990. *Healthy People 2000: National Health Promotion and Disease Prevention Objectives* (Washington, D.C.: U.S. Government Printing Office, DHHS Pub. (PHS) 91–50213).

being. Back pain, for example, plagues a large percentage of the population. In most cases, it can be directly traced to weak abdominal and spinal muscles with poor muscular endurance; inadequate flexibility in the spine, hips, and legs; and chronically poor posture.

A basic principle in physical training is "Use it or lose it!" If muscles aren't used, they degenerate. If joints aren't moved, they become stiff. But if you do specific exercises for strength and flexibility, your functioning both in sports and in everyday life is improved. Muscular

strength, for example, is an advantage whether you're hitting a baseball, unscrewing the lid of a jar, or moving your furniture into a new apartment. Stronger muscles make it easier to move the body, and they're also less susceptible to injury and disability, especially in the long term. Similarly, flexible joints that are pain-free and capable of normal movement are less likely to impede your activities, whether you're sprinting to class or running a marathon. Good posture helps to keep your spine properly aligned, which helps keep your back and neck pain-free. And an attractive, fit, healthy-looking body helps you feel good about yourself and project self-confidence and radiant well-being.

Improved Health over the Life Span

Exercising regularly may be the single most important thing you can do in your twenties to improve the quality of your life in your forties, fifties, sixties, and beyond. All the benefits of exercise continue to accrue but gain new importance as the resilience of youth begins to wane. Physically fit individuals are less likely to develop the diseases and disabilities now associated with middle age in our society, including heart disease, stroke, diabetes, and high blood pressure. They may be able to avoid fatigue, weight gain, memory loss, and other problems associated with aging. Their cardiorespiratory systems tend to resemble those of people 10 or more years younger than themselves. With flexible spines, strong hearts and muscles, lean bodies, and a repertoire of physical skills they can call on for exercise and enjoyment, these people have the potential to maintain their physical and mental well-being throughout their entire lives. People with disabilities also benefit immensely from exercise (see the box "Fitness and Disability: From Wheelchair Racing to Workout Videos").

A specific benefit of exercise, especially for women, is protection against **osteoporosis,** a disease that results in loss of bone density and poor bone strength (see Chapter 12). Weight-bearing exercise, which includes almost everything except swimming, helps build bone during the teens and twenties, when bones are still growing. Older people with denser bones can endure the bone loss that comes with osteoporosis better than can people whose bones are not as dense. With stronger bones, they're less likely to suffer the bone fractures that debilitate so many older people.

DESIGNING YOUR EXERCISE AND FITNESS PROGRAM

The best exercise and fitness program has two primary characteristics: It promotes your health and it's fun for you to do. Exercise doesn't have to be a chore. On the contrary, it can provide some of the most pleasurable moments of your day, once you make it a habit. A little thought and planning will help you achieve these goals.

If you are over 35 or have questions about your health, get a medical examination before beginning an exercise program. Diabetes, asthma, heart disease, or extreme obesity are conditions that may call for a modified program. If you have an increased risk of heart disease because of smoking, high blood pressure, or obesity, have an exercise **electrocardiogram (ECG)** before beginning a program. This checkup can help ensure that your program is a benefit to your health rather than a potential hazard.

As discussed earlier, fitness has many components—each has value and requires specific exercises. Lifting weights develops muscle strength, for example, but it doesn't condition the heart and lungs. Running is excellent for increasing cardiorespiratory capacity, but it contributes little to upper body strength and power. In addition, different sports and activities call for different skills; and to become proficient in them, you have to practice the specific movements they require. Therefore, to develop all the fitness components, you must participate in a variety of activities.

Consider your choice of activities carefully. First, be sure the activities you choose contribute to your general health and well-being, especially your cardiorespiratory endurance (as discussed in detail in the next section). Second, choose activities that make sense for you. Are you competitive? If so, try racquetball, basketball, or squash. Do you prefer to exercise alone? Then consider cross-country skiing or road running. If you think you may have trouble sticking with an exercise program, find a structured activity that you can do with a buddy or a group. If you don't have any favorite sports or activities, try something new. Take a physical education class, join a health club, sign up for jazz dancing. You're sure to find an activity that's both enjoyable and good for you.

Third, be realistic about the constraints presented by some sports, such as accessibility, expense, and time. For example, if you have to travel for hours to get to a ski area, skiing may not be a good choice for your regular exercise program. If you don't have large blocks of time available, you may have trouble squeezing in eighteen holes of golf. And if you've never played tennis, it will probably take you a fair amount of time to reach a reasonable skill level; you may be better off with a program of walking or jogging to get good workouts while you're improving your tennis game (see the box "Walking to Fitness" for suggestions).

It's difficult to stay in shape for all the activities in which you might want to participate—swimming, skiing, tennis, ice skating, roller skating, dancing, hiking, golf, volleyball, basketball, and so on. What you can do instead is choose a few activities and exercises and do them regularly as part of a general conditioning program. Then if you want to add an activity or try a new sport, you'll be in good shape to begin. A general conditioning program that supports an active lifestyle and promotes good health should contain the following components: cardiorespiratory endurance exercises, flexibility exercises, muscle strengthening exercises, and training in specific skills.

Osteoporosis A bone disease characterized by the loss of bone mineral. It is particularly prevalent in postmenopausal women.

Electrocardiogram (EKG or ECG) A recording of the changes in electrical activity of the heart.

TERMS

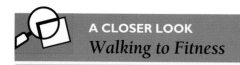

If you're someone who doesn't like jogging or swimming, who never learned to ski or play tennis, or who refuses to spend money on a health club, don't despair. You can still get into great shape—by walking!

Many people aren't aware that the physical conditioning value and aerobic effects of walking approach those of more strenuous exercise. If done briskly or long enough, walking can be as beneficial as jogging or any other endurance exercise for developing cardiorespiratory fitness. Walking promotes increased lung action, stimulates blood circulation, lowers elevated blood pressure, activates many large muscle groups, and even strengthens bones, perhaps lowering the risk of osteoporosis. Walking also tones the body and promotes weight loss, especially when combined with a low-fat diet. And like many other forms of exercise, walking helps reduce the effects of stress.

Perhaps the best news is that these benefits come with very little cost. Compared with other forms of exercise, walking has a very low injury rate, and the potential for pleasure is high. Also encouraging is the fact that even a modest program of 20 minutes of walking three times a week produces health benefits, as long as the pace puts your heart rate in the target range (see the box on determining your target heart rate). To check your heart rate while you're walking, carefully count your pulse at your wrist or throat (count for 15 seconds and multiply by 4). If necessary, stop walking long enough to do this and then resume, adjusting your pace as required to keep your heart rate in the target range.

You can vary the intensity of your workouts by walking briskly on level ground, taking to the hills, and then finishing on the flats. When walking uphill, try leaning forward slightly—it's easier on your leg muscles. Surprisingly, walking downhill can be harder on your body than walking uphill; it can jar the joints, especially the knees, and cause muscle soreness.

Walking uphill burns more calories than walking on flat land. If you weigh 150 pounds, walking at 3.5 miles an hour on flat terrain burns about 300 calories per hour. On a gentle incline (a 4 percent grade), the same pace burns almost 400 calories an hour. On a slightly steeper incline (an 8 percent grade), nearly 500 calories per hour are consumed. If you walk on a treadmill, you can elevate the grade mechanically, although you should do so gradually to minimize soreness.

To increase the physical benefits of your walking program and to avoid boredom, try these variations:

- Choose diverse terrains. Walking on grass or gravel burns more calories than walking on a dirt track. Walking on sand increases calorie consumption dramatically.

- Walk up and down stairs every day; skip all escalators and elevators.

- Swing or pump your arms for an upper body workout.

- Use hand weights while you walk to boost your heart rate and calorie consumption (but not if you have high blood pressure or heart disease). Begin with 1-pound weights and increase gradually, if you wish, but the weights shouldn't add up to more than 10 percent of your body weight. Don't use ankle weights; they increase the risk of injury.

- Stride-walk—lengthen your stride, swing your arms more, and pick up your pace.

- Retrowalk—walk backwards to work your back, abdominal, and thigh muscles. (Be sure to choose a smooth, unobstructed surface, such as a track.)

- Walk in water. The deeper the water and the faster the pace, the higher the calorie-burning value. Waist-high water is ideal, but you can achieve the same benefits in shallow water by walking faster and longer.

- Use walking poles to work the muscles in your chest, arms, and abdomen. Think of it as cross-country skiing without the skis. You can buy lightweight, rubber-tipped walking poles in sporting goods stores. Choose them carefully; you should be able to grip the pole and keep your forearm about level as you walk.

- Learn racewalking, a sport that involves moving your body forward as quickly as possible without breaking into a run. It eliminates the up-down motions of regular walking. Racewalking takes study, practice, and, at competitive levels, intensive training.

As a form of regular exercise, walking offers many advantages over other activities. It's comfortable, convenient, affordable, and safe. It also lends itself to socializing, sharing, and enjoying nature. And because it's so easy and pleasurable, you're likely to continue walking long after you've dropped more exotic or strenuous sports.

Adapted from E. E. Esckilsen. 1992. "The Short Walk to Health." *Take Care.* Summer, pp. 1–3; "Better Walking Workouts," *University of California at Berkeley Wellness Letter,* September 1992, pp. 4–5.

TABLE 14-2 Recommended Quantity and Quality of Exercise for Healthy Adults

Mode of activity	Cardiorespiratory endurance exercises such as running-jogging, walking-hiking, swimming, skating, bicycling, rowing, cross-country skiing, rope skipping, and various game activities
Frequency of training	3 to 5 days per week
Intensity of training	60 to 90 percent of maximum heart rate or 50 to 85 percent of maximum oxygen uptake
Duration of training	20 to 60 minutes of continuous aerobic activity; duration dependent on the intensity of the activity
Resistance training	At least one set of 8 to 12 repetitions of 8 to 10 exercises that condition the major muscle groups; recommended minimum frequency—at least two days per week

Source: American College of Sports Medicine. 1990. *ACSM Position Stand. The Recommended Quantity and Quality of Exercise for Developing and Maintaining Cardiorespiratory and Muscular Fitness in Healthy Adults.*

Personal Insight Do you exercise because you like it or because you think you should? Is there any form of exercise that you do just for the love of it?

Cardiorespiratory Endurance Exercises

Exercises that condition your heart and lungs should have a central role in your fitness program. The best exercises for developing **cardiorespiratory endurance** are those that stress a large portion of the body's muscle mass for a prolonged period of time. These include walking, jogging, running, swimming, bicycling, and aerobic dancing. Games such as racquetball, tennis, basketball, and soccer are also good if the skill level and intensity of the game are sufficient to provide a vigorous workout.

Specific recommendations have been made by the American College of Sports Medicine for the kind and amount of exercise that provide the optimal workout for your heart and lungs. They have defined three dimensions of training that should be taken into consideration: frequency, intensity, and duration of exercise. Frequency refers to the number of times per week you exercise; intensity refers to how hard you work; and duration refers to the length of your exercise session. Basic recommendations for quantity and quality of exercise are outlined in Table 14-2.

Frequency of Training The optimal workout schedule for endurance training is three to five days per week. Beginners should start with three and work up to five days. Training more than five days a week often leads to injury for recreational athletes. While recent evidence suggests that you get some health benefits from exercising from only one or two days per week, you risk injury because your body never gets a chance to adapt fully to regular exercise training.

Intensity of Training The most misunderstood aspect of conditioning, even among experienced athletes, is training intensity. Intensity is the crucial factor in attaining a training effect—that is, in increasing the body's cardiorespiratory capacity. A primary purpose of endurance training is to increase **maximal oxygen consumption (MOC)**. MOC represents the maximum ability of the cells to use oxygen and is considered the best measure of cardiorespiratory capacity. Intensity of training is the crucial factor in attaining a training effect—that is, in increasing the body's cardiorespiratory capacity—and in improving MOC.

However, it's not true that the harder you work, the better it is for you. Working too hard can cause injury, just as not working hard enough provides little benefit. One of the easiest ways to determine exactly how intensely you should work involves measuring your heart rate. It is not necessary or desirable to exercise at your maximum heart rate—the fastest heart rate possible before exhaustion sets in—in order to improve your cardiorespiratory capacity. Beneficial effects occur at lower heart rates with a much lower risk of injury. To find out how you can determine the intensity at which you should exercise, refer to the box "Determining Your Target Heart Rate."

After you begin your fitness program, you may improve quickly, because the body adapts readily to new exercises at first but slows after the first month or so. The more fit you become, the harder you will have to work to improve. By monitoring your heart rate, you will always know if you are working hard enough to improve, not

Cardiorespiratory endurance The extent to which the heart and lungs can respond to physical exercise.
Maximal oxygen consumption (MOC) The body's maximum ability to transport and use oxygen.

TERMS

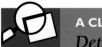

Your *target heart rate* is the rate at which you should exercise to experience cardiorespiratory benefits. Your target heart rate is based on your maximum heart rate, which can be estimated from your age. (If you are a serious athlete or face possible cardiovascular risks from exercise, you may want to have your maximum heart rate determined more accurately through a treadmill test in a physician's office, hospital, or sports medicine laboratory.) Your target heart rate is actually a range—the lower value corresponds to moderately intense exercise while the higher value is associated with high-intensity activities. Target heart rates for people in the age groups between 20 and 60 are shown in the accompanying table.

You can monitor the intensity of your workouts by measuring your pulse either at your wrist or at one of your carotid arteries, located on either side of your Adam's apple. Your pulse rate drops rapidly after exercise, so begin counting immediately after you have finished exercising. You will obtain the most accurate results by counting beats for 15 seconds and then multiplying by 4 to get your heart rate in beats per minute. To build cardiorespiratory endurance, you must exercise at your target heart rate for a minimum of 20 minutes, at least three times per week.

Maximum and Target Heart Rates Predicted from Age

Age (in years)	Predicted Maximum Heart Rate (in beats per minute)	Target Heart Rate Range (in beats per minute)
20–24	200	149–174
25–29	200	149–174
30–34	194	145–170
35–39	188	142–165
40–44	182	138–160
45–49	176	134–155
50–54	171	131–151
55–59	165	128–146
60–64	159	124–142
60+	153	121–137

Adapted from Metropolitan Life Insurance Company charts and Karvonen formula
(target heart rate = 0.6 or 0.8 × [$HR_{max} - HR_{rest}$] + HR_{rest}).

hard enough, or too hard. For most people, a fitness program involves attaining an acceptable level of fitness and then maintaining that level. There is no need to keep working indefinitely to improve; doing so only increases the chance of injury. After you have reached the level you want, you can maintain fitness by exercising at the same intensity approximately three times per week, 20 minutes per session.

Many people work out using a technique known as **periodization of training**, or *cycle training*. This technique involves varying the intensity of the workout from one session to the next so that you're rested on the days you exercise the hardest. For example, the intensity schedule of a week-long series of workouts might be (1) hard, (2) easy, (3) moderate, (4) easy, (5) moderate, (6) rest, and (7)

rest. A hard workout might be practiced at the high end of the target heart rate range, a moderate workout in the middle of the range, and an easy workout at the low end of the range (see the box "Determining Your Target Heart Rate.") Cycle training allows your body to adapt rapidly to intense workouts by giving it time to recover between strenuous sessions. Competitive athletes also use yearly cycles—varying workouts during different times of the year and competitive season.

Duration of Training The length of time you should spend on a workout depends on its intensity. If you are walking, swimming slowly, or playing a stop-and-start game like tennis, you should participate for 45 to 60 minutes. High-intensity exercises such as running that keep

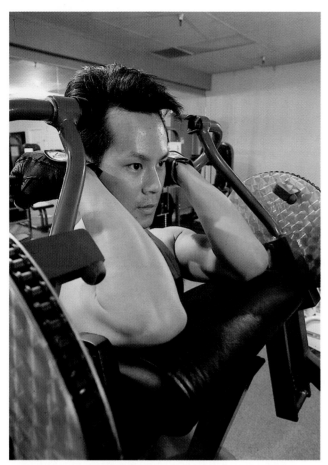

Building muscular strength is an important component of a fitness program. Weight training is just one way to increase strength, improve muscle tone, and enhance the overall appearance of the body.

your heart rate in the target zone for at least 20 minutes can be practiced for a shorter period of time. The recreational athlete should start off with less vigorous activities and only gradually increase intensity. For most people, continuous endurance exercise should last from 20 minutes (high-intensity activities) to 60 minutes (low-intensity activities).

You can use these three dimensions of cardiorespiratory endurance training—frequency, intensity, and duration—to construct a fitness program that strengthens your heart and lungs and provides all the benefits described earlier in this chapter. Build your program around at least 20 minutes of continuous aerobic activity at your target heart rate three to five times a week. Then add exercises that develop the other components of fitness.

Flexibility Exercises

Flexibility, or stretching, exercises are perhaps the most neglected part of fitness programs, but they are extremely important. They are necessary to maintain the normal range of motion in the major joints of the body. Some exercises, such as running, actually decrease flexibility be-

cause they require only a partial range of motion. It's important to do stretching exercises at least three to five times a week to develop this component of fitness.

Stretching should be performed statically. "Bouncing" (ballistic stretching) is dangerous and counterproductive. Stretch to the point of tightness in the muscle and hold the position 10 to 30 seconds (up to 60 seconds if your muscles are tight). You should feel a pleasant, mild stretch as you let the muscles relax; stretching shouldn't be painful. There are large individual differences in flexibility, so don't feel you have to compete with others during stretching workouts. Flexibility increases gradually over a period of time as you incorporate stretching exercises into your fitness program. You can set apart a special time for these exercises or do them before or after your aerobic exercise. You may develop more flexibility if you do them after exercise, because your muscles are warmer then and can be stretched farther. A sequence of appropriate stretching exercises is given in the box "Exercises for Flexibility."

Muscle Strengthening Exercises

Exercises that develop muscular strength and muscular endurance should also be included in any program designed to promote health. Your ability to maintain correct posture and to move efficiently depends in part on adequate muscle fitness. Strengthening exercises also increase muscle tone, which improves the appearance of your body. A lean, healthy-looking body is certainly one of the goals and one of the benefits of an overall fitness program.

Muscular strength and endurance can be developed in many ways, from weight training to calisthenics. (Taking **anabolic steroids** is *not* a safe or healthy way to increase muscle strength or endurance; in fact, it runs counter to all the practices that promote good health discussed in this chapter. See the box "The Dangers of Anabolic Steroids"). Common exercises such as sit-ups, push-ups, pull-ups, and wall-sitting (leaning against a wall in a seated position and supporting yourself with your leg muscles) maintain the muscular strength of most people if they practice them three to five days a week. To condition and tone your whole body, choose exercises that work the major muscles of the shoulders, chest, back, arms, abdomen, and legs.

To increase strength, you must do **resistive exercise**—exercises in which your muscles must exert force

Periodization of training A training technique that systematically varies the volume and intensity of the workouts.

Anabolic steroids Synthetic male hormones used to increase muscle size and strength.

Resistive exercise Exercise that forces muscles to contract against increased resistance; for example, weight training.

TERMS

1. **Shoulder blade scratch** (shoulders, arms)
   Reach back with one arm as if to scratch your shoulder blade. Use your other hand to extend the stretch. Alternate arms.

2. **Towel stretch** (arms, shoulders, chest)
   Grasp a rolled towel at both ends and slowly bring it back over your head as far down as possible. Keep your arms straight. (The closer your hands are, the greater the stretch.)

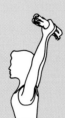

3. **Alternate knee-to-chest** (lower back)
   With hands behind your knees, bring one knee up to your chest. Curl your head toward your knee. Keep the other leg on the floor. Alternate knees.

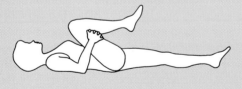

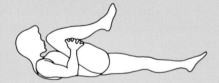

4. **Double knee-to-chest** (buttocks, lower back)
   Same as alternate knee-to-chest (3), except bring both knees up to your chest.

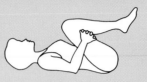 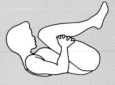

5. **Sole stretch** (groin)
   With the soles of your feet pressed together, pull your feet toward you while pressing your knees down with your elbows.

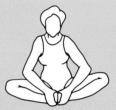

6. **Seated toe touch** (hamstrings)
   Sit with your legs straight. Fold one leg in front and gradually reach for the toes of your other foot. Eventually you will be able to grasp your feet at the instep. Keep your head down. Alternate legs.

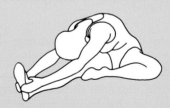

7. **Seated foot-over-knee twist** (hips)
   Seated as depicted, turn at the hips to face the rear. Hold your ankle to keep your foot on the floor. Alternate legs.

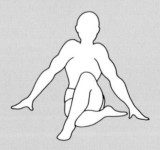 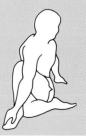

8. **Prone knee flexion** (quadriceps)
   Lying on your side with one arm tucked behind your head, use the other arm to slowly pull one foot up toward your buttocks. Flex the leg up until you feel the stretch in your quadriceps. Alternate legs.

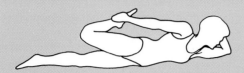

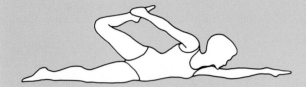

9. **Wall lean** (lower legs)
   Lean against the wall with one leg bent and the other straight. Keep your back straight and your heels on the floor. Bend the knee of the straight leg—this changes the stretch from the calf muscle to the Achilles tendon. Alternate legs.

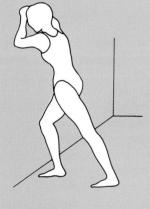

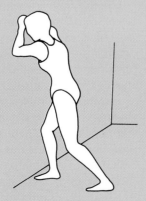

10. **Stride stretch** (hips, hamstring)
    Assume the racer's starting position and stretch one leg backward. Keep your head down. Alternate legs.

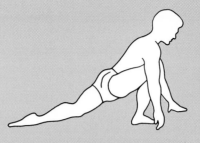

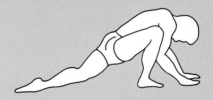

Source: I. Kusinitz and M. Fine. 1992. *Your Guide to Getting Fit.* 2nd ed. (Mountain View, Calif.: Mayfield).

The Dangers of Anabolic Steroids

Anabolic steroids are drugs that resemble male hormones such as testosterone and are widely used by athletes in sports like track and field, weight lifting, and football. Athletes take them in the hope of gaining weight, strength, power, speed, endurance, and aggressiveness. Recently young people who are not athletes have begun taking these drugs to improve their appearance. Studies indicate that as many as 400,000 American teens may have experimented with steroids. Steroid use is costly both to athletic careers and to health: Steroid use cost Ben Johnson his Olympic gold medal in 1988, and pro football player Lyle Alzado blamed long-term steroid use for the brain cancer that eventually led to his death.

Steroids work by enhancing the anabolic (tissue-building) properties of male hormones. These include accelerated growth of muscle, bone, and red blood cells and enhanced neural conduction. Most experts feel that anabolic steroids are effective in improving some types of athletic performance—but only at a cost to health, because they have dangerous side effects.

The physiological side effects of steroid use include reduced testosterone production, testicular function, and sperm cell production, which in turn can lead to atrophy of the testes. These changes may reverse themselves after use stops, but prolonged use may permanently disturb the delicate hormone regulatory system. Anabolic steroids also increase fluid retention and may harm the immune system. Libido (sex drive) may increase or decrease.

Steroid use by women and children may have masculinizing effects, including hair growth on face and body, deepening of the voice, oily skin, increased sweat gland activity, acne, and baldness. In women, some of these changes are irreversible. Women may also experience clitoral enlargement and menstrual irregularity. Children initially experience accelerated maturation followed by premature closure of growth centers in the long bones.

Taken orally, anabolic steroids also present a risk of toxicity, particularly to the liver. Prolonged use has been linked to severe liver disorders such as blood-filled cysts, liver cancer, and bile duct obstruction.

Several factors associated with steroid use are linked to increased risk of coronary heart disease: high levels of blood cholesterol and triglycerides, high blood pressure, and low levels of high-density lipoproteins (HDLs). Many athletes use steroids for long periods of time (10 to 20 years), risking premature death from atherosclerosis. High blood pressure is also common, probably due to fluid retention.

A variety of other side effects has been reported, including psychological disorders, muscle cramps, gastrointestinal distress, headache, dizziness, sore nipples, and abnormal thyroid function. Some of these side effects even show up in people who have taken only low doses for short periods of time.

---

against a significant resistance. Resistance can be provided by weights, exercise machines, or your own body weight. Your muscles become stronger when you subject them to **overload,** an exercise stress that is more severe than what they are used to. By pushing your muscles to temporary fatigue and by gradually increasing the amount of resistance or the number of times they must resist, you force them to adapt to greater physical stress. If you use heavy resistance with few repetitions (1 to 10), you build muscle strength and size. If you use lighter resistance and do more repetitions, you improve muscular endurance (the ability to exert force over a longer period of time). Strength training improves performance in most sports and has become a prominent part of the training program of many athletes. In general, you have to train at least twice a week for an hour to experience significant results. You also have to allow recovery time between workouts—two to four days—to train properly and avoid injury.

There are three different kinds of strengthening exercises. **Isometric exercises** involve applying force without movement, such as when you contract your abdominal muscles. This static type of exercise is valuable for toning and strengthening muscles. Isometrics can be practiced anywhere and don't require any equipment. Try holding your stomach in for 10 to 30 seconds several times during the day (but don't hold your breath—that can restrict blood flow to your heart and brain). Within a few weeks, you'll notice the effect of this exercise. Isometrics are particularly useful when recovering from an injury.

Isokinetic exercises involve exerting force at a constant speed against an equal force exerted by a specialized strength training machine. Proponents of this type of exercise claim that training at faster speeds produces a training effect more specific to the rapid movements used in sports. Isokinetic machines are considerably more expensive than traditional weight training equipment and so are not as widely available.

Isotonic exercises involve applying force with movement, as, for example, in weight training exercises such as the bench press. These are the most popular type of exercises for increasing muscle strength and seem to be most valuable for developing strength that can be transferred to other forms of physical activity. They include exercises using barbells, dumbbells, weight machines, and the body's own weight, as in push-ups or sit-ups.

Examples of isotonic exercises for various muscle groups include the bench press for the chest; the overhead press, the behind-the-neck press, and upright rowing for the shoulders; barbell and dumbbell curls for the arms; pull-ups and chin-ups for the upper back; sit-ups and crunches for the abdominals; and squats and leg presses for the legs. Exercises are repeated until the muscles are fatigued, and muscle contraction—the lifting or pushing part of the exercise—is always accompanied by an exhalation. Begin with a weight that you can lift fairly easily for 10 repetitions, and do three sets (groups) of 10 repetitions of each exercise. Increase your level of exertion gradually over a period of weeks. To learn how to do these exercises properly so they increase your muscle strength and don't cause injury, you should receive instruction from a trainer in a gym, a health club, a physical education class, or a Y or community recreation department.

Training in Specific Skills

The fourth element in your fitness program is learning the skills required in the sports or activities in which you choose to participate. Taking the time and effort to acquire competence means that instead of feeling ridiculous, becoming frustrated, and giving up in despair, you achieve a sense of mastery and add a new physical activity to your repertoire.

The first step in learning a new skill is to get help. Sports like tennis, golf, sailing, and skiing require mastery of basic movements and techniques, so instruction from a qualified teacher can save you hours of frustration and increase your enjoyment of the sport.

Skill is also important in conditioning activities such as jogging, swimming, and cycling. Know your own capacity and learn to gauge the intensity of exercise that will result in improvement without injury. Some instruction on technique from a coach or fellow participant can often help you to move and train more efficiently. Even if you learned a sport as a child, additional instruction now can help you refine your technique, get over stumbling blocks, and relearn skills that you may have learned incorrectly.

Finally, as discussed earlier, choose activities and sports that suit your personal tastes, your time constraints, and your pocketbook. Be sure to vary your program enough so you don't get bored.

Putting It All Together

Now that you know the basic components of a fitness program, you can put them all together in a program that works for you. Remember to include the following:

- Cardiorespiratory endurance exercise—do at least 20 minutes of aerobic exercise at your target heart rate three to five times a week

- Muscle strengthening exercise—work the major muscle groups two to three times a week
- Flexibility exercise—do stretches three to five times a week
- Skill training—incorporate some or all of your aerobic or strengthening exercise into an enjoyable sport or physical activity

A summary of the fitness benefits of a variety of activities is provided in Table 14-3 to help you plan your program.

In any program, it's important to *warm up* before you exercise and *cool down* afterwards. Warming up enhances your performance and decreases your chances of injury. Your muscles work better when their temperature is elevated slightly above resting level. Warming up helps your body's physiology gradually progress from rest to exercise. Blood needs to be redirected to active muscles, and your heart needs time to adapt to the increased demands of exercise. Warm-up helps spread **synovial fluid** throughout joints, which helps protect surfaces from wear and tear. (This is like an automobile: Warming up a car spreads oil through the engine parts before you shift into gear.)

A warm-up session should include low-intensity movements similar to those in the activity that will follow. Low-intensity movements include hitting forehands and backhands before a tennis game and running a 12-minute mile before progressing to an 8-minute one. Some experts also recommend warm-up stretching exercises for flexibility after the warm-up and before intense activity.

Cooling down after exercise is important to restore circulation to its normal resting condition. When you are at rest, a relatively small percentage of your total blood volume is directed to muscles, but during exercise as much as 85 percent of the heart's output is directed to them. During recovery from exercise, it is important to continue exercising at a low level to provide a smooth transition to the resting state. Cooling down helps maintain the return of blood to your heart.

There are as many different adequate fitness programs as there are different individuals. Consider these examples:

Maggie is a person whose life revolves around sports. She's been on volleyball teams, softball teams, and

Overload Subjecting the body to more stress than it is accustomed.
Isometric exercise Application of force without movement. Also called *static exercise*.
Isokinetic exercise Application of force at constant speed. A form of isotonic exercise.
Isotonic exercise Application of force with movement.
Synovial fluid Fluid found within many joints that provides lubrication and nutrition to the cells of the joint surface.

TERMS

TABLE 14-3 Fitness Benefits of Selected Activities

Sports and activities are classified here as high (H), moderate (M), or low (L) for their ability to develop five different components of physical fitness: cardiorespiratory endurance (CRE), body composition (BC), muscular strength (MS), muscular endurance (ME), and flexibility (F). In the Skill Level column, low (L) means little or no skill is required to obtain fitness benefits from the activity; moderate (M) means average skill is required; and high (H) means much skill is required. In the Fitness Prerequisite column, low (L) means there is little or no fitness prerequisite; moderate (M) means some preconditioning is required; and high (H) means substantial fitness is required. In the How Paced column, 1 means the activity is self-paced; 2 means pacing is by a combination of yourself and others; and 3 means it's paced by someone other than yourself. The last two columns give the calorie cost of each activity. To determine how many calories you burn when you engage in a particular activity, multiply the value in the appropriate column by your body weight and then by the number of minutes you exercise.

Sports and Activities	Components					Skill Level	Fitness Prerequisite	How Paced	Approximate Calorie Cost (calories/lb./min.)	
	CRE	BC	MS	ME	F				Moderate	Vigorous
Aerobic dance	H	H	M	H	H	L	L	3	.046	.062
Backpacking	H	H	H	H	M	L	M	1	.032	.078
Badminton (skilled, singles)	H	H	M	M	M	M	M	2	-	.071
Ballet (floor combinations)	M	M	M	H	H	M	L	3	-	.058
Ballroom dancing	M	M	L	M	L	M	L	3	.034	.049
Baseball (pitcher and catcher)	M	M	M	H	M	H	M	3	.039	-
Basketball	H	H	M	H	M	M	M	3	.045	.071
Bicycling	H	H	M	H	M	M	L	1	.049	.071
Bowling	L	L	L	L	L	L	L	1	-	-
Calisthenic circuit training	H	H	M	H	M	L	L	1	-	.060
Canoeing and kayaking	M	M	M	H	M	M	M	1	.045	-
Cross-country skiing	H	H	M	H	M	M	M	1	.049	.104
Fencing	M	M	M	H	H	M	L	3	.032	.078
Field hockey	H	H	M	H	M	M	M	3	.052	.078
Folk and square dancing	M	M	L	M	L	L	L	3	.039	.049
Football/touch	M	M	M	M	M	M	M	3	.049	.078
Frisbee/ultimate	H	H	M	H	M	M	M	2	.049	.078
Golf (riding cart)	L	L	L	L	M	L	L	1	-	-
Handball (skilled singles)	H	H	M	H	M	M	M	3	-	.078
Hiking	H	H	M	H	L	L	M	1	.051	.073
Hockey/ice and field	H	H	M	H	M	M	M	3	.052	.078
Horseback riding	M	M	M	M	L	M	M	1	.052	.065
Interval circuit training	H	H	H	H	M	L	L	1	-	.062

TABLE 14-3 *Fitness Benefits of Selected Activities (continued)*

Sports and Activities	Components CRE	BC	MS	ME	F	Skill Level	Fitness Prerequisite	How Paced	Approximate Calorie Cost (calories/lb./min.) Moderate	Vigorous
Jogging and running	H	H	M	H	L	L	L	1	.060	.104
Judo	M	M	H	H	M	M	L	3	.049	.090
Karate	H	H	M	H	H	L	M	3	.049	.090
Modern dance (moving combinations)	M	M	M	H	H	L	L	3	-	.058
Popular dancing	M	M	L	M	M	M	L	3	-	.049
Racquetball (skilled, singles)	H	H	M	M	M	M	M	2	.049	.078
Rock climbing	M	M	H	H	H	H	M	1	.033	-
Rope skipping	H	H	M	H	L	M	M	1	.071	.095
Rowing	H	H	H	H	H	L	L	1	.032	.097
Sailing	L	L	L	M	L	M	L	1	-	-
Skating/ice and roller	M	M	M	H	M	H	M	1	.049	.065
Skiing/alpine	M	M	H	H	M	H	M	1	.039	.078
Soccer	H	H	M	H	M	M	M	3	.052	.097
Squash (skilled, singles)	H	H	M	M	M	M	M	2	.049	.078
Stretching	L	L	L	L	H	L	L	1	-	-
Surfing (including swimming)	M	M	M	M	M	H	M	2	-	.078
Swimming	H	H	M	H	M	M	L	1	.032	.088
Table tennis	M	M	L	M	M	M	L	3	-	.045
Tennis (skilled, singles)	H	H	M	M	M	M	M	2	-	.071
Volleyball	M	M	L	M	M	M	M	3	-	.065
Walking	H	H	L	M	L	L	L	1	.029	.048
Water skiing	M	M	M	H	M	H	M	2	.039	.055
Weight training	L	BC	MS	ME	H	L	L	1	-	-
Wrestling	H	H	H	H	H	H	H	3	.065	.094
Yoga	L	L	L	M	H	H	L	1	-	-

Adapted from I. Kusinitz and M. Fine. 1991. *Your Guide to Getting Fit.* 2nd ed. (Mountain View, Calif.: Mayfield).

swim teams, and now she's on her college varsity soccer team. She follows a rigorous exercise regimen established by her soccer coach. Soccer practice is from four to six four afternoons a week. It begins with warm-ups, drills, and practice in specific skills, and it ends with a scrimmage and then a jog around the soccer field. Games are every Saturday. Maggie likes team sports, but she also enjoys exercising alone, so she goes on long bicycle rides whenever she can fit them in. She can't imagine what it would be like not to be physically active every day.

Janine is a young mother of twins. Her life is so busy caring for them that she hardly has time to comb her hair, much less spend a lot of time exercising. To keep in shape, she joined a health club with a weight room, exercise classes, and child care. Every Monday, Wednesday, and Friday morning, she takes the twins to the club and attends the seven o'clock "wake-up" low-impact aerobics class. The teacher leads the class through warm-ups; a 20-minute aerobic workout; exercises for the arms, legs, abdomen, buttocks, and legs; stretches; and a relaxation exercise. Janine is exhilarated and ready for the rest of the day before nine.

Tom is an engineering student with a lot of studying to do and an active social life as well. For exercise, he plays tennis. He likes to head for the courts around 6 P.M., when most people are eating dinner. He warms up for 10 minutes practicing his forehand and backhand against a backboard, and then plays a hard, fast game with his regular partner for 45 minutes to an hour. After he walks back to his room, he does some stretching exercises while his muscles are still warm. Then he showers and gets ready for dinner. Twice a week he works out at the gym, with particular attention to keeping his arms strong and his elbows limber. On Saturday nights, he goes dancing with his girlfriend.

Each of these people has worked an adequate or more-than-adequate fitness program into a busy daily routine. How can you include exercise in your life?

Personal Insight In our society, boys and men tend to be more active in sports and physical activities than do girls and women. Why do you think that is? How do you feel about it?

GETTING STARTED AND KEEPING ON TRACK

Once you have a program that fulfills your basic fitness needs and suits your personal tastes, adhering to a few basic principles will help you improve at the fastest rate,

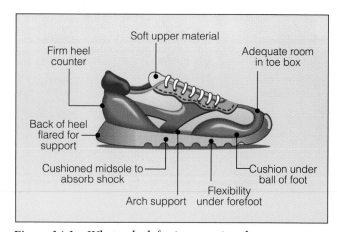

Figure 14-1 *What to look for in a running shoe.*

have more fun, and minimize the risk of injury. These principles include buying appropriate equipment, eating and drinking properly, and managing your program so it becomes an integral part of your life.

Selecting Equipment

When you're sure of the activities you're going to do, buy the best equipment you can afford. Good equipment will enhance your enjoyment and decrease your risk of injury. Part of the "fitness fad" has been a wave of new equipment and clothing. Some of it is truly revolutionary: New skis allow you to go faster with better control, new tennis racquets make it easier to hit the ball over the net, and new materials make sports clothing more comfortable and fashionable. Unfortunately, some new products are either overpriced or of poor quality. A flashy but overweight tennis racquet can produce an elbow injury, and a shoe that can't absorb shock can cause leg pains.

Before you invest in a new piece of equipment, investigate it. Is it worth the money? Does it produce the results its proponents claim for it? Is it safe? Does it fit properly and is it in good working order? Look for equipment that provides a genuine workout, such as stationary bicycles, cross-country skiing machines, or stair-climbers, not passive devices such as massage machines and rubberized suits. Ask the experts (coaches, physical educators, and sports instructors) for their opinion. Better yet, educate yourself. Every sport, from running to volleyball, has its own magazine. A little effort to educate yourself will be well rewarded.

Footwear is perhaps the most important piece of equipment for almost any sport. Buy shoes that fit properly and that are appropriate for the activity. Running shoes, court shoes (for tennis, racquetball, basketball, and so on), and shoes for aerobic dance and exercise have different characteristics. Figure 14-1 shows the characteristics of an ideal running shoe.

Manipulation of the diet in hopes of enhancing athletic performance has a long and checkered history. As recently as 20 years ago, football players were encouraged on hot practice days to "toughen up" for competition by consuming salt tablets and by not drinking water—a practice now recognized as potentially fatal. Today's athletes still search for ways to maximize their potential, but they can now take advantage of scientific evidence that some substances—notably carbohydrates—may enhance athletic performance in some situations without posing a threat to their health.

Carbohydrate is an indispensable fuel for essentially all types of athletic performance. Depletion of stored carbohydrate (glycogen) is a cause of fatigue in endurance exercise that lasts longer than 60 to 90 minutes; it may diminish performance in brief, high-intensity activities as well. Reduced levels of sugar (glucose) in the blood during endurance activities may also cause fatigue.

One of the better known ways to manipulate carbohydrates in the diet is *carbohydrate loading,* the practice of gradually reducing the duration of training sessions during the week before an important competition while progressively increasing the consumption of dietary carbohydrates. For example, an athlete may consume 40 percent of dietary calories as carbohydrate for the first three days of the carbohydrate-loading regimen and then increase to 70 to 85 percent during the rest of the week. This procedure maximizes the storage of glycogen before competition and has been shown to significantly increase endurance time for the average athlete. It is a safe procedure, although some people experience gastrointestinal discomfort or a feeling of sluggishness with high-carbohydrate diets.

Performance can also be improved by increasing the level of glucose in the blood *during* competition. Carbohydrate drinks that contain glucose, fructose, or sucrose, for example, supply the athlete with a continuous source of energy. Drinks containing about 5 to 8 percent carbohydrates are usually ideal. Average athletes usually show about a 5 to 7 percent improvement in endurance when using carbohydrate drinks; elite athletes may experience up to a 30 percent improvement.

Other substances have been investigated for their effect on athletic performance, including sodium bicarbonate, caffeine, and various vitamins and minerals, but none of them has proven as safe or useful as have carbohydrates.

Eating and Drinking for Exercise

Most people do not need to change their eating habits when they begin a fitness program. Many athletes and other physically active people are lured into buying aggressively advertised vitamins, minerals, and protein supplements. The truth is that in almost every case a well-balanced diet (see Chapter 12) contains all the energy and nutrients needed to sustain an exercise program.

A balanced diet is also the key to improving your body composition when you begin to exercise more. One of the promises of a fitness program is a decrease in body fat and an increase in lean, muscular body mass. As mentioned earlier, the control of body fat is determined by the balance of energy in the body. If more calories are consumed than are expended through metabolism and exercise, then fat increases. If the reverse is true, fat is lost. The best way to control body fat is to follow a diet containing adequate but not excessive calories and to exercise.

The one change in diet that some long-distance runners and other athletes make is to increase the proportion of carbohydrates they consume. Diets that are higher than average in carbohydrates can benefit athletes because carbohydrates increase the amount of **glycogen** present in the body. Glycogen, a carbohydrate stored in muscles and the liver, is vitally important for sustaining physical activity over long periods of time. When levels of this substance are low, the athlete feels sluggish, weak, and tired. One exciting discovery in sports medicine in recent years has been that consuming carbohydrate drinks during exercise can improve performance and that drinking them immediately after exercise rapidly replenishes glycogen. For a more detailed discussion of the role of carbohydrates and other substances in exercise and athletic performance, see the box "Carbohydrate Loading."

One of the most important principles to follow when you're exercising is to drink enough water. Your body depends on water to sustain many chemical reactions and to maintain correct body temperature. Sweating during exercise depletes your body's water supply and can lead to dehydration if fluids aren't replaced. Serious dehydration can cause reduced blood volume, increased heart rate, raised body temperature, muscle cramps, heat stroke, and other serious problems. Drinking water before and during exercise is important to prevent dehydration and enhance athletic performance.

Thirst alone is not a good indication of how much you need to drink, because thirst is quickly depressed by drinking even small amounts of water. Most of your weight loss immediately after exercise is from loss of fluids. If you rely on thirst, it can take 24 hours or more to

Glycogen   A complex carbohydrate, found largely in the liver and skeletal muscle, that serves as a carbohydrate storage depot.

TERMS

Here a student is taking a maximum endurance test on a treadmill. His cardiovascular fitness is assessed by monitoring his heart rate, heart function, oxygen intake, and blood pressure.

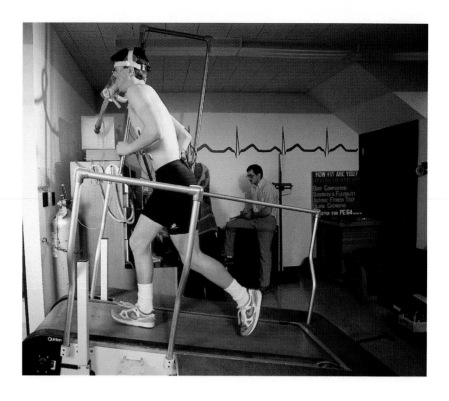

replace these fluids. Ideally, you should restore your body fluids before you exercise vigorously again. As a rule of thumb, try to drink about 8 ounces of water (more in hot weather) for every 30 minutes of heavy exercise. Bring a water bottle with you when you exercise so you can replace your fluids while they're being depleted. Water—preferably cold—or diluted carbohydrate drinks such as Cytomax or Gatorade are the best fluid replacements. Carbohydrate drinks are good because they also supply energy and electrolytes, such as sodium and potassium. You don't need to take salt pills—your body is very efficient at sparing electrolytes during exercise.

Managing Your Fitness Program

How can you tell when you're in shape? When do you stop improving and start maintaining? How can you stay motivated? These are important questions if your program is going to become an integral part of your life and if the principles behind it are going to serve you well in the years ahead.

Consistency: The Key to Physical Improvement It's important to be able to recognize when you have achieved the level of fitness that is adequate for you. This level will vary, of course, depending on your goals, the intensity of your program, and your natural ability. Your body gets into shape by adapting to increasing levels of physical stress. If you don't push yourself by increasing the intensity of your workout—by adding weight or running a little faster or a little longer—no change will occur in your body.

But if you subject your body to overly severe stress, it will break down and become distressed, or injured. Overdoing exercise is just as bad as not exercising hard enough. No one can become fit overnight. Your body needs time to adapt to increasingly higher levels of stress. The process of improving fitness, of training, involves a countless number of stresses and adaptations. If you feel extremely sore and tired the day after exercising, then you have worked too hard. Injury will slow you down just as much as a missed workout.

Consistency is the key to getting into shape without injury. Steady fitness improvement comes when you overload your body consistently over a long period of time. The best way to ensure consistency is by keeping a training journal in which you record the details of your workouts—how far you ran, how much weight you lifted, how many laps you swam, and so on. This record will help you evaluate your progress and plan your workout sessions intelligently. Don't increase your exercise volume by more than 5 to 10 percent per week.

Assessing Your Fitness When are you "in shape"? It depends. One person may be out of shape running a mile in 5 minutes; another may be in shape running a mile in 12 minutes. As mentioned earlier, your ultimate level of fitness depends on your goals, your program, and your natural ability. The important thing is to set goals that make sense for you.

If you are interested in finding out exactly how fit you are before you begin a program, the best approach is to get an assessment from a modern sports medicine laboratory. Such laboratories can be found in university physical

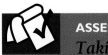

You can obtain a general rating of your cardiorespiratory fitness by taking the 1.5-mile run-walk test. Don't attempt this test unless you have completed at least six weeks of some type of conditioning activity. Also, if you are over age 35 or have questions about your health, check with your physician before taking this test.

You'll need a stopwatch, clock, or watch with a second hand and a running track or course that is flat and provides measurements of up to 1.5 miles. You may want to practice pacing yourself prior to taking the test to avoid going too fast at the start and becoming fatigued before you finish. Allow yourself a day or two to recover from your practice run before taking the test.

Warm up before taking the test with some walking, easy jogging, and stretching exercises. The idea is to cover the distance as fast as possible, at a pace that is comfortable for you. You can run or walk the entire distance, or use some combination of running and walking. If possible, monitor your own pace or have someone call out your time at various intervals to help you determine whether your pace is correct. When you have completed the test, refer to the table for your cardiorespiratory fitness rating. Be sure to cool down by walking or jogging slowly for about 5 minutes.

Standards for the 1.5 Mile Run-Walk (min:sec)

	High	Good	Fair	Poor
Males				
20–29	9:45	12:00	13:00	15:00
30–39	10:00	12:15	13:30	16:00
40–49	10:30	12:30	14:00	16:30
50–59	11:00	13:30	15:00	18:30
60+	11:15	14:30	16:30	19:00
Females				
20–29	11:00	13:15	14:15	16:15
30–39	11:15	13:30	14:45	17:15
40–49	11:45	13:45	15:15	17:45
50–59	12:15	14:45	16:15	19:45
60+	12:30	15:45	17:45	20:15

education departments and medical centers. Here you will receive an accurate profile of your capacity to exercise. Typically, your endurance will be measured on a treadmill or bicycle, your body fat will be estimated, and your strength and flexibility will be tested. This evaluation will reveal whether your physical condition is consistent with good health, and the personnel at the laboratory can suggest an exercise program that will be appropriate for your level of fitness.

Assessing your own fitness is more difficult because endurance, strength, coordination, agility, and other components of fitness are specific to activities or tasks. It's meaningless to count how many pull-ups or push-ups you can do when you're interested in having the muscle strength to play tennis, ski, or jog. Endurance for running

doesn't translate directly into endurance for swimming or bicycling—you have to practice the activities themselves to improve in them. Nevertheless, a very rough estimate of your cardiorespiratory fitness can be obtained by checking your time in the 1.5-mile run or walk. Use the table in the box "Taking the 1.5-Mile Run-Walk Test" to find out in general terms whether your level of fitness is consistent with good health.

Dealing with Athletic Injuries Injuries can happen even to the most careful physically active person. Although annoying, most are neither serious nor permanent. However, an injury that isn't cared for properly can escalate into a chronic problem, sometimes serious enough to permanently curtail the activity. It's important

Evaluating Health and Fitness Clubs

Are you looking for a health and fitness club to help you get or stay in shape? If so, some general guidelines will help you weed out the clubs that are in it just for the profit and find one that can really meet your needs. The general advice that follows is offered by *Consumers Guide.*®

High-Pressure Selling

When you enter a health club, you can expect a tour followed by a high-pressure sales pitch. Be ready for it. Instructors and managers are well schooled in making an effective representation. They want your business.

Consumers Guide® sees nothing wrong with the health club manager's making a strong case emphasizing the value of exercise. But that's it. Under no circumstances should you feel badgered, embarrassed, belittled, threatened, detained, or mocked. If you feel any excessive amount of pressure, leave or at least ask for more time. If you are told this is a once-in-a-lifetime deal or that the rates go up tomorrow, forget it. It's a high-pressure outfit interested in the dollar figure, not yours.

The Contract

Read the contract carefully. If you want more time, take it. If you feel you should read it at home or want to discuss it with anyone else, do so. If the health club won't permit you to take the contract home, steer clear of that organization. Make sure the contract commits you to no more than two years; one year is preferable. All contracts should provide for a minimum three-day cooling-off period; look for a "use of facility" clause permitting you to use the club during those three days.

Key Considerations

During the tour, explanation of facilities, and closing, you should be aware of the following:

1. Is there a discussion of your individual problems? This should take place prior to signing the contract. Is there a discussion of your physical limitations, risk factors, and the possibility of stress tests? Do they recommend that you talk to your doctor before you embark on an exercise program?

2. Is the person conducting the tour an instructor, a manager, or what? Does he or she seem to be well trained and not just well built? Ask if he or she is a physical education or physical therapy graduate with additional training in fitness. If not, does the club have an in-service training program emphasizing cardiovascular fitness? Do you sense that the person has a genuine interest in you? Is he or she able to explain how the machines operate, their value and limitations? Are the aerobics instructors safety conscious and concerned about their students? Do they teach them how to monitor their heart rates?

3. Does the spa manager or instructor emphasize cardiovascular fitness, or is the focus on muscle strength and endurance? If the emphasis is on muscle strength and endurance, you can eliminate that club. The primary focus should be on cardiovascular fitness.

4. Visit the club *at a time of day when you plan to use it*. This is crucial. Every club has a peak usage time. Waiting in line to run on the treadmill, ride a bicycle, or lift weights can be a serious inconvenience. Consider time and use of facilities as important factors.

5. Before signing anything, talk to several of the people who are exercising (or who have just finished, if you don't want to interrupt their work). Ask what they think of the program, what the emphasis is, and whether personal attention is given.

6. Observe the facility. Is it clean, well ventilated, and properly maintained? Is equipment in good condition? Is there shock-absorbent flooring for aerobics workouts—a suspended wood floor, high-density matting, or carpet over cushioning? High-impact activity should never be done on tile, linoleum, or cement.

7. Find out how long the club has been in your area. The longer the better, and if under the same management, that's another plus. Approach a new club with caution—especially "pre-opening" sales. There have been cases where con artists have held pre-opening sales for clubs that never opened.

8. Find out if the club belongs to the Association of Physical Fitness Centers. This trade association for full-service health spas is dedicated to upgrading the industry. The Association has established a code of ethics that covers programs, facilities, employees, and consumers' rights. You can also check on the club with the Better Business Bureau to see if any complaints have been filed against it.

Adapted from Carol Krucoff. 1989. "Joining the Club." *Washington Post Health.* 5 September, p. 20.

---

to learn how to deal with injuries so they don't derail your fitness program.

Some injuries require medical attention. Consult a physician for head and eye injuries, possible ligament in-juries, broken bones, and internal disorders such as chest pain, fainting, and intolerance to heat. Also seek medical attention for apparently minor injuries that do not get better within a reasonable amount of time.

For minor cuts and scrapes, stop the bleeding and clean the wound with soap and water. Treat soft tissue injuries (muscles and joints) immediately with ice packs. Elevate the affected part of the body above the level of the heart, and compress it with an elastic bandage to minimize swelling. Take care not to wrap the bandage too tightly—it can cut off circulation. Use ice for 48 hours after the injury or until all swelling is gone. (Because of the danger of frostbite, don't leave ice on one spot for more than 20 minutes at a time.) Over-the-counter medication that decreases inflammation, such as aspirin or ibuprofen, is also helpful in treating soft tissue injuries.

Don't use heat on an injury at first because heat draws blood to the area and increases swelling. However, after the swelling has subsided (usually about 24 to 48 hours after the injury occurred), apply heat to speed up healing. Heat helps relieve pain, relax muscles, and reduce stiffness. Check with your physician about whether moist heat (hot towels, heat packs) or dry heat (heating pads) is better for your particular injury. Whirlpools are a good way to combine heat and gentle massage.

To rehabilitate your body after a minor athletic injury, follow these four steps: (1) reduce the initial inflammation using the RICE principle (rest, ice, compression, elevation), (2) restore normal joint motion, (3) restore normal strength and endurance, and (4) restore normal function. This fourth step involves gradually reintroducing the stress of the activity until you are capable of returning to full intensity. Before returning to full exercise participation, you should have a full range of motion in your joints, normal strength and balance among your muscles, normal coordinated patterns of movement, with no injury compensation movements, such as limping, and little or no pain.

To prevent injuries in the future, follow a few basic guidelines: (1) stay in condition; haphazard exercise programs invite injury; (2) warm up thoroughly before exercise; (3) use proper body mechanics when lifting objects or executing sports skills; (4) don't exercise when you're ill or overtrained (extreme fatigue due to over-exercising); (5) use the proper equipment; and (6) don't return to your normal exercise program until athletic injuries have healed. Professional athletes appear to recover quickly from their injuries because they treat them promptly and correctly. You can keep your fitness program on track by doing the same.

Staying with Your Program

Once you have attained your desired level of fitness, you can maintain it by exercising on a regular basis at a consistent intensity, three to five times a week. You must work at the intensity that brought you to your desired fitness level. If you don't, your body will become less fit because less is expected of it. In general, if you exercise at the same intensity over a long period, your fitness will level out and can be maintained easily. Sometimes it's easiest to stay with a program

if you spend money to take a class or join a club. Community and Y programs are affordable for nearly anyone, but health clubs can be overpriced and their services of questionable value; see the box "Evaluating Health and Fitness Clubs" for some hints on choosing a good one. Exercising with a friend is also a good motivator.

What if you run out of steam? Although good health is an important *reason* to exercise, it's a poor *motivator* for consistent adherence to an exercise program. If you don't enjoy your program, you won't continue it for very long. It's easy to say, "Missing this workout isn't going to matter." Unfortunately, that missed workout can stretch into several weeks or months. But if you *select a physical activity that you like and look forward to, you will be much more faithful*. A variety of specific suggestions for staying with your program are given in the Behavior Change Strategy at the end of this chapter. It's also a good idea to have a goal, anything from fitting into the same size jeans you used to wear to successfully skiing down a new slope. Remember, you can have goals without striving to improve your fitness.

Varying your program is another way to stay interested. Some people alternate two or more activities—swimming and jogging, for example—to improve a particular component of fitness. The practice, called **cross-training**, can help prevent boredom and overuse injuries. It's a good idea to explore many exercise options. Consider competitive sports at the recreational level—swimming, running, racquetball, volleyball, golf, and so on. Find out how you can participate in an activity you've never done before—canoeing, hang gliding, windsurfing, backpacking. Try new activities, especially ones that you will be able to do for the rest of your life. Get maps of the park, recreational, or wilderness areas near you and go exploring. Fill a canteen, pack a good lunch, and take along a wildflower or bird book. Every step you take will bring you closer to your ultimate goal—fitness and health that last a lifetime.

Personal Insight Was exercise part of your family life when you were growing up? How much do your parents exercise? Do you think you're influenced by their attitudes and habits? How will you motivate your own children to exercise?

Cross-training Participating in two or more activities to develop a particular component of fitness.

TERMS

What Is Physical Fitness and Why Is It Important?

- The components of overall *physical fitness* include cardiorespiratory endurance; flexibility; muscular strength, power, and endurance; and body composition. Components of fitness for a specific activity might include coordination, speed, agility, balance, and skill.

- The body can improve its functioning; the level of physical fitness generally reflects the amount and intensity of physical activity.

- The body works best when it is active. By improving the overall functioning of the body, exercise can help in managing stress, maintaining emotional well-being, controlling weight, boosting the immune system, and protecting against serious diseases.

Why Is Exercise So Good for You?

- Cardiorespiratory endurance (or aerobic) exercise improves the ability of the heart, lungs, and circulatory system to carry oxygen to the body's tissues. This efficiency means that the heart doesn't have to work as hard in daily life and can meet emergency needs.

- Exercise has a positive effect on the balance of lipids in the blood; exercise increases HDLs and lowers LDLs. Exercise also decreases the secretion of hormones triggered by emotional stress and helps diffuse hostility.

- Endurance exercise improves the efficiency of the body's metabolism, helping to regulate energy balance and body weight.

- Exercise has social, psychological, and emotional benefits. Endorphins, secreted by the brain during exercise, help decrease pain, produce euphoria, and suppress fatigue.

- Exercises designed to improve muscular strength and endurance, joint flexibility, and posture are also essential to fitness.

- Beginning to exercise regularly can improve health over the life span. Physical fitness helps prevent heart disease, stroke, diabetes, and high blood pressure; it may help prevent fatigue, weight gain, memory loss, and other problems associated with aging. Exercise is especially helpful in preventing osteoporosis.

Designing Your Exercise and Fitness Program

- The best exercise and fitness programs develop all fitness components, promote health, and are fun to do. Activities should fit the personality; accessibility, expense, and time need to be considered as well.

- Cardiorespiratory endurance exercises stress a large portion of the body's muscle mass for a prolonged period of time.

- To be effective, endurance exercise should be undertaken three to five days a week and last from 20 minutes (high-intensity activities) to 60 minutes (low-intensity activities).

- Intensity of training is crucial to increasing the body's maximal oxygen capacity; monitoring the heart rate helps ensure that a workout is done at the appropriate intensity.

- Flexibility, or stretching, exercises are necessary to maintain the normal range of motion in the major joints of the body.

- Exercises to develop muscular strength and endurance are necessary for correct posture, efficient movement, and muscle tone. Resistive exercises are necessary to increase muscle strength.

- Learning the skills required for specific sports or activities helps people achieve a sense of mastery and adds new physical activities to their exercise programs.

- Warming up exercises decrease chances of injury by helping the body gradually progress from rest to exercise as blood is redirected to active muscles.

- Cooling down after exercise involves continuing to exercise at a low level to provide a smooth transition to the resting state.

Getting Started and Keeping on Track

- Good equipment enhances enjoyment and decreases risk of injury. Footwear is especially important; it should fit properly and be appropriate for the activity.

- A well-balanced diet contains all the energy and nutrients needed to sustain a fitness program. Increasing the proportion of carbohydrates can benefit some athletes.

- When exercising, it's important to drink enough water, which is necessary to prevent dehydration and maintain correct body temperature.

- Subjecting the body to severe stress will cause injury. Consistency leads to steady improvement.

- The ultimate level of fitness depends on the goals, the program, and natural ability. Fitness levels can be evaluated at sports medicine laboratories.

- Injuries that require medical attention include head and eye injuries, possible ligament injuries, broken bones, and internal disorders such as chest pain, fainting, and intolerance to heat.

- Rest, ice, compression, and elevation (RICE) are the appropriate treatments for muscle and joint injuries. Heat can be used after swelling has subsided.

- A desired level of fitness can be maintained by exercising three to five times a week at a consistent intensity. Ways to stay motivated include having specific goals, enjoying the activity, working out with a friend or group, and maintaining interest by varying the program.

TAKE ACTION

1. Go to your school's physical education office and ask for a comprehensive listing of all the exercise and fitness facilities available on your campus. Visit the facilities you haven't yet seen and investigate the activities that are done there. If there are sports or activities you'd like to try, consider doing so.
2. Investigate the fitness clubs in your community. How do they compare with each other, and how do they measure up in terms of the guidelines provided in this chapter?

JOURNAL ENTRY

1. In your health journal, list the positive behaviors and attitudes that help you avoid a sedentary lifestyle and stay fit. How can you strengthen these behaviors and attitudes? Then list the negative behaviors and attitudes that block a physically active lifestyle. Which ones can you change? How can you change them?
2. Habit helps us conserve energy as we go through our daily lives, but it also blinds us to areas we could change. Make a list of 10 ways you can incorporate more physical activity into your life by changing a habit, such as walking instead of riding the bus, taking the stairs in a certain building instead of the elevator, and so on.

3. *Critical Thinking:* Study the ads for fitness products and clubs on television, in popular magazines, and in your local newspaper. What markets are they targeting? How do they try to appeal to their audience? What other messages are they sending? Write a short essay describing your findings.

BEHAVIOR CHANGE STRATEGY

PLANNING A PERSONAL EXERCISE PROGRAM

Although most people recognize the importance of incorporating exercise into their lives, many find it difficult to do. No single strategy will work for everyone, but the general steps outlined here should help you create an exercise program that fits your goals, preferences, and lifestyle. A carefully designed contract and program plan can help you convert your vague wishes into a detailed plan of action. And the strategies for program compliance outlined here and in Chapter 1 can help you enjoy and stick with your program for the rest of your life.

Step 1: Set Goals

Setting specific goals to accomplish by exercising is an important first step in a successful fitness program because it establishes the direction you want to go. Your goals might be specifically related to health, such as lowering your blood pressure and risk for heart disease, or they might relate to other aspects of your life, such as improving your tennis game or the fit of your clothes. If you can decide why you're starting to exercise, it can help you to keep going.

Think carefully about your reasons for incorporating exercise into your life, and then fill in the goals portion of the Personal Fitness Contract.

Step 2: Select a Sport or Activity

As discussed in the chapter, the success of your fitness program depends upon the consistency of your involvement. You should select activities that encourage your commitment: The right program will be its own incentive to continue; poor activity choices provide obstacles and can turn exercise into a chore.

When choosing activities for your fitness program, you should consider the following:

- Is this activity fun? Will it hold my interest over time?
- Will this activity help me reach the goals I have set?
- Will my current fitness and skill level allow me to participate fully in this activity?
- Can I easily fit this activity into my daily schedule? Are there any special requirements (facilities, partners, equipment, etc.) that I must plan for?
- Can I afford any special costs required for equipment or facilities?
- (If you have special exercise needs due to a particular health problem.) Does this activity conform to my special health needs? Will it enhance my ability to cope with my specific health problem?

Refer to Table 14-3, which summarizes the fitness benefits and other characteristics of many activities. Using the guidelines listed above, select a number of sports and activities. Fill in the "Program Plan" portion of the Fitness Contract, using Table 14-3 to include the fitness components your choices will develop and the intensity, duration, and frequency standard you intend to meet for each activity. Does your program meet the criteria of a complete fitness program discussed in the chapter?

Personal Fitness Contract

I, _____ , am contracting with myself to follow an exercise program to work at the following goals.

Fitness Goals

(Note as many as appropriate)

1. _____
2. _____
3. _____
4. _____
5. _____

Program Plan

Activities	Components (Check ✓)					Intensity	Duration	Frequency (Check ✓)						
	CRE	BC	MS	ME	F			M.	Tu.	W.	Th.	F.	Sa.	Su.
1. _____														
2. _____														
3. _____														
4. _____														
5. _____														
6. _____														
7. _____														
8. _____														
9. _____														
10. _____														

I will begin my program on _____ .

I agree to maintain a record of my activity, assess my progress periodically, and, if necessary, revise my goals.

Signed _____   Date _____

Witness _____

Note: You should conduct activities for achieving CRE goals at your target heart rate.

Adapted from Ivan Kusinitz and Morton Fine. 1991. *Your Guide to Getting Fit*, 2nd ed. Mountain View, Calif.: Mayfield.

Step 3: Make a Commitment

Complete your Fitness Contract and Program Plan by signing your contract and having it witnessed and signed by someone who can help make you accountable for your progress. By completing a written contract you will make a firm commitment and will be more likely to follow through until you meet your goals.

Step 4: Begin and Maintain Your Program

Start out slowly to allow your body time to adjust. Be realistic and patient—meeting your goals will take time. The following guidelines may help you to start and stick with your program:

- Set aside regular periods for exercise. Choose times that fit in best with your schedule and stick to them. Allow an adequate amount of time for warm-up, cool-down, and a shower.

- Take advantage of any opportunity for exercise that presents itself (for example, walk to class, take the stairs instead of the elevator).

- Do what you can to avoid boredom. Do calisthenics to music or watch the evening news while riding your stationary bicycle.

- Exercise with a group that shares your goals and general level of competence.

- Vary the program. Change your activities periodically. Alter your route or distance if biking or jogging. Change racquetball partners or find a new volleyball court.

- Establish minigoals or a point system and work rewards into your program. Until you reach your main goals, a system of self-rewards will help you stick with your program. Rewards should be things you enjoy and that are easily obtainable.

Step 5: Record and Assess Your Progress

Keeping a record that notes the daily results of your program will help remind you of your ongoing commitment to your program and give you a sense of accomplishment. Create daily and weekly program logs that you can use to track your progress. You should record the activity type, frequency, and duration. Keep your log handy and fill it in immediately after each exercise session. Post it in a visible place to both remind you of your activity schedule and offer incentive for improvement.

Here are some additional tips to help make your program a success:

- If in the first few weeks you find that your program is unrealistic, revise the goals and activity information on your contract. Expect to make many adjustments in your program along the way.

- Don't expect your progress to be even and regular. You will notice fluctuations: On some days your progress will be excellent, while on others you will barely be able to drag yourself through the scheduled activities.

- Don't rush yourself. Overzealous exercising can result in discouraging discomforts and injuries. Your program is meant to last a lifetime, so begin slowly and increase your activity level gradually.

- If you notice that you are slacking off, try to list the negative thoughts and behaviors that are causing noncompliance. Devise a strategy to decrease the frequency of negative thoughts and behaviors. Adjust your program plan and reward system to help renew your enthusiasm and commitment to your program.

- Review your goals. Visualize what it will be like to reach them, and keep these pictures in your mind as an incentive to stick to your program.

SELECTED BIBLIOGRAPHY

American College of Sports Medicine. 1991. *Guidelines for Exercise Testing and Prescription*. Philadelphia: Lea and Feibiger.

Armstrong, R. B., G. L. Warren, and J. A. Warren. 1991. Mechanisms of exercise-induced muscle fibre injury. *Sports Medicine* 12:184–207.

Bielen, E., R. Fagard, and A. Amery. 1990. Inheritance of heart structure and physical exercise capacity: A study of left ventricular structure and exercise capacity in 7-year-old twins. *European Heart Journal* 11:7–16.

Blair, S. N., and H. W. Kohl. 1988. Physical activity or physical fitness: Which is more important for health? *Medical Science Sports Exercise* 20:S8.

Blair, S. N., H. W. Kohl, R. S. Paffenbarger, D. G. Clark, K. H. Cooper, and L. W. Gibbons. 1989. Physical fitness and all-cause mortality: A prospective study of healthy men and women. *Journal of the American Medical Association* 262:2395–2401.

Brooks, G. A., and T. D. Fahey. 1987. *Fundamentals of Human Performance*. New York: Macmillan.

Convertino, V. A., G. W. Mack, and E. R. Nadel. 1991. Elevated central venous pressure: A consequence of exercise training-induced hypervolemia? *American Journal Physiological* 29:R273–77.

DeLorme, R., and F. Stransky. 1990. *Fitness and Fallacies*. Dubuque, Iowa: Kendall/Hunt.

Fahey, T. D., ed. 1986. *Athletic Training: Principles and Practice*. Mountain View, Calif.: Mayfield.

Hickson, J. F., and I. Wolinsky. 1989. *Nutrition in Exercise and Sport*. Boca Raton, Fla.: CRC Press.

Jett, M., K. Sidney, and J. Campbell. 1988. Effects of a twelve-week walking programme on maximal and submaximal work output indices in sedentary middle aged men and women. *Journal of Sports Medicine and Physical Fitness* 28:59–66.

Komi, P. V., ed. 1992. *Strength and Power in Sports*. London: Blackwell Scientific Publications.

Manning, R. J., J. E. Graves, D. M. Carpenter, S. H. Leggett, and M. L. Pollock. 1990. Constant vs. variable resistance knee extension training. *Med. Sci. Sports Exerc.* 22:397–401.

Nieman, D. C. 1990. *Fitness and Sports Medicine: An Introduction*. Palo Alto, Calif.: Bull Publishing.

Noakes, T. D. 1988. Implications of exercise testing for prediction of athletic performance: A contemporary perspective. *Medicine and Science in Sports and Exercise* 20:319–30.

Porcari, J. P., C. B. Ebbeling, A. Ward, P. S. Freedson, and J. M. Rippe. 1989. Walking for exercise testing and training. *Sports Medicine* 8:189–200.

Rippe, J. M., A. Ward, and P. S. Freedson. 1987. Walking: Nothing pedestrian about it. *1988 Medical Health Annual*. Chicago: Encyclopedia Britannica.

Rogers, H. B., T. Schroeder, N. H. Secher, and J. H. Mitchell. 1990. Cerebral blood flow during static exercise in humans. *Journal of Applied Physiology*. 68:2358–61.

Rowell, L. B., and D. S. O'Leary. 1990. Reflex control of the circulation during exercise: Chemoreflexes and mechanoreflexes. *Journal of Applied Physiology*. 69:407–18.

Safran, M. R., A. V. Seaber, and W. E. Garrett. 1989. Warm-up and muscular injury prevention. *Sports Medicine* 8:239–49.

Sale, D. G. 1988. Neural adaptation to resistance training. *Medicine and Science in Sports and Exercise*. 20 (suppl.):S135–45.

Smith, M. L., D. L. Hudson, H. M. Graitzer, and P. B. Raven. 1989. Exercise training bradycardia: The role of autonomic balance. *Medicine and Science in Sports and Exercise*. 21:40–44.

United States Olympic Committee. 1989. *USOC Drug Education Handbook*. Colorado Springs: USOC.

RECOMMENDED READINGS

Anderson, B. 1980. *Stretching*. Bolinas, Calif.: Shelter Publications. *A complete guide to stretching that includes stretching programs for general fitness, for many sports and activities, and for care of the back.*

Cooper, K. 1983. *The Aerobics Program for Total Well-Being*. New York: Bantam Books. *A comprehensive guide to shaping up your heart and lungs.*

Fahey, T. 1994. *Basic Weight Training for Men and Women,* 2nd ed. Mountain View, Calif.: Mayfield. *A practical guide to developing training programs tailored to individual needs.*

Fahey, T. D., and G. Hutchinson. 1992. *Weight Training for Women.* Mountain View, Calif.: Mayfield. *A practical guide to developing a healthier, stronger body that contains complete coverage of topics of special interest to women.*

Kan, E., and M. Kraines. 1991. *Keep Moving! It's Aerobic Dance.* 2nd ed. Mountain View, Calif.: Mayfield. *Discusses the fitness principles and techniques every aerobic dancer should know.*

Kusinitz, I., and M. Fine. 1991. *Your Guide to Getting Fit.* 2nd ed. Mountain View, Calif.: Mayfield. *A step-by-step guide to developing a personalized fitness program.*

Maglischo, E. W., and C. F. Brennan. 1984. *Swim for the Health of It.* Mountain View, Calif.: Mayfield. *Includes discussions of conditioning and stroke techniques for people who want to use swimming to improve their health and physical fitness.*

Meyers, C. 1992. *Walking: A Complete Guide to the Complete Exercise.* New York: Random House. *Offers strategies for putting together individualized walking programs for weight control and cardiovascular fitness.*

Nokes, T. D. 1991. *Lore of Running.* 3rd ed. Champaign, Ill.: Human Kinetics. *A comprehensive guide that includes discussions of the physiology of running; training for running; and recognizing, avoiding, and treating running injuries.*

Van der Plas, R. 1990. *The Bicycle Fitness Book: Riding Your Bike for Health and Fitness.* Rev. ed. Mill Valley, Calif.: Bicycle Books. *Includes practical advice on choosing equipment, riding safely, and putting together a personal training program.*

15

Cardiovascular Health

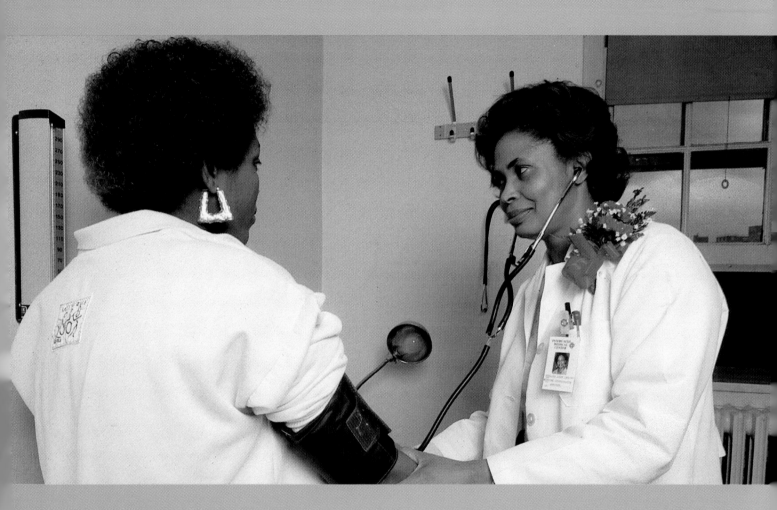

CONTENTS

The student health center sponsored a health fair on campus last week, and just for fun you decided to have your blood pressure tested. It turned out to be high. The nurse said you should see a physician so you can repeat the test and, if necessary, set up a program to lower it. You're tempted to ignore the whole episode. You're young and in good shape and you feel great. You figure it will be another 20 or 30 years before you have to start worrying about blood pressure and heart disease. Are you right? Could someone who feels as good as you do actually have high blood pressure? Should you see a physician just in case?

You've tried, but your busy college schedule won't accommodate the rigorous, five-day-a-week, 90-minute running and weight training program you followed in high school. You figure it's okay to quit exercising for a while now—you'll resume your exercise regimen after graduation, when you'll have more free time. But one of your housemates thinks differently—she says that not exercising is bad for your health and that even a small amount of easy exercise is better than none. She walks everywhere, plus takes a half-hour bike ride around campus several times a week. To you, that hardly sounds like exercise and certainly doesn't seem worth the time. You've always believed in doing something right or not at all. Is what your housemate says true? Could such a small amount of exercise be good for your health?

Your roommate had to fly home last week because his father had a heart attack and was in intensive care at the hospital. When he came back, he told you that his father's condition was quite serious, partly because he had waited several hours after the attack before going to the hospital. Your roommate says his father had some pain in his arm and felt dizzy but didn't connect these symptoms with his heart. You're surprised. Isn't it obvious when you're having a heart attack? What are the signs of a heart attack anyway?

One day when you were visiting your grandmother, a strange thing happened. She was standing in the kitchen when suddenly she became so dizzy she had to sit down. When you asked her what was wrong, she was able only to mumble some sounds you couldn't understand. Then just as suddenly, she was fine again. You were greatly relieved that she recovered but concerned about what had happened. You wanted her to call her physician, but she said it was just one of her spells and nothing to be alarmed about. Is she all right? What should she do if it happens again? What should you do?

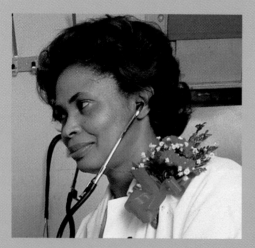

MAKING CONNECTIONS

Cardiovascular disease is so common in our society that you or someone you know is very likely to fall victim to it. The habits you adopt now can make a big difference in whether you keep your healthy heart or develop one of the debilitating cardiovascular diseases. In each of the scenarios presented on this page, all related to cardiovascular health, individuals have to use information, make a decision, or choose a course of action. How would you act in each of these situations? What response or decision would you make? This chapter provides information about cardiovascular health and disease that can be used in situations like these. After finishing the chapter, read the scenarios again. Has what you've learned changed how you would respond?

Cardiovascular disease (CVD) is the leading cause of death in the United States, claiming one life every 34 seconds. More Americans die from diseases of the heart and blood vessels than from cancer, accidents, emphysema, pneumonia, influenza, suicide, and HIV infection combined (Figure 15-1). In fact, almost half of all Americans living today will die from CVD. Though we typically think of CVD as primarily affecting men and the elderly, heart attack is the number one killer of American women. And 45 percent of heart attacks and 28 percent of strokes occur in people younger than 65 years of age (see the box "CVD in America: A Statistical Summary").

Not all the news about CVD is bad, however. The lifestyle changes and medical advances that have occurred in recent years have led to significant progress in the fight against CVD. Since 1979, the death rate from heart attack in this country has fallen 30 percent; deaths from strokes have dropped by 31.5 percent. Because lifestyle is such an important factor in the development of CVD, there is a great deal you can do to reduce your risk of developing CVD. People who are most vulnerable to early heart attacks or strokes are smokers, those with uncontrolled high blood pressure, those with unhealthy cholesterol profiles, and those who are overweight and inactive.

Exactly what is CVD, and how does it do its damage? More important, what steps can you take now to make sure you keep your heart healthy throughout your life? This chapter provides some answers to these questions.

THE CARDIOVASCULAR SYSTEM

The **cardiovascular system** consists of the heart and the blood vessels (veins, arteries, and capillaries); together they pump and circulate blood throughout the body. Blood travels through two separate circulatory systems, the right and left sides of the heart. The right side pumps blood to and from the lungs; this is called the **pulmonary circulation.** The left side pumps blood through the rest of the body; this is called the **systemic circulation** (Figure 15-2). A person weighing 150 pounds has about 5 quarts of blood, which is circulated about once every minute.

The heart is a four-chambered muscle, shaped like a cone and about the size of a fist (Figure 15-3). It is located just beneath the ribs, under the left breast. Its role is to pump oxygen-depleted blood to the lungs and to pump oxygenated blood to the rest of the body. Used, oxygen-depleted blood enters the right upper chamber, or **atrium,** of the heart through the **vena cava,** the largest vein in the body. Valves prevent it from flowing the wrong way. As it fills, the right atrium contracts and pumps blood into the right lower chamber, or **ventricle,** which, when it contracts, pumps blood through the **pulmonary artery** into the lungs. There blood picks up oxygen and discards carbon dioxide. Cleaned, oxygenated blood then

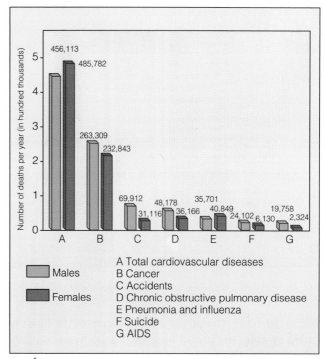

 VITAL STATISTICS

Figure 15-1 *Leading causes of death for men and women.*

flows through the pulmonary veins into the left atrium. As this chamber fills, it contracts and pumps blood into the powerful left ventricle. When the left ventricle contracts, blood is pumped through the **aorta,** the body's largest artery, which feeds into the rest of the blood ves-

Cardiovascular disease (CVD) Diseases of the heart and blood vessels.

Cardiovascular system The heart and blood vessels.

Pulmonary circulation The portion of the circulatory system governed by the right side of the heart; the circulation of blood between the heart and the lungs.

Systemic circulation The portion of the circulatory system governed by the left side of the heart; the circulation of blood between the heart and the rest of the body.

Atria The two upper chambers of the heart in which blood collects before passing to the ventricles; also called auricles (*sing.* atrium).

Vena cava Large vein through which blood is returned to the right atrium of the heart.

Ventricles The two lower chambers of the heart from which blood flows through arteries to the lungs and other parts of the body.

Pulmonary artery The artery that receives blood from the right ventricle and carries it to the lungs.

Aorta The large artery that receives blood from the left ventricle and distributes it to the body.

TERMS

- *CVD* in all its forms kills about 930,000 Americans per year. That's one death every 34 seconds. One in two Americans dies of CVD. One-fifth of the victims are under age 65.

- *High blood pressure* afflicts about 63.6 million Americans. About 33,000 die from it each year.

- *Coronary heart disease* afflicts 6.2 million Americans. 1.5 million will have a heart attack this year. 500,000 of them will die.

- *Stroke* strikes about 500,000 Americans each year. It kills 150,000 a year.

- *Rheumatic heart disease* afflicts 1.3 million Americans. It kills about 6,000 every year.

- *CVD* is not an equal-opportunity disease. The death rate for African American men is 37 percent higher than for white men. The death rate for African American women is 64 percent higher than for white women.

- *CVD* will cost the nation about $117.4 billion in 1993 for medical services and lost productivity.

Source: The American Heart Association. 1993. *Heart and Stroke Facts.*

---

sels in the body. The period of contraction of the heart is called **systole;** the period of relaxation between contractions is called **diastole.**

The action of the heart is controlled by electrical impulses that trigger the split-second sequence of contractions of the heart's four chambers—what we call the heartbeat. The electrical signal originates in a bundle of specialized cells located in the right atrium. The signal from this natural **pacemaker** moves across both atria, causing the muscle cells to contract. After both atria have contracted, the electrical message travels over specialized fibers in the ventricles, causing them to contract together in a wringing motion. The heart produces electrical impulses at a steady rate unless the brain signals it to speed up or slow down in response to such stimuli as danger or exhaustion.

Blood vessels are classified by size and function. Veins carry blood *to* the heart, arteries carry it *away* from the heart. Arteries have thick elastic walls that enable them to expand and relax as blood is pumped into them under pressure from the heart. Veins have thinner walls. After leaving the heart, the aorta branches into smaller and smaller arteries. Two vital arteries branch off the aorta to carry blood back to the tissues of the heart itself; these are the **coronary arteries** (Figure 15-4). The smallest arteries, called **arterioles,** branch still further into **capillaries,** tiny vessels only one cell thick.

An exchange of nutrients and waste products takes place between the capillaries and the tissues, so that the oxygen- and nutrient-rich blood becomes oxygen-poor, waste-carrying blood. This blood empties out of the capillaries into small veins called **venules,** then into the larger veins that return it to the heart. From there the cycle is repeated.

TERMS

Systole   Contraction of the heart.

Diastole   Relaxation of the heart.

Pacemaker   The natural "pacemaker" is a small bundle of specialized cells in the right atrium; it emits electrical signals that cause the heart to contract. An artificial pacemaker is an electrical device that can regulate heartbeat by emitting rhythmic electrical impulses.

Coronary arteries   Two arteries branching from the aorta that provide blood to the heart muscle.

Arterioles   The smallest arteries that end in capillaries.

Capillaries   Very small blood vessels that distribute blood to all parts of the body.

Venules   Small veins.

High-density lipoproteins (HDLs)   Blood fats that help transport cholesterol out of the arteries and thus protect against heart diseases.

Platelets   Microscopic disk-shaped cell fragments in the blood. These disintegrate on contact with foreign objects and release chemicals that are necessary for the formation of blood clots.

Hypertension   Sustained abnormally high blood pressure.

Atherosclerosis   The principal form of arteriosclerosis; in atherosclerosis, the inner layers of artery walls are made thick and irregular by deposits of a fatty substance. The internal channel of arteries becomes narrowed, and blood supply is reduced.

RISK FACTORS FOR CARDIOVASCULAR DISEASE

Researchers have identified a variety of factors associated with increased risk for cardiovascular disease. Some of these, such as age and gender, are beyond an individual's control. But many of them are linked to controllable lifestyle factors such as diet, exercise habits, and ways of dealing with stress. CVD can begin in childhood, so to protect yourself you need to intervene early to change those risk factors you can control.

Major Risk Factors

The American Heart Association has identified four major risk factors linked to the development of CVD. These are tobacco use, high blood pressure, unhealthy blood cholesterol levels, and physical inactivity.

Tobacco Use People who smoke a pack of cigarettes a day have twice the risk of heart attack that nonsmokers have; smoking two or more packs a day triples the risk. And when smokers do have heart attacks, they are two to four times more likely than nonsmokers to die from them. Women who smoke and use oral contraceptives are up to 39 times more likely to have a heart attack and up to 22 times more likely to have a stroke than are women who neither smoke nor take the pill.

Smoking harms the cardiovascular system in several ways. Smoking can reduce levels of **high-density lipoproteins (HDL)**, the so-called "good cholesterol," in the bloodstream. The psychoactive drug in tobacco, nicotine, is a central nervous system stimulant, causing increased blood pressure and heart rate. The carbon monoxide in cigarette smoke displaces oxygen in the blood, reducing the amount of oxygen available to the heart and other parts of the body. Cigarette smoking also causes the **platelets** in blood to become sticky and cluster, shortens platelet survival, decreases clotting time, and increases blood thickness. All these effects increase a person's risk of heart attack and other cardiovascular disease.

You don't have to smoke to be affected. Environmental tobacco smoke (ETS) in high concentrations has been linked to the development of cardiovascular disease. One recent study found that nonsmokers who are regularly exposed to cigarette smoke have significantly more blockage in their coronary arteries than do nonsmokers with no exposure to ETS. Living or working with smokers for a long period of time may be a significant risk factor for CVD.

Smokers' risk for CVD drops rapidly after quitting, regardless of how long or how much they've smoked. Ten years after quitting, a former smoker has about the same risk for CVD as a person who has never smoked. (For more on the effects of tobacco use and suggestions for quitting, see Chapter 9.)

High Blood Pressure High blood pressure (**hypertension**) is a risk factor for many types of cardiovascular disease but is also considered a form of disease itself. High blood pressure occurs when too much force or pressure is exerted against the walls of the arteries. If your blood pressure is high, your heart has to work harder to push the blood forward. Over time, a strained heart weakens and tends to enlarge, which weakens it further. Increased blood pressure also scars and hardens arteries and arterioles, making them less elastic. Heart attacks, strokes, **atherosclerosis,** and kidney failure can result. High blood

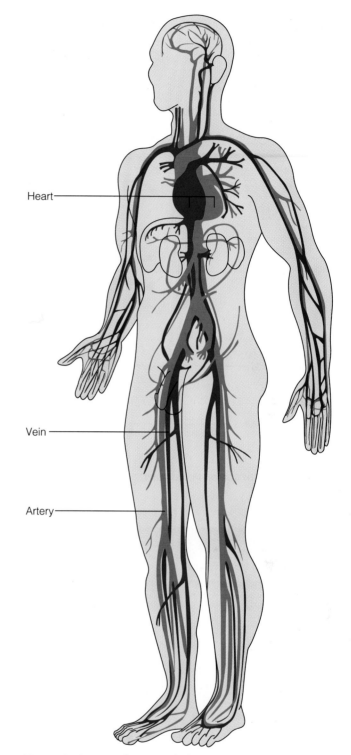

Heart

Vein

Artery

Figure 15-2 *Circulation in the body.*

pressure usually has no early warning signs, so it's important to have your blood pressure tested at least once a year. If yours is high, your physician can help you lower it through diet, weight management, exercise, and, if necessary, medication. (High blood pressure and atherosclerosis are discussed in greater detail later in the chapter.)

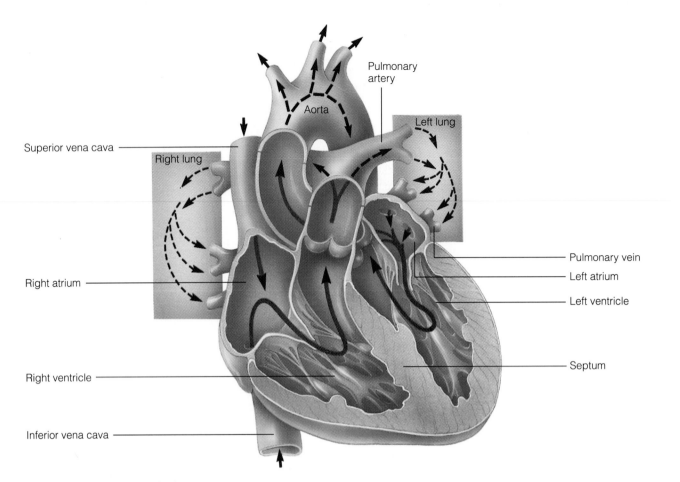

Figure 15-3 *Circulation in the heart.*

TABLE 15-1 Cholesterol Guidelines	
Total blood cholesterol	
Less than 200 mg/dl	Desirable
200–239 mg/dl	Borderline high
240 mg/dl or more	High
LDL cholesterol	
Less than 130 mg/dl	Desirable
130–159 mg/dl	Borderline high
160 mg/dl or more	High
HDL cholesterol	
The higher the level of HDL cholesterol, the lower the risk of CVD. Average HDL levels are 45 mg/dl for American men and 55 mg/dl for American women; levels below 35 mg/dl are considered undesirable.	

Source: The National Cholesterol Education Program.

Cholesterol   Cholesterol is a fatty, waxlike substance, or lipid, that circulates through the bloodstream and is an important component of cell membranes, sex hormones, vitamin D, **lung surfactant,** and the protective sheaths around nerves. Adequate cholesterol is essential for the proper functioning of the body. However, excess cholesterol can clog arteries and increase the risk of cardiovascular disease. New evidence also suggests that very low levels of cholesterol may be associated with an increased risk of death from other causes.

Our bodies obtain cholesterol in two ways: from the liver, which manufactures it, and from the foods we eat. If our blood contains more of the "bad" type of cholesterol than we can use or dispose of, the excess is deposited on artery walls.

Cholesterol Testing   The first step in controlling cholesterol is to have your total blood cholesterol level tested. The National Cholesterol Education Program (NCEP) recommends testing for all adults at least once every five years, beginning at age 20, or at least every three years if there is a family history of heart disease. However, some experts feel that women under age 50 do not need to have their cholesterol tested unless they have at least one CVD

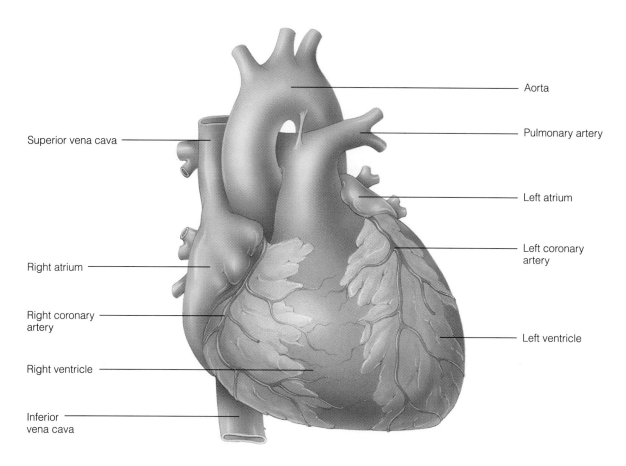

Superior vena cava

Right atrium

Right coronary
artery

Right ventricle

Inferior
vena cava

Aorta

Pulmonary artery

Left atrium

Left coronary
artery

Left ventricle

Figure 15-4 *Blood supply to the heart.*

risk factor. "Desirable" total cholesterol readings are 200 milligrams per deciliter of blood (mg/dl) or lower. Readings of 240 mg/dl or above are considered "high"; readings between 200 and 240 mg/dl are "borderline high" (Table 15-1). An estimated 30.4 percent of women and 26.7 percent of men ages 20 to 24 have total cholesterol levels of 200 mg/dl or higher.

The NCEP advises people with borderline high or high cholesterol levels to begin a cholesterol-lowering diet immediately (see below). Experts calculate that people can cut their heart attack risk by 2 percent for every 1 percent that they reduce their total blood cholesterol levels. People who lower their total cholesterol from 250 to 200 mg/dl, for example, reduce their risk of heart attack by 40 percent. In addition, studies indicate that lowering total blood cholesterol levels not only reduces the likelihood that arteries will become clogged, but it can also reverse deposits on artery walls, actually helping to clean out diseased arteries.

It's recommended that people with high total cholesterol, as well as those with borderline high readings who have other risk factors for CVD, have an additional test to determine the proportions of different types of cholesterol in their blood.

Good Versus Bad Cholesterol   Cholesterol is carried in the blood in protein-lipid packages called lipoproteins. Lipoproteins can be thought of as one-way shuttles that transport cholesterol to and from the liver through the circulatory system (Figure 15-5). **Low-density lipoproteins (LDLs)** are known as "bad" cholesterol because they shuttle cholesterol from the liver to the organs and tissues that require it. If the LDLs transport more cholesterol than the body can use, the excess is deposited in the blood vessels. When it accumulates, it can block arteries and cause heart attacks and strokes. High-density lipoproteins (HDLs), or "good" cholesterol, shuttle unused cholesterol back to the liver for recycling. High LDL levels and low HDL levels are associated with high risk for CVD; low levels of LDL and high levels of HDL are associated with lower risk (see Table 15-1).

Lung surfactant   Chemical fluid coating the surface of the lungs that lowers surface tension, aids in gas exchange, and helps keep the lungs from collapsing.

Low-density lipoproteins (LDLs)   Blood fats that transport cholesterol from the liver to organs and tissues; excess is deposited on artery walls, where it can eventually block the flow of blood to the heart and brain.

TERMS

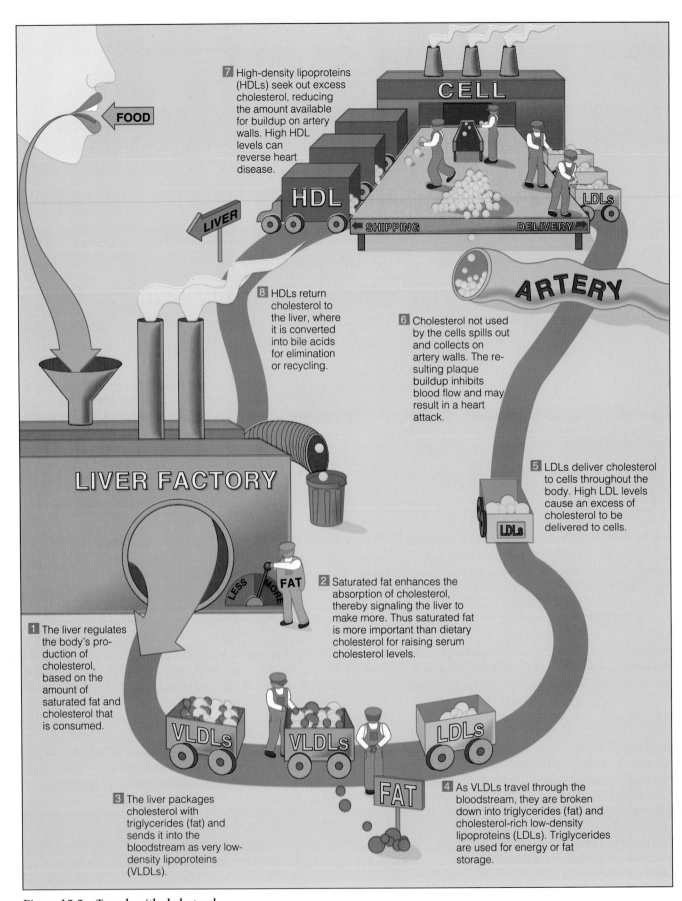

FOOD

7 High-density lipoproteins (HDLs) seek out excess cholesterol, reducing the amount available for buildup on artery walls. High HDL levels can reverse heart disease.

CELL

HDL

LIVER

SHIPPING

DELIVERY

LDLs

ARTERY

8 HDLs return cholesterol to the liver, where it is converted into bile acids for elimination or recycling.

6 Cholesterol not used by the cells spills out and collects on artery walls. The resulting plaque buildup inhibits blood flow and may result in a heart attack.

LIVER FACTORY

5 LDLs deliver cholesterol to cells throughout the body. High LDL levels cause an excess of cholesterol to be delivered to cells.

LDLs

LESS MORE FAT

2 Saturated fat enhances the absorption of cholesterol, thereby signaling the liver to make more. Thus saturated fat is more important than dietary cholesterol for raising serum cholesterol levels.

1 The liver regulates the body's production of cholesterol, based on the amount of saturated fat and cholesterol that is consumed.

VLDLs   VLDLs   LDLs

FAT

3 The liver packages cholesterol with triglycerides (fat) and sends it into the bloodstream as very low-density lipoproteins (VLDLs).

4 As VLDLs travel through the bloodstream, they are broken down into triglycerides (fat) and cholesterol-rich low-density lipoproteins (LDLs). Triglycerides are used for energy or fat storage.

Figure 15-5 *Travels with cholesterol.*

The national plan to educate people about cholesterol has come under fire from various quarters almost since it began. Critics point out that the studies on which the National Cholesterol Education Program's guidelines are based involved only middle-aged men with very unhealthy levels of cholesterol. They question the applicability of the guidelines for other groups. Women, for example, generally have a different cholesterol and heart disease profile than men, with high levels of HDL and lower rates of heart attack, especially before menopause. The elderly were also excluded from most of the clinical trials, even though they suffer the vast majority of heart attacks. Cholesterol rises with age, and many older people do have elevated cholesterol; but the link between cholesterol level and coronary disease weakens with age, particularly in men.

Some prominent heart experts question whether the elderly, children, and those not at high risk ought to follow the dietary recommendations for lowering cholesterol. Other countries with similar rates of CVD have not adopted such a far-reaching strategy, which involves testing a huge number of seemingly healthy people and adopting long-term treatments in order to avoid a possibly modest number of heart attacks. There is concern about potential long-term side effects if patients resort to a lifetime of cholesterol-lowering drugs. Critics point out that although lowering cholesterol is associated with a lowered number of heart attacks, it isn't associated with reduced mortality. Very low cholesterol levels may actually increase the death rate from causes other than heart disease.

Critics also believe the emphasis on cholesterol diverts attention from other factors like cigarette smoking, which is the number one risk factor for CVD. In addition, preliminary research suggests that iron may deserve as much attention as cholesterol as a risk factor for cardiovascular disease (see box elsewhere in this chapter).

Proponents of the cholesterol-lowering plan concede that not every aspect of their advice is based on irreproachable data, and they do not recommend that people focus on cholesterol to the exclusion of other risk factors. However, they argue that cholesterol reduction does no harm, that reducing saturated fats in the diet has other benefits, and that the guidelines may well prevent heart attacks in many people. They believe that early lifestyle changes are the only way to change the rate of heart disease in the United States. Many people can reduce their cholesterol levels by an average of 10 percent if they follow a diet low in saturated fat and so will never have to resort to drugs to lower cholesterol.

What is the average American to make of all this? First of all, the focus on cholesterol shouldn't distract people from the importance of other risk factors, such as smoking, high blood pressure, and a sedentary lifestyle. Second, although not everyone needs to make dietary changes (genetic and other factors allow some people to eat just about anything they want without raising their cholesterol levels), most people do not benefit from a diet high in calories and saturated fat. A diet low in fat and high in fiber is a reasonable goal for every American.

Adapted from G. Kolata. "Cholesterol's New Image: High Is Bad; So Is Low." *The New York Times*, 11 August 1992, p. C1, and 26 September 1989, p. C1; T. Johnson. "The Cholesterol Controversy." *Harvard Medical School Health Letter*, December 1989.

Can Cholesterol Be Too Low?   Some recent evidence suggests that very low levels of cholesterol may be unhealthy. Studies have found that the death rate for people with total cholesterol levels below 160 mg/dl is equivalent to the death rate for people with very high cholesterol levels. For example, very low cholesterol is associated with an increased risk of certain strokes. The reason may be that blood needs a minimum concentration of cholesterol and fats to clot effectively, and impaired clotting ability is a risk factor for this type of stroke. People with very low cholesterol levels also have an increased risk of certain cancers, liver disease, and lung disease. It's possible that lack of adequate cholesterol interferes with the production of crucial materials such as sex hormones and lung surfactant. The findings about very low cholesterol levels are still preliminary, and no guidelines regarding low cholesterol have been established. However, some cardiovascular disease experts suggest that cholesterol levels between 180 and 200 mg/dl may be optimal. (See the box "Cholesterol: Crusades and Controversies" for more information on this and other cholesterol-related issues.)

A Dietary Plan for Controlling Cholesterol   For most Americans, changing their diets to lower their total cholesterol level means cutting total fat intake and substituting unsaturated fats for saturated fats. The NCEP recommends that all Americans over the age of 2 adopt a diet in which total fat consumption is no more than 30 percent of total daily caloric intake. No more than one-third of those fat calories should come from saturated fat, which is found in animal products, palm and coconut oil, and hydrogenated vegetable oils. Saturated fat influences the production and excretion of cholesterol by the liver, so decreasing your saturated fat intake is the most important dietary change you can make to control your cholesterol.

One-third or more of your fat calories should come from monounsaturated fats, such as olive or canola oil; intake of these oils may raise HDL levels. And up to one-third of your fat calories should come from polyunsaturated fats, which may help you lower your total cholesterol level without reducing HDL.

Animal products contain cholesterol as well as saturated fat. The NCEP recommends limiting dietary choles-

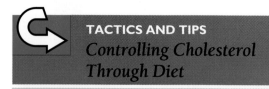
A diet that improves cholesterol levels is high in dietary fiber and low in fat, saturated fat, and cholesterol. To lower your risk for CVD, try some of these dietary changes.

Decrease Intake	Increase Intake
Whole milk	Nonfat and low-fat milk
Hard cheeses, cream cheese	Cottage cheese, low-fat yogurt
Beef, pork, sausage, bacon	Fish, skinless chicken, turkey
Butter, high-fat mayonnaise	Mustard, vegetable oil
Ice cream	Sherbet, frozen yogurt
Palm and coconut oils	Olive and vegetable oils
Many luncheon meats	Turkey, chicken meats
Many prepared baked goods	Fruits, vegetables
Egg yolks (egg whites are OK)	Beans, cereals, pasta, bread

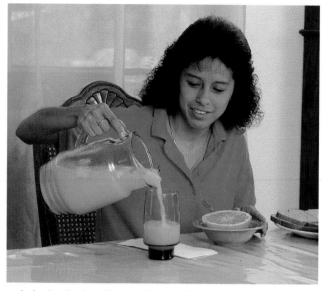

A daily diet high in fiber and low in fat and saturated fat can help lower levels of total cholesterol and LDLs. This young woman is off to a good start with a low-fat breakfast of whole wheat toast, fruit, and juice.

terol to 300 mg or less per day, slightly more than the amount in one egg. (Vegetable products do not contain cholesterol.)

Research has linked other dietary factors to improving cholesterol levels. Dietary fiber can help reduce cholesterol by trapping the bile acids the liver needs to manufacture cholesterol and carrying them to the large intestine, where they are excreted. Good sources of fiber include wheat bran, oatmeal, psyllium, barley, legumes, apples, pears, figs, and the pulp of citrus fruits. Omega-3 fatty acids, found in fish and shellfish, may also be helpful in lowering cholesterol. Some experts recommend eating fish or seafood two or three times a week; fish-oil capsules are not recommended, however, because they have not been proven effective and they add calories and fat to the diet. Alcohol, particularly certain components of red wine, has been shown to increase HDL cholesterol levels. However, experts don't recommend alcohol consumption as a strategy for preventing CVD either. The other risks of alcohol, including automobile crashes and alcoholism, outweigh any potential benefits.

No Quick Fix   Some people seize on a particular food as a "magic bullet" against heart disease. They may begin frying everything in olive oil, popping fish-oil capsules, or eating half a dozen oat bran muffins a day. However, if they don't reduce their fat and saturated fat consumption,

they won't be doing themselves any good. Substituting a tablespoon of olive or canola oil for a tablespoon of butter may be helpful; but adding a tablespoon of new oil to your diet—without subtracting a tablespoon of fat elsewhere—will not. The box "Controlling Cholesterol Through Diet" summarizes nutrition advice for improving cholesterol levels; refer back to Chapter 12 for additional hints on lowering fat intake and including more fiber in your diet.

Two other steps in cholesterol control are regular exercise and smoking cessation. Smoking lowers your HDL. Exercise, which is the closest thing to a "magic bullet" against disease, raises HDL.

Physical Inactivity   In 1992, the American Heart Association elevated a sedentary lifestyle to the ranks of major risk factors for CVD, putting it on a par with smoking, unhealthy cholesterol levels, and high blood pressure. Lack of exercise had previously been considered only a contributing factor. Exercise lowers CVD risk by helping to decrease blood pressure, increase HDL levels, maintain desirable weight, and prevent or control diabetes.

An estimated 35 to 50 million Americans are so sedentary that they are at high risk for developing CVD. They can reduce their risk significantly with as little as 90 minutes a week of mild exercise like walking, gardening, or bowling. Moving from a mild exercise program to a moderate one—say 30 minutes to an hour of brisk walking or cycling, four or more times a week—reduces risk even more. Moving from a moderate to an intense program provides little added benefit in terms of CVD prevention, although intense exercise can improve your strength, endurance, and athletic performance. See Chapter 14 for information on developing a complete, personalized exercise program.

Contributing Risk Factors

Various other factors have been identified as contributing to risk for cardiovascular disease, including overweight, diabetes, responses to stress, personality type, and social factors.

Overweight   A person whose body weight is more than 30 percent above the recommended level is at higher risk for heart disease and stroke even if no other risk factors are present. Excess weight increases the strain on the heart by contributing to high blood pressure and high cholesterol. It can also lead to diabetes, another CVD risk factor (see below). As discussed in Chapter 13, the distribution of body fat is also significant: Fat that collects in the torso is more dangerous than fat that collects around the hips. A prudent diet and regular exercise are the best ways to achieve and maintain a healthy body weight. Avoid yo-yo dieting—evidence suggests that repeatedly losing and regaining weight may be more harmful to the cardiovascular system than living with some excess weight.

Diabetes   As described in Chapter 12, diabetes is a nutrition-related disorder in which the body produces insufficient insulin to metabolize glucose. People with diabetes are at increased risk for CVD because the disease affects the levels of cholesterol in the blood. Diabetes appears to have both a genetic component and a behavioral component. The best way to avoid diabetes is to exercise regularly and control body weight.

Stress   Excessive stress may contribute to CVD over time. If the alarm reaction (the "fight-or-flight" response) is triggered repeatedly, it can put a strain on the heart and blood vessels. In addition, people sometimes adopt unhealthy habits as a means of dealing with severe stress; they may start smoking, overeating, or skipping meals. (See Chapter 2 for information on effective strategies for managing stress.)

Psychological and Social Factors   In the 1970s, two astute cardiologists noticed that people with hard-driving, aggressive personalities had a high incidence of heart disease. They dubbed this heart-attack-prone personality "Type A"; its laid-back, healthier counterpart was termed "Type B." In the 1980s, further research found that only certain traits in the Type A personality—hostility, cynicism, and anger—increase the risk for heart disease. For more information on this connection, see the box "Hostility and CVD."

Other links between personality and CVD are the subject of ongoing research. Several recent studies suggest that people who hide psychological distress—even from themselves—have a higher rate of heart disease than people who experience similar distress but share it with others. Lack of social support has also been linked with an increased risk for CVD. Low socioeconomic status and low educational attainment are other risk factors. These associations are probably due to a variety of factors, including lifestyle and access to health care.

Risk Factors That Can't Be Changed

Not everyone is equal when it comes to cardiovascular disease. Some segments of the population have a much higher risk than others.

- *Heredity.* The tendency to develop CVD seems to be inherited. If your father or mother has had heart or blood vessel disease, you are at greater risk of developing CVD yourself. High cholesterol levels, abnormal blood clotting problems, diabetes, and obesity are other CVD risk factors that have genetic links. It's important to remember that people who inherit a tendency for CVD aren't destined to develop it. They may, however, have to work harder than other people to prevent cardiovascular problems.

- *Age.* The risk of heart attack increases dramatically after age 65. About 55 percent of all heart attack victims are age 65 or older, and almost four out of five who suffer fatal heart attacks are over 65. But cardiovascular disease is no longer considered a disease solely of old age. Many people in their thirties and forties, especially men, have heart attacks (Figure 15-6).

- *Gender.* Although CVD is the leading killer of both men and women in the United States, rates are three to four times higher for men than women during the middle decades of life. Later in life, CVD is twice as common in men than in women. Estrogen production, which is highest in the childbearing

Current research indicates that individuals who have a persistently hostile outlook, a quick temper, and a mistrusting, cynical attitude toward life are more likely to develop heart disease than are individuals with a calmer, more trusting attitude. Why should this be the case? What is the link between chronic hostility and the heart?

The connection is most likely to be found in the physiological mechanism of the stress response (see Chapter 2). Studies show that people who are prone to chronic hostility experience the stress response more intensely and frequently than do more relaxed individuals. When they encounter the irritations of daily life, their blood pressure increases much more than is the case for less hostile people. They also seem to have trouble shutting down the stress response. Less hostile people tend to calm down much more quickly, taking the stress off their bodies—especially their hearts.

Are You Hostile?

How hostile do you think you are? To get an idea, read the following questions and respond to each with *never, sometimes, often,* or *always.*

- When people do things (or fail to do things) that prevent you from doing what you want to do, do you begin to think that they are selfish, mean, inconsiderate, incompetent, or stupid?

- When people do things that strike you as messy, selfish, inconsiderate, incompetent, or stupid, do you quickly experience feelings of frustration, irritation, anger, or rage?

- When you experience the feelings mentioned above, are they accompanied by physical sensations like increases in heart rate, breathing rate, perspiration, and so on?

- When you have these experiences, are you likely to express your feelings, whether in words, body language, facial expression, or action, to the person you see as responsible?

If you answer *often* or *always* to two or more of these questions, it's likely that your level of hostility is creating a health risk for you.

Developing a "Trusting Heart"

According to Redford Williams, noted researcher and author of *The Trusting Heart* and *Anger Kills,* hostile people can learn to change their attitudes and, in doing so, reduce their risk of heart disease. Just as hostility increases the risk of heart disease, having a trusting heart—being slow to anger, expecting the best of others, and spending minimal time feeling resentful, irritable, and angry—appears to prevent heart disease. Williams has created a 12-point behavior modification plan for developing a more trusting—and healthier—heart:

1. Monitor your cynical thoughts, recording them in a journal, and then analyze the record to learn more about the situations that trigger these responses.

2. Acknowledge your cynicism and hostility, and seek support for change from a friend or family member.

3. Stop hostile thoughts when you notice them coming on. Silently shout "STOP!" or, if you're alone, go ahead and yell out loud.

4. Use reason to talk yourself out of your hostile thoughts. Is it really likely, for example, that the person driving so slowly up ahead is doing so simply to torment you?

5. Put yourself in the other person's shoes. Empathy and anger are incompatible.

6. Learn to laugh at yourself when you're getting hostile.

7. Practice the relaxation response, using one of the methods described in Chapter 2, to calm yourself down.

8. Practice trust—look for opportunities to entrust yourself to others. Begin with simple situations in which you have little to lose, such as letting a friend choose a restaurant or pick your seats at a movie.

9. Learn to listen. If you're in the habit of interrupting, force yourself to let others finish before you speak.

10. Learn to be assertive without being aggressive. Situations do occur in which you're treated unfairly and an appropriate response is justified. To be assertive without being aggressive, follow these guidelines: (a) Take a moment to collect your thoughts and plan what you'll say; (b) don't lash out at the person; focus instead on the behavior that's bothering you; (c) describe the behavior and the feelings it is arousing in you; (d) suggest a solution to the problem, such as a change in the offensive behavior; (e) tell the other person what the consequences will be if the behavior doesn't change; (f) ask for a response to your proposal; (g) wait for the answer and listen carefully to it, trying to understand the other person's point of view.

11. Pretend this is the last day of your life. Put your angry thoughts in perspective.

12. Practice forgiveness. Anger, resentment, and blame are weights you carry around. Let go of them and allow yourself to experience more contentment and joy in life.

Begin today to try out some of these simple steps; they could give your heart a whole new lease on life.

years, may offer premenopausal women some protection against CVD. However, when heart attacks occur, they are more deadly for women than for men: 39 percent of women who have heart attacks die within a year compared to 31 percent of men. After age 65, this disparity is more dramatic—older women who have heart attacks are twice as likely as men to die from them within a few weeks (see the box "Women and CVD").

- *Race/Ethnicity.* The chance that African American men and women will have high blood pressure is one-third higher than the chance for whites, putting blacks of both sexes at greater risk of heart disease and stroke (see box "African Americans and CVD"). Puerto Ricans, Cuban Americans, and Mexican Americans are also more likely to suffer from high blood pressure and angina (a warning sign of heart disease) than are non-Hispanic white Americans. These differences may be due in part to differences in education, income, and other socioeconomic factors. Asian Americans historically have had far lower rates of CVD than white Americans. However, recent studies indicate that cholesterol levels among Asian Americans are rising, presumably because of the adoption of a high-fat American diet.

MAJOR FORMS OF CARDIOVASCULAR DISEASE

The chief forms of CVD are atherosclerosis, high blood pressure, stroke, congestive heart failure, congenital heart disease, and rheumatic heart disease. Except for congenital heart disease and rheumatic heart disease, the various forms are interrelated and have elements in common; we treat them separately here for the sake of clarity.

Atherosclerosis

One of the most common cardiovascular diseases is atherosclerosis, the principal form of arteriosclerosis, or hardening of the arteries. Atherosclerosis is a slow, progressive process that often begins in childhood. Arteries become narrowed by deposits of fat, cholesterol, and other substances. As these deposits, called **plaques,** accumulate on the walls of the arteries, the arteries lose their elasticity and are unable to expand and contract (Figure 15-7). The flow of blood through the narrowed arteries is restricted. Platelets in the blood may get stuck on a plaque and form a blood clot (**thrombus**), which further restricts the flow of blood, blocking the artery and depriving the heart, brain, or other organ of the vital oxygen carried by the blood. When a coronary artery is blocked, the result is a *coronary thrombosis,* which is one type of heart attack. When a cerebral artery (leading to the brain) is blocked, the result is a *cerebral thrombosis,* a type of stroke.

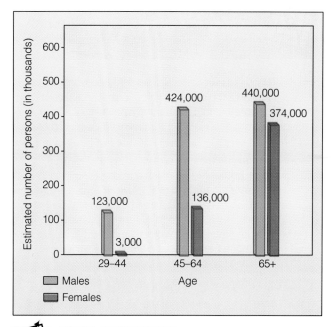

VITAL STATISTICS

Figure 15-6 *Estimated number of Americans who have a heart attack each year. Source:* American Heart Association. 1993. *Heart and Stroke Facts.*

What causes atherosclerosis? Although there are many possible contributing factors, four of the main factors are cigarette smoking, high levels of blood cholesterol, hypertension (high blood pressure), and physical inactivity. Of these, the most important risk factor for atherosclerosis is smoking. Recent studies indicate that high levels of iron in the blood may also contribute to the formation of plaques (see the box "The Iron Question").

Hypertension

Every time the heart contracts, or beats (systole), blood pressure increases. When the heart relaxes between beats (diastole), the pressure decreases. Blood pressure can fluctuate considerably, depending on different factors. For example, when you're excited or when you're exercising, the heart pumps more blood into your arteries and your blood pressure rises. But when blood pressure exceeds normal limits most of the time, a person is considered to have high blood pressure, or hypertension. It can result from either increased output of blood by the heart due to overweight or increased resistance to blood flow in the arteries due to narrowing and hardening. Either way,

Plaque   A deposit of fatty (and other) substances on the inner wall of the arteries.

Thrombus   A blood clot that forms in a blood vessel and remains attached there.

TERMS

- *CVD* in all its forms kills about 500,000 women a year. That's twice the number who die from all forms of cancer combined. One in nine women aged 45 to 64 has some form of CVD. One in three women 65 and older has CVD.

- *Heart attack* is the number one killer of American women. It kills 22,000 women under age 65 each year; one quarter are under age 55. African American women over age 35 have a death rate from heart attack that is twice that of white women and three times that of women of other races. Women are more likely than men to die from a heart attack. Women who survive are more likely than men to suffer a second attack.

- *High blood pressure* afflicts more than one in four women.

- *High cholesterol* is a problem for 55 million women. It affects 60 percent of white women, 54 percent of African American women, and 14 million girls under age 20.

- *Stroke* kills 90,000 women per year. Breast cancer kills only about half that many.

- *Smokers* who take birth control pills are up to 39 times more likely to have a heart attack than women who neither smoke nor use oral contraceptives. They are up to 22 times more likely to have a stroke.

Source: National Center for Health Statistics; The American Heart Association. 1993. *Heart and Stroke Facts.*

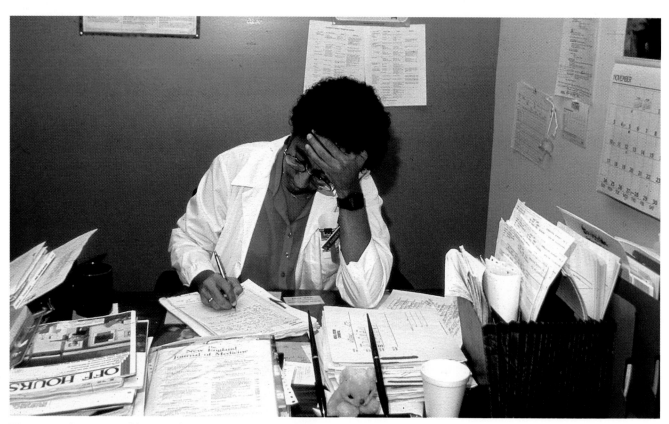

Women are less susceptible to cardiovascular disease than men. Even though this woman has to cope with the same on-the-job stresses as men in her profession, she is less likely to have a heart attack in middle age than they are.

Although cardiovascular disease is the leading cause of death for all Americans, African Americans are far more likely to experience CVD than white Americans. In 1987 the death rate from coronary heart disease was 208 per 100,000 for black males, compared to 185 per 100,000 for white males. The death rate for black females was 129 per 100,000, compared to 90 per 100,000 for white females. Black men are 50 percent more likely to die from a heart attack than white men, even if they make it to a hospital. Death from stroke is five times more common in African Americans than in other Americans. And hypertension is twice as common among African Americans as among Caucasians. Hypertension, which is both a disease in and of itself and a risk factor for other forms of CVD, damages blood vessels and is a major contributor to heart attacks and strokes.

What accounts for these higher levels of CVD among African Americans? Contributing factors can be grouped into three areas—biological/genetic factors; low income and discrimination; and lifestyle factors.

Biological/genetic risk factors

Researchers are investigating a number of genetic factors that may contribute to CVD in blacks. One is heightened sensitivity to lead, a toxic heavy metal that was once commonly used in house paint, gasoline, and water pipes and that causes a variety of serious health problems when ingested. Evidence suggests that lead in the bloodstream interacts with the hormones that regulate blood pressure. A recent study indicated that African Americans may be more sensitive to the damaging effects of lead than are other groups. Other researchers are investigating the hypothesis that some African Americans may have an inherited hypersensitivity to salt, which causes blood pressure to be elevated in many people.

Genetics also plays a role in cholesterol levels and may be involved in the cholesterol profile of African Americans. A recent study of cholesterol levels among black physicians and white physicians found that even when income level and lifestyle factors are similar (all physicians presumably have access to health care and to information about diet, exercise, and stress management), African Americans tend to have higher levels of LDLs, the "bad" form of cholesterol. The study suggests that there may be underlying genetic factors contributing to the less healthy cholesterol profiles typical of African Americans.

Another genetic condition associated with CVD is sickle-cell anemia, which occurs almost exclusively among African Americans (see Chapter 8). Sickle-cell anemia damages organs by impairing blood flow, and this damage can lead to heart failure.

Low income and discrimination

Another factor in the high incidence of CVD among African Americans is low income. One-third of African Americans live below the official poverty line. Economic deprivation usually means reduced access to adequate health care and health insurance. Associated with low income are poorer educational opportunities, which often mean less information about preventive health measures, such as diet and stress management.

Discrimination may also play a role in CVD among blacks. Research has shown that many physicians and hospitals treat the medical problems of African Americans differently than they do those of whites. Studies found, for example, that African Americans are half as likely as whites to receive bypass operations for heart disease and one-third less likely to receive kidney transplants. Discrimination, along with low income and other forms of deprivation, may also increase stress, which is linked with hypertension and CVD.

Lifestyle factors

Lifestyle choices also play a role in CVD rates. People with low income tend to smoke more, use more salt, and exercise less than those with higher incomes. In addition, almost half of African American women and one-third of African American men are severely overweight. According to Louis Sullivan, Secretary of Health and Human Services and the highest-ranking black official during the Bush administration, quitting smoking and losing weight could eliminate up to 45 percent of deaths due to CVD among African Americans.

Some of these risk factors are far beyond the individual's control, but others are not. Medical experts advise all Americans to have their blood pressure checked regularly, exercise, eat a healthy diet, manage stress, and avoid tobacco. These preventive strategies may be particularly important for African Americans.

Sources: C. Gorman, "Why Do Blacks Die Young?" *Time* 16 September 1991, pp. 50–52; J. Raloff, "Lead Heightens Hypertension Risk in Blacks," *Science News,* 28 April 1990, p. 261; M. F. Goldsmith, "African Lineage, Hypertension Linked," *Journal of the American Medical Association* 266(15): 2049; W. Alexander, 1991. "Study links status, pressure," *Black Enterprise* 21(11): 40.

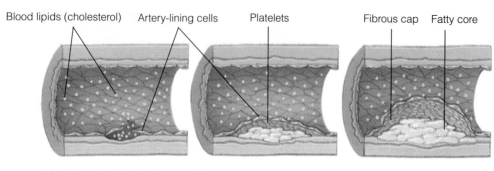

Blood lipids (cholesterol)   Artery-lining cells   Platelets   Fibrous cap   Fatty core

(a)   Plaque buildup begins when excess fat particles, called lipids, collect beneath cells lining the artery that have been damaged by smoking, high blood pressure, or other causes.

(b)   Platelets, one of the body's protective mechanisms, collect at the damaged area and cause a cap of cells to form, isolating the plaque within the artery wall.

(c)   The narrowed artery is now vulnerable to blockage by clots that can form if the cap breaks and the fatty core of the lesion combines with the clot-producing factors in the blood.

Figure 15-7   *Stages of plaque development.*

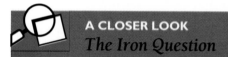

A CLOSER LOOK
The Iron Question

Iron may prove to be a major risk factor for heart disease. In a recent study of 2,000 Finnish men, researchers found heart attacks were twice as common among those with high iron levels as among those with lower readings, and four times as common among those with both high iron and high cholesterol levels. Of 19 CVD risk factors examined in the study, only smoking proved to be a stronger predictor of cardiovascular disease than was iron level.

The study, published in 1992, provided the first empirical evidence for the theory advanced in the early 1980s that iron helps form the plaques that harden artery walls and lead to heart attacks. If further research confirms the theory, it will help explain why the risk of heart disease for premenopausal women is so much lower than that of men. It could be that menstrual bleeding, rather than estrogen production, protects women's hearts. Regular monthly bleeding reduces the amount of iron in women's bodies. After menopause, a woman's cholesterol level usually doesn't change much, but her iron level rises sharply, along with her risk for heart attack.

This theory would also offer a possible explanation for why the heart attack rate among Seventh-day Adventist men is half that of other nonsmoking men with average cholesterol counts: As vegetarians, Seventh-day Adventists eat no iron-rich meats.

Therapy for high iron levels might include a prescription to donate a pint of blood three times a year. However, until the Finnish findings are confirmed by further studies, experts caution that it is too early to make any recommendations. They warn that too great a reduction in iron can cause anemia, an energy-sapping blood disorder.

Source: G. Cowley and M. Hager. 1992. "Bad News for the Geritol Set." *Newsweek,* 21 September, p. 69.

the heart is working harder than normal and the arteries are under greater strain.

High blood pressure is often called a "silent killer" because it usually has no early warning signs. It's possible to have high blood pressure for years without realizing it. During those years, it may be causing damage to vital organs and blood vessels, including the heart and coronary arteries. Blood vessels in the kidneys, for example, may rupture from constant pressure, causing kidney damage or failure. In the eyes, pressure on capillaries in the retina may cause tiny hemorrhages, resulting in blindness.

An estimated 63 million Americans have high blood pressure, and only a small percentage have it under control. There is no cure. Having your blood pressure checked at least once a year is the key to avoiding the complications of hypertension.

Measuring Your Blood Pressure   Blood pressure is measured with a stethoscope and an instrument called a **sphygmomanometer,** which consists of an inflatable cuff and a column of mercury marked off in millimeters. The cuff is wrapped around the upper arm and inflated. This depresses the brachial artery in the arm, stopping the flow of blood. As air is slowly released from the cuff, the ex-

TABLE 15-2 Blood Pressure Classification

Classification	*Systolic	*Diastolic	What to Do
Normal	Below 130	Below 85	Recheck in 2 years
High normal	130–139	85–89	Recheck in 1 year
Mild hypertension	140–159	90–99	Confirm within 2 months
Moderate hypertension	160–179	100–109	See physician within a month
Severe hypertension	180 or above	110 or above	See physician immediately

Examples

120/80	Normal
135/85	High normal
145/95	Mild hypertension
160/105	Moderate hypertension
180/115	Severe hypertension

Adapted from The National High Blood Pressure Education Program and the fifth report of the Joint National Committee on Detection, Evaluation, and Treatment of High Blood Pressure, *Archives of Internal Medicine,* 25 January 1993.

*Based on an average of two or more readings on two or more occasions.

aminer will hear a thudding sound with the stethoscope as blood flow resumes. The height of the mercury when the sound is first heard is the reading of the *systolic* blood pressure, the pressure when the ventricular heart contraction is occurring. The pressure at the point when the sound can no longer be heard is *diastolic* blood pressure, the pressure when the heart is relaxed. Blood pressure is expressed as two numbers—for example, 120/80; the first is systolic pressure, and the second is diastolic pressure. The unit of measurement is millimeters of mercury (mm Hg).

Blood pressure readings can be quite variable, depending on such factors as anxiety, excitement, and setting. For this reason, it's best to compute an average based on at least three measurements on different days. Average blood pressure readings for young adults in good physical condition are 110 to 120 mm Hg systolic over 70 to 80 mm Hg diastolic. Elevated blood pressure in adults is defined as a systolic pressure of 140 mm Hg or more and/or a diastolic pressure of 90 mm Hg or more (Table 15-2).

What Causes Hypertension?

In up to 95 percent of the cases of hypertension, the cause is unknown. High blood pressure of unknown cause is called **essential hypertension,** which most likely involves many factors, including diet, obesity, alcohol abuse, physical and emotional stress, and psychological and genetic factors.

Environmental factors alone probably do not produce hypertension in someone without a genetic predisposition to it.

In the remaining cases, the condition is a symptom of another problem, such as a defect in a kidney or other organ. In these cases, referred to as **secondary hypertension,** blood pressure usually returns to normal when the underlying problem is corrected surgically.

Treating Hypertension

Cases of mild hypertension (see Table 15-2) can frequently be treated by changes in diet alone, such as restricted salt intake in salt-sensitive people, reduced caloric intake, or both. Although not everyone's blood pressure is affected by salt consumption, blood pressure in some people goes up as soon as they consume salt. These salt-sensitive people must restrict their salt intake to control their blood pressure. Restricting salt intake tends to curb fluid retention, thus reducing blood volume.

Sphygmomanometer An instrument for measuring blood pressure.

Essential hypertension Persistent elevated blood pressure without known or specific cause.

Secondary hypertension High blood pressure caused by disease such as kidney dysfunctioning or tumor.

TERMS

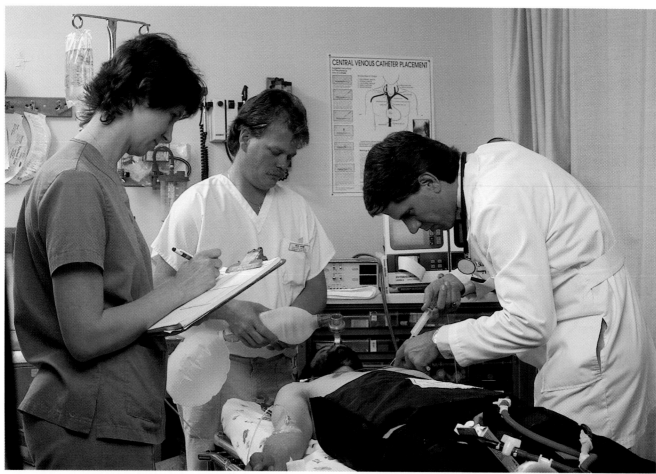

Heart attack victims who receive prompt attention from trained personnel have the best chance of survival. This emergency room physician is injecting epinephrine to stimulate the patient's heart.

Overweight people are more susceptible to elevated blood pressure because added weight places greater demands on the cardiovascular system. Adipose (fatty) tissue requires blood to nourish it, so in overweight people, the heart must pump blood through a more extensive system of blood vessels.

Treatment of more severe hypertension often also involves the use of **antihypertensive drugs.** One group of antihypertensive drugs is the **diuretics,** which increase fluid secretion by the kidneys. Use of diuretics is recommended for patients whose hypertension is thought to be due primarily to increased blood volume. Beta-blockers, another group of antihypertensive drugs, block certain

sympathetic nerves that cause arteries to narrow. These vasodilators cause the muscle in the walls of the arteries to relax, permitting the artery to dilate (widen). ACE inhibitors, a relatively new group of drugs, interfere with the body's production of **angiotensin,** a protein that causes arteries to contract.

Heart Attacks

Every year over a million Americans have a heart attack. (see Figure 15-6). Although a heart attack may come without warning, it is the end result of a long-term disease process. The most common form of heart disease is coronary artery disease caused by atherosclerosis. When one of the coronary arteries—the arteries that branch off the aorta and supply blood directly to the heart muscle—becomes blocked by a blood clot, a heart attack results. A heart attack caused by a clot is called a **coronary thrombosis,** a **coronary occlusion,** or a **myocardial infarction.** In myocardial infarction, part of the heart muscle (myocardium) may die from lack of oxygen.

If the heart attack is not fatal—that is, if enough of the muscle is undamaged to permit life to continue—the

TERMS

Antihypertensive drugs   Prescribed drugs that lower blood pressure.

Diuretics   Drugs that increase the secretion of salts and water by the kidneys.

Angiotensin   A naturally occurring substance that constricts blood vessels.

Coronary thrombosis   A clot in a coronary artery, often causing sudden death.

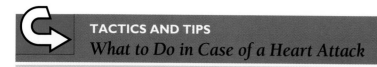

muscle begins to repair itself. It does so through a process called **collateral circulation,** in which small blood vessels open to take over the functions of the blocked artery and to move more blood through the damaged area. As healing takes place, scar tissue replaces part of the injured muscle.

Angina   Arteries narrowed by disease may still be open enough to deliver blood to the heart. At times, however— chiefly during emotional excitement, stress, or physical exertion—the heart requires more oxygen than narrowed arteries can accommodate. When the need for oxygen exceeds the supply, the heart's electrical system may be disrupted, also causing a heart attack. Chest pain, called **angina pectoris,** is a signal that the heart is not getting enough blood to supply the oxygen it needs. Angina pain is felt as an extreme tightness in the chest and heavy pressure behind the breastbone or in the shoulder, neck, arm, hand, or back. This pain, although not actually a heart attack, is a warning that the load on the heart must be reduced. Angina may be controlled in a number of ways (with diet and drugs), but its course is unpredictable. Over a period of months or years, the narrowing often goes on to full blockage and a heart attack.

Arrhythmias   Of the roughly 500,000 heart attack deaths each year, about 60 percent happen within the first hour from an abnormal heartbeat called an arrhythmia, which usually results from damaged heart muscle. Sudden death can be caused by failure of the heart's natural pacemaker, which normally sends electrical impulses through the heart at a rate of 60 to 100 times per minute. A normal heart rhythm can often be restored using a defibrillator, which gives an electrical shock to the heart. This must be done within three to four minutes unless blood flow is restored through **cardiopulmonary resuscitation (CPR).**

Helping a Heart Attack Victim   Most people who suffer a fatal heart attack do so within two hours from the time they experience the first signals. And half of all heart attack victims wait more than two hours before getting help. This accounts for some of the 300,000 heart attack deaths that occur each year among people who never make it to the hospital. Therefore, recognizing the signals and responding immediately by getting to the nearest

Coronary occlusion   Partial or total obstruction of a coronary artery, as by a clot; usually resulting in myocardial infarction.

Myocardial infarction   A heart attack in which the heart muscle is damaged through lack of blood supply.

Collateral circulation   The movement of blood by a system of smaller blood vessels when a main vessel is blocked.

Angina pectoris   A condition in which the heart muscle does not receive enough blood, causing severe pain in the chest and often in the left arm and shoulder.

Cardiopulmonary resuscitation (CPR)   A technique involving mouth-to-mouth breathing and chest compression to keep oxygen flowing to the brain.

TERMS

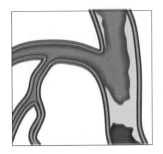
(a) Thrombus

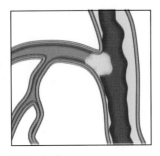
(b) Embolism

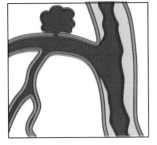
(c) Hemorrhage

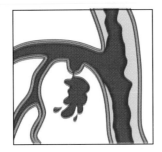
(d) Aneurysm (ruptured)

Figure 15-8 *Causes of stroke.*
Five out of six strokes are caused by blood clots, either a thrombus (a) or an embolism (b). A hemorrhagic stroke (c) is more serious and occurs when a blood vessel in the brain bursts. When an aneurysm ruptures (d), a stroke results.

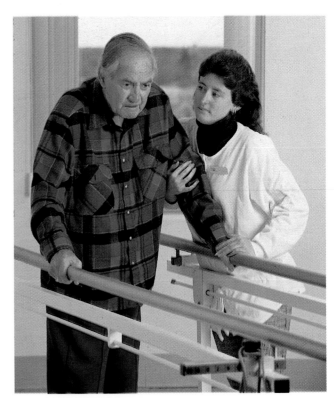

Rehabilitation after a stroke can be a long and arduous process. Complete recovery eludes many stroke victims.

hospital or clinic with 24-hour emergency cardiac facilities is critical (see the box "What to Do in Case of a Heart Attack"). If the person loses consciousness, emergency cardiopulmonary resuscitation (CPR) should be initiated by a qualified person. Damage to the heart muscle increases with time. If the victim gets to the emergency room quickly enough, a clot-dissolving agent can be injected to dissolve a clot in the coronary artery. These relatively new "clot-busting" drugs, such as streptokinase, urokinase, and tissue plasminogen activator (TPA), are being used successfully to treat not only heart attacks but also some types of stroke. The sooner these drugs are used, the more effective they are.

Detecting and Treating Heart Disease Physicians have a variety of diagnostic tools to evaluate the condition of the heart and the arteries. To determine whether a person is at risk of a heart attack, physicians order a stress or exercise test, in which the patient runs on a treadmill while being monitored for heart rhythm abnormalities with an **electrocardiogram (ECG)**. Certain characteristic changes in the heart's electrical activity while under stress can reveal particular heart problems, such as restricted blood flow to the heart muscle.

Other tools allow the physician to visualize the patient's heart and arteries. **Magnetic resonance imaging (MRI)**, also called **nuclear magnetic resonance imaging**

(NMR), uses powerful magnets to look inside the heart. **Radionuclide imaging** involves injecting radioactive markers into the bloodstream. The markers are taken up by the heart in areas where there is adequate blood flow. Sensitive cameras can then be used to determine if the heart is well-supplied with blood and its chambers are functioning properly. Other tests involve threading a catheter through arteries and into the heart. Dye is injected through the catheter; x-rays are used to trace the liquid's flow. The resulting pictures, called **angiograms** or **arteriograms**, reveal the presence of any obstructions. A newer test uses a catheter tipped with a tiny ultrasound transducer. The transducer sends out a beam of sound waves that bounce off the tissue of the arteries and create pictures of the artery walls.

A variety of treatments, ranging from changes in diet to major surgery, is available if a problem is detected. Along with a low-fat diet, regular exercise, and smoking cessation, one frequent nonsurgical recommendation for people at high risk of CVD is for them to take one-half an aspirin tablet a day. Aspirin has an anticlotting effect; it discourages platelets in the blood from sticking to arterial plaque and forming clots. Too much aspirin, however, may increase risks of certain types of stroke and cause ulcers or gastrointestinal bleeding.

The most common surgical procedure performed today for coronary disease is **balloon angioplasty**, or **per-**

cutaneous transluminal angioplasty (PCTA). This technique involves threading a catheter with an inflatable balloon tip through the artery until it reaches the area of blockage. The balloon is then inflated, flattening the fatty plaque and widening the arterial opening. However, repeat clogging of the artery, known as *restenosis,* is common.

New variations on this technique are being tried to decrease the occurrence and severity of restenosis. Surgeons have put lasers, rotating blades, drill bits, and even miniature ultrasound "jackhammers" on the tips of catheters and threaded them into blocked arteries, where they vaporize, shave, drill, or pulverize plaques. To keep arteries open, some surgeons are testing laser-heated balloons that "weld" artery walls in place. Others are using catheters to install tiny springs, called stents, which remain in place as a framework to keep the artery open.

Coronary bypass surgery is performed on nearly 400,000 men and women a year. Surgeons remove a healthy blood vessel, usually a vein from one of the patient's legs, and graft it to one or more coronary arteries to bypass a blockage. A heart-lung machine maintains circulation during the surgery.

Whatever treatment is used, the person with heart disease is also advised to make behavior and lifestyle changes, such as changing the diet to improve blood cholesterol levels and quitting smoking. Otherwise, the arteries simply become clogged again, and the same problems recur a few years later.

Stroke

For brain cells to function as they should, they must have a continuous and ample supply of oxygen-rich blood. If brain cells are deprived of blood for more than a few minutes, they die. A **stroke,** also called a *cerebrovascular accident* (CVA), occurs when the blood supply to the brain is cut off. Stroke can be particularly serious because injured brain cells, unlike those of other organs, cannot regenerate.

Types of Strokes   There are three major types of stroke. The most common is the *thrombotic stroke,* caused by a blood clot, or *thrombus,* that forms in one of the cerebral arteries (Figure 15-8). This condition, called **cerebral thrombosis,** is likely to occur when the cerebral arteries become narrowed or damaged by atherosclerosis. If a cerebral artery is clogged with plaque, the formation of clots is more likely. The risk of stroke is much higher among people with hypertension than among those with normal blood pressure, since high blood pressure accelerates the process of atherosclerosis.

A second type of stroke, the *embolic stroke,* occurs when a wandering blood clot, or **embolus,** is carried in the bloodstream and becomes wedged in one of the cerebral arteries. This event is called a **cerebral embolism.**

The third type of stroke, the *hemorrhagic stroke,* is the least common but most severe type of stroke. It occurs when a blood vessel in the brain bursts, spilling blood into the surrounding tissue and causing damage to it. When a **cerebral hemorrhage** occurs, cells normally nourished by the artery are deprived of blood and cannot function. People who suffer from both atherosclerosis and high blood pressure are more likely to suffer cerebral hemorrhage than are those who have only one condition or neither. About one in ten strokes is caused by a brain hemorrhage rather than a blood clot.

Bleeding of an artery in the brain may also be caused by a head injury or by the bursting of an **aneurysm.** An aneurysm is a blood-filled pocket that bulges out from a weak spot in an artery wall. Aneurysms in the brain may remain stable and never break. But when they do, the result is a stroke.

Effects of a Stroke   The interruption of the blood supply to any area of the brain prevents the nerve cells there from functioning, in some cases causing death. Of the 500,000 Americans who have strokes each year, approxi-

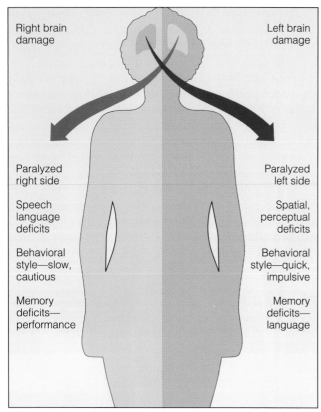

Right brain damage

Left brain damage

Paralyzed right side

Speech language deficits

Behavioral style—slow, cautious

Memory deficits—performance

Paralyzed left side

Spatial, perceptual deficits

Behavioral style—quick, impulsive

Memory deficits—language

Figure 15-9 *Damage caused by strokes. Source:* American Heart Association. 1993. *Heart and Stroke Facts.*

mately 150,000 die. Those who survive usually have some lasting disability. Which parts of the body are affected by the stroke depends on the area of the brain affected (Figure 15-9). Nerve cells control sensation and most of our bodily movements, so a stroke may cause paralysis, walking disability, speech impairment, or memory loss. The severity of the stroke and its long-term effects depend on which brain cells have been injured, how widespread the damage is, how effectively the body can restore the blood supply, and how rapidly other areas of the brain can take over.

Detecting and Treating Stroke   Strokes can be treated, but effective treatment requires prompt recognition of symptoms and correct diagnosis of the type of stroke that has occurred. Warning signs of a stroke include the following:

- Sudden numbness or weakness of the face, arm, and leg on one side of the body
- Loss of speech or difficulty speaking or understanding speech
- Dimming or loss of vision, especially in only one eye
- Unexplained dizziness, particularly if other symptoms are present

Some stroke victims have a **transient ischemic attack**

(TIA), or ministroke, days, weeks, or months before they have a full-blown stroke. TIAs produce temporary stroke-like symptoms, such as weakness or numbness in an arm or leg, speech difficulty, or dizziness, but these symptoms are brief and don't seem to cause permanent damage. TIAs should be taken as warning signs of a stroke and reported to a physician.

Until recently, there was very little that could be done to treat strokes, but now they are treated with the same urgency as heart attacks. A person who has had or is having a stroke should be rushed to the hospital for diagnosis and treatment. Tests may include an electrocardiogram (which measures the electrical activity of the heart), an **electroencephalogram** (which measures nerve cell activity in the brain), and a **computerized tomography (CT)** scan (a painless technique that can assess brain damage). The CT scan uses a computer to construct a picture of the brain from x-rays beamed through the head.

If the tests reveal that the stroke was caused by a blood clot, the person can be treated with the same kind of clot-dissolving drugs that are being used to treat coronary artery blockages. If the clot is dissolved quickly enough, damage to the brain is minimized and symptoms may disappear. The longer the brain goes without oxygen from a blood clot, the greater the risk of permanent brain damage.

If tests reveal that the stroke was caused by a cerebral hemorrhage, drugs may be prescribed to lower the blood pressure, which is usually high. Careful diagnosis is crucial, since administering clot-dissolving drugs to a person suffering a hemorrhagic stroke would cause more bleeding and potentially more brain damage.

If detection and treatment of stroke come too late, rehabilitation is the only treatment. Although damaged or destroyed brain tissue cannot regenerate, the brain can find new pathways, and some functions can be taken over by other parts of the brain. Some spontaneous recovery starts immediately after a stroke and continues for a few months.

Rehabilitation consists of various types of therapy: physical therapy, which helps strengthen muscles and improve balance and coordination; speech and language therapy, which helps those whose speech has been damaged; and occupational therapy, which helps improve hand-eye coordination and everyday living skills. Progress varies from person to person and can be unpredictable. Some people recover completely in a matter of days or weeks, but most stroke victims who survive struggle with disability for the rest of their lives.

Congestive Heart Failure

A number of conditions, including high blood pressure, heart attack, atherosclerosis, rheumatic fever, and birth defects, can damage the heart's pumping efficiency. When the heart cannot maintain its regular pumping rate and force, fluids begin to back up. When this extra fluid seeps through capillary walls, edema (swelling) results, most commonly in the legs and ankles, but sometimes in other parts of the body as well. Fluid can collect in the lungs and interfere with breathing, particularly when a person is lying down. This condition is called **pulmonary edema;** the entire process is **congestive heart failure.**

Congestive heart failure can be controlled. Treatment includes reducing the workload on the heart, modifying salt intake, and using drugs that help the body eliminate excess fluid. Drugs used to treat congestive heart failure include digitalis, which increases the pumping action of the heart; diuretics, which help the body eliminate excess salt and water; and vasodilators, which expand the blood vessels, decrease the pressure, and allow blood to flow more easily, which in turn makes the heart's work easier.

Heart Disease in Children

Although most cardiovascular disease occurs in adults— and usually in middle-aged or older adults at that—it can occur in children, usually as congenital heart disease or as a result of rheumatic fever.

Congenital Heart Disease About 30,000 children born each year in the United States have a defect or malformation of the heart or major blood vessels. These conditions are referred to collectively as **congenital heart disease.** They cause 5,800 deaths a year.

The most common congenital defects are holes in the wall that divides the lower chambers of the heart. Holes may also occur in the wall between the upper chambers. With these defects the heart produces a distinctive sound, making diagnosis relatively simple. Another defect is **coarctation of the aorta,** which is a narrowing, or constriction, of the aorta. Heart failure may result unless the constricted area is repaired by surgery.

Most of the common congenital defects can now be accurately diagnosed and treated with medication or surgery. Important in saving lives is the early recognition that the newborn infant who shows blue appearance, respiratory difficulty, or failure to thrive may be suffering from congenital heart disease.

Rheumatic Heart Disease A leading cause of heart trouble in children is **rheumatic fever,** a consequence of untreated strep throat. Rheumatic fever can damage the heart muscle and heart valves. Symptoms of strep throat are the sudden onset of a sore throat, painful swallowing, fever, swollen glands, headache, nausea, and vomiting. Strep infections can be diagnosed by rapid laboratory detection tests. The symptoms of rheumatic fever are generally vague, making diagnosis difficult. Symptoms in children include loss of weight or failure to gain weight; a low but persistent fever; poor appetite; repeated nose-bleeds without apparent cause; jerky body movements; pain in the arms, legs, or abdomen; fatigue; and weakness. Rheumatic fever can usually be prevented by treating strep throat, when it occurs, with antibiotics.

PROTECTING YOURSELF FROM CARDIOVASCULAR DISEASE

What can you do now, while you're still young, to improve your chances of avoiding CVD? Here are a number of important steps you can take:

- Have your blood pressure measured by a physician or other health care provider at least once a year, even if your blood pressure has been normal in the past. Self-administered blood pressure tests in pharmacies and other public places may be misleading and are no substitute for a test performed by a trained professional. If your blood pressure is high, follow your physician's advice on how to lower it.

- Have your blood cholesterol measured if you've never had it done. Finger-prick tests at health fairs and other public places are generally fairly accurate, especially if they're offered by a hospital or other reputable health group. When you know your "number," follow these guidelines from the National Cholesterol Education Program:

  If your cholesterol is under 200 mg/dl, maintain a healthy lifestyle—including eating a low-fat diet, getting regular exercise, maintaining a healthy body weight, and not smoking—and get another test within five years.

  If your cholesterol is between 200 and 239 mg/dl, have a second test performed and average the results. If that number falls in the same range, and if you do

Transient ischemic attack (TIA) A small stroke; usually a temporary interruption of blood supply to the brain, causing numbness or difficulty with speech.

Electroencephalogram (EEG) A test that measures nerve cell activity in the brain.

Computerized tomography (CT) scan A test using computerized x-ray images to create a cross-sectional depiction of tissue density.

Pulmonary edema Accumulation of water in the lungs.

Congestive heart failure A condition resulting from the heart's inability to pump out all the blood that returns to it. Blood backs up in the veins leading to the heart, causing an accumulation of fluid in various parts of the body.

Congenital heart disease Disease present at birth due to malformation of the heart or its major blood vessels.

Coarctation of the aorta A congenital defect in which the aorta is narrowed or constricted.

Rheumatic fever A disease, mainly of children, characterized by fever, inflammation, and pain in the joints; often damages the heart muscle.

TERMS

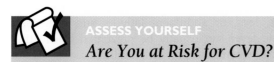
Your chances of suffering an early heart attack or stroke depend on a variety of factors, many of which are under your control. The best time to identify your risk factors and change your behavior to lower your risk is when you are young. You can significantly affect your future health and quality of life if you adopt healthy behaviors. To help identify your risk factors, circle the response for each risk category that best describes you.

1. Gender

   0 Female

   2 Male

2. Heredity

   0 Neither parent suffered a heart attack or stroke before age 60.

   3 One parent suffered a heart attack or stroke before age 60.

   7 Both parents suffered a heart attack or stroke before age 60.

3. Smoking

   0 Never smoked

   1 Quit more than 2 years ago

   2 Quit less than 2 years ago

   8 Smoke less than ½ pack per day

   13 Smoke more than ½ pack per day

   15 Smoke more than 1 pack per day

4. Environmental Tobacco Smoke

   0 Do not live or work with smokers

   2 Exposed to ETS at work

   3 Live with smoker

   4 Both live and work with smokers

5. Blood Pressure

   The average of the last three readings:

   0 130/80 or below

   1 131/81 to 140/85

   5 141/86 to 150/90

   9 151/91 to 170/100

   13 Above 170/100

6. Total Cholesterol

   The average of the last three readings:

   0 Lower than 190

   1 190 to 210

   2 Don't know

   3 211 to 240

   4 241 to 270

   5 271 to 300

   6 Over 300

7. HDL Cholesterol

   The average of the last three readings:

   0 Over 65 mg/dl

   1 55 to 65

   2 Don't know HDL

   3 45 to 54

   5 35 to 44

   7 25 to 34

   12 Lower than 25

8. Exercise

   0 Aerobic exercise three times per week

   1 Aerobic exercise once or twice per week

   2 Occasional exercise less than once per week

   7 Rarely exercise

9. Diabetes

   0 No personal or family history

   2 One parent with diabetes

   6 Two parents with diabetes

   9 Non-insulin-dependent diabetes (Type 2)

   13 Insulin-dependent diabetes (Type 1)

10. Weight

   0 Near ideal weight

   1 Six pounds or less above ideal weight

   3 Seven to 19 pounds above ideal weight

   5 Twenty to 40 pounds above ideal weight

   7 More than 40 pounds above ideal weight

11. Stress

   0 Relaxed most of the time

   1 Occasional stress and anger

   2 Frequently stressed and angry

   3 Usually stressed and angry

Scoring

Total your risk factor points. Refer to the list below to get an approximate rating of your risk of suffering an early heart attack or stroke.

Score	Estimated Risk
Less than 20	Low risk
20–29	Moderate risk
30–45	High risk
Over 45	Extremely high risk

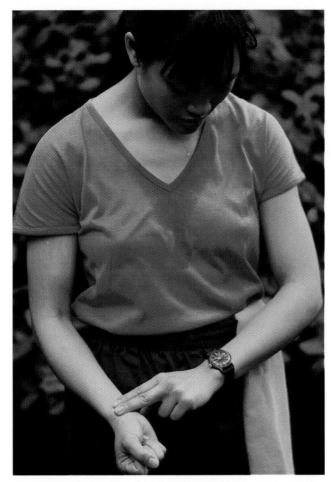

One of the primary benefits of endurance exercise is its conditioning effect on the heart and lungs. A lifetime of sensible exercise habits offers protection against cardiovascular disease later in life.

not have any form of CVD or two other risk factors for CVD, change your diet to improve your cholesterol. In addition, eliminate any other risk factors you have and get tested again in about one year. If you have CVD or other risk factors for CVD, your physician should order a more detailed cholesterol analysis, including measurement of HDL and LDL. You should begin a cholesterol-improving diet and follow any other therapy recommended by your physician.

If your cholesterol is 240 mg/dl or more, your physician should order a more detailed cholesterol analysis and recommend therapy based on the results. You should begin a cholesterol-improving diet immediately.

• Get regular exercise. Sedentary people can significantly reduce their risk of premature death from CVD just by walking a dog every day, taking up gardening, playing golf on weekends, enrolling in a weekly dance class, or joining a bowling league.

People who have already built mild exercise into their weekly routines can reduce their CVD risk even further by exercising a little harder, a little more often, or both. Exercise programs needn't be rigid or strenuous to provide protection from CVD. The American Medical Association recommends exercising a total of between 90 minutes and four hours each week.

• If you smoke, quit. If you live or work with people who smoke, encourage them to quit—for their sake and yours (see Chapter 9).

• Bring your diet into line with the guidelines of the National Cholesterol Education Program. Consume fewer than 30 percent of your total daily calories as fat; fewer than 10 percent should come from saturated fat. Eat fewer than 300 milligrams of dietary cholesterol a day. Choose foods high in fiber and complex carbohydrates. And adjust your caloric intake to achieve or maintain a healthy body weight.

• Develop effective ways to handle stress and anger. Refer to Chapter 2 for suggestions about how to manage stress and avoid its negative consequences.

• Follow your physician's advice about any medical problems you may have, such as diabetes.

• Know your CVD risk factors. Take the quiz in the box "Are You at Risk for CVD?"

In a sense, some of us choose our diseases when we choose the way we live. On the other hand, sometimes it's difficult to see that other choices are possible. Our competitive society fosters certain values and behaviors. When there's still work to do, it's not always easy to leave the desk or computer terminal and take the time to exercise and eat a healthy meal instead of fast food. But if we can see that we have choices, if we can learn to mediate the negative effects of the "fast track," we can perhaps make cardiovascular disease less inevitable in our lives.

Personal Insight   Have you taken any steps to lower your chances of developing cardiovascular disease later in life, such as cutting back on fat or exercising regularly? If you haven't, why haven't you? When do you think you will?

SUMMARY

• Cardiovascular disease is the number one killer of both men and women in the United States.

The Cardiovascular System

• The cardiovascular system pumps and circulates blood throughout the body; the pulmonary and systemic circulation systems are controlled by the right and left sides of the heart.

- The heart beats when the ventricles contract (systole), pumping blood to the lungs via the pulmonary artery and to the body via the aorta and the entire arterial system. When the heart relaxes between beats (diastole), blood flows from the atria into the ventricles. The action of the heart is controlled by electrical impulses.

- The exchange of nutrients and waste products takes place between the capillaries and the tissues.

Risk Factors for Cardiovascular Disease

- Smoking greatly increases the risk for cardiovascular disease; it lowers HDL levels, increases blood pressure and heart rate, reduces the amount of oxygen available to the body, and increases the likelihood of blood clots. ETS has also been linked to cardiovascular disease.

- High blood pressure weakens the heart and scars and hardens blood vessels; it often has no early warning signs.

- Cholesterol is crucial to the body's functioning, but high levels contribute to clogged arteries and increase the risk for CVD. High LDL and low HDL levels are associated with high risk. Very low levels of cholesterol may be associated with an increase in death rates.

- Dietary changes that can help improve cholesterol levels include limiting intake of fat, saturated fat, and cholesterol and increasing intake of fiber.

- Physical inactivity increases risk for CVD; as little as 90 minutes a week of mild exercise can reduce this risk.

- Other risk factors that contribute to CVD include overweight, diabetes, high levels of stress, a hostile personality, lack of social support, and low income and educational attainment.

- Risk factors for CVD that can't be changed include being over 65, being male, being African American, and having a family history of CVD.

Major Forms of Cardiovascular Disease

- Atherosclerosis is the process whereby arteries become narrowed by deposits of fat, cholesterol, and other substances. As plaques accumulate, arteries lose elasticity and the ability to expand and contract. Platelets may get stuck on a plaque and form a blood clot, which can block the artery and deprive organs of blood.

- Hypertension occurs when blood pressure exceeds normal limits most of the time. It can damage vital organs, including the heart, eyes, and kidneys.

- High blood pressure is defined as systolic pressure of 140 mm Hg or higher and/or diastolic pressure of 90 mm Hg or higher.

- Mild hypertension can sometimes be treated by restricting salt intake and losing weight. More severe hypertension may require treatment with antihypertensive drugs.

- Heart attacks are the end result of a long-term disease process.

- Angina pectoris is the chest pain that occurs when—because of narrowed arteries—the heart doesn't get enough blood to supply the oxygen it needs.

- Arrhythmia is an abnormal heartbeat; if the heart's electrical system fails, sudden death can occur.

- Heart disease can be diagnosed through use of stress or exercise tests, electrocardiograms, magnetic resonance imaging, angiograms, and radioactive tracers.

- Nonsurgical treatments include a low-fat diet, regular exercise, smoking cessation, and small, regular doses of aspirin. Surgical treatments include balloon angioplasty and coronary bypass surgery.

- A stroke occurs when the blood supply to the brain is cut off; injured brain cells cannot regenerate themselves. A stroke can be caused by a thrombus, an embolism, or a hemorrhage. Head injuries and burst aneurysms also cause bleeding in the brain.

- Strokes usually lead to some lasting disability, such as paralysis, walking disability, speech impairment, or memory loss.

- Transient ischemic attacks are warning signs of a stroke. Diagnostic tests include electrocardiograms, electroencephalograms, and CT scans.

- Congestive heart failure occurs when the heart's pumping efficiency is reduced and fluids build and collect in the lungs or other part of the body. The extra fluids cause swelling; pulmonary edema causes shortness of breath.

- Defects or malformations of the heart or major blood vessels at birth constitute congenital heart disease. These include holes in the wall that divides the chambers of the heart and a constricted aorta.

Protecting Yourself from Cardiovascular Disease

- To avoid CVD, it's important to have blood pressure checked regularly; have blood cholesterol measured; exercise regularly; quit smoking; alter diet to reduce intake of fat and saturated fat; increase intake of fiber; learn to handle stress and anger; monitor medical problems; and know personal and familial risk factors.

1. The CPR courses given by the Red Cross and other groups provide invaluable training that may help you save a life some day. Anyone can take these courses and become qualified to administer CPR. Investigate CPR courses in your community and sign up to take one.

2. Do some research into your family medical history. Is there cardiovascular disease in your family, as indicated by premature deaths from heart attack, stroke, or congestive heart failure? Such a history is a risk factor for you. Keep that in mind as you consider whether you need to make lifestyle changes to avoid CVD.

JOURNAL ENTRY

1. If the hostility assessment in the chapter indicates that you may have a hostile personality, examine your thoughts and behavior more carefully. In your health journal, keep track of your cynical thoughts, angry feelings, and aggressive acts. For each entry, include the time, place, and cause of your cynical thoughts; what thoughts actually went through your head; the emotions you felt; and any actions you took. Review your journal at the end of a week to learn more about the frequency and kinds of situations that trigger these thoughts and behaviors.

2. *Critical Thinking:* How much responsibility does an individual have for his or her health? Do people have an obligation to take care of themselves as best they can to help avoid becoming a burden on their family and on society? Do people have a right to choose whatever lifestyle they want—no matter how unhealthy? In your health journal, write an essay describing your opinion about individual responsibility for health. Be sure to explain your reasoning.

BEHAVIOR CHANGE STRATEGY

REDUCING THE SATURATED FAT IN YOUR DIET

The American Heart Association recommends that no more than 10 percent of the calories in your diet come from saturated fat. The biggest sources of saturated fats are animal products, such as red meat, cheese, milk, cream, yogurt, and butter; the "tropical oils," such as palm and coconut oil; and heavily hydrogenated vegetable oils. To see how your diet measures up, monitor yourself for a week, keeping track of everything you eat. Keep your record in your health journal, writing the foods you eat (including meals and snacks) on the left side of the page and leaving room on the right for information about each food.

Information about the calorie and fat content of the foods you eat is available on many food labels and in books available in libraries and bookstores. You can use the appendix to Chapter 12 of this book to look up nutritional information for fast foods.

Each day, after you have noted the foods you ate, enter the calories and the grams of saturated fat, and then compute the percentage of saturated fat for each food using the formula explained in Chapter 12. (Multiply grams of saturated fat by 9 and divide the product by the total calories. The result is the percentage of saturated fat.) Repeat the calculations for each day (based on total grams of saturated fat and total calorie intake) and for the week. How close do the daily and weekly percentages you have calculated come to the goal of 10 percent or fewer calories from saturated fat?

You can also monitor and compute the percentages of monounsaturated and polyunsaturated fats in your diet. Foods high in polyunsaturated fat include corn oil, cottonseed oil, safflower oil, soybean oil, mayonnaise made with any of these oils, margarine, sunflower seeds, and walnuts. Foods high in monounsaturated fat include olive oil, peanut oil, sesame oil, almonds, cashews, hazelnuts, peanuts, pecans, pistachio nuts, and avocados. Try to keep each of these groups at or below about 10 percent of your total calories too.

If your diet includes more than your fair share of saturated fat, you can take steps to reduce it. Begin by looking at the tips in the box "Controlling Cholesterol Through Diet." Start to become more aware of what type of food you order in restaurants, buy at the supermarket, and prepare for meals. Do you usually go for hamburgers, hot dogs, steaks, and chops? Choose lean meat, chicken, or fish instead, and broil or bake it instead of frying it. Do you have salami and cheese on rye for lunch? Try turkey for a change. Is ice cream your downfall? Sliced fruit in season with low-fat yogurt and honey is a delicious alternative.

If there is a lot of saturated fat in your diet, you may have to change some of your habits for a while—you may have to avoid fast food restaurants or forgo pizza at night with your friends. Put your best effort into finding attractive, satisfying, and enjoyable activities as substitutes, such as trying out restaurants that serve low-fat dishes. If you can recruit some friends to join you in your campaign, it will be easier to stick with it. Remember, cardiovascular disease often starts when people are in their teens or early twenties. By making a conscious effort to establish a healthy diet and cut down on saturated fat now, you'll be doing yourself a favor that will give you benefits your whole life.

SELECTED BIBLIOGRAPHY

Alexander, W. 1991. Study links status, pressure. *Black Enterprise* 21(11): 40.

American College of Cardiology. 1992. 41st Annual Scientific Session, Dallas, Texas. *Supplement A:* 1A–395A.

American Heart Association. 1993. *Heart and Stroke Facts.*

———. 1992. *Physicians' Cholesterol Education Handbook.*

American Medical Association. 1992. *Position Paper on Exercise.*

Caralis, P. V. 1991. Coronary artery disease in Hispanic Americans: How does ethnic background affect risk factors and mortality rates? *Postgraduate Medicine* 91(4): 179–82, 185–88, 193.

Centers for Disease Control. 1992. Trends in ischemic heart disease and mortality—United States. *Morbidity and Mortality Weekly Report* 41(30): 548–49.

Douglas, P. S., and others. 1992. Exercise and atherosclerotic heart disease in women. *Medicine and Science in Sports and Exercise* 6 Suppl.: S266–76.

Fletcher, G. F., and others. 1990. Exercise standards: A statement for health professionals from the American Heart Association. *Circulation* 82(6): 2286–2322.

Goldsmith, M. F. 1991. African lineage, hypertension linked. *Journal of the American Medical Association* 26(15).

Gorman, C. 1991. Why do blacks die young? *Time,* 16 September, 50–52.

Haskell, W. L., and others. 1992. Cardiovascular benefits and assessment of physical activity and physical fitness in adults. *Medicine and Science in Sports and Exercise* 6 Suppl.: S201–20.

———. 1992. Role of water-soluble dietary fiber in the management of elevated plasma cholesterol in healthy subjects. *American Journal of Cardiology* 69(5): 433–39.

Keil, J. E., and others. 1992. Does equal socioeconomic status in black and white men mean equal risk of mortality? *American Journal of Public Health* 82(8): 1133–36.

Leaf, A. 1992. Health claims: Omega-3 fatty acids and cardiovascular disease. *Nutrition Reviews* 50(5): 150–54.

Liebson, P. R. 1992. Intravascular ultrasound in coronary atherosclerosis: A new approach to clinical assessment. *American Heart Journal* 123(6): 1643–60.

Musante, L., and others. 1992. Hostility: Relationship to lifestyle behaviors and physical risk factors. *Behavioral Medicine* 18(1): 21–26.

Pinnelas, D., and others. Total serum cholesterol levels in Asians living in New York City: Results of a self-referred cholesterol screening. *New York State Journal of Medicine* 92(6): 245–49.

Raloff, J. Lead heightens hypertension risk in blacks. *Science News,* 28 April, 261.

Shakespeare, C. F. 1992. Recent advances in cardiology. *Postgraduate Medical Journal* 68(799): 327–37.

Williams, R. 1989. *The Trusting Heart.* New York: Times Books.

Wood, P. D., and others. 1991. The effects on plasma lipoproteins of a prudent weight-reducing diet, with or without exercise, in overweight men and women. *New England Journal of Medicine* 325(7): 461–66.

RECOMMENDED READINGS

Donahue, P. J. 1989. *How to Prevent a Stroke.* Emmaus, Penn.: Rodale Press. *Neurologist Mark L. Dyken, M.D., past chairman of the American Heart Association's Stroke Council, was the medical adviser for this comprehensive look at recommended lifestyle changes for people at risk for stroke.*

Fletcher, A. 1990. *Eat Fish, Live Better.* New York: Harper and Row. *The author reviews the findings related to fish and heart disease. It includes an extensive glossary describing common and uncommon varieties of fish.*

Grundy, S. 1989. *American Heart Association Low-Fat, Low-Cholesterol Cookbook: An Essential Guide for Those Concerned About Their Cholesterol Levels.* New York: Random House. *Recipes and easy-to-follow advice for heart-healthy eating.*

Healthline, July 1990. *Entire issue is devoted to preventing heart disease.* 830 Menlo Avenue, Suite 100, Menlo Park, Ca. 94025

Moser, M. 1989. *Lower Your Blood Pressure and Live Longer: A Simple and Effective Program Developed by a Leading Specialist in Hypertension.* New York: Villard Books. *Comprehensive advice on lifestyle changes to reduce blood pressure without drugs. Helpful charts list sodium content of common foods. Also covers hypertension medications, their uses, and side effects.*

Ulene, A. 1989. *American Medical Association Campaign Against Cholesterol: Count Out Cholesterol, A Program to Help Lower Your Cholesterol in 30 Days!* New York: Random House. *Offers a step-by-step plan for changing your eating habits, with useful tables and charts that break out the fat composition of foods.*

Williams, R. and V. Williams. 1993. *Anger Kills: Seventeen Strategies for Controlling the Hostility that Can Harm Your Health.* New York: Times Books. *Dr. Williams, an expert in behavioral medicine, discusses the biological correlates of anger and hostility that can lead to heart disease and suggests strategies for recognizing and controlling hostility.*

16

Cancer

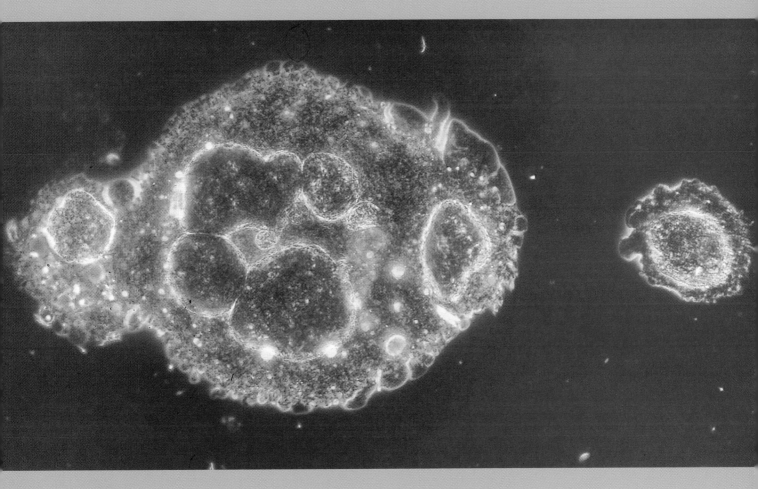

CONTENTS

◗ You and a group of friends are going for a hike today. As you get ready, your room-mate puts sunscreen on her face, neck, and arms and then asks if you want to use some. You tell her you don't need it, since you have the kind of skin that always tans. She says the sun damages your skin whether you tan or burn and can even cause skin cancer. Is she right? Are suntans bad for your skin?

◗ A friend of yours tells you that her recent Pap test was abnormal. She's supposed to have minor surgery to remove some cells or, she says, they could turn into cancer. Her gynecologist told her that in the future she can help protect herself against cancer of the cervix by making sure her sexual partner uses a condom. You're surprised. Is her gyne-cologist suggesting that cervical cancer is a sexually transmissible disease? How can condoms protect you against cancer?

◗ Your grandmother had breast cancer, so your mother has always been very careful to do breast self-exams and have regular checkups. Her physician recently advised her to cut down on her alcohol consumption to lower her risk of breast cancer. Your mother enjoys having a few glasses of wine with dinner every night, and she doesn't know what drinking alcohol has to do with her breasts. Is her physician giving her good advice? How could alcohol consumption affect her risk of breast cancer?

◗ Lately it seems that everywhere you go—the supermarket, the gas station, the liquor store, your favorite restaurants—you notice signs warning that certain chemicals and other substances are "known to cause cancer." You know your state recently passed a law that these signs have to be posted where carcinogens are present, but you're shocked at how often you see them. Are there really that many carcinogens around? How dangerous are they? What can you do to avoid them?

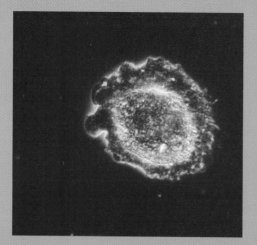

MAKING CONNECTIONS

Although cancer is not the leading cause of death among Americans, it is a particularly dreaded disease that many people fear above all others. Cancer-causing agents and risks seem to abound in our society, but there are steps you can take to protect yourself. In each of the scenarios presented on this page, all related to cancer, individuals have to use information, make a decision, or choose a course of action. How would you act in each of these situations? What response or decision would you make? This chapter pro-vides information about cancer that can be used in situations like these. After finishing the chapter, read the scenarios again. Has what you've learned changed how you would respond?

The word *cancer* comes to us from the Greek word for crab, *karkinos*. We are all familiar with cancer as a tumor—an invasive and malignant growth. The ancient Greek physicians who first described cancer noticed that some malignant tumors resemble a crab—a hard mass with clawlike extensions. In modern times, cancer has retained its reputation as an alien invader and is perhaps the most feared of all noninfectious diseases. Cancer is not the most common cause of death, but it is correctly seen as a progressive, often fatal, condition that cannot always be successfully treated.

WHAT IS CANCER?

Cancer is a group of diseases characterized by uncontrolled growth of abnormal cells. If the spread of these abnormal cells is not controlled, cancer can cause death. Most cancers take the form of tumors, although not all tumors are cancers. A tumor is simply a mass of new tissue that serves no physiological purpose. It can be benign, like a wart, or malignant, like most lung cancers; the terms **malignant tumor** and **malignant neoplasm** are synonymous with *cancer*. **Benign tumors** are made up of cells similar to the surrounding normal cells and are enclosed in a membrane that prevents them from penetrating neighboring tissues. They are dangerous only if their physical presence interferes with bodily functions. A benign brain tumor, for example, can cause death if it blocks the blood supply to the brain. A malignant tumor, or cancer, is capable of invading surrounding structures, including blood vessels, the **lymph system**, and nerves. It can also spread, or *metastasize,* to distant sites via the blood and lymphatic circulation and so can produce invasive tumors in almost any part of the body. A few cancers, like the **leukemias,** or cancers of the blood, don't produce a mass and so aren't properly called tumors. But since the leukemic cells do have the fundamental property of rapid, uncontrolled growth, they are still malignant and therefore cancers.

Metastasis occurs because cancer cells do not stick to each other as strongly as normal cells do and so may not remain at the site of the original or *primary tumor.* They break away and can pass through the lining of lymph or blood vessels to invade nearby tissue. They can also drift to distant parts of the body, where they establish new colonies of cancer cells. This traveling and seeding process is called metastasizing, and the new tumors are called *secondary tumors,* or *metastases.*

Traveling cancer cells can follow two courses. They can produce secondary tumors in the lymph nodes and be carried through the lymph system to form secondary sites elsewhere, or they can invade blood vessels and circulate through the vessels to colonize other organs. This ability of cancer cells to metastasize makes early cancer detection critical. To control the cancer and prevent death, every cancerous cell must be removed. Once cancer cells enter either the lymph or the blood system, it is extremely difficult to stop their spread to other organs of the body.

Every case of cancer begins as a change in a cell that allows it to grow and divide when it should not. Normally (in adults), cells divide and grow at a rate just sufficient to replace dying cells. When you cut your finger, for example, the cells around the wound divide more rapidly to heal the wound. When the wound is healed, the rate of cell growth and division returns to normal. In contrast, a malignant cell divides without regard for normal control mechanisms and gradually produces a mass of abnormal cells, or a tumor. It takes about a billion cells to make a mass the size of a pea, so a single tumor cell must go through many divisions, often taking years, before the tumor grows to a noticeable size. Eventually it produces a sign or symptom that is determined by its location in the body. In the breast, for example, a tumor may be felt as a lump and diagnosed as cancer by x-ray or **biopsy.** In less accessible locations, like the lung, ovary, or bowel, a tumor may be noticed only after considerable growth has taken place and may then be detected only by an indirect symptom—for instance, a persistent cough or unexplained bleeding or pain. In the case of leukemia, there is no lump, but the changes in the blood will eventually be noticed as increasing fatigue, infection, or abnormal bleeding.

Types of Cancer

The behavior of tumors arising in different body organs is characteristic of the tissue of origin. (Figure 16-1 shows the major cancer sites and the incidence of each type.) Since each cancer begins as a single (altered) cell with a specific function in the body, the cancer will retain some of the properties of the normal cell for a time. So, for instance, a cancer of the thyroid gland may produce too much thyroid hormone and cause hyperthyroidism as

---

Malignant tumor A tumor that is cancerous and capable of spreading.

Malignant neoplasm A cancerous growth. A new growth of abnormal cells.

Benign tumor A tumor that is not malignant or cancerous.

Lymph system A system of vessels that returns proteins, lipids, and other substances from fluid in the tissues to the circulatory system.

Leukemias Malignant diseases of the blood-forming system.

Metastasis The spread of cancer cells from one part of the body to another.

Biopsy The removal and examination of a small piece of body tissue. A needle biopsy, usually done in a physician's office, uses a needle to remove a small sample; some biopsies require surgery.

TERMS

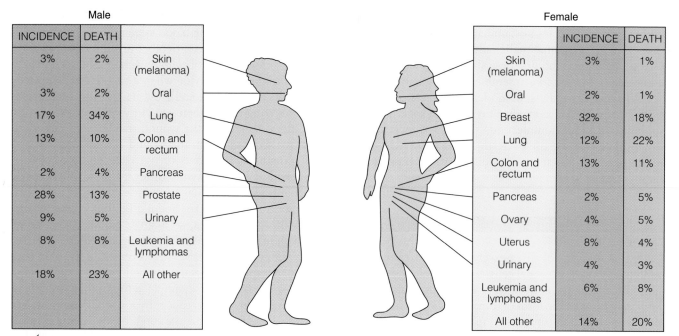

Male		
INCIDENCE	DEATH	
3%	2%	Skin (melanoma)
3%	2%	Oral
17%	34%	Lung
13%	10%	Colon and rectum
2%	4%	Pancreas
28%	13%	Prostate
9%	5%	Urinary
8%	8%	Leukemia and lymphomas
18%	23%	All other

Female		
	INCIDENCE	DEATH
Skin (melanoma)	3%	1%
Oral	2%	1%
Breast	32%	18%
Lung	12%	22%
Colon and rectum	13%	11%
Pancreas	2%	5%
Ovary	4%	5%
Uterus	8%	4%
Urinary	4%	3%
Leukemia and lymphomas	6%	8%
All other	14%	20%

VITAL STATISTICS

Figure 16-1 *Cancer incidence by site and sex, and cancer deaths by site and sex.* Percentages shown are estimates for 1993, excluding nonmelanoma skin cancer. The "incidence" column indicates what percentage of all cancers occurred in each site; the "death" column indicates what percentage of all cancer deaths were attributed to each type. Note: Columns do not all total 100 percent due to rounding. *Source:* American Cancer Society, 1993. *Cancer Facts and Figures, 1993.*

well as cancer. Usually, however, a cancer loses its resemblance to normal tissue as it continues to divide, and it becomes a group of rogue cells with increasingly unpredictable behavior.

Malignant tumors are classified according to the types of cells that give rise to them. The most common cancers are carcinomas, sarcomas, lymphomas, and leukemias (the suffix *-oma* means "tumor"). **Carcinomas,** the most common form of cancer, arise from the **epithelial layers** (outside layers) of cells, which are usually the most actively growing cells in the adult body. Important epithelial layers include the skin, the epithelium of glandular organs (breast, uterus, prostate), and cells lining the respiratory tract (lungs, bronchial tubes), gastrointestinal tract (mouth, stomach, colon, rectum), and urinary tract. Carcinomas metastasize primarily via the lymph vessels. In breast cancer, cells that break away from the tumor metastasize to the nearby lymph nodes. In fact, counting the number of lymph nodes that contain cancer cells is one of the principal methods of predicting the outcome of the disease; the probability of a cure is much greater when the lymph nodes do not contain cancer cells.

Sarcomas occur less often than carcinomas. They arise from connective and fibrous tissue like muscle, bone, cartilage, and the membranes covering muscles and fat. Sarcomas have the reputation of metastasizing primarily by

way of the blood vessels. **Lymphomas** are cancers of the lymph nodes, part of the body's infection-fighting system. They are closely related to leukemias, and like leukemias, they arise from changes in the white blood cells.

Leukemias are cancers of the blood-forming cells, which reside chiefly in the bone marrow; these cancers are due to an abundance of abnormal white cells. Rapid growth of these cells displaces the red blood cell precursors from the bone marrow and can lead to anemia. Because malignant white cells no longer fight infection, the immune system also loses its ability to defend against bacteria, viruses, and other infectious organisms.

There is a great deal of variation in how easily different cancers can be detected and how well they respond to treatment (Figure 16-2). For instance, basal cell skin cancer (one type of skin cancer) is easily detected, grows slowly, and is very accessible. Although there are almost 700,000 cases per year in the United States, virtually all are cured. On the other hand, cancer of the pancreas, fortunately far less frequent, is difficult to detect and only rarely approachable surgically. Only about 3 percent of patients are alive 5 years after diagnosis. In general, the ability of the **oncologist** to predict how a specific tumor will behave is imperfect; since every tumor arises from a unique set of changes in a single cell, predicting the course of the disease is always uncertain.

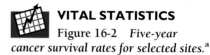

VITAL STATISTICS

Figure 16-2 *Five-year cancer survival rates for selected sites.*[a]

Source: National Cancer Institute. [a](The five-year survival rate is defined as the ratio of the survival rate of the cancer patients to the survival rate for a comparable group [same age and sex] of people not suffering from cancer.)

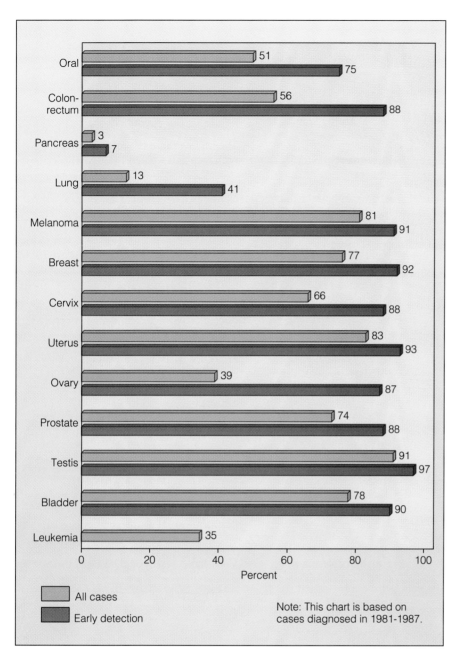

Incidence of Cancer

In 1993, about 1,170,000 people in the United States were diagnosed as having cancer. More than half will be cured, but about 44 percent will eventually die as a result of their cancer. These grim statistics exclude more than 700,000 cases of the curable types of skin cancer. About 85 million Americans now living will eventually develop cancer, or about one in three, according to present rates. Cancer is second only to heart disease as a cause of death in the United States.

Is the incidence of cancer increasing or decreasing? The question must be answered carefully, because the American population is aging and cancer strikes more frequently with advancing age. As the nation improves its

Site	Estimated New Cases 1993	Estimated Deaths 1993	Warning Signals	Comment
Lung	170,000	149,000	Persistent cough or lingering respiratory ailment	The leading cause of cancer death among both men and women.
Colon and rectum	152,000	57,000	Change in bowel habits; bleeding	Considered a highly curable disease when digital and proctoscopic examinations are included in routine checkups.
Breast	183,000	46,300	Lump or thickening in the breast	Until recently, the leading cause of cancer death in women; now surpassed by lung cancer.
Prostate	165,000	35,000	Urinary difficulty	Occurs mainly in men over 60; the disease can be detected by digital rectal exam at annual checkup.
Kidney and bladder	79,500	20,800	Urinary difficulty; bleeding—in which case consult physician at once	Protective measures for workers in high-risk industries are helping to eliminate one of the important causes of these cancers.
Stomach	24,000	13,600	Unexplained indigestion continuing for more than a week	A 40 percent decline in mortality in 25 years, for reasons unknown.
Uterus (including cervix)	44,500[b]	10,100	Unusual bleeding or discharge	Cervical cancer mortality has declined 70 percent during the last 40 years with wider application of the Pap smear. Postmenopausal women with abnormal bleeding should be checked.
Oral (including pharynx)	29,800	7,700	Sore that does not heal; difficulty in swallowing	Many more lives should be saved because the mouth is easily accessible to visual examination by physicians and dentists.
Skin (melanoma)	32,000[c]	6,800	Sore that does not heal; change in wart or mole	Melanoma is readily detected by observation and diagnosed by simple biopsy.
Leukemia	29,300	18,600	Leukemias are cancers of blood-forming tissues and are characterized by the abnormal production of immature white blood cells. Acute leukemia strikes mainly children and is treated by drugs that have extended life from a few months to as much as 10 years. Chronic leukemia strikes usually after age 25 and progresses less rapidly.	
Other blood and lymph tissues	63,700	31,400	These cancers arise in the lymph system and include Hodgkin's disease and lymphosarcoma. Some patients with lymphatic cancers can lead normal lives for many years. Five-year survival rate for Hodgkin's disease increased from 40 percent to 77 percent in 20 years.	

Source: Incidence estimates are based on rates of cancer in the United States from American Cancer Society. 1993. *Cancer Facts and Figures—1993.* (New York: American Cancer Society).

[a]All figures rounded to nearest 100 and include both sexes.
[b]Totals do not include cases in which the carcinoma is confined to the epithelium.
[c]Totals do not include nonmelanoma skin cancers (700,000 new cases annually).

cardiovascular health through better eating and exercise habits, people are living longer and so are increasingly likely to die of cancer rather than of heart attack or stroke. When cancer death rates are adjusted for the effects of an older population, death rates from major types of cancer appear to be leveling off or decreasing. The only major exception to this trend is lung cancer, which is increasing rapidly in women. The rate of death from lung cancer in women today parallels the increased rate of smoking in women about twenty years ago.

Could more people be saved from cancer? The American Cancer Society estimates that 90 percent of skin cancer could be prevented by protecting the skin from the rays of the sun and 87 percent of lung cancer could be prevented by avoiding exposure to tobacco smoke. Thousands of cases of colon, breast, and uterine cancer could be prevented by decreasing dietary fat intake, increasing dietary fiber intake, and controlling body weight. Regular screenings and self-examinations have the potential to save an additional 100,000 lives per year. This information makes it clear that although cancer is primarily a disease of older individuals, your behavior now will determine your cancer risk in the future. Damage to the **DNA** in your cells today may lead to a cancer 20 to 30 years in the future. What you need to know about cancer now is (1) which cancers are avoidable and (2) what precautions can be taken to prevent cancer-producing changes in DNA. In this chapter we will put strongest emphasis on the risk factors for specific cancers, where they are known, and on the lifestyle changes that can help you prevent the "cancer fuse" from being lit.

Personal Insight   Has anyone in your family had cancer or died of cancer? If so, how was it handled? What were you told about it? How do you think it has affected you?

COMMON CANCERS

A discussion of all types of cancer would be beyond the scope of this book, but in this section we look at some of the most common cancers and their causes, prevention, and treatment.

Lung Cancer

Lung cancer is the most common cause of cancer death in the United States and is responsible for over 140,000 deaths each year. (Table 16-1 lists the leading cancer sites in Americans.) For over 40 years breast cancer was the major cause of cancer death in women, but since 1987, lung cancer has surpassed breast cancer as a killer of women. The chief risk factor in lung cancer is tobacco smoke, which accounts for 87 percent of cancers. (Other negative effects of tobacco smoke on the lungs were discussed in detail in Chapter 9.) When smoking is combined with exposure to other environmental carcinogens, such as radioactive radon gas present in some residences or asbestos particles from insulation installed prior to 1970, the risk of cancer can be multiplied by a factor of 10 or more. (See Chapter 24 for more information on radon gas and asbestos.)

The smoker is not the only one at risk. In early 1993, the Environmental Protection Agency classified environmental tobacco smoke (ETS) as a human **carcinogen**—that is, a substance that causes cancer in humans. Long-term exposure to ETS increases risk for lung cancer. The smoke from the burning end of the cigarette, called secondhand or sidestream smoke, has significantly higher concentrations of the toxic and carcinogenic compounds found in mainstream smoke, including nitrosamines, ammonia, and nicotine. It's estimated that ETS causes about 4,000 lung cancer deaths each year.

Lung cancer is difficult to detect at an early stage, and it is difficult to cure even when detected early. Symptoms of lung cancer don't usually appear until the disease has advanced to the invasive stage. Signals such as a persistent cough, chest pain, or recurring bronchitis may be the first indication of the tumor's presence. A diagnosis can usually be made by chest x-ray or by studying the cells in sputum. Because almost all lung cancers arise from the cells that line the bronchi, tumors can sometimes be visualized by fiber-optic bronchoscopy, a test in which a flexible lighted tube is inserted into the windpipe and the surfaces of the lung passages are directly inspected. Lung cancer is most often treated by surgery; if all the tumor cells can be removed, a cure is possible. Unfortunately, lung cancer is usually detected only after it has begun to spread, and lung cancer cells are resistant to almost all forms of **chemotherapy**. It isn't surprising that only about 13 percent of lung cancer patients are alive 5 years after diagnosis. The rate of survival has improved only slightly during the past 10 years.

There is a ray of hope. About 25 percent of lung cancers, those known as small cell lung cancers, are susceptible to chemotherapy. These tumors can now be treated fairly successfully without surgery, using modern chemotherapy combined with radiation. A large percentage of cases respond with **remission**, and in some cases the remission lasts for years.

DNA   Deoxyribonucleic acid, a chemical substance that carries genetic information.

Carcinogen   Any substance that causes cancer.

Chemotherapy   Treatment of cancer with chemicals that selectively destroy cancerous cells.

Remission   Condition in which there are no symptoms or other evidence of disease.

Colon and Rectal Cancer

Another common cancer in the United States is colon and rectal cancer (also called colorectal cancer). It is the second leading cause of cancer death, after lung cancer. You are at moderate risk of developing colorectal cancer once you reach the age of 40. But the majority of cases occur in individuals over 50. This cancer is clearly linked both to diet and to genetic susceptibility (discussed in the next section). In countries where diets are low in fat and high in fiber, the incidence of this cancer may be only 10 or 20 percent of that seen in the United States. Probably one-quarter to one-third of the population is uniquely susceptible to colon cancer because of heredity, but we don't yet know enough to be able to accurately identify those at greatest risk. Even for those of us most susceptible, however, attention to diet can make a significant difference. Decreasing the amount of fat and increasing the amount of insoluble fiber (found in fruits, vegetables, and whole grains) in your diet can minimize your risks of colon cancer. Just as cessation of smoking can reverse precancerous changes in the lung, a high-fiber diet can slow or even reverse precancerous changes in colon cells.

Colon cancer rarely occurs before the age of 40, but to have the best chance of preventing it, you should begin to make dietary changes now. Most colon cancers arise from preexisting **polyps**, small growths on the wall of the colon that may gradually drift toward malignancy over a period of years. The tendency of an individual to form colon polyps appears to be determined by specific genes, so you should be particularly vigilant if colon cancer has occurred among your close relatives. Polyps may bleed as they progress. A polyp may be directly visualized using a **sigmoidoscope,** a flexible fiber-optic device inserted through the rectum. The sigmoidoscope and related instruments allow both visualization and biopsy of the polyp, or even its removal, without the need for major surgery.

The standard warning signs of colon cancer are bleeding from the rectum or a change in bowel habits, but early detection requires more aggressive measures than simply waiting for danger signs. A rectal examination can detect some rectal tumors, and a stool occult blood test, done during a routine physical exam, can detect small amounts of blood in stool long before obvious bleeding would be noticed. The American Cancer Society recommends that this examination be performed annually after age 40. Colon and rectal cancer is more curable than lung cancer, particularly if it is caught before it spreads beyond the bowel to other parts of the body. The 5-year survival rate is 55 percent overall—about 88 percent if the tumor is localized, but only 40 percent if it has spread.

Breast Cancer

Breast cancer is the most common cancer in women and causes almost as many deaths in women as lung cancer.

In men, breast cancer occurs only rarely. In the United States, about one woman in nine will develop breast cancer during her lifetime. In 1993, breast cancer was diagnosed in approximately 183,000 American women, and about 46,000 died from the disease. About 77 percent of patients survive at least 5 years after the diagnosis is made, and most of these achieve a complete cure. The incidence of breast cancer has been increasing at the rate of about 3 percent per year since 1980 and at a slower rate for the past 40 years. Some of this increase is due to simple demographics—the increase in average age of the female population—and some is due to improvements in screening. Environmental and lifestyle factors probably account for the remainder of the increase.

TABLE 16-2 Established and Probable Risk Factors for Breast Cancer

Risk Factor	Relative Risk[a]
Family history of breast cancer	
Two first-degree relatives affected[b]	4–6
Mother affected before age 60	2
Age at birth of first child	
Under 20 years	1
20–24 years	1.3
25–29 years	1.6
30 years or older	1.9
No children	1.9
Benign breast disease	1.5–4
Oral contraceptive use	
Current use	1.5
Past use	1.0
Alcohol use	
None	1.0
1 drink per day	1.4
3 drinks per day	2.0

Adapted from J. R. Harris and others. 1992. "Breast Cancer: Medical Progress." *New England Journal of Medicine* 327(5): 321.

[a]Relative risk means the risk of breast cancer for a woman with a specific risk factor compared to a woman without that risk factor.
[b]First-degree relatives are parents and siblings.

Only a small percentage of breast cancer cases occurs before the age of 30, but a woman's risk doubles every five years between the ages of 30 and 45 and then increases more slowly, by 10 to 15 percent every five years after age 45. The majority of breast cancers are diagnosed in women over 50. When breast cancer does occur, a cure is most likely if the tumor is detected when it is still small. Since this is an increasingly common cancer, attention to screening is a good investment even for younger women.

Risk Factors for Breast Cancer Breast cancer has been called a "disease of civilization," because incidence is high in industrialized Western countries but remains low in less developed non-Western countries. This pattern has led some researchers to point to a link between breast cancer and the Western lifestyle, which is sedentary and includes a diet high in calories and fat and low in fiber. There is also a strong genetic factor in breast cancer. A woman who has two close relatives with breast cancer is four to six times more likely to develop the disease than is a woman who has no close relatives with breast cancer (Table 16-2). However, even though genetic factors do increase the risk of breast cancer, only about 20 percent of cancers occur in women with a family history of it.

Other risk factors include alcohol use, certain kinds of benign breast disease, obesity, use of oral contraceptives, early first menstruation, late menopause, and late first childbirth. The unifying factor for many of these risk factors may be the female sex hormone estrogen. Estrogen circulates in a woman's body in high concentrations during the years between puberty and menopause, and it promotes the growth of responsive cells in a variety of sites. Fat cells also produce estrogen, and estrogen levels are higher in obese women. Alcohol can interfere with metabolism of estrogen in the liver and increase its levels in the blood. The evidence suggests that estrogen is a promoter of cancer in sites that are estrogen-responsive, including breast tissue and the uterus.

The links between breast cancer and diet and exercise habits are still being investigated. Recent studies indicate that a high-fat diet alone may not increase the risk of breast cancer. However, research suggests that women may be more likely to get breast cancer if their diets are low in fiber, if they have a sedentary lifestyle, or if they are obese.

Although some of the risk factors for breast cancer—including heredity and some hormonal factors—cannot be changed, important lifestyle factors for breast cancer are under the control of the individual. Maintaining a normal weight by exercising regularly and eating a low-fat, high-fiber diet can minimize the chance of breast cancer. This is true even for women at risk due to family history or other factors.

Detecting and Treating Breast Cancer The American Cancer Society advises a three-part personal program for early detection of breast cancer. Monthly breast self-examination is recommended for all women over 20 (see the box "Breast Self-Examination"), and a clinical breast exam performed by a physician should be part of a regular health checkup every three years. For women over 40, the odds of finding a tumor early can be improved by having the breasts examined with a sensitive low-dose x-ray technique called **mammography.** (Mammograms are not recommended for women in their twenties and thirties because at that age breast tissue is too dense for this screen to be effective.) Mammograms are recommended every one to two years for women over 40 and once a year after 50, although a woman's individual health history and risk factors need to be considered along with these recommendations. These steps, consistently followed, will detect a majority of tumors at an early stage.

If a lump is detected, it may be scanned by **ultrasonography** and biopsied to see if it is cancerous. The biopsy may be done either by needle in the physician's office or surgically. Nine times out of ten, the lump is found to be a cyst or other harmless growth and no further treatment is needed. If the lump does contain cancer cells, a variety of surgeries may be called for, ranging from a lumpectomy (removal of the lump and surrounding tissue) to a mastectomy (removal of the breast). To determine if the cancer has spread, lymph nodes from the armpit may be removed and examined. If cancer cells are found, tumor cells remaining in the body can often be slowed or killed by additional therapy, such as radiation, chemotherapy, or both.

The chance of survival in cases of breast cancer varies, depending both on the nature of the tumor and whether it has metastasized. If the tumor is discovered early, before it has spread to the adjacent lymph nodes, the patient has about a 92 percent chance of surviving more than 5 years.

Personal Insight How do you feel about performing self-examinations for cancer? Do you do them regularly? If not, why not? Are you reluctant? If so, what do you think underlies your reluctance?

Polyp A small, usually harmless mass of tissue that projects from the inner surface of the colon or rectum.

Sigmoidoscope A flexible fiber-optic probe used for examination of the lower bowel.

Mammography Low-dose x-rays of the breasts used to check for early signs of breast cancer.

Palpation Examination by touch.

Ultrasonography An imaging method in which sound waves are bounced off body structures to create an image on a TV monitor.

TERMS

All women over 20 should practice monthly breast self-examination (BSE) to assist in early detection of breast cancer. Examine your breasts when they are least tender, usually seven days after the start of your menstrual period. If you discover a lump or detect any changes, seek medical attention. Most breast changes are not cancerous.

For a complete BSE, remember these seven P's: positions, perimeter, **palpation**, pressure, pattern, practice with feedback, and plan of action.

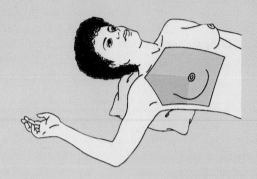

1. *Positions.* The first part of BSE is a visual inspection while standing in front of a mirror. Examine your breasts with your arms raised. Look for changes in contour and shape of the breasts, color and texture of the skin and nipple, and evidence of discharge from the nipple. Repeat the visual examination with your arms at your side, with your hands on your hips, and while bending slightly forward.

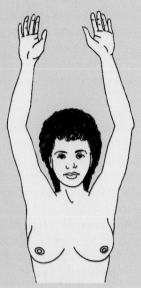

The remainder of the examination involves palpation of your breasts. Two positions are possible: *side-lying* or *flat.* The side-lying position is particularly recommended for women with large breasts: Lie on your side and rotate one shoulder back to the flat surface. You will be examining the breast on the side that is rotated back. If you use the flat position, place a pillow or folded towel under the shoulder of the breast to be examined.

2. *Perimeter.* The area you should examine is bounded by a line which extends down from the middle of the armpit to just beneath the breast, continues across along the underside of the breast to the middle of the breast bone, then moves up to and along the collar bone and back to the middle of the armpit. Most cancers occur in the upper outer area of the breast (shaded area).

3. *Palpation.* Use your left hand to palpate the right breast, while holding your right arm at a right angle to the rib cage, with your elbow bent. Repeat the procedure on the other side. Use the pads of three or four fingers to examine every inch of your breast tissue. Move your fingers in circles about the size of a dime. Do not lift your fingers from your breast between palpations. You can use powder or lotion to help your fingers glide from one spot to the next.

4. *Pressure.* Use varying levels of pressure for each palpation, from light to deep, to examine the full thickness of your breast tissue. Using pressure will not injure the breast.

5. *Pattern of search.* Use one of the following search patterns to examine all of your breast tissue:

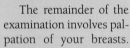

Prostate Cancer

The prostate gland is situated at the base of the bladder in men. It produces seminal fluid; if enlarged, it can block the flow of urine. Prostate cancer is the most common cancer in men and, after lung and colon cancer, the cause of the most deaths. There are over 160,000 new cases of prostate cancer in the United States each year. Prostate cancer is a disease that increases with age, and 80 percent of cases are diagnosed in men over the age of 65. One of

11 men will be diagnosed with prostate cancer during his lifetime. Diet and lifestyle probably influence the occurrence of this cancer, but compared to the other cancers we have discussed, the risk factors are somewhat obscure. For reasons not completely understood, African Americans have the highest incidence of prostate cancer in the world.

The best method for controlling prostate cancer is through early detection, and the methods of screening are becoming increasingly sophisticated. Most cases are first

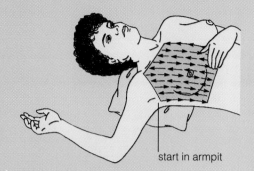

start in armpit

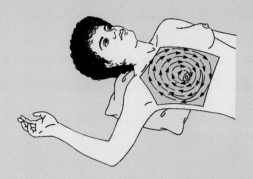

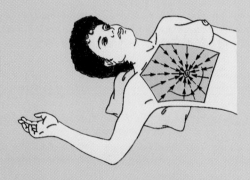

Vertical Strip: Start in the armpit and proceed downward to the lower boundary. Move a finger's width toward the middle and continue palpating upward until you reach the collarbone. Repeat this until you have covered all breast tissue. Make at least six strips before the nipple and four strips after the nipple.

Wedge: Imagine your breast divided like the spokes of a wheel. Examine each separate segment, moving from the outside boundary toward the nipple. Slide fingers back to the boundary, move over a finger's width and repeat this procedure until you have covered all breast tissue. You may need between 10 and 16 segments.

Circle: Imagine your breast as the face of a clock. Start at 12 o'clock and palpate along the boundary of each circle until you return to your starting point. Then move down a finger's width and continue palpating in ever-smaller circles until you reach the nipple. Depending on the size of your breast, you may need 8 to 10 circles.

Once you have completed the pattern, perform two additional exams: (1) squeeze your nipples to check for discharge (some women have a normal discharge), and (2) examine the breast tissue that extends into your armpit while your arm is relaxed at your side.

6. *Practice with feedback.* Have your BSE technique checked by your physician or another health care professional. Practice under supervision until you feel comfortable and confident.

7. *Plan of action:* Your personal breast health plan of action should include the following: (1) discuss the American Cancer Society breast cancer detection guidelines with your physician, (2) schedule clinical breast examinations and mammograms as appropriate, (3) do monthly BSEs, and (4) report any changes to your health care professional.

Source: American Cancer Society. 1992. *Breast Self-Examination: A New Approach,* May.

detected by rectal examination during a routine physical exam. The physician can feel the prostate gland through the rectum and determine whether it is enlarged and whether lumps are present. Although a rectal exam is unpleasant, it is a quick, inexpensive, and practical way to detect the early stages of both prostate and rectal cancers.

A new blood test that measures the amount of prostate-specific antigen (PSA) in the blood can also be used to help diagnose prostate cancer. An elevated level or a rapid increase in PSA can signal trouble. A single measurement of PSA can help catch early prostate cancer, but it also registers benign conditions (about two-thirds of men over 50 have benign prostate disease). The PSA test is probably most useful if it is repeated over time to chart a rate of change; used in this way, it can more accurately distinguish between cancer and benign prostate disease.

Ultrasound is used increasingly as a follow-up, to detect lumps too small to be felt and to determine their size, shape, and properties. A needle biopsy of suspicious

Unlike most cancers, which have their peak incidence after the age of 60, cancer of the cervix often occurs in younger women in their thirties or even in their twenties. Since there is an excellent system of diagnosis and treatment for very early cervical cancer, all women should take advantage of the effective screening methods for this cancer.

Screening for the changes in cervical cells that precede cancer is done chiefly by means of the Papanicolaou test, commonly known as the Pap test. In this procedure, loose cells are scraped from the uterine cervix with a flat plastic probe. They are then spread on a slide, stained for easier viewing, and examined under a microscope to see whether they are normal in size and shape. If cells are abnormal, additional Pap tests are done at intervals. Sometimes the cells spontaneously return to their normal size and shape, but in about one-third of cases, the changes progress toward malignancy. If this happens, the abnormal cells must be removed, either by removing them surgically or by destroying them with a cryoscopic probe (ultracold) or localized laser treatment. When the abnormal cells are in a precancerous state, called cervical carcinoma in situ, the patch of dangerous cells is small and can be completely removed by one of these methods.

Without timely surgery, the malignant patch of cells goes on to invade the wall of the cervix and spreads to adjacent lymph nodes and to the uterus. At this stage cytotoxic (cell-killing) chemotherapy may be used to kill the fast-growing cancer cells, but chances for a complete cure are much lower. Even when a cure can be achieved, it often means surgical removal of the uterus and therefore sterility.

How does cervical cancer get started, and what can be done to prevent it? A great deal of clinical and epidemiological data suggests that the critical event may be infection of the cervical cells by one of the human papillomaviruses (HPV). This is a large group of viruses that cause common warts as well as venereal, or genital, warts. These viruses can cause normally well-behaved cells to divide and grow rapidly. The initial infection probably begins when the virus is introduced into the cervix by an infected sexual partner.

As noted in the text, cervical cancer is strongly associated with early sexual activity and multiple partners; women who do not have sexual relations are not at risk for cervical cancer. Although few studies have been done, it seems likely that regular use of condoms reduces the risk of transmitting papillomavirus infection, as well as other infectious agents that may be important in cervical cancer.

Only a very small fraction of HPV-infected women ever get cervical cancer. There must be added factors, or cofactors, working in parallel with the HPV infection to produce a cancer. All the data are not yet in, but it seems that the most important cofactors are (1) smoking and (2) infection with another common sexually transmitted virus, the genital type of herpesvirus. Both smoking and herpesvirus can cause cancerous changes in cells in the laboratory, and they can speed and intensify the cancerous changes begun by the papillomaviruses. It has recently been shown that nicotine and other mutagenic chemicals, carried from the lungs by the circulation of blood, can be identified in the cervical secretions of women who smoke.

Another important system controls the potential damage done by viral infections, and that is the immune system. It is very likely that normal cellular immunity plays the most important role in controlling the initial HPV infection and in preventing progression from a symptomless infection to cervical dysplasia and then on to malignancy. Chemicals that suppress the immune system, as substances in tobacco appear to do, are associated with an increase in dysplasia and cancer. Stress, poor nutrition, and frequent infections are additional factors that can inhibit normal immune function; these all appear to be secondary risk factors in cancer of the cervix.

The incidence of cervical cancer has steadily decreased in the United States over the years, due to wide availability of Pap test screening. At present, the 5-year survival rate for all cervical cancer is 66 percent. However, in patients who have yearly Pap tests, the cancer is almost always diagnosed at the stage of carcinoma in situ, and survival in these cases is virtually 100 percent.

lumps can be performed relatively painlessly, and a **pathologist** can determine whether the biopsied cells are malignant or benign by examining them under a microscope. If they are malignant, the prostate is usually removed surgically; alternative or additional treatments include radiation, hormones, or anticancer drugs. Of course, early detection leads to a better outcome. Survival rates for all stages of this cancer have improved steadily since 1940—in the last 30 years, 5-year survival has increased from 50 percent to 76 percent.

Uterine, Cervical, and Ovarian Cancer

The uterus, uterine cervix, and ovaries are subject to similar hormonal influences, so the cancers of these organs can be discussed as a group. The cervix is the neck of the

TERMS

Pathologist   A specialist in the study of the origins, nature, and course of disease.

Endometrium   Tissue lining the uterus.

Pap test (Papanicolaou test)   A scraping of cells from the cervix for examination under a microscope to detect cancer.

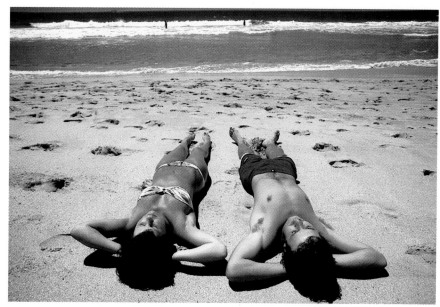

Cumulative exposure to sunlight, beginning in childhood, increases the risk of skin cancer later in life. Blistering sunburns are particularly dangerous, but tanning also poses a hazard. Sunscreens help protect the skin from the sun's radiation.

uterus, the narrow end that opens into the vagina, and the uterus itself is in contact with the ovaries, which are deep in the abdomen. Uterine cancer is the most common cancer of the reproductive system, but ovarian cancer and cervical cancer are more deadly. Most early detection, however, is directed at cervical cancer.

Cancer of the body of the uterus, or **endometrium,** is usually a disease of mature women, and diagnosis is most often made between the ages of 55 and 69. The risk factors are a history of infertility, obesity, and prolonged estrogen therapy. Fortunately, endometrial cancer is often detectable during a standard pelvic exam, and it is curable by surgery. About 83 percent of patients are living and apparently healthy 5 years after diagnosis.

Cervical cancer, in contrast, attacks younger women and eventually kills about one-third of those who are diagnosed with it. In a sense, cervical cancer is one of the great success stories of cancer control during the last few decades. As the use of the **Pap test** has become almost universal in the United States during the past 40 years, the death rate from cervical cancer has dropped by over 70 percent. Cells for the Pap test are collected during a routine gynecologic pelvic exam. Cells scraped from the cervix are placed on a slide and observed under the microscope. The early noninvasive form of cervical cancer can be identified by the presence of abnormal cells in these Pap tests. If abnormal cells are present, they can then be removed before they reach a dangerous invasive stage. The risk factors for cervical cancer are different from those for uterine cancer. They include early age at first intercourse, multiple sex partners, cigarette smoking, and a history of sexually transmissible diseases. Some re-

cent insights into cervical cancer are discussed in the box "Cervical Cancer and Papillomavirus: Evidence for a Link?"

Even though ovarian cancer is rare compared to uterine and cervical cancer, it causes more deaths than the other two combined. It cannot be detected by a Pap test or any other simple screening method and is often noticed only late in its development, when surgery and other therapies are unlikely to be completely successful. Ovarian cancer incidence increases with age, as does the incidence of most cancers, and reaches its peak at ages over 60 years. For women at high risk, particularly those with a family history of ovarian cancer, more frequent pelvic examinations and ultrasound imaging of the ovaries may be helpful. However, a significant improvement in mortality from ovarian cancer will occur only if a sensitive new screening test or a much more effective therapy is developed.

Skin Cancer

Skin cancer is the most common cancer of all when cases of the highly curable forms are included in the count. (Usually these forms are not included, precisely because they are easily treated.) There were over 700,000 cases of all skin cancer in 1993, but only about 32,000 of these were the most serious type. Treatments are usually simple and successful when the cancers are caught early.

Almost all cases of skin cancer can be traced to excessive exposure to the ultraviolet rays of the sun, especially during the childhood years. Skin cancer may also be caused by exposure to coal tar, pitch, creosote, arsenic, and radioactive materials; but compared to sunlight,

Protecting Your Skin from the Sun

Experts are becoming more and more convinced that there is no such thing as a "safe tan," and more people are getting the message that the sun causes skin cancer and premature aging of the skin. But that doesn't mean you shouldn't lead an active outdoor life. Proper clothing and use of sunscreens can protect your skin against most sun-induced damage.

Clothing

- Wear long-sleeved shirts made of closely woven cotton fabric to protect the forearms, chest, and back. Thin, white shirts and wet clothing that clings to the body will not protect you sufficiently.

- Wear a wide-brimmed hat to protect the ears, forehead, and upper cheeks.

Sunscreen

- Use a sunscreen with an SPF (sun protection factor) of 15 or higher. (An SPF rating refers to the amount of time you can stay out in the sun before you burn, compared to using no sunscreen; for example, a product with an SPF of 15 would allow you to remain in the sun without burning 15 times longer, on average, than if you didn't apply sunscreen.) If you're fair-skinned or will be outdoors for long hours, use a sunscreen with a high SPF. Look for the seal of approval from the Skin Cancer Foundation, which tests sunscreens with SPF 15 or higher for safety and effectiveness.

- Choose Photoplex or a "broad spectrum" sunscreen for maximum protection against the full range of ultraviolet radiation from the sun. Many ingredient combinations

work together to block a broader range of light waves and also wash off less easily.

- Apply sunscreen 30 to 45 minutes before exposure. This allows time for the sunscreen to penetrate the skin.

- Reapply sunscreen frequently and generously. Use a water-resistant sunscreen if you swim or sweat quite a bit.

- If you're taking medication, ask your physician or pharmacist about possible reactions to sunlight and interactions with sunscreens.

Time of Day/Location

- Try to avoid sun exposure between 10 A.M. and 3 P.M. when the sun's rays are most intense.

- Ultraviolet rays can penetrate at least three feet in water, so swimmers should wear water-resistant sunscreen.

- Locations near the equator have more intense sunlight, and so stronger sunscreens should be used and applied often. High elevations also have intense sunlight, because there is less atmosphere to filter the ultraviolet rays.

- Snow reflects the sun's rays, so don't forget to apply sunscreen before skiing and other snow activities. Sand and water also reflect the sun's rays, so you still need to apply a sunscreen if you are under a beach umbrella.

Adapted from "Protecting Yourself Against the Sun," *Healthline*, June 1992; "Sunscreens: The Full Spectrum," *University of California at Berkeley Wellness Letter*, February 1989.

---

these agents account for only a small proportion of cases. Because of the link between severe sunburns in childhood and greatly increased risk of **melanoma** in later life, children in particular should be protected from traumatic sunburns. Men and women are equally at risk for skin cancer, but individuals with naturally heavy skin pigmentation have a considerable degree of protection. Conversely, people with fair skin have lower natural protection against skin damage from the sun and have a higher risk of developing certain skin cancers. Both severe, acute sun reactions (sunburns) and chronic low-level sun reactions (suntans) can lead to skin cancer.

Because of damage to the ozone layer (discussed in Chapter 24), there is a chance that we may all be exposed to increasing amounts of ultraviolet radiation in the future. Take time now to understand the risks of excessive sun exposure, because the precautions suggested here will become increasingly critical if the ozone shield continues to thin.

Types of Skin Cancer There are three main types of skin cancer, named for the types of skin cell from which they develop:

- **Basal cell** and **squamous cell carcinomas** together account for about 95 percent of the skin cancers diagnosed each year. They are usually found in chronically sun-exposed areas, such as face, neck, hands, and arms. They usually appear as pale, waxlike, pearly nodules, or red, scaly, sharply outlined patches. These cancers are often painless, although they may bleed, crust, and form an open sore on the skin.

- Melanoma is by far the most dangerous skin cancer because it spreads so rapidly. Since 1973, the incidence of melanoma has increased about 4 percent per year. It can occur anywhere on the body, but the most common sites are the back, chest, abdomen, and lower legs. A melanoma usually appears at the

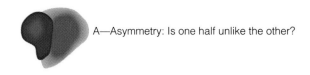
A—Asymmetry: Is one half unlike the other?

B—Border irregularity: Does it have an uneven, scalloped edge rather than a clearly defined border?

C—Color variation: Is the color uniform, or does it vary from one area to another—from tan to brown to black, or from white to red to blue?

D—Diameter larger than one-fourth inch: At its widest point, is the growth as large as or larger than a pencil eraser?

Figure 16-3 *ABCD test for melanoma.*

site of a preexisting mole. The mole may begin to enlarge, become mottled or varied in color (colors can include blue, pink, and white), or develop an irregular surface or irregular borders. Tissue invaded by melanoma may also itch, burn, or bleed easily.

Preventing and Detecting Skin Cancer   One of the major steps you can take to protect yourself against all forms of skin cancer is to avoid lifelong overexposure to sunlight. Blistering, peeling sunburns from unprotected sun exposure are particularly dangerous, but suntans also increase your risk of developing skin cancer later in life. Tanning salons cannot offer safe tanning because tanning in any form increases the risk of skin cancer. People of every age, including babies and children, need to be protected from the sun with **sunscreens** and protective clothing. For a closer look at sunlight and skin cancer, see the box "Protecting Your Skin from the Sun."

The only sure way to avoid a serious outcome from skin cancers is to make sure they are recognized and diagnosed early. In most successfully treated cases, patients themselves bring their melanoma or other skin cancer to their physician's attention. Make it a habit to examine your skin regularly. Most of the spots, freckles, moles, and blemishes on your body are normal; you were born with some of them, and others appear and disappear throughout your life. As you age, you may develop "liver" spots, patches of darkened skin that look like freckles—these

are harmless. But if you notice an unusual growth, discoloration, or sore that does not heal, see your physician or a dermatologist immediately. The characteristics that may signal that a lesion is a melanoma—asymmetry, border irregularity, color change, and a diameter greater than 6 mm—are illustrated in Figure 16-3. Additionally, if someone in your family has had numerous skin cancers or melanomas, you may want to consult a dermatologist for a complete skin examination and discussion of your particular risk.

If you do have an unusual skin lesion, your physician will sometimes be able to determine whether it is benign, precancerous, or cancerous by a physical examination. In other cases, a biopsy is necessary for a definite diagnosis. If the lesion is cancerous, it is usually removed surgically, a procedure that can almost always be performed in the physician's office using local anesthesia. Occasionally, other forms of treatment may be used. Even for melanoma, the outlook after removal in the early stages is good, with a 5-year survival rate of 95 percent and a 10-year rate of 90 percent. If the tumor is removed later, after it has begun to invade the surrounding tissues or other areas of the body, the survival rate drops sharply. Since prevention requires a minimum of time and attention, it pays to be alert.

Oral Cancer

Oral cancer—cancers of the lip, tongue, mouth, and throat—can be traced principally to cigarette, cigar, or pipe smoking, use of smokeless or chewing tobacco, and excess use of alcohol. These risk factors work together to multiply the risk of oral cancer in an individual. The incidence of oral cancer is twice as great in men as in women and most frequent in men over 40. Some prominent sufferers of oral cancer have included Sigmund Freud and Fidel Castro, both notorious cigar smokers. Sports figures who have cultivated a taste for smokeless tobacco or "dipping snuff" are now also increasingly being diagnosed with oral cancer. Although cigarette smoking has declined over the past 25 years, there has been a resurgence in the use of all forms of smokeless tobacco (see Chapter 9). Among long-term snuff users, the excess risk of cancers of cheek, tongue, and gum is nearly fiftyfold.

Oral cancers do have the virtue of being fairly easy to detect, but they are often hard to cure. The principal methods of treatment are surgery and radiation. The

Melanoma   A malignant tumor of the skin that arises from pigmented cells, usually a mole.

Basal cell carcinoma   Cancer of the deepest layers of the skin.

Squamous cell carcinoma   Cancer of the surface layers of the skin.

Sunscreen   Substance used to protect the skin from ultraviolet rays; usually applied as an ointment or a cream.

TERMS

To detect testicular cancer, the American Cancer Society recommends the following self-examination:

1. The best time to perform the examination is after a warm bath or shower, when the scrotal skin is most relaxed. (*Scrotal* refers to the scrotum, the pouch in which the testicles normally lie.)

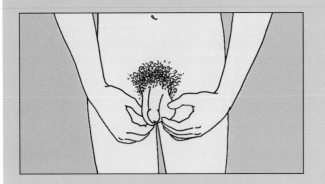

2. Roll each testicle gently between the thumb and fingers of both hands. A normal testicle is smooth, egg-shaped, and somewhat firm to the touch. At the rear of each testicle is a tube called the *epididymis,* which carries sperm away from the testicle; this is a normal part of your body.

3. If you find any hard lumps or nodules, or if there is any change in the shape, size, or texture of the testicles, consult a physician promptly. These signs may not indicate a malignancy, but only your physician can make a diagnosis.

Repeat this examination every month. It is important that you know what your own testicles feel like normally so that you will recognize any changes.

Source: American Cancer Society. 1990. *For Men Only: Testicular Cancer and How to Do TSE (a Self-Exam).*

5-year survival rates vary from 91 percent for lip cancer to 26 percent for throat cancer. Overall 5-year survival is about 51 percent.

Testicular Cancer

Testicular cancer is relatively rare, accounting for only 1 percent of cancer in men, but it is the most common cancer in men 29 to 35 years of age. Self-examination helps in early detection of testicular cancer (see the box "Testicle Self-Examination"). Men with undescended testicles are at increased risk for testicular cancer, and for this reason the condition should be corrected in early childhood. Treatment of this cancer has improved dramatically in the past 20 years; 5-year survival rates have risen from 63 percent to 91 percent.

Other Cancers

There were about 52,300 cases of bladder cancer in the United States in 1993. Bladder cancer is four times as common in men as in women, and smoking is responsible for about half of all cases in men. People living in urban areas and workers exposed to dye, rubber, or leather are at increased risk. The first symptoms are likely to be blood in the urine and/or increased frequency of urination. These symptoms should motivate a quick trip to your physician for a thorough exam, since the survival rate for early-stage bladder cancer is 88 percent.

Pancreatic cancer is the fifth leading cancer killer, with about 27,700 deaths in the United States in 1993. This cancer is both hard to detect and almost always deadly. The major environmental risk factor is, again, smoking. In addition, countries where the diet is high in fat have higher rates of pancreatic cancer. The disease often has a "silent" course, and by the time symptoms occur, the disease is usually far advanced. Very little is known about this disease or how to prevent it. Better methods of imaging, as discussed in the final section of this chapter, may eventually allow earlier diagnosis.

A rare form of skin cancer, Kaposi's sarcoma, is seen almost exclusively in people with HIV infection, apparently as a result of the immune system's inability to function properly. It is discussed further in Chapter 17.

WHAT CAUSES CANCER

Although scientists don't know everything about what causes cancer, they have identified genetic, environmental, and lifestyle factors. (For information on possible factors involved in cancer incidence, see the box "Can Poverty Cause Cancer?") There are usually several steps in the transformation of a normal cell into a cancer cell, and in many cases, different factors may work together in the development of cancer.

Take Good Care of Your DNA

Mutational damage to a cell's DNA, particularly to the DNA of the genes that control cell growth, can lead to

Along with the well-publicized seven warning signs of cancer, an eighth might be added—an empty bank account. As if the inner-city scourges of crime, drug abuse, and neglect weren't enough, Americans with low incomes are also afflicted with more than their share of cancer and cancer deaths. Not only are they more susceptible to cancer, but they are also more likely to die of it—even if the extent of their condition and treatment is similar to that of wealthier cancer victims. As National Cancer Institute director Samuel Broder has stated, "Poverty is a carcinogen."

Why does cancer afflict the economically disadvantaged so disproportionately? Some of the reasons are known, and others are under investigation. A principal factor is lifestyle—people in low-income brackets are more likely to smoke, abuse alcohol, and eat high-fat diets, all of which have been associated with cancer. Another reason is lack of knowledge and information. Studies have found that low-income people are less exposed to information about cancer, less aware of its early warning symptoms, and less likely to seek medical care when they have such symptoms.

A third reason may be an inability to respond to health information and health needs. "Just because you know you should get annual checkups doesn't mean you are able," points out Angelo Alonzo, an associate professor of sociology at Ohio State University and an expert in medical sociology. Many low-income people know they should eat nutritious foods and get regular checkups, but they still may not be able to afford such foods and may not have transportation or access to health clinics.

In fact, many of the cancer-related threats that people with low incomes face are difficult or impossible to avoid. They may be forced to live and work in unsafe or unhealthy environments. They may have jobs, for example, in which they come into daily contact with carcinogenic chemicals, and they may not have been trained in handling them properly. They face similar risks in their homes and schools, where they may be exposed to asbestos or other cancer-causing hazards on a daily basis. The environments in which economically disadvantaged people find themselves are simply less conducive to good health than are those of wealthier people.

But even poor health habits and dangerous living and working conditions don't completely explain the high cancer mortality rates among the disadvantaged. Although scientists don't have a full explanation for it, there's something about economic deprivation that makes cancer deadlier. In a study of various income groups in Boston, researchers found that low-income people had substantially lower 1- and 3-year cancer survival rates than did wealthier individuals, even though they were treated at the same clinics and hospitals. The results had no relation to differences in the stage of cancer at diagnosis, age of patients, or type of treatment they received. In a study of cancer patients at two New York City hospitals, it was found that chemotherapy was less effective on the tumors of the poorer patients. They had a lower rate of cancer remission than wealthier patients, even when the latter had more extensive disease.

One possible explanation for these statistics can be found in the high levels of stress associated with poverty. Studies have found that stress can dampen the immune system, the body's first line of defense against cancer, and experiments with animals have shown that a stressful environment can enhance the growth of a variety of tumors. The link between poverty, stress, and cancer mortality in humans has not been proven, but studies have shown a link between stress and other illnesses.

What can be done about reducing the rate of cancer and cancer mortality among low-income populations? Educating people about prevention is clearly important, and elementary and high schools are places where people can be reached in time to encourage healthy habits and prevent bad habits before they begin. However, people from lower socioeconomic groups are less likely to value education, and they tend to have high dropout rates. Furthermore, most people have a difficult time worrying about a disease they might get in 10 or 20 years when their immediate concern is survival.

For these reasons, some medical scientists look to policymakers for solutions. They maintain that living and working conditions in the inner cities must be improved. Then, even without new miracle drugs or medical breakthroughs, the United States will see a real decrease in cancer rates among low-income populations.

Adapted from Jeff Grabmeier. 1992. "Poverty Can Cause Cancer." *USA Today*, July.

rapid and uncontrolled division of cells. Environmental agents that produce mutational damage, known as **mutagens,** include radiation, viral infection, and chemical substances in the air we breathe and the food we eat. When these agents also cause cancer, we call them carcinogens. We know that several mutational changes are required before a normal cell takes on the properties of a cancer cell. Almost every month researchers identify new genes in which mutational changes are associated with the conversion of a normal cell into a cancer cell; these critical genes are known as **oncogenes.** Careful study of oncogenes will

Mutagen   Any factor (chemical, radiation, and so on) that can cause mutation.

Oncogene   A gene involved in the transformation of a normal cell into a cancer cell.

TERMS

TABLE 16-3 Selected Foods That May Have a Role in Cancer

Substance	Major Dietary Sources	Suspected Role in Cancer	Comment
Possible Protectors			
Beta-carotene (transformed into vitamin A by the body)	Yellow, orange, and green leafy vegetables and fruit, such as carrots, cantaloupe, broccoli, yams, spinach	Deficiency may increase risk of lung, stomach, cervical, bladder, and other cancers.	This antioxidant is thought to be more anticarcinogenic than dietary vitamin A. Extra carotene is stored in most tissue for future use. Not toxic.
Vitamin A	Liver, butter, milk, cheese, egg yolk, fish oil	Deficiency may cause abnormal cell growth, possibly leading to cancerous tumors.	Much of its protectiveness is due to beta-carotene (above). Avoid vitamin A supplements— megadoses can be toxic.
Vitamin C	Citrus fruits, tomatoes, broccoli, strawberries, potatoes, peppers, kale (C is destroyed by improper storage or long cooking)	Deficiency of this antioxidant may increase risk of cancer of stomach and esophagus. Presence may block conversion of nitrites and nitrates to cancer-causing agents.	Adult RDA is 60 milligrams, supplied by 4 ounces of fresh orange juice. Unused C is excreted. Megadoses (over 1 gram daily) can cause diarrhea and may result in kidney stones.
Vitamin E	Nuts, vegetable oils, liver, margarine, whole grains, wheat germ, dried beans	An antioxidant. Shown to protect lab animals against some cancers.	Adult RDA is supplied by one tablespoon of margarine.
Selenium	Seafood, liver, meats, grains, egg yolks, tomatoes	An antioxidant. Shown to protect lab animals against some cancers.	No RDA. Plentiful in most diets. Supplements can be extremely dangerous.
Fiber	Found only in plant foods, such as fruits, vegetables, whole grains, legumes	Promotes healthy bowel function. May lower risk of colon and rectal cancer.	Choose whole-grain breads and cereals. Eat fruit and vegetables with skins when possible.
Cruciferous vegetables	Vegetables of the cabbage family, e.g., broccoli, kale, brussels sprouts, cauliflower	Contain antioxidants and other anticarcinogens that may block production of potential cancer-causing agents.	Eat at least 2–3 servings each week. Excellent sources of fiber, minerals, and vitamins.

eventually lead to more precise and sensitive methods of determining who is at risk for certain cancers and to new methods of diagnosis and treatment.

Although much still needs to be learned about oncogenes, it's clear that minimizing mutational damage to our DNA will lower our risk of many cancers. Unfortunately, a great many substances produce cancer-causing mutations, and we can't escape them all. By identifying the important carcinogens and understanding how they produce their effects, we can help keep our DNA intact and avoid activating "sleeping" oncogenes.

Cancer Initiators and Cancer Promoters Carcinogenic agents that cause mutational changes in the DNA of oncogenes are known as "initiators" of cancer. Ultraviolet rays from the sun or tanning lamps are an example of a cancer initiator. Other chemical agents are not capable of producing DNA mutations directly but can instead act as "promoters" of cancer. Promoters accelerate the growth of cells without damaging or permanently altering the cell's DNA. An example of a cancer promoter is estrogen, the female sex hormone, which acts as a growth stimulus to cells of female reproductive organs. By speeding up cell growth, promoters increase the odds that any damage done to DNA by initiators will be permanently preserved; they do so by stimulating the cell to replicate before damage can be repaired.

Colon cancer provides a good example of how the combination of initiators and promoters contributes to the development of cancer. Cells in the colon tend to divide more rapidly if your diet is high in fat and low in fiber. Under these circumstances of growth *promotion,* a cell with preexisting mutation in an oncogene has an increased chance of progressing toward cancer. Increasing your intake of dietary fiber will tend to reverse this effect and slow the growth of the cells that line the colon. This

TABLE 16-3 Selected Foods That May Have a Role in Cancer (continued)

Substance	Major Dietary Sources	Suspected Role in Cancer	Comment
Possible Villains			
Fats	Meats, poultry skin, whole milk and milk products, vegetable oils	Excess consumption of fats may contribute to cancers of the digestive and reproductive systems and to obesity, another risk factor for cancer.	Choose low-fat dairy products and lean meats; trim all visible fat and discard poultry skin; don't fry meats. Eat fish. Avoid high-fat processed foods.
Alcohol	Beer, wine, liquor	Heavy drinking, especially combined with smoking, contributes to cancers of the mouth, throat, liver, and bladder. May also be a factor in breast cancer.	Drink only in moderation, if at all: no more than two drinks a day.
Nitrites	Used to preserve cured meats, such as bacon, hot dogs, sausages, ham	Promotes cancers of stomach and esophagus in lab animals.	Avoid eating cured meats habitually. Use low-temperature cooking methods; for example, microwaved bacon is lower in carcinogens, especially if you drain the fat.
Aflatoxins	Poisons formed in moldy peanuts, peanut butter, seeds, corn, and other crops	If eaten in large amounts, can cause liver cancer, a rare disease in this country.	Discard moldy, shriveled, discolored peanuts. Refrigerate freshly ground peanut butter; discard entire jar if moldy.
Browned foods	Meats grilled, barbecued, or fried at high temperatures	These cooking methods create cancer-causing agents. Most dangerous when cooking fatty meat over a heat source.	As often as possible, choose other cooking methods—steam, bake, roast, or microwave. Scrape off charred material.

Source: University of California at Berkeley Wellness Letter, October 1987.

directly lessens the possibility that a cancer may develop. As more relationships of this kind are identified, we can expect major changes in the incidence of certain cancers.

Hereditary Cancer Risks   Certain types of cancer have a genetic basis; in other words, an individual who has inherited a damaged or activated oncogene from one or both parents is at increased risk of developing cancer. In their undamaged form, many oncogenes play a role in controlling and restricting cell growth; they are called **suppressor genes.** These growth-controlling suppressor genes normally act as a brake on the growth of cells. They are inherited as a pair, one from each parent, with one gene copy on each **chromosome** of a chromosome pair. Some individuals are born with one of these suppressor genes already damaged; loss of the second suppressor gene through a later mutation will then "release the brake" on cell division and lead directly to more rapid cel-

lular growth and division. As discussed earlier, this is a precondition for development of cancer.

Colon cancer provides an example of the consequences of inheriting an altered suppressor gene. About one-quarter of all Americans have inherited an alteration in one or both copies of a pair of suppressor genes vital for control of growth of colon cells. As these individuals age, they tend to form colon polyps, which can progress to cancer. As our understanding increases, we should be able to identify these individuals by testing for the pres-

Suppressor gene   A type of oncogene that normally functions to restrain growth of tissue cells.

Chromosomes   Material in the nucleus of a cell that transmits genetic information. Abnormal chromosomes are common in cancer cells.

TERMS

ence of the suppressor gene's altered DNA. Their risk of cancer can then be reduced by careful attention to diet and increased monitoring.

Dietary Factors in Cancer

As noted above, agents that cause cancer are called carcinogens. **Anticarcinogens** are substances that protect us from cancer. The foods we eat contain both (Table 16-3).

Fat and Fiber   A "fatty" diet, high in saturated fats such as those found in red meats, appears to contribute to colon, prostate, and other cancers. People in Scotland, for example, consume a great deal of fatty red meat (over 40 percent of calories from fat), and Scotland has the highest incidence of colorectal cancer in the world. The Japanese, by contrast, eat much less fat (less than 20 percent of total calories) because fish, rather than fatty meat, is the staple dietary protein; and colorectal cancer is uncommon in Japan. These patterns cannot be explained by genetic or racial susceptibility. Japanese who have emigrated to the United States, where fatty meats are a major part of the diet, are as susceptible to colorectal cancer as other Americans.

Recent studies have shed some light on the mechanism by which dietary fats promote colorectal cancer. Dietary fats stimulate the production of bile acids, which are necessary to break down and digest material in the colon. Once produced, these bile acids remove layers of cells from the intestinal epithelium, which in turn are replaced by growth of new cells. Newly formed and rapidly growing cells are particularly susceptible to cancer-causing agents. In addition, the animal fat we consume may contain fat-soluble synthetic pesticides, like dioxin and PCBs, that are themselves carcinogenic.

Some groups of people, particularly vegetarians, have little colorectal cancer. The vegetarian diet is typically low in fat and high in insoluble fiber. This link, backed up by laboratory evidence, suggests that colorectal cancer may also be related to lack of fiber in the diet. While fiber does not supply nutrition, it has many other useful properties. It provides bulk, which dilutes any carcinogens that may

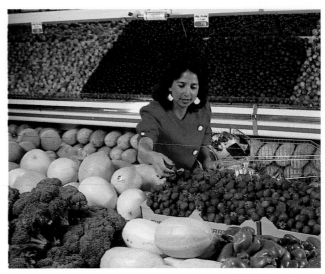

The American Cancer Society recommends a high-fiber diet containing cruciferous vegetables and rich in vitamins A and C. Broccoli, strawberries, and red and green peppers are all excellent choices.

be present. It reduces the transit time of waste through the intestine, so that carcinogens have less time to act on the epithelial cells. Fiber also binds bile acids and other lipids that promote the development of colorectal cancer.

Alcohol   Alcohol is associated with an increased incidence of several cancers. The link between alcohol intake and breast cancer is not well understood, but it is dramatic. An average alcohol intake of three drinks per day is associated with a doubling in the risk of breast cancer (see Table 16-2). As mentioned earlier, alcohol and tobacco (cigarettes or smokeless tobacco) interact as risk factors for oral cancer. The combination of the two multiplies the carcinogenic effect of each substance. Heavy users of both alcohol and tobacco have a risk for oral cancer up to 15 times greater than that of people who don't drink or smoke.

Anticancer Agents in the Diet   Some dietary compounds have the ability to prevent carcinogenesis by environmental agents and so are known as anticarcinogens. An example is **beta-carotene,** a precursor of vitamin A that is present in carrots and other yellow and orange vegetables and in leafy green vegetables. Beta-carotene, carotenoids, and vitamin A itself seem to act as antipromoters, slowing the growth of epithelial cells throughout the body. Beta-carotene looks so promising in cancer prevention that the National Cancer Institute has set up longterm clinical trials to determine its efficacy. Other anticarcinogens in your diet act at the level of cancer initiation. For example, **antioxidants** such as vitamin C and vitamin E can intercept and render harmless many of the chemical agents capable of causing mutagenic damage to DNA. Because it takes so long for most cancers to de-

The National Cancer Institute estimates that about one-third of all cancers are in some way linked to what we eat. This means that you can affect your risk of developing cancer by changing your diet in certain ways. The following changes in diet are recommended as a way to reduce your chances of getting cancer:

- Eat a varied diet.
- Eat more high-fiber foods such as fruits, vegetables, and whole-grain cereals, breads, and pasta.
- Eat dark-green and deep-yellow fruits and vegetables rich in vitamins A and C.
- Eat cruciferous vegetables such as cabbage, broccoli, brussels sprouts, and cauliflower.
- Be moderate in your consumption of salt-cured, smoked, and nitrite-cured foods.
- Cut down on your intake of fat and saturated fat.
- Maintain a healthy body weight.
- Be moderate in your consumption of alcoholic beverages.

Using the list of food components that offer protection from cancer, Susan Zarrow with the Rodale Food Center compiled a list of the 50 top anti-cancer foods. To make the list, a food had to be extremely high in one factor believed to prevent cancer, a good source of several factors, or a low-fat substitute for a common high-fat item. Her list includes the following foods:

Apricots	Broccoli
Bran cereal	Brown rice
Brazil nuts	Brussels sprouts
Butternut squash	Papaya
Cabbage	Peas (with edible pods)
Cantaloupe	Popcorn
Carrots	Potatoes
Cauliflower	Prunes
Chard	Pumpkin
Chicken breast	Raisins
Collard greens	Salmon (canned)
Corn and canola oil	Sardines (canned)
Evaporated skim milk	Skim milk
Figs (dried)	Spinach
Grapefruit	Strawberries
Great northern beans	Sunflower seeds
Kale	Sweet peppers
Kidney beans	Sweet potatoes
Kiwis	Swordfish
Mangoes	Tofu
Nonfat yogurt	Tuna (canned)
Nonfat yogurt cheese	Turnips and rutabagas
Oatmeal	Wheat germ
Oranges	Whole-wheat bread

Sources: American Cancer Society; S. Zarrow with the Rodale Food Center. 1989. "Eat to Beat Cancer: Our 50 Food Picks." *Prevention,* February.

velop, it may be 10 to 20 years before the outcome of the NCI trials can tell us whether we should add these supplements to our diet; in the meantime, be sure to include the RDAs of these vitamins in your diet (see Chapter 12).

People whose diet includes broccoli and other members of the **cruciferous** (cabbage) family of vegetables have a lower risk of a number of cancers. A potent anticarcinogen, **sulforaphane,** has recently been purified from broccoli. Sulforaphane can induce, or turn on, the body's natural detoxifying enzymes, which are made by the colon, liver, and other tissues. These detoxifying enzymes are able to render many natural and synthetic dietary carcinogens harmless.

Additional protection against some cancers may be provided by vitamin D and calcium. In one recent study, men whose diets contained the most vitamin D and calcium were almost three times less likely to develop cancer of the large intestine than were those whose diets contained the lowest amounts of these nutrients. Although the mechanism is still unclear, it appears that the combined presence of vitamin D and calcium slows the growth of cells in the bowel, thereby having an antipromoting effect on potentially cancerous cells. Low- and nonfat milk and milk products are excellent sources of both vitamin D and calcium.

Some general dietary guidelines for protecting yourself from cancer are given in Table 16-3 and in the box "A Dietary Defense Against Cancer."

Personal Insight Although many people are aware that certain behaviors help prevent cancer—such as using sunscreen and modifying their diets—a large percentage of them don't act on their knowledge. Do you follow through with behavior changes when you learn that certain things you do increase your risk of cancer? If so, how do you make the changes? If not, why do you think you don't?

TABLE 16-4 Occupational and Environmental Carcinogens: Ten Suspects

Agents	Where Found	Cancers They May Cause
Arsenic	Mining and smelting industries	Skin, liver, lung
Asbestos	Brake linings, construction sites, insulation, powerhouses	Lung, pleura, peritoneum
Benzene	Solvents, insecticides, gasoline	Bone marrow
Benzidine (outlawed in Great Britain and former Soviet Union, still used widely in U.S.)	Manufacturing rubber, dyestuffs	Bladder
Coal combustion products	Steel mills, petrochemical industry, asphalt, coal tar	Lung, bladder, scrotum
Nickel compounds	Metal industry, alloys	Lung, nasal sinuses
Radiation	Ultraviolet rays from the sun, medical treatments	Bone marrow, skin, thyroid
Synthetic estrogens	Drugs	Vagina, cervix, uterus
Tobacco	Cigarettes, cigars, pipes	Lung, bladder, mouth, esophagus, pharynx, larynx
Vinyl chloride	Plastics industry	Liver, brain

Carcinogens in the Environment

Some carcinogens occur naturally in the environment, like the ultraviolet rays from the sun or the radioactive radon gas that seeps out of the earth and into houses in some regions. Others are manufactured or synthetic substances that show up occasionally in the general environment but more often in the work environments of specific industries.

Ingested Chemicals Since World War II, new methods of distributing and marketing foods have greatly increased the length of time it takes food to travel from its source to the consumer. To prevent food from becoming spoiled or stale during this time, the food industry adds preservatives and numerous other additives, including stabilizers, binders, and emulsifiers (see Chapter 12). Some of these compounds are antioxidants and may actually decrease any cancer-producing properties the food might have. Other compounds, like the nitrates and nitrites found in processed meat, are potentially more sinister.

Nitrosamines Chemical substances that can cause cancer.

Nitrates and nitrites are added to foods like beer and ale, ham, bacon, hot dogs, bologna, and other luncheon meats. The nitrates inhibit the growth of bacteria, which could otherwise cause food poisoning. They also preserve the pink color of the meat, which has no bearing on taste but looks more appetizing to many people. While nitrates and nitrites are not themselves carcinogenic, they can combine with dietary amines in the stomach and be converted to **nitrosamines,** which are highly potent carcinogens. Foods cured with nitrites, as well as those cured by salt or smoke, have been linked to esophageal and stomach cancer, and they should be eaten only in modest amounts.

Environmental and Industrial Pollution Pollutants in urban air have long been suspected of contributing to the incidence of lung cancer. Fossil fuels and their combustion products, such as complex hydrocarbons, have been of special concern, and most gas stations are now required to provide special nozzles to reduce the amount of gasoline vapor released when you fill your tank. The effect of air pollutants has been difficult to study, due to the overwhelmingly greater influence of smoking on lung cancer rates. Urban air pollution appears to have a measurable but limited role in causing lung cancer.

The best available data indicate that less than 2 percent of cancer deaths are caused by general environmental pollution, such as substances in our air and water. Exposure to carcinogenic materials in the workplace is a more serious problem. Occupational exposure to specific carcinogens may account for up to 5 percent of cancer deaths. Some of the more important environmental carcinogens are listed in Table 16-4.

Workers in the rubber, plastics, paint and dye, cable, and petroleum industries have historically been at greater risk of cancer than the rest of the population. Shipyard workers, for instance, who were exposed to high levels of asbestos while building ships during World War II, have experienced a very high incidence of lung cancer; those who also smoked have even higher rates. With increasing industry and government regulatory control, we can anticipate that these industrial sources of cancer risk will continue to diminish, at least in the United States. By contrast, in the former Soviet Union and Eastern European countries, where environmental concerns were sacrificed to industrial productivity for decades, cancer rates due to industrial pollution continue to climb.

Radiation   All sources of radiation are potentially carcinogenic—including medical x-rays, radioactive substances (radioisotopes), and the ultraviolet rays of the sun. The most striking historical example of this has been the increased rates of cancer seen in the survivors of the atomic bombings of Hiroshima and Nagasaki in 1945. Excess new cancers, chiefly leukemias, are still occurring nearly 50 years later. A recent review of excess deaths from the bombings has caused authorities to again raise the estimates of cancer and leukemia risk from exposure to radiation. The excess of leukemias seen in survivors of Hiroshima is a warning to us that any unnecessary exposure of children or fetuses to ionizing radiation should be strictly avoided. Most physicians and dentists are quite aware of the risk of radiation, and successful efforts have been made to reduce the amount of radiation needed for mammograms, dental x-rays, and other necessary medical x-rays.

Another source of environmental radiation is radon gas. Radon is a radioactive decomposition product of radium, which is found in small quantities in some rocks and soils. Since radon is inhaled with the air we breathe, it comes into intimate contact with the cells of the lung, where its radiation can produce mutations. Radon and smoking together create a more-than-additive risk of lung cancer. Fortunately, in most of our homes and classrooms, radon is rapidly dissipated into the atmosphere, where it presents no threat. But in certain kinds of enclosed spaces, such as mines, some basements, and airtight houses built of brick or stone, it can rise to dangerous levels (see Chapter 24).

Sunlight is a very important source of radiation, but since its rays penetrate only a millimeter or so into the skin, it could be considered a "surface" carcinogen. Most cases of skin cancers are the relatively benign and highly curable basal cell cancers, but a substantial minority are the potentially deadly malignant melanomas. As discussed earlier, all types of skin cancer are increased by early and excessive exposure to the sun, and severe sunburn early in childhood appears to carry with it excessive risk of melanoma later in life.

DETECTING, DIAGNOSING, AND TREATING CANCER

Early cancer detection often depends on our willingness to be aware of changes in our own body or to make sure we keep up with recommended diagnostic tests. Although treatment success varies with individual cancers, cure rates have increased—sometimes dramatically—in this century.

Detecting Cancer

Unlike those of some other diseases, early signs of cancer are usually not apparent to anyone but the victim. Even pain is not a reliable guide to early detection, since the initial stages of cancer may be painless. Self-monitoring is the first line of defense, and the American Cancer Society recommends that you pay close attention to the following signs, which you can remember with the acronym "CAUTION":

- **C**hange in bowel or bladder habits
- **A** sore that does not heal
- **U**nusual bleeding or discharge
- **T**hickening or lump in the breasts or elsewhere
- **I**ndigestion or difficulty in swallowing
- **O**bvious change in a wart or mole
- **N**agging cough or hoarseness

Although none of these signs is a sure indication of cancer, the appearance of any one should send you to see your physician. By being aware yourself of the risk factors in your own life, including the cancer history of your immediate family and your own past history, you can often bring a problem to the attention of a physician long before it would have been detected at a routine physical (see the box "What Is Your Risk of Developing Certain Cancers?").

The American Cancer Society is probably the best authority on which tests for cancer detection should be made routine. Their recommendations are summarized in Table 16-5. These routine tests are intended for people who have no signs of cancer. Self-examination of breast or testicles is probably the most useful self-screening procedure and should be performed on a regular basis. Men and women over 40 should have a yearly rectal examination by a physician and a stool occult blood test every year after age 50.

For each question, select the response that best describes you; record the point value in the space provided. Total your points for each section separately.

Lung Cancer

1. Sex   _____
   2   Male
   1   Female

2. Age   _____
   1   39 or less
   2   40–49
   5   50–59
   7   60 and over

3. 8   Smoker   _____
   1   Nonsmoker

4. Type of smoking   _____
   10   Current smoker of cigarettes or little cigars
   3   Pipe and/or cigar, but not cigarettes
   2   Ex-cigarette smoker
   1   Nonsmoker

5. Amount of cigarettes smoked per day   _____
   1   0
   5   Less than 1/2 pack
   9   1/2–1 pack
   15   1–2 packs
   20   2 or more packs

6. Type of cigarette*   _____
   10   High tar/nicotine
   9   Medium tar/nicotine
   7   Low tar/nicotine
   1   Nonsmoker

7. Duration of smoking   _____
   1   Never smoked
   3   Ex-smoker
   5   Up to 15 years
   10   15–25 years
   20   25 or more years

8. Type of industrial work   _____
   3   Mining
   7   Asbestos
   5   Uranium and radioactive products

Lung total   _____

*Tar/nicotine levels:
High: 20 + mg. tar/1.3 + mg. nicotine
Medium: 16–19 mg. tar/1.1–1.2 mg. nicotine
Low: 15 mg. or less tar/1.0 mg. or less nicotine

Colon and Rectal Cancer

1. Age   _____
   10   39 or less
   20   40–59
   50   60 and over

2. Has anyone in your immediate family ever had: _____
   20   Colon cancer
   10   One or more colon polyps
   1   Neither

3. Have you ever had: _____
   100 Colon cancer
   40   One or more colon polyps
   20   Ulcerative colitis
   10   Cancer of the breast or uterus
   1   None

4. Bleeding from the rectum (other than obvious hemorrhoids or piles)   _____
   75   Yes
   1   No

Colon and rectal total   _____

Skin Cancer

1. Frequent work or play in the sun   _____
   10   Yes
   1   No

2. Work in mines, around coal tars, or around radioactivity   _____
   10   Yes
   1   No

3. Complexion—fair skin and/or light skin   _____
   10   Yes
   1   No

Skin total   _____

Breast Cancer (Women Only)

1. Age group   _____
   10   20–34
   40   35–49
   90   50 and over

2. Racial group   _____
   5   Asian
   20   African American
   25   Non-Hispanic White
   10   Hispanic

3. Family history   _____
   30   Mother, sister, aunt, or grandmother with breast cancer
   10   None

4. Your history   _____
        25 Previous lumps or cysts
        10 No breast disease
       100 Previous breast cancer
5. Maternity   _____
        10 1st pregnancy before 25
        15 1st pregnancy after 25
        20 No pregnancies

Breast total   _____

Cervical Cancer (Women Only)

1. Age group   _____
        10 Less than 25
        20 25–39
        30 40–54
        30 55 and over
2. Racial group   _____
        10 Asian
        20 African American
        10 Non-Hispanic White
        20 Hispanic
3. Number of pregnancies   _____
        10 0
        20 1 to 3
        30 4 and over
4. Viral infections   _____
        10 Herpes and other viral infections
            or ulcer formations on the vagina
         1 Never
5. Age at first intercourse   _____
        40 Before 15
        30 15–19
        20 20–24
        10 25 and over
         5 Never
6. Bleeding between periods or
    after intercourse   _____
        40 Yes
         1 No

Cervical total   _____

Analysis

If your *lung* total is:

24 or less   You have a low risk for lung cancer.
24–49   You may be a light smoker and would
             benefit from quitting.
50–74   As a moderate smoker, your risks for lung
             and upper respiratory tract cancer are
             increased. If you stop smoking now, these risks
             will decrease.

75 or over   As a heavy cigarette smoker, your risks for lung
             and upper respiratory tract cancer are greatly
             increased. You should stop smoking now. See
             your physician if you have possible signs of
             lung cancer (nagging cough, hoarseness,
             persistent sore in the mouth or throat).

If your *colon and rectal* total is:

29 or less   You are at low risk for colon and rectal cancer.
30–69   You are at moderate risk. Testing by your
             physician may be indicated.
70 or over   You are at high risk. You should see your
             physician for the following tests: digital rectal
             exam, stool occult blood test, and (where
             applicable) proctoscopic exam.

Numerical risks for *skin* cancer are difficult to state. For instance, a person with a dark complexion can work longer in the sun and be less likely to develop cancer than a light-complected person. Furthermore, a person wearing a long-sleeved shirt and wide-brimmed hat may work in the sun and be less at risk than a person who wears a bathing suit for only a short period. The risk goes up greatly with age. If you answered "yes" to any question, you need to protect your skin from the sun or any other toxic material. Changes in moles, warts, or skin sores are very important and need to be seen by your physician.

If your *breast* total is:

100 or less You are at low risk. You should practice
             monthly BSE and have your breasts examined
             by a physician as part of a cancer-related
             checkup.
100–199   You are at moderate risk. You should practice
             monthly BSE and have your breasts examined
             by a physician as part of a cancer-related
             checkup. Periodic mammograms should be
             included as directed by your physician.
200 or over You are at high risk. You should practice
             monthly BSE and have professional
             examinations more often. See your physician
             for the examinations recommended for you.

If your *cervical* total is:

40–69   You are at low risk. Your physician will advise
             you about how often you should have a Pap
             test.
70–99   You are at moderate risk. More frequent Pap
             tests may be required.
100 or more You are at high risk. You should have a Pap test
             and pelvic exam as advised by your physician.

Source: American Cancer Society

TABLE 16-5 Summary of Tests Recommended by the American Cancer Society for the Early Detection of Cancer in Asymptomatic People

Site of Cancer	Test or Procedure	Sex	Age	Frequency
			Population	
Colon or rectum	Sigmoidoscopy	M & F	Over 50	Every 3–5 years
	Stool occult blood test	M & F	Over 50	Every year
	Digital rectal examination	M & F	Over 40	Every year
Prostate	Digital rectal examination	M	40 and over	Every year
	PSA blood test	M	50 and over	Every year
Uterus or cervix	Pap smear	F	18–65; under 18, if sexually active	At least every three years after 3 negative exams 1 year apart
	Pelvic examination	F	18–39; under 18, if sexually active	Every 3 years
			40 and over	Every year
	Endometrial tissue sample	F	At menopause; women at high risk[a]	At menopause
Breast	Breast self-examination	F	20 and over	Every month
	Breast physical examination	F	20–40	Every 3 years
			Over 40	Every year
	Mammography	F	under 40	Baseline
			40–49	Every 1–2 years
			50 and over	Every year
Lung	Chest x-ray		Not recommended	
	Sputum cytology		Recommended for people at risk	
Other[b]	Health counseling and cancer checkup	M & F	20–39	Every 3 years
		M & F	40 and over	Every year

[a]History of infertility, obesity, failure of ovulation, abnormal uterine bleeding, or estrogen therapy
[b]To include examination for cancers of the thyroid, testicles, prostate, ovaries, lymph nodes, oral region, and skin

Trends in Diagnosis and Treatment

Detection of a cancer by physical examination is only the beginning, and further diagnosis and treatment of cancer has become increasingly individualized. Methods for determining the exact location, type, and degree of malignancy of a cancer are sophisticated, and they continue to improve. Knowledge of the exact location and size of a tumor is necessary for precise and effective surgery or radiation therapy. This is especially true in cases where the tumor may be hard to reach, as in the brain. New high-technology diagnostic imaging techniques have replaced exploratory surgery for some patients. In **magnetic resonance imaging (MRI)**, a huge electromagnet is used to detect hidden tumors by mapping, on a computer screen, the vibrations of different atoms in the body. **Computerized tomography (CT)** scanning uses x-rays to examine the brain and other parts of the body. The process allows the construction of cross sections, which show a tumor's shape and location more accurately than is possible with conventional x-ray technique. For patients undergoing radiation therapy, CT scanning enables the

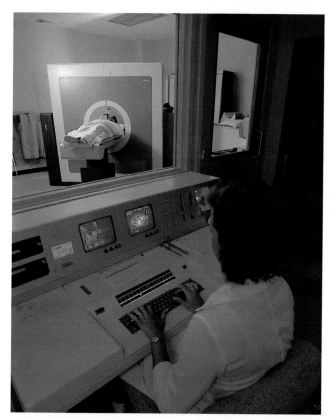

Computerized tomography—also known as CT or CAT scanning—is a diagnostic technique that provides a computer-assisted image of a relatively inaccessible part of the body, such as the brain.

therapist to pinpoint the tumor more precisely and so provide more accurate radiation dosage while sparing normal tissue. Ultrasonography has also been used increasingly in the past few years to visualize tumors. It has several advantages: It can be used in the physician's office, it is less expensive than other imaging methods, and it is completely safe. Prostate ultrasound (a rectal probe using ultrasonic waves to produce an image of the prostate gland) is currently being investigated for its ability to increase the early detection of small, hidden tumors that would be missed by a digital rectal exam.

Treatment methods for cancers are based primarily on surgery (removing the tumor), chemotherapy, and radiation therapy. In the last two techniques, cancer cells that can't be surgically removed are killed either by interfering chemically with their growth or by killing them directly with concentrated ionizing radiation. Newer and still experimental methods of treatment are also showing promise. **Immunotherapy,** for instance, uses the body's own immune system to control cancer; interferon, interleukin-2, and several other biological-response modifiers that stimulate the immune system are under study. They have already been shown more effective than conventional therapy in treating certain leukemias, kidney can-

cer, and melanoma. Several laboratories are also working on vaccines for melanoma, which have been shown to be effective in animal models and are now being used in clinical trials. New technologies have made it possible to use **bone marrow transplantation** as a treatment option in patients with leukemia, lymphoma, and breast cancer, when their own bone marrow must be destroyed by radiation to purge the body of cancer cells. Other potent natural substances recently made available in quantity through genetic engineering include factors that stimulate the growth of both red and white blood cells (erythropoietin and colony-stimulating factors, respectively). These substances allow chemotherapy patients, whose blood-forming cells have been severely reduced, to replace these vital cells much faster than formerly.

All of these newer techniques offer the hope of reducing mortality from the common cancers and extending the lives of those who do have cancer. However, we should keep in mind that there are no technologies on the horizon that promise an all-encompassing cancer cure. As is the case with so many diseases, prevention remains your best protection against cancer.

PREVENTING CANCER

Because your behaviors and behavior changes can radically lower your cancer risks, you can take a very practical approach to cancer prevention. Primary prevention involves measures you can take to avoid cancer-causing agents in the environment, such as those in the following list. Secondary prevention involves having cancers that do develop discovered as quickly as possible by following the cancer test recommendations of the American Cancer Society, particularly for breast, colorectal, testicle, and cervical cancers (see Table 16-5). Both levels of prevention are important to your long-term health. The primary prevention measures recommended by the American Cancer Society include the following:

- Stop smoking and avoid breathing the smoke from other people's cigarettes. Smoking is responsible for 80 to 90 percent of all lung cancers and for about 30

Magnetic resonance imaging (MRI)   A method of visualizing body structures in cross section without radiation by detecting the vibration of atoms in a magnetic field; used to detect tumors.

Computerized tomography (CT) scan   A test using computerized x-ray images to create a cross-sectional depiction of tissue density.

Immunotherapy   Experimental cancer treatment that uses various methods to stimulate the immune system to kill cancer cells.

Bone marrow transplantation   Replacement of one individual's bone marrow with that of another.

TERMS

percent of all cancer deaths. People who smoke two or more packs of cigarettes a day have lung cancer mortality rates 15 to 25 times greater than those of nonsmokers. The carcinogenic chemicals in smoke are transported throughout the body in the bloodstream, making smoking a cocarcinogen for many forms of cancer other than lung cancer.

- Protect your skin from the sun. Almost all cases of nonmelanoma skin cancer are considered to be sun-related, and sun exposure is a major factor in the development of melanoma as well. Wear protective clothing when you're out in the sun and use a sunscreen with an SPF rating of 15 or higher. Don't go to tanning salons; they do not provide "safe tans."

- Drink alcohol only in moderation, if at all. Oral cancer and cancers of the larynx, throat, esophagus, and liver occur more frequently among heavy drinkers of alcohol. Risk is even higher among heavy drinkers who smoke.

- Avoid smokeless tobacco. Chewing tobacco and snuff, both highly habit-forming because of their nicotine content, are associated with cancer of the mouth, larynx, throat, and esophagus.

- Avoid excessive exposure to radiation. Most medical x-rays are adjusted to deliver the lowest dose possible without sacrificing image quality. Radiation from radon, on the other hand, may pose a threat. The American Cancer Society believes there is a problem with exposure to radon in some homes. Remedial steps should be taken in these cases.

- Avoid occupational exposure to carcinogens. A number of industrial agents are associated with cancer, including nickel, chromate, asbestos, vinyl chloride, and others. Risks increase greatly when combined with smoking.

- Watch your weight and exercise regularly. The risk for colon, breast, and uterine cancers increases for obese people. A high-fat diet may be a factor in the development of certain cancers, although the link between obesity and cancer hasn't been fully explained. Maintaining normal weight through a healthy diet and regular exercise lowers the risk.

- Control your diet. Based on hundreds of studies, the National Cancer Institute estimates that about one-third of all cancers are in some way linked to what we eat. Choose a low-fat, high-fiber diet containing cruciferous vegetables and foods rich in vitamins A and C; avoid salt-cured, smoked, and nitrite-cured foods. See the specific suggestions in the box and table on dietary factors in cancer.

Although other factors are important, lifestyle is a strong predictor of cancer risk. Mormons and Seventh-day Adventists, for example, are much less likely to develop cancer than is the general population. Church doc-

trine of both groups forbids tobacco and alcohol use. Members also maintain a strong support network, which may influence both the incidence and the outcome of disease. A recent study determined that middle-aged Mormon men in the lay priesthood of that faith have reduced their risk of cancer to less than half that of the general population. Important factors in this risk reduction appear to be avoidance of tobacco and alcohol, regular exercise, and proper sleep. By making similar changes in lifestyle, other groups have every reason to expect to achieve the 50 percent cancer mortality reduction seen among Mormons and set as a goal for the nation by the National Cancer Institute for the year 2000.

SUMMARY

What Is Cancer?

- A malignant tumor can invade surrounding structures and spread to distant sites via the blood and lymphatic system, producing additional tumors.

- A malignant cell divides without regard for normal growth. As tumors grow, they produce signs or symptoms that are determined by their location in the body.

- Carcinomas begin in the epithelial layers of cells, which are the most actively growing cells in the adult body. They metastasize primarily via the lymph vessels.

- Sarcomas, which metastasize primarily via blood vessels, arise from connective and fibrous tissue. Lymphomas, cancers of the lymph nodes, result from changes in the white blood cells.

- Leukemias are cancers of blood-forming cells in the bone marrow.

- One person in three will develop cancer, but more than half will be cured.

Common Cancers

- Lung cancer is the most common cancer in the United States, and it kills more people than any other type of cancer. Smoking, the primary cause of lung cancer, also intensifies the effects of other causes like radon gas or asbestos.

- Long-term exposure to environmental tobacco smoke increases the risk of lung cancer for nonsmokers.

- Because lung cancer is usually detected only after metastasis has begun, treatment is difficult and survival rates are low.

- Colorectal cancer is clearly linked to both diet and heredity. High-fiber diets can prevent and even reverse precancerous changes in colon cells. Most colon cancers arise from preexisting polyps.

- Breast cancer affects about one in nine women in the United States. Although there is a genetic component to breast cancer, diet and hormones are also risk factors.

- Early detection of breast cancer depends on monthly self-examination, clinical breast exams, and regular mammograms. Malignancies are treated by surgery and—if the cancer has spread—chemotherapy or hormonal therapy.

- Prostate cancer is chiefly a disease of aging; diet and lifestyle probably are factors in its occurrence. Early detection is possible through rectal examinations, blood tests, and sometimes ultrasound. Surgery is performed to remove malignancies; chemotherapy and radiation may also be used.

- Endometrial cancer is highly curable; risk factors include infertility, obesity, and prolonged estrogen therapy.

- Because use of Pap tests has become nearly universal, the death rate from cervical cancer has dropped by 70 percent in 40 years. Abnormal cells can be detected and removed before they reach the invasive stage.

- Ovarian cancer is dangerous because it can't be detected by a Pap test or any simple screening method.

- Abnormal cellular changes in the epidermis, often a result of exposure to the sun, cause skin cancers, as does chronic exposure to certain chemicals. Skin cancers occur as basal cell carcinoma, squamous cell carcinoma, and melanoma.

- Skin cancer prevention means avoiding overexposure to the sun. Early diagnosis leads to more successful treatment. Survival rates are high if the cancer is caught in its early stages.

- Oral cancer is caused primarily by cigarette and cigar smoking, excess alcohol consumption, and use of smokeless tobacco. Oral cancers are easy to detect, but often hard to treat.

- Testicular cancer can be detected early through self-examination. Bladder cancer, often associated with smoking, has a high survival rate if detected at an early stage. Pancreatic cancer is hard to detect and usually fatal. Kaposi's sarcoma has become more common as a result of the spread of HIV infection.

What Causes Cancer?

- Mutational damage to a cell's DNA can lead to rapid and uncontrolled growth of cells; mutagens include radiation, viral infection, and chemical substances in food and air.

- Cancer initiators cause mutations in DNA; cancer promoters accelerate the growth of cells. If cell growth is speeded up, the cell replicates damaged DNA before it can be repaired.

- The genetic basis of some cancers appears to be related to suppressor genes, which normally limit cell growth; people can inherit altered suppressor genes.

- Food contains both carcinogens and anticarcinogens. A diet high in fat and low in fiber contributes to colon, prostate, and other cancers. Alcohol is associated with breast and oral cancers. Elements of the diet that seem to protect against cancer include beta-carotene; vitamin C, vitamin E, and other antioxidants; cruciferous vegetables; dietary fiber; and vitamin D and calcium.

- Some carcinogens occur naturally in the environment; others are manufactured substances.

- Additives and preservatives are added to food to preserve freshness, but a few react with other substances to become carcinogenic. Exposure to carcinogenic chemicals in the workplace puts workers in some industries at increased risk for cancer. All sources of radiation are potentially carcinogenic including x-rays, radioisotopes, radon gas, and the ultraviolet rays of the sun.

Detection, Diagnosis, and Treatment

- Self-monitoring is essential to early cancer detection; the appearance of any early signs necessitates a visit to a physician. (The signs can be remembered by using the acronym CAUTION.)

- The most important cancer screening tests include self-examination of breasts and testicles, yearly rectal exams (after age 40), and yearly stool blood tests (after age 50).

- Magnetic resonance imaging and computerized tomography allow more precise visualization of tumors than do standard x-rays. Ultrasound is also being used more frequently in cancer detection.

- Treatment methods consist of surgery, chemotherapy, and radiation therapy. Immunotherapy, vaccines, and genetic engineering also hold promise as effective treatments.

Preventing Cancer

- Primary prevention involves avoiding cancer-causing agents in the environment. Secondary prevention involves early detection of cancers that do occur.

- Primary prevention includes (1) not smoking and avoiding smoke, (2) protecting skin from the sun,

(3) drinking alcohol in moderation, if at all, (4) avoiding smokeless tobacco, (5) avoiding excessive exposure to radiation, (6) avoiding occupational exposure to carcinogens, (7) watching one's weight and exercising, and (8) controlling one's diet.

- Lifestyle is a strong predictor of cancer risk. Studies have shown that an altered lifestyle can reduce cancer risk as much as 50 percent.

TAKE ACTION

1. Look through the list of foods in the box "A Dietary Defense Against Cancer" and choose four or five that you don't typically eat. During the next week, make a point of trying each of the foods you've chosen.

2. Devise a plan for incorporating regular self-examinations for cancer (breast self-examination or testicle self-examination) into your life. What strategies will help you remember to do your monthly exam? How can you keep yourself motivated?

3. Interview your parents or grandparents about your family medical history. Are there any cases of cancer in your family, and has anyone died of cancer? Do you see any patterns?

JOURNAL ENTRY

1. In your health journal, list the positive behaviors that help you avoid cancer. How can you strengthen these behaviors? Also list the behaviors that tend to increase your risk. What can you do to change these behaviors?

2. *Critical Thinking:* Smoking is responsible for 85 to 90 percent of all lung cancers. Are tobacco companies in any way responsible for the high number of deaths from lung cancer each year? Or is each individual entirely responsible for his or her own behavior and health? In your health journal, write a brief essay outlining your position on this issue. Then write a brief essay that supports the opposite viewpoint.

3. Make a list of risk factors for cancer over which you have no control, including heredity and personal history. Do these risk factors increase your risk for any cancers? If so, make a list of behaviors you can adopt that will lower your risk for these cancers.

BEHAVIOR CHANGE STRATEGY

PHASING IN A HEALTHIER DIET

Is it hard to break bad eating habits? Of course, and it doesn't happen in a day. But two nutritional scientists at the Oregon Health Sciences University in Portland have devised a plan for improving eating habits in three phases. Although Dr. William Connor and Sonja Conner designed their diet (described in their book *The New American Diet*) to reduce the risk of heart disease, their plan and many of their specific suggestions work as an anticancer diet as well. The guiding principle is to avoid doing anything radical, but instead to increase gradually your consumption of fruits, vegetables, and grains while you reduce your intake of fat, cholesterol, and known and suspected carcinogens.

Begin by monitoring your diet for one or two weeks, noting in your health journal both the health-protecting and the cancer-promoting foods you eat. (See Table 16-3 and the box "A Dietary Defense Against Cancer").

After you have recorded your diet, analyze it to see how often you consume the foods listed. Do you have cruciferous vegetables two or three times a week? Are carrots, peaches, or apricots part of your diet? Do you eat bacon only occasionally? Do you limit your intake of alcohol? Once you have some idea of how much your diet protects you against cancer and how much it puts you at risk, try implementing the following three-phase diet-change plan:

Phase I: Substitutions

Avoid egg yolks, butter, lard, organ meats, bacon and other cured meats, and any burnt meat. Start using vegetable oils for all purposes rather than animal fats. Switch to low-fat or nonfat milk products and other low-fat foods. Discard chicken skin and meat fat. Reduce consumption of beer and wine. Keep using favorite recipes, but decrease salt and fat content.

Phase II: New Recipes

Reduce the amount of red meat and cheese you eat; replace with chicken and fish. Cut down on fats, including vegetable fats. Begin to replace meats and fats with grains, beans, fruits, and vegetables, especially those high in vitamins A and C and members of the cabbage family. Choose low-fat dishes when eating out. Replace recipes that cannot be altered.

Phase III: A New Way of Eating

Eat meats and cheeses as side dishes, in small amounts, rather than as main courses. Increase consumption of beans and grains as protein and fiber sources. Save rich foods such as chocolate and bakery goods for special treats only, no more than once a month. Make a habit of trying new grains and beans, fruits, and vegetables (select some from the lists given in the chapter, or see what the supermarkets and ethnic stores in your community offer). Keep developing a new repertory of recipes.

A diet like this can provide benefits to your cardiovascular system, help you lose weight gradually and permanently, and give you some insurance against cancer later in life. Try making these changes over the course of a few months to improve your overall health and your chances for a cancer-free future.

Adapted from "Phasing in a Healthier Diet." *University of California at Berkeley Wellness Letter,* October 1987.

SELECTED BIBLIOGRAPHY

Ames, B. N., and L. S. Gold. 1992. Animal cancer tests and cancer prevention. *Monographs/National Cancer Institute* 12:125–132.

Andriole, G. L., and W. J. Catalona. 1991. The diagnosis and treatment of prostate cancer. *Annual Reviews of Medicine* 42:9–15.

Banks, B. A., and others. 1992. Attitudes of teenagers toward sun exposure and sunscreen use. *Pediatrics* 89(1): 40–42.

Bates, M. N. 1991. Extremely low frequency electromagnetic fields and cancer: The epidemiologic evidence. *Environmental Health Perspectives* 95:147–56.

Colditz, G. A., and others. 1990. Prospective study of estrogen replacement therapy and risk of breast cancer in postmenopausal women. *Journal of the American Medical Association* 264:2648–53.

Connolly, G. N., and others. 1992. Snuffing tobacco out of sport. *American Journal of Public Health* 82(3): 351–53.

"Fat and Cancer: A Clear Picture at Last." *Consumer Reports on Health.* December 1992.

Glantz, S. A., and W. W. Parmley. 1992. Passive smoking causes heart disease and lung cancer. *Journal of Clinical Epidemiology* 45(8): 815–919.

Glover, E. D., and others. 1989. Smokeless tobacco use among American college students. *Journal of American College Health* 38(2): 81–85.

Harris, J. R., and others. 1992. Breast cancer: Medical progress. *New England Journal of Medicine* 327(5): 319–27 (a detailed and critical three-part review).

Hirayama, T. 1992. Life-style and cancer: From epidemiological evidence to public behavior change to mortality reduction of target cancers. *Monographs/National Cancer Institute* 12:65–74.

Howard, J., and others. 1992. A collaborative study of differences in the survival rates of black patients and white patients with cancer. *Cancer* 69(9): 2349–60.

Howe, G. R., and others. 1991. A cohort study of fat intake and breast cancer. *Journal of the National Cancer Institute* 83: 336–340.

Keinan, G., and others. 1992. Predicting women's delay in seeking medical care after discovery of a lump in the breast: The role of personality and behavior patterns. *Behavioral Medicine* 17(4): 177–83.

Kolonel, L. N., and M. T. Goodman. 1992. Racial variation in cancer incidence: Fact or artifact? *Journal of the National Cancer Institute* 84(12): 915–16.

La Vecchia, C. 1992. Cancers associated with high-fat diets. *Monographs/National Cancer Institute* 12:79–85.

Mattson, M. E., and D. M. Winn. 1989. Smokeless tobacco: Association with increased cancer risk. *Monographs/National Cancer Institute* 8:13–16.

NIH Consensus Development Panel. 1988. Health implications of smokeless tobacco use: NIH consensus statement. *Biomedicine and Pharmacotherapy* 42(2): 93–98.

Schapira, D. V., and others. 1991. Estimate of breast cancer risk reduction with weight loss. *Cancer* 67(10): 2622–25.

Truhan, A. P. 1991. Sun protection in childhood. *Clinical Pediatrics* 30(12): 676–81.

Vail-Smith, K., and D. M. White. 1992. Risk level, knowledge, and preventive behavior for human papillomaviruses among sexually active college women. *Journal of American College Health* 40(5): 227–30.

Wynder, E. L. 1992. Cancer prevention: Optimizing life-styles with special reference to nutritional carcinogenesis. *Monographs/National Cancer Institute* 12:87–91.

Zhang, Y., and others. 1992. A major inducer of anticarcinogenic protective enzymes from broccoli: Isolation and elucidation of sulforaphane structure. *Proceedings of the National Academy of Sciences of the United States of America* 89(6): 2399–2403.

RECOMMENDED READINGS

American Cancer Society. 1993. *Cancer Facts and Figures— 1993.* New York: American Cancer Society. *Available in every library, this is a condensed and authoritative summary of the current cancer statistics, renewed each year.*

Dollinger, M., E. H. Rosenbaum, and G. Cable. 1991. *Everyone's Guide to Cancer Therapy: How Cancer Is Diagnosed, Treated, and Managed Day to Day.* Toronto: Somerville House. *An authoritative lay guide to cancer diagnosis and treatment written by top cancer specialists.*

Love, S. M. 1990. *Dr. Susan Love's Breast Book.* Reading, Mass.: Addison-Wesley. *A comprehensive guide to breast cancer written by one of the country's leading breast surgeons.*

National Cancer Institute. 1992. *National Cancer Institute Fact Book.* Bethesda, Md.: Office of Cancer Communications. *A source book of detailed and up-to-date information on the cancer problem.*

Moore, M., and E. Potts. 1987. *Choices: Realistic Alternatives in Cancer Treatment.* New York: Avon Books. *An exploration of the current choices in cancer therapy, from the patient's perspective.*

Prescott, D. M., and A. S. Flexner. 1986. *Cancer: The Misguided Cell.* Sunderland, Mass.: Sinauer Associates. *A widely used text describing recent advances in cancer research, with insight into the psychosocial and political aspects of the disease.*

Sohn, W., and S. Corngold. 1992. *Colorectal Cancer: Reducing Your Risk.* New York: Bantam Books. *A guide to understanding the hereditary factors in bowel cancer and to controlling environmental risk factors.*

American Cancer Society (1-800-ACS-2345) publishes a wide range of materials on the prevention and treatment of cancer, all available free of charge. Titles include: *Nutrition and Cancer, How to Examine Your Breasts, Cancer Facts for Women, Facts on Ovarian Cancer,* and *Sexuality and Cancer.*

The National Cancer Institute (NCI) maintains a database of the latest published information about cancer. Operators will perform a search for callers on specific subjects and send along relevant materials (1-800-4-CANCER). NCI also publishes a wide range of cancer materials, available free of charge. Sample titles: *Cancer Prevention, Cancer Rates and Risks, Breast Biopsy: What You Should Know, What You Need to Know About Colon and Rectal Cancer, When Someone In Your Family Has Cancer, The Future of Cancer Therapy*. Publications may be ordered by writing: Public Inquiries Section, Office of Cancer Communications, NCI, Bldg. 31, Room 10A16, 9000 Rockville Pike, Bethesda, MD 20892.

17

Sexually Transmissible Diseases

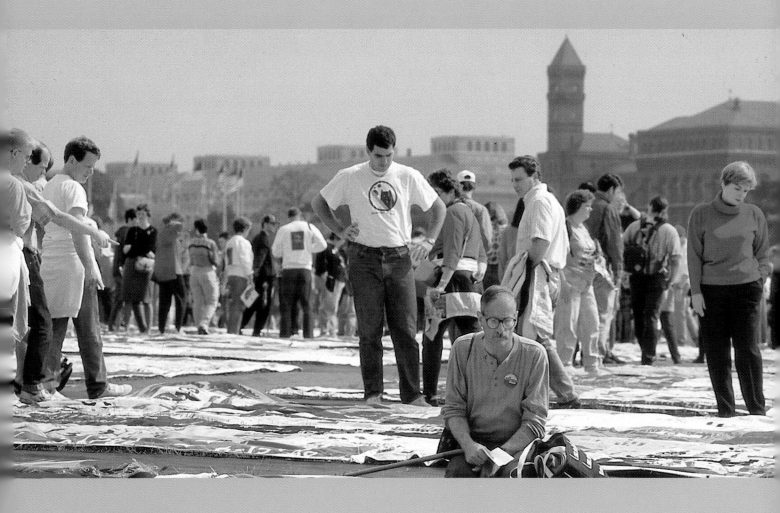

CONTENTS

The Major STDs

Other STDs

What Can You Do?

BOXES

◗ Your brother and his wife have been trying to have a baby for three years, without success. It seems that your sister-in-law had pelvic inflammatory disease while she was in college and her oviducts were permanently damaged. How did she get this disease, and how can it be avoided?

◗ You've been dating someone whom you know has been involved in sexual relationships before. As you get closer to an intimate sexual relationship with him, you find yourself wondering about his previous experience. You'd really like to ask him if he's ever been exposed to any sexually transmissible diseases and if he's sure he doesn't have any now. Is it acceptable to bring up this subject? How? What if your questions offend him or make him angry?

◗ A friend of yours just found out that her former boyfriend is being treated for gonorrhea. He told her he doesn't know where he got it or how long he's had it, but his doctor advised him to inform his former sexual partners and tell them they should be examined also. Your friend feels fine and has no symptoms of any kind, so she's pretty sure she's not infected. She's not inclined to bother seeing a doctor. Is she making a mistake?

◗ One of your housemates does volunteer work for a community service group that provides help for AIDS patients. Once a week he buys groceries, cleans house, helps with laundry, and runs errands for a homebound person with AIDS. He enjoys his volunteer work and doesn't seem worried about having so much contact with someone infected with HIV. You've heard that HIV isn't spread through "casual contact," but you wonder about things like washing dishes or cleaning up around the house. Is your friend taking a big risk?

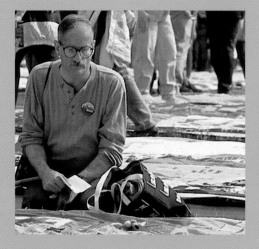

MAKING CONNECTIONS

Although everyone knows about the AIDS epidemic, many people think that diseases like syphilis and gonorrhea are a thing of the past. But in fact, cases of all the sexually transmissible diseases are increasing, and it's more important than ever to know how to protect yourself from these infections. In each of the scenarios presented on this page, all related to sexually transmissible diseases, individuals have to use information, make a decision, or choose a course of action. How would you act in each of these situations? What response or decision would you make? This chapter provides information about sexually transmissible diseases that can be used in situations like these. After finishing the chapter, read the scenarios again. Has what you've learned changed how you would respond?

No single health issue has commanded as much public attention in recent years as **acquired immunodeficiency syndrome,** or **AIDS.** This fatal, incurable disease currently ranks ninth as a cause of death among Americans, and the epidemic of **HIV infection** is considered the number one health priority in the United States. Although recent public education campaigns have focused primarily on HIV infection, they deserve to be repeated for all the **sexually transmissible diseases (STDs)**—gonorrhea, chlamydia, herpes, syphilis, and others—because their incidence also continues to climb among Americans.

STDs are a particularly insidious group of diseases. People can become infected and pass the infection on to a sexual partner without ever feeling sick or even knowing they have a disease. Not until years later does the cost of unprotected sex practices become apparent. Then an infected person may find that an undiagnosed STD has caused infertility, contributed to the development of cancer, or caused a birth defect in a child. In the case of HIV infection, the immune system becomes fatally weakened and can no longer provide protection from disease.

Why is the incidence of STDs continuing to rise? One factor is the sheer number of sexually active people. The "baby boom" generation came of age and passed through their most active sexual years in the 1960s, 1970s, and 1980s. Many people became sexually active at a younger age than earlier generations had, and they tended to have more partners. American society began to show greater acceptance of premarital sex, the media promoted more open attitudes toward sexuality, and contraceptive information and services became more generally available. Oral contraceptives (which don't provide protection against STDs) grew in popularity and largely replaced condoms (which do provide some protection). Finally, there was an increase in alcohol and drug abuse, which has a powerful influence on sexual behavior.

The seriousness of STDs is compounded and magnified by other concerns, such as the extent of undetected infections, reduced government funding for STD-related programs, limited access to affordable health care for many people, and a growing population of people who exchange sex for drugs without regard for whether they're spreading disease. It has probably never been so important for people to have a clear understanding of what the STDs are, how they are transmitted, and, most important, how they can be prevented. The crucial message is that they *can* be prevented. This chapter is designed to provide information about healthy, safe sexual behavior and to help you develop responsible attitudes toward prevention, diagnosis, and treatment of STDs.

Personal Insight How would you feel if your sexual partner told you he or she exposed you to an STD? How would you feel if you contracted an STD?

What are the most severe and dangerous STDs? In general, seven different diseases pose major health threats: HIV infection/AIDS, hepatitis, syphilis, chlamydia, gonorrhea, herpes, and human papillomavirus (HPV), which causes genital warts. These diseases are considered "major" because they are serious in themselves, cause serious complications if left untreated, and/or pose risks to a fetus or newborn. Additionally, pelvic inflammatory disease (PID) is a common complication of gonorrhea and chlamydia and merits discussion as a separate disease.

HIV Infection/AIDS

HIV infection is one of the most serious and challenging problems facing the United States and the world today. By the year 2000, HIV infection could become the largest epidemic of the century, surpassing the influenza epidemic of 1918 that killed 20 million people. Despite the intense efforts of health professionals all around the world, HIV infection continues to spread and a cure is yet to be found. By the end of 1992, over 250,000 Americans had been diagnosed with AIDS, and over a million were believed to be infected with HIV (see the box "AIDS Milestones"). In 1989, the Centers for Disease Control and Prevention (CDC) reported that more than 25,000 American college students were probably already infected with HIV; other estimates put the figure as high as 1 out of every 10 students. Worldwide, over 2 million people are believed to have AIDS; and by the year 2000, it's estimated that 40 to 120 million people will be infected with HIV. According to the World Health Organization, someone is infected with HIV every 15 to 20 seconds.

While education has slowed the rate of infection in developed countries, the disease continues to spread rapidly in poorer nations (see the box "Changing Patterns of HIV Infection Around the World"). Research indicates that there are different strains of HIV in different parts of the world, each with slightly different characteristics. This fact makes controlling the epidemic even more difficult.

What Is HIV Infection? HIV infection is a chronic disease that progressively damages the body's immune system, making an otherwise healthy person susceptible to a variety of infections and disorders. Under normal condi-

AIDS, acquired immunodeficiency syndrome A fatal, incurable, sexually transmissible viral disease.

HIV infection A chronic, progressive disease that damages the immune system; caused by the human immunodeficiency virus (HIV).

Sexually transmissible diseases (STDs) Diseases that can be transmitted by sexual contact; some can also be transmitted by other means.

TERMS

In January 1993, the AIDS epidemic reached a milestone of sorts when the Centers for Disease Control expanded the definition of AIDS. Their revised system of classification of HIV infection will cause an increase in the number of AIDS cases reported each year in the United States.

1. June 1981: An unusual type of immune-system failure primarily among gay men is first reported in the United States; similar outbreaks seen in other parts of the world.

2. April 1982: Cases among injecting drug users are reported.

3. July 1982: The new disease, now named acquired immune deficiency syndrome or AIDS, is first reported among hemophiliacs.

4. December 1982: First AIDS case linked to blood transfusion is detected.

5. January 1983: Two women whose sexual partners had AIDS contract the disease, thus adding heterosexuals to the list of risk groups.

6. May 1983: French research team at the Pasteur Institute in Paris, headed by Luc Montagnier, reports the isolation of a virus believed to cause AIDS.

7. April 1984: Robert Gallo at the National Cancer Institute isolates the AIDS virus, which is the same as that identified by the French.

8. March 1985: The first test to detect HIV antibodies is approved in the United States. Blood banks begin testing.

9. October 1985: Rock Hudson dies of AIDS. The disclosure of his illness touches off major media attention to the disease.

10. September 1986: Surgeon General C. Everett Koop releases his controversial report on the AIDS epidemic.

11. March 1987: AZT, the first drug shown to fight HIV infection, is

approved for experimental use by the FDA.

12. January 1988: Number of AIDS cases in the United States reaches 50,000.

13. June 1988: The President's AIDS commission turns in report calling for expanded research and prevention programs and a federal ban on AIDS discrimination.

14. July 1989: Number of AIDS cases in the United States surpasses 100,000.

15. April 1990: Teenage spokesperson Ryan White dies from AIDS.

16. October 1991: The FDA approves a second anti-HIV drug, ddI.

17. November 1991: Magic Johnson announces he is HIV-positive.

18. December 1991: The 200,000th case of AIDS in the United States is reported.

19. June 1992: A third anti-HIV drug, ddC, is approved by the FDA. Number of deaths from AIDS in the United States surpasses 150,000.

20. December 1992: Number of AIDS cases in the United States surpasses a quarter of a million.

21. January 1993: The CDC expands its definition of AIDS. Dancer Rudolf Nureyev and tennis player Arthur Ashe die from AIDS.

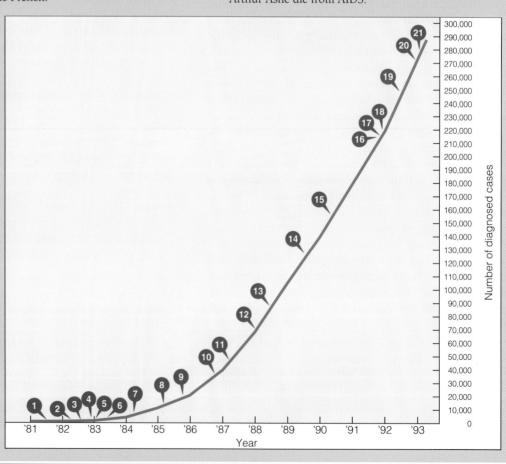

Changing Patterns of HIV Infection Around the World

Although first detected among heterosexuals in Africa, AIDS captured world attention in the early 1980s as a disease occurring primarily among homosexual men in the United States and Europe. Since then, AIDS has spread around the world. HIV infections have been reported in virtually all countries of the world, and actual AIDS cases have been documented in 164 countries. Over 12 million people worldwide have been infected with HIV since the epidemic began. The World Health Organization predicts that 30 to 40 million people will be infected with HIV by the year 2000. The Harvard-based Global AIDS Policy Coalition predicts that the number will be much higher, perhaps as high as 110 million.

As AIDS education and prevention programs take hold in developed countries, the vast majority—70 to 90 percent—of new infections are expected to occur in developing countries, where heterosexual contact is the main means of transmission. In the developed world, too, the pattern of infection is shifting away from homosexual males and toward the larger heterosexual population. Women are the fastest-growing group of newly infected people in the industrialized world.

Currently, more than 7 million of those infected with HIV are in Africa, where, in some cities, one-third of all adults carry the virus. Sub-Saharan Africa remains the hardest hit of all areas of the world. However, experts believe that Asia is now at the same stage of the disease that Africa was 10 years ago. As in Africa, the principal means of transmission is heterosexual contact. In Asia, however, many more people are at risk, since Asia accounts for more than 50 percent of the world's population. The World Health Organization hopes that education campaigns can prevent India, China, and Southeast Asia from following the same path followed in Africa.

Efforts to combat AIDS are complicated by political, economic, and cultural barriers in many parts of the world. Education and prevention programs are often hampered by resistance from social and religious institutions and by taboos on open discussion of sex. Condoms are unfamiliar in many countries, for example, and when their use has been proposed as a way to prevent disease, responses have ranged from hostility on the part of political leaders to confusion and indignation on the part of members of the general population. Additionally, women in many societies do not have sufficient power over their lives to demand that men use condoms during sex.

Despite these obstacles, education and prevention remain the best hope for slowing the spread of AIDS. Although many countries still deny the extent of infection among their populations, many others are overcoming their reluctance to discuss sensitive subjects and embracing campaigns that include graphic descriptions of safer sex practices. Some leaders are aggressively leading discussions about AIDS and encouraging their governments to set up national educational programs. In some Asian countries, strategies to block the disease are already in place. Until there is a cure for AIDS, efforts must continue to focus on widespread educational campaigns and prevention through behavior change.

Sources: D. C. Weeks. 1992. "The AIDS Pandemic in Africa." Current History, May; J. Frank. 1992. "Focus of World AIDS Prevention Is Shifting from Africa to Asia." San Francisco Chronicle, 16 December; "AIDS Crisis Hits Asia, Grows Rapidly," The Wall Street Journal, 30 December 1991; L. Garrett. 1992. "The Call for an Aggressive New AIDS Strategy." Washington Post, 21 July.

Projection of Adult HIV Infections for 1995
(Cumulative Numbers)

Geographic Area	Estimated Number of Adult HIV Infections, 1995
North America	1,495,000
Western Europe	1,186,000
Oceania	40,000
Latin America	1,407,000
Sub-Saharan Africa	11,449,000
Caribbean	474,000
Eastern Europe	44,000
Southeast Mediterranean	59,000
Northeast Asia	80,000
Southeast Asia	1,220,000
Total	17,454,000

Source: Global AIDS Policy Commission

tions, when a virus or other disease-causing agent enters the body, it is targeted and destroyed by the body's immune system. But the human immunodeficiency virus (HIV) attacks the immune system itself, invading and taking over the cells that initiate and control the body's entire system of defense. Once these cells have been sidetracked from their duties, the immune system can no longer respond adequately to infection. (See Chapter 18 for a more detailed explanation of the process by which HIV disarms the immune system.)

The incubation period of HIV—the time between the initial infection with the virus and the onset of disease

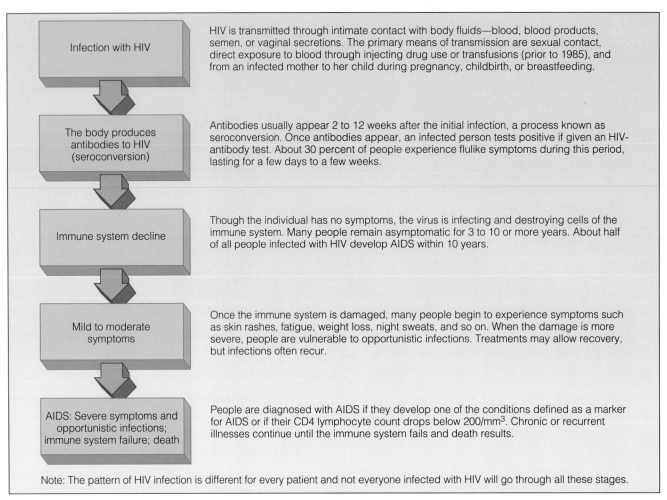

Infection with HIV	HIV is transmitted through intimate contact with body fluids—blood, blood products, semen, or vaginal secretions. The primary means of transmission are sexual contact, direct exposure to blood through injecting drug use or transfusions (prior to 1985), and from an infected mother to her child during pregnancy, childbirth, or breastfeeding.
The body produces antibodies to HIV (seroconversion)	Antibodies usually appear 2 to 12 weeks after the initial infection, a process known as seroconversion. Once antibodies appear, an infected person tests positive if given an HIV-antibody test. About 30 percent of people experience flulike symptoms during this period, lasting for a few days to a few weeks.
Immune system decline	Though the individual has no symptoms, the virus is infecting and destroying cells of the immune system. Many people remain asymptomatic for 3 to 10 or more years. About half of all people infected with HIV develop AIDS within 10 years.
Mild to moderate symptoms	Once the immune system is damaged, many people begin to experience symptoms such as skin rashes, fatigue, weight loss, night sweats, and so on. When the damage is more severe, people are vulnerable to opportunistic infections. Treatments may allow recovery, but infections often recur.
AIDS: Severe symptoms and opportunistic infections; immune system failure; death	People are diagnosed with AIDS if they develop one of the conditions defined as a marker for AIDS or if their CD4 lymphocyte count drops below 200/mm^3. Chronic or recurrent illnesses continue until the immune system fails and death results.

Note: The pattern of HIV infection is different for every patient and not everyone infected with HIV will go through all these stages.

Figure 17-1 *The general pattern of HIV infection.*
Adapted from: R. Schwartz, 1992. *AIDS Medical Guide.* San Francisco: San Francisco AIDS Foundation;
and Centers for Disease Control. 1991. *HIV Infection and AIDS: Are You At Risk?*

symptoms—is usually from 3 to 10 or more years (Figure 17-1). About 30 percent of infected people experience flulike symptoms shortly after the initial infection, but the rest have no symptoms at all. Most people infected with the virus remain generally healthy for years; but during this time, the virus is progressively infecting and destroying the cells of the immune system. People infected with HIV can pass the virus to others—even if they have no symptoms and even if they do not know they have been infected.

The destruction of the immune system by HIV is signaled by the loss of a certain type of white blood cell, called the **CD4 lymphocyte,** or T4 cell, which is vital to the functioning of the immune system. As the number of CD4 cells declines, an infected person may begin to experience mild to moderately severe symptoms. A person is diagnosed with "full blown" AIDS when he or she develops one of the conditions defined as a marker for AIDS or when the number of CD4 cells in the blood drops below a certain level (200/mm^3). People with AIDS are vulnera-

ble to a number of serious, often fatal secondary, or "opportunistic," infections.

How Is the Virus Transmitted? HIV lives only within cells and body fluids, not outside of the body. It is transmitted by blood and blood products, semen, and vaginal and cervical secretions. It cannot live in air, in water, or on objects or surfaces such as toilet seats, eating utensils, or telephones. The three main routes of HIV transmission are (1) from particular kinds of sexual contact, (2) from direct exposure to infected blood, and (3) from an HIV-infected woman to her fetus during pregnancy or childbirth or, possibly, to her infant during breastfeeding.

Among different types of sexual contact, HIV is more likely to be transmitted by unprotected anal or vaginal intercourse than by other sexual activities. Oral-genital contact carries some risk of transmission, although less than anal or vaginal intercourse. HIV can be transmitted through minute tears in the fragile lining of the vagina, cervix, penis, anus, and mouth and through direct infec-

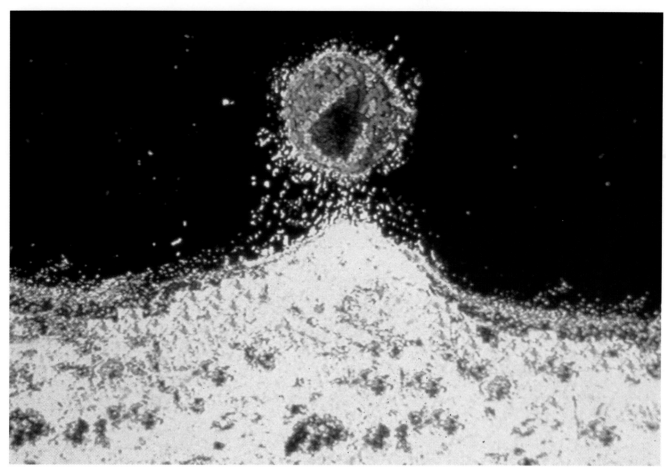

The human immunodeficiency virus attacks the body's immune system, using immune cells to reproduce itself and destroying them in the process. This micrograph shows an HIV virus as it bursts out of an infected lymphocyte (white blood cell), ready to attack another cell.

tion of cells in some of these areas. The presence of lesions or blisters from other sexually transmissible diseases in the genital, anal, or oral areas makes it easier for the virus to be transmitted. During vaginal intercourse, male-to-female transmission is more likely to occur than female-to-male transmission. HIV has been found in pre-ejaculatory fluid, so transmission can occur before ejaculation.

Direct, bloodstream contact with the blood of an infected person is the second major route of HIV transmission. Needles used to inject drugs (including heroin, cocaine, and anabolic steroids) are routinely contaminated by the blood of the user. If needles are shared, small amounts of one person's blood are directly injected into another person's bloodstream. HIV may also be transmitted through subcutaneous and intramuscular injection as well, from needles or blades used in acupuncture, tattooing, ritual scarring, and piercing of the earlobes, nose, lip, or nipple.

HIV has been transmitted in blood and blood products used in the medical treatment of **hemophilia,** injuries, and serious illnesses. The blood supply in all licensed blood banks and plasma centers in the United States is now screened for HIV. However, the Centers for Disease Control estimate that more than 20,000 cases of AIDS will be attributed to contaminated blood and blood products received by people before 1985, when widespread screening began.

A small number of health care workers who participated in the care of people with HIV infection acquired HIV on the job. Most of these cases involve needle sticks—in which a health care worker accidentally sticks him or herself with a needle used on an infected patient. The only case of transmission *to* patients is that of a Florida dentist who infected five of his patients; the CDC

CD4 lymphocyte   A type of white blood cell that helps coordinate the activity of the immune system; it is the primary target for HIV infection. A decrease in the number of these cells correlates with the risk and severity of HIV-related illness.

Hemophilia   A hereditary blood disease in which blood fails to clot and abnormal bleeding occurs, which requires transfusions of blood with a specific factor to aid coagulation.

TERMS

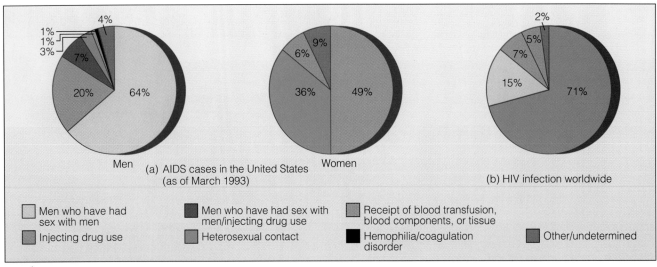

Men (a) AIDS cases in the United States Women
(as of March 1993)

(b) HIV infection worldwide

| Men who have had sex with men | Men who have had sex with men/injecting drug use | Receipt of blood transfusion, blood components, or tissue |
| Injecting drug use | Heterosexual contact | Hemophilia/coagulation disorder | Other/undetermined |

VITAL STATISTICS

Figure 17-2 *Routes of HIV transmission among adults.*

Sources: Centers for Disease Control and Prevention. 1993. *HIV/AIDS Surveillance Report*, May, pp. 7–8; Mann, J., D. J. M. Tarantola and T. W. Netter, eds. 1992. *AIDS in the World.* Cambridge, Mass.: Harvard University Press, p. 33.

is not yet sure exactly how the virus was transmitted in this case. In general, the risk of infection is far greater for health care workers and dentists than it is for patients because they are more likely to be exposed to infected body fluids.

The final major route of HIV transmission is mother-to-child, also called *vertical transmission.* About 25 to 30 percent of infants born to HIV-infected mothers are also infected with the virus. Most of these infections seem to occur during pregnancy, but a few may happen during childbirth. In addition, HIV has been found in breast milk, and a few babies have apparently been infected through breastfeeding. By the end of 1992, over 4,000 cases of AIDS among children infected by their mothers had been reported in the United States.

What about contact with other body fluids? Trace amounts of HIV have been found in the saliva and tears of some infected people. However, researchers believe that these fluids don't carry enough of the virus to infect another person, and no cases of HIV infection have been traced to exposure to tears or saliva. HIV has been found in urine and feces, and contact with the urine or feces of an infected person may carry some risk. Contact with an infected person's sweat is not believed to carry any risk.

Among Americans with AIDS, the most common means of exposure to HIV has been sexual activity between men; injecting drug use and heterosexual contact are the next most common (Figure 17-2). Changes in the sexual behavior of homosexual men and the screening of all donated blood have slowed the rate of infection from these sources. Women—infected through injecting drug use or sexual activity—and children born to infected mothers make up an increasingly large proportion of new cases of HIV infection.

HIV is not spread through casual contact. A person is not at risk of getting HIV infection by being in the same classroom, dining room, or even household with someone who is infected. Before this was generally known, many people with HIV infection, including children, were the targets of ostracism, hysteria, and outright violence. Today, it is an acknowledged responsibility of all to treat people with HIV infection with respect and compassion, regardless of their age or how they became infected.

Symptoms of HIV Infection/AIDS Signs and symptoms suggesting HIV infection include persistent swollen glands; lumps, rashes, sores, or other growths on or under the skin or on the mucous membranes of the eyes, mouth, anus, or nasal passages; persistent yeast infections; unexplained weight loss of more than 10 pounds or 10 percent of body weight in less than two months (unrelated to illness, dieting, or increased physical activity); fever and drenching night sweats; dry cough and shortness of breath; persistent diarrhea; easy bruising and unexplained bleeding; profound fatigue, sometimes accompanied by lightheadedness or dizziness; loss of memory; loss of sense of balance, tremors, or seizures; changes in vision, hearing, taste, or smell; difficulty in swallowing; changes in mood and other psychiatric symptoms; and persistent or recurrent pain. Obviously some of these symptoms can also occur with minor colds or flu.

Because the immune system is weakened, people with HIV infection are highly susceptible to infections, both common and uncommon (Table 17-1). The infection most often seen among people with HIV is ***Pneumocystis carinii***, a protozoal infection that produces pneumonia. **Kaposi's sarcoma**, a rare form of cancer, is common among HIV-infected men. More and more cases of

TABLE 17-1 Infections/Disorders Commonly Associated with HIV/AIDS

Condition	Symptoms
Pneumocystis carinii pneumonia (PCP)	Shortness of breath, a persistent dry cough, sharp chest pains, difficulty breathing
Kaposi's sarcoma (KS)	Purple or brownish lesions that resemble bruises but are painless and do not heal
Tuberculosis (TB)	Fever, night sweats, fatigue, cough, weight loss
AIDS dementia (AD)	Sensory disturbances, impairment of memory and judgment, loss of intellectual, social, or occupational abilities
Lymphadenopathy syndrome (LAS)	Persistent swollen glands in the absence of other illness
Cytomegalovirus (CMV) retinitis	Blurred vision, visual impairment, "floaters" (vision partially blocked by shapes that seem to float), blindness
Mycobacterium avium complex (MAC)	High fever, night sweats, weakness
Cryptosporidiosis	Severe diarrhea, abdominal cramping, weight loss, vomiting, loss of appetite
Invasive cervical cancer	Bleeding from the vagina between menstrual periods or after menopause, dull backache, general ill health

tuberculosis (TB) are also being reported among people with HIV; in Africa, drug-resistant strains of TB are now the most deadly infection among people with AIDS. Most of the infections associated with HIV are rare among people with healthy immune systems and are not contagious; however, tuberculosis is spread through the air and may pose a risk for non-HIV-infected people, especially medical personnel (see Chapter 18 for more information on tuberculosis).

Diagnosis Early diagnosis of HIV infection is important to minimize the impact of the disease, medically, psychologically, and socially. Up until a few years ago, there were no known ways to combat the disease. Now, drugs exist that can be used to slow the progress of the virus and to fight specific infections, especially if they are discovered early.

The surest diagnosis of HIV infection is the detection of the virus itself in human tissues through laboratory tissue culture procedures, but the techniques for this method are expensive and not available everywhere. The most commonly used screening test is the **HIV antibody test.** This test, developed by the National Cancer Institute, consists of an initial screening called an **ELISA test,** and a more specific confirmation test called the **Western blot.** These tests determine whether a person has **antibodies** to HIV circulating in the bloodstream, a sign that the virus is present in the body. If an individual repeatedly tests positive on the HIV antibody test and the diagnosis is confirmed in follow-up tests, the person is considered both infected (**HIV-positive**) and infectious. (For a discussion of the issues involved in testing, see the box "Who Needs an HIV Test?")

The FDA has recently approved the HIV-1 antigen test for use. This test measures the HIV particles in the bloodstream and is known as the P-24 antigen test. It can be used as a diagnostic tool for the presence of HIV and as a way for physicians to monitor the effectiveness of treatments.

TERMS

Pneumocystis carinii An organism that causes a particular type of pneumonia common in people infected with HIV.

Kaposi's sarcoma A form of cancer characterized by purple or brownish lesions that are generally painless and occur anywhere on the skin; usually appears in men infected with HIV.

HIV antibody blood test A test currently being used to determine if an individual has been infected by the human immunodeficiency (HIV) virus.

ELISA (or Enzyme Linked Immune Sorbant Assay) A test that detects the presence of antibodies produced against HIV by an infected person's immune system.

Western blot A test that detects the presence of HIV antibodies. It is a more accurate and more expensive test, so it is used to confirm positive results from an ELISA test.

Antibody A globular protein produced in the blood in response to a foreign substance with which it combines.

HIV-positive A person who has tested positive for the presence of HIV in his or her bloodstream; also referred to as seropositive.

If you are at risk for HIV infection, it is important that you consider being tested. Early treatment for HIV infection can slow the progress of the disease and help keep you free of symptoms for a longer period of time. If you know you are HIV-positive, you can inform any partners and encourage them to consider testing and, if necessary, to obtain treatment. You can also avoid transmitting HIV to others by abstaining from sex or limiting your sexual activity to safer practices.

How can you tell if you are at risk for having HIV? Researchers believe that HIV has been in the United States since the middle to late 1970s. You are potentially at risk if any of the following apply to you since that time.

- You have had unprotected sexual contact with more than one partner or with a partner who was not in a mutually monogamous relationship with you.

- You have used or shared syringes, bulbs, works, cookers, or needles for injecting drugs (including steroids).

- You received a transfusion of blood or blood products prior to 1985.

If any of these statements are true for you, there are secondary risk factors that can increase your risk for HIV. These include living in a heavily populated area such as New York, Chicago, Miami, Los Angeles, or San Francisco and having chronic or recurrent episodes of other sexually transmissible diseases.

Should you decide to be tested for HIV, look for a testing program that offers both pre- and post-test counseling about the interpretation of the results, the emotional impact of the test results, and the actions you may want to consider taking in response to the outcome of the test. If you have doubts about whether to be tested, get counseling; then you can decide whether to go ahead with testing. Some states offer anonymous testing, where no one asks your name and you are the only one who can reveal your test result to others; other states provide confidential testing, where your record is kept secret from everyone except medical personnel and, in some states, the state health department. To find out where you can receive counseling and testing, check with your physician, your local or state health department, or the national AIDS hot line (800-342-AIDS, or 800-344-SIDA for Spanish speakers).

The test itself is fairly simple. A blood sample is drawn and analyzed in the laboratory for the presence of antibodies to HIV. If the first stage of testing, the ELISA test, proves positive, it is followed by a confirmatory test, the Western blot. The accuracy of the combined tests is high. However, it usually takes about 2 to 12 weeks (possibly longer in some individuals) after exposure to HIV for antibodies to appear (a process called **seroconversion**); so a person may need to be retested at a later date to be absolutely certain of his or her HIV status. False-positive results are also possible, but most labs do a second set of tests to confirm the accuracy of any positive test result.

As mentioned earlier, AIDS is the most severe form of HIV infection. The criteria for a diagnosis of AIDS were recently revised by the CDC to more accurately reflect the stage of HIV infection at which a person's immune system becomes dangerously compromised. As of January 1993, a diagnosis of AIDS is made if a person is HIV-positive and either has developed an infection defined as an AIDS indicator or has a severely damaged immune system (as measured by CD4 cell counts). Three new illnesses have been added to the list of marker conditions—tuberculosis, recurrent bacterial pneumonia, and invasive cervical cancer. These three conditions are particularly prevalent among women and drug users infected with HIV.

Reporting All cases of AIDS, as defined by the CDC, must be reported to public health authorities. This measure is meant to help public health officials track the disease and keep their records of its progress up-to-date. Reporting requirements vary from state to state; although all states require that cases of AIDS be reported, most do not require that incidences of positive HIV tests alone be reported.

The issue of confidentiality is an important one. Despite public education campaigns, people who have AIDS or who have tested HIV-positive are often stigmatized and subjected to discrimination. For this reason, physicians, hospitals, and public health departments must keep all information about testing, diagnosis, and treatment of AIDS completely confidential. If people believe they are risking their jobs, friends, or social acceptability by being tested, they are unlikely to come forward. At the same time, it is essential that sufficient information be disclosed through reporting to protect individuals and society at large. People have a right to know the incidence of the disease in their community or city, for example, and the CDC has to keep accurate records of the epidemic.

Treatment Early hopes for a cure faded as the complexity and virulence of HIV became apparent. There is no known cure for HIV infection, but new drugs have been developed to slow the advance of the virus and to treat some of the opportunistic infections. People infected with HIV may now live ten years before becoming sick with AIDS. Researchers hope that before too long, AIDS

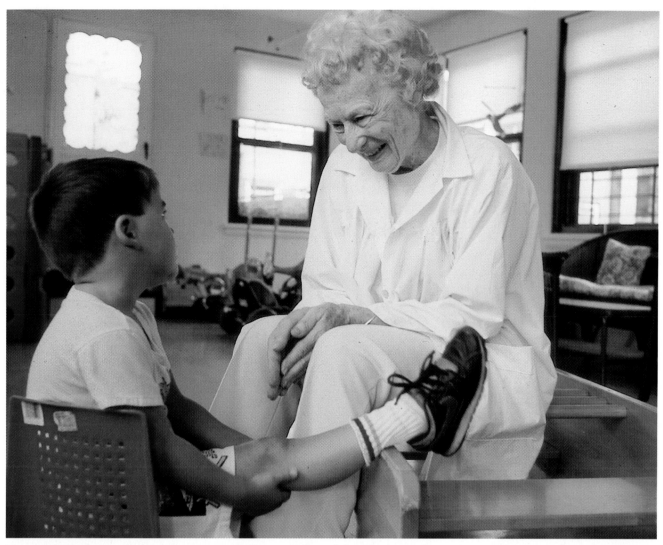

The ever-widening net cast by STDs ensnares children as well as adults. This boy with AIDS, being cared for in a group home for children infected with HIV is part of a growing population of children infected with HIV in the womb.

may be a manageable chronic disease that people will be able to control with medication.

Current research is focused on two categories of anti-HIV drugs—antivirals and drugs that stimulate or regulate the immune system. Antivirals are agents that kill the virus directly or limit its growth. To date, none of these agents has been able to eradicate HIV from an infected person, but they can help delay the onset of severe symptoms. The most widely known and used is **zidovudine (AZT),** and many people with HIV take AZT regularly. In addition to helping to delay the onset of symptoms, AZT has also been found to prolong the lives of some HIV-infected people suffering from PCP. However, AZT does have some disadvantages, including severe side effects in some people and a high price tag. Other antivirals include didanosine (ddI), dideoxycytidine (ddC), and Compound Q.

Another group of drugs under study is those designed to stimulate, regulate, or modulate the immune system. These include naltrexone, anti-interferon, globulin, disulfiram (antabuse), and interleukin-2. Many of these drugs have adverse effects and are potentially dangerous.

Depending on the type of infection, treatment for HIV-related conditions may include antibiotics, chemotherapy, and radiotherapy. Researchers are also working to develop drugs to help prevent the occurrence of some common HIV-related infections. For example, Septra

Seroconversion   The appearance of antibodies to HIV in the blood of an infected person.

Zidovudine (AZT)   A drug used in the treatment of HIV infection that inhibits the reproduction of HIV.

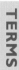

TERMS

(Bactrim), Dapsone, or aerosolized pentamidine can help prevent *Pneumocystis carinii* pneumonia. To treat pneumonia and tuberculosis, antibiotics are typically used; chemotherapy may be used for Kaposi's sarcoma and cervical cancer.

The cost of treatment for HIV continues to be an area of major concern. Medications alone for a person with AIDS average about $3,000 to $4,000 per month. The average cost of treatment for a person infected with HIV is about $10,000 per year; for someone diagnosed with AIDS, treatment may cost more than $40,000 per year.

What about a vaccine? No vaccine has ever been developed for a virus like HIV, and the difficulties—scientific, political, industrial, and financial—are considerable. The virus's ability to mutate poses a major challenge to researchers attempting to develop a vaccine. Successful vaccines have been developed against the simian version of HIV, but a vaccine for the human version is not expected to be ready for at least five or ten years.

With treatments still limited, most efforts right now are being directed to offering care for people with AIDS. Volunteer agencies and groups have rallied to this cause and are the core of local and national efforts. Many of them provide counseling, long-term emotional support, and assistance with the increasing difficulties of daily life for those with the disease. A highly visible and moving effort has been the "Names Project," a quilt put together from panels made by individuals in memory of their loved ones. When displayed in cities across the United States, the quilt brings together thousands upon thousands of otherwise diverse people whose lives have been touched and torn apart by the devastation of AIDS.

Prevention   Although AIDS is currently fatal and incurable, it is a preventable disease. You can protect yourself by avoiding behaviors that may bring you into contact with HIV. This means making careful choices about sexual activity and not sharing needles to inject drugs.

Make Careful Choices About Sexual Activity   In a sexual relationship, it is your behavior and you and your partner's past behaviors that determine the amount of risk involved. If you are uninfected and in a mutually monogamous relationship with another uninfected person, you are not at risk for HIV.

For anyone not involved in a long-term, mutually monogamous relationship, abstinence from any sexual activity that involves the exchange of body fluids is the only sure way to prevent HIV infection. Safer sex includes many activities that carry virtually no risk of HIV infection, like hugging, massaging, closed-lip kissing, rubbing bodies together, kissing your partner's skin, and mutual masturbation.

Anal and vaginal intercourse are the sexual activities associated with the highest risk of HIV infection. If you have intercourse, always use a latex condom with a sper-micide containing **nonoxynol-9.** Condoms are not perfect, and they do not provide risk-free sex; however, used properly, a latex condom provides a high level of protection against HIV. The use of a spermicide containing nonoxynol-9 may increase the protection provided by a condom, but it should never take the place of condom use. Condoms should also be worn during oral sex. Some experts also suggest the use of latex squares and dental dams, rubber devices that can be used as barriers during oral-genital or oral-anal sexual contact.

Limiting the number of sexual partners you have—particularly partners who have engaged in risky behaviors in the past—can also lower your risk of exposure to HIV. Take the time to talk with a potential new sexual partner about HIV and safer sex. Talking about sex may seem embarrassing and uncomfortable, but good communication is critical for your health. Asking a partner about past sexual experiences can also be helpful, but you cannot always depend on that information. It is much safer to take precautions with every partner. Don't agree to have intercourse or give up precautions as a way to show your love or commitment to a relationship. Your specific sexual practices can be just as important as the number of partners you have.

Removing alcohol and other drugs from sexual activity is another crucial component of safer sex. The use of alcohol and mood-altering drugs may lower inhibitions and affect judgment, making you more likely to engage in unsafe sex. The use of drugs is also associated with sexual activity with multiple partners.

Remember, you can't tell if someone is infected by looking at him or her. Researchers believe that HIV has been in the United States since the mid- to late-1970s; anyone who has engaged in an unsafe behavior since that time is potentially at risk for HIV. Consider in advance what you will say and do in particular situations. Be assertive with your sexual partners and negotiate for safer sex practices.

Surveys of college students indicate that the majority of students are not engaging in safer sex. Although most students know that condom use can protect against HIV infection, this knowledge is often not translated into action. Many students also report a willingness to lie about past sexual activity in order to obtain sex. In addition, many students believe their risk of contracting HIV depends on "who they are" rather than on their sexual behavior. These attitudes and behaviors place college students at continued high risk for contracting HIV.

Don't Share Drug Needles   People who inject drugs should avoid sharing needles, syringes, or anything that might have blood on it. Any injectable drug, legal or illegal, can be associated with HIV transmission. Needles can be decontaminated with a solution of bleach and water, but it is not a foolproof procedure. (Boiling needles and syringes does not necessarily destroy HIV either.) If you

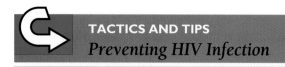

For those who don't have a long-term monogamous relationship with an uninfected partner, abstinence is the only truly safe option. Individuals should remember that it is OK to say no to sex and drugs.

"Safer sex" activities that allow intimate skin-to-skin contact without exposure to body fluids carry virtually no risk of HIV infection. These include fantasy, hugging, massage, rubbing bodies together, mutual masturbation, and kissing with lips closed. (Although no cases of HIV infection have been traced to kissing, transmission of HIV through deep-mouth kissing is thought to be possible.)

If you choose to be sexually active, talk with potential sexual partners about HIV, safer sex, and the use of condoms before you begin a sexual relationship. The following behaviors will help lower your risk of exposure to HIV during sexual activities:

- Limit the number of your sexual partners. Avoid sexual contact with people who have HIV or who have engaged in risky behaviors in the past, including unprotected sex and injecting drug use.

- Use latex condoms during every act of intercourse and oral sex.

- Use condoms properly to obtain maximum protection (refer back to the detailed instructions for condom use given in Chapter 6). Use a water-based lubricant containing the spermicide nonoxynol-9; don't use oil-based lubricants such as petroleum jelly or baby oil. Unroll condoms gently to avoid tearing them, and smooth out any air bubbles.

- Avoid sexual contact that could cause cuts or tears in the skin or tissue.

- Get prompt treatment for any STDs you contract.

- Don't drink or use drugs in sexual situations. Mood-altering drugs can affect your judgment and make you more likely to engage in risky behaviors.

If you inject drugs of any kind, don't share needles, syringes, or anything that might have blood on it. Decontaminate needles and syringes with household bleach and water.

If you are at risk for HIV infection, don't donate blood, sperm, or body organs. Don't have unprotected sex or share needles or syringes. Consider being tested for HIV.

---

are an injecting drug user, your best protection against HIV is to obtain treatment and refrain from using drugs (see Chapter 11 for more information about treatment for drug abuse).

Participate in an HIV Education Program   The cornerstone of all efforts to prevent the continued spread of HIV is education—in schools, homes, communities, and the media. In the absence of a vaccine against the virus or any effective therapy for the disease, behavior change is the only defense against HIV. Educational efforts mounted in the earlier days of the epidemic met with partial success. Efforts at behavior change were particularly effective in the gay community, where the rate of new infections has dropped sharply. But other segments of the population have been harder to reach. Injecting drug users, the poor, homeless, people of color, women, and prostitutes worldwide remain at higher risk for HIV infection. The rate of infection is increasing most rapidly among women and children.

What can you do to reinforce what you know about HIV? Many schools and colleges have peer counseling and education programs about preventing HIV. These programs give you a chance to practice skills in communicating with potential sexual partners and negotiating safer sex, to engage in role-playing to build self-confidence, and, although controversial, even to learn about how to use condoms.

Many young people still believe that they are invulnerable to most kinds of harm and persist in thinking of themselves as not being at risk for HIV. The attitude of "it won't happen to me" is pervasive among high school and college students and is a major stumbling block to HIV prevention. Until there is a vaccine and a cure, HIV infection will remain one of the biggest challenges of this generation. Education and individual responsibility can lead the way to controlling this devastating epidemic (see the box "Preventing HIV Infection").

Hepatitis

An inflammation of the liver, **hepatitis** is usually caused by one of three common hepatitis viruses. Infection with hepatitis viruses can be transmitted sexually as well as through nonsexual contact. The Centers for Disease Control and Prevention estimate that between 200,000 and 300,000 Americans become infected with hepatitis each year and that between 750,000 and 1 million people are carriers (capable of infecting others) of the most common

---

Nonoxynol-9   A spermicide that may kill some forms of disease-causing organisms, including HIV.

Hepatitis   Inflammation of the liver caused by one of a group of viruses that can be transmitted through certain types of sexual and nonsexual contact.

TERMS

form—hepatitis B. There is no known cure for hepatitis, and hepatitis can cause death in severe cases. The disease is preventable, however, and a vaccine for hepatitis B is available.

Transmission   Three different agents have been identified as primary causes of viral hepatitis. Hepatitis A virus causes the mildest form of the disease and is usually transmitted by food or water contaminated by sewage or an infected person. Anal-oral contact is the primary means of sexual transmission of hepatitis A.

The hepatitis B virus is found in all body fluids, including blood and blood products, semen, saliva, urine, and vaginal secretions. Hepatitis B is easily transmitted through any sexual activity that involves the exchange of body fluids, the use of contaminated needles, and any blood-to-blood contact, including the use of contaminated razor blades, toothbrushes, and eating utensils. The primary risk factors for acquiring hepatitis B are heterosexual exposure and injecting drug use; having multiple sexual partners greatly increases risk. A decade ago, male homosexual activity was the leading risk factor for hepatitis B, but changes in sexual behavior due to HIV infection have greatly reduced this risk. In addition, a pregnant woman can transmit hepatitis B to her unborn child.

The hepatitis C virus used to be the leading cause of hepatitis following blood transfusions, but the blood supply is now screened for both hepatitis B and C. As a result, the risk of hepatitis infection is now only about 3 per 10,000 units of blood transfused. Hepatitis C virus is transmitted in the same way as hepatitis B, but sexual transmission has not been confirmed.

Symptoms   Many people infected with hepatitis never develop symptoms; they have what are known as "silent" infections. The normal incubation period for hepatitis ranges from about 40 to 110 days. Mild cases of hepatitis cause flulike symptoms such as fever, body aches, chills, and loss of appetite. As the illness progresses, there may be nausea, vomiting, dark-colored urine, abdominal pain, and **jaundice.** Some people with hepatitis also develop a skin rash and joint pain or arthritis.

Most cases of hepatitis A tend to be of short duration, although relapses do occur. People with hepatitis B or C sometimes recover completely, but they can also become chronic carriers of the virus, capable of infecting others for the rest of their lives. Some chronic carriers remain asymptomatic, while others develop chronic liver disease. Chronic hepatitis can cause cirrhosis of the liver, liver failure, and a deadly form of liver cancer. Hepatitis kills about 6,000 Americans each year.

Diagnosis and Treatment   Blood tests can be used to diagnose hepatitis through analysis of liver function and detection of the specific organism causing the infection. There is no cure for hepatitis, and treatment is designed to minimize damage to the liver. Researchers are investigating the use of corticosteroids and interferon.

Treatment with gamma globulin within two weeks of exposure to hepatitis A is about 80 to 90 percent effective in preventing the disease; household members and sexual partners of anyone who becomes infected with hepatitis A should receive gamma globulin. For people exposed to hepatitis B, treatment with hepatitis B immunoglobulin can provide temporary protection against the virus. The limitation with both of these treatments is that people often do not know they have been exposed to hepatitis.

Prevention   To reduce your risk of contracting hepatitis A, avoid contaminated water and infected food, wash your hands frequently, and avoid oral-anal sexual contact. Preventive measures for the B and C forms of hepatitis are similar to those for HIV infection: Avoid sexual contact that involves sharing of body fluids, including saliva; use condoms during intercourse; and don't share hypodermic needles.

The vaccine for hepatitis B is safe and highly effective. All pregnant women should be tested for hepatitis B and infants of infected mothers vaccinated immediately after birth. Many physicians recommend routine immunization of all infants and adolescents as part of the normal set of childhood vaccinations. Immunizations are also recommended for adults in high-risk groups, including health care workers, homosexually active men, injecting drug users, and heterosexually active individuals with multiple partners. A vaccine for hepatitis A is currently being tested and may be available within the next five years.

Syphilis

Dreaded throughout history but not well understood, syphilis has been known by a variety of names, including the "evil pox," the "great pox" (as distinguished from smallpox), and the "great imposter" (because its symptoms resemble those of so many other ailments). Syphilis affected millions until drugs developed in the twentieth century finally provided relief. Before World War I, arsenic compounds were used; and then, beginning in the 1940s, penicillin.

Death and disability from syphilis declined dramatically after penicillin treatment was introduced, but in recent years there has been an upsurge in the number of cases, especially among teenagers, homosexuals, and minority populations. There are about 100,000 new cases every year, including congenital cases (infants infected by their mothers), which increased fourfold in the 1980s.

What Is Syphilis?   Syphilis is caused by a spirochete (pronounced "spy-ro-keet") called ***Treponema pallidum,*** a thin, corkscrew-shaped bacterium that moves by rotating on its long axis. It requires warmth and moisture to survive and dies very quickly outside the human body. The disease is usually acquired through sexual contact, although unborn children can contract it through the placenta from an infected mother. The organism passes through any break or opening in the skin or mucous membranes and can be transmitted by kissing, vaginal or anal intercourse, or oral-genital contact.

Syphilis is characterized by sores or lesions known as **chancres** (pronounced "shang-kers") containing large numbers of bacteria; they make the disease highly contagious when they are present. Left untreated, an individual can remain contagious for as long as 18 months. In later stages, when the lesions have disappeared and the person is no longer contagious, the disease can cause devastating damage to almost any system of the body.

Symptoms   Syphilis progresses through three stages as the organism becomes established in the body.

First Stage: Primary Syphilis   Within 10 to 90 days (usually about three weeks) of contact with an infected partner, a single chancre about the size of a dime appears at the site where the organism entered the body, most commonly the genital area. Chancres can also appear in the mouth or armpit or on the tongue, lips, breasts, or fingers. These sores are painless unless they become infected and may not even be noticed. They generally heal within a few weeks.

Second Stage: Secondary Syphilis   Approximately six weeks after a chancre first appears, an untreated person begins to show signs and symptoms of secondary disease. These include fever, malaise, sore throat, headache, hoarseness, a depressed appetite, swollen lymph glands, and loss of hair. The second stage may also be characterized by a rash that appears anywhere on the body but most typically on the palms of the hands and the soles of the feet. The rash may also affect the mucous membranes of the lips, cheeks, tongue, tonsils, throat, and vocal chords, where grayish-white patches of mucus surrounded by dull red borders appear. These sores break down and ooze a clear fluid that contains large numbers of bacteria, making this stage highly contagious. With or without antibiotic treatment, skin lesions of secondary syphilis usually heal in two to ten weeks. However, if the disease remains untreated, relapses can occur.

Third Stage: Latent Syphilis   By definition, people without symptoms but with evidence of having had syphilis in the past have latent syphilis. In this stage of the disease, the organism invades the internal organs and the central nervous system. The principal manifestation of central nervous system damage is a condition called **paresis,** which involves partial or complete paralysis and chronic, progressive mental degeneration leading to death. Symptoms may include facial tremors, slurred speech, impaired vision, headaches, epileptic convulsions, exaggerated reflexes, defective memory, delusions, depression, and dementia (insanity).

In infected pregnant women, the syphilis organism can cross the placenta after the tenth week of gestation. If the mother is not treated before the eighteenth week, the probable result is stillbirth or congenital deformity. The infected child may be crippled, blind, or deaf or have facial abnormalities such as cleft lip and palate.

Diagnosis and Treatment   To diagnose primary syphilis, clinicians take a specimen from the surface of the chancre and examine it under the microscope. A special microscopic examination, called the dark field, permits direct visualization of the *Treponema* organism if it is present. Diagnosis of secondary syphilis is made from blood tests and clinical observation of the symptoms.

Penicillin remains the drug of choice for the treatment of syphilis in all stages. For those allergic to penicillin, tetracycline and erythromycin can be effective substitutes. Sexual partners must be treated as well. Follow-up tests should be performed four weeks after the completion of treatment and every three months thereafter for one year to ensure that the bacterium has been eradicated.

A person who has had syphilis should not have sexual contact with others until at least one month after treatment is completed. As with any serious disease, it is absolutely vital that the entire course of prescribed medication be completed and not discontinued when the symptoms have disappeared. As with all STDs, it makes sense to avoid it by practicing responsible sexual behavior.

Chlamydia

Gonorrhea and chlamydia have similar symptoms and are often mistaken for each other, but chlamydia is now the more common disease. In fact, *Chlamydia trachomatis* currently causes the most prevalent bacterial infection in the United States, with 3 to 4 million new cases reported every year. The rise in the incidence of chlamydia may be

Jaundice   Increased bile pigment levels in the blood, characterized by yellowing of the skin and the whites of the eyes.

Syphilis   A sexually transmissible disease caused by a spiral-shaped, corkscrew bacteria called a spirochete.

Treponema pallidum   The spiral-shaped organism that causes syphilis.

Chancre   The sore produced by syphilis in its earliest stage.

Paresis   Central nervous system damage, sometimes a result of syphilis, involving paralysis and mental degeneration.

Chlamydia trachomatis   A sexually transmissible organism that produces a wide variety of sometimes acute infections; now reaching epidemic scale in the United States.

TERMS

a matter not only of more actual cases but also of increased awareness and improved diagnostic techniques.

Although men, women, and children are all susceptible to chlamydia, women bear the greatest burden because of the possible complications and consequences of the disease. In men, chlamydia is the leading cause of urinary tract infection and is also responsible for approximately 50 percent of the 500,000 cases of **epididymitis** (inflammation of the testicles) seen annually in the United States. *In most women, chlamydial infection produces no early symptoms,* a factor that contributes to the devastation it can cause (see the box "Myths About STDs"). If left undetected for two months or more, it can lead to severe symptoms and cause extensive damage, such as inflammation of the cervix and oviducts (fallopian tubes), a condition known as pelvic inflammatory disease (PID). PID is a leading cause of infertility. (PID is discussed in greater detail later in this chapter.)

Infants of infected mothers can acquire the infection through contact with the organism in the birth canal during delivery. In newborns, chlamydia can cause eye infections, pneumonia, and (less often) ear infections. Chlamydia is the most common cause of eye infections and pneumonia in infants under 6 months of age. Over 150,000 babies are born each year to infected mothers, and these infants are at high risk for contracting chlamydia infections.

Symptoms   In men, chlamydia symptoms include painful urination and a slight watery discharge from the penis. In women, symptoms include a discharge from the cervix, painful urination, and painful inflammation of the oviducts, which is symptomatic of PID at this point. However, most people experience few or no symptoms, increasing the likelihood that they will inadvertently spread the infection to their partners.

Diagnosis   Physicians often diagnose chlamydia only after they have excluded the presence of gonorrhea during an examination. A definitive diagnosis is made after the organism is grown in tissue culture or through a microscopic antibody test. Because of the seriousness of an undetected infection, some physicians may add a laboratory test for chlamydia to a routine Pap test. Screening pregnant women and treating those with chlamydia is a highly effective way to prevent infection of babies during birth.

Treatment   Once chlamydia has been diagnosed, the infected person and his or her sexual partner or partners are given antibiotics, either tetracycline, doxycycline, or erythromycin. *Penicillin is not effective against chlamydia.* As with all antibiotics, it is essential that the entire course of medication be completed by all infected individuals, regardless of whether the symptoms have disappeared. Otherwise, reinfection and complications are likely. It is also important to refrain from sexual intercourse until the treatment is completed.

Chlamydia is an expensive disease. In the United States, costs associated with the infection run to more than $1 billion a year, mostly for the treatment of PID and the care of infants hospitalized with chlamydial pneumonia. And on an individual level, the physical and emotional costs—damaged reproductive organs, sterility, or an infected infant—can be even more devastating.

Gonorrhea

In the United States, between 300,000 and 400,000 new cases of **gonorrhea** are reported every year. The highest incidence is among 20- to 24-year-olds.

Like chlamydia, untreated gonorrhea can cause PID in women and epididymitis in men, leading to sterility. It can also cause **dermatitis** (inflammation of the skin) and a type of arthritis. An infant passing through the birth canal of an infected mother may contract **gonococcal conjunctivitis,** an infection in the eyes that can cause blindness if left untreated. In some states, all newborn babies are routinely treated with antimicrobial eye drops to prevent infection.

Like syphilis and chlamydia, gonorrhea is a bacterial disease, caused by the bacterium *Neisseria gonorrhoeae,* which grows well in mucous membranes, including the moist linings of the mouth, throat, vagina, cervix, urethra, and anal canal. It cannot live long outside the warm, moist environment of the human body and dies within moments of exposure to light and air. Consequently, gonorrhea cannot be contracted from toilet seats, towels, or other objects.

Symptoms   In men, the incubation period for gonorrhea is brief, generally about five days. The first symptoms are a form of urethritis (inflammation of the urethra) that causes discomfort on urination and a thick, yellowish-white or yellowish-green discharge from the penis. The lips of the urethral opening may become inflamed and swollen. In some men, the lymph glands in the groin become enlarged and swollen. A small percentage of men—10 to 30 percent—will have very minor symptoms or none at all.

Approximately 80 percent of women with gonorrhea have no symptoms whatsoever and therefore don't know when they are infected. Additionally, some women with symptoms mistake the discharge from a gonorrhea infection for a normal preovulation mucus discharge. When symptoms do appear in women, they are similar to those in men, including an irritating discharge and discomfort on urination. When the infection has been established for a longer period of time, generally two months or more, symptoms may include lower abdominal cramping or pain, fever, and vaginal bleeding, indicating that the woman may have PID. Any woman with discomfort and an unusual discharge should see a physician immediately to be tested for gonorrhea.

Gonorrhea bacteria can also infect the throat or rectum in individuals with the disease who engage in oral or anal sex. The symptoms of gonorrhea in the throat may be a sore throat or pus on the tonsils, and those of gonorrhea in the rectum may be pus in the feces or rectal irritation, pain, and itching. As with other infections, gonorrhea is often accompanied by a fever and swollen glands.

Diagnosis   The test for gonorrhea consists of a smear test or a culture of the discharge. In men, a positive smear is generally sufficient to make the diagnosis. Asymptomatic people who suspect they might have the infection can have cultures taken. Women who suspect they may have the infection should seek examination and testing seven to ten days after they were exposed to the disease. Accurate diagnosis of gonorrhea is especially important

because new strains of the gonococcal organism are antibiotic-resistant. The exact strain causing a gonorrheal infection must be accurately identified before proper treatment can be given.

Treatment   When gonorrhea is diagnosed early, treatment is relatively easy. Broad-spectrum antibiotics used in combination are the preferred drugs for treating acute, uncomplicated gonorrhea. For those allergic to penicillin, tetracycline is effective. *Using drugs prescribed for friends or sexual partners or left over from other illnesses is not a safe and effective way to treat gonorrhea or any other STD.* As mentioned earlier, the entire course of medication must be taken, and if two people share a prescription, neither will be cured.

After completion of the course of medication, follow-up testing should be done to ensure that all traces of the infection have been eradicated. Sexual activity should not be resumed until the results of follow-up testing have been obtained. As mentioned earlier, if gonorrhea is untreated and allowed to become chronic, it can spread internally and lead to infertility as a consequence of PID.

Pelvic Inflammatory Disease

A major complication in 10 to 15 percent of women who have been infected with either gonorrhea or chlamydia, or both, is **pelvic inflammatory disease (PID).** An infection of the oviducts that may extend to the ovaries, PID is often serious enough to require hospitalization and sometimes surgery. Even if the disease is treated successfully, the woman has a continuing susceptibility to recurrent infection, ectopic (tubal) pregnancy, sterility, and chronic menstrual problems. PID is the leading cause of infertility in young women, often undetected until later when the desire to have a child leads to further testing.

Both infectious agents may be transmitted sexually by an infected partner. During or just after menstruation, these organisms appear to rise into the uterine cavity, where they may cause inflammation, or they may pass directly into the oviducts. This inflammatory process spreads easily into the pelvic cavity, causing further infection and in some cases pelvic abscess.

Epididymitis   An inflammation of the small body of ducts that rests on the testes.

Gonorrhea   A sexually transmissible disease caused by a type of bacteria that usually affects mucous membranes.

Dermatitis   An inflammation of the skin evidenced by itching, redness, and various skin lesions.

Gonococcal conjunctivitis   An inflammation of the mucous membrane lining of the eyelids, caused by the gonococcus bacterium.

Pelvic inflammatory disease (PID)   An infection that progresses from the vagina and cervix to infect the pelvic cavity and oviducts.

TERMS

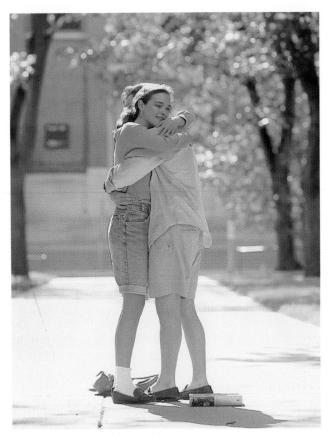

By taking a responsible attitude toward STDs, people show respect and concern for themselves and their partners. This couple's plans for the future could be seriously disrupted if one of them contracted an STD like gonorrhea or chlamydia. Either of these diseases, if untreated, could result in pelvic inflammatory disease, the leading cause of sterility in young women.

Symptoms Following infection with either organism, most women remain asymptomatic for some time, usually until the next menstrual cycle. Once the organisms reach the oviducts, the rate of the development of symptoms varies from one to seven days. Women with rapid onset of symptoms most often have chills, fever, loss of appetite, nausea, and/or vomiting. Most complain of abdominal pain on both sides, although the pain may be greater on one side than the other. The pain may be caused by sudden movements like sneezing or coughing. Some women may also have abnormal vaginal bleeding, prolonged menstruation, or abnormal vaginal discharge.

Diagnosis Diagnosis of PID is usually made on the basis of symptoms. Laparoscopy may be used to isolate the suspected organism and grow it in a culture medium. Cultures from the rectum or cervix may also be taken to assist in identifying the specific organism. Treatment is more effective when the causative organism is identified, but since gonorrhea and chlamydia are often both present, a broader-spectrum approach to treatment is usually initiated. It is also very helpful in diagnosing the disease

and choosing a treatment to examine and test the woman's sexual partner(s).

Treatment Beginning treatment of PID as quickly as possible is important in order to avoid severe damage to the reproductive organs. Antibiotics are usually started immediately; in severe cases, the woman may be hospitalized and antibiotics given intravenously. Commonly used drugs include penicillin and tetracycline. Repeat cultures are done to ensure that the bacteria have been eradicated.

When a woman has PID, it's especially important that her sexual partners be treated for infection. As many as 60 percent of the male contacts of women with PID are asymptomatic, and many men believe that unless they have symptoms, they are not infected.

Effects of PID are serious and irreversible. Scarring of the oviducts, often a result of abscesses, can result in adhesions, chronic pelvic pain, and ectopic pregnancies.

Genital Warts

The incidence of **genital warts,** or condyloma, has increased rapidly in recent years and is now exceeded only by that of gonorrhea and chlamydia. Condyloma is the most common STD for which diagnosis and treatment is sought in student health services; the disease appears to be most prevalent in young people aged 16 to 25.

Condyloma presents a new challenge to the medical community because of its known relationship to cervical cancer. The precancerous condition known as cervical dysplasia often occurs among women with untreated genital warts. (See the discussion of this topic in Chapter 16.) Identification of the causative agent of condyloma has revealed a family of viruses known as **human papillomavirus (HPV),** of which there may be as many as 65 different strains. Five of these are commonly isolated from genital warts; the strains most often implicated in cervical cancer are HPV16 and HPV18.

A genital wart infection is very contagious through contact with the lesions. Early diagnosis and effective treatment are often impeded by a long incubation period (which averages two to three months), a lack of awareness of symptoms in women, and a complex approach to treatment, which may not always work.

Symptoms Genital warts look like the warts that might develop on any other part of the body. They're dry, painless growths, rough in texture and gray or pink in color. They can be flat or raised, and they vary in size. Untreated warts can grow together to form a cauliflowerlike mass. In males, they appear on the penis, more commonly in circumcised men. They often involve the urethra, appearing first at the opening and then spreading as a complication. The growth may cause irritation and bleeding, leading to painful urination and a urethral discharge. Warts may also appear around the anus or within the rectum.

In women, warts may appear on the labia, vulva, and may spread to the perineum, the area between the vagina and the rectum. They may also appear on the cervix. If the warts are small and flat, they can be difficult for the physician to see.

The incubation period for condyloma has been estimated at four to six weeks from the time of contact, and it can be as long as two to three months before any symptoms are identified. People can be infected with the virus and be capable of transmitting it to their sex partners without having any symptoms at all. This is one reason why it's essential that people who do have symptoms inform their sex partners that they may be infected. In addition, although the risk to newborns is not clear, they can be infected during delivery.

Diagnosis   To treat genital warts effectively, the physician has to differentiate the lesions from those of other diseases, particularly those of secondary syphilis. Sometimes both diseases are present, and each requires a different treatment. The virus lives within the lesion itself and does not travel throughout the body. Therefore, HPV is diagnosed by the physical appearance of the lesion and the presence of the virus in it.

Treatment   Treatment focuses on individual lesions. The traditional and long-standing treatment for genital warts is application of **podophyllin,** a toxic agent, directly to the lesion. The drug can burn surrounding tissue, so careful application is necessary. Repeat applications are often required.

Other treatment options include removal of the lesion by electrocautery, cryosurgery (freezing), surgery, and, recently, CO_2 laser therapy. In 1989 the FDA approved a new drug, alpha interferon, to treat genital warts. The drug is administered in a series of injections; the long-term effects of the treatment are still being studied.

Even when treated, however, genital warts can recur, probably because the treatment has eradicated the wart but not the viral infection. Follow-up care is especially important with this condition, as are avoidance of sexual contact until healing is complete, and continuing open communication with sexual partners. Because of the relationship of HPV to increased risk of cervical cancer, women who have had genital warts should have Pap tests every six months.

Herpes

Infection with herpesvirus type II is considered a serious STD in part because of its extremely high incidence—more than 500,000 new cases each year and over 20 million total cases in the United States—and in part because of its serious impact on newborns. Additionally, there is no cure, nor is there a vaccine available. Despite research and efforts to develop treatments, vaccines, and specific preventive approaches, the "arsenal" to combat this relatively common STD remains quite small.

After an initial herpes infection is over, new outbreaks can be triggered by a variety of factors. Each time the infection recurs, the person is contagious again, making it a difficult disease to deal with and to prevent from spreading to others. Adding to the complexity of the infection and to the confusion about its transmissibility is the fact that there are six different viruses in the herpes family that infect human beings, all with different manifestations:

- *Herpes simplex, type I,* which causes cold sores and fever blisters around the lips, mouth, and facial area; as a result of oral-genital contact, it is sometimes also responsible for infections in the genital area
- *Herpes simplex, type II,* also known as genital herpes, which is usually seen in the genital area; as a result of oral-genital contact, it is sometimes also responsible for infections of the lips, mouth, and facial area
- *Varicella-zoster,* which causes chicken pox in children and shingles in adults
- *Epstein-Barr virus (EBV),* which is implicated as the cause of infectious mononucleosis and has recently been linked with Burkitt's lymphoma and a type of nasopharyngeal cancer
- *Cytomegalovirus (CMV),* which can cause severe infections of the lungs, brain, colon, and eyes in people with suppressed immune systems (including people with HIV) and can also cause birth defects
- *Human herpesvirus 6 (HHV 6),* which has only recently been identified

All of these organisms have the unique ability to adapt to their human hosts, and they are widespread in the population. Of the six, herpes simplex I and II, cytomegalovirus, and HHV6 are considered sexually transmissible. Although varicella-zoster and Epstein-Barr virus occasionally seem to be transmitted through sexual contact, they appear to play no significant role in STD incidence.

Symptoms   Typically, herpes infections (both types I and II) appear two to twenty days after initial exposure. Both types are highly contagious. Symptoms can include one or more blisterlike sores on or around the mouth, the

---

Genital warts   A sexually transmissible disease caused by a virus and characterized by the appearance of growths on the genital area of men and women.

Human papillomavirus   The organism that causes genital warts.

Podophyllin   An acid used in the treatment of warts.

Herpes   A type of virus, or the disease produced by the virus, such as cold sores; considered sexually transmissible.

TERMS

face, or the genitals. The sores are painful, fluid-filled lesions and may be accompanied by swollen glands, general muscle aches and pains, fever, a mild burning sensation during urination in men, and a vaginal discharge in women. Some women may have internal lesions on the vagina or the cervix. Because the cervix has no nerve endings, an infected woman may be completely unaware that lesions are present.

Although a direct relationship between the herpesvirus and cancer is yet to be established, women with genital herpes are five times more likely to develop cancer of the cervix. It is recommended that women who have had genital herpes inform their physicians and be sure to have a Pap test every six months.

Herpes infections are particularly dangerous to newborns because of their immature immune systems and their somewhat restricted ability to fight off a virulent virus like herpes simplex I or II. Newborns should not have direct contact with adults with cold sores, and pregnant women with herpes have to be monitored near the time of delivery to ensure that the newborn isn't exposed to the virus. If the woman's infection becomes active, the baby will usually be delivered by cesarean section to protect it from contact with lesions in the birth canal or genital area. There is no effective treatment for babies who contract the herpesvirus, which can cause severe brain damage and sometimes death in newborns.

One of the most frustrating aspects of a herpes infection is its ability to recur. After the first infection, which can last as long as three to four weeks, the virus lies dormant along nerve pathways in the area of initial infection. (It does not travel from one location to another; rather, it tends to recur at the site of the original lesion.) Dormancy lasts for different lengths of time in different individuals. An active infection may be triggered by exposure to sun, temperature extremes, high levels of stress, certain foods (chocolate, seeds, and nuts, for example), acute illness, lowered resistance from poor general health, or some other factor. Because herpes is chronic, it has a long-lasting effect on sexuality. A person with an active infection is contagious and has an obligation to prevent the spread of the disease to others. Maintaining good general health and avoiding factors that may trigger new outbreaks can help prevent repeated bouts of infection.

Diagnosis Of the herpes cases seen by medical practitioners, 90 percent are diagnosed on the basis of the presence of lesions, medical history, and other symptoms. If doubt exists that the infection is caused by the herpesvirus, a sample smear can be obtained from the lesion and grown in live tissue culture to determine the type of virus.

Treatment At present, there is no cure for herpes. Research has yet to solve the puzzle of how to intercept and destroy a virus that can lie dormant in the body without also damaging healthy surrounding tissues and organs. As scientists learn more about the characteristics of viruses in general, cures will be developed and effective preventive approaches identified. For the time being, treatment of herpes is directed at relieving pain, itching, and burning, avoiding secondary infection of lesions, and preventing the infection from spreading to other parts of the body. Bathing with soap and water or other drying agents, such as Epsom salts or Burrow's solution, is helpful in preventing secondary infection and speeds drying of the lesions.

For more than ten years, the drug **acyclovir** has been used to treat genital herpes, with varying degrees of effectiveness for different individuals. The long-term effects of acyclovir have yet to be evaluated, and the issue of viral resistance to the drug is being explored. Additional treatments include zinc compounds, a variety of ointments, and ultrasound. The use of L-lysine has been thought to damage the virus, and an alteration in diet to shift the balance between lysine and arginine is sometimes considered in treating herpes. None of these has stood the test of time or clinical trials, so individuals need to work closely with their personal physician to develop the best treatment for their case.

OTHER STDs

Although they are far less serious than the diseases already described, a few other diseases are transmitted sexually and are therefore included in this discussion. More annoying than threatening, these STDs still require responsible sexual behavior to prevent their spreading to others. They include trichomoniasis, a protozoal infection; *Candida albicans,* a fungal (yeast) infection; and pubic lice and scabies, parasitic infections.

Trichomoniasis, commonly called "trich," is one of the most common protozoal infections in North America. The one-celled organism that causes trich, ***Trichomonas vaginalis,*** thrives in warm, moist conditions, making women particularly susceptible to these infections in the vagina. This organism can remain alive on external objects for as long as 60 to 90 minutes, in urine for three hours, and in seminal fluid for six hours. Thus it is possible to contract trich by nonsexual means. However, it is rare; the most likely means of transmission is sexual contact with an infected partner.

Women who become symptomatic with trich develop a greenish, foul-smelling vaginal discharge within four days of the time of contact with the organism. The discharge also causes severe itching and irritates the vagina and vulva, causing redness and pain. Although most males do not have any symptoms, some may experience slight itching, clear discharge, and sometimes painful urination.

Diagnosis of trich can be done through microscopic

examination of the discharge. The drug of choice is metronidazole (Flagyl). Sexual partners should be treated as well to prevent the "Ping-Pong" effect that occurs when partners pass infection back and forth to each other.

Candida albicans is an extremely common organism normally found in the vaginal tract. The problem occurs when there is an increased production of the fungus, resulting in discomfort and itching (often referred to as a "yeast infection"); symptoms can then be transmitted to a male partner. A Ping-Pong effect is common, since males do not generally experience symptoms but are capable of giving the infection back to their sexual partner. Candidiasis is also a common opportunistic infection in people with HIV infection.

Various factors may contribute to the increased production of fungus in the vaginal tract, and often a runaway yeast infection is a symptom of a more extensive problem. These include diabetes, metabolic changes due to pregnancy, use of oral contraceptives (in some women), antibiotic therapy, and general lowering of body resistance to infection.

Intense vaginal and vulval itching and a thick, cottage cheese-like discharge are common symptoms of candidiasis. This infection can also manifest itself in the mouth (thrush) and show as whitish patches on the mucous membrane of the insides of the cheeks and back of the throat, making eating very difficult. The two manifestations require very different approaches to treatment.

Vaginal suppositories of the antibiotic mycostatin have proven very effective in women, but other methods of treatment are dependent on a complete medical evaluation of the individual. Over-the-counter remedies should not replace medical diagnosis and treatment. As with any infection, following medical advice and completing the course of medication are as vital as refraining from sexual intercourse until the infection is cleared up.

Pubic lice, most commonly known as "crabs," are included here because they are so highly contagious, both sexually and nonsexually. Called pubic lice because they are attached to the pubic hairs of the body, these parasites have three claws in front and four pairs of small legs in back. They are often difficult to see but are the color and size of small freckles until they have fed, and then they become dark brown in color. Like mosquitoes, lice feed on human blood. Although usually found in pubic hair, they have been known to attach themselves to hair on the head, eyelashes, underarms, and even mustaches and beards. (Head lice belong to a different species than pubic lice.) Separated from their human hosts, lice are able to survive about 24 hours.

Easily passed from person to person, lice can also be transmitted via infested bedding, towels, clothing, sleeping bags, and even toilet seats. Intense itching is the usual symptom, and with careful examination, both the parasite and its eggs, or nits, can be seen.

Treatment is generally easy, although the infestation can require repeated applications of over-the-counter medications. These preparations are in lotion or shampoo form and include a fine comb for removing any remaining lice or nits from body hair. Washing clothing and linen carefully is also essential for preventing reinfestation. If the infestation persists, a stronger medication is available by prescription.

Scabies is another fairly common infestation. A burrowing parasite, the scabies mite deposits eggs beneath the skin in the creases of the body. These hatch in a few days, and the new mites congregate around hair follicles. Any burrowing parasite produces intense itching, especially at night. The usual sites of infestation are between the fingers, on wrists, in armpits, underneath the breasts, along the inner surfaces of the thighs, penis, scrotum, and occasionally the female genitals.

Scabies is easily spread from person to person, not only through sexual contact but also through any direct or close contact. Diagnosis is made by actual identification of the mite, the eggs, or the larvae in scrapings taken from the burrows in the skin of the human host. Standard treatment is prolonged hot baths with vigorous scrubbing of infected areas and the application of benzyl benzoate emulsion or Kwell lotion, available by prescription only. Itching and inflammation may occur as a result of secondary infection and should be checked by a physician.

WHAT CAN YOU DO?

You can take responsibility for your health and contribute to a general reduction in the incidence of STDs in three major areas: education, prevention, and diagnosis and treatment. To assess your current level of responsibility about STD prevention, complete the quiz in the box "Do Your Attitudes and Behaviors Put You at Risk for STDs?"

Education

Since the AIDS epidemic began, public and private agencies have grown more serious about educating the public and increasing their awareness of all the STDs. This campaign may already be paying off in changing attitudes and sexual behaviors, at least among certain segments of the

TERMS

Acyclovir   A drug used in the treatment of recurrent herpes infection.

Trichomonas vaginalis   The one-celled organism (protozoa) that causes a vaginal infection in women; may be carried by male sexual partners.

Candida albicans   The organism that causes the candida (or yeast) infection.

Pubic lice   Parasites that infest the hair of the pubic region.

Scabies   A contagious skin disease caused by a type of mite.

Do Your Attitudes and Behaviors Put You at Risk for STDs?

All sexually transmissible diseases are preventable. You have control over the behaviors and attitudes that place you at risk for contracting STDs and for increasing their negative effects on your health. To identify your risk factors for STDs, read the following list of statements and identify whether they're true or false for you.

T or F

_____ 1. I have never been sexually active. (If false, continue. If true, you are not at risk; respond to the remaining statements based on how you realistically believe you would act.)

_____ 2. I am in a mutually faithful relationship with an uninfected partner or am not currently sexually active. (If false, continue. If true, you are at minimal risk now; respond to the remaining statements according to your attitudes and past behaviors.)

_____ 3. I have only one sexual partner.

_____ 4. I always use a latex condom for each act of intercourse.

_____ 5. I use a lubricant containing the spermicide nonoxynol-9.

_____ 6. I discuss STDs and prevention with new partners before having sex.

_____ 7. I do not use alcohol or another mood-altering drug in sexual situations.

_____ 8. I would tell my partner if I thought I had been exposed to an STD.

_____ 9. I am familiar with the signs and symptoms of STDs.

_____ 10. I regularly perform genital self-examination.

_____ 11. When I notice any sign or symptom of any STD, I consult my physician immediately.

_____ 12. When diagnosed with an STD, I inform all recent partners.

_____ 13. When I have a sign or symptom of an STD that goes away on its own, I still consult my physician.

_____ 14. I do not use drugs prescribed for friends or sexual partners or left over from other illnesses to treat STDs.

_____ 15. I do not share syringes or needles to inject drugs.

False answers indicate attitudes and behaviors that may put you at risk for contracting STDs or for suffering serious medical consequences from them.

---

populations. Recent surveys indicate that condom use is increasing, and the number of new cases of HIV infection among the gay population has been smaller in recent years than was originally feared. On the other hand, surveys also reveal that there are often lapses in safer sex practices, times when individuals revert to unprotected sex. Such lapses are dangerous because they can mean exposure to a serious or fatal disease. Also discouraging is the fact that the number of cases of HIV infection among harder-to-reach groups, such as intravenous drug abusers and their sexual partners and children, is still increasing.

Education efforts targeted at increasing public awareness about AIDS through the media have included public service announcements, dramatic presentations, and support from well-known public figures. However, the continuing controversy over the proper timing and nature of sex education still hinders active discussion of sexuality in schools, in churches, and on television. From a public health perspective, it has become a public health risk not to talk about sexuality, including the risks of STDs and the use of condoms.

In addition to public awareness campaigns, there are other opportunities for education about STDs in our society. Colleges offer courses in human sexuality. Free pamphlets and other literature are available from public health departments, health clinics, physicians' offices, student health centers, and Planned Parenthood; and easy-to-understand books are available in libraries and bookstores. Several national hot lines have been set up to provide free, confidential information and referral services to callers anywhere in the country.

- *National STD hot line,* sponsored by the Centers for Disease Control and the American School Health Association, provides confidential information and referrals about sexually transmissible diseases. Call 1-800-227-8922, between 8 A.M. and 11 P.M. (Eastern time), Monday through Friday.

- *National AIDS hot line,* sponsored by the Centers for Disease Control, provides confidential information about HIV infection and referrals for testing and treatment. Call 1-800-342-AIDS or 1-800-344-SIDA (Spanish).

Information about STDs is widely disseminated, but learning about STDs is still up to the individual. You must assume responsibility for learning about the causes and

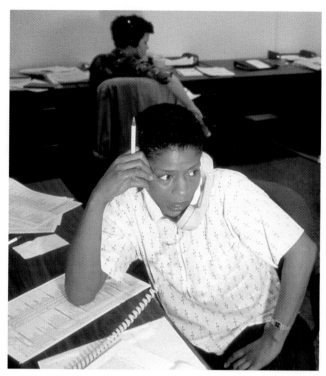

Accurate, confidential answers to personal questions are available from local and national STD hot lines. Separate AIDS hot lines, such as the one shown here, provide referrals, information, and updates on the success of the latest AIDS treatments.

nature of STDs and their potential effects on you, the children you may have, and others with whom you have relationships. Once you know about STDs—their symptoms, how they're transmitted, how they can be prevented—you are in a position to educate others. Providing information to your friends and partners, whether in casual conversation on in more serious decision-making discussions, is an important way that you can make a difference in your own and others' health.

Diagnosis and Treatment

Early diagnosis and treatment of STDs can help you and your sexual partner(s) avoid unnecessary complications and help prevent the spread of STDs. If you are sexually active, be alert for any sign or symptom of disease, such as a rash, a discharge, sores, or unusual pain (see the box "Genital Self-Examination Guide"), and don't hesitate to have a professional examination if you notice such a symptom. Be alert for these signs or symptoms in your sexual partner too, and don't hesitate to question him or her if you notice something unusual.

Testing for STDs is done through private physicians, public health clinics, community health agencies, and some student health services. If you are diagnosed as having an STD, you should begin treatment as quickly as possible. Inform your partner(s) to prevent further spread of the infection and to protect him or her from the com-

plications that can occur when treatment is delayed. Avoid any sexual activity until your treatment is complete and testing indicates that you are cured. If your sexual partner tells you that he or she has contracted an STD, you need to be tested immediately, even if you don't have any symptoms. Sometimes uninfected partners are treated to ensure that an STD won't spread or recur.

Telling a sexual partner that you have exposed him or her to an STD isn't easy. You may be afraid your partner will be angry or resentful, or you may worry that your partner will think less of you or reject you. At the same time, you may be feeling afraid, ashamed, embarrassed, or angry yourself. Feelings like these can block communication and lead to lies ("I caught it from a toilet seat"), half-truths ("No one knows how I got it, but you have to be treated too"), or rationalizations ("He'll find out sooner or later if he's got it, even if I don't tell him").

Despite the awkwardness and difficulty, it's crucial that your partners be informed about a disease they may have been exposed to and urged to seek testing and/or treatment as quickly as possible. Because it is awkward and difficult, you can get help telling your partner if you should need it. Public health departments will notify sexual partners of their possible exposure while maintaining your confidentiality and anonymity. Peer counseling and student health programs often assist students with practice in role-playing in these circumstances, and concerned health care personnel can also provide assistance.

As stressed throughout this chapter, undetected and untreated STDs can lead to serious medical complications and even death. In asymptomatic cases, the only way infected people can find out they have a disease is by being told they need to be tested. Uninformed sexual partners can go on to spread the disease to others, contributing to anguish for others as well as spiraling public health problems. The responsibility of informing partners is an ethical task too important to shirk.

With the exception of AIDS treatment, available treatments are safe, effective, and generally inexpensive. If you are being treated, follow instructions carefully and complete all the medication as prescribed. Don't stop taking the medication just because you feel better or your symptoms have disappeared. Above all, don't give any of your medication to your partner or to anyone else. Doing so will only make your treatment incomplete and reinfection more likely. Being cured of an STD doesn't mean that you will not get it again; exposure to STDs doesn't convey lasting immunity, nor does it prevent you from getting any other STD. This is all the more reason to be informed, to inform your partners, and to practice safer sex.

Personal Insight   How do you feel about seeking examination or treatment for an STD? Do you feel differently than you would about other symptoms?

Although only a physician can make a proper diagnosis of an STD, you can examine yourself to determine if you have any of the signs or symptoms that might indicate an infection. The instructions that follow are excerpted from the genital self-examination (GSE) guide developed by Burroughs Wellcome Company. To receive a copy of the guide in English or Spanish, call 1-800-234-1124.

General Instructions

If you're sexually active, see your physician and get an examination on a regular basis. Between checkups, use GSE periodically to check yourself for early warning signs. Throughout the exam, look for bumps, sores, blisters, or warts on the skin. Bumps or blisters may be red or light-colored; they may look like pimples or they may develop into open sores. Genital warts may appear as very small bumpy spots or they may have a fleshy, cauliflowerlike appearance. You should see your physician if you see anything that resembles a sore, blister, bump, or wart; if you feel any bumpy growth; or if you have any of the other symptoms described below. In addition, if you've had contact with someone who you think might have an STD, see your physician even if you don't have any symptoms.

GSE for Women

Undress and assume a comfortable position. You may want to use a mirror—position it so you can see your entire genital area. You may find it difficult to see the area from your urinary opening down—do the best you can without making yourself uncomfortable.

Start by spreading your pubic hair apart and examining the area covered by pubic hair (the mons and the outer lips). Look for any bumps, sores, blisters, or warts. Next, spread your outer vaginal lips apart and take a close look at the hood of your clitoris. Then gently pull the hood up to examine your clitoris.

Next look at both sides of your inner lips for the same signs. Then move on to examine the area around your urinary and vaginal openings. This is as far up as we recom-

mend that you look. Signs of STDs may appear out of view (up in your vagina or on your cervix), so it's important to see your physician if you think you've been exposed to an STD, even if you don't discover any signs or symptoms during GSE.

In addition to examining your entire genital area, be alert to other symptoms that can be associated with STDs: abnormal vaginal discharge (possibly thicker than usual, yellow, or with an unpleasant odor), a painful or burning sensation when urinating, pain in your pelvic area, bleeding between menstrual periods, or an itchy rash around the vagina.

GSE for Men

Once undressed, hold your penis in your hand. Start by examining the head of the penis from the urinary opening down to where it extends out a little just above the shaft. If you are not circumcised, pull down the foreskin to examine the head. Look over the entire head of the penis in a clockwise direction, checking carefully for any bumps, sores, blisters, or warts on the skin.

Next move down the shaft and look for the same signs. Then go on to the base. At the base, try to separate your pubic hair with your fingers so you can get a good look at the skin underneath. After careful examination here, move on to the underside of the penis. You may want to use a mirror to be sure that you've seen the entire underside. A mirror can also be helpful as you examine the scrotum. Handling each testicle gently, examine the scrotum for bumps, blisters, sores, and warts. Also be aware of any lump, swelling, or soreness in the testicle.

In addition to examining your entire genital area, be alert to other symptoms that can be associated with STDs. STDs may cause burning or pain when you urinate. Some STDs cause a drip or discharge from the penis. The discharge may be thick and yellow, or it could be watery or very slight.

Adapted from: *Genital Self-Examination Guide.* Research Triangle Park. N.C.: Burroughs Wellcome Co.

Prevention

STDs *are* preventable. As discussed earlier, the only sure way to avoid exposure to STDs is to abstain from sexual activity. Should you decide not to abstain, the key is to think about prevention *before* you have a sexual encounter or find yourself in the "heat of the moment." Find out what your partner thinks before you become sexually involved. Remember, you can become infected with an STD from just one unprotected encounter.

Most people don't want to think, talk, or ask questions about STDs for a variety of reasons. They may think it de-

tracts from the appeal and excitement of the moment, that it takes away from the spontaneity of the experience, or that it will be perceived as a personal insult. For others, simply not knowing how to talk about STDs and safer sex may prevent them from bringing up the issue with a partner. (For some advice on communicating with potential sexual partners, see the box "Talking About Condoms and Safer Sex.")

Plan ahead for safer sex. Know what sexual behaviors are risky. Find out about your partner's sexual history and practices. Be honest and ask your partner to do the same. You may find that your partner is just as concerned as you

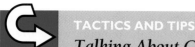

The only sure way to prevent STDs, including HIV infection, is to abstain from sexual activity. If you choose to be sexually active, you should do everything possible to protect yourself from STDs. This includes good communication with your sexual partner(s).

For most of us, talking about sex, STDs, and condoms is difficult. But it's vital for preventing the spread of STDs. Your partner may be just as concerned about STDs as you are and may bring up the subject first. However, you can't count on other people to protect you from STDs; it's up to you to make a commitment to have only protected sex and then to plan ahead for it.

The time to talk about safer sex is before you begin a sexual relationship. (However, even if you've been having unprotected sex with your partner, it is still worth it to start practicing safer sex now.) You'll feel less nervous talking about safer sex if you practice talking about it first. Decide ahead of time what you will say and how you will say it. You can rehearse in front of a mirror or with a friend until you find the words you feel most comfortable with. (You can also practice using condoms so you'll be able to use them correctly and to incorporate them into your sexual activity.)

There are many ways to bring up the subject of safer sex and condom use with your partner. Be honest about your concerns and stress that protection against STDs means that you care about yourselves. Here are a few suggestions about how to bring up the subject of condom use.

- "A lot of people are using condoms now and I think it's a good idea. How about you?"

- "I'm not going to give up sex, but the risk of AIDS has me scared. I'm going to use condoms whenever I have sex."

- "I'd like to make love with you, but I always use condoms to be safer."

- "I've been hearing a lot lately about all the diseases we can get. But if we use condoms, we can prevent them."

Your partner may say, "Yes, I want to use condoms, too." But if he or she resists the idea of using condoms, you may need to negotiate for safer sex. Stress that you both deserve to be protected and that sex will be more enjoyable when

you aren't worrying about STDs. Try some of these approaches:

If your partner says . . .	Try saying . . .
"They're not romantic."	"Worrying about AIDS isn't romantic, and with condoms we won't have to worry." OR "If we put one on together, a condom could be fun."
"You don't trust me."	"I do trust you, but how can I trust your former partners or mine?" OR "It's important to me that we're both protected."
"I don't like the way they feel."	"They might feel different, but let's try." OR "Sex won't feel good if we're worrying about diseases."
"I don't use condoms."	"I use condoms every time." OR "I don't have sex without condoms."
"But I love you."	"Being in love can't protect us from STDs." OR "I love you, too. We still need to use condoms."
"But we've been having sex without condoms."	"I want to start using condoms now so we won't be at any more risk." OR "We can still prevent infection or reinfection."

If, no matter what you say, your partner won't agree to use a condom, you owe it to yourself to say "no" to sex. There's no good reason for you to give in to a partner who doesn't care enough to use a condom. There's nothing wrong with saying "no."

Sources: Krames Communication. 1988. *Understanding Safer Sex.* (312 90th Street, Daly City, CA 94015); and San Francisco AIDS Foundation. 1988. *Condoms for Couples.* (IMPACT AIDS, 3692 18th Street, San Francisco, CA 94110).

are. By thinking and talking about STDs, you are expressing a sense of caring for yourself, your potential partner, and your future children. Taking STDs seriously is practical, courageous, and loving; it means giving yourself the respect you deserve.

Everyone can reduce the risk of infection by practicing responsible sexual behaviors. After abstinence, the next most effective approach to preventing STDs is having sex with one mutually faithful uninfected partner. If you are

sexually active, use a condom lubricated with the spermicide nonoxynol-9 during every act of intercourse to reduce your risk of contracting a disease. Although not foolproof, a properly used condom provides an effective barrier against disease-causing organisms, including HIV. A disease can be transmitted if there is contact with an infected area that isn't protected by the condom, however, such as the scrotum, the perineum, or the anal area. The use of a barrier over the cervix (diaphragm, cervical cap,

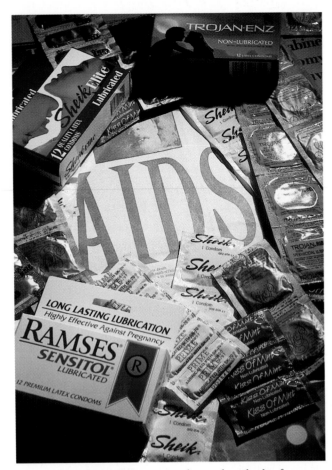

The use of condoms fell as more advanced methods of contraception, such as birth control pills and IUDs, became available. But condoms are once again gaining in popularity because of the protection they afford against STDs, especially when lubricated with the spermicide nonoxynol-9 or used in combination with spermicidal foam.

or sponge) in addition to a condom can help further lower the risk of STDs for women; as discussed in Chapter 6, these methods may provide some protection against the organisms that cause gonorrhea, genital warts, and chlamydia.

Approaches to STD prevention that are not safe include urinating or douching after intercourse, engaging in oral sex, or practicing genital play without full penetration. Birth control pills and sterilization protect you against conception and unwanted pregnancy but not against STDs. Further preventive measures include knowing the signs and symptoms of STDs, seeking treatment of any infections that do occur, and communicating openly with health care professionals and sexual partners.

The decision to have a sexual relationship carries with it certain uncertainties and risks, both physical and emotional. It also carries the responsibility of safeguarding one's own health and that of others. You and your partner need mutual respect and honesty to make good decisions together. Caring about yourself and your partner means

asking questions and being aware of signs and symptoms. It may be a bit awkward, but the temporary embarrassment of asking intimate questions is a small price to pay to avoid contracting or spreading disease. If your partner thinks less of you for being concerned, you may want to reconsider the relationship in terms of your personal values. Concern about STDs is part of a sexual relationship, not an intrusion into it, just as sexuality is part of life, not separate from it.

Personal Insight   Do you feel comfortable about having a frank discussion with a new sexual partner about your sexual histories? Under what circumstances do you feel such a discussion would be appropriate or inappropriate?

SUMMARY

The Major STDs

- The seven major STDs are serious in themselves, cause serious complications if untreated, and/or pose risks to a fetus or newborn.

- Over 250,000 Americans have been diagnosed with AIDS and over a million are believed to be infected with HIV, many without knowing it.

- HIV affects the immune system, making an otherwise healthy person susceptible to a variety of infections.

- HIV is carried in blood and blood products, semen, and vaginal and cervical secretions. HIV is transmitted through the exchange of these fluids.

- Because HIV weakens the immune system, infected people are susceptible to serious opportunistic infections.

- Diagnosis of HIV infection depends upon detecting antibodies to HIV circulating in the bloodstream. AIDS is diagnosed when an infected individual develops an AIDS indicator condition or has a CD4 cell count below 200/mm^3.

- There is currently no cure or vaccine for HIV infection. Drugs have been developed to slow the course of the disease and to prevent and treat particular infections.

- HIV infection can be prevented by making careful choices about sexual activity, not sharing drug needles, and learning as much as possible about protecting yourself from the disease.

- Hepatitis is usually caused by a viral infection of the liver transmitted through sexual and nonsexual contact. The most common form, hepatitis B, is transmitted through exchange of infected body fluids.

- Hepatitis commonly causes flulike symptoms and

jaundice. Most people recover, but some become chronic carriers of the virus. A few develop a chronic, progressive form of the disease that can lead to cirrhosis, liver failure, liver cancer, and death.

- There is no cure for hepatitis, but there is a vaccine for hepatitis B.

- Syphilis is contracted through sexual contact or through the placenta of an infected mother. If untreated, syphilis can lead to mental degeneration, paralysis, and death.

- Syphilis is diagnosed from a chancre specimen or blood tests; all three stages are treated with penicillin.

- Chlamydia is the most prevalent bacterial infection in the United States. It causes urinary tract infection and epididymitis in men; in women, it can lead to PID if untreated. Many infected people are symptom-free. Chlamydia is treated with antibiotics.

- Untreated, gonorrhea can cause PID in women and epididymitis in men, leading to sterility; infants exposed to the bacteria during birth may develop an infection that can cause blindness if untreated. Many people, especially women, have no symptoms.

- Gonorrhea can be diagnosed from a smear test and treated with appropriate antibiotics.

- Pelvic inflammatory disease, a complication of untreated gonorrhea or chlamydia, is an infection of the oviducts that may extend to the ovaries. It can lead to chronic infections and sterility.

- Genital warts, caused by the human papillomavirus, are associated with cervical cancer. An infection is contagious through contact with the dry, painless growths. Genital warts are diagnosed through examination of lesions and treated with toxic agents.

- Herpes has a high incidence in the United States, can be fatal to newborns, and is incurable. After an initial infection, the herpesvirus lies dormant in the area of the infection. Recurrences can be triggered by environmental, health, and personal factors.

- Herpes is usually diagnosed on the basis of medical history and the presence of lesions and other symptoms. The drug acyclovir offers relief to some patients.

Other STDs

- Trichomoniasis is usually contracted sexually, although the organism that causes it can live on external objects for up to 90 minutes. Trich is diagnosed through a microscopic examination of the discharge and treated with the drug metronidazole.

- *Candida albicans* causes discomfort and itching (a so-called yeast infection) if production of the organisms increases. Men rarely have symptoms. Mycostatin is usually used to treat the infection.

- Pubic lice are parasites that attach to the pubic hair and feed on human blood. They can be transmitted sexually, but also through infested bedding, towels, clothing, and surfaces. Treatment consists of over-the-counter medications.

- The scabies mite is a burrowing parasite that deposits eggs beneath the skin surface. Scabies can be contracted through any close contact. Diagnosis is made through identification of the organism; treatment consists of hot baths and applications of prescription lotions.

What Can You Do?

- Successful treatment of STDs on an individual basis means being alert to symptoms in oneself and one's partners, seeing a physician if symptoms occur, getting treatment, informing partners, and avoiding sexual activity until treatment is complete.

- Informing a partner can be awkward and difficult but is crucial to preventing the spread of STDs.

- All STDs are preventable; the key is practicing responsible sexual behaviors—which requires planning. Those who are sexually active are safest with one mutually faithful uninfected partner. Using a condom, especially one lubricated with nonoxynol-9, helps protect against STDs.

TAKE ACTION

1. Go to a drugstore and examine the over-the-counter contraceptives. Which ones contain nonoxynol-9? Which ones provide protection against STDs? If you are sexually active, make sure you use the best protection available.

2. More and more communities have treatment and support programs for people with HIV infection. Look in the yellow pages or contact local health agencies to find out what services are available where you live. If any of these agencies use volunteers, consider donating some of your time to help.

JOURNAL ENTRY

1. In your health journal, list the positive behaviors that help you avoid exposure to sexually transmissible diseases. Consider what additions you can make to this list or how you can strengthen your existing behaviors. Then list the behaviors that may block your positive behaviors or put you at risk of contracting an STD. Consider which ones you can change and how you can begin doing so.

2. *Critical Thinking:* What responsibility do you think the federal government has for funding programs for prevention and treatment of HIV infection? Do you think the government should pay for national prevention programs or increase financial aid to cities bearing the medical costs of caring for people with HIV; or should these costs be borne by individuals, families, communities, or private insurance companies? Write an essay describing what role, if any, you think the government should play; explain your reasoning.

SELECTED BIBLIOGRAPHY

American College Health Association. 1990. *HIV Infection and AIDS: What Everyone Should Know.* Baltimore, Md.: American College Health Association.

Aral, S. O., and K. K. Holmes. 1990. Epidemiology of STDs. In *Sexually Transmitted Diseases,* 2nd ed., ed. K. K. Holmes and others, 19–36. New York: McGraw-Hill.

Basen-Enquist, K. 1992. Psychosocial predictors of safer sex behaviors in young adults. *AIDS Education and Prevention* 4(2): 120–34.

Brunham, R. C., and F. A. Plummer. 1990. A general model of STD epidemiology and its implications for control. *Medical Clinics of North America* 74:1339.

Cates, W., Jr. 1990. The epidemiology and control of STDs in adolescents. *Adolescent Medicine: State of the Art Reviews* 3:409.

Centers for Disease Control. 1988. Condoms for the prevention of STDs. *Mortality and Morbidity Weekly Report* 37:133.

Corey, L. 1990. Genital herpes. In *Sexually Transmitted Diseases,* 2nd ed., ed. K. K. Holmes and others, 391–414. New York: McGraw-Hill.

Darrow, W. W., and K. Siegel. 1990. Preventive health behavior and STDs. In *Sexually Transmitted Diseases,* 2nd ed., ed. K. K. Holmes and others, 85–94. New York: McGraw-Hill.

Doucett, M., M. Perry, and B. Winterbottom. 1992. AIDS education of college students: The effect of an HIV positive lecturer. *AIDS Education and Prevention* 4(2): 160–71.

Felts, W. M., and S. M. Knight. 1992. The nature and prevention of viral hepatitis: What health educators should know. *Journal of Health Education* 23(5): 267–74.

Goldsmith, M. F. 1992. Critical moment at hand in HIV/AIDS pandemic, new global strategy to arrest its spread proposed. *Journal of the American Medical Association* 268(4): 445.

Hatcher, R. A., and others, eds. 1990. *Contraceptive Technology, 1990–1992. With Two Special Sections: AIDS and Condoms,* 15th rev. ed. New York: Irvington Press.

Holmes, K. K., P. March, P. F. Sparling, and P. J. Weisner, eds. 1990. *Sexually Transmitted Diseases,* 2nd ed. New York: McGraw-Hill.

Hook, E. W. III, and H. Handsfield. 1990. Gonorrhea infection in the adult. In *Sexually Transmitted Diseases,* 2nd ed., ed. K. K. Holmes and others, 149–60. New York: McGraw-Hill.

Lemon, S. M., and J. E. Newbold. 1990. Viral hepatitis. In *Sexually Transmitted Diseases,* 2nd ed., ed. K. K. Holmes and others, 449–66. New York: McGraw-Hill.

Minuk, G. Y. 1986. Condoms and prevention of AIDS. *Journal of the American Medical Association* 256:1443.

O'Leary, A., F. Goodhart, L. S. Jermmott, and D. Boccher-Lattimore. 1992. Predictors of safer sex on the college campus: A social-cognitive theory analysis. *Journal of American College Health,* vol. 40, May.

Oriel, D. 1990. Genital human papillomavirus infection. In *Sexually Transmitted Diseases,* 2nd ed., ed. K. K. Holmes and others, Chap. 38. New York: McGraw-Hill.

Paavonen, J., L. A. Koutsky, and N. Kiviat. 1990. Cervical neoplasia and other STD related genital and anal neoplasias. In *Sexually Transmitted Diseases,* 2nd ed., ed. K. K. Holmes and others, Chap. 48. New York: McGraw-Hill.

Russell, S. 1992. Definition of AIDS broadens tomorrow. *San Francisco Chronicle,* 31 December.

San Francisco AIDS Foundation. 1992. *AIDS Medical Guide,* 3rd ed. San Francisco: Impact AIDS.

Smith, K. V., and D. M. White. 1992. Risk level knowledge and prevention behavior for human papillomaviruses among sexually active college women. *Journal of American College Health,* vol. 40, March.

Spear, P. G. 1990. Biology of herpes viruses. In *Sexually Transmitted Diseases,* 2nd ed., ed. K. K. Holmes and others, Chap. 34. New York: McGraw-Hill.

Squires, S. 1992. Hepatitis B vaccinations. *Washington Post Health,* 5 May.

Sroka, S. R. 1989. *Educators Guide to AIDS and Other STDs.* Lakewood, Ohio: Health Education Consultants.

Teen-agers high risk behavior courts AIDS. 1992. *USA Today,* 22 July, 9A.

Voeller, B., J. M. Reinisch, and M. Gottlieb, eds. 1990. *AIDS and Sex: An Integrated Biomedical and Behavioral Approach.* New York: Oxford University Press, Kinsey Institute Series.

RECOMMENDED READINGS

Burroughs Wellcome Co. 1990. *What You Need to Know About Sexually Transmitted Diseases, HIV Disease and AIDS.* Distributed at the American Medical Association Conference on STDs: Risk Assessment, Diagnosis and Treatment. Research Triangle Park, N.C.: Burroughs Wellcome, November. *An easy-to-read survey of the STDs.*

Burroughs Wellcome Co. 1991. *Important Information for All People About HIV/AIDS: An Update.* Research Triangle Park, N.C.: Burroughs Wellcome, September. *Contains basic information, written for the general public.*

Mass, L. 1989. *Medical Answers About AIDS.* New York: Gay Men's Health Crisis. *A comprehensive, well-written, understandable book about AIDS.*

Oates, J. K. 1983. *Herpes: The Facts.* New York: Penguin Books. *A small, readable book about herpes that provides information without being intimidating.*

Sacks, S. L. 1989. *The Truth About Herpes.* West Vancouver: Gordon Soules. *A complete overview of the disease that makes a good reference for self-care information.*

Shilts, R. 1987. *And the Band Played On: Politics, People and the AIDS Epidemic.* New York: St. Martin's Press. *A highly readable account of the AIDS epidemic and the political response it has evoked, written by a concerned and committed reporter.*

18

Immunity and Infection

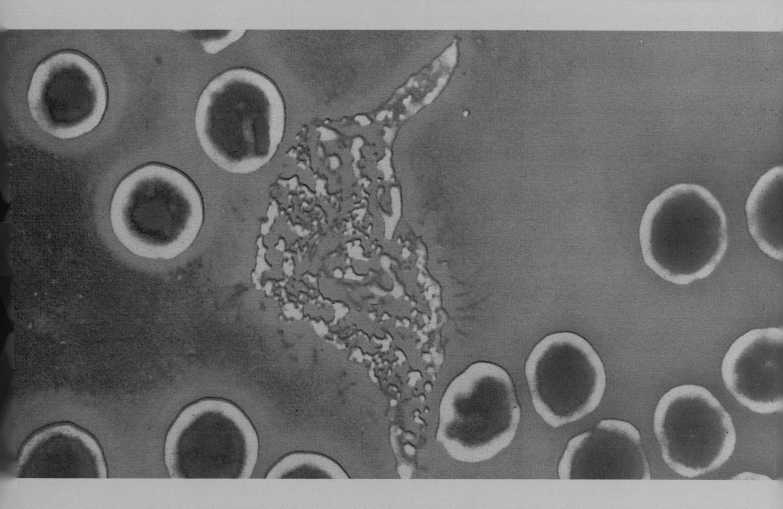

CONTENTS

You've had a cold for five days and have forgone your daily run to give your body a chance to get well. One of the people you normally run with says you're making a mistake. "Exercise is always good for you," your friend claims. "It'll help you recover more quickly." You're feeling kind of weak, and your throat is still irritated. Should you get out there and run, or should you wait until you feel better?

You've come down with a sore throat, slight fever, and runny nose, and you ache all over. You figure it's a cold or the flu, and you go to bed with a box of tissues and a good book. But your roommate thinks you ought to go to the student health center to get a prescription for an antibiotic. "Why be sick for a week when you can be well in two days?" your roommate says. You're not sure an antibiotic would help. Is your roommate giving you good advice?

You return from a hike in the woods one Saturday to discover a tick attached to your ankle. It appears to be bloated and full of blood. One of your friends says you should grab it and turn it counterclockwise to release it from your skin; another says you should burn it with a cigarette to make it drop off. A third thinks you should go to the emergency room to have it removed and to get some antibiotics in case you've been infected with a disease. You've never had a tick bite before. Are they dangerous? Do you need an antibiotic? What should you do?

You're playing Frisbee with some friends in a park when you step on something sharp. It turns out to be a nail, which has pierced the sole of your shoe and punctured your foot. It doesn't bleed when you pull it out, so you decide to continue playing. But one of your friends asks when you last had a tetanus shot, and since you're not sure, he suggests you go to the health center for a booster shot. Should you act on your friend's suggestion?

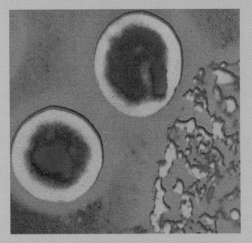

MAKING CONNECTIONS

One consequence of the AIDS epidemic has been to make many people more aware of the incredible job constantly being performed by the human immune system—and of the equally incredible devastation that occurs when the system falters. Clearly, it's better to keep your immune system working well than to try to heal it after it's damaged. In each of the scenarios presented on this page, all related to immunity and infection, individuals have to use information, make a decision, or choose a course of action. How would you act in each of these situations? What response or decision would you make? This chapter provides information about the immune system that can be used in situations like these. After finishing the chapter, read the scenarios again. Has what you've learned changed how you would respond?

Most of the time we go about our daily lives thinking of the world as a place inhabited by beings more or less like ourselves. We seldom think of the countless, unseen microscopic organisms that live around, on, and in us. Many of them would like nothing better than to consume the very tissues and organs they call home. Only constant vigilance on the part of our immune system keeps these microorganisms at bay and our bodies intact and healthy.

Even without these "invaders," our bodies have a tendency to develop problems and diseases. The natural aging process of the human body is a prime example of the second law of thermodynamics—all things, living and otherwise, have a tendency to disintegrate or fall apart. The immune system works to keep the body from being overwhelmed not just by invaders from the outside (infection) but also by changes on the inside, such as cancer.

Most people don't pay much attention to any of these internal skirmishes unless they become sick and find themselves deprived of their usual feelings of well-being. But many people today are more knowledgeable about the complexities of immunity because they've read or heard about HIV infection, which directly attacks the immune system. This chapter provides information that will help you understand immunity, infection, and how you can keep yourself well in a world of hungry microorganisms.

THE BODY'S DEFENSE SYSTEM

Our bodies have very effective ways of protecting themselves against invasion by foreign organisms, especially **pathogens,** microorganisms that cause disease. The body's first line of defense is a formidable array of physical and chemical barriers. When these barriers are breached, the body's immune system comes into play. Together, these defenses provide an effective response to nearly all the challenges and invasions our bodies will ever experience.

Physical and Chemical Barriers

The skin, the body's largest organ, prevents many microorganisms and particles from entering the body. Although many bacterial and fungal organisms live on the surface of the skin, very few can penetrate it except through a cut or break. Wherever there is an opening in the body, or an area without skin, other barriers exist. The mouth, the main entry to the gastrointestinal system, is lined with mucous membranes, which contain cells designed to prevent the passage of unwanted organisms and particles. These surfaces and the fluids that cover them (for example, tears, saliva, and vaginal secretions) are rich in antibodies (discussed in detail later in the chapter) and in **enzymes** that break down and destroy many microorganisms.

The respiratory tract is lined not only with mucous membranes but also with cells having hairlike protrusions called **cilia.** The cilia sweep foreign matter up and out of the respiratory tract. Particles that are not caught by this mechanism may be expelled from the system by a cough. If the ciliated cells are damaged or destroyed, as they are by smoking tobacco, a cough is the body's only way of ridding the airways of foreign particles. This is one reason why smokers generally have a chronic daily cough— they're compensating for damaged airways.

Routes of Infection

Despite the body's defenses, pathogens do manage to enter the body. Disease is transmitted in one of three ways: (1) by penetration of the skin (for example, through an insect bite or cut) or by direct contact (for example, when mucous membranes come into contact with a herpes or syphilis lesion), (2) by inhalation of particles, or (3) by ingestion of contaminated food or water.

Bacteria and viruses that enter the skin or mucous membranes can cause a local infection of the tissue, or they may penetrate into the bloodstream or **lymphatic system** to cause more extensive **systemic infection.** Agents that cause STDs usually enter the body through the mucous membranes lining the urethra (in the male) or the cervix (in the female).

Organisms that are transmitted via respiratory secretions (such as the tuberculosis and pertussis bacteria and the influenza virus) may cause upper respiratory infections or pneumonia, or they may enter the bloodstream and cause systemic infection. Most respiratory infections, however, are contracted through direct contact, from hand to hand and then to mouth or nose, rather than through the inhalation of airborne droplets.

Food- and water-borne organisms enter the mouth and travel to the location that will best support their reproduction. They may attack the cells of the small intestine or the colon, causing diarrhea and other symptoms, or they may enter the bloodstream via the digestive system and travel to other parts of the body. Certain bacteria, on the other hand, are present in massive quantities in the

Infection Disease caused by a pathogen.

Pathogens Organisms that cause disease.

Enzymes Chemicals necessary for energy production and protein synthesis in normal animal cells.

Cilia Microscopic hairlike structures that sweep mucus and foreign substances up out of the bronchial tubes.

Lymphatic system A system of vessels and organs that picks up excess fluid, proteins, lipids, and other substances from the tissues; filters out disease-causing organisms and other waste products; and returns the cleansed fluid to the general circulation.

Systemic infection An infection of large portions of the body.

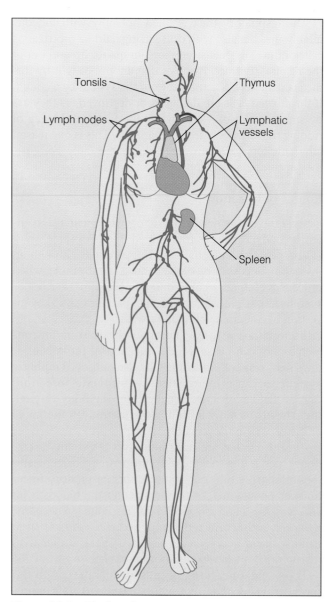

Figure 18-1 *The lymphatic system.*
The lymphatic system consists of a network of vessels and organs, including the spleen, lymph nodes, thymus, and tonsils. The vessels pick up excess fluid and proteins, lipids, and other particles from body tissues. These pass through the lymph nodes, where lymphocytes and macrophages help clear the fluid (called lymph) of debris and bacteria and other disease-causing organisms. The system then returns the cleansed fluid to the circulatory system. The lymphatic organs are production centers for infection-fighting cells and sites for some immune responses.

Toxins Poisons.

Neutrophil A type of white blood cell that engulfs foreign organisms and infected, damaged, or aged cells; they are particularly prevalent during the inflammatory response.

Macrophages Large phagocytic ("cell-eating") cells that devour foreign particles.

gut. (Did you know that a large portion of your daily stool is made of bacteria?) These "normal" bacteria are necessary for digestion and cause disease only when the integrity of the bowel is compromised, as when an appendix ruptures. Other "unfriendly" bacteria, such as those that cause food poisoning or botulism, disrupt the normal harmony by invading the cells that line the bowel or by producing **toxins** that cause damage.

Personal Insight How do you feel when you get sick? Do you feel "weak"? Guilty? Angry? Are you impatient to get back on your feet, or do you want to prolong the time you can legitimately be excused from your normal obligations? When you were sick as a child, was it unpleasant or did it have certain pleasant aspects, such as getting extra attention or staying home from school? How have your childhood experiences affected your current feelings about being sick?

The Immune System

Once the body has been invaded by a foreign organism, an elaborate system of responses is activated. The immune system operates through a remarkable information network involving billions of cellular defenders who rush to protect the body when a threat arises. We discuss here two of the body's responses: the inflammatory response and the immune response. But before we cover these specific defenses, let's turn to a brief description of the defenders themselves and the mechanisms by which they work.

The Immunological Defenders and How They Work
The immune response is carried out by different types of white blood cells, all of which are continuously being produced in the bone marrow. **Neutrophils,** one type of white blood cell, travel in the bloodstream to areas of invasion, attacking and ingesting pathogens. **Macrophages,** or "big eaters," take up stations in tissues and act as scavengers, devouring pathogens and worn-out cells. **Natural killer cells** directly destroy virus-infected cells and cells that have turned cancerous. **Lymphocytes,** of which there are several types, are white blood cells that travel in both the bloodstream and the lymphatic system. At various places in the lymphatic system there are lymph nodes (or glands), where macrophages congregate and filter bacteria and other substances from the lymph (Figure 18-1). When these nodes are actively involved in fighting an invasion of microorganisms, they fill with cells; physicians use the location of swollen lymph nodes as a clue to the location and cause of an infection.

The two kinds of lymphocytes are known as **T-cells** and **B-cells.** T-cells are further differentiated into **helper T-cells, killer T-cells,** and **suppressor T-cells.** B-cells are lymphocytes that produce **antibodies.** The first time T-cells and B-cells encounter a specific invader, some of them are reserved as **memory T- and B-cells,** enabling the body to mount a rapid response should the same invader appear again in the future. These cells and cell products—macrophages, natural killer cells, T-cells (helper T-cells, killer T-cells, and suppressor T-cells), B-cells and antibodies, and memory cells—are the principal players in the body's immune response.

The immune system is built on a remarkable feature possessed by these defenders—the ability to distinguish foreign cells from the body's own cells. Since the lymphocytes are capable of great destruction, it's essential that they not attack the body itself. When they do, they cause **autoimmune diseases,** such as lupus and rheumatoid arthritis.

How do the lymphocytes know when they've encountered an enemy? All the cells of an individual's body display markers on their surfaces—tiny molecular shapes—that identify them as "self" to lymphocytes who encounter them. Lymphocytes also recognize the markers displayed on the surfaces of invading microorganisms and know they've encountered "not self." Markers that are recognized by lymphocytes as foreign and that trigger the immune response are known as **antigens.**

Lymphocytes recognize all these markers through their own sets of complementary surface markers, which work with antigens like a lock and key (Figure 18-2). When an antigen appears in the body, a lymphocyte with a complementary pattern locks onto it, triggering a series of events designed to destroy the army of invaders. The truly astonishing thing is that the body doesn't synthesize the appropriate lymphocyte lock after it comes in contact with the antigen key. Rather, lymphocytes already exist in the body with complementary markers for millions, if not billions, of possible antigens. When any of these antigens enters the body, a matching lymphocyte appears to bind with it.

The Inflammatory Response   When the body has been injured or infected, one of the body's responses is the inflammatory response. Special cells in the area of invasion or injury release **histamine** and other substances that cause blood vessels to dilate and fluid to flow out of capillaries into the injured tissue. This produces increased heat, swelling, and redness in the affected area. White blood cells, including neutrophils and macrophages, are drawn to the area and attack the invaders, in many cases destroying them. At the site of infection there may be pus, a collection of dead white blood cells and debris resulting from the encounter.

The Immune Response   Another bodily response to invasion is the immune response (Figure 18-3). For convenience, we can think of this response as having four phases: (1) recognition of the invading pathogen, (2) am-

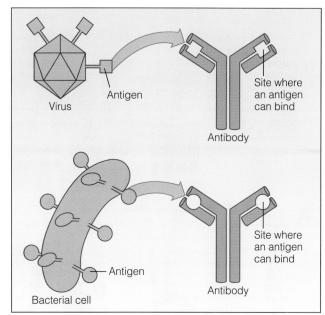

Figure 18-2   *The binding of antigen and antibody.*
The binding sites on the tips of Y-shaped antibodies are specific to a single kind of antigen. When an antibody encounters a corresponding antigen, the two bind together in a kind of lock-and-key fit.

Natural killer cell   A type of white blood cell that directly destroys virus-infected cells and cancer cells.

Lymphocytes   White blood cells continuously made in lymphoid tissue as well as in bone marrow.

T-cell   One kind of lymphocyte; arises in bone marrow, and some progeny move into thymus (giving its name).

B-cells   Lymphocytes that produce antibodies.

Helper T-cells   Lymphocytes that stimulate other lymphocytes to increase.

Killer T-cells   Lymphocytes that kill cells of the body that have been invaded by foreign organisms; also can kill cells that have turned cancerous.

Suppressor T-cells   Lymphocytes that discourage the growth of other lymphocytes.

Antibodies   Specialized proteins, produced by white blood cells, that can recognize and neutralize specific microbes.

Memory T- and B-cells   Lymphocytes that are generated during an initial infection and circulate in the body for years, "remembering" the specific antigens that caused the infection and quickly destroying them if they appear again.

Autoimmune disease   Disease in which an individual's immune system attacks the individual's own body or body parts.

Antigen   A molecule that marks an invading particle; can be recognized and neutralized by an antibody.

Histamine   A chemical responsible for the dilation and increased permeability of blood vessels in allergic reactions.

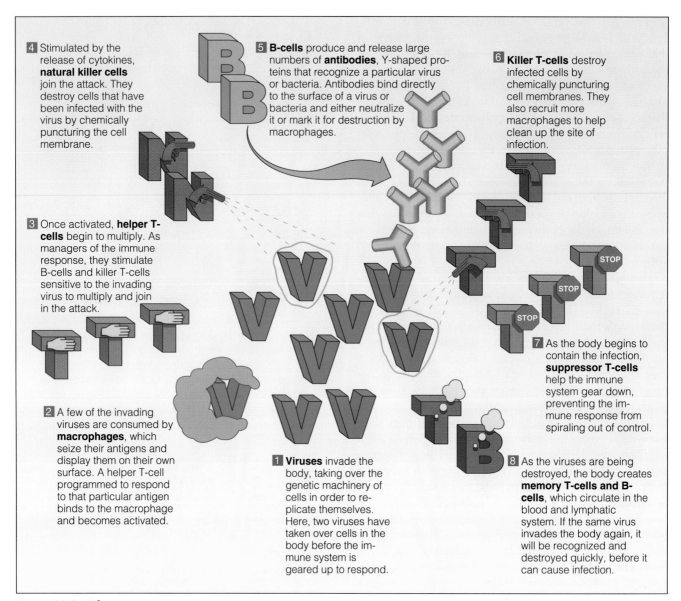

4 Stimulated by the release of cytokines, **natural killer cells** join the attack. They destroy cells that have been infected with the virus by chemically puncturing the cell membrane.

5 **B-cells** produce and release large numbers of **antibodies**, Y-shaped proteins that recognize a particular virus or bacteria. Antibodies bind directly to the surface of a virus or bacteria and either neutralize it or mark it for destruction by macrophages.

6 **Killer T-cells** destroy infected cells by chemically puncturing cell membranes. They also recruit more macrophages to help clean up the site of infection.

3 Once activated, **helper T-cells** begin to multiply. As managers of the immune response, they stimulate B-cells and killer T-cells sensitive to the invading virus to multiply and join in the attack.

2 A few of the invading viruses are consumed by **macrophages**, which seize their antigens and display them on their own surface. A helper T-cell programmed to respond to that particular antigen binds to the macrophage and becomes activated.

1 **Viruses** invade the body, taking over the genetic machinery of cells in order to replicate themselves. Here, two viruses have taken over cells in the body before the immune system is geared up to respond.

7 As the body begins to contain the infection, **suppressor T-cells** help the immune system gear down, preventing the immune response from spiraling out of control.

8 As the viruses are being destroyed, the body creates **memory T-cells and B-cells**, which circulate in the blood and lymphatic system. If the same virus invades the body again, it will be recognized and destroyed quickly, before it can cause infection.

Figure 18-3 *The immune response.*
Once invaded by a pathogen, a complex series of reactions takes place to eliminate the invader. Pictured here are the principal elements of the immune response to a virus; not shown are the many types of cytokines that help coordinate the actions of the different types of defenders.

plification of defenses, (3) attack, (4) slowdown. In each phase, crucial actions occur that are designed to destroy the invader and restore the body to health.

1. In the first phase, macrophages are drawn to the site of the injury and consume the foreign cells; they then provide information about the enemy by displaying its antigen on their surfaces. Helper T-cells, the "commanders-in-chief" of the immune response, read this information and rush to respond.

2. Now the second phase of the immune response gets under way. Multiplying rapidly, helper T-cells trigger the production of killer T-cells and B-cells in the spleen and lymph nodes. **Cytokines**, chemical

messengers secreted by lymphocytes, help regulate and coordinate the immune response. **Interleukins** and **interferons** are two examples of cytokines. They stimulate increased production of T- and B-cells and antibodies, promote the activities of natural killer cells, produce fever, and have special antipathogenic properties themselves.

3. With its forces constantly amplifying, the immune system launches its attack, the third phase of its response. Killer T-cells strike at foreign cells and cells of the body that have been invaded and infected, identifying them by the antigens displayed on the surface of the cells. (They destroy body cells that have

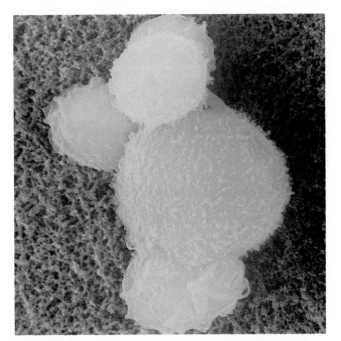

Killer T-cells can recognize the antigens of both foreign cells and mutated body cells. In this electron micrograph magnified 2,300 times, four killer T-cells are in the process of attacking a cancer cell.

mutated and become cancerous in the same way.) Puncturing the cell membrane, they sacrifice body cells in order to destroy the foreign organism within. This type of action is known as a *cell-mediated immune response,* because the attack is carried out by cells. Killer T-cells also trigger an amplified inflammatory response and recruit more macrophages to help clean up the site.

B-cells work in a different way. Stimulated to multiply by helper T-cells, they produce large quantities of antibody molecules, which are released in the bloodstream and tissues. Antibodies are Y-shaped protein molecules that bind to antigen-bearing targets and mark them for destruction by macrophages. This type of response is known as an *antibody-mediated immune response.* Antibodies work against bacteria and against viruses and other substances when they are in the body but outside cells. They don't work against infected body cells or viruses that are replicating inside cells.

4. Now that the invading microorganism has been destroyed or incapacitated, the body has to call off the attack. The last phase of the immune response is the slowdown of activity. A third type of T-cell, the suppressor T-cell, regulates the levels of lymphocytes in the body and controls their activities. When the danger is over, suppressor T-cells halt the immune response and restore homeostasis. Dead cells, killed pathogens, and other debris that result from the immune response are scavenged by certain types of white blood cells; filtered out of circulation by the liver, spleen, and kidneys; and excreted from the body. (The box "HIV: The Immune System Under Siege" explains how the body's response to pathogens is disrupted by HIV.)

Immunity In many infections, survival confers **immunity;** that is, an infected person will never get the same illness again. This is because some of the lymphocytes created during the amplification phase of the response are reserved as memory T- and B-cells. They continue to circulate in the blood and lymphatic system for years or even for the rest of the person's life. If the same antigen enters the body a subsequent time, the memory T- and B-cells recognize and destroy it before it can cause illness. This subsequent response takes only a day or two, whereas the original response lasted several days, during which time the individual suffered the symptoms of illness. The ability of memory lymphocytes to remember previous infections is known as **adaptive** or **acquired immunity.**

Symptoms and Contagion The immune system is operating at the cellular level within your body all the time, maintaining its vigilance when you're well and fighting invaders when you're sick. How does it all feel to you, the host and playing field for these activities? How do your symptoms relate to the course of the infection and the immune response?

During **incubation**—when a virus is multiplying in the body or when bacteria are actively multiplying before the immune system has gathered momentum—you may not have any symptoms of the illness, but you may be contagious. During the second and third phases of the immune response, you may still be unaware of the infection, or you may "feel a cold coming on."

Cytokines   Chemical messages released by immune system cells that help amplify and coordinate the immune response.

Interleukins   A class of cytokines that alert immune system cells to the presence of foreign organisms and stimulate them into action.

Interferons   A class of cytokines that bind to cell membranes, increasing their resistance to many viruses; they also stimulate the activities of macrophages and natural killer cells.

Immunity   Mechanisms that defend the body against infection; or the status of those mechanisms in general; or specific immunity or defenses against specific pathogens.

Adaptive or acquired immunity   The body's ability to mobilize the cellular "memory" of an attack by a pathogen to throw off subsequent attacks. This ability can be acquired through vaccination as well as the normal immune response.

Incubation   Period when a bacteria or virus is actively multiplying inside the body's cells; usually a period without symptoms of illness.

TERMS

The human immunodeficiency virus (HIV) destroys the immune system, short-circuiting its responses before they can be mobilized. Normally, viruses that have entered the blood or lymphatic system are engulfed by helper T-cells, which then trigger the immune response. But when a helper T-cell encounters and engulfs a human immunodeficiency virus, the HIV takes over part of the cell's reproductive system and uses it to produce more viruses. Eventually, the helper T-cell is destroyed, and the immune system begins to wane. In a healthy person, there are normally about twice as many helper T-cells as suppressor T-cells; in a person with HIV infection, this ratio is often reversed.

People infected with HIV become susceptible to many secondary infections that people with healthy, intact immune systems have no problem overcoming. It is these **opportunistic diseases** that cause most of the serious illnesses and deaths in people with HIV infection. Although T-cell immunity is severely affected by HIV infection, B-cell production of antibodies continues and the body remains protected against many common diseases. The infections that most often prove deadly for people with HIV seldom occur in people with healthy immune systems.

B-cells do produce antibodies against HIV, but unfortunately these antibodies do not protect against the spread of the virus. HIV antibodies are the basis for most of the tests for HIV infection (see Chapter 17). For other diseases, a blood test that reveals an antibody against a particular pathogen may indicate protective immunity—that is, the body would be protected from the organism. In the case of HIV, the presence of the antibody indicates an active case of the disease.

The only situation in which an HIV antibody could be present in the body without indicating ongoing infection is if the antibodies themselves are from another source. For example, HIV antibodies can pass through the placenta of an infected mother to her child, regardless of whether the virus itself has been transmitted. In fact, most babies born to infected mothers have HIV antibodies in their blood at birth and would test HIV-positive if given an HIV-antibody test. Additional tests that screen for the presence of the virus itself must be done to determine whether a baby with HIV antibodies is actually infected.

Many of the symptoms of an illness are actually due to the immune response of the body rather than to the actions or products of the invading organism. For example, fever is thought to be caused by the release and activation of certain cytokines in macrophages and other cells during the immune response. Cytokines travel in the bloodstream to the brain, where they cause the body's thermostat to be "reset" to a higher level. The resulting elevated temperature is thought to assist the body in its fight against pathogens by enhancing many of the immune responses.

Similarly, you get a runny nose when your lymphocytes destroy infected mucosal cells, leading to increased mucus production. You get a sore throat when your lymphocytes destroy infected throat cells. The general malaise and fatigue of the "flu" are probably caused by interferons.

You are contagious when there are active organisms replicating in your body and they can gain access to another person. This may be before a vigorous immune response has occurred, so at times you may be contagious before experiencing any symptoms. This means that you can transmit an illness to another person without knowing you're infected or catch an illness from someone who doesn't appear to be sick. On the other hand, your symptoms may continue after the invading organisms have been mostly destroyed, when you are no longer infectious.

Personal Insight How do you feel when you hear that someone has HIV infection? Herpes? Chickenpox? Bronchitis? If you feel differently about these cases, what is the basis for the difference?

Immunization

The ability of the immune system to remember previously encountered organisms and retain its strength against them is the basis for immunization. When a person is immunized against a disease, the immune system is "primed" with an antigen that's similar to the disease-causing organism but not as dangerous. The body responds by producing antibodies to the organism, which prevent serious infection when and if the person is exposed to the disease itself. These preparations used to manipulate the immune system are known as **vaccines.**

Vaccines were first used by English physician Edward Jenner late in the eighteenth century. He had noticed that people who milked cows occasionally showed an infection similar to smallpox. These victims of cowpox—a relatively mild disease—never contracted the lethal smallpox. He rubbed scrapings from infected cow udders into the skin abrasions of people who had not had smallpox to see if this procedure would protect them. It did: None of these people—the first to be vaccinated—contracted smallpox.

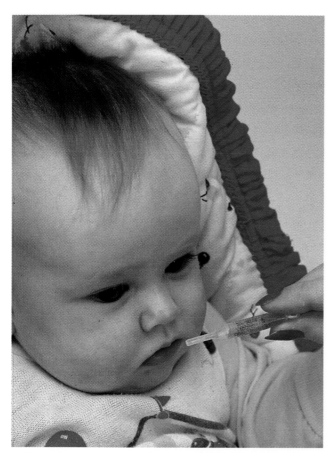

Before polio vaccines were developed by Jonas Salk and Albert Sabin in the 1950s, many people, especially children, were paralyzed or killed by this viral infection. This 1-year-old is being given oral polio vaccine as part of the standard series of childhood immunizations.

Smallpox and cowpox are caused by closely related viruses. Cowpox virus doesn't cause severe illness, but it does stimulate the lymphocytes to produce antibodies against smallpox. Without knowing the specifics of how the immune system works, Jenner had grasped the essence of the body's immune response. In the middle of the nineteenth century, French chemist Louis Pasteur developed similar procedures against other diseases, such as rabies.

Today, vaccines are made in several ways. In some cases, organisms are cultured in the laboratory in a way that weakens (attenuates) them. These "live, attenuated" organisms are used in vaccines against such diseases as measles, mumps, and rubella (German measles). In other cases, when it's not possible to breed attenuated organisms, vaccines are made from pathogens that have been killed in the laboratory but that still retain their ability to stimulate the production of antibodies. Vaccines composed of "killed" viruses are used against influenza viruses, among others. A third type of vaccine has been developed to protect against tetanus. This disease is caused by a bacterium that thrives in deep puncture wounds and produces a deadly toxin. The vaccine is made from a "toxoid" that resembles the toxin—that is, lymphocytes recognize it as being the same—but that doesn't produce the same effects. Tetanus shots are normally needed every ten years, but in the case of a deep wound, a tetanus shot may be needed if five years have elapsed since the last shot. Immunizations available in the United States are listed in Table 18-1.

Vaccines confer what is known as *active immunity*—that is, the vaccinated person produces his or her own antibodies to the microorganism. Another type of injection confers *passive immunity*. In this case, a person exposed to a disease is injected with the antibodies themselves, produced by other human beings or animals who have recovered from the disease. Injections of **gamma globulin**—a product made from the blood plasma of many individuals, containing all the antibodies they have ever made—are sometimes given to people exposed to a disease against which they haven't been immunized. Such injections create a rapid but temporary immunity and are useful against certain viruses, such as hepatitis A. Gamma globulin is also sometimes used to treat antibody deficiency syndromes.

Allergy—The Body's Defense System Gone Haywire

You probably know someone with **allergies,** or perhaps you have an allergy yourself. Allergic reactions are a response of the immune system, but in this case the response is inappropriate, annoying, and sometimes even life-threatening. Allergic reactions occur when the body recognizes a relatively harmless substance, such as dust, pollen, or animal hair, as a dangerous antigen and mounts an immune response to it. B-cells multiply, antibodies are produced, and quantities of histamine and other substances are released from cells near the location of the invasion. The resulting inflammatory response produces such symptoms as runny nose, red, itchy eyes, sneezing, congestion, hives, and asthma. The full course of the allergic reaction, as well as the latest research into this still-

Opportunistic disease Illnesses caused when organisms take the opportunity presented by a primary (initial) infection to multiply and cause a secondary (additional) infection. For example, *Candida albicans* frequently infects people weakened by HIV infection.

Vaccines A preparation of killed or weakened pathogens injected or taken orally, thereby arousing the body's natural adaptive immune system to produce specific antibodies.

Gamma globulin Serum containing specific antibodies, injected to provide temporary immunity to specific antigens.

Allergies Diseases caused by the body's own exaggerated response to foreign chemicals and proteins.

TERMS

TABLE 18-1 Immunizations Available in the United States

Type of Immunization	Who Should Be Immunized	Effectiveness of Immunization and Frequency of Booster Doses
Diphtheria	All children	Highly effective; renew every 10 years
Gamma globulin	Travelers to nonindustrialized countries	Effective for 6 months
German measles (rubella)	All children	Highly effective; need for boosters not established
Hemophilus influenza	All children	Very effective against meningitis
Hepatitis B	All health care workers; sexual partners and newborns of hepatitis B carriers (recommendation may be extended to all children in the future)	Very effective; may need booster if exposed
Influenza	Adults over age 65; anyone with chronic disease of the heart, respiratory tract, or endocrine system	Renew every year (because viral strains change easily)
Measles	All children. Adults born after 1956 should get a booster.	Highly effective; some states now require booster for school entry
Mumps	All children	Believed to confer lifetime immunity
Pneumococcus	Adults over age 65; anyone with chronic heart or lung disease or who doesn't have a spleen	About 70 percent effective
Polio	All children; all adults, particularly travelers, those exposed to children, and those in health and sanitation industries	Long-lasting immunity; no booster necessary unless exposure anticipated
Rabies	Only those bitten by rabid animal	A vaccination each day for 14 to 21 days beginning soon after the bite
Tetanus (lockjaw)	Everyone	Very effective, renew every 10 years or when treated for a contaminated wound if more than 5 years have elapsed since last booster
Typhoid fever	Travelers to endemic areas	About 80 percent effective
Whooping cough (pertussis)	Essential for children by age 3 to 4 months	Highly effective
Yellow fever	Travelers to endemic areas	Highly effective; provides immunity for at least 17 years

mysterious overreaction of the immune system, is described in the box "Sneezing and Wheezing: Allergies and Asthma."

THE TROUBLEMAKERS— PATHOGENS AND DISEASE

Now that we've discussed the beautiful and intricate system that protects us from disease, let's consider some

pathogens, those disease-producing organisms that live within us and around us. When they succeed in gaining entry to body tissue, they can cause illness and sometimes death to the unfortunate host. They include bacteria, viruses, fungi, protozoa, and parasitic worms.

Bacteria

Among the microorganisms that exist everywhere in our environment are one-celled organisms called **bacteria.**

Sneezing and Wheezing: Allergies and Asthma

If you have ever experienced the itchy eyes, runny nose, and sneezing of hay fever or the swelling and itching of hives, you know how uncomfortable an allergy can make you. And though you might blame pollen, dust, or cat hair, the problem is not so much the allergy trigger, or allergen, as your body's reaction to it.

Allergies arise when the immune system—so efficient at identifying and destroying viruses and bacteria—gets all worked up over a harmless invader such as a particle of pollen. This oversensitivity involves an excess of one or more antibodies belonging to the broad class known as immunoglobin E, or IgE. IgE antibodies tend to take up residence on the surface of *mast cells*, which congregate in the soft tissue surrounding blood vessels in the lungs, sinuses, skin, and other areas. Mast cells contain reservoirs of the chemical *histamine*, which they are ready to release on the proper signal. If a person's mast cells are well stocked with IgE antibodies against a particular allergen, and that allergen comes along and binds to them, the histamine floodgates open and the trouble begins.

Histamine's main effect is to render nearby blood vessels more porous, allowing fluid and cells from the blood to flood the local tissue. Histamine also stimulates mucus production and, primarily in the lungs, can cause smooth muscle to contract. The precise symptoms that result depend on what part of the body is affected. In the nose, histamine causes flushing, congestion, and sneezing; in the eyes, it can produce itching, tearing, and inflammation; in the skin it can cause redness, swelling, and itching; and in the lungs it can cause the muscles surrounding air passages to contract, making breathing difficult. The most serious kind of allergic reaction—fortunately very rare—involves a release of histamine throughout the body, causing a life-threatening loss of blood pressure known as anaphylactic shock.

Many triggers can provoke an allergic reaction in a sensitive individual, including animal dander, dust mites (microscopic insects found in the home), pollen, molds, insect stings, and certain foods. The most effective treatment for an allergy is total avoidance of the allergen, but very often this is impossible. Medications include antihistamines, decongestants, and anti-allergy nasal sprays. Many over-the-counter medications cause drowsiness, but newer, nonsedating antihistamines, as well as synthetic steroid sprays, are available by prescription.

Asthma is a condition that may or may not be associated with allergies. The symptoms of asthma—shortness of breath, wheezing, coughing, and a feeling of tightness in the chest—are all related to the obstruction of air flow in the lungs. Asthma is caused by both a spasm of the muscles surrounding the airways and by inflammation of the airways. The spasm causes constriction, and the inflammation causes the airway linings to swell and to secrete extra mucus, which further obstructs the passages.

An asthma attack begins when something sets off a spasm in the bronchial tubes. Usually it's an allergic reaction to an inhaled trigger, most commonly dust mites, mold, animal dander, or pollen. Anything that irritates or overtaxes the bronchial airways can also trigger spasms: exercise, cold air, environmental pollutants, smoking or secondhand smoke, infection, emotional stress, or even a hearty laugh. These instigators also cause inflammation of the airways. The bronchial tubes swell and become plugged with mucus. The inflammation can become chronic, making the airways even more sensitive to the triggers. Inhaling a muscle-relaxing medication from a bronchodilator can relieve an asthma attack immediately by opening the bronchial tubes. Newer medications—inhaled anti-inflammatory drugs—are designed to treat the underlying inflammation. Both treatments may be needed to get asthma under control.

The incidence of asthma is increasing throughout the world, for reasons not completely understood. Over the last ten years, the number of Americans with asthma increased by one-third, and deaths from asthma nearly doubled. Particularly affected are African Americans living in inner cities, people over 65, and children. Several theories have been proposed for this increased incidence, including poorer indoor ventilation, higher levels of outdoor air pollution, smoking among mothers, and better diagnosis of asthma cases. A combination of factors may well be responsible.

As with allergies, the best way to treat asthma is to avoid the triggers when possible and to manage the condition with medications. Asthma was once a debilitating illness, but it no longer has to be. In fact, 70 athletes in the 1984 Olympics suffered from exercise-induced asthma, and 40 of them won medals. With early recognition of symptoms and proper medical care, asthma can be kept under control.

Sources: Allergy and asthma 1992. 1992. *Healthline;* Treating the real cause of asthma attacks. 1992. *Consumer Reports on Health,* October; White, M. W., and R. Bonheim. 1987. Allergy research: Stalking the sneezemakers. *Rx Being Well,* March-April.

Essential for life as we know it, bacteria break down dead organic matter, allowing it to be restructured for use by other organisms so that life can go on. They also perform a similar task in our intestines, helping digest food for better absorption by the body. If we view the entire digestive tract as a long hollow tube beginning in the mouth and moving down the esophagus, stomach, small and large intestine to the anus, we see that even though bacteria reside inside the intestine, they are not really a part of the body. Underneath the skin, within the bloodstream, tissues and organs, the body is devoid of bacteria, or "sterile." Bacteria found in these areas are almost always pathogenic, or disease-producing. It is here that the immune system keeps up its constant surveillance, seeking out and destroying any invaders.

Bacteria can cause infection almost anywhere in or on the body. They can cause meningitis, an infection of the spinal fluid and tissue surrounding the brain; conjunctivitis, infection of the layer of cells surrounding the eyes; pharyngitis or "sore throat"; bronchitis, infection of the airways (bronchi); pneumonia, infection of the lung itself; gastroenteritis or enterocolitis, infections of the gastrointestinal tract; cellulitis, infection of the soft tissues; osteomyelitis, infection of the bones; and so on, for each tissue and organ.

Because of their tiny size, bacteria cannot be seen with the naked eye. It was only in the seventeenth century that Anton van Leeuwenhoek used the microscope to show what had been suspected since biblical times; namely, that many diseases are transmitted by "invisible creatures." Van Leeuwenhoek also described the major forms of bacteria, which he called "animalcules." Today we know them as bacilli (rods), cocci (spheres), and spirochetes (spirals).

In the 1880s, a Danish microbiologist, Christian Gram, devised a special stain to help identify some of these organisms. Today, this same stain is still used to visualize and classify bacteria and thus to help diagnose disease. Organisms that stain dark blue are called "gram-positive"; those that stain red are "gram-negative."

Gram-positive Bacteria

In the laboratory, specimens from diseased patients are cultured; that is, they are placed on special media to aid the growth of bacteria. It is the job of the microbiologist to discover which particular bacterium is responsible for the underlying illness. This detective work frequently starts with the gram stain. For example, the bacterium that often inflames the tonsils and throat is the **streptococcus,** a gram-positive (stains blue) coccus (sphere) that often grows in chains. This same organism often causes skin infections such as impetigo and erysipelas; other species of streptococci are implicated in pneumonia and endocarditis (infection of the heart valve).

Another gram-positive coccus is **staphylococcus,** which appears in small clusters under the microscope. Its name means "cluster of grapes." These bacteria reside on the skin even in healthy individuals, but can cause many diseases, including boils and other skin infections. A species of these bacteria, *Staphylococcus aureus,* is responsible for toxic shock syndrome. The bacteria produce a deadly toxin that causes shock (potentially life-threatening low blood pressure), high fever, a peeling skin rash, and inflammation of several organ systems. The disease was first diagnosed in women using highly absorbent tampons, which appear to deplete the vaginal environment of magnesium, allowing the growth of staphylococci. It has more recently been found in women not using tampons and in men as well.

Gram-negative Bacteria

Gram-negative organisms (those that stain red) are more commonly bacilli (rod-shaped). Many types of gram-negative rods inhabit the intestines of all of us but generally are not present in the mouths or on the skin of healthy people. These organisms most often cause disease when there is a breakdown in the normal immune system or when the gut integrity is breached. The vagina normally contains gram-negative bacteria, but if these bacteria travel up the urethra to the bladder, they can cause urinary tract infections.

Though they stain poorly, *Legionella* species are usually classified as gram-negative bacilli. These organisms were discovered in 1976 during the investigation of an outbreak of severe pneumonia at an American Legion convention in Philadelphia. *Legionella* flourish in the moist environment of air conditioning systems and have been responsible for outbreaks of disease in hospitals and other large buildings.

Spirochete Infections

Spirochetes, the spiral-shaped organisms, are very difficult to grow in culture. As a result, researchers have had difficulties in understanding their life cycle as well as in diagnosing infections caused by these pathogens. Syphilis is caused by the spirochete *Treponema pallidum* (see Chapter 17). A different spirochete, *Borrelia burgdorferi,* causes the illness known as Lyme disease. Here, the spirochete is transmitted by the deer tick *Ixodes,* which makes its home on deer and mice, except in California, where the culprit is the closely related black-legged tick, which also lives on wood rats. Ticks acquire the spirochete by feasting on the blood of an infected animal and then may transmit it to their next meal. Lyme disease has been reported in 46 states and is most common in New York, Connecticut, Pennsylvania, and other Atlantic states; in some areas in the East, up to 75 percent of deer ticks carry the spirochete.

Symptoms of Lyme disease vary from person to person, but like syphilis the disease manifests in three stages. In the first stage an expanding red rash develops from the area of the tick bite, usually about two weeks after the bite occurs. (A rash that occurs within three days is probably just a reaction to the bite itself.) Some people develop flu-like symptoms as well. The second stage occurs weeks to months later in about 10 to 20 percent of untreated patients. Symptoms involve the nervous or cardiovascular systems and can include impaired motor coordination, partial facial paralysis, and heart rhythm abnormalities. These symptoms usually disappear within a few weeks. The third stage, which occurs in about half of untreated people, can occur years after the tick bite and usually consists of chronic or recurring arthritis (an inflammation of the joints), almost always affecting the knees. Lyme disease can also cause fetal damage or death at any stage of pregnancy. See the box "Protecting Yourself from Lyme

If you live in an area where Lyme disease is prevalent and spend time in the woods or even in your yard—especially between May and September—take these steps:

- Cover your body as much as possible; wear long pants (tucked into your shoes or socks), a long-sleeved shirt, and closed shoes. It's easier to spot ticks on light-colored clothes. Wear a hat to protect your scalp.

- Check yourself occasionally for ticks, especially if you're in the underbrush or forest. When you get home, do a thorough check of your entire body, clothes, and gear. Deer ticks and black-legged ticks are smaller than dog ticks (see below); when engorged with blood these eight-legged ticks look like blood blisters. The immature ticks, called nymphs, are even smaller (about the size of a pinhead) and are responsible for up to 90 percent of all cases of Lyme disease. A nymph will feed on you for two to three days, an adult tick for up to a week. *The sooner you remove it, the better your chance of avoiding infection. Recent studies reveal that if the tick is on you for less than 24 hours, it is improbable that you'll develop the disease.*

Deer tick (actual size)

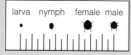

- Inspect children daily, especially during the summer, when they spend lots of time outdoors.

- Check pets after they've been outdoors. They can carry ticks to your home or property or develop the disease themselves.

- Use an insect repellent containing DEET (short for N, N-diethyltoluamide) or a clothing spray containing the insecticide permethrin. DEET has caused allergic reactions in some children (and should be used with caution.)

- Remove a tick with thin-lipped tweezers—always carry a pair with you when outdoors. (It is almost impossible to remove a small tick with your fingers.) Exert a slow, steady pull. Don't twist the tick. This may break off the mouthparts and lead to a secondary infection.

- Put the tick in a small jar containing alcohol (carry one with you if you're out hiking) so you can take it to your doctor or health department for identification.

- If you have been in an area where Lyme disease is a problem and you notice any symptoms—a rash or a flulike illness within the next two to three weeks—call your physician (see the text for a full description of symptoms). Lyme disease is treatable and almost always curable with antibiotics, especially in its early stages.

If you take these precautions and know what to watch for, you can still enjoy the outdoors without taking a chance of getting Lyme disease.

Source: "Lyme Disease Update," *University of California at Berkeley Wellness Letter, August 1992;* "Nervous About Ticks?" *Consumer Reports on Health, July 1993.*

Disease" for some guidelines on avoiding this disease.

As mentioned earlier, spirochetes are difficult to grow in culture; therefore, diagnosis in these diseases usually depends on the measurement of specific antibodies to the organisms in the patient's blood. This can be confusing, because once we develop antibodies we often retain them for life, regardless of whether the organism is causing disease.

Other Bacteria and Bacterialike Organisms
A multitude of organisms aren't easily categorized by gram stain. **Tuberculosis** (TB) is caused by a bacterium that requires a special stain called "acid fast." The infection is transmitted via the respiratory route and almost always manifests as a pneumonia, an infection of the lungs. Early in this century TB was a major killer, but it is now treatable. Unfortunately, today we are seeing a resurgence, rather than a disappearance, of this disease (see the box "Tuberculosis—A Killer Returns").

Mycoplasma is an organism like other bacteria, but with an incomplete cell wall. It will not grow on the usual laboratory culture media, so special techniques are required to culture it. It is the most common cause of pneumonia in young adults and may also cause ear infections

Bacteria Organisms about 100–1,000 times larger than viruses, about 100 species of which can cause disease in humans.

Streptococci Bacteria that cause infections such as strep throat, which can lead to serious cardiac damage.

Staphylococci Bacteria, found on the skin, that can cause infection if allowed to multiply in food and then ingested.

Tuberculosis A bacterial disease almost always infecting the lungs.

Mycoplasma One of the smallest bacteria; has an incomplete cell wall.

TERMS

A scourge once considered under control in the United States is again posing a major health threat, particularly for people infected with HIV, recent immigrants, and those who live in inner cities. Tuberculosis, or TB, is a contagious disease with symptoms that include coughing, fatigue, night sweats, weight loss, and fever. TB is caused by rod-shaped bacteria known as tubercle bacilli. Although TB can attack other organs, the bacteria usually attack patches of tissue in the lungs, killing cells and making breathing difficult. Sometimes the attack extends to adjacent blood vessels, and patients cough up blood. Eventually the lungs become too riddled with infection to function, and the patient dies by suffocation.

TB is spread through prolonged contact with someone who has the disease in its active form. Coughing spreads droplets carrying the bacteria, and when these are inhaled, the bacteria multiply in the lungs.

About 10 million Americans are infected with TB, but only about 10 percent of them will actually come down with the disease. In the rest, although their skin tests for TB antibodies register positive, the immune system keeps the disease under control. Nevertheless, 3 million people worldwide die of the disease each year. Before the turn of the century, TB was the leading cause of death in the United States, and between 1900 and 1950, 5 million Americans died of the disease. At that point, though, with improved sanitation and treatment facilities and the advent of antibiotics, the number of cases in the United States fell steadily for 30 years.

But now TB is back. Since 1989, the United States has been experiencing a wave of tuberculosis that threatens to return pockets of American society to a time when antibiotics were unknown. The resurgence has been swift and forceful within the inner cities, where conditions encourage the proliferation of the disease. Urban crowding, homelessness, poor nutrition, drug abuse, and the rapid disappearance of preventive-medicine clinics and other health care services are all factors that increase susceptibility.

Additionally, a strong relationship exists between tuberculosis and HIV infection. HIV impairs the immune system, allowing TB to become active and to spread throughout the body. In some cities, nearly half the TB patients are infected with HIV.

Tuberculosis responds to antibiotics, but only over a long course lasting at least six months. Under the stressful conditions of poverty, however, many people—the homeless, for instance—go untreated. Others fail to complete their treatment, taking antibiotics only until the symptoms of the disease go away. Not only does such an interruption result in relapses, but it also encourages the development of strains of bacteria resistant to antibiotics. The spread of TB cases that are completely resistant to treatment is the most alarming aspect of this public health crisis.

Many physicians are urging the government to restore funding for the old TB-control programs and even to revive the notion of TB sanatoriums so that infectious patients can be quarantined and their treatment monitored. Cuts in such programs may have laid the groundwork for the recent outbreaks. "We've not been too wise over the years," concedes Dr. Dixie Snider of the Centers for Disease Control and Prevention.

Snider points out that almost everything about the science of TB is too old or too slow. Simply diagnosing the drug-resistant strains can take three months or more; and treatment efforts, which succeed only half the time, last an average of three years. It may therefore require a fresh infusion of research funds as well as public health measures to catch up with an old killer that has learned some dangerous new tricks.

and sore throats. **Rickettsiae** are the agents of Rocky Mountain spotted fever and typhus and are transmitted by ticks, fleas, and lice.

The body's immune system can fight off many, if not most, bacterial infections. However, while the body musters its defenses, some bacteria can cause a great deal of damage: Inflammation, caused by the gathering of white blood cells, may lead to scarring and permanent damage of tissues. In helping the body deal with these infections, science and medicine have made what is possibly their greatest contribution to humankind: antibiotics.

Antibiotics   Antibiotics are both naturally occurring and synthetic substances having the ability to kill bacteria. Most of the natural antibiotics are produced by molds. **Penicillin,** for example, was discovered by Alexander Fleming in 1929 when he noticed that bacteria growing on a culture were inhibited by a mold left in the laboratory overnight. Since that time thousands of naturally occurring substances have been screened for antibiotic activity, and many have been marketed for use in treating infected patients. Other antibiotics have been created completely in the test tube.

However they originated, most antibiotics work in a similar fashion: they interrupt the production of new bacteria by damaging some part of their reproductive cycle or by causing faulty parts of new bacteria to be made. Penicillins (plural because there are now a great many similar compounds used for this purpose) inhibit the formation of the cell wall when bacteria divide to form new cells. Other antibiotics inhibit the production of certain necessary proteins by the bacteria, and still others interfere di-

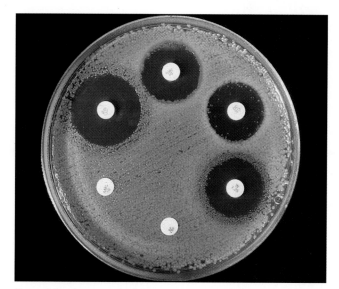

One of the dangers of antibiotic overuse is the development of bacteria resistant to drugs. Cultures of *E. coli* (a bacterium normally present in the human intestine) in this laboratory dish are sensitive to four different types of antibiotics, as indicated by the wide circles where no bacteria are growing, but they are resistant to two other types, which have no effect on their growth.

rectly with the reading of genetic material (DNA) during the process of bacterial reproduction.

When antibiotics inhibit a specific bacteria's growth, these bacteria are said to be "sensitive." Unfortunately, when bacteria are repeatedly exposed to small doses of antibiotics, a few develop a resistance to the drug and can survive and multiply even when the drug is present. Antibiotic-resistant bacteria can develop if antibiotics are overused or if people don't finish their entire course of medication. In recent years, antibiotic-resistant strains of gonorrhea, salmonella, tuberculosis, streptococcus, and many other bacteria have been identified. Because of extensive antibiotic use, many bacterial infections—particularly those acquired in a hospital setting—can be very resistant to antibacterial therapy, and hence very difficult to treat. In treating each particular bacterial infection, a physician must keep in mind just what particular bacterium might be causing the disease; otherwise, the antibiotic might not help fight the infection at all. Antibiotics are useful mainly against bacteria; against most viruses (which we discuss next), they are ineffective.

Viruses

Visible only with an electron microscope, **viruses**, the smallest of the pathogens, are on the borderline between living and nonliving matter. The pure virus particle appears to have no metabolism of its own. Viruses lack all the enzymes essential to energy production and protein synthesis in normal animal cells, and they cannot grow or reproduce by themselves. They must lead a **parasitic** ex-

istence inside a cell, borrowing what they need for growth and reproduction from the cells they invade. Once a virus is inside the host cell, it sheds its protein covering and its genetic material takes control of the cell and tricks it into manufacturing more viruses like itself (Figure 18-4). The normal functioning of the host cell is thereby disrupted.

Different viruses affect different kinds of cells, and the seriousness of the disease they cause depends greatly on which kind of cell is affected. The viruses that cause colds, for example, attack upper respiratory tract cells, which are constantly cast off and replaced. The disease is therefore mild. Poliovirus, in contrast, attacks nerve cells that cannot be replaced and the consequences, such as paralysis, are severe.

Illnesses caused by viruses are the most common forms of **contagious disease.** They include most of the minor ailments that cause short-lived illness and are rarely precisely diagnosed. Among these are the common cold, a variety of brief and undiagnosed respiratory infections, **influenza**, gastrointestinal upsets that cause diarrhea, and assorted aches and pains. More serious are the diseases that occur mainly in childhood and frequently cause a severe rash, such as measles, chickenpox, and mumps. Smallpox, which used to be the most severe of these diseases, has now been eliminated, thanks to a worldwide vaccination program carried out by the World Health Organization (WHO) in the 1960s and 1970s.

The herpesviruses are a large and important group of viruses. They are remarkable in that, once infected, the host is never again free of the virus (see Chapter 17). The virus lies latent within certain cells and ventures forth from time to time to produce symptoms. Normally the immune system keeps these viruses in check. However, when the immune system is depressed—for instance, by drugs used to aid organ transplantation or by immune deficiency disease, such as HIV infection—the herpesviruses may cause life-threatening disease.

Infectious mononucleosis (mono) is caused by a herpesvirus called **Epstein-Barr virus (EBV).** This disease is

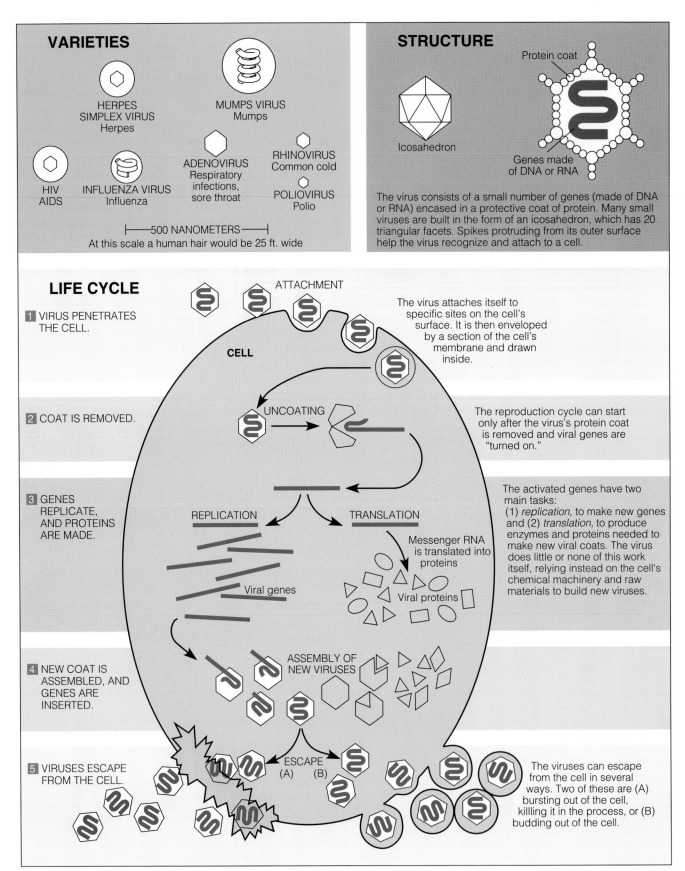

VARIETIES

HERPES
SIMPLEX VIRUS
Herpes

MUMPS VIRUS
Mumps

HIV
AIDS

INFLUENZA VIRUS
Influenza

ADENOVIRUS
Respiratory
infections,
sore throat

RHINOVIRUS
Common cold

POLIOVIRUS
Polio

├──── 500 NANOMETERS ────┤
At this scale a human hair would be 25 ft. wide

STRUCTURE

Protein coat

Icosahedron

Genes made
of DNA or RNA

The virus consists of a small number of genes (made of DNA or RNA) encased in a protective coat of protein. Many small viruses are built in the form of an icosahedron, which has 20 triangular facets. Spikes protruding from its outer surface help the virus recognize and attach to a cell.

LIFE CYCLE

ATTACHMENT

1 VIRUS PENETRATES
THE CELL.

The virus attaches itself to specific sites on the cell's surface. It is then enveloped by a section of the cell's membrane and drawn inside.

CELL

2 COAT IS REMOVED.

UNCOATING

The reproduction cycle can start only after the virus's protein coat is removed and viral genes are "turned on."

3 GENES
REPLICATE,
AND PROTEINS
ARE MADE.

REPLICATION

TRANSLATION

Messenger RNA
is translated into
proteins

Viral genes

Viral proteins

The activated genes have two main tasks: (1) *replication*, to make new genes and (2) *translation*, to produce enzymes and proteins needed to make new viral coats. The virus does little or none of this work itself, relying instead on the cell's chemical machinery and raw materials to build new viruses.

4 NEW COAT IS
ASSEMBLED, AND
GENES ARE
INSERTED.

ASSEMBLY OF
NEW VIRUSES

5 VIRUSES ESCAPE
FROM THE CELL.

ESCAPE
(A)   (B)

The viruses can escape from the cell in several ways. Two of these are (A) bursting out of the cell, killling it in the process, or (B) budding out of the cell.

Figure 18-4 *Viruses: varieties, structure, and life cycle.*

spread by close contact and usually affects children and young adults. The virus attacks white blood cells, and its symptoms may even look like leukemia. About three weeks after contact, the infected person has a severe sore throat with painful swelling of lymph nodes in the neck, lethargy, and fever. Antibiotics have no effect on the disease process, which is usually self-limited. Some infected people may be troubled by fatigue for weeks, even several months.

Several years ago, EBV was implicated as the cause of chronic fatigue syndrome, a long-term illness characterized by extreme fatigue, mental depression, and sometimes fever and swelling of the lymph nodes. Further research has indicated that EBV is probably not the cause of the disease; however, people with this disease have elevated levels of antibodies for many viruses. Controversy remains concerning the cause of chronic fatigue syndrome. Some researchers propose that it is the result of a chronic active viral illness. Many others believe it is caused by a problem with the immune system itself—specifically, a malfunction of the suppression stage of the immune response. If the immune system is activated by one or more viruses and the immune response continues even after the virus is cleared from the body, feelings of infection continue. Over time, factors of immune stimulation, physical deconditioning, and psychological depression combine to produce a thoroughly miserable person. Researchers continue to study this disease, seeking effective treatments.

More severe infections caused by viruses include HIV infection and hepatitis. Both of these are transmitted through contact with infected body fluids (see Chapter 17). There is no cure for either HIV infection or hepatitis, but there is an effective vaccine for the most common type of hepatitis (hepatitis B). Another serious viral infection is **poliomyelitis,** or polio, which attacks muscle-controlling nerves; in some cases, it leads to permanent paralysis. Fortunately, there is an effective vaccine for polio and the disease is now rare in the United States.

Certain viruses can also cause cell proliferation. The human disease resulting from this property is warts, which generally is very mild but can become extremely severe if the resistance of the infected person breaks down. There are many members of the human wart virus family, and some of them appear to be responsible for cervical cancer in women (see Chapter 16). Another virus, called HTLV-1 and related to HIV, causes a rare leukemia in adults (T-cell leukemia). As our knowledge of the molecular biology of cancer increases, other tumors may turn out to be caused by viruses, but the majority of human cancers are thought to be caused by other factors.

Although most viruses cannot be treated medically, there are a few "antiviral" agents. Influenza A, for example, can be treated with a drug that actually helps cure the patient. Herpes can be treated with acyclovir, an antiviral agent that helps alleviate symptoms and decrease the

length of each recurrence. However, it cannot eradicate the latent virus, so it must be taken at each recurrence. If taken daily, it can prevent recurrences as well. HIV infection can be treated with AZT (zidovudine) or other antivirals that inhibit the virus and slow its progress. These antivirals afford no cure, but people tend to feel better and live longer if they take them.

Most other viral diseases cannot be treated and must simply run their course. Over-the-counter cold remedies and pain relievers treat symptoms, not their viral cause (see the box "The Common Cold"). If you want to take an OTC medication for your cold or flu, it's probably better to avoid the "shotgun" approach—taking all medications at once. Take medication only for those symptoms you actually have. Sometimes it's difficult to determine whether your symptoms are due to a virus, a bacteria, or an allergy, but this information is important for appropriate treatment (Table 18-2).

Fungi, Protozoa, and Parasitic Worms

The organisms referred to as **fungi** are primitive plants that may be multicellular (like molds) or unicellular (like yeasts). Mushrooms and the molds that form on bread and cheese are all examples of fungi. Only about 50 fungi out of many thousands of species cause disease in humans, and these diseases usually are restricted to the skin, mucous membranes, and lungs. Some fungal diseases are extremely difficult to treat. To defend themselves against treatments, some fungi form spores, which are an especially resistant dormant stage of the organism.

The most common fungal malady is **candidiasis,** a yeast infection of the vagina that can also occur in other areas of the body, especially in the mouth in infants **(thrush).** Candidiasis, which begins as a relatively mild disease that causes itching, should be treated by a physician. When untreated and persistent, the disease can become severe and inflame the mucous membranes on which it normally exists.

Another common group of fungal diseases affects the skin, including athlete's foot, jock itch, and ringworm, a disease of the scalp. These three mild conditions are usually easy to cure and rarely give rise to major problems.

Fungi can also cause systemic disease, infecting large portions of the body. Such disease is severe, life-threatening, and extremely difficult to treat. Among the systemic

---

Poliomyelitis A disease of the nervous system, sometimes crippling; vaccines now prevent most polio.

Fungi Molds, mushrooms, and yeasts—primitive plants.

Candidiasis A sexually transmissible disease caused by the fungus *Candida albicans,* producing vaginitis and infant thrush (mouth sores); an opportunistic infection often accompanying AIDS.

Thrush A yeast infection of the mouth.

TERMS

TABLE 18-2 Is It a Virus, Bacteria, or Allergy?

	Virus	Bacteria	Allergy
Runny nose	Often	Rare	Often
Aching muscles	Usual	Rare	No
Headache	Often	Rare	No
Dizziness	Often	Rare	Rare
Fever	Often	Often	No
Cough	Often	Sometimes	Rare
Dry cough	Often	Rare	Sometimes
Raising sputum	Rare	Often	Rare
Hoarseness	Often	Rare	Sometimes
Recurs at a particular season	No	No	Often
Only a single complaint (sore throat, earache, sinus pain, or cough)	Unusual	Usual	Unusual
Do antibiotics help?	No	Yes	No
Can your physician help?	Sometimes	Yes	Sometimes

Source: R. Baxter. 1988. "Uncommon Facts About the Common Cold." *Healthline,* October.

forms of fungal disease are **cryptococcosis** and **coccidioidomycosis.** The latter disease is also known as "valley fever" because it is most frequently seen in the San Joaquin Valley of California. Fungal infections can be especially virulent (deadly) in people without a completely functioning immune system.

Another group of pathogens are the **protozoa,** microscopic single-celled animals, which are associated with such tropical diseases as **malaria, African sleeping sickness,** and **amoebic dysentery.** Many protozoa-based diseases are recurrent. The pathogen remains in the body, alternating between activity and inactivity. Hundreds of millions of Asians, Africans, and South Americans suffer from protozoal infections (for more information on infectious diseases in developing countries, see the box "Patterns of Disease and Death Around the World"). The most common protozoal disease in the United States is trichomoniasis, a relatively mild vaginal infection (see Chapter 17). Another protozoal disease, which can be contracted by drinking untreated water even in pristine wild areas, is giardiasis, characterized by diarrhea, nausea, and abdominal cramps.

Finally, the parasitic worms are the largest organisms that can enter the body to cause infection. The tapeworm, for example, can grow to a length of several feet. Worms, including such intestinal parasites as the tapeworm, hookworm, and pinworm cause a great variety of relatively mild infections. Smaller worms known as **flukes** infect such organs as the liver and lungs and, in large numbers, can be deadly. Generally speaking, worm infections originate from contaminated food or drink and can be controlled by careful attention to hygiene.

TERMS

Cryptococcosis   Severe systemic fungal disease.

Coccidioidomycosis   Valley fever; life-threatening systemic fungal disease.

Protozoa   Microscopic single-celled animals, often producing recurrent, cyclical attacks of disease.

Malaria   Severe, recurrent, mosquito-borne protozoal disease.

African sleeping sickness   Severe, recurrent, insect-borne protozoal disease marked by lassitude.

Amoebic dysentery   Protozoal infection of the intestines.

Flukes   Parasitic worms that can infest lungs and liver; can cause death.

A cold is an inflammation of the upper respiratory tract caused by a viral infection. More than 200 different viruses cause colds, but many cold-causing viruses fall into one of three families—rhinoviruses, coronaviruses, and adenoviruses. Like all viruses, those that cause colds trick cells in the body into ingesting them and then take over the cells' reproductive machinery to make new viruses. When an infected cell dies, new virus particles are released and go on to infect other cells.

Some of the symptoms of a cold are caused by the actions of the virus. For example, destruction of cells lining the respiratory tract or throat can cause sore throat, cough, and runny nose. Other symptoms are caused by the body's immune reaction to the virus. When the body recognizes the viruses as foreign, immune cells release interferons and leukotrienes, which help mobilize the body's defenses but also cause fever, aches, and fatigue.

Colds are usually spread by simple hand-to-hand contact with another person or with inanimate objects such as doorknobs and telephones. People with colds often touch their mouth or nose, contaminate their hands, and then unknowingly infect others. The best way to interrupt this mode of transmission is to wash your hands frequently with soap and warm water. Viruses can also be transmitted in the small airborne particles produced by a cough or sneeze, but this requires very close contact and is relatively rare. Whether you come down with a cold once you've been exposed to the virus depends on a variety of factors, including age, genetics, type and amount of exposure, whether you smoke, and whether you've developed antibodies to that particular virus.

There is no cure for the common cold. Consumers spend more than $1 billion every year on nonprescription treatments for coughs and colds, but these products provide only temporary relief:

- *Antihistamines* decrease nasal secretions by blocking the effects of histamine, which causes swelling of small blood vessels and results in sneezing and runny nose. Antihistamines are most useful in treating allergies, which are associated with high levels of histamine. Caution—antihistamines can make you drowsy.

- *Decongestants* shrink nasal blood vessels, relieving swelling and congestion caused by colds. However, they may dry out mucous membranes in the throat and make a sore throat worse.

- *Cough medicines* may be helpful when your cough is nonproductive (not bringing up mucus) or if it disrupts your sleep or work. Expectorants make coughs more productive by increasing the volume of mucus and decreasing its thickness; this helps remove irritants from the respiratory airways. Suppressants (antitussives) reduce the frequency of coughing.

- *Analgesics*—aspirin, acetaminophen (the ingredient in Tylenol), and ibuprofen (the ingredient in Advil and Motrin)—help lower fever and relieve muscle aches. Some evidence suggests that aspirin may prolong the time a person sheds the virus in his or her secretions, thereby lengthening both the contagious phase and the duration of the illness. Aspirin is also associated with an increased risk for Reye's syndrome in children; for this reason, aspirin should not be given to children. Some studies suggest that ibuprofen in combination with a decongestant actually decreases the time of viral shedding and reduces the duration of symptoms.

- *Antibiotics* aren't necessary for a cold unless a bacterial infection such as strep throat is present.

What about chicken soup? This favorite home remedy is an effective treatment for some of your cold symptoms—the steam soothes a sore throat and loosens secretions, and the liquid and salt help prevent dehydration.

So, although there's no cure for a cold, you can make yourself more comfortable while you wait for your body to fight off the infection. When you have a cold, the best plan may be to rest, drink plenty of hot liquids, and get what relief you can from appropriate nonprescription cold remedies.

Adapted from: "The Common Cold." *Mayo Clinic Health Letter,* September 1992; and R. Baxter. 1988. "Uncommon Facts About the Common Cold." *Healthline,* October.

Other Immune Disorders: Cancer and Autoimmune Diseases

The immune system has evolved to protect the body from invasion by foreign microorganisms. Sometimes, as in the case of cancer, the body comes under attack by its own cells. Cancer cells cease to cooperate normally with the rest of the body and multiply uncontrollably. The exact causes of all cancers are mostly unknown. However, scientists are aware of several mechanisms whereby cancer cells can arise.

One of these mechanisms, simply put, is alteration of the genetic structure of a cell by a carcinogen, a substance or energy from outside the body that can predispose cells to becoming cancerous, or malignant (see Chapter 16). The immune system can often detect cells that have recently become malignant and then destroy them just as they would a foreign microorganism. But if the immune system breaks down, as it may when people get older, when they have certain immune disorders (including HIV infection), or when they are receiving chemotherapy for other diseases, the cancer cells may multiply out of con-

One hundred years ago, the vast majority of all deaths worldwide were caused by infectious diseases. Today, developed countries have largely conquered infectious disease, but the developing world still struggles with this scourge. Among the 3.6 billion people living in developing countries (one-half of them in China and India), 45 percent of all deaths are caused by infectious and parasitic diseases.

Nearly 40 percent of all deaths in these countries occur among children age five or younger and 72 percent of children's deaths are caused by infectious and parasitic diseases. Diarrhea kills 3 to 4 million people a year, mostly children below the age of five; acute respiratory infection kills 5 million; tuberculosis, 3 million; measles, 2 million; whooping cough, 1.6 million; and malaria, 1 million. Additionally, there are more than 6 million people infected with HIV in Africa alone, and the World Health Organization expects the number to rise to more than 10 million by the year 2000.

In contrast, only about 5 percent of all deaths in the developed world (Europe, North America, Australia, New Zealand, and Japan) are caused by infectious and parasitic diseases. Two-thirds of these deaths are due to acute respiratory infections (mainly pneumonia) among the elderly. HIV infection accounts for many other deaths. The leading causes of death in the developed world are heart disease, cancer, stroke, and respiratory disease—chronic, degenerative diseases associated with older populations and unhealthy lifestyles.

As the developing countries work to defeat infectious diseases through improvements in public health and immunization and treatment programs, they are also starting to see an increase in deaths from cardiovascular disease and cancer. This pattern indicates not only that people are living longer but also that they are adopting the lifestyles—and the health burdens—of the developed world. They are eating more refined diets, drinking more alcohol, leading more sedentary lives, experiencing more stress, and, most critically, smoking more cigarettes. World Health Organization statistics point to a worldwide increase in cancer due largely to increases in tobacco use. WHO notes with great concern the aggressive marketing of cigarettes to nonsmoking populations in Asia and Latin America, particularly women and young people.

At current rates, heart disease and cancer will surpass infectious diseases as the leading causes of death in the developing world by the year 2000, according to WHO. If preventive measures aren't taken, these diseases could have devastating consequences on the health and economies of developing countries. The challenge for these countries is to continue their efforts to eradicate infectious and parasitic diseases at the same time that they adopt educational measures and public policies aimed at preventing lifestyle diseases.

Sources: C. Mathers. 1991. "Who Dies of What (These Days)?" *The Medical Journal of Australia* 154:227–28; J. Maurice. 1990. "Development Kills." *World Press Review,* August.

trol before the immune system recognizes the danger. By the time the immune system gears up to destroy the cancerous cells, it may be too late.

Another immune disorder occurs when the body confuses its own cells with foreign organisms. As described earlier, the immune system must be able to recognize many thousands of antigens as foreign and then be able to recognize the same antigens again and again. Our own tissue cells also are antigenic; that is, they would be recognized by another person's immune system as foreign. A delicate balance must be maintained to ensure that one's immune system recognizes only truly foreign antigens as enemies; erroneous recognition of one's own cells as foreign produces havoc.

This is exactly what happens in what are known as "autoimmune" disorders. In this type of malady, the immune system seems to be a bit too sensitive and begins to misapprehend itself as "not-self." Rheumatoid arthritis is one such disease; the immune system attacks the joints, sometimes causing crippling arthritis. Systemic lupus erythematosus is another autoimmune disease, in which blood vessels, or the lining of the heart, lungs, or brain become inflamed when the body attacks itself.

These diseases and a number of similar disorders are treated with medicines called **anti-inflammatory medications,** which counteract some of the immune effects. In large doses, over a period of time, anti-inflammatory drugs like aspirin, ibuprofen, and certain prescription medications can slow the autoimmune process. Steroids such as prednisone have a more powerful effect on the immune system and cause the immune response to diminish to the point where the patient can actually have an immune deficiency and become susceptible to a number of serious diseases.

GIVING YOURSELF A FIGHTING CHANCE: WHAT YOU CAN DO TO SUPPORT YOUR IMMUNE SYSTEM

Pathogens pose a formidable threat to human health and lives, but many steps can be taken to prevent them from

Many people believe, on an intuitive level, that stress makes them more vulnerable to illness. Studies have shown that rates of illness are higher for weeks or even months among people who have experienced the severe emotional trauma of divorce or the death of a loved one. Can more commonplace anxieties and stresses also cause significant, measurable changes in the immune system? In 1981, psychologist Janice Kiecolt-Glaser and immunologist Ronald Glaser, both of Ohio State University, set out to answer this question.

The two researchers recruited 75 medical students for their study. They gave them psychological tests to determine their stress levels and drew blood samples to assess their immune strength during the regular school year. Then they repeated the tests during exam week. The researchers found that the students' immune defenses—the number of natural killer cells that attack viruses and cancer—had dropped significantly under the stress of exams. In students who carried herpes, there were clear signs that the virus had become more active. The students who were loneliest and most socially isolated according to the psychological profiles suffered the biggest drop in immune function.

In seeking to explain these effects, researchers looked at the connections among emotions, stress, hormones, and immunity. They were particularly interested in the corticosteroids—the "stress" hormones released into the bloodstream when we're alarmed or anxious. Some hormones, such as cortisol, have been found to impair the ability of immune cells to multiply and function. Others, such as prolactin, seem to give immune cells a boost.

Since 1981, the Ohio State researchers have studied later classes of medical students; people in the midst of divorce; people mourning the death of a spouse; people caring for a family member with Alzheimer's disease, and newly married couples. In almost every case, they found that emotional stress had a measurable dampening effect on the body's defenses. They also found that relaxation training improved the immune functioning of both elderly individuals and medical students.

Over the past few years, the Glasers have followed a group of students around during exam week, sampling their blood every hour. They also conduct experiments in which they invite couples into the laboratory and, by means of a question or two about money or in-laws, instigate a quarrel. The researchers then take blood samples every 15 minutes to check on the status of each person's immune cells. By matching stress levels and hormonal changes to the ups and downs of immune function, they hope to gain a better grasp of the shifting chemistry of mind and immunity.

Adapted from: P. Jaret. 1992. "Mind over Malady." *Health,* November/December.

---

getting a foothold. Public health measures and environmental controls protect people from many diseases that are carried in water or food or by insects. A clean water supply and adequate sewage treatment help control typhoid fever and cholera, for example; and mosquito eradication programs control malaria and encephalitis. Proper food preparation prevents illness caused by food-borne pathogens. These include the parasitic roundworm *Trichina spiralis,* which causes trichinosis and is found in some uncooked meat, especially pork; the salmonella bacterium, which causes food poisoning and is often found in chicken; and the deadly toxin botulinum, which causes botulism and is produced by certain bacteria in improperly canned food (usually foods canned at home). (See Chapter 12 for guidelines on preparing food safely.)

But what can you do as an individual to "beef up" your immune system to help prevent infection? The most important thing you can do is to take good care of your body, with adequate diet, rest, and moderation in lifestyle. There are no special vitamins or diets that have been shown conclusively to boost the immune system. A balanced diet that includes the recommended daily amounts of vitamins and minerals helps keep all your cells functioning at their best. Medical science has come

up with nothing that can better the millions of years of evolution that have culminated in your complex system of immunity. Of course, once infection has begun, some diseases can be fought with the aid of antibiotics and antiviral agents. But these medications are not helpful in *preventing* infection, except in circumstances where normal immunity is breached, such as in surgery.

Scientists have discovered, however, that even the strongest immune system (as measured by the number of helper T-cells) waxes and wanes throughout a person's life. You are most susceptible to disease at the extremes of life, namely when first born, before you have developed active immunity against most pathogens, and in old age, when the immune system, like the rest of the body, starts to deteriorate. Now, you can't avoid being young or old, but you can make sure you get appropriate vaccinations, those given to aid the immune system in case of invasion

Anti-inflammatory medications Drugs like aspirin, ibuprofen, and corticosteroids that are often used to treat autoimmune diseases.

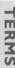

- Eat a balanced diet and maintain moderate weight. Consume a variety of low-fat foods to obtain the recommended amount of nutrients every day (see Chapter 12). No particular vitamin or mineral, including vitamin C, has been shown conclusively to prevent or cure the common cold or any other infectious disease.

- Get enough sleep—six to eight hours per night. Sleep is extremely important in helping the body replenish itself. Adequate sleep allows the proper production of all immune-related cells and products. Insufficient sleep predisposes you to a great number of illnesses and more severe infections.

- Exercise (but not while you're sick). Moderate aerobic exercise is an excellent way to reduce stress and strengthen the body, thereby preventing infection. However, exercise while you are sick—such as with a virus causing an upper respiratory infection—actually decreases your immunity and can prolong the infection,

probably by facilitating the replication of the viruses. The exact mechanism of this process is unknown.

- Don't smoke—smoking decreases the levels of some immune cells.

- Drink alcohol only in moderation. Heavy and long-term drinking interferes with the normal functioning of the immune system.

- Wash your hands. Since most viral illnesses are transmitted by hand-to-hand contact, proper hand washing with soap and hot water can often prevent transmission of disease.

- Avoid contact with people who are infectious with diseases transmitted via the respiratory route, such as influenza, chickenpox, and tuberculosis.

- Practice "safer sex" (see Chapter 17) and don't inject drugs to protect yourself against diseases such as hepatitis and HIV infection.

by specific pathogens. Infants should receive all required immunizations, such as diphtheria, pertussis, tetanus, measles, mumps, rubella, and polio (see Table 18-1). Adults over 65 years of age or people with chronic respiratory diseases should receive both the pneumococcal vaccine (only once) and the influenza vaccine (every year).

One factor that is known to influence the immune response and that can also be affected by lifestyle and attitudes is that nebulous entity called stress. Research has shown that the actual number of helper T-cells rises and falls inversely with stress; that is, the higher the stress, the lower the T-cell count. (For more on the effects of stress on the immune response, see the box "Immunity and Stress.") The term *stress* encompasses many variables ranging from emotional stressors, such as anger, anxiety, depression, and grief, to physical stressors, such as poor nutrition, sleep deprivation, overexertion, and addictions. Obviously, there's no magic potion you can take to relieve stress, since it is an integral and necessary part of life. But developing effective ways of coping with the stress in your life is essential to your overall good health (see Chapter 2).

In addition to managing the stress in your life and getting all your immunizations, you can help your body defend itself against disease by following the tips in the box "To Keep Yourself Well . . ." As is the case with all your body systems, your immune system works best when you support it with a healthy lifestyle.

Personal Insight Have you ever noticed an association between high levels of stress in your life and a tendency to get sick? Do you feel that the two are linked?

SUMMARY

The Body's Defense System

- The body's defense system against outside organisms consists of physical and chemical barriers, backed up by the immune system.

- Physical and chemical barriers to microorganisms include skin, mucous membranes, and the cilia lining the respiratory tract.

- Foreign organisms still manage to enter the body by penetration of the skin, inhalation, or ingestion.

- The immune response is carried out by white blood cells that are continuously produced in the bone marrow. These include neutrophils, macrophages, natural killer cells, and lymphocytes.

- B-cells are lymphocytes that produce antibodies. T-cell lymphocytes are divided into helper T-cells, killer T-cells, and suppressor T-cells.

- Lymphocytes recognize the antigens of invading organisms as foreign. When a foreign organism appears in the body, the appropriate lymphocyte locks onto it and sets off the immune response.

- The inflammatory response occurs when cells in the area of invasion or injury release histamines and other substances that cause blood vessels to dilate and fluid to flow out of capillaries.
- The immune response has four stages: recognition of the invading pathogen; rapid replication of killer T-cells and B-cells; attack by killer T-cells and macrophages; suppression of the immune response.
- Memory T- and B-cells recognize and destroy an antigen that enters the body a subsequent time.
- Contagion exists when active organisms are replicating in the body and can gain access to another person.
- Immunization is based on the body's ability to remember previously encountered organisms and retain its strength against them. Vaccines are preparations made of antigens similar to a disease-causing organism but not so dangerous.
- Vaccines confer active immunity; injections of antibodies themselves confer passive immunity.
- Allergic reactions occur when the immune system responds to harmless substances as if they were dangerous antigens.

The Troublemakers—Pathogens and Disease

- Bacteria are one-celled organisms that break down dead organic matter; in the human digestive tract, they help digest food. Anywhere else in the body they are pathogenic. They occur as bacilli, cocci, and spirochetes.
- Gram-positive bacterial organisms like streptococcus and staphylococcus reside on the skin even in healthy individuals, but they can cause infections when they enter the body.
- Gram-negative bacteria inhabit the intestines of healthy people but cause disease when the normal immune system breaks down or when gut integrity is breached.
- Both syphilis and Lyme disease are caused by spirochetes.
- Tuberculosis is caused by a bacterium identified by an acid fast stain.
- The mycoplasma organism causes many cases of pneumonia, ear infections, and sore throats in young adults. Rickettsiae are organisms that cause Rocky Mountain spotted fever and typhus.
- Although the immune system can fight off many bacterial infections, damage can be caused by both the bacteria and the body's immune defenses.
- Most antibiotics work by interrupting production of new bacteria. Bacteria can become resistant to antibiotics, which do not work against viruses.

- Viruses, the smallest pathogens, cannot grow or reproduce by themselves; they live a parasitic existence in the cells they invade. The seriousness of diseases caused by viruses depends on which kind of cell is infected.
- Some viruses, like herpesvirus, never leave the host but lie latent and reemerge from time to time.
- Viruses cause HIV infection, polio, and hepatitis. Some viruses cause cell proliferation; both warts and T-cell leukemia are caused by viruses.
- About 50 species of fungi can cause diseases in humans, usually restricted to the skin, mucous membranes, and lungs.
- Protozoa cause several tropical diseases as well as giardiasis and trichomoniasis.
- Parasitic worm infections generally originate in contaminated food or drink.
- The immune system often detects malignant cells and destroys them as if they were pathogens. If the immune system breaks down, cancer cells can multiply before the immune system recognizes danger.
- Autoimmune diseases occur when the body identifies its own cells as foreign.

Giving Yourself a Fighting Chance

- Public health measures protect people from pathogens carried by water, food, and insects.
- The immune system needs little help other than adequate nutrition and rest, a moderate lifestyle, and protection from excessive stress. Appropriate vaccinations help protect against disease during infancy and old age.

TAKE ACTION

1. Find out from your parents or your health records which immunizations you have had, including when you last had a tetanus shot. Are your immunizations up-to-date? If they aren't, or if you're not sure, check with the health center about what they recommend.
2. Go to your local pharmacy and examine the cold and cough remedies. Exactly which symptoms does each one claim to alleviate, and with what active ingredient? If possible, ask the pharmacist which ones he or she recommends for various symptoms.

JOURNAL ENTRY

1. In your health journal, list the positive behaviors that help you avoid or resist infection. Consider how you can strengthen those behaviors. Then list the

behaviors that tend to block your positive behaviors and put you at risk for contracting infection. Consider which of these you can change.

2. *Critical Thinking:* Does the government have the right to quarantine people who have serious infectious diseases such as tuberculosis or measles? Which should take precedence—concerns about public safety or the rights of individuals? Are there aspects of an illness—such as the seriousness of the illness or the mode of transmission—that should be considered in making this decision? Write an essay outlining your position on this issue; describe what circumstances, if any, you feel would warrant quarantining an infectious person.

3. Monitor yourself the next time you feel a cold coming on, keeping a record like the one shown in Chapter 1 for eating behavior. Note the symptoms, how they felt, the time and date of their occurrence, what you were doing, how you were feeling emotionally, and what you did in response to the symptoms. Keep the record until the cold is gone, noting how long it takes to run its course. Is there an association between your emotional state and how you experienced the symptoms? Between your emotional state and the length of the cold? Does taking medication (decongestant, cough syrup, etc.) make a difference in the symptoms or the duration of the cold?

SELECTED BIBLIOGRAPHY

Balows, A., W. J. Hausler, and E. H. Lennette, eds. 1988. *Laboratory Diagnosis of Infectious Disease, Principles and Practice.* New York: Springer-Verlag.

Barnes, P. F., A. B. Bloch, P. T. Davidson, and D. E. Snider, Jr. 1991. Tuberculosis in patients with human immunodeficiency virus infection. *New England Journal of Medicine* 324:1644–50.

Caldwell, M. 1992. Resurrection of a killer. *Discover,* December, 59–64.

Centers for Disease Control. 1991. *Health Information for International Travel.* Atlanta: Centers for Disease Control, Bureau of Epidemiology.

———.1991. Lyme disease surveillance—U.S., 1989–90. *Morbidity and Mortality Weekly Report* 40(25).

Cohen, S., D. A. J. Tyrrell, and A. P. Smith. 1991. Psychological stress and susceptibility to the common cold. *New England Journal of Medicine* 325:606–12.

Evans, A. S., ed. 1991. *Bacterial Infections of Humans: Epidemiology and Control,* 2nd ed. New York: Plenum.

———. ed. 1991. *Viral Infections of Humans: Epidemiology and Control,* 3rd ed. New York: Plenum.

Fischi, M. A., G. L. Daikos, R. B. Uttamchandani, R. B. Poblete, and J. N. Moreno. 1992. Outcome of patients with HIV infection and multidrug-resistant tuberculosis. *Annals of Internal Medicine* 117:191–96.

Goldsmith, M. F. 1990. Forgotten (almost) but not gone, tuberculosis suddenly looms large on domestic scene. *Journal of the American Medical Association* 264(2):165–66.

Holmes, K. K., P. Mardh, P. F. Sparling, and P. J. Weisner, eds. 1990. *Sexually Transmitted Diseases,* 2nd ed. New York: McGraw-Hill.

A killer returns. 1992. *American Health,* April, 9–10.

Mandell, G. B., and others. 1990. *Principles and Practice of Infectious Diseases,* 3rd ed. New York: Churchill Livingstone.

Markell, E. K., M. Voge, and D. T. John. 1992. *Medical Parasitology,* 7th ed. New York: W. B. Saunders.

Murphy, J. W., H. Friedman, and M. Bendinelli, eds. 1992. *Fungal Infections and Immune Responses.* New York: Plenum.

Neglected for years, TB is back. 1992. *The New York Times,* 11 October.

Rahn, D. W., and S. E. Malawista. 1991. Lyme disease: Recommendations for diagnosis and treatment. *Annals of Internal Medicine* 114:472–81.

Stoeckle, M. Y., and R. G. Douglas, Jr. 1992. Infectious diseases. *Journal of the American Medical Association* 268(3).

TB takes a deadly turn. 1991. *Time,* 2 December, 85.

Warren, K. S., and A. F. Mahmoud. 1990. *Tropical and Geographical Medicine,* 2nd ed. New York: McGraw-Hill.

RECOMMENDED READINGS

Bollet, A. J. 1987. *Plagues and Poxes: The Rise and Fall of Epidemic Diseases.* New York: Demos Publications. *Includes descriptions of the history and epidemiology of famous epidemics.*

Brock, T., ed. 1990. *Microorganisms—From Smallpox to Lyme Disease: Readings from Scientific American Magazine.* New York: W. H. Freeman. *A collection of articles from* Scientific American *on medical microbiology and communicable diseases.*

Chase, A. 1982. *Magic Shots: A Human and Scientific Account of the Long and Continuing Struggle to Eradicate Infectious Diseases by Vaccination.* New York: William Morrow. *An entertaining historical and medical account of the discovery and use of vaccinations.*

Dowling, H. F. 1977. *Fighting Infection: Conquests of the Twentieth Century.* Cambridge, Mass.: Harvard University Press. *Tales of medical drama and breakthroughs, including diseases such as tuberculosis, diphtheria, and measles.*

Levy, S. B. 1992. *The Antibiotic Paradox: How Miracle Drugs Are Destroying the Miracle.* New York: Plenum. *An easy-to-understand description of the effects of misuse and overuse of antibiotics, with suggestions for changing current practices to protect the effectiveness of antibiotics.*

Oliver, W. W. 1970. *Stalkers of Pestilence: The Story of Man's Ideas of Infection.* College Park, Md.: McGrath. *First published in 1930, this is a historical account of the search for the causes of infectious diseases.*

19

Aging: A Vital Process

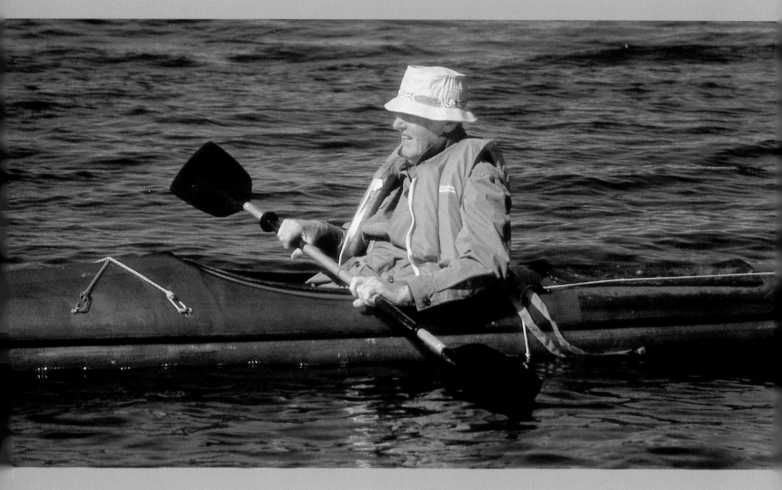

CONTENTS

▶ Your mother and her sister are only two years apart, but your mother looks about ten years younger than her sister. Your aunt, an avid golfer, has deep wrinkles in her face and her skin is leathery and dry. Are her wrinkles the result of too much exposure to the sun? What other habits or behaviors could account for her appearance? Can you avoid them?

▶ Your brother's wife has been upset lately because her parents are trying to decide whether to put her elderly grandfather into a nursing home. He's recovering from a hip injury and needs help getting around, but his mental faculties are fine and he feels he can care for himself. Your sister-in-law's parents are afraid he'll fall again and be unable to get help. The decision is traumatic for everyone involved. Are there any alternatives besides placing him in a nursing home? What advice can you give them?

▶ When you were home the last time, you were shocked to see a neighbor whom you had known your whole life wandering down the street in his pajamas. As you watched through the window, another neighbor ran out of her house and led him back home. When you asked your parents about it they said he had become senile in his old age. "He's become increasingly confused and forgetful," your father says. What has happened to your neighbor? Is this what aging leads to in everyone? Is there anything you can or should do to avoid it yourself?

▶ You were looking at some family photos with your grandmother and came on a snapshot of her taken when she was just about your age. As you peer at it, you recognize her dark eyes, her smile, and the contours of her face. Even the way she holds her head hasn't changed. "It looks like me, doesn't it," she says, "minus all the wrinkles and gray hair. I remember clearly how I felt when that picture was taken. Inside, I'm still the same person." You hadn't thought about it very much, but what she says makes you realize you think old people are qualitatively different from young people. Something happens when you become elderly, doesn't it? Isn't there a big change of some kind that transforms you into an old person?

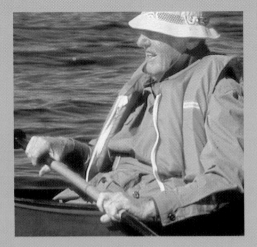

MAKING CONNECTIONS

You are aging throughout your life, right from the moment of birth, but the aging process gains momentum in the second half of life. Then the lifestyle behaviors that you adopted earlier begin to pay off, for better or for worse, and you start to experience the consequences of your choices—good health and vigor or poor health and debilitation. In each of the scenarios presented on this page, all related to aging, individuals have to use information, make a decision, or choose a course of action. How would you act in each of these situations? What response or decision would you make? This chapter provides information about aging that can be used in situations like these. After finishing the chapter, read the scenarios again. Has what you've learned changed how you would respond?

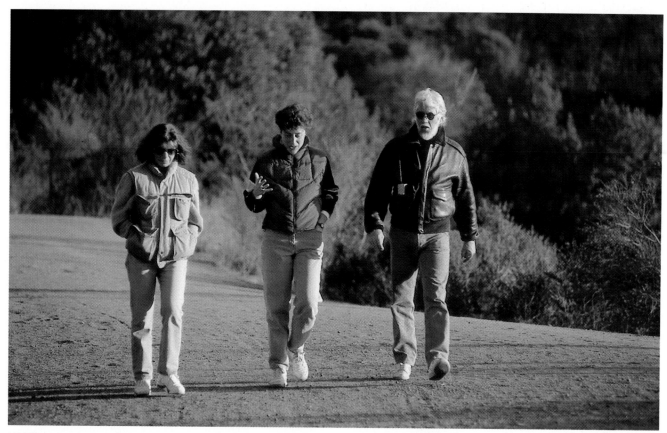

Middle age is a time of reassessment and readjustment in preparation for the second half of life. Many people in their forties and fifties who have cultivated healthy lifestyles will continue to lead vigorous lives well into old age.

Many people would like to live for a long time and never grow old. When we see that old age has taken us in its grip, we're stunned. We regard old age as something alien, a foreign species: Can I become a different being while I still remain myself? Yes. And no. Life is like a river. The flow is continuous and so you can never step in the same place twice.

Aging does not begin on the sixty-fifth birthday, and there is no precise age at which a person becomes "old." Rather, aging is a normal process of development that occurs over the entire lifetime. It happens to everyone, but at different rates for different people. Some people are "old" at 25; others are still young at 75.

Although youth is not entirely a state of mind, your attitude toward life and your attention to your health significantly influence the satisfaction you will derive from life, especially when new physical, mental, and situational challenges occur in later years. If you take charge of your health during young adulthood, you can exert great control over the physical and mental aspects of aging, and you can better handle your response to events that might be out of your control. With foresight and energy you can shape a creative, graceful, and even triumphant old age.

GENERATING VITALITY AS YOU AGE

Circumstances, bodies, and mental faculties change. Some changes occur gradually, over a lifetime. **Biological aging**, for example, includes all the normal, progressive, irreversible changes to one's body that begin at birth and continue until death. Psychological and social aging usually involve more abrupt changes in circumstance and emotion: relocating, changing homes, losing a spouse and friends, retiring, having a lower income, and changing roles and social status. These changes represent opportunities for growth throughout life. Not all of these changes happen to everybody, and their timing varies, partly depending on how people have prepared for their later days. Some never have to leave their homes and appear to be in good health until the day they die. Others have tremen-

Biological aging Changes in body structure and function that result from the passage of time.

Aging and Changing: Your Body Through Time

Skin   Skin becomes looser as you get older—it stretches more easily and doesn't snap back as well after stretching. Long-term exposure to ultraviolet light from the sun produces wrinkles and areas of spotty pigmentation ("age spots"). Skin also becomes drier as you age, as sweat and oil glands quit working. Overuse of soaps and antiperspirants can worsen dry skin.

Body Fat   You can expect an increase in body fat and reduction in body size from a decrease in muscle mass and body water content. However, changes in muscle tone and body composition (the ratio of fat to muscle) can be kept to a minimum through regular exercise. Deposits of fat in the waist are associated with a higher incidence of disease (see Chapter 13). Weight management is important throughout life.

Hearing   The ability to hear high-pitched and sibilant (hissing) consonant sounds such as s, z, sh, and ch declines for most people as they age, enough so that hearing loss is now the fourth most common chronic physical disability in the United States. Even by age 35, you may not hear as well as you did at 25. Most people don't notice the progressive muffling until their sixties, when they may begin to have difficulty following speech. These losses may be due to abuse rather than to aging, however. Extremely loud noise, such as from stereo earphones or loud machines may contribute to hearing loss. In less industrialized and quieter societies, hearing is almost as keen in old age as it is in youth. A high-fat diet has been linked to clogging of the blood vessels that nourish the hearing organs.

Eyesight   By your mid-forties you will develop **presbyopia**—a gradual decline in the ability to focus on objects close to you or to see small print. This occurs because the ocular lens no longer expands and contracts as readily. You will need brighter lights for reading and cooking. Glare may be a problem. Seeing in the dark becomes more difficult and depth perception weakens. Color clarity changes, especially in the blue-green range. **Cataracts**, the clouding of the lens that may dim vision by the sixties, are the result of lifelong oxidation damage, a by-product of normal body chemistry. Smoking and exposure to radiation and the sun may also contribute to the development of cataracts.

Taste and Smell   Sensations of taste and smell diminish with age. About two-thirds of the taste buds in the mouth die by age 70, as do many of the sensory receptors in the nose. Some medications can further interfere with taste, and long-term exposure to smoke lessens the ability to smell.

Hair   As you age, cells at the base of hair follicles produce progressively less pigment and eventually die. By age 50 half of Americans are partially gray, and hair loss in men becomes apparent. Twelve percent of men are balding by age 25; 65 percent by age 65. Thickest at age 20, individual hair shafts shrink after that; by age 70, your hair will probably be as fine as when you were a baby.

Bones, Muscles, and Teeth   Bones maintain themselves through a cyclic process called remodeling in which old bone is absorbed and new bone develops. By the mid-thirties, more bone is being absorbed than developed. Loss of bone mass is generally not a problem for men because they have denser bones than women to begin with. For women, bone loss accelerates after menopause. One out of every four women over age 60 develops **osteoporosis**, in which bones become weaker, more porous, and more prone to fractures. Adequate calcium in your diet and regular weight-bearing exercise will help build strong bones while you're young and slow the loss of bone as you age (see Chapter 12).

Muscles become weaker, too, although you can retard your loss of muscle strength and mass through regular physical work and play. As you age, more protein is being broken down and less is being synthesized, so muscle fibers atrophy and lose their ability to contract; some are lost; fat and collagen accumulate. Aging muscles are less flexible and more susceptible to strains, pulls, and cramps. After the mid-forties, strength usually declines: A man may lose 10 to 20 percent of his maximum strength by age 60, and a woman even more.

Height also decreases with age—about 1 to 4 inches are lost after young adulthood. Factors contributing to this decrease in height include loss of bone mass, weakening back muscles, and deterioration of the discs between the bones in the spine.

Your teeth, with proper care, can last a lifetime. Not aging, but disuse, abuse, and chronic degenerative disease

---

TERMS

Presbyopia   The inability of the eyes to focus sharply on nearby objects, caused by a loss of elasticity of the lens that occurs with advancing age.

Cataracts   Opacity of the lens of the eye that impairs vision and can cause blindness.

Osteoporosis   Loss of bone density that causes bones to become weak, porous, and more prone to fractures.

dous adjustments to make—to entirely new surroundings with fewer financial resources, to new acquaintances, to decreasing mobility, to the changing physical condition of their bodies and new health problems, and possibly to loneliness and loss of self-esteem.

Successful aging requires preparation. People need to establish good health habits in their teens and twenties. In their twenties and thirties they usually develop important relationships and settle into particular lifestyles. By their mid-forties they know how much money they need to cause teeth problems. Teeth and all their support systems respond well to the stress and stimulation of chewing crunchy foods. **Periodontitis** is a common agent in tooth loss after age 35; it is caused by the buildup of plaque. You can prevent it with proper dental care, including brushing and flossing each day, as described in Chapter 21.

Heart Your resting heartbeat stays about the same throughout your life, but the heart pumps less blood with each beat as you get older. This effect is most pronounced during exercise because your pulse can no longer rise as high, nor return as rapidly to its resting rate, as it once did. The dramatic problems of the cardiovascular system associated with aging—heart attack and stroke—are usually caused by atherosclerosis and high blood pressure, which can be largely controlled by eating right and exercising regularly.

Lungs Good news: Your respiratory system resists change, and your respiratory tract actually grows stronger with age. After a lifetime of exposure to viruses, people build up immunity and catch fewer and less severe colds by middle age. Your vital capacity—the amount of air you can expel from your lungs—should not decline if you keep fit and healthy and don't smoke. Regular and vigorous exercise can increase vital capacity in young people and reverse losses in older ones.

Digestive System and Kidneys With age, your stomach will secrete less acid and smaller amounts of the enzymes that aid digestion. Digesting a meal takes longer and may be more difficult, but your small intestines won't lose the power to absorb nutrients. Kidneys deteriorate, eventually filtering wastes more slowly.

Immune System With age your defense system may become less efficient, but the decline varies greatly among people. Only the progressive atrophy of the thymus gland seems invariably linked to advancing age. The consequences of immune system decline are increased rates of cancer and autoimmune and infectious diseases but better tolerance of tissue and organ transplants. Both good diet and exercise benefit the immune system. People who are in good physical shape rid themselves of respiratory infections much faster than do those who are not.

Brain and Nervous System Only half as much blood travels to the brain of a 50-year-old as to that of a 10-year-old, with most of the reduction occurring before age 30. By age 85, the brain has lost 10 to 20 percent of its weight, mainly through nerve cell atrophy. These **neuron** losses are selective: Some sites show no loss, while in the **cerebral cortex,** the site of higher mental activities, loss is significant. Your mental ability will not necessarily decline with the loss of neurons, partly because the brain continues to sprout new **dendrites,** communication lines to other neurons. They may be one way the brain compensates for neuron loss.

Sleep patterns change with age, although troubled sleep may be a sign of an emotional or physical disorder rather than of age. The deepest stage of non-REM sleep decreases as you age, which may explain why older people are considered light sleepers. Reliance on sleeping medications should be avoided because they interfere with REM sleep (see Chapter 2 for more information on sleep).

Sexual Organs and Sexual Response An active and satisfying sex life can continue as you age. Women do not ordinarily lose their capacity for orgasm nor men their capacity for erection and ejaculation. A slowing of response, especially in men, is considered a part of the normal aging process.

For women, menopause (cessation of menstruation) usually occurs between the ages of 47 and 50. The common symptoms of menopause, including hot flashes and sweating, can be treated with hormone therapy. Women may experience a drying and thinning of the vaginal walls due to lower levels of estrogen after menopause; use of an estrogen cream and/or a water-soluble lubricant can usually treat the problem. A hysterectomy or mastectomy does not have to affect sexual activity.

As they age, men may take longer to attain an erection and the erection may not be as firm or as large as when they were younger. The prostate gland may become enlarged after middle age, causing problems with urination. This condition can now usually be treated without affecting sexual response.

support the lifestyle they've chosen. They need to assess their financial status and perhaps adjust their savings so they continue enjoying that lifestyle after retirement. In their mid-fifties, they need to reevaluate their health plans and may want to think about retirement housing. Throughout life, people should cultivate interests and hobbies they enjoy, both alone and with others so that they can continue to live an active and rewarding life after retirement. All of these actions help to prepare them for life in their later years.

Periodontitis Disease of the bone, tissue, and gum that support the teeth, caused by the accumulation of plaque.

Neuron A nerve cell.

Cerebral cortex The outer layer of the brain, which controls the behavior and mental activity of humans.

Dendrites A branched part of a nerve cell that transmits impulses toward the cell body.

TERMS

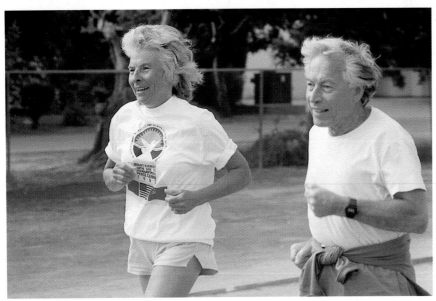

Regular exercise throughout life is an important key to graceful aging. By keeping fit, this vigorous couple in their 60's have maintained a high level of physical functioning. Regular exercise also helps prevent depression, boredom, and losses in fluid intelligence typically associated with aging.

Personal Insight How do you envision your old age? How will it resemble the old age of elderly people you know now, and how will it differ? What external events could affect your control of your lifestyle when you're older?

What Happens as You Age?

Many of the characteristics associated with aging aren't due to aging at all. They are due rather to neglect and abuse of our bodies and minds. These assaults lay the foundation for later mental problems and chronic conditions like arthritis, heart disease, diabetes, hearing loss, and high blood pressure. We sacrifice our optimal health by smoking, eating a poor diet and overeating, abusing alcohol and drugs, bombarding our ears with excessive noise, and exposing our bodies to too much ultraviolet radiation from sun rays. We also jeopardize our bodies through inactivity, encouraging our muscles and even our bones to wither and deteriorate. And we endure abuse from the toxic chemicals in our environment.

But even with the best behavior in the best environment, aging does occur. It results from biochemical processes that we don't yet fully understand. The physiological changes in organ systems are caused by a combination of gradual aging and injury from disease. Thanks to redundancy in most organ systems, the body's ability to function is not affected until damage is fairly extensive. Studies of healthy people indicate that functioning remains essentially constant until after age 70. Look at the box "Aging and Changing: Your Body Through Time" for a summary of the bodily changes that accompany aging.

Life-enhancing Measures: Age Proofing

You can prevent, delay, lessen, or even reverse some of the changes associated with aging through good health habits. A few simple things you can do every day will make a vast difference to your appearance, your health, your energy and vitality. The following suggestions have been mentioned throughout this text, but are profoundly related to health in later life and so are highlighted here.

Challenge Your Mind Creativity and intelligence remain stable in healthy individuals. Develop interests and hobbies that you can enjoy throughout your life. Staying involved in learning as a lifelong process can help you remain sharp and keep your mental abilities.

Develop Physical Fitness Exercise enhances both mental and physical health. Enough cannot be said for the positive effects of appropriate exercise throughout your life, particularly when weighed against the physical and mental deterioration of the elderly who have not kept their minds and bodies fit.

The benefits of an active and vigorous lifestyle include the following:

- Increased resiliency and suppleness of arteries
- Better protection against heart attack and much increased chance of survival should one occur
- Sustained capacity of lungs and respiratory reserves

- Weight control through less accumulation of fat
- Maintenance of physical flexibility, balance, agility, reaction time
- Greatly preserved muscle strength
- Protection against ligament injuries, dislocation strains in the knees, spine, shoulders
- Protection against osteoporosis
- Increased effectiveness of the immune system
- Maintenance of mental agility and flexibility, response time, memory, hand-eye coordination

Many functional losses are actually due to lack of exercise rather than to aging. Part of the decline in pulmonary function that often occurs may be due to preventable declines in muscle strength. Opera singers trained in diaphragmatic breathing show fewer changes in pulmonary function with age. Older men who continue with racquet sports and running show faster reaction times than do their sedentary counterparts. The stimulus that exercise provides also seems to protect against the loss of some **fluid intelligence**—the ability to find solutions when confronted with a new problem. fluid intelligence depends on rapidity of responsiveness, memory, and alertness. Contrary to former notions that this capability necessarily declines with age, studies reveal that older people who are highly fit score better on tests of intelligence than do their less fit counterparts. Exercise also appears to have some power against depression, apathy, and boredom.

You need to find a variety of activities that you enjoy and can do on a regular basis. Your exercise program should be moderate in its intensity and frequency and should include a warm-up and stretching exercises to protect against injury. Read Chapter 14 for ideas, and build physical activity into your daily routine.

Eat Wisely   Health at every age is helped by a varied diet with special attention to lower fat and calorie intake.

- Eat meals low in fat and high in complex carbohydrates. Concentrate on fresh fruits and vegetables; high-fiber, whole-grain cereals and breads; potatoes; brown rice; pasta.
- Eat fish, preferably salmon, tuna, mackerel, swordfish, and rainbow trout, and poultry (no skin) instead of eggs and fatty meats.
- Use no-fat or low-fat dairy products. Substitute olive oil for other oils and fats. Say no to all but the occasional fatty, rich dessert.
- Control caloric intake so that it does not exceed your needs in maintaining healthy body weight.
- If you frequently salt your food, reduce your intake.

Maintain Healthy Weight   People can control their weight, although it takes time and can be stressful; it's es-

pecially difficult for people who have been overweight most of their lives. A sensible program of using more calories through exercise and perhaps cutting calorie intake or a combination of both will work for most people who want to lose weight, but there is no magic formula. Obesity is not physically healthy, and it leads to premature aging.

Control Drinking   Alcohol impairs both liver and kidney function; heavy drinkers suffer brain damage as well.

Don't Smoke   The average pack-a-day smoker can expect to live about 12 years less than a person who doesn't smoke. Worse, smokers suffer more illnesses that last longer, and they are subject to respiratory disabilities that limit their total vigor for many years before their death. Even young cigarette smokers suffer respiratory impairment, some within a year of starting to smoke. Premature balding and skin wrinkling have been linked to cigarette smoking. Smokers at age 50 have the wrinkles of a person of 60. See Chapter 9 for more details, and remember that smoking is not part of the long or good life.

Schedule Physical Examinations to Detect Treatable Diseases   Some diseases that escape notice during early stages can nevertheless take a terrible toll in premature disability and death. But when detected early, many can be successfully controlled by medication and lifestyle changes. Hypertension, diabetes, and many types of cancer are examples of diseases that, when diagnosed early, often can be successfully treated. Regular testing for **glaucoma** after age 40 can prevent blindness from this treatable eye disease. And keeping your immunizations up-to-date can protect you from preventable infectious diseases. Look at the medical tests for healthy people listed in Chapter 21 and the immunizations recommended in Chapter 18. Guidelines are provided for how frequently you should have them throughout your life.

Recognize and Reduce Stress   Stress-induced physiological changes increase wear and tear on your body. Cut down on the stresses in your life, perhaps by riding a bicycle instead of driving a car or by avoiding noisy environments. Don't wear yourself out too fast through lack of sleep, abuse or misuse of drugs, or workaholism. Practice relaxation, using the techniques described in Chapter 2. If you contract a disease, consider it your body's attempt to interrupt your life pattern and permit you to reevaluate your lifestyle, perhaps to slow down.

Fluid intelligence   The ability to develop a solution when confronted with a new problem.

Glaucoma   Disease in which fluid inside the eye is under abnormally high pressure; can lead to blindness.

TERMS

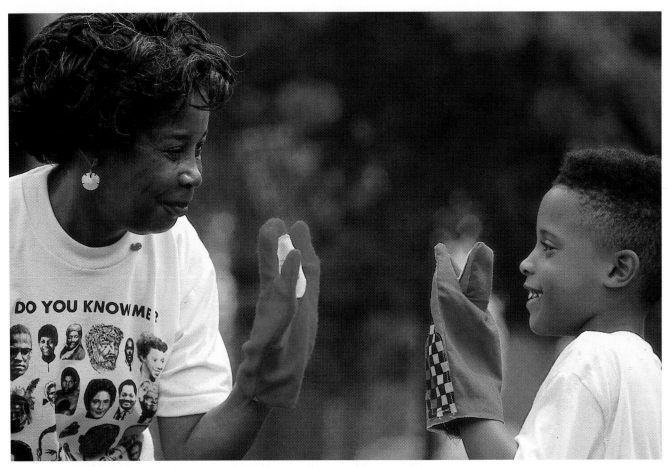

One of the challenges of aging is finding satisfying activities that provide meaningful connections with others. This retired woman is using hand puppets to help teach refusal skills as part of a substance abuse prevention project.

Ironically, the health behaviors you practice now weigh more heavily in determining how long you will live than will your behaviors at a later age. Retiring from your life's occupation with a physically healthy body will allow far more options for enjoying yourself than will retiring with frail health or disabilities. Poor health that could have been prevented drains finances, emotions, and energy and contributes to poor mental health. By attending to yourself now, you're buying some insurance for the future.

CONFRONTING THE CHANGES OF AGING

The changes that occur with aging have repercussions that must be grappled with and resolved. Just as you can act now to prevent or limit the physical changes of aging, you can also begin preparing yourself mentally, socially, and financially for changes that may occur later in life. These developmental tasks of aging are determined by biological, social, and perhaps economic changes and may require significant lifestyle adjustments. Although aging puts unique demands on each person, the changes cut across ethnic and socioeconomic variables. If you have aging parents, grandparents, and friends, the following information may give you insight into their lives and encourage you to begin cultivating appropriate and useful behaviors now.

Planning for Social Changes

Retirement marks a major change in the second half of life. As the longevity of Americans has increased, individuals spend a larger proportion of their lives in retirement—25 years or more. This has implications for reestablishing important relationships, developing satisfying interests outside work, and saving for an adequate retirement income.

Changes in social roles are a major feature of middle age. Children become young adults and leave home, putting an end to day-to-day parenting. Parents experiencing this "empty nest syndrome" must adapt to changes in their customary responsibilities and personal identities. And though retirement is a wished-for landmark for most people, it may also be viewed as a threat to prestige, purpose, and self-respect—the loss of a valued or customary role—and will probably require a period of adjustment.

Retirement and the end of child rearing also bring about changes in the relationship between marriage partners. The amount of time a couple spend together will increase and activities will change. Couples may need a period of adjustment, in which they get to know each other as individuals again. Discussing what types of activities each partner enjoys can help couples set up a mutually satisfying routine of shared and independent activities.

Planning ahead for retirement is crucial. What kinds of things do you enjoy doing? How will you spend your days? Although retirement confers the advantages of leisure time and freedom from deadlines, competition, and stress, many people do not know how to enjoy their free time. If you have developed diverse interests, retirement can be a joyful and fulfilling period of your life. Retirement can provide opportunities for expanding your horizons by giving you the chance to try new activities, take classes, and meet new people. Volunteering in your community can enhance self-esteem and allow you to be a contributing member of society.

Retirement often also brings a new economic situation. It may mean a severely restricted budget or possibly even financial disaster if you don't take stock of finances and plan ahead. Planning for retirement is especially difficult during inflationary periods that erode the dollars saved toward retirement. Almost twice as many men as women are covered by **pension** plans, reflecting the fact that many women have lower-paying jobs or work part-time during their childbearing years. And although the gap is closing, women currently outlive men by about seven years; consequently, their needs for financial stability require careful planning.

Financial planning for retirement should begin early in life. People in their twenties and thirties should estimate how much money they need to meet their standard of living, calculate their projected income, and begin a savings program. The earlier such a program is begun, the more money will be saved for retirement.

Adapting to Physical Changes

As described earlier in the chapter, there are many things an individual can do to avoid or lessen the physical changes associated with aging. However, some changes in physical functioning are inevitable, and successful aging involves anticipating and accommodating these changes.

Decreased energy and changes in health mean that older people have to develop priorities for how to use their energy. Rather than curtailing activities to conserve energy, they need to learn how to generate energy. This usually involves saying "yes" to enjoyable activities and paying close attention to needs for rest and sleep.

Adapting, rather than giving up, favorite activities may be the best strategy for dealing with physical limitations. For example, if **arthritis** interferes with piano playing, a person can continue to enjoy music by attending concerts or checking out music from the local library. Obtaining treatment for medical problems such as arthritis and glaucoma can also help limit the effects of aging on day-to-day activities (see the box "Arthritis" for more information).

One common physical disability—hearing loss—can have a particularly strong effect on the lives of elderly people. Hearing loss affects a person's ability to interact with others and can lead to a sense of isolation and depression. If someone you know complains that words are difficult to understand, that another person's speech sounds slurred or mumbled, or that people are not speaking loudly enough, that person may have suffered some hearing loss. You may also notice that the person sets the volume of a radio or TV very high. Hearing loss should be assessed and treated by a health care professional; in some cases, hearing can be completely restored by dealing with the underlying cause of hearing loss. In other cases, hearing aids may be prescribed to help with hearing. The following strategies can help improve communication with a hearing-impaired person:

- Speak at your normal rate; do not shout or overarticulate. This distorts speech sounds and makes visual clues more difficult to follow.

- Speak to the person at a distance of 3 to 6 feet. Stand near a good light so that your lip movements, facial expressions, and gestures may be seen more clearly.

- If the person does not understand you, rephrase your ideas. Use short, simple sentences.

- Don't leave hearing-impaired people out of conversations. Practice can improve their ability to communicate.

There are many strategies for dealing with the gradual decline in vision that occurs with aging. The first is to treat any underlying medical problems, such as cataracts or glaucoma. Older people may need about a 30 percent increase in light in order to work more effectively; increasing the number of light sources and painting rooms in a lighter, paler color helps. Increasing light sources in darkened areas such as stairwells can reduce falls from the slower light-to-dark accommodation that occurs with age. Hats and sunglasses worn outside help reduce glare. If visual losses are more severe, large-print books, magnifying glasses, and a variety of electronic devices are available to help an individual adapt to limitations in eyesight.

Pension   A sum of money paid regularly as a retirement benefit.
Arthritis   Inflammation of a joint or joints causing pain and swelling.

TERMS

Over 50 percent of all people age 65 and older have some form of arthritis. Arthritis is a chronic disease that causes pain and loss of movement in joints. Warning signs of arthritis include the following:

- Swelling in one or more joints
- Early morning stiffness
- Recurring pain or tenderness in any joint
- Changes in joint mobility
- Obvious redness or warmth in a joint
- Unexplained weight loss, fever, or weakness in combination with joint pain

There are over 100 different types of arthritis. Three of the most common are osteoarthritis, rheumatoid arthritis, and gout. Osteoarthritis is a degenerative joints disease most often affecting the hands and the weight-bearing joints of the body—knees, ankles, and hips. Initially, pain occurs after activity, and rest brings relief; later, pain can occur with minimal movement or even during rest. Osteoarthritis in the hands or hips sometimes seems to run in families and may have a genetic component. Being overweight has been linked to osteoarthritis in the knees; overuse of a joint during recreational or work-related activities is associated with the disease in knees, hips, and elbows.

Rheumatoid arthritis is the most disabling form of arthritis because the nerve degeneration associated with the disease ultimately causes loss of movement at the muscular level. In this disease, the synovial membrane that surrounds a joint gradually becomes inflamed, causing inflammation in other parts of the joint and destruction of bone. Rheumatoid arthritis can also cause inflammation of the heart, blood vessels, and body tissues. Rheumatoid arthritis affects all age groups; women are affected three times more often than men. Its exact cause is unknown, but it may be brought on by an autoimmune disorder, in which the body mistakenly identifies its own cells as foreign and destroys them. Other possible causes include infection by a microorganism, stress, and environmental toxins; there may also be a genetic component.

Gout is a painful form of arthritis that usually affects the toes, ankles, knees, elbows, wrists, and hands; it occurs most frequently in older men. Swelling and extreme tenderness develop around the affected joint(s). Medication can stop gout attacks and prevent future attacks and damage to the joints.

The goal of treatment for arthritis is to reduce pain and inflammation, keep joints moving safely, and avoid further damage to joints. The medications most often used to relieve pain and reduce inflammation are aspirin and nonsteroidal anti-inflammatory drugs such as ibuprofen. These drugs block the production of prostaglandins, which cause the pain and inflammation experienced by arthritis sufferers. Over-the-counter and prescription drugs for arthritis should always be taken under the supervision of a health professional. Nondrug treatments include applying hot or cold compresses, soaking in a warm bath, swimming in a heated pool, or applying ice packs to relieve the pain.

Exercise is also an important part of treatment for arthritis. Exercise helps keep joints moving and reduces pain. It also strengthens muscles around the affected joints and helps control body weight, which reduces the stress on joints. During an acute episode of the disease, rest may be important for a joint. A physical therapist can help develop a personal program that balances exercise and rest.

If joints become severely damaged and activity is limited, surgery may be considered as a treatment option. Damaged joints can be repaired or replaced. Because of their importance in maintaining mobility, hip and knee joints are those most commonly replaced.

Adapted from National Institute of Aging. 1991. "Arthritis Advice". In *Age Pages*. U.S. Department of Health and Human Services, National Institutes of Health.

Handling Psychological and Mental Changes

Many people associate old age with forgetfulness, and slowly losing one's memory was once considered an inevitable part of growing old. However, we now know that most elderly people in good health remain mentally alert.

Slight confusion and occasional forgetfulness may indicate only a temporary overload of facts on the brain or fatigue. Many people become smarter as they become older and more experienced.

Severe and significant brain deterioration in elderly individuals, called senility or **dementia,** affects about 7 percent of people under age 80 (the incidence rises sharply for people in their eighties and nineties). Early symptoms include slight disturbances in a person's ability to grasp the situation he or she is in; as dementia progresses, memory failure becomes apparent and people may forget conversations, the events of the day, or how to perform simple tasks. Dementia can be caused by many different factors, some of which are treatable, so it's important to

In the early 1900s, a German neurologist named Alois Alzheimer performed an autopsy on a patient in her mid-fifties whom he had diagnosed several years earlier with presenile dementia, a condition marked by mental deterioration, loss of memory, and unpredictable behavior and occurring before aging has advanced very far. Alzheimer had assumed that the cause was hardening of the arteries. On autopsy, however, he discovered no signs of arteriosclerosis. What he did discover was massive damage to nerve cells in the brain. The condition known as presenile dementia is now referred to as Alzheimer's disease.

Alzheimer's is a fatal brain disorder that causes physical and chemical changes in the brain. As nerve cells are destroyed in the brain, the system that produces the neurotransmitter acetylcholine breaks down, and communication among parts of the brain deteriorates. Autopsies reveal two other important characteristics: Nerve cells are packed with shriveled filaments known as tangles, and the tips of their branches are mired in plaques, clusters of degenerating nerve fibers.

To the layperson, Alzheimer's disease is synonymous with dementia, which literally means "deprived of mind." Among the elderly, Alzheimer's probably accounts for most cases of dementia, but there are at least 50 known disorders that can cause this condition. Many cases can be attributed to strokes or to Parkinson's disease. Deterioration from all three of these disorders is irreversible. Less common causes of dementia include brain injuries or tumors, chronic alcoholism, depression, vitamin B-12 deficiency, thyroid disease, and reaction to drugs taken for kidney or heart disease. Dementia from many of these causes can be reversed with treatment.

The first symptom of Alzheimer's disease is loss of memory. This doesn't mean that simple forgetfulness—forgetting a friend's birthday or where you left the car keys—is a sign. Rather, an afflicted person is likely to forget the identity of a familiar person or how to operate a familiar appliance such as a washing machine.

Other symptoms of the disease include confusion or disorientation, depression, anxiety, sleep disorders, and aggressive behavior. As the disease progresses, afflicted people lose the ability to function mentally. They experience a change in personality, a loss of identity. Eventually, they lose control of physical functioning, becoming incontinent and completely dependent on caregivers to feed and clothe them. On average, a person will live eight to ten years from the development of the first symptoms. Autopsy is the only certain way currently of diagnosing the disease.

Scientists do not yet know what causes Alzheimer's disease. Some researchers believe that a slow-acting virus is the cause. Others are investigating a link to environmental toxins; abnormal accumulations of aluminum found in the brain cells offer evidence for this theory. Still others believe that Alzheimer's is caused by a prion—a "proteinaceous infectious particle" that affects the genetic structure of cells.

Indeed, the disease does seem to have a genetic link, especially the form known as early-onset Alzheimer's disease (also called "familial Alzheimer's disease"). People who have early-onset Alzheimer's usually show symptoms before the age of 57; people with late-onset Alzheimer's on the other hand, may not show symptoms until well into their sixties. The early-onset form of the disease accounts for 10 to 30 percent of all cases. The chance of inheriting early-onset Alzheimer's disease is much greater than that of inheriting late-onset Alzheimer's.

According to the National Institute on Aging, about 10 percent of the adult population over the age of 65 has Alzheimer's disease, and about 47 percent of people over 85 have the disease. At any given time, an estimated 1.5 million to 4 million Americans suffer from the disease. Currently, it is the fourth leading cause of death for adults. As the population of aging Americans continues to grow, the disease will become more significant. By the year 2050 there may be 14 million Americans with Alzheimer's. Although there is no cure or treatment right now, research holds promise. Scientists are working on drugs to slow the progress of the disease and thus halt the decline of mental ability. When such drugs are developed, the burden of this tragic disease will be eased for both families and society.

Sources: K. Flieger. 1992. "Despite New Clues, Alzheimer's Mystery Remains Unsolved." *Healthline,* September; S. B. Prusiner. 1991. "Molecular Biology of Prion Diseases." *Science,* June; D. Chase and D. Lumpe. 1991. "Not All Memory Loss is Alzheimer's." *New Choices,* September.

have any symptoms evaluated by a health professional. Even for **Alzheimer's disease** and other incurable forms of dementia, appropriate treatment may greatly improve an afflicted person's quality of life (see the box "Alzheimer's Disease" for more information).

You can improve communication with a person suffering from dementia. Slow down and simplify what you are saying—dementia often means a person processes information more slowly. Avoid correcting mistakes in memory, and be patient with any repetition of ideas. Listen to the meaning behind the communication and be supportive.

Repeatedly telling stories about the past—something older people often do—doesn't necessarily indicate dementia. Reminiscence, the recollection of past personal experiences and significant events, is a normal part of development. Repeatedly telling the same stories allows an older person to integrate life by making past events

Year	Both Sexes	Men	Women
At birth:			
1900	47.3	46.3	48.3
1950	68.2	65.6	71.1
1960	69.7	66.6	73.1
1970	70.9	67.1	74.8
1980	73.7	70.0	77.4
1987	75.0	71.5	78.4
At age 65:			
1900–02	11.9	11.5	12.2
1950	13.9	12.8	15.0
1960	14.3	12.8	15.8
1970	15.2	13.1	17.0
1980	16.4	14.1	18.3
1987	16.9	14.8	18.7

Sources: 1900 to 1980 data: National Center for Health Statistics. 1989. *Health, United States, 1988.* Washington, D.C.: Department of Health and Human Services, DHHS Pub. No. (PHS)89–1232; 1987 data: National Center for Health Statistics. 1990. "Life Tables." *Vital Statistics of the United States, 1987,* vol.II, section 6. Washington, D.C.: Department of Health and Human Services.

meaningful in the present. Reminiscence can be of great significance to members of the younger generations because it is a rich source of social, cultural, and family history.

Another psychological and emotional challenge of aging is dealing with grief and mourning. Aging is associated with losses—friends, peers, physical appearance, possessions, and health. Grief is the work of getting through the pain of loss, and it can be one of the most lonely and intense times in a person's life. It can take a year or two to completely come to terms with the loss of a loved one and to establish a new model of the self without the loved one. (See Chapter 20 for more information about responses to loss and how to support a grieving person.)

Unresolved grief can have serious physical and mental health consequences and may require professional help. Signs of unresolved grief include hostility toward people connected with the death (physicians or nurses, for example), talking about the death as if it occurred yesterday, and unrealistic or harmful behavior (such as giving away all of one's own belongings). Many people become depressed after the loss of a loved one or when confronted with retirement or a chronic illness. But after a period of grieving, people are generally able to resume their lives.

Unresolved grief can lead to depression, a common problem among the elderly (see Chapter 3). If you notice the signs of depression in yourself or someone you know, consult a mental health professional. Listen carefully when an older friend or relative complains about being depressed—this may be a request for help. Suicide rates are relatively high among the elderly, so depression should be taken seriously. It is a mistake to believe that a depressed person will "snap out of it" or that people are too old to be helped. Both professional treatment and support groups can help people deal successfully with major life changes, such as retirement, moving, health problems, or loss of a spouse. If someone refuses help, be reassuring and stress that treatment helps make people feel better; in some cases, a mental health professional can make a home visit.

One of the most important ways of dealing with the changes associated with aging is to adopt a flexible attitude toward whatever life brings you. Self-enjoyment and acceptance can help make the later years more meaningful and enjoyable. The right attitude can also help stave off the negative effects of some circumstances. Acceptance of limitations, an optimistic outlook, and a sense of humor are tools that can help you cope with all of life's changes.

AGING AND LIFE EXPECTANCY

Human **life expectancy** is the average length of time we can expect to live. It is calculated by averaging mortality statistics—the ages of death of a group of people over a certain period of time. A woman born in the United States today has a longer life expectancy (78.3 years) than does her male counterpart (71.1 years). Individuals who reach their sixty-fifth birthday can expect to live even longer—17 more years or longer—because they have already survived hazards to life in the younger years (Table 19-1). The reason for the gender gap in life expectancy is not known, but estrogen production and other factors during a woman's fertile years appear to protect her from heart disease. Her risks increase after menopause. Increased male mortality can also be traced to smoking (lung cancer, heart, and respiratory disease), more accidents, and more alcoholism. Where these factors are not operative, as among the Amish, men live as long as women. Life expectancy also varies among racial and ethnic groups; reasons for these differences include socioeconomic, genetic, and lifestyle factors.

Life expectancy from birth in the United States has increased dramatically in this century, as described in

Chapter 1. This does not mean that every American now lives longer than in 1900; rather, far fewer people die young now, because childhood and infectious diseases are better controlled and diet and sanitation are much improved since 1900. In 1900 only 30 percent of the population lived to be 70 years old. In 1990 closer to 65 percent live to be 70.

How long can humans expect to live in the best of circumstances? It now seems possible that our maximum potential **life span** is about 100 or 110 years. (Although there are reports of very long-lived individuals, there is little evidence that anyone lives past age 110.) Failure to achieve that span in good health results to some degree from destructive environmental and behavioral factors—factors over which we can exert considerable control. Long life doesn't necessarily mean a longer period of disability, either. People often live longer because they have been well longer. A healthy, productive old age is very often an extension of a healthy, productive middle age. However, behavior changes cannot extend the maximum human life span, which seems to be built into our genes.

Throughout history people have searched for and invented a great variety of "magic" preparations, devices, and practices for preserving youth. None has ever worked. More recently, science has entered the arena and directed research toward aging. Researchers would like to break through the riddles of hormones and the cell to enable people to live longer and maintain much of their youthful vigor.

What causes the eventual breakdown of the body? No existing theory of aging accommodates all the facts, and it may be that aging is caused by a variety of different processes and affected by a variety of factors, both environmental and biological.

Biological theories can be divided into cellular and noncellular explanations for aging. Some aging processes may be built into individual cells; others seem to involve whole systems, such as the nervous system, the endocrine system, and the immune system. A cellular theory based on the genetic makeup of cells suggests that a cell contains "aging" genes that specify the exact number of times the cell can duplicate itself. The limiting number varies from species to species. This is why the maximum life span for fruit flies is about 100 days, for dogs about 25 to 30 years, for humans about 110 years, and for giant tortoises about 180 years. Another cellular theory suggests that errors in RNA/DNA protein synthesis cause structural or functional defects. These defects disable normal cell functioning, causing the cell to deteriorate. Errors in synthesis may occur randomly or through the effects of environmental factors such as radiation.

A theory of aging involving the immune system suggests that the body begins to err in synthesizing protein and produces proteins that the immune system cannot recognize. The immune system then attacks them as it would any foreign substance, destroying cells and impairing body functions. Alternatively, the immune system itself may weaken in old age, producing fewer antibodies to fight disease. Researchers are testing drugs that would reinforce faltering immune systems.

A theory of aging that focuses on metabolic function helps explain the immobility seen in old age. Connective tissue all over the body, such as collagen and elastic fibers, becomes stiffer and chemically immobilized with age. This is because by-products of metabolism, called cross-links, form between parallel collagen fibers, making it impossible for the two fibers to slip past each other or stretch.

Brain chemistry and hormones have also been implicated in aging. Levels of certain neurotransmitters—chemicals that transmit nerve impulses—are reduced in old age, preventing the brain from coordinating the functions of various glands and tissues. Experiments aimed at maintaining levels of certain neurotransmitters are being conducted to help slow down pathological aging. Changes in body hormones are also associated with the aging process. Although the use of testosterone has not been found useful in men, estrogen replacement therapy has been used successfully to treat problems associated with menopause and osteoporosis.

Is aging associated with decline in all areas of functioning? Some social theorists maintain that while the biological processes tend to break down with aging, psychological and social development continues. In his theory of psychosocial development, Erik Erikson described the last phase of life as one in which people look back over their lives in an attempt to integrate and accept who they are and what they've accomplished. This review of life and integration of events can be a catalyst for personal growth. Despite possible physical limitations, many of your elderly friends and relatives may be role models for the successful personal integration of life's experiences and the ability to adapt to life's changes and challenges.

Personal Insight What kinds of contact with older people did you have when you were growing up? Were these experiences positive or negative? How have they affected your current attitudes toward aging and elderly people?

Life expectancy The average length of life of members of a species.
Life span Theoretically projected length of life based on maximum potential of the human body in the best environment.

TERMS

As life expectancies increase, a larger proportion of the population will be in the later years; this change will necessitate new government policies and changes in our general attitudes toward elderly people.

America's Aging Minority

People over 65 are a large minority in the American population—over 30 million people, 12 percent of the total population in the 1990s. (For a statistical look at the elderly in America, see Figure 19-1.) As birth rates drop, the percentage is increasing dramatically. Many older people are happy, healthy, and self-sufficient. Changes that come with age, including negative ones, normally occur so gradually that most people adapt, some even gracefully.

Today the status of the aging is improving more than ever before. People now in their forties and fifties will probably benefit from new knowledge about the aging process. And the enormous increase in the over-55 population is markedly affecting our stereotypes of what it means to grow old. The misfortunes associated with aging—frailty, forgetfulness, poor health, isolation—occur to fewer people in their sixties and seventies and are shifting instead to burden the very old, those over 85.

The "younger" elderly who are in good physical and mental health are gaining status in our society; politicians are listening to them; advertisers have targeted them as a good market. The elderly are, in general, better off than they have ever been in the past. They have more money than they did 20 years ago. The poverty rate of the elderly dropped from 28.5 percent in 1966 to 11.4 percent in 1989, largely from the effects of Social Security payments and health care benefits from Medicare. About three-quarters of elderly Americans own their homes. Their living expenses are lower after retirement because they no longer support children and have fewer work-related expenses; they consume and buy less food. They are more likely to continue practicing their expertise for years after retirement and to be paid in cash. Thousands of retired consultants, teachers, technicians, and craftspeople work until their middle and late seventies. They receive greater amounts of assistance, such as Medicare, pay proportionately lower taxes, and have greater net worth from lifetime savings.

As the aging population increases proportionately, however, the number of older people who are ill and dependent rises. Health care remains the largest expense for older adults. On average, they visit a physician eight times a year and are hospitalized more frequently and require twice as many prescription drugs as the general population. Tens of thousands of older Americans live in poverty, particularly minorities and women living alone. These other elderly—poverty-stricken, isolated, lonely—are just as ignored as they ever were. Their numbers are increasing: Of all people above the age of 65, more than 12 percent live below the "official" poverty line. About a fifth of the poor elderly live in central city poverty areas. Single black women fare worst: About 64 percent are poor.

Retirement finds many older people with their incomes reduced to subsistence levels. This is especially true of the very old. The majority of older Americans live with fixed sources of income, such as pensions, that are eroded by inflation. Expenses tend to increase more rapidly, especially those due to circumstances over which people have little or no control, such as deteriorating health. Many elderly Americans rely on **Social Security** payments as their only source of income; they are not covered by other types of retirement plans. Social Security was intended to serve as a supplement to personal savings and private pensions, not as a sole source of income. A number of pension plans do provide adequate incomes to retirees; these include the Federal Retirement system, the Teachers Insurance and Annuity Association, and many union and company plans. However, if a company closes down, an employee is laid off, or the pension plan is not adequately managed, an individual could face many years of poverty. For this reason, it is vital that people plan early for an adequate retirement income.

Family and Community Resources for the Elderly

With help from friends, family members, and community services, elderly people can remain active and independent. About 70 percent of elderly Americans live with a spouse or other family member; 25 percent live alone or with a nonrelative. Only 5 percent of people over age 65 live in nursing homes or other institutional settings.

Family Involvement in Caregiving Most families do not abandon their elderly relatives when they need help. Studies show that in about three out of four cases, a grown daughter or daughter-in-law assumes a caregiving role for elderly relatives. This may mean bringing them into the home, helping them remain in their own homes, or arranging for alternative housing (see the box "Living and Care Options for the Elderly"). With more parents living into their eighties and with fewer children per family, many people, especially women, will face the choice of how to care for an aging relative. Recent surveys indicate that the average woman will spend about 17 years raising children and 18 years caring for an aging relative.

TERMS

Social Security A government program that provides financial assistance to people who are unemployed, disabled, or retired (and over a certain age); financed through taxes on business and workers.

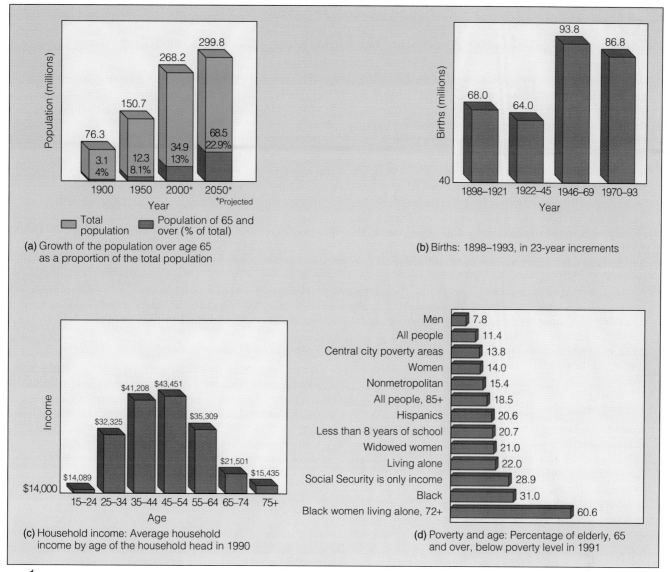

VITAL STATISTICS

Figure 19-1 *A statistical look at the elderly in America.*

Sources: U.S. Bureau of the Census. 1992. *Statistical Abstract of the United States,* 112th ed. (Washington, D.C.: U.S. Government Printing Office.) U.S. Senate Special Committee on Aging. 1991. *Aging America: Trends and Projections.* (Washington, D.C.: U.S. Department of Health and Human Services.) U.S. Bureau of the Census. 1989. *Historical Statistics of the United States, Colonial Times to 1970,* 3rd ed. (Washington, D.C.: U.S. Government Printing Office).

Caregiving can bring moments of closeness and joy, but it is also hard work. If the experience is stressful and continues over a long period of time, family members may become emotionally exhausted ("burned out"). Caregivers should avail themselves of available community services and be sure to consider their own needs for relaxation and relief from caregiving duties. A rested and relaxed caregiver is better able to provide care. Professional health care advice regarding the physical and mental well-being of the person being cared for is another critical part of successful home care.

The best thing a family can do to prepare for the task of caring for aging parents is to talk frankly about the future. What does everyone expect will happen? What living and caring options are available and which do family members prefer? What community resources are available? Planning ahead can reduce the stress on everyone involved and help ease difficult transitions.

Community Resources Different kinds of community resources are available to help elderly people remain active and in their own homes. The key to success is matching services with the needs of the individual person. Typical services include the following:

When we think of living and care options for the elderly, nursing homes usually come to mind. However, there are several alternatives to nursing homes. Choosing the option that is right for you or an elderly family member depends on income, level of functioning, and personal preferences. Let's take a look at these options.

Living Independently

Some elders prefer to remain in their own homes. This is a good choice for those who would benefit from familiar surroundings; however, it calls for adequate financial resources, good health, a safe neighborhood, and a stimulating social life. And since few elders manage to remain completely independent until death, they and their families must consider the availability of community resources such as home assistance programs. Home assistance programs may include adult day programs that provide social and rehabilitative health care services, delivered meals, and transportation services. Programs such as these, along with paid caregivers, can extend the period of time elders can remain in their own homes.

Homesharing

Homesharing, shared living situations arranged by agencies that specialize in recruiting and matching like-minded individuals, is an option for elders who find it difficult to maintain their own homes due to financial, social, or personal constraints. Homesharing offers elders who are mobile and in fairly good health the opportunity for stimulating new relationships, either with peers or with a younger family. In addition, intergenerational homesharing may relieve elders of transportation problems, chores, and other physical tasks which can be taken care of by younger household members.

Reassembling

Reassembling refers to aging parents and adult children who decide to live together again for economic or health reasons, the death of a spouse, or other circumstances. Reassembling requires a great deal of time, energy, and discussion. For one thing, as parents live longer, reassembling is likely to take place when the adult child is at or near retirement age. And if the aging parent is in poor health, families must consider the burden of constant care. Home assistance programs, like respite care, which allows temporary relief for caregivers, may alleviate some of this burden. On the positive side, however, elders in good health can help busy, working families with household duties and child care.

Retirement Communities

Retirement communities present a good option for individuals in good health, with a good income, who want to maintain home ownership. These communities typically offer social and recreational activities and maintenance services to their residents. There are many types of retirement communities available to the elderly, varying in cost and atmosphere. Personal preference and financial concerns dictate the type of retirement home an elder may choose.

- Senior citizens' centers or adult day care centers, which may offer meals, group social activities, and some health services for seniors unable to be alone during the day
- Homemaker services, which may include light housekeeping, cooking, running errands, doing shopping, and providing escort service
- Visiting nurses, who provide some basic health care services
- Household services, which may include basic household repairs and seasonal work
- Friendly visitor or daily telephone reassurance services, which provide daily contacts for elderly who live alone and may feel isolated
- Home food delivery services, which provide daily meals to homebound seniors
- Adult day hospital care, which provides day care plus physical therapy and treatment for chronic illnesses

- Low-cost legal aid, which can help in management of finances and health care

Sometimes elderly people refuse services. They may worry about the cost, be confused about what the service offers, be unwilling to accept "charity," or want to avoid feeling dependent on others. You can help an elderly friend or relative to accept needed services by providing accurate information about the services and stressing that they are designed to help the person remain independent. It may help to have an older friend of your relative suggest the service. When cost is a problem, some people offer to make arrangements for payment or to pay part or all of the cost of the service as a gift. Services can usually be located by looking in the phone book under local government agencies or in the yellow pages under "Senior Citizens' Services."

Transportation   Driving a car is an important status symbol in our society. It is one of the rites of passage com-

Living and Care Options for the Elderly (continued)

Nursing Homes

The decision to place a family member in a nursing home often brings feelings of grief and remorse. These days, however, the picture is not so grim—considerable evidence suggests that the typical nursing home has improved in quality over the past several decades. Quality has a price tag, however—nursing homes are very expensive, costing as much or more than the average household income for a 45- to 54-year-old per year. And only nursing homes with certified skilled care are eligible for Medicare coverage.

There are several options available in nursing home care. Residential care facilities provide room and board, and some offer social and recreational programs. Continuing care communities include room and board plus personal and health care and social activities. Assisted living facilities include retirement homes and board and care homes. Services range widely from place to place but usually include meals and help with personal care. Skilled nursing facilities provide 24-hour nursing care and supervision with emphasis on improving or maintaining personal care skills.

How do you go about finding a good nursing home? If you need help, seek out the little-known ombudsperson service in your state—it helps families find the right nursing home for aging parents at no cost. To get further information, call your state office on aging. If you are looking for a nursing home on your own, plan ahead—the best nursing homes have long waiting lists. And don't start *after* you or your aging relative is too sick to function independently. Once you are sure nursing home placement is necessary, ask physicians, friends, clergy, or the health department for rec-

ommendations. Then start visiting the homes, keeping the following evaluation points in mind:

- First, determine what you want in a nursing home. Level of care required, proximity to a hospital or family members, and the kind and number of activities offered are typical issues to consider.

- To get a realistic picture, visit the facility during meal or activity times, not on open house days, or drop in unannounced on a weekday.

- Check the rooms—look at the quality and condition of furnishings and notice whether personal possessions have been brought from home.

- Look for friendly interactions among residents and a friendly and supportive staff.

- Notice the physical, emotional, and mental condition of the residents. Talk to them and/or their visitors. Ask if they are satisfied with the home. Ask if residents have access to a staff person to help them resolve complaints.

- Be wary of any home where more than a few residents are restrained. Also be wary if a lot of residents seem drugged or overmedicated, and keep an eye out for residents who appear dehydrated (with very dry skin and mouth and sunken eyeballs).

Making decisions about living and care options for the elderly can seem overwhelming, but proper planning will result in finding the best situation for you or a loved one.
Sources: T. Adams and K. Armstrong. 1992. "What Children Can Do for Elderly Parents." *San Francisco Chronicle,* 20 October. "Help Finding a Nursing Home." *Changing Times,* May 1990.

---

pleted by teenagers and maintained throughout adulthood. Older drivers usually have safe driving records compared with young adults because they tend to be more cautious; however, accidents in the older age group are more likely to be fatal. Many states require special driver's testing for people over age 70 and may restrict some drivers as to the time, area, and distances they may drive. Because of changes in vision or other health problems, some older drivers may be required to give up their license before they feel ready. Elderly people report that the loss of a driver's license and the loss of independence that it brings is one of the most severe hardships they face.

Older people who no longer have a driver's license must investigate and use other forms of transportation. These include buses, some of which are specially designed for people with disabilities; friends and family members with cars; taxis; dial-a-ride services; and volunteer drivers for seniors. Community agencies can help match seniors with appropriate forms of transportation.

Whatever their circumstances, elderly people have the same needs as people at any other stage of life, including the need to feel that their lives have meaning. Becoming dependent on others for daily care and transportation is difficult for many people to accept. Most caregivers are motivated by love and responsibility and want to do the best they can for their aging friend or relative. However, some situations can lead to abuse, physical or economic (see the box "Abuse of the Elderly"). Assistance for both caregivers and seniors is available, including respite care for caregivers and legal and protective services for abused elders.

Personal Insight How do you think you would react if you had to care for an elderly parent or grandparent? Could you be patient or would you lose your temper frequently? What experiences make you answer the way you do?

Before 1979, elder abuse was scarcely an issue in the public mind. But that year, a federally funded research project in Boston published its study on the subject, and what it revealed shocked the nation. Reports of battering, neglect, and mistreatment by family members and other caregivers led to the creation of an extensive system of laws designed to protect older individuals from abuse.

Abuse of the elderly is a serious problem in America among all ethnic and economic groups. More than 140,000 cases of physical abuse are reported each year, although health care workers suggest that fewer than 20 percent of all cases are reported. It is estimated that 1.1 million older Americans experience abuse of some kind. Most victims are 75 or older.

Typically, abusers are family members. Roughly half of all abusers are children or other relatives of the elderly person. The victim's spouse is the abuser in about 40 percent of cases.

Types of Abuse

Abuse by close family members is likely to take the form of verbal abuse, moderate physical abuse (slapping, pushing, hitting with objects), or psychological abuse, such as ignoring the person's presence. Victims may feel too ashamed and humiliated to do anything about it; they may fear reprisal or the possibility of abandonment; or they may not even recognize that they are being abused.

About 75 percent of all abuse cases involve elders who are dependent on others for daily care (bathing, dressing, eating, and so on). Often, the person has lost mental and physical functions as a result of stroke, Alzheimer's disease, or other brain disorder. In these instances, neglect is probably the most serious type of abuse. The victim may suffer malnutrition, dehydration, mismanaged medication, or infection due to poor hygiene.

Physical abuse is the most serious form of abuse, but financial exploitation may be the most common. This includes taking control of financial assets, stealing government benefit checks, and conning the victim to make investments. Distant relatives and acquaintances often are responsible for this form of abuse.

Abandonment may be considered another form of abuse. An estimated 100,000 to 200,000 elderly are abandoned at hospitals each year. "Dumping" of the elderly in public places happens rarely but usually makes the news. These are acts of desperate caregivers, frustrated by the economic and physical demands of caring for an aged friend or relative.

Why Does Abuse Occur?

Caring for a dependent adult can be stressful, especially if the elder is incontinent, has suffered mental deterioration, or is violent. Abuse may become an outlet for frustration. Typically, however, some or all of the following characteristics are present:

- A pattern of physical abuse already exists in the family.
- The caregiver abuses alcohol or drugs.
- The caregiver suffers mental illness.
- The caregiver is the least capable member of the family—the least financially secure, the least skilled, or the most distant relative.

What Can Be Done?

During the 1980s, 43 states passed laws requiring health care workers to report any injuries or conditions suggesting elder abuse to state authorities. Most of these laws are patterned after child abuse laws. But these laws are coming under scrutiny, especially by special interest groups representing the elderly. Some experts say the laws strip the elderly of their right to a confidential relationship with their physician, as well as their right to make their own decisions. They believe that most older Americans do not need such protection and that it wastes time and money. And in fact, about 40 percent of elderly Americans are independent, and most are financially secure; they can speak for themselves and make their own decisions.

In spite of differing opinions over elder abuse laws, there seems to be widespread agreement on the real solution to the problem of elder abuse. The solution is support—that is, greater social assistance. Adult day-care centers, for example, provide needed relief for caregivers. What families need most of all is financial help in caring for aged relatives. They need to be able to earn a living while simultaneously providing round-the-clock care, if necessary. Some officials believe that preventing abuse is the solution, and that education and public care programs are steps toward prevention.

Adapted from J. S. Shapiro. 1992. "The Elderly Are Not Children." *U.S. News and World Report.* 13 January.

Government Aid and Policies

The government assists elderly people through several programs, such as food stamps, housing subsidies, Social Security, Medicare, and Medicaid. Social Security, the life insurance and old-age pension plan, has saved many from destitution, although it is intended not as a sole source of income but as a supplement to other income. Social Security funds are currently being used to cover other government financial deficits, so the future solvency of the program is uncertain.

Medicare is a major health insurance program for the elderly and the disabled. It has two parts—Part A is financed by part of the payroll FICA) tax that also pays for

Social Security; Part B is financed by monthly premiums paid by people who choose to enroll. Part A helps pay for inpatient hospital care, some inpatient care in a skilled nursing facility, and some types of home and hospice care. Medicare Part B helps pay for physicians' services and other medical supplies and services not covered by Part A.

Medicare pays about 30 percent of the medical costs of the elderly. But serious gaps in Medicare coverage require elderly people to pay for some health care expenses out of their own pockets. Medicare provides basic health care coverage for acute episodes of illness that require skilled professional care; it does not pay for custodial or preventive care, including most expenses for routine checkups, dental care and dentures, immunizations, and prescription drugs. Over a million elderly people currently live in nursing homes; but Medicare pays less than 2 percent of nursing home costs, and private insurers pay less than 1 percent, creating a tremendous financial burden for elderly nursing home residents and their families. People on Medicare need to inquire whether their physician will accept Medicare payments and whether they will be responsible for additional payments. Due to these gaps in coverage, many elderly are joining managed health care plans to get more health care for their money.

When their financial resources are exhausted, elderly people may apply for the Medicaid program. Medicaid is run and funded by individual states; it is designed to help those with low incomes and few resources. The federal government helps pay for Medicaid, but each state has its own rules regarding coverage and eligibility.

A crucial question in aid for the elderly is, "Who will pay for it?" The government picks up a substantial share of the health expenses of the elderly, primarily through Medicare and Medicaid. Personal health care expenditures are about 12 percent of the U.S. gross national product, and about one-third of these expenditures go to care for the elderly. The average government expenditure for personal health services for those over age 65 is three to four times greater than that for people under age 65.

Many health planners believe that instead of adding stopgap measures to Medicare and Medicaid, the government should address the issue of health insurance for the elderly in the context of an overall national health care policy. Many difficult and complex issues need attention, including the lack of health insurance for more than 30 million Americans, the rising cost of nursing home care, the declining condition of the hospital system, and the high rate of infant mortality. Since resources are ultimately limited, difficult decisions have to be made and priorities have to be established.

In the meantime, health policy planners hope that rising medical costs for the elderly will dwindle dramatically through education and prevention. Health professionals, including **gerontologists** and **geriatricians**, are beginning to practice preventive medicine, just as pediatricians

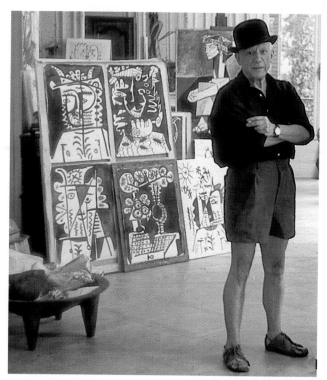

Some extraordinary individuals defy all preconceived ideas about old age. Picasso, in his seventies when this picture was taken, lived an intensely vigorous and creative life right up until his death at the age of 92.

do. They advise older people on how to avoid and, if necessary, how to manage disabilities. They try to instill an ethic of bodily and mental maintenance that will prevent chronic disease and allow older people to live long, healthy, vigorous lives.

Changing the Public's Idea of Aging

Aging people may be one of our least used and least appreciated resources (for another view of aging and elderly people, see the box "Words of Wisdom: Attitudes Toward Aging Among Native Americans and Hispanic Americans"). How can we employ the knowledge and productivity of our growing numbers of older citizens, particularly those now leaving the workforce through mandatory early retirement?

First, we must change our thinking about what aging means. We must learn to judge productivity rather than age. Capacity to function should replace age as a criterion for usefulness. Instead of singling out 65 as a magic num-

Gerontologist   One who studies the biological, psychological, and social phenomena associated with aging and old age.
Geriatrician   A physician specializing in the diseases, disabilities, and care of the elderly.

TERMS

DIMENSIONS OF DIVERSITY

Words of Wisdom: Attitudes Toward Aging Among Native Americans and Hispanic Americans

The following is excerpted from an article written by Dr. Robert Coles, a professor of psychiatry and medical humanities at Harvard Medical School.

Why are so many Americans afraid of growing old? This question occurred to me often during the three years my wife and I lived in New Mexico and Arizona. Not a day went by when we weren't reminded of how much Native American and Hispanic families value old age. These are cultures that grant dignity and authority to their elders.

One young Hispanic woman described to us her relationship with her parents, both in their seventies, in this way: "When I am wondering what to do about a problem, I turn to my mother or my father. Even if they are not here, I still turn to them. I picture them in my mind and I hear them saying words that make good sense." One day, this woman's father made a show of his humorous and practical good sense before his young grandson. "You know what my son said to me that night when he was going to bed?" the woman asked. "He told me he wished he could be old like his grandpapa!"

In another town, a Pueblo woman told us, "When my children ask me what it means to be a Pueblo Indian, I point to my parents, and I don't even talk." The woman went on to describe how her mother enhanced her own life. "She wants me to remember that the land, our land, was here before I came, and it will be here after I have left. 'We are visitors,' she always says, 'so we should be grateful for every day and

not waste time with stupid things.' That is why old people are here, to remind us of what is important and what is not."

To be old is to "last" oneself—to go through ups and downs, to survive bad luck and avoid successfully all sorts of hazards. To be old, then, is to be blessed by fate, by chance and circumstance. Pueblo Indians know that. One Hopi child drew me a picture of an old woman shaking hands with the moon. Then she explained, "When you're old, you're a full moon; you make the night a little less dark." For Hopi children, an older person is a source of encouragement, instruction, inspiration, a part of nature's awesome presence.

For many young people living in other parts of America, old age is regarded not as a major achievement but rather as a last, sad, brief way station. One boy in Boston commented, "It's no fun to be old; it's the worst thing in the world, except to die." To many of us, old age means abandonment, rejection, loneliness, a loss of respect from others, and subsequently a loss of self-respect. This is not the case, though, in Hispanic and Native American cultures. The elders we met in New Mexico and Arizona showed a great deal of self-confidence, and in general they seemed contented with their lives. In their contentment and harmony with nature lies a lesson for all of us.

Adapted from: R. Coles. 1989. "Full-Moon Wisdom." In *New Choices for the Best Years,* September.

---

ber, we could consider ages 50 to 75 as the third quarter of life. Changes occur around 50 that signal a new era: Children are usually grown and gone; a person has reached the maximum level of advancement in employment and highest real earnings. The upper end of the quarter is determined by the fact that most people today are vigorous, in good health, mentally alert, and capable of making a productive contribution until they are at least 75 years old. That age estimate may be a bit high for some, but not for most. About 20 percent of the population—50 million people—falls within the third quarter. But 25 years from now, about 85 million will be in their third quarter.

Other formulas have been suggested for drawing the boundary line between middle and old age. Rather than counting from birth, we could count back a fixed number of years from the expected age at death. Using a current life table, we could calculate the age at which the average number of remaining years of life is 15. That would place old age around 67 today and 72 in the year 2030. Another way to decide who is old would be to limit the

group to the most elderly 10 percent of the population, which would fix the age at 75 in 2030.

Whatever way we define old age, the costs of losing what these people can contribute to our national productivity and quality of life are too high. Through their early retirement we forfeit substantial income-tax and Social Security tax revenues on their earnings. Those who retire at 62 start using their Social Security benefits earlier than otherwise.

A far better arrangement would be to make available full- and part-time volunteer and paid employment. We would benefit by providing retraining programs for both occupational and leisure time activities. We need more community-sponsored classes in remunerative activities such as real estate selling and management, horticulture, and library work, and in recreational and self-improvement activities such as music, writing, and health maintenance. Volunteer opportunities, such as preparing recordings for the blind, helping with activities for the retarded, and performing necessary tasks in hospitals, could be expanded. At the same time we could possibly change both public and private pension programs to make partial retirement possible. In such cases we could allow people to borrow against their Social Security benefits to finance their retraining or enrollment in wholly new educational programs.

There can be benefits to aging, but they don't come automatically. They require planning and wise choices earlier in life. One octogenarian, Russell Lee, founder of a medical clinic in California, perceived the advantages of aging as growth: "The limitations imposed by time are compensated by the improved taste, sharper discretion, sounder mental and esthetic judgment, increased sensitivity and compassion, clearer focus—which all contribute to a more certain direction in living. . . . The later years can be the best of life for which the earlier ones were preparation."

SUMMARY

- People who take charge of their health in youth have greater control over the physical and mental aspects of aging.

Generating Vitality as You Age

- Biological aging takes place over a lifetime, but some of the other changes associated with aging are more abrupt. The more people prepare for aging, the more likely they are to be satisfied with their middle and old ages.

- Many characteristics traditionally considered to be consequences of aging are due rather to neglect and abuse of body and mind. Nevertheless, aging is inevitable, a result of biochemical processes.

- A lifetime of interests and hobbies helps maintain creativity and intelligence.

- Exercise throughout life enhances physical and mental health; it may prevent deterioration of fluid intelligence with age.

- A low-fat, high-carbohydrate diet that includes a variety of foods promotes health at every age. Obesity leads to premature aging.

- Alcohol impairs liver and kidney function; tobacco use not only shortens life but also may cause severe health impairment for many years.

- Regular physical examinations help detect conditions that can shorten life and make old age less healthy. Immunizations protect against preventable infectious diseases.

- Stress increases wear and tear on the body; getting enough sleep, avoiding drugs, and practicing relaxation help reduce stress.

Confronting the Changes of Aging

- Retirement can be a fulfilling and enjoyable time of life for those who adjust to their new roles, enjoy participating in a variety of activities, and have planned ahead for financial stability.

- Decreased energy levels require older people to set priorities for their activities. Successful aging involves anticipating and accommodating physical limitations.

- Slight confusion and forgetfulness are not signs of a serious illness; severe symptoms may indicate Alzheimer's disease or another form of dementia. Reminiscing about past events can help older people integrate these events into their lives.

- Resolving grief and mourning and dealing with depression are important tasks for older adults; adopting a flexible attitude can help.

Aging and Life Expectancy

- Life expectancy, which has risen dramatically in the 1900s, is generally greater among women. Life expectancy increases with age.

- The maximum potential human life span seems to be 100 to 110 years; environmental and behavioral factors prevent most people from achieving it.

- Cells may contain "aging" genes or may begin synthesizing defective proteins after a certain point. The immune system may attack proteins it doesn't recognize, or it may itself become weaker in old age.

- Connective tissue in the body becomes stiffer with age and leads to some of the inflexibility of old age.

- Neurotransmitters and hormones seem to be involved in the aging process.

- Elderly people can be role models for the successful integration of life's experiences and the ability to adapt to challenges.

Life in an Aging America

- People over 65 form a large minority in the United States, and their status is improving.

- Those of the aged who are ill and dependent—often those who were already poor—experience major social and economic problems.

- About three-quarters of all elderly people are cared for by their spouse or by family members, usually daughters and daughters-in-law.

- Community resources for the elderly can help them stay active and independent. Programs include day activities, help with household chores, meal delivery, medical services, legal aid, and transportation.

- Government aid to the elderly includes food stamps, housing subsidies, Social Security, Medicare, and Medicaid. Medicare does not cover all medical expenses, especially those related to chronic diseases and nursing homes. The question of paying for medical care for the elderly has received much attention, but difficult decisions still need to be made.
- Preventive medicine is as important for the elderly as for the rest of the population and may help reduce medical costs.
- The aged represent an underused resource; society needs to learn to consider productivity and capacity to function rather than age.

TAKE ACTION

1. Interview your parents or grandparents to find out how they want to spend their old age. Do they want to live at home, in a retirement community, with a relative? Do they plan to live on a pension, retirement account, Social Security? Have they made any concrete plans, or have they not yet confronted those decisions?

2. Investigate and if possible visit the different facilities in your community for the elderly—nursing homes, hospitals, senior citizen centers, recreational programs. What do you like about them and what do you dislike? Do you have suggestions for improvement?

3. Interview several people from different cultural backgrounds about their attitudes toward aging and elderly people. How do they view the aging process? How are elderly people treated or viewed in their culture? Do you notice any significant differences between their attitudes and yours?

JOURNAL ENTRY

1. Imagine that you are very old and are looking back on your life. What will have given you satisfaction—a successful career, parenthood, happiness, travel, self-knowledge? Make a list in your health journal of your life goals and priorities. What actions can you take now to work toward your goals? Choose one goal and take an action this week that moves you toward it.

2. *Critical Thinking:* Assuming that government funding for medical care is limited, should more money be allocated for children's services or for medical care for elderly people? Write a brief essay making a case for each side of the debate. Provide evidence to support each position.

SELECTED BIBLIOGRAPHY

Adler, L. 1991. *Centenarians: People over 100 a Triumph of Will and Spirit.* New York: Heal Press

Aging: It ain't necessarily so. 1989. *University of California at Berkeley Wellness Letter*, June.

Aging successfully: How to succeed at the business of growing older. 1992. *Mayo Clinic Health Letter*, November.

Cole, T. R., and S. A. Gadow, eds. 1986. *What Does It Mean to Grow Old? Reflections from the Humanities.* Durham: Duke University Press.

Cox, H. 1991. *Annual Editions: Aging.* New York: Dushkin.

Dychtwald, K., and J. Flower. 1989. *Age Wave.* Los Angeles: Jeremy P. Tarcher.

Enders, R. 1991. *A Country Lawyer's Essays on Estate Planning and Aging.* New York: SOS.

Late-life love. 1992. *Harvard Health Letter*, November.

Pifer, A., and L. Bronte. 1986. *Our Aging Society.* New York: W. W. Norton.

Porter, S. 1991. *Planning Your Retirement.* New York: Prentice-Hall.

Porterfield, J. D., and R. St. Pierre. 1992. *Healthful Aging.* New York: Dushkin.

Rosenfeld, A. 1985. *Prolongevity II.* New York: Alfred A. Knopf.

Sherman, C. 1992. The aging process: How to cope with growing older. *San Francisco Chronicle*, 20 October, G1, G6.

U.S. Department of Health and Human Services. 1992. *The Medicare Handbook.* Washington, D.C.: Health Care Financing Administration.

RECOMMENDED READINGS

Biracree, T., and N. Biracree. 1991. *Over 50: The Resource Book for the Better Half of Your Life.* New York: HarperCollins. *Offers comprehensive advice and information on finances, health care, recreation, housing, and social life; includes directories of government agencies and private organizations.*

Goldsmith, S. 1990. *Choosing a Nursing Home.* Englewood Cliffs, N.J.: Prentice-Hall. *A practical guide for families seeking the best possible nursing home for an elderly relative.*

Humphreys, H. 1989. *Take Charge! A Step-by-Step Guide to Managing Your Money.* Ashland, Oreg.: Gatehouse Books. *A workbook with worksheets and information to help people plan for retirement.*

McGivney, S. A., and J. H. McGivney. 1989. *Eternally Young: A Guide to Aging Well.* New York: Ageless Publishing. *A practical guide to optimizing quality of life for people over age 50 and their families.*

Silverstone, B. and H. K. Human. 1989. *You and Your Aging Parent: A Family Guide to Emotional, Physical and financial Problems,* 3rd ed. New York: Pantheon Books. *Contains essential information for families of aging parents; includes extensive coverage of community services and financial and medical assistance programs.*

For more information about retirement planning and other issues that affect the lives of older people, contact the American Association of Retired Persons, 601 E Street, N.W., Washington, D.C. 20049.

20

Dying and Death

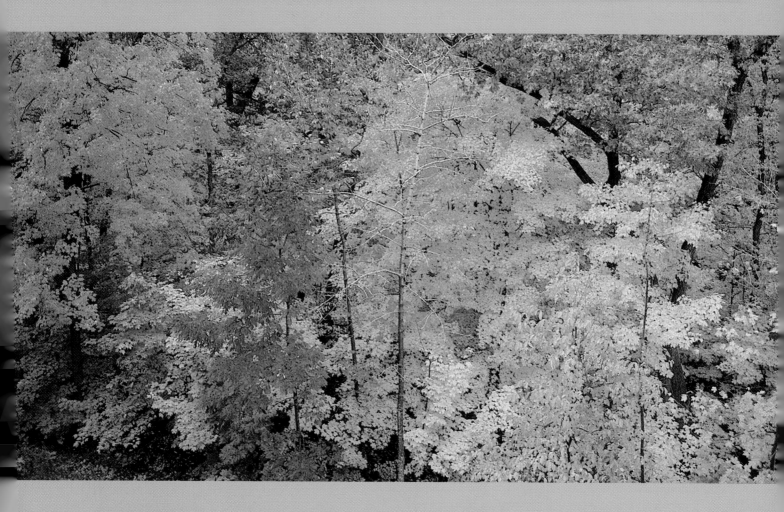

An older neighbor has asked you to witness the signing of a document he calls a "living will." He says it tells a hospital not to take any extraordinary measures to keep him alive if he's ever critically injured or ill and has no hope of recovery. "You know," he says, "it tells them to go ahead and pull the plug." You're hesitant about witnessing the document. Is it legal? Is it really ethical to make or carry out such a request? What should you do?

Your parents are in their sixties, and your sister says she wants to talk to them sometime soon about planning for death. She wants to know how they want their bodies disposed of, whether they want to die in a hospital or at home, whether they want heroic measures taken to keep them alive, and what kinds of funerals they want. You feel extremely uncomfortable about discussing these topics with your parents, and you think they would be offended if you brought them up. Your sister reminds you that both your grandfathers died of heart attacks before they were 60. She thinks it's important to talk to your parents now, while they're still healthy, but she won't if you strongly disagree. Are you right to want to protect your parents from this discussion, or is your sister right to bring it up? What should you do?

Your parents recently found out that your grandmother is terminally ill and has only about four months to live. Your mother wants to bring her to your home to spend her last days with your family. Your father is against the idea—he thinks that it would be too disruptive of family life, that caring for your grandmother full-time would place too great a burden on your mother, and that the family lacks the necessary skills and experience to provide adequate care. As far as you know, are there any alternatives or resources that might be helpful to your parents in this situation? What information or advice can you offer?

Your cousin's wife died recently after being ill for only a few weeks. At first your cousin didn't seem to be having any emotional reaction to her death at all. Surrounded by friends and relatives, he kept busy by arranging her funeral and taking care of legal and business arrangements. Now that he's finishing those tasks, he's showing some emotion but not the emotion you expected. Instead of being sad he seems angry—at the world, at himself, even at his late wife. At a recent family dinner, he said things that seem unrealistic to you, such as: "She wouldn't have died if she really loved me" and "It's my fault that she got sick and died." Is your cousin all right? You wonder if you should suggest that he try to calm down and not talk about things that upset him so much. How should you respond, and what can you do to help?

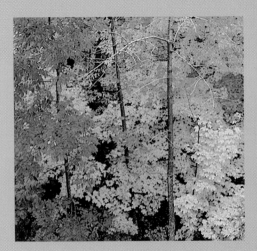

MAKING CONNECTIONS

No one gets out of this world alive, but many of us act as if we will. Learning to accept and deal with death is a difficult but important part of life, a process that requires information, insight, and commitment, just as simpler life tasks do. In each of the scenarios presented on this page, all related to dying and death, individuals have to use information, make a decision, or choose a course of action. How would you act in each of these situations? What response or decision would you make? This chapter provides information about dying and death that can be used in situations like these. After finishing the chapter, read the scenarios again. Has what you've learned changed how you would respond?

A man hiking a high mountain trail suddenly lost his footing and found himself hurtling toward certain death. As he plummeted past a small bush growing out of the sheer rock wall, he caught a berry in his hand and ate it. It was the most delicious berry he had ever eaten. We are each that man, hurtling toward certain death. How we deal with our mortality has a lot to do with how we live our lives.

If you suddenly discovered you had a terminal illness, how would you spend your last year or months? What kind of final ceremony would your family have? How would you wish to dispose of your possessions? Have you ever discussed these things with your family?

WHAT IS DEATH?

Death, like life, is change. When the body is no longer able to resist unhealthy changes in itself or is mechanically broken beyond repair, it ceases to function and dies.

Defining Death

Traditionally, death has been defined in clinical terms as occurring when the heart stops beating and breathing ceases. Defining death in this way—as cessation of the flow of vital bodily fluids—is adequate for determining death in most cases. However, the use of respirators and other **life-support systems** in modern medicine allows some bodily functions to be artificially sustained. To determine death in such cases requires investigating the presence or absence of a physical response other than heartbeat or breathing.

Medical scientists now agree that the brain is the physical locus for determining whether a person is alive or dead. Thus, when a body is being kept alive on a respirator, for example, death is determined by measuring brain-wave activity. According to the standards published in 1968 by a Harvard Medical School committee, four characteristics describe **brain death:** (1) lack of receptivity and response to external stimuli, (2) absence of spontaneous muscular movement and spontaneous breathing, (3) absence of observable reflexes, and (4) absence of brain activity, signified by a flat **electroencephalogram** (EEG). The Harvard criteria call for a second set of tests to be performed after 24 hours have elapsed. They also exclude cases of hypothermia (body temperature below 90° F) as well as situations involving the presence of central nervous system depressants, such as barbiturates. Most states have adopted legislation that redefines death according to these criteria when conventional methods of determining death prove inconclusive.

In contrast to **clinical death,** which is determined according to the criteria just discussed, **cellular death** refers to a gradual process that takes place when heartbeat, respiration, and brain activity have stopped. It encompasses the breakdown of metabolic processes in the cells, resulting in the complete cessation of function at the cellular level. Death can be defined biologically as the cessation of life resulting from irreversible changes in cell metabolism.

The definition of death can have legal and social consequences in areas such as criminal prosecution, inheritance, taxation, treatment of the corpse, even mourning. It also directly affects the practice of organ transplantation. Some organs—hearts, most obviously—must be taken from a human being whose heart is undamaged but who is legally determined to be dead. Critical timing is needed to remove a heart from someone who has been declared dead and to transplant it into a person whose life can thereby be saved. The definitions of death currently in use provide strict safeguards to ensure that the determination of death takes place separate from and without regard to any subsequent transplantation of the deceased's organs.

Why Is There Death?

Ultimately, no answer to the question of why death exists can be completely satisfying. Although we acknowledge that every living thing eventually dies, that recognition is of little comfort. Nor are we comforted by being told that matter and energy are never destroyed but simply changed. Most of us want our conscious self to continue. The notion of being reborn, with another consciousness, is not especially attractive.

Looking at the big picture, we see that death promotes variety. It permits the renewal and evolution of species. The average human life span is long enough to allow us to reproduce ourselves and to ensure that the lineage of our species continues. Yet it is brief enough to allow for new genetic combinations. As a species, this mechanism provides a means of adaptation to changing conditions in the environment. Thus, looked at from the perspective of species survival and evolution, the cycle of life and death makes sense. From a personal point of view, however, death challenges our sense of emotional and intellectual security—especially when it involves seemingly needless, accidental, or sudden death or the deaths of children or adults in the prime of life.

Consequently, theories abound concerning what happens when we die. Most religions are founded on the issue of death and what, if anything, follows. Some promise a better life after death if adherents accept the beliefs and behave according to the rules of the group and its god(s). Other religions or philosophies teach that everyone is evolving toward divinity and is reborn over and over again until eventually reaching perfection. Other views suggest that we cannot know what happens after death and that any judgment about whether life is worth living must be made on the basis of rewards we find or create for ourselves in this life.

Attitudes Toward Death

Death is absolute loss. The death of a best friend, parent, mate, or child typically evokes feelings of confusion and pain. The prospect of our own death can be emotionally devastating. We prefer not to think about it—not so much because we don't know what will happen after death, but because death is the relinquishment, the letting go, of everything and everyone dear to us. Death forces us to puzzle out an understanding of its meaning in our lives. We may choose not to ponder some issues, such as the possibility of an afterlife, but we cannot refrain from facing the reality of death itself. Regardless of our explanations and efforts to minimize its effect, death is painful—both to the person who is dying and to those left behind.

Our attitudes toward death change as we grow and mature, as does our understanding of it. Very young children recognize death as an interruption and an absence, but their lack of a mature time perspective means they don't understand death is final. This view of death evolves considerably from about ages 5 to 9. Children come to understand that death is final, although initially this recognition applies only to others, not to themselves. They think they will somehow escape the universality of death (an illusion that even adults sometimes display by their risk-taking activities). By age 10 or so, most children do recognize that death is universal, inescapable, and irreversible. During the years of adolescence and young adulthood, the mature understanding of death is further refined by contemplating the impact of death on close relationships and the value of religious or philosophical answers to the enigma of death.

Still, possessing a mature understanding of death does not mean that one never experiences anxiety about the deaths of loved ones or the prospect of one's own death. Among couples who have shared nearly a lifetime together, thoughts of death may elicit fears about being left alone. Attending the funeral of a friend or coworker may bring to the surface an underlying anxiety about death.

The news of a friend's or loved one's terminal illness can shock us into an encounter with mortality, creating the need to cope not just with the painful reality of our friend's or loved one's illness, but also with the prospect of our own death. In these and many other situations, our ability to find meaning and comfort depends not only on our understanding the facts of death, but also on our attitude toward it.

Denying Death Over the past several generations, Americans have generally engaged in denial about death. We know that death is an unavoidable reality, yet we try fervently to avoid any thought or mention of it. Rather than speak the words "die" or "dead," we describe the deceased as having "passed away" or "gone to glory," or we use some other euphemism that distances us from death. As if acknowledging the fact of death might prove to be traumatic for us, the sick and old are isolated in hospitals or nursing homes. Few Americans have been present at the death of a loved one. Death is rarely a home event. Instead, death takes place in a hospital or nursing home. Usually, we don't want to be told the details, or we are happy to allow the details to be tastefully edited. Such practices foster the notion that death happens to others, not to you or me.

The reality of death, its finality and its aftermath of grief, is largely a taboo subject in our culture. Instead, we amuse ourselves with unrealistic pictures of death. When death is faked on television and movie screens, it is often presented as reversible. Violent deaths are repeated in television show after television show, night after night. These deaths, occurring to characters we barely know, do not force us to confront the reality of death as it is portrayed in the great dramatic tragedies or experienced in real life. Our children watch a daily fare of superhuman heroes and robots, invincible to bullets and other weapons, as well as characters traveling through time to thwart inevitable death. In their games, children reenact these ideas of death—falling down "dead" and jumping up again. Video games, like cartoons, present death in a two-dimensional world where one can "die" and then be "reborn" to play another day. (For another perspective on death, see the box "Día de los Muertos.")

Welcoming Death Although denial of death constitutes the predominant attitude in American society, death is sometimes welcomed as a relief or release from insufferable pain. This attitude toward death is associated with people who suffer mental and emotional anguish related to depression or physical pain caused by terminal illness. The physical debility and social isolation that may accompany old age can also give rise to a welcoming attitude toward death. It is important to recognize that individuals may hold conflicting or ambivalent attitudes toward death—denying its reality while simultaneously seeking the release or relief it seems to offer.

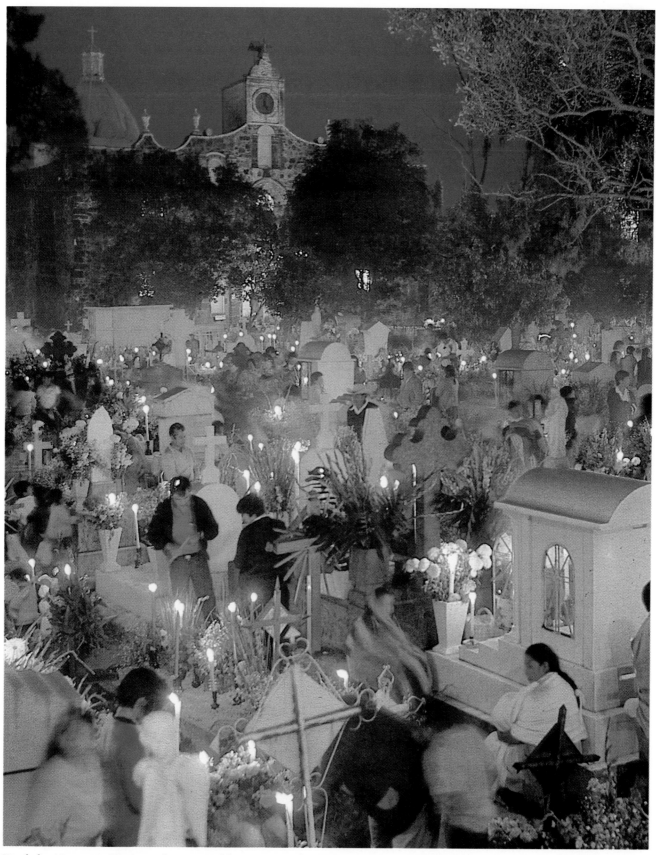

Día de los Muertos in Mexico is characterized by a mixture of reverent remembrance of the departed, festivity to make them happy upon their return, and irony and mockery to defy the fear of death itself. After cleaning the graves and decorating them with candles and flowers, these families will spend the night in the graveyard eating, singing, praying, and talking with the departed.

In contrast to the solemn attitude toward death so prevalent in the United States, a familiar and even ironic attitude is more common among Mexicans and Mexican Americans. In the Mexican world view, death is another phase of life, and those who have passed into it remain accessible. Ancestors are not forever lost, nor is the past dead. This sense of continuity has its roots in the culture of the Aztecs, for whom regeneration was a central theme. When the Spanish came to Mexico in the sixteenth century, their beliefs about death, along with such symbols as skulls and skeletons, were absorbed into the native culture.

Today, symbols of death are visible everywhere in Mexico and in the Mexican American communities of the United States. Mexican artists and writers confront death with humor and even sarcasm, depicting it as the inevitable fate that all—even the wealthiest—must face. At no time is this attitude toward death livelier than at the beginning of each November on the holiday known as *Día de los Muertos,* "the Day of the Dead." This holiday coincides with All Soul's Day, the Catholic commemoration for the dead, and represents a unique blending of indigenous ritual and Church dogma.

Festive and gay, the celebration in honor of the dead typically spans two days—one day devoted to dead children, one to adults. It reflects the belief that the dead return to earth in spirit once a year to rejoin their families and partake of holiday foods prepared especially for them. The fiesta usually begins at midday on October 31, with flowers and food—candies, cookies, honey, milk—set out on altars in each house for the family's dead children. The next day family groups stream to the graveyards, where they have cleaned and decorated the graves of their loved ones, to celebrate and commune with the dead. They bring games, music, and special food—chicken with *mole* sauce, enchiladas, tamales, and *pan de muertos,* the "bread of the dead," sweet rolls in the shape of bones. People sit on the graves, eat, sing, and talk with the departed ones. Tears may be shed as the dead are remembered, but mourning is tempered by the festive mood of the occasion.

Perhaps the greatest contrast between the solemn North American attitude toward death and the livelier Mexican way is found in the colors associated with death. In Mexico it is yellow, not black, that colors the rituals of death. During the season of the dead, graveyards and family altars are decorated with yellow candles and yellow marigolds—the "flower of death." In some Mexican villages, yellow flower petals are strewn along the ground, connecting the graveyard with all the houses visited by death during the year.

As families cherish memories of their loved ones on this holiday, the larger society satirizes death itself—and political and public figures. The impulse to laugh at death finds expression in what are called *calaveras*—a word meaning "skeleton" or "skull" but also referring to humorous newsletters that appear during this season. The *calaveras* contain biting, often bawdy, verses caricaturing well-known public figures, often with particular reference to their deaths. Comic skeletal figures march or dance across these pages, portraying the wealthy and influential as they will eventually become.

Wherever Mexican Americans have settled in the United States, *Día de los Muertos* celebrations keep the traditions alive, and the cultural practices associated with the Day of the Dead have found their way into the nation's culture. Books and museum exhibitions have brought to the public the "art of the dead," with its striking blend of skeletons and flowers, bones and candles. Even the schools in some areas celebrate the holiday. Students create paintings and sculptures depicting skeletons and skulls with the help of local artists.

Does this more familiar attitude toward death help people accept death and come to terms with it? Keeping death in the forefront of consciousness may provide solace to the living, reminding them of their loved ones and assuring them that they themselves will not be forgotten when they die. Yearly celebrations and remembrances may help people keep in touch with their past, their ancestry, and their roots. The festive atmosphere may help dispel the fear of death, allowing people to look at it more directly. Although it is possible to deny the reality of death even when surrounded by images of it, such natural practices as *Día de los Muertos* may help people face death with more equanimity.

Adapted from T. Puente. 1991. "Día de los Muertos," *Hispanic,* October; J. Milne. 1965. *Fiesta Time in Latin America.* (Los Angeles: Ward Ritche Press); and L. Despelder and A. Strickland. 1992. *The Last Dance,* 3rd ed. (Mountain View, Calif.: Mayfield).

This ambivalence toward death is seen most clearly in cases of **suicide,** the intentional taking of one's own life. The motive for suicide commonly involves despair over one's life situation coupled with a sense of hopelessness about the future. Often, the specific motives that lead to a person's decision to end his or her life are not altogether clear, and a **psychological autopsy** is needed to uncover them. Initiated by a coroner or medical examiner when the circumstances surrounding a death are unclear, the psychological autopsy provides a method for determining the thoughts, feelings, and actions of the victim prior to his or her death. Information is gathered by interviewing the deceased's friends and relatives, with particular attention to the role of stressful circumstances, psychiatric and medical histories, and lifestyle. Both social context and individual factors are examined. The goal of such an investigation is to provide a picture of a person's state of mind prior to suicide.

Analysis of suicidal behavior often reveals the presence of conflicting forces that compete for the greater share of the person's mental energies. At issue is the will to live versus the will to die. In this sense, a suicidal act can be characterized as risk-taking behavior, and an otherwise minor incident can tip the scales one way or the other—toward life or death. Plans for self-destruction often proceed simultaneously with fantasies of rescue.

Given this ambivalence, one way to assist people who are experiencing a suicidal crisis is to help them discover something about themselves that matters, however small or insignificant it may seem. Suicidal thoughts and behaviors indicate a critical loss of a person's belief in himself or herself. Nevertheless, the desire to help a suicidal person should be tempered by the recognition that the sustaining motive to survive cannot come from outside; it must be generated from within the potentially suicidal person. For a discussion of assistance and treatment for suicidal people, see Chapter 3.

The death-welcoming attitude exemplified by suicide is an affront to the death denial that pervades our culture. Suicide reminds us of the awesome fact that each of us has the power to choose whether we continue to live. It forces us to contemplate our own mortality and to assess our attitudes toward death. Few people wholly avoid death or wholly seek death. The fear of death and the wish to deny its reality usually coexist more or less peaceably with a sense of resignation, even acceptance. While perhaps consciously wishing to postpone the inevitable, our behavior—especially in the context of taking risks—reveals that we actually hold a considerable range of attitudes toward death.

> **Personal Insight**   Think back to your first encounter with dying and death in your childhood. Who or what died—a pet, a relative, a neighbor? What were your feelings at the time, and what are your feelings as you recall the incident now? What were you told about death when you were a child? What would you tell your own children?

PLANNING FOR DEATH

Once we acknowledge the inevitability of death, we can plan for it and thereby ease what otherwise could be difficult decisions for both our survivors and ourselves. Preparing for death requires completing unfinished business, dealing with medical care needs, allocating our time and other resources, and helping our survivors plan tasks that will be carried out after we die. People who unexpectedly find themselves in the midst of a painful and debilitating terminal illness may be so drained physically and emotionally that they are unable to make prudent de-

cisions that could have easily been made before the onset of crisis.

Indeed, some decisions can be made while you are young. Decisions about a will, for example, can and should be made as early as the college years. Adequate planning can help to ensure that a sudden, unexpected death is not made even more difficult for survivors. Although some decisions cannot be made until one is actually in a particular situation, other decisions can be anticipated and discussed with close relatives and friends.

Making a Will

It is estimated that seven out of ten Americans die without leaving a will. Perhaps the failure to make a will is attributable to the discomfort we feel about death. Whatever the reason, dying without a will creates added hardships for survivors, even when an estate is quite modest. If the estate is substantial, the complications can be formidable.

A will is a legal document expressing a person's intentions and wishes for the disposition of his or her property after death. It is a declaration of how a person's estate—that is, everything he or she owns—will be distributed upon that person's death (Figure 20-1). During the life of the **testator** (the person making the will), a will can be changed, replaced, or revoked. Upon the testator's death, it becomes a legal instrument governing the distribution of the testator's estate.

The right or privilege to determine how one's property will be distributed following death is not available in all societies, nor is it entirely without limitations. For instance, state laws usually stipulate that a surviving spouse cannot be disinherited and that the will must make provision for the deceased's dependent children. Anything that conflicts with ordinary standards of social policy may be deemed invalid if the will is contested.

When a person dies **intestate**—that is, without having left a valid will—his or her property is distributed according to rules set up by the state. A court-appointed administrator supervises the distribution and is awarded a commission taken directly from the estate. The failure to provide a will may cause the welfare of one's spouse and children to be considered separately, resulting in a distribution of property that may not be compatible with one's own wishes or best suited to the interests and needs of

Suicide   The act of taking one's own life, voluntarily and intentionally.

Psychological autopsy   An investigation to determine the thoughts, feelings, and actions of a suicide victim prior to his or her death.

Testator   A person who dies with a will in force.

Intestate   Situation in which a person dies having made no legal will.

Last Will and Testament

I, _____ , of the city of _____ and state of _____ , being of sound mind, memory, and understanding, declare this to be my last will and testament, as follows:

1. **Debts and Funeral Expenses**. I direct that all debts enforceable against my estate, and funeral expenses, be paid as soon as possible.

2. **Executor and Trustee**. I nominate and appoint _____ _____ as executor and trustee of my estate. My executor and trustee shall have the full power at his discretion to do all the things necessary for the liquidation of my estate.

3. **Spouse**. I give and bequeath to my_____ [husband or wife] all my interest in real estate and 50% of all money that I have in banks, savings and loans, certificates of deposit, and similar institutions.

4. **Children**. I give and bequeath the following items to my children. To my son, _____ _____ , I give _____ . To my daughter,_____ , I give _____ _____ . To my_____ , I give _____ _____ .

5. **Charity**. I give and bequeath the following items to charitable organizations. To _____ _____ , I give _____ _____ . To _____ _____ , I give _____ .

6. **Remainder of Estate**. I direct that the remainder of my estate be sold and that the proceeds be divided as follows: _____ _____ .

7. **Death of Beneficiaries**. In the event that any of the beneficiaries named in this will die before me, or at approximately the same time as me, I direct that their children shall take their share, equally. In the event that any of the beneficiaries die before me without leaving children, I direct that the remaining beneficiaries shall take their share, equally.

8. **Revocation of Other Wills**. I hereby revoke all prior wills, codicils, and testamentary dispositions made by me.

IN WITNESS TO THIS WILL I HAVE SET MY HAND TO THIS WILL THIS _____DAY OF_____, 19___.

This will, consisting of_____pages, each bearing the signature of_____ was signed on this date, and declared by_____ to be the last will and testament.

The will was signed in the presence of the following three witnesses

WITNESS	WITNESS	WITNESS
SIGNATURE	SIGNATURE	SIGNATURE
ADDRESS	ADDRESS	ADDRESS

Figure 20-1 *A sample will.*

heirs. Although the distribution may be just the way you would have done it, chances are it will not be.

To avoid having property undergo **probate**—the process of settling an estate—in addition to making a will, you might want to consider transferring title to property or adding names for joint ownership. Sensible, legal steps can be taken to avoid probate or at least minimize its cost.

Arranging that fewer assets fall under the rules of probate can make the process of settling an estate briefer and less complex. However, plans to avoid or minimize probate should be adopted only after careful consideration and after availing oneself of competent legal and financial advice. It is usually helpful to involve family members in the process of will making and financial planning to prevent problems that might arise when such actions are taken without the knowledge of those who will be affected.

Choosing Where to Die

Would you prefer to spend your last days at home tended by relatives and friends? Or would you rather have access to the sophisticated medical techniques available in the hospital setting? Would hospice care, with its emphasis on alleviation of pain and family involvement, be your choice for care at the end of life? Although the place where we die is not always something we can choose, we can and should consider the alternatives. If our death is not unexpected, perhaps coming as the final chapter of a long illness, some degree of choice can probably be exercised about where our death will occur. The more we know about options, the more likely we and our families will be to make the most appropriate and personally satisfying choice.

Home   Until well into the early decades of this century, virtually everyone died at home. Now, however, most deaths occur in an institutional setting, usually a hospital or nursing home. Although few Americans now spend their last days at home, advocates of home care believe that a person's home is the preferred setting for terminal care at the end stage of an illness. Among the advantages of home care, the most obvious is that the dying person is in a familiar setting, one intimately connected with family and friends. Compared to institutional settings such as hospitals and nursing homes, home care makes it easier to sustain relationships with loved ones and to exercise self-determination about the details of care. Rather than being forced to follow a schedule of visiting hours and caregiving determined by institutional routine, the patient and his or her family can set their own timetable.

The advantages of home care come at a price, however. Support must be available not only from the patient's family and friends, but also from skilled, professional caregivers who supervise the care being provided at home and provide relief when necessary. Since home care is a full-time job, its success depends on adequate preparation and commitment. If a patient requires sophisticated medical procedures, cannot afford the professional staff needed to make home care work, or intends to donate organs, hospital care may be more appropriate. Similarly, unless family members or friends can dedicate themselves to the necessary continuity of care, other alternatives should be considered. It is not always possible to make a home into a hospital. Still, for those who wish to provide home care to a loved one, resources are available for educating oneself about every facet of tending a dying patient (see, for example, Deborah Duda's *A Guide to Dying at Home,* listed at the end of the chapter). When appropriate, home care is probably the most satisfying option for caring for a loved one as his or her life comes to a close.

Hospital   Hospitals are organized to provide short-term intensive treatment for acute injury and illness. Highly specialized care is provided to patients who usually stay in the hospital only briefly before returning to normal life. Because of this emphasis on acute care, hospitals are generally not well suited to meet the needs of patients expected to die from terminal disease. Staff and equipment are oriented toward saving life, not providing comfort during a patient's final days or weeks. Because carrying out its primary mission of saving life requires highly trained staff and expensive medical technologies, the costs of hospital care are high.

Nevertheless, some medical institutions have instituted **palliative care** programs to care for patients who are not expected to recover. Unlike acute care, which involves active measures to sustain life, palliative care is focused on providing relief from pain while acknowledging that further treatment would be futile. In some hospitals, a separate ward is created for terminal patients; in others, the care of dying patients is integrated within the general hospital population. A comprehensive program of hospital-based palliative care offers counseling support to dying patients and their families as well as care by specially trained staff.

Hospice   The concept of **hospice** care grew out of the perception that care of the dying within conventional hospital settings was inadequate. Intravenous apparatuses, respirators, and related devices for prolonging life are absent from hospices. In their place is a peaceful atmosphere wherein the process of dying is accepted. An alternative to both home care—especially when families need relief—and hospital care, the hospice philosophy of care has met with rapid and widespread acceptance (see the box "Hospice: Comfort and Care for the Dying").

Although hospice groups can now be found in most areas of the United States, few are equipped to provide full-time care. Most hospice organizations provide support services to patients who are either at home or in an institutional care setting. Initially, hospices were focused on meeting the needs of terminal cancer patients, and this remains the major focus. Since the early 1980s, however, ministering to the needs of patients dying from AIDS-related illnesses has claimed an increasing share of hospice resources. In addition, hospice programs have been initiated to provide care specifically for terminally ill children. In a relatively brief time, the hospice philosophy of care—

Probate   The legal process of establishing a will as valid and settling an estate.

Palliative care   Measures taken to reduce the intensity of a disease, especially those involving control of pain and other symptoms.

Hospice   A facility or program designed to provide care and support for terminally ill patients.

TERMS

Hospice: Comfort and Care for the Dying

If you have a relative or friend who died of a terminal illness in recent years, you may be familiar with hospice care. Hospice is a special kind of care for people in the final phase of a terminal illness. Its goals are to help provide a dignified, comfortable death and to care for the patient and family together.

Although institutions dedicated to the care of the dying have existed throughout history, the modern hospice movement began in 1967 when Dr. Cicely Saunders began St. Christopher's Hospice in England. The principles on which St. Christopher's was founded form the basic standards of hospice care today:

- Effective control of pain and symptoms
- Care of the patient and family as a unit
- An interdisciplinary approach to care
- The use of trained volunteers
- A continuum of care, including home care, and continuity of care across different settings
- Follow-up care of the family after the patient's death

Most hospice programs are based on home care and offer support to the family members and friends who are providing the primary care. Included are the coordinated services of physicians, nurses, counselors, therapists, aides, and volunteers, as well as medical supplies and medications for pain and symptom management. Hospice programs can also be administered in a hospital or other institutional setting.

How does hospice care differ from other types of health care? The goal of hospice care is to relieve pain and symptoms rather than to cure disease. Sophisticated pain management techniques are used to maximize comfort and alertness. The emphasis is on enhancing the quality of life rather than extending its length. Thus, many disorders and conditions related to the disease are not aggressively treated with the techniques of acute care medicine, except to control pain.

The focus is also on the person—the whole person—rather than the disease. The hospice team addresses the medical, emotional, psychological, and spiritual needs of the patient. The hospice team also addresses the needs of the family. Caring for a dying family member is stressful, and illness and death may uncover unresolved family problems. Hospice programs provide counseling and help in coping with conflict, guilt, anger, and grief both before and after the patient dies.

Several studies have found that hospice care in the last year of life is less expensive than conventional care. More than 20 percent of Medicare expenditures are for terminally ill patients, with a high percentage of those costs occurring in the last month of life. For this reason, a Medicare hospice option was passed in 1982, making hospice care eligible for reimbursement. Many private insurance companies also cover hospice care.

Despite these trends, hospices serve only a small percentage of terminally ill patients. Of the more than 2,000 hospices in the United States, only about two-thirds are Medicare-certified due to the difficulty of working within Medicare parameters. An example is the Medicare requirement of diagnosing a terminal illness, which is difficult, and then setting a six-month ending point, harder still. As a result, many qualified hospices do not seek certification, which limits the number of patients who have access to hospice care through Medicare. Most terminal patients continue to die in hospitals in this country, and an increasing number die in nursing homes, where hospice care is uncommon.

This is unfortunate because studies show that quality of life is significantly better for hospice patients, and patients themselves express greater satisfaction with the care. The hospice approach is also an alternative to legalized euthanasia, which some people are promoting as an alternative to conventional care for the dying in hospitals. Many medical experts are calling for an expansion of hospice programs and the development of innovative ways of using the hospice approach in conventional settings. Such changes would ensure more humane care for people near death and better support for families in a time of severe stress.

Adapted from J. Rhymes. 1990. "Hospice Care in America." *Journal of the American Medical Association* 264(3) and "A Guide to Hospice Care." *Harvard Health Letter Special Supplement*, April 1993.

---

with its emphasis on alleviation of pain and acceptance of death—has made important contributions to methods of caring for dying patients and assisting their families.

Asking for Help: Granting Power of Attorney

Just as making a will is a responsible way to plan for the eventuality of one's own death, a person may delegate authority over certain matters to a trusted friend or relative who can thereby act on his or her behalf. This trusted person, or agent, is granted **power of attorney,** the legal authority to act in another person's name. This delegation of authority can be general, allowing the agent to take action on any matters affecting the patient, or for a specified purpose. A time limit on the power of attorney can also be stipulated. Depending on the authority being delegated, it may be important to acquaint one's agent with any survivor benefits that are expected (such as Social Security, pensions, and life insurance) as well as with important documents such as:

- Will
- Birth and adoption certificates
- Marriage and divorce papers
- Citizenship papers
- Military service papers
- Social Security numbers
- Organizational memberships and benefits
- Life and accident insurance policies
- Bank accounts, stocks, and bonds
- Safe deposit box
- Deeds and other real estate papers

The power of attorney to make health care decisions is of particular importance to patients with a life-threatening condition, though it is useful for any of us who wish to express our wishes about the kind of care we would want if we could no longer act on our own behalf. Such a situation could arise, for example, if one were severely injured in an automobile accident and in a coma, unable to speak or respond. The power of attorney for health care allows a person to designate an agent who is empowered to make health care decisions on the delegator's behalf, including those that pertain to the withholding or withdrawing of life-sustaining treatment. The agent must act consistently with the patient's wishes as stated in the document or as otherwise made known. A number of states have enacted legislation that gives legal sanction to the power of attorney for health care and similar proxies.

Deciding Whether to Prolong Life

If you were diagnosed with a terminal illness, would you want to be kept alive on life-support systems? Framing an answer to this question could determine the quality of the final phase of your life. Many people are alive today because of advanced medical technology, such as the heart pacemaker and the kidney dialysis machine. In spite of successes, however, modern medical innovations do not always clearly confer benefits.

The medical approach that strives to keep people alive by all means and at any expense is being questioned. The human organism often can be kept alive despite the cessation of normal heart, brain, respiratory, or kidney function. Should a patient without any hope of recovery be kept alive by means of artificial life support? What if the patient has fallen into a **persistent vegetative state**—that is, profound unconsciousness, lacking any sign of normal reflexes and unresponsive to external stimuli, with no reasonable hope of improvement?

Ethical questions about the "right to die" have become widespread in American society since the landmark case of Karen Ann Quinlan; in 1975 at age 22 she was admitted in a comatose state to an intensive care unit where her breathing was soon being sustained by a respirator. When she remained unresponsive in a persistent vegetative state, her parents requested that the respirator be disconnected, but this request was denied by the medical staff responsible for Karen's care. Eventually, the request reached the New Jersey Supreme Court, which ruled that artificial respiration could be discontinued.

More recently, courts in various parts of the country have ruled on requests to remove other forms of life support, including artificial feeding mechanisms that provide nutrition and hydration to comatose patients who are able to breathe on their own. The case of Nancy Beth Cruzan was heard before the U.S. Supreme Court in 1990. As a result of injuries she received in 1983, Cruzan was in a persistent vegetative state. Physicians had implanted a feeding tube to provide nourishment, the only form of life support she was receiving. As in the case of Karen Quinlan, when Nancy Cruzan's parents requested that artificial life support be withdrawn, hospital personnel refused, arguing that the state had an inherent interest in preserving life.

The Supreme Court ruled that states are justified in making a requirement that only the patient can decide to withdraw treatment. Since Nancy apparently had not provided a clear expression of her wishes on the matter before her accident, the state was not bound to honor the wishes of her parents. However, a few months later, in light of new testimony from several of Nancy's friends that she had expressed her wishes "not to live like a vegetable," a state court ruled that the "clear and convincing" evidence standard now had been met and permission was obtained for removal of the feeding tube. This case points up the value of expressing one's wishes regarding life-sustaining measures, preferably in writing, before the need for such a statement arises.

Allowing Someone to Die When suffering outweighs the benefits of continued existence, many people argue that individuals have a "right to die," whether or not they choose to exercise that right. Withdrawing or not initiating treatments that could potentially sustain life is sometimes termed **passive euthanasia,** although many medical practitioners and ethicists reject this term because it

TERMS

Power of attorney   A legal instrument allowing one person to act as the agent of another person.

Persistent vegetative state   A condition of profound unconsciousness caused by disease or injury in which an individual lacks normal reflexes and is unresponsive to external stimuli, lasting for an extended period with no reasonable hope of improvement.

Passive euthanasia   The practice of withholding (not initiating) or withdrawing (removing) life-prolonging but ultimately futile treatment, thereby allowing a terminally ill person to die naturally.

A CLOSER LOOK
Helping Terminally Ill Patients Die: Is It Legal? Is It Ethical?

In 1990, a 54-year-old teacher named Janet Adkins was diagnosed with Alzheimer's disease. Although the disease was still in its early stages, Adkins decided she could not face a future of increasing dementia and personality loss. With the help of Jack Kevorkian, a Detroit physician, Adkins ended her own life swiftly and calmly with a lethal injection of potassium chloride. The device she used, often referred to as a "suicide machine," was invented by Kevorkian and is endorsed by some advocates of the "right to die" movement. Kevorkian's role in Adkins's death, and in others since then, has been hotly debated in the medical and legal communities, fueling the arguments for and against legalized euthanasia.

Many patients facing a terminal illness may wish to end their pain and suffering by refusing medical treatment that prolongs life. As of 1990, this choice is sanctioned by law. In the case of *Cruzan vs. Missouri*, the Supreme Court decided that a person has the right, according to the Constitution, to refuse life-sustaining medical treatment. Subsequently, Congress passed the Patient Self-Determination Act, which requires that all government-funded health care providers inform patients of their right to refuse medical treatment. Hospitals and physicians, then, are permitted to withhold or withdraw treatment when a patient is in a persistent vegetative state, with no chance of recovery, and when there is evidence that the person wants no life-prolonging treatment— for example, if the person communicated these wishes through a living will or other advance directive. In fact, perhaps as a result of the *Cruzan vs. Missouri* case, living wills have become more popular.

Although the 1990 Supreme Court ruling permits withdrawal or non-initiation of treatments, it does not enable health care workers to assist actively in a patient's choice to die, as in the case of Janet Adkins. Many "right to die" advocates want physician-assisted suicide to be legalized, and the issue of euthanasia has found a political forum. In 1991 and 1992, voters in Washington and California rejected initiatives that would legalize physician-assisted suicide. Oregonians may consider a similar initiative in 1994. Currently, 27 states consider assisted suicide to be a crime. In other states, there are no legal statutes that define the act of assisted suicide.

The issue of suicide—whether assisted or not—is a complex one. On the whole, Americans value quality of life, humane treatment for pain and suffering, and the right of free choice for individuals. At the same time, society places a high value on the very nature of life, and Americans tend to fear the consequences of condoning suicide. To many people, it simply seems unethical to accept death as a solution, because it devalues human life. Attitudes toward suicide are also shaped by religion. Christian doctrine holds that humans have no inherent right to control their own death. So suicide, whether assisted or not, runs contrary to most religious belief in America.

Attitudes are also shaped by our views toward physicians and the health care system in America. Some people fear that if assisted suicide becomes legal, health care workers may abuse patients' trust or that errors in judgment will result in unnecessary deaths. Many people believe that sanctioning assisted suicide will negate the advances in medical science that offer hope to terminally ill patients. Cures may arrive before a patient dies, or advances in pain management may sufficiently relieve a patient's discomfort and enhance his or her quality of life. Finally, there is concern that the growing "right to die" movement may be a response to rising health care costs: Patients may look to death as a solution only because the expense of medical treatment may be burdensome.

In spite of these attitudes, many Americans seem to believe that people have the right to terminate their lives and to seek help in doing so. In a January 1991 Gallup Poll, 58 percent of the respondents said that a person with an incurable disease has the moral right to end his or her life; 66 percent said that a person in great pain and with no hope of improvement has such a right; and 65 percent said that physicians should be allowed to end a patient's life if requested to do so by the patient and the patient's family. With strong feelings on both sides of this issue, physician-assisted suicide is certain to remain a subject of heated debate in the years ahead.

Adapted from R. L. Worsnop. 1992. "Assisted Suicide." *CQ Researcher*, 21 February, pp. 147–51 and "Euthanasia: What Is the 'Good Death'?" *The Economist*, 20 July 1991, pp. 21–24.

tends to confuse the generally unacceptable and unlawful practice of actively causing death with the fairly well-established practice of withholding or withdrawing useless treatments. It is increasingly considered good medical practice not to artificially prolong the life and suffering of a person whose condition is inevitably fatal. Courts also seem to be coming to a consensus that mentally competent, informed patients have the right to refuse medical treatment, including life support provided by mechanical or artificial means.

Active Euthanasia　In contrast to withdrawing or withholding treatment, **active euthanasia** refers to the practice of intentionally hastening the death of a terminal patient who requests it in order to avoid a painful and prolonged dying. Death in such cases is usually hastened by a **lethal injection.** The distinction between passive and active euthanasia is sometimes characterized as the difference between "letting die" and "killing" (although advocates of active euthanasia prefer the phrase "helping to die").

In most countries, including the United States, taking active steps to end someone's life is a crime, even if the motive is based on good intentions. Thus, active euthanasia, which has been called "the most compassionate of crimes," must also be the most secret. As a result, few cases of active euthanasia are reported. Also, because dying patients are often heavily dosed with painkilling drugs that have potentially lethal side effects, the immediate cause of death may not be entirely certain.

The greatest acceptance of active euthanasia is currently found in the Netherlands. There, in terminal cases that meet strict guidelines, a physician may give a lethal injection to a dying person who has requested it, without fear of judicial punishment. The standards set out by the Dutch courts for noncriminal aid in dying include these requirements:

1. There must be physical or mental suffering that the patient finds unbearable.

2. The suffering and the desire to die must be lasting, not temporary.

3. The decision to die must be the voluntary decision of an informed patient.

4. The patient must have a correct and clear understanding of his or her condition and of other possible treatments, must be capable of weighing these options, and must have done so.

5. There must be no other reasonable (acceptable to the patient) remedy to improve the situation.

6. The time and manner of death should be such that it will not cause avoidable misery to others. If possible, the next of kin should be informed beforehand.

7. The decision to give aid in dying should not be made by only one person. According to the circumstances of the case, the physician must consult another medical professional, social worker, or psychologist.

8. A medical doctor must be involved in the decision to prescribe the lethal drug.

9. The decision-making process and the act of giving aid must be done with the utmost care.

Many people who endorse the philosophy of hospice and palliative care argue that adequate treatment for pain and depression usually eliminates the need to consider active measures to end a patient's life. According to this view, the distinction between active euthanasia and allowing to die ought to be maintained. However, a patient who is surrounded by an array of machinery and tubes may seem less a human being than an extension of medical technology. In such situations the claims in favor of a human being's "right to die" are most clearly and emotionally rendered. If we wish to avoid the burden on ourselves and on medical practitioners of actively hastening patients' deaths, it follows that we must actively seek better ways of lifting the burden of suffering experienced by the dying. (For information on physician-assisted suicide, see the box "Helping Terminally Ill Patients Die: Is It Legal? Is It Ethical?")

Living Wills Since the mid-1970s, most American states have enacted legislation that allows people to complete a **living will** or other form of advance directive to express their wishes regarding medical care in the event of a terminal condition. Most such documents state that if the person is suffering from a terminal illness or injury that is certified by one (sometimes two) physicians, his or her life should not be sustained by artificial means or heroic measures.

In some cases, before a living will is presumed to be valid, a person must be declared a "qualified patient"— that is, he or she must be in a terminal condition. Some advance directives remain in force only for a specified number of years. Although living wills do not universally have the force of law, they can nevertheless be an important source of information about a person's wishes. In addition, they may protect physicians from liability for acting in accordance with such wishes.

In light of the increasingly widespread judicial standard of "clear and convincing evidence" of a patient's wishes regarding life-sustaining treatment, it may be prudent to complete both a living will and a power of attorney for health care (Figure 20-2). While the living will, as an advance directive, allows you to specify your wishes in case you become unable to speak for yourself, the power of attorney for health care allows you to designate a proxy—that is, a trusted friend or relative—who can act on your behalf to make a broad range of medical decisions and to see that your wishes are carried out should the need arise.

> *Personal Insight* How do you think you would feel if someone you loved were terminally ill and in pain and asked to be allowed to die? What would you do? How do you think you would feel if a friend told you he or she wanted to die because of depression and an inability to cope with life's problems? What would you do?

Active euthanasia The practice of intentionally hastening the death of a person who requests it to avoid a painful or prolonged dying.

Lethal injection The administering, by injection, of a drug intended to result in death.

Living will A document enabling individuals to provide instructions about the kind of medical care they wish to receive or refuse, including the use of life-sustaining procedures, should they become unable to participate in treatment decisions. A living will often states that the individual's life should not be sustained by artificial means or medical heroics if recovery is impossible.

TERMS

ADVANCE DIRECTIVE
Living Will and Health Care Proxy

Death is a part of life. It is a reality like birth, growth, and aging. I am using this advance directive to convey my wishes about medical care to my doctors and other people looking after me at the end of my life. It is called an advance directive because it gives instructions in advance about what I want to happen to me in the future. It expresses my wishes about medical treatment that might keep me alive. I want this to be legally binding.

If I cannot make or communicate decisions about my medical care, those around me should rely on this document for instructions about measures that could keep me alive.

I do not want medical treatment (including feeding and water by tube) that will keep me alive if:
- I am unconscious and there is no reasonable prospect that I will ever be conscious again (even if I am not going to die soon in my medical condition), *or*
- I am near death from an illness or injury with no reasonable prospect of recovery.

I do want medicine and other care to make me more comfortable and to take care of pain and suffering. I want this even if the pain medicine makes me die sooner.

I want to give some extra instructions: *[Here list any special instructions; e.g., some people fear being kept alive after a debilitating stroke. If you have wishes about this or any other conditions, please write them here.]*

The legal language in the box that follows is a health care proxy.
It gives another person the power to make medical decisions for me.

I name _____ , who lives at _____
_____ , phone number _____
to make medical decisions for me if I cannot make them myself. This person is called a health care "surrogate," "agent," "proxy," or "attorney in fact." This power of attorney shall become effective when I become incapable of making or communicating decisions about my medical care. This means that this document stays legal when and if I lose the power to speak for myself, for instance, if I am in a coma or have Alzheimer's disease.

My health care proxy has power to tell others what my advance directive means. This person also has power to make decisions for me, based either on what I would have wanted, or if this is not known, on what he or she thinks is best for me.

If my first choice health care proxy cannot or decides not to act for me, I name _____
_____ , address _____ ,
phone number _____ , as my second choice.

I have discussed my wishes with my health care proxy, and with my second choice if I have chosen to appoint a second person. My proxy(ies) has(have) agreed to act for me.

I have thought about this advance directive carefully. I know what it means and want to sign it. I have chosen two witnesses, neither of whom is a member of my family, nor will inherit from me when I die. My witnesses are not the same people as those I named as my health care proxies. I understand that this form should be notarized if I use the box to name (a) health care proxy(ies).

_____	_____	_____
SIGNATURE	WITNESS' SIGNATURE	WITNESS' SIGNATURE
_____	_____	_____
DATE	WITNESS' PRINTED NAME	WITNESS' PRINTED NAME
_____	_____	_____
ADDRESS	ADDRESS	ADDRESS

_____
NOTARY [to be used if proxy is appointed]

Figure 20-2 *Sample advance directive containing both a living will and a power of attorney for health care.*
Source: Choice in Dying (formerly Concern for Dying/Society for the Right to Die), 200 Varick St., New York, NY 10014 (212-366-5540)

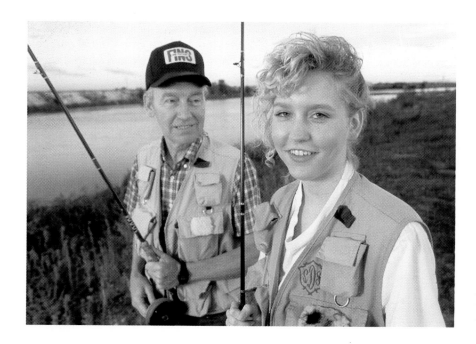

Organ transplants give hope to those who would otherwise have died. This young woman is on a camping trip with her father after recovering from a heart-lung transplant.

Donating Organs

A human body is a valuable resource. Of all the recent advances in medical techniques for helping patients who were formerly considered beyond recovery, probably the best known and most widely accepted is the transplantation of human organs. Eye corneas can be transplanted to give sight to the blind. Kidneys can give years of vigorous life to people whose own have stopped working. Human skin is the best dressing for burn wounds. Bones can be used for grafting. In some parts of the world, undiseased blood from dead bodies is used for transfusions. Perhaps the most dramatic organ transplants are those involving the heart. Although some people may find the thought of donating organs unsettling, the procedures aren't very different from those used in routine autopsies and normal preparation for burial.

The Uniform Anatomical Gift Act, approved in 1968 and enacted in some form in all 50 states, provides for the donation of the body or specific body parts upon the donor's death. The most widely used method for donating body parts is through the **Uniform Donor Card,** which is available from the National Kidney Foundation (Figure 20-3). In some states, the desire to donate organs can be communicated by use of a card attached to a person's driver's license. Besides specifying how one's body may be used after death, the donor may also specify the final disposition of his or her remains once the donation has been completed. Many donations are authorized by relatives at the time of a loved one's death. Plans for organ or body donation should be discussed with members of your family so that they are aware of your wishes and can help see that they are fulfilled.

Deciding What to Do with the Body

Most people have a preference about how their body will be disposed of when they die. For Americans, this decision usually involves either burial or cremation. Burial can be in a single grave dug into the soil or entombment in a multitiered mausoleum. Cremation involves burning a body to its bones by intense heat. Cremated remains can be buried, entombed, kept by the family, or scattered at sea or on land, in accordance with state and local laws. If a body or organ donation has been made, burial or cremation will take place once the donation procedures have been completed. Depending on the type of funeral ceremony desired, a body destined for burial or cremation may or may not be embalmed.

Plans for body disposition may be made explicit by executing a preplanned (or "pre-need") arrangement with a funeral home or memorial society. Decisions about how one's body will be disposed of after death are best considered early in life while a person is healthy and able to gather the necessary information about available choices.

Thought should also be given to how funeral and body disposition costs will be paid. Depending on the options selected, costs range upwards from $500. The average cost of a traditional funeral is now about $3,500. Help with funeral costs may be available from governmental sources, such as Social Security insurance and the Veter-

Uniform Donor Card A consent form authorizing the use of the signer's body parts for transplantation or medical research upon his or her death.

TERMS

UNIFORM DONOR CARD

of ______________________________
(print or type name of donor)

In the hope that I may help others, I hereby make this anatomical gift, if medically acceptable, to take effect upon my death. The words and marks below indicate my wishes.

I give: (a)________any needed organs or parts

(b)________only the following organs or parts

____
(specify the organ(s), tissue(s) or part(s))

for the purposes of transplantation, therapy, medical research or education;

(c)________my body for anatomical study if needed

Limitations or special wishes, if any: ______________________

Signed by the donor and the following two witnesses in the presence of each other:

Signature of Donor ______________ Date of Birth of Donor ______________

Date Signed ______________ City and State ______________

Witness ______________ Witness ______________

This is a legal document under the Anatomical Gift Act or similar laws.

☐Yes, I have discussed my wishes with my family.

For further information consult your physician or

THE NATIONAL KIDNEY FOUNDATION

30 East 33rd Street New York, NY 10016

Figure 20-3 *A sample organ donor card.*

ans Administration. Veterans may be eligible for burial in a national cemetery, a choice that can reduce costs. Unions, fraternal societies, and ethnic or service organizations sometimes provide lump-sum payments to help defray the costs of members' funerals. In addition to a preplanned arrangement with a funeral home or memorial society, it is also possible to earmark a special bank account for funeral expenses so that relatives will not have to assume the financial burden at a time of grief. If the estate is large enough, funds may simply come out of the estate's assets.

In the United States, most people choose some form of traditional funeral service followed by burial. However, concerns about the cost of this traditional approach to body disposal have created an interest in alternatives. One response has been the rise of **memorial societies**—nonprofit groups that help members prearrange simple, economical burial or cremation. Those who choose this plan often prefer a no-frills funeral service or perhaps only a simple memorial service. (Unlike traditional funerals, which typically have the body of the deceased present for viewing by mourners, memorial services forgo the presence of the body and are often held after burial or cremation has already taken place.) Although one can join a memorial society at any time, it is best to investigate the services they offer before the need becomes urgent.

Conventional funeral establishments have also responded to the widespread desire for a less costly alternative to the traditional funeral by offering burial and cremation plans that are similar to those available through memorial societies. The result is a wide range of choices to meet the diverse needs and wishes of consumers.

Planning a Funeral or Memorial Service

It is generally agreed that bereaved persons benefit from participating in a ceremony to mark the death of a loved one. The choice of funeral rites may involve a traditional funeral ceremony or a simple memorial service. The tone of the rites might reflect a somber remembrance of the deceased or a more upbeat wake or party. Some people express the preference for no services, although bereaved friends and relatives generally benefit from the opportunity to mark their grief through ritual and ceremony. Ideally, last rites and body disposition will be planned in agreement with the wishes and needs of one's survivors.

A typical American Christian funeral ceremony involves **embalming** the corpse, viewing the body in the funeral home before the funeral service, a religious ceremony with the body present, and a processional to the graveside where a brief final ceremony is held. Other religious traditions follow different practices, as do other ethnic groups. In a pluralistic society like the United States, there are many ways of constructing a meaningful funeral or memorial service.

Some people choose a minimal role in caring for their dead loved ones; others seek more active participation. A ceremony can develop in whatever way is appropriate and meaningful for those involved. It may be held indoors or outside in natural surroundings. The participants may choose to voice their feelings about the deceased or simply share their loss in silence. A member of the clergy or other leader may be called upon to officiate, or the participants may create their own form of ritual to mark the deceased's passing from the community. The sharing of grief may be expressed in a common meal, dancing, singing, or prayer.

Previewing Tasks for Survivors

Following death, the deceased's family must obtain copies of the death certificate signed by a physician, medical examiner, or **coroner.** Required by all legal jurisdictions in the United States, the death certificate constitutes legal proof of death and affects disposition of property rights, life insurance benefits, pension payments, and so on. If a person dies unexpectedly (even of natural causes) or from a rare or highly researched disease, the medical staff may request an **autopsy,** which involves surgically opening the body, examining the organs of interest, and perhaps removing certain body parts for further study. If the cause of death is not known, unexplained, or accidental, or if the death occurred under questionable or suspicious circumstances, the coroner will require an autopsy. Other-

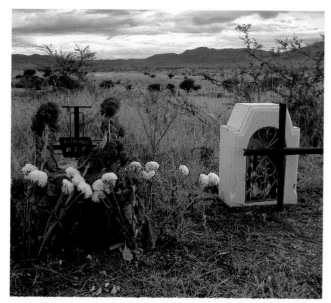

Death can challenge our sense of emotional and intellectual security, particularly the sudden death of a young person. These roadside markers were placed in memory of people killed in an automobile crash at this site.

wise, permission of the next of kin must be obtained before an autopsy is performed.

Notification of the death should be made promptly to close friends and relatives. If possible, a list of telephone numbers and addresses should be prepared beforehand. Friends can be asked to help with the notification process.

The following checklist for survivors is adapted from Ernest Morgan's *A Manual of Death Education and Simple Burial*. While some of these tasks must be attended to soon after the death occurs, others take weeks or months to complete. Many of these tasks—especially those that need to be dealt with in the first hours and days following the death—can be taken care of by friends and relatives of the immediate survivors.

- Prepare a list of relatives, close friends, and business colleagues, and arrange to telephone them about the death as soon as possible.

- If flowers are to be omitted from the funeral or memorial service, choose an appropriate charity or other memorial to which gifts may be made.

- Write the obituary. Include the deceased's age, place of birth, cause of death, occupation, degrees held, memberships, military service record, outstanding accomplishments, the names and relationships of nearest survivors, and an announcement of the time and place of funeral or memorial services.

- Arrange for family members or close friends to take turns welcoming those who come to express their condolences in person and responding to those who

telephone their condolences. Keep a record of the condolence calls so that acknowledgments can be sent later.

- Arrange for child care, if necessary.

- Ask friends to help coordinate the supplying of meals for the first days following the death.

- Consider asking friends to help with household needs.

- Arrange hospitality for relatives and friends who are visiting from out of town.

- If a funeral ceremony is planned, choose the persons who are to be pallbearers and notify them that you would like their participation.

- Notify the lawyer, accountant, and other personal representatives who will be helping to settle the deceased's estate.

- If flowers will be a part of the funeral, arrange for their disposition afterwards (perhaps they can be sent to a convalescent hospital or rest home).

- Prepare a list of the people who should be notified of the death by letter or printed notice and prepare a suitable message.

- Send handwritten or printed notes of acknowledgment to the people who have provided assistance or who have sent flowers or their condolences.

- With the aid of your attorney or accountant, review all life and casualty insurance policies as well as other sources of potential death benefits, such as Social Security, military service, fraternal organizations, and unions. Be sure to check whether any of these sources have provisions for income to assist survivors.

- Promptly review all debts, mortgages, and installment payments. Some may carry clauses that cancel the debt in the event of death. If payments must be delayed, contact creditors to arrange for a grace period.

TERMS

Memorial societies   Nonprofit membership groups that offer consumers no-frills, economical burial or cremation.

Embalming   Removing blood and other fluids from a body and replacing them with chemicals to disinfect and temporarily retard deterioration of the corpse.

Coroner   An elected public official charged with investigating the causes of deaths occurring within a specific legal jurisdiction and providing assistance to law enforcement personnel in the event of criminal violations involving death.

Autopsy   The detailed dissection and examination of a body after death to determine the cause of death or to investigate the extent and nature of changes caused by disease; also performed in connection with medical research and training.

People with life-threatening illness face costly medical care, loss of earnings, repeated and often lengthy hospitalization, and the emotional havoc that accompanies the news of a potentially terminal condition. The emotional response to life-threatening illness can include anguish, a sense of hopelessness, depression, and feelings of isolation and loneliness. Gathering information about the disease and its treatment, sharing one's experience in settings where mutual support can be provided, and finding ways of communicating more clearly with caregivers as well as with family and friends are all examples of positive approaches to dealing with life-threatening illness.

Coping with Dying

How do individuals come to terms with the prospect of dying? In his book *Dying*, John Hinton noted that about half of the dying people he observed openly acknowledged their death and accepted it. Of the remaining half, about a quarter spoke with undisguised anguish about their impending death, and the other quarter denied it entirely and did not speak about it at all. When death confronts us squarely, even if we have come to some degree of acceptance, we may yet hope for a last-minute reprieve. The way each of us copes with dying will likely resemble the ways we've coped with living and with other losses in our lives.

After talking with hundreds of dying people, Elisabeth Kübler-Ross identified several common, although not inevitable, psychological stages that people experience while coping with the prospect of imminent death. She described this coping process in her landmark study *On Death and Dying*. In an idealized model, an early period of shock, disbelief, and denial eventually gives way to some degree of acceptance. It should be emphasized that not everyone experiences each of the psychological stages, or states, listed below, nor are they necessarily experienced in the same order or for the same duration. Indeed, some reactions may be experienced simultaneously, and there is a cycling between the various states during different phases of the illness. Dealing with these intense emotions can enable the dying person eventually to arrive at a personal sense of acceptance with respect to his or her impending death.

- *Denial and isolation.* The initial stage of coping with terminal illness is characterized as a temporary state of shock in which people deny the fact of death and isolate themselves from further confrontation with it. They say "Not me" and insist "It can't be." Denial is a useful coping mechanism because it acts as a buffer against shock and allows time for the mobilization of other defenses.

- *Anger.* When the truth can no longer be denied, anger often follows. People ask "Why me?" and may lash out at family members, their physicians, and the hospital staff—blaming them for the situation. Anger is a normal response to disability and the loss of control over one's life and situation.

- *Bargaining.* As a means of marshaling what hope remains, people often try to find a way out. A common scenario involves making promises to God in exchange for a prolonged life. The intense desire to find an "out" can also cause people to grasp at straws, becoming vulnerable to so-called miracle cures promoted by quacks and charlatans.

- *Depression.* When people begin to accept their fate and face the reality of their impending death, they may become depressed about things that will be left unfinished in their lives and all they are leaving behind. Depression is a natural part of grief as a person strives to prepare for separation from this world. Although depression is emotionally painful, it is an appropriate step in the process of coming to terms with loss; it is eased when people are allowed to express their sorrow in an atmosphere of nonjudgmental support and compassion.

- *Acceptance.* People facing their own death may eventually come to some resolution about their situation. They are no longer angry or depressed, nor are they searching for some kind of miracle to change their fate. They accept the reality that nothing is certain until it happens, and they are willing to live to the fullest extent possible in the time that remains to them. It often seems that they are able to suspend judgment or expectations about the future and simply appreciate the present. Acknowledging that they are ultimately not in control of their future, they seem content to make the best of what comes their way. At the end, when death is near, they may choose not to talk much with visitors, even family members and close friends. This, too, is part of letting go.

Again, this list is a general description of the coping process, not a schedule to be strictly followed or imposed on a particular situation. In actuality, the way a person will live his or her final weeks and days cannot be predicted. Changing circumstances may make it seem as if the dying person is tossed from one emotion to another and then back again. Edwin Shneidman observed that the dying process often displays a seesaw effect, shaped somewhat by personality: "a waxing and waning of anguish, terror, acquiescence and surrender, rage and envy, disinterest and ennui, pretense, taunting and daring, and even yearning for death—all these in the context of bewilderment and pain." The point to remember is that a dying person will not and should not behave in some prescribed fashion; rather, each person's patterns of coping should be respected.

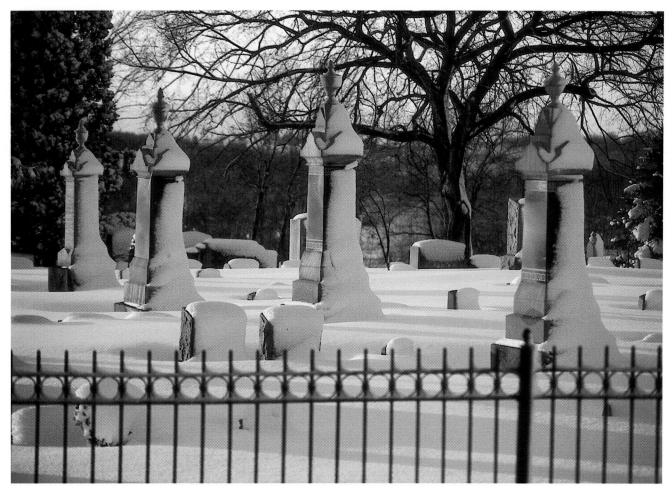

Death awaits all of us at the end of our lives, and accepting and dealing with death is a difficult but important task. Some people have found that facing the prospect of death makes them more aware of the preciousness of life.

Supporting a Dying Person

Most people feel somewhat uncomfortable in the presence of a person who has been diagnosed with a terminal illness. What can we say? How should we act? It may seem that any attempt to provide comfort results in words that are little more than stale platitudes. Nevertheless, we want to express our concern and make meaningful contact. Perhaps the most important gift we can bring to the person who is confronting his or her own death is the gift of listening. Giving the person an opportunity to speak honestly and openly about his or her experience is crucial, even though talking about death may be painful at first.

Although we sometimes tend to place dying people in a special category, the reality is that their needs are not fundamentally different from anyone else's, although their situation is perhaps more urgent. As is true of anyone, dying people want to know that they are valued, that they are not alone, that they are not being unfairly judged, and that those close to them are also trying to come to terms

with a difficult situation. As with any relationship, there are opportunities for growth on both sides.

Besides friends and family, the dying person may want access to other supportive resources. These might include the family physician, counselors, and clergy. Not all therapists are equally effective in dealing with issues relating to death, and it might take some time to find one who seems right. To be effective with the dying, a counselor must be compassionate, have professional training in the principles of caring for the dying, be comfortable with the idea of death, and have a nonjudgmental philosophy. As a benevolent outsider, the counselor can run interference for patients and serve as liaison between patients, their families, and physicians. Referrals to death-related counselors in most areas of the country can be provided by the Association for Death Education and Counseling, which can be contacted by writing to 638 Prospect Avenue, Hartford, CT 06105.

Many hospitals, hospices, and other health care organizations sponsor group programs for dying patients. These groups are usually chaired by a professional counselor and are designed to help patients express their concerns in a supportive atmosphere. You can make contact with groups of this kind by inquiring among hospital staff or other medical personnel. In addition, local chapters of support groups affiliated with organizations such as the American Cancer Society and Make Today Count can be found in many cities.

COPING WITH LOSS

Even if we have not experienced the death of someone close, all of us are survivors of the various losses that have occurred in our lives. Death is not the only kind of loss that calls upon our resources for coping; everyone experiences the losses that accompany changes and endings. The loss of a job, the ending of a relationship, transitions from one neighborhood or school to another—all these are examples of the kinds of losses that fill our lives. Some people call these losses "little deaths," and our response to them, although less painful perhaps, includes many of the mental and emotional reactions that occur in connection with the deaths of loved ones.

Grieving

Grief encompasses a person's emotional response to the event of loss. It can include feelings of sadness, longing, loneliness, and sorrow, as well as feelings of guilt, anger, and rage. When we recognize that many kinds of feelings occur in grief—not just feelings of sadness—then we are likely to be better able to accept our grief and move toward its resolution. Grieving is the means to healing.

When a loved one dies after a long period of illness, survivors may experience feelings of relief that the ordeal is over as well as anguish at the ending of a beloved relationship. When death takes someone close to you, anger may be felt over unresolved issues in the relationship. The emotions that occur in grief are much like those experienced by a dying person: shock, disbelief, denial, anger, guilt, vulnerability, depression. The bereaved person is likely to experience many different feelings, often conflicting ones.

Talking and crying, even yelling in rage, are ways of resolving the intense feelings of grief. Don't try to hold back feelings or to be "strong" and "brave." Those who offer such advice do not understand the dynamics of grief, nor the necessity for grief to be expressed as a way of healing. On the other hand, you needn't pretend to grieve or exaggerate your emotions if the strong feelings that often accompany grief simply aren't present in your particular experience.

Although various models have been proposed to summarize the processes associated with grief, each person's actual experience is highly individual. We can use such models as an aid to understanding grief, but it is impor-

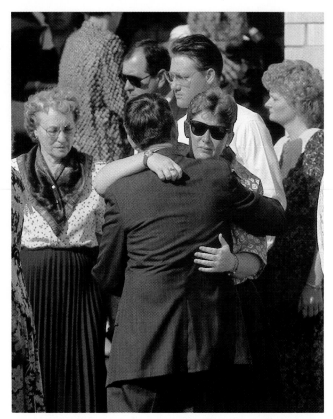

Funeral or memorial services give friends and relatives of the deceased the opportunity to mark their grief through ritual and ceremony.

tant that we do not try to superimpose a rigid structure on our own or another's experience.

In the aftermath of a death, the early period of grief is characterized by shock and numbness, often with strong feelings of disbelief and denial. We can't believe that the devastating loss has happened; it can't be real. The sense of disorganization that pervades our mental and emotional life during this period is challenged by the need to attend to the various actions and decisions surrounding the disposition of the deceased's body. Being forced to engage in such activities is therapeutic; it helps us accept the reality of the death, thereby taking us beyond the initial period of shock and into the intense grief work that is at the heart of coping with loss.

The middle phase of grief, then, is a period of intense grief work as we experience the pain of separation. The bustle of activities that takes place immediately after a death begins to lessen, and friends are usually not as accessible as they had been during the initial crisis. This is often a time of intense yearning for the lost loved one, an intense reexamination of the whole relationship as the bonds of attachment are slowly relinquished. Survivors experience fantasies of somehow "undoing" the loss, making everything as it was before. Varying considerably

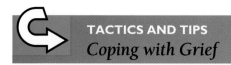

- Realize and recognize the loss.
- Take time for nature's slow, sure, stuttering process of healing.
- Give yourself massive doses of restful relaxation and routine busy-ness.
- Know that powerful, overwhelming feelings will lessen with time.
- Be vulnerable, share your pain, and be humble enough to accept support.
- Surround yourself with life: plants, animals, and friends.
- Use mementos to help your mourning, not to live in the dead past.
- Avoid rebound relationships, big decisions, and anything addictive.

- Keep a diary and record successes, memories, and struggles.
- Prepare for change, new interests, new friends, solitude, creativity, growth.
- Recognize that forgiveness (of ourselves and others) is a vital part of the healing process.
- Know that holidays and anniversaries can bring up the painful feelings you thought you had successfully worked through.
- Realize that any new death-related crisis will bring up feelings about past losses.

Source: The Centre for Living with Dying

among survivors and depending, too, on the circumstances of the loss, this phase of grief generally lasts from several weeks to several months. It is during this period that many physiological symptoms associated with intense grief are experienced: lethargy, restlessness, disturbed sleep, lack of appetite, and weight loss.

As survivors and as caring helpers, we need to keep in mind that social support is every bit as critical during this phase of grief as during the early days following the loss. To go through the psychological process of mourning, the bereaved person needs to express his or her feelings. As the reality of the loss is absorbed, the predominant feeling will likely be sadness. By gradually undoing the bonds of the lost relationship through intense grieving, emotions are slowly freed for reinvestment in life (see the box "Coping with Grief").

The last phase of "active" grief is characterized as a period of resolution, a time of reestablishing our physical and emotional balance, of reintegration. The acute feelings and emotional turmoil of grief are no longer experienced constantly. Our sadness doesn't go away completely, but it recedes into the background. Reminders will stimulate the pain of loss from time to time, but we begin to move ahead with life and focus more on present concerns, not past memories. This new-found sense of freedom can be difficult to admit at first; it may feel like a betrayal of the deceased loved one. In fact, it indicates a healthy willingness to engage once again in the outside world. Coming to terms with grief does not mean forgetting the loved one or denying the significance of the lost relationship. At various times throughout our lives, reminders of the loss can stimulate a recurrence of grief; as

time passes, however, this happens with diminishing frequency and intensity.

Supporting a Grieving Person

A variety of activities, rituals, and social institutions can help survivors cope with loss. Social support provided by relatives and friends can be a major source of strength for the bereaved. The simple gift of listening can be extremely helpful, since talking about a loss is an important way that survivors cope with their changed reality. The key to being a good listener is to refrain from making judgments about whether the feelings expressed by the survivor are "right" or "wrong," "good" or "bad." The feelings generated by a loss are not necessarily the ones we might expect. However, they are valid in terms of a particular survivor's total response to bereavement. We have two ears and one mouth, a ratio between listening and speaking that can guide our conversations with the recently bereaved.

Funerals and similar leave-taking rituals can help provide a sense of closure on the deceased's life, helping survivors integrate the loss into their ongoing lives. Among some societies, funerals provide an opportunity for the bereaved not only to express their sadness at losing a loved one, but also to vent their anger at the deceased's abandonment of them: "Why did you leave me? I need you!" This practice of scolding the corpse stands in contrast to the Western cultural notion that one should not speak ill of the dead. In modern American society, there are different styles of mourning behavior among different regional or ethnic groups. For one group, funerals are occasions of weeping and wailing; for another, stoic expressions and subdued emotions are the rule. Whatever its characteristics, the funeral provides a social framework for expressing grief and provides closure that helps survivors cope with the fact of death.

Although family and friends may be very supportive during the initial period following a death, the extended need for support that continues throughout the first year or two of mourning may not be met by relying solely on those traditional sources of support. Organized support groups offer a helpful way for bereaved persons to share their concerns and empathy with one another as they come to terms with loss. Perhaps the best known of the organized support groups are those focused on concerns of widows and widowers. Other support groups provide support for particular types of loss. The Compassionate Friends organization, for example, serves parents who have experienced a child's death. Hospital or hospice social workers and community service organizations can provide referrals to appropriate support groups.

COMING TO TERMS WITH DEATH

For many of us death has been kept out of view, a fearful possibility that we avoid at all costs. With the death of a friend or a relative, or perhaps with news of a major disaster, we are forced to confront our emotions, our relationship with the experience that awaits all of us at the end of life. Encountering death can help make us more aware of the preciousness of life. Prisoners incarcerated in the Nazi death camps during World War II have repeatedly expressed this theme in their writings. Many had been condemned to death and were awaiting execution. Yet, they found that the confrontation with death liberated them from petty personal concerns that had once seemed overwhelming. People who have come very near death as a result of accident or other catastrophe report a similar awakening to what is ultimately valuable in life.

In facing death, we find that relationships are more important than things; priorities are reordered as we cope with the painful reality of loss. Realizing that life offers no guarantees, we find ourselves able to overcome our own anxieties and petty concerns as well as the social structures that stop us from living more fully.

Examining our assumptions about death leads us to a discovery of its meaning in our own lives. Denying death eventually results in denying life. This denial is inherent in our news reports, where only the deaths of the famous or violent deaths get attention, and then only for a moment. In societies where each individual is considered important and irreplaceable, death is not ignored but is marked by community-wide grief for a genuine social loss. When we stop avoiding death, we find that it is an event whose significance touches not only the individual and his or her immediate family and friends, but also the wider community of which we are all part.

SUMMARY

- How people deal with death affects how they live their lives.

What Is Death?

- The use of respirators and other life-support systems allows some bodily functions to be artificially sustained, thereby requiring a definition of death that goes beyond the traditional criteria that focus only on vital signs of breathing and heartbeat.

- Brain death is characterized by lack of receptivity and response to external stimuli; absence of spontaneous muscular movement and spontaneous breathing; absence of observable reflexes; and absence of brain activity, signified by a flat electroencephalogram.

- Clinical death refers to a determination of death made according to either the traditional signs of death or the criteria used in defining brain death. Cellular death refers to the breakdown of metabolic processes in the cells when heartbeat, respiration, and brain activity cease.

- Although death makes logical sense in terms of species survival and evolution, no answer to the question of why death exists can ever be completely satisfying.

- From about age 10, most children understand that death is universal, inescapable, and irreversible.

- For most of the present century, Americans have engaged in denial of death by practices that seek to blunt its impact.

- Ambivalence toward death is a common component of suicide. The psychological autopsy is used to uncover the factors that led to a particular suicide.

Planning for Death

- Some decisions about death can and should be made while one is young.

- A will is a legal instrument governing the distribution of a person's property after his or her death. A person who dies intestate may have his or her estate distributed in a manner contrary to what would have been wanted.

- Dying at home requires considerable time and energy

from relatives or friends who must also learn the techniques of home care.

- Palliative care devoted to making dying patients comfortable and pain-free is available in many hospitals.

- The hospice philosophy of care stresses a team approach in providing palliative care to dying patients and relies to a large extent on volunteer help.

- A terminal patient can grant power of attorney to a trusted friend or relative to handle matters affecting the patient if he or she becomes incapacitated or otherwise unable to attend to legal matters.

- Passive euthanasia refers to the practice of withdrawing or withholding life-sustaining treatment; it has become a fairly well-established practice in modern medicine.

- Active euthanasia refers to the practice of intentionally hastening the death of a patient; it is unlawful and generally unacceptable in the United States.

- Living wills, powers of attorney for health care, and other advance directives are vehicles for expressing one's wishes about the use of life-sustaining measures.

- All states have legal provisions that allow people to donate their bodies or individual organs for use after death.

- For Americans, the decision about what to do with the body after death usually involves either burial or cremation.

- It is generally agreed that bereaved persons benefit from participating in a funeral ceremony or memorial service to commemorate a loved one's death.

The Experience of Life-threatening Illness

- Facing death is a difficult and painful experience. Although the dying must find their own way of adapting to the changes they face, they can benefit from the help of others.

- Responses to one's own imminent death vary greatly, although periods of denial and isolation, anger, bargaining, depression, and acceptance are commonly experienced.

- Those who wish to offer support to a dying person should consider that person's unique needs. Giving the dying person opportunities to speak openly is crucial.

Coping with Loss

- Grieving is the emotional process of healing the pain of loss, and it can include a variety of feelings.

- At various times throughout one's life, reminders of a loss can stimulate a recurrence of grief; as time passes, this happens with diminishing frequency and intensity.

- Social support provided by relatives and friends is a major source of strength for the bereaved.

Coming to Terms with Death

- Encountering death can help make a person more aware of the preciousness and precariousness of life.

- Death touches not only the individual and his or her family and friends, but also the wider community.

TAKE ACTION

1. In some states, the motor vehicle department now sends organ donor forms to residents along with auto registration materials. Individuals can fill them out and keep them with their driver's license. If your state doesn't provide them, you can also request a Uniform Donor Card from the National Kidney Foundation (30 East 33rd St., New York, NY 10016). When you receive the donor form, consider the advantages and disadvantages of being a donor. If you decide to be a donor, fill out the card and keep it with your driver's license.

2. Investigate the services available in your community to care for the dying, including hospitals, hospices, and counseling resources. Visit one or more of them and evaluate their services.

3. Obtain sample copies of a living will and a durable power of attorney for health care that are appropriate for the state you live in. Check with your local hospital or health services organization for these forms or request them from Choice in Dying (200 Varick Street, New York, NY 10014). After you have reviewed the forms, consider the advantages and disadvantages of their use. If you decide to execute a living will or durable power of attorney for health care, discuss your decision with members of your family to make them aware of your wishes.

4. Talk with your spouse, parents, grandparents, or other family members about their wishes for how they would want things to be at the end of their lives. Ask if they have made out wills, living wills, or powers of attorney for health care decisions. If they do not wish to discuss these matters, let them know that you are open to such a discussion in the future.

JOURNAL ENTRY

1. What do you believe happens after death—heaven or hell, eternal sleep, nothingness, return to life in another form, union with a higher consciousness,

something mysterious and unknowable? Write a brief essay explaining your concept or belief. Where did it come from? Is it what you wish would happen after death?

2. *Critical Thinking:* Research the issue of physician-assisted suicide (active euthanasia). Write a brief essay that presents the main arguments on both sides of the issue; conclude your essay with a statement of your own opinion. Be sure to explain your reasoning. What are the most important factors in your decision? Why do you think you hold the opinion you do?

SELECTED BIBLIOGRAPHY

Annas, G. J. 1991. *The Rights of Patients: The Basic ACLU Guide to Patients Rights,* 2nd ed. Clifton, N.J.: Humana Press.

Badham, P., and L. Badham, eds. 1986. *Death and Immortality in the Religions of the World.* New York: Paragon House.

Callahan, D. 1990. *What Kind of Life: The Limits of Medical Progress.* New York: Simon and Schuster.

Carroll, D. 1985. *Living with Dying: A Loving Guide for Family and Close Friends.* New York: McGraw-Hill.

DeSpelder, L. A., and A. L. Strickland. 1992. *The Last Dance: Encountering Death and Dying,* 3rd ed. Mountain View, Calif.: Mayfield.

Doka, K. J., ed. 1989. *Disenfranchised Grief: Recognizing Hidden Sorrow.* Lexington, Mass.: Lexington Books.

Duda, D. 1982. *A Guide to Dying at Home.* Santa Fe, N. Mex.: John Muir.

Feinstein, D., and P. E. Mayo. 1990. *Rituals for Living and Dying: From Life's Wounds to Spiritual Awakening.* San Francisco: HarperCollins.

Gervais, K. G. 1986. *Redefining Death.* New Haven, Conn.: Yale University Press.

Hinton, J. 1972. *Dying,* 2nd ed. Baltimore, Md.: Pelican.

Kapleau, P. 1989. *The Wheel of Life and Death: A Practical and Spiritual Guide.* New York: Doubleday.

Kübler-Ross, E. 1968. *On Death and Dying.* New York: Macmillan.

LeGrand, L. E. 1986. *Coping with Separation and Loss as a Young Adult.* Springfield, Ill.: Charles C. Thomas.

Macklin, R. 1987. *Mortal Choices: Bioethics in Today's World.* New York: Pantheon Books.

Mor, V., D. S. Greer, and R. Kastenbaum, eds. 1988. *The Hospice Experiment.* Baltimore: Johns Hopkins University Press.

Morgan, E. 1988. *Dealing Creatively with Death: A Manual of Death Education and Simple Burial,* 11th ed. Burnsville, N.C.: Celo Press.

Osterweis, M., F. Solomon, and M. Green, eds. 1984. *Bereavement: Reactions, Consequences, and Care.* Washington, D.C.: National Academy Press.

Sanders, C. M. 1989. *Grief, the Mourning After: Dealing with Adult Bereavement.* New York: John Wiley.

Shneidman, E. S., ed. 1984. *Death: Current Perspectives,* 3rd ed. Mountain View, Calif.: Mayfield.

Stillion, J., E. McDowell, and J. May, eds. 1989. *Suicide Across the Life Span: Premature Exits.* New York: Hemisphere.

Winslade, W. J., and J. W. Ross. 1986. *Choosing Life or Death: A Guide for Patients, Families, and Professionals.* New York: Free Press.

Zeleski, C. G. 1988. *Otherworld Journeys: Accounts of Near-Death Experiences in Medieval and Modern Times.* New York: Oxford University Press.

RECOMMENDED READINGS

Beresford, L. 1993. *The Hospice Handbook: A Complete Guide.* Boston: Little, Brown. *Addresses practical questions, such as knowing when hospice care is needed, insurance coverage, and Medicare benefits, and describes different kinds of hospice care.*

Enright, D. J. 1983. *The Oxford Book of Death.* New York: Oxford University Press. *Attitudes toward death are revealed through a wide-ranging selection of quotations from literary and philosophical sources.*

Kastenbaum, R., and B. Kastenbaum, eds. 1989. *Encyclopedia of Death.* Phoenix: Oryx Press. *Provides broad coverage of topics relating to dying and death; most entries include references for further study.*

Rando, T. A. 1988. *Grieving: How to Go on Living When Someone You Love Dies.* Lexington, Mass.: Lexington Books. *An outstanding and sensitive guide to coping with loss.*

Veatch, R. M. 1989. *Death, Dying, and the Biological Revolution: Our Last Quest for Responsibility,* rev. ed. New Haven, Conn.: Yale University Press. *Provides a comprehensive and useful discussion of the issues important to an understanding of medical ethics.*

Weisman, A. D. 1984. *The Coping Capacity: On the Nature of Being Mortal.* New York: McGraw-Hill. *A practical and intellectually stimulating discussion of coping strategies that can be applied in confronting death as well as the losses encountered in daily life.*

21

Medical Self-Care: Skills for the Health Care Consumer

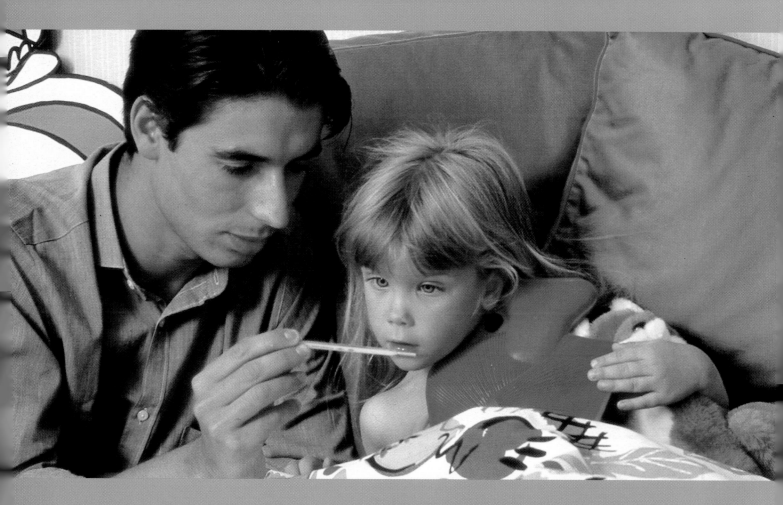

When you were playing volleyball yesterday, you landed awkwardly on your right foot and twisted your ankle. It seemed to be OK at the time and you continued playing. But when you woke up this morning, your ankle was swollen, and you couldn't put your weight on it. You're not sure what to do. Should you wait for it to get better by itself? Elevate it and apply an ice pack? Soak it in Epsom salts? Go to the clinic to see a physician?

You took a home pregnancy test three weeks ago and it indicated that you weren't pregnant. But since your period still hasn't started, you called the clinic to see if they might know what was wrong. The nurse said that your test result might have been a false negative and you should come in for an examination. Does that mean you might be pregnant after all?

You've had a lot of sore throats in the past year, and your family physician wants you to have your tonsils removed. You've heard that tonsillectomies are unnecessary, but you don't feel comfortable questioning the medical opinions of a physician who has known you your whole life. Should you seek a second opinion? Follow his recommendation? What are your rights and responsibilities in this situation?

You're getting a cold—your nose is running, you're sneezing, and you feel tired and feverish. You stop at the pharmacy for something to relieve your symptoms. But when you get home, your roommate says, "Why did you get a combination cold remedy? You have just a runny nose and a fever. This stuff also has a cough suppressant and an antihistamine for allergies." You reply that you thought you'd be better off with a comprehensive treatment, something that would cover any symptoms you might develop. She says that by taking more drugs, you're multiplying the number of side effects you might experience. Is she right? Is it better to take a medication with only a single ingredient? Or is it better to try to cover all the bases?

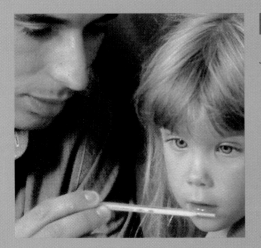

MAKING CONNECTIONS

Just as people have been changing personal habits to maintain and improve their health, they have also been taking greater responsibility for self-care when they get sick. This shift means people have to acquire the information and skills required for managing illnesses and injuries. In each of the scenarios presented on this page, all related to self-care, individuals have to use information, make a decision, or choose a course of action. How would you act in each of these situations? What response or decision would you make? This chapter provides information about self-care and the effective use of the health care system that can be used in situations like these. After finishing the chapter, read the scenarios again. Has what you've learned changed how you would respond?

When you think of the health care system, do you envision physicians, nurses, clinics, hospitals, and medical laboratories? This is an accurate picture as far as it goes, but don't forget your own role in the health care system—as a self-care provider. Even with today's dazzling medical technology, highly effective medications, and wide variety of skilled practitioners, the individual plays a crucial role in the health care system. In fact, the professional medical care system depends on the functioning of nonprofessional care. If people were to stop practicing self-care and seek professional care for even a small percentage of the complaints they usually manage themselves—colds, backaches, stomach aches, headaches, fatigue, and so on—the professional health care system would be overwhelmed. The average person has about four new medical symptoms each *month* yet consults a physician only four times a *year.* At least 80 percent of medical symptoms are self-diagnosed and self-treated.

Until recently, this critical role of people as the *primary* providers of health care for themselves and their families went largely unnoticed. With attention focused on the "delivery" of professional services, many individuals remained unaware of how important a part they played in their own health care. Today, people are becoming more confident of their own ability to solve personal health problems. With increased knowledge of when and how to self-treat and when to seek professional care, they can become even more competent in self-care.

Even a small increase in appropriate self-care could result in billions of health care dollars saved. For example, in one study, simply providing people with a book of information about self-care and when to contact a health professional reduced overall visits to physicians by 17 percent and visits for minor illnesses by 35 percent. When people are provided with clear, simple information, they can prevent and treat most common health problems in their own homes—earlier, more cheaply, and often better than health professionals.

The key element in this transition is the recognition that people can *manage* their own health care. Managers don't do everything themselves; they use others—consultants, advisers, experts—to help them get the job done. Once they have all the information they need, they make decisions and take responsibility for follow-through. People who manage their own health gather information—whether from physicians, friends, classes, books, magazines, or self-help groups—solicit opinions and advice, and then make their own decisions. They recognize that everyday choices about diet, exercise, and other habits are critical determinants of health. They participate in every phase of their health care and accept personal responsibility for it. They realize that the choices are theirs.

Health promotion and a healthy lifestyle include being an informed partner in medical care and practicing safe, effective self-care. How can you develop this self-care attitude and take a more active role in your health care? The first step is to learn the skills you need to identify and manage medical problems. The second step is to learn how to make the health care system work effectively for you. This chapter provides information that will help you become competent in both these areas.

MANAGING MEDICAL PROBLEMS

Effectively managing medical problems involves developing several skills. First, you need to learn how to be a good observer of your own body and assess your symptoms. Second, you need to be able to decide when to seek professional advice and when you can safely deal with the problem on your own. Third, you need to know how to safely and effectively self-treat common medical problems.

Self-Assessment

Self-care begins with careful observation of your own body. We are constantly observing our bodies, scanning for unusual sensations, aches, or pains. Symptoms are signals from our bodies. They alert us that something may be wrong.

Symptoms are often an expression of the body's attempt to heal itself. For example, the pain and swelling that occur after an ankle injury immobilize the injured joint to allow healing to take place. A fever may be an attempt to make the body less hospitable to infectious agents. A cough can help clear the airways and protect the lungs. Understanding what a symptom means and what is going on in your body helps reduce anxiety about symptoms and allows you to practice safe self-care that supports your body's own healing mechanisms.

Carefully observing symptoms also helps you identify those signals that suggest you need professional assistance to help your body heal. You should begin by noting when the symptom began, how often and when it occurs, what makes it worse, what makes it better, and if you have any associated symptoms. You can also monitor your body's "vital signs" such as temperature and pulse rate. These signs may give important clues as to how your body is managing an illness.

Not too long ago, the thermometer was the only tool available to evaluate medical problems at home. Now a new generation of medical self-tests are available: home blood pressure machines, home blood glucose tests for diabetics, pregnancy tests, self-tests for urinary tract infections, and over a dozen other do-it-yourself kits and devices. All these tools are designed to help you make a more informed decision about when to seek medical help and when to self-treat.

Home medical tests offer several advantages: cost savings, convenience, privacy, an increased sense of control, and sometimes more comprehensive information. Blood

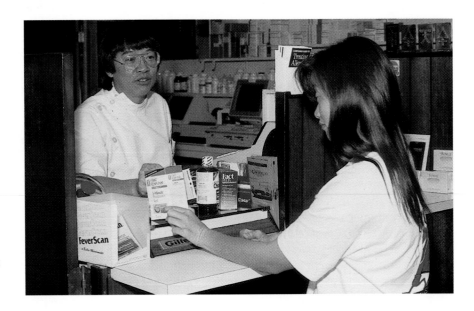

Home pregnancy test kits are just one type of self-test that can be obtained without a prescription in a pharmacy or even your supermarket. Using one of these kits, a woman can determine if she is pregnant within a week of having missed her period.

pressure measurements taken at home can give a more complete picture of what your blood pressure is like throughout the day, not just during visits to the physician. Many people suffer from "white-coat hypertension"—their blood pressure may go up during the stress of a visit to the physician. Home blood pressure checks can also help hypertensives under medical supervision try non-drug treatments such as diet, exercise, or relaxation. One study even suggests that home blood pressure monitoring *itself* may lower blood pressure. Why? One theory is that checking your own blood pressure may be a form of biofeedback—as you become aware of pressure changes you can voluntarily control them. It may be that over time you experience less anxiety while checking your pressure. Or you may begin, unconsciously, to change your diet and other factors that affect blood pressure.

For diabetics, home blood glucose monitoring can be a more efficient, less expensive way to check blood glucose levels, because it allows frequent, rapid measurements without interrupting normal daily activities to go to a laboratory. With home monitoring, diabetics can work in partnership with their physicians to keep their blood sugar levels under better control by adjusting their insulin doses, diet, and exercise. Sometimes tighter control can reduce the need for frequent visits to the laboratory or hospitalization to manage unstable diabetes.

Privacy and convenience are also important factors in the growth of home medical tests. For example, a self-test for pregnancy lets a woman find out for herself whether she is pregnant.

Careful reading of the instructions with home test kits, including when *not* to test, as well as coaching from your physician, will help maximize the accuracy and usefulness of home tests. If you do find an abnormal test result, repeat the test. If it is still abnormal, if you are at all doubtful about the test results, or if your symptoms persist even if the tests are normal, consult your physician.

Careful self-observation and selective use of self-tests may help provide you with the type of information you need to make informed self-care decisions and participate more actively in your care.

> ***Personal Insight*** How do you feel about taking responsibility for your health? Do you feel confident about self-care? Are there ways you can increase your confidence?

Decision Making: Knowing When to See a Physician

To self-treat or not self-treat, that is the question. When confronted with a symptom, a person must ask a series of questions: "What's going on in my body?" "Is this dangerous?" "Have I or anyone else I know had something like this before?" Some of the answers you give to these questions are conscious and rational; others are more unconscious, emotional responses.

People often make two kinds of mistakes in deciding what to do when faced with symptoms. They may rush to their physician too often or too quickly for minor complaints they could easily and effectively manage on their own. Or they may ignore symptoms and self-treat when they should be seeking professional assistance.

For example, suppose you develop diarrhea and some mild abdominal cramping. If you immediately rush off to a clinic, you are likely to waste your time and the physician's. However, if you knew what key signs to look for (such as blood in the stool, high fever, and dehydration) and how to practice effective self-care for the symptoms (clear liquid diet and so on), you would be in a position to make a more informed choice.

At the other extreme, people too often ignore symptoms that *should* trigger a visit to the doctor. For example, any breast lump should be medically evaluated. Although 80 to 90 percent of breast lumps turn out to be noncancerous, early treatment of the few that are cancerous can save lives. Informed self-care involves knowing how to evaluate symptoms so that you don't go to a physician either too early *or* too late.

Your decision to seek professional assistance for a symptom is generally guided by your history of medical problems and the nature of the symptom you are experiencing. In general, you should check with a physician for symptoms that are

1. *Severe.* If the symptom is very severe or intense, medical assistance is advised. Examples include severe pains, major injuries, and other emergencies.

2. *Unusual.* If the symptom is very peculiar and unfamiliar, it is wise to check it out with your physician. Examples include unexplained lumps, changes in a skin blemish or mole, problems with vision, difficulty swallowing, numbness, weakness, unexplained weight loss, and blood in sputum, urine, or bowel movement.

3. *Persistent.* If the symptom lasts longer than expected, seek medical advice. Examples in adults include fever for more than five days, a cough lasting longer than two weeks, a sore that doesn't heal within a month, and hoarseness lasting longer than three weeks.

4. *Recurrent.* If a symptom tends to return again and again, medical evaluation is advised. Examples include recurrent headaches, stomach pains, and backache.

Sometimes a single symptom is not a cause for concern; but when the symptom is accompanied by other symptoms, the combination suggests a more serious problem. For example, a fever with a stiff neck suggests meningitis. A cough with green sputum and a high fever might mean pneumonia.

If you evaluate your symptoms and think that you need professional assistance, then you must decide how urgent the problem is. If it is a true emergency, then you should go (or be taken) to the nearest emergency room. Emergencies would include

• Major trauma or injury, such as head injury, suspected broken bone, deep wound, severe burn, eye injury, or animal bite

• Uncontrollable bleeding or internal bleeding, as indicated by blood in the sputum, vomit, or a bowel movement

• Intolerable and uncontrollable pain

• Severe chest pain

• Severe shortness of breath

• Persistent abdominal pain, especially if associated with nausea and vomiting

• Poisoning or drug overdose

• Loss of consciousness or seizure

• Stupor, drowsiness, or disorientation that cannot be explained

• Severe or worsening reaction to an insect bite or sting, or to a medication, especially if breathing is difficult

Unfortunately, many visits to the emergency room are not true emergencies. And there are many reasons not to go to a hospital emergency room if it is not a true emergency. Emergency rooms do not operate on a first-come first-served basis. Patients are **triaged,** a screening process in which those patients with the most urgent needs are treated first. So if your problem is not a true emergency, you may have to wait hours while more critically ill patients are seen before you. Your medical records are usually not available in the emergency room, and it is harder to get appropriate follow-up care. Also, many insurance policies do not cover nonemergency visits to emergency rooms, so if you go to an ER with a mild symptom, you could end up paying the bill. And emergency room medical bills are much higher than office or urgent care center visits.

If your problem is not an emergency, but still requires medical attention, consider a call to your physician's office. Often you can be given medical advice over the phone without the inconvenience of a visit. If you do require a visit, it can often be arranged at the most convenient and appropriate time and place. Nearly 16 percent of all outpatient medical advice and 30 percent of pediatrics advice is now dispensed by telephone.

To help you make wise medical decisions, a "Self-Care Guide for Common Medical Problems" is provided in Appendix I. This guide includes some specific guidelines on when to call a physician for certain medical problems and on when and how to self-treat. To know whom to call see Chapter 22, where the different types of health care professionals are discussed.

Self-Treatment

When confronted with a new symptom, many people try to find some pill or potion that will relieve or cure it. However, other self-treatment options are available. In most cases, your body can itself relieve your symptoms and heal the disorder. The prescriptions filled by your body's internal pharmacy are frequently the safest and most effective treatment. So patience and careful self-observation are often the best choices in self-treatment. Nondrug treatments are also sometimes highly effective.

> **Triage** A screening and sorting out of people who are sick or injured so that the most seriously ill can be treated first or so that the patient is directed to the most appropriate type of medical practitioner.

The longer life expectancy of Americans today is partly due to advances in the use of medications designed to prevent or fight disease. Drugs are an essential part of modern medical care, but they are also powerful chemicals that have the potential for harm. Being an informed consumer can help ensure that you receive the maximum benefit from the medications you take, while minimizing your risks.

How Are Drugs Classified?

Drugs are classified as prescription or over-the-counter (OTC). Prescription drugs are those you buy with a physician's prescription from a licensed pharmacy. OTC medicines are available without a prescription and include everything from aspirin to medicated shampoo.

Generic versus Brand-Name Drugs

When a drug is first developed, it's given a patent and a generic name. The patent gives the firm that discovers it the sole right to sell the drug while the patent is in effect. When the drug comes on the market, it is usually given a brand name by the manufacturer. After the patent expires (usually in about 17 years), the drug becomes public property and other companies can make and sell the drug under its generic name or their own brand name. Generic drugs contain the same active ingredients as the original brand-name drug but may contain different inactive ingredients. Generic drugs usually cost less than their brand-name counterparts, and they can often be substituted at a substantial savings to the patient. However, for some drugs it may be important that you use a particular brand; ask your physician whether a generic drug is available and suitable for you.

Side Effects

All drugs cause changes in your body's chemistry; usually these changes are helpful, but they can also harm you. Side effects can occur with all drugs. Most often side effects are mild—such as a slight headache or drowsiness—but they can also be serious. Ask your physician or pharmacist what side effects you might expect from a drug. If you suffer an unexpected or severe side effect, contact your physician.

Drug Interactions

Medications can interact with other drugs and with what you eat. If you take two or more drugs at the same time, the medications may interact and cause undesirable effects. Food can delay or reduce the absorption of many drugs; other drugs are better absorbed or less irritating to your stomach when you take them with food. Unless otherwise directed by your physician, it's best to take drugs with a full glass of water at least one hour before, or two hours after, a meal. Your physician or pharmacist will tell you if a drug should be taken with food. Alcohol and other drugs may either enhance or reduce the effect of a medication. Combining alcohol with a medication that causes sedation can result in dangerous depression of the central nervous system. Don't take medications with alcohol.

Using the same pharmacy on a continuing basis is an important health care decision. A pharmacist who knows about your medical conditions and the drugs you are taking can alert you to possible interactions and answer questions about your medications.

Communicate Before You Medicate

To safely prescribe medications for you, your physician(s) must know your medical condition, what medications you are currently taking (including OTCs), whether you are allergic to any drugs, how much and how often you use alcohol, and whether you are pregnant or plan to become pregnant in the near future. Never hesitate to ask your physician or pharmacist questions about any prescription or OTC drug. You should know why you are taking it, what action you can expect it to have, what the proper dosage is, how and when you should take it, and whether there are any restrictions or side effects.

Be Informed and Act Wisely

In addition to discussing your medications with your physician and pharmacist, read all drug labels carefully—both prescription and OTC. Pay close attention to all directions, warnings, and precautions, and take all your medications exactly as directed. Don't stop taking a drug unless directed to do so by your physician. Keep a list of all the prescription and OTC drugs you are taking.

Taking medications is a big responsibility. For your own health and safety, listen, read, ask questions, and understand your medications.

Source: "Medications: Know What You're Taking and Why." *Medical Essay: Supplement to Mayo Clinic Health Letter,* October 1992.

For example, massage, ice packs, and neck exercises may be, at times, more helpful than drugs in relieving headaches and other aches and pains. For a variety of disorders either caused or aggravated by stress, relaxation and stress management strategies may be the treatment of choice (see Chapter 2). So before reaching for medications, consider *all* your options for self-treatment.

Self-Medication Self-treatment with nonprescription medications is an important and valuable part of our health care system. Within every two-week period, nearly 70 percent of people self-medicate with one or more drugs. If even a small percentage of people stopped using such **over-the-counter (OTC)** drugs and began making appointments with physicians for their colds, sore

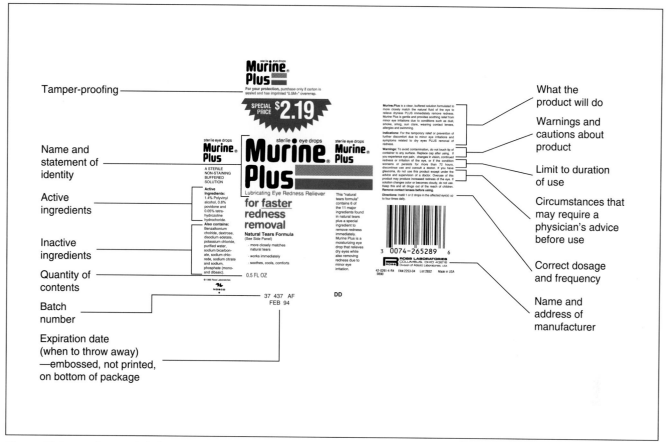

Figure 21-1 *Looking at labels: OTCs.*

throats, backaches, and headaches, the physicians could not possibly handle the load. Many OTC drugs are highly effective in relieving symptoms and sometimes in curing illnesses. Physicians themselves may recommend OTC products when they can be helpful. About 60 percent of all medications are sold over the counter.

The Food and Drug Administration (FDA) has undertaken a massive review of the safety, effectiveness, and labeling of OTC products. As a result, many ineffective or unsafe OTC medications have been taken off the market. Other medications that formerly required a physician's prescription are now available without prescription. So you can now walk into any pharmacy and purchase without prescription such drugs as hydrocortisone cream and antifungal agents. But with this increased consumer choice comes increased responsibility to use these medications wisely (see the box "Safe and Effective Use of Medications").

You need to be aware of the barrage of drug advertising aimed at you. The implicit message of such advertising is that every symptom, every ache and pain, every problem, can be solved by a product. Many of the OTC products *are* effective, but many simply waste your money and divert your attention from better ways of coping. Many ingredients in OTCs—perhaps 70 percent—have not been proven to be effective, a fact the FDA does not dispute.

It is important to remember that any drug, whether bought in the supermarket or prescribed by a physician, may have side effects. However, following some simple guidelines will improve your chances of safely and effectively self-medicating:

1. Always read drug labels and follow directions carefully. By law, the label must include the names and quantities of the active ingredients, precautions, and adequate directions for safe use. Carefully reading the label and reviewing the individual ingredients may help prevent you from taking medications that have caused problems for you in the past. If you don't understand the information on the label, ask a pharmacist or physician before using a product (Figure 21-1).

2. Do not exceed the recommended dosage or length of treatment unless you discuss this change with your physician.

OTC (over-the-counter) Medications and products that can be purchased by the consumer without a prescription.

TERMS

TABLE 21-1 Your Home Self-Care Kit

Symptom or Problem	Medication or Supplies
Allergies/hay fever	Antihistamine
Coughs	Expectorant or cough suppressant (dextromethorphan)
Constipation	Milk of Magnesia Bulk laxative (psyllium seed)
Diarrhea	Kaolin/pectate Loperamide
Eye irritations	Eyedrops and artificial tears Eyecup
Fever	Thermometer Acetaminophen (children or adults) Aspirin (adults)
Fungal infections of skin (athlete's foot, ringworm)	Antifungal preparations
Heartburn and indigestion	Antacids (nonabsorbable, such as magnesium hydroxide or aluminum hydroxide)
Hemorrhoids	Hemorrhoid preparations
Nasal congestion	Decongestant tablets, nose sprays, or drops
Pain (minor)	Aspirin, acetaminophen, or ibuprofen
Poisoning (to induce vomiting)	Syrup of ipecac
Skin rashes and irritations	Hydrocortisone cream Sodium bicarbonate (baking soda) Burrow's solution
Sore throat	Anesthetic lozenges, gargle, or spray
Splinters	Needle-nosed tweezers
Sprains and strains	Elastic bandages Ice pack Heating pad/hot water bottle
Sunburn (preventive)	Sunscreen (15+ SPF)
Wounds (minor)	Povidone iodine (Betadine) Antibacterial creams/ointments Adhesive bandages Gauze Cotton balls Adhesive tape

3. Use caution if you are taking other medications—OTC and prescription drugs can interact. If you have questions about drug interactions, ask your physician or pharmacist *before* you mix medicines.

4. Try to select medications with one active ingredient rather than combination ("all-in-one") products. A product with multiple ingredients is likely to include drugs for symptoms you don't even have, so why risk the side effects of medications you don't need? Using single-ingredient products also allows you to adjust the dosage of each medication separately for optimal symptom relief with minimal side effects.

5. When choosing medications, try to buy **generic drugs,** which contain the same active ingredient as

the brand-name product but generally at a much lower cost.

6. Never take or give a drug from an unlabeled container or in the dark when you can't read what the label says.

7. If you are pregnant, nursing, or have a chronic disease such as kidney disease, consult your physician before self-medicating.

8. Many medications have an expiration date of about two to three years. Dispose of all expired medications. Don't flush medications down the toilet or toss them into the trash—they can be toxic to the environment. The safest way to dispose of unwanted medications is to take them to a pharmacy, clinic, or hospital.

9. Store your medications in a safe place away from the reach of children. Poisoning with medications is a common and preventable problem. The usual bathroom medicine chest is usually not a secure or dry place to store medications. Consider a lockable tool chest or fishing box that can be stored out of reach of children—preferably not in a bathroom or other location where dampness or heat might ruin medications.

10. Use special caution with aspirin. Because of information indicating an association with a rare but serious problem known as Reye's syndrome, aspirin should not be used for children or adolescents who may have the flu, chickenpox, or any other viral illness.

The Home Pharmacy If you were to survey home medicine chests, what would you find? On average, there would be 22 medications, including 17 OTC products. You would probably find an oversupply of expired medications, leftover prescription drugs, and useless medications. At the same time, certain essential medications and equipment would be absent. Most people wait until a crisis arises. They then search frantically through a poorly stocked medicine chest and often have to make an inconvenient midnight dash to a pharmacy, if they can find one open.

Only a few supplies are essential; additional items depend upon the particular health problems you or your family are likely to face (Table 21-1). Since many of the medications deteriorate, buy small quantities of infrequently used medications and replace them about every three years.

GETTING THE MOST OUT OF YOUR MEDICAL CARE

Self-care involves more than self-diagnosis and self-treatment. It includes knowing when to seek professional care and how to get the most out of your medical care. The key to making the health care system work for you lies in good communication with your physician and with the other members of the health care team. Studies show that patients who are more active in interacting with physicians, who ask more questions, enjoy better health outcomes such as lower blood glucose levels in diabetics and lower blood pressure measurements in hypertensive patients.

Unfortunately, many people are intimidated by their physicians and afraid to communicate freely. Medical jargon can be very confusing. One survey revealed that 20 to 30 percent of college-educated people had significant misunderstandings about the meaning of such common medical terms as *hypertension, virus, herpes, tumor, Pap test, strep throat,* and *uterus.* Yet patients tend not to ask their physicians what such medical jargon means, because they fear appearing stupid (see the box "How Well Do You Understand Medispeak?"). Others are afraid to ask why a test or treatment is needed for fear of appearing to challenge the authority of the physician. Patients often conceal personal concerns about sexuality, drug abuse, emotional problems, and cancer. All these fears and others block open communication with the physician.

Physicians share the responsibility for poor communication. They may feel they are too busy or important to take time to talk with patients. They may ignore questions, use incomprehensible medical jargon, and respond in an unsupportive way to patients' attempts to assert themselves.

The Physician-Patient Partnership

The physician-patient relationship is undergoing an important transformation. The image of the physician as a God-like, all-knowing authority and the patient as a passive supplicant is slowly fading. What is emerging is more of a physician-patient *partnership,* in which the physician acts more like a consultant and the patient participates more actively. The necessary ingredients in a successful physician-patient partnership are a sympathetic, caring physician and a prepared, assertive patient. As one observer commented, "It is not enough for the doctor to stop playing God. You've got to get off your knees."

Generic drug Non-brand-name drug that is not registered or protected by a trademark.

TERMS

Did you ever wonder why your physician says "edema" instead of "swelling" and "hemorrhage" instead of "bleed"? Whether you call it medispeak or medicalese, the overuse of medical terminology and medical jargon can result in confusion, misinterpretation, and apprehension rather than compliance and trust. In some cases, unnecessary jargon may be used to ward off questions and challenges from listeners. In other cases, the physician may simply not be aware of what you do and don't understand.

Whatever the situation, you can avoid communication problems by becoming fluent in some basic medical terminology yourself. Begin by testing yourself on the following commonly used terms. Cover the column on the right to see how many terms you know.

1.	Adipose	Fatty
2.	Ambulatory	Able to walk
3.	Analgesic	Painkiller
4.	Antipyretic	Fever reducer
5.	Atropy	Shrinkage or wasting of muscle or tissue
6.	Benign	Noncancerous
7.	Congenital	Condition present at birth
8.	Contraindicated	To be avoided
9.	Dermatitis	Irritation of the skin
10.	Diaphoresis	Perspiration
11.	Etiology	Pertaining to the causes of disease
12.	Febrile	Feverish
13.	Hemorrhage	Bleeding
14.	Idiopathic	Of unknown cause
15.	Lesion	Any sore or wound
16.	Malignant	Cancerous
17.	Negative test result	The patient doesn't have a disorder
18.	Parenteral	Medicine given by injection
19.	Prognosis	Expected outcome of a disease
20.	Pruritus	Itching
21.	Psychogenic	Having an emotional origin
22.	Q.I.D.	Take four times a day
23.	Sepsis	Infection
24.	Sequela	Aftereffect of a disease
25.	Subclinical	Having no symptoms
26.	Subcutaneous	Beneath the skin
27.	Syndrome	A specific collection of symptoms
28.	Systemic	Affecting the whole body
29.	Topical	On the surface
30.	Urticaria	Hives, usually from an allergic reaction

How did you do? If you knew 24 to 30 of the terms, you probably understand your physicians' explanations and instructions most of the time. If you knew 12 to 23, you're on your way to medical fluency. If you knew fewer than 12 of the terms, you may want to invest in a medical dictionary for laypeople. Ask for explanation of terms you don't know and repeat instructions back to your physician to make sure you've understood them properly. Knowing the language is one of the keys to self-confidence when it comes to dealing with professional health care providers.

You should try to remember that physicians are human: They have off days, and they make mistakes just as everyone else does. You don't have to "love" your physician as a best friend, but you should expect someone who is attentive, caring, able to listen, and able to clearly explain things to you. You also have to do your part. You need to be assertive in a firm but not aggressive manner. You need to express your feelings and concerns, ask questions, and, if necessary, be persistent. If your physician is unable to communicate clearly with you in spite of your best efforts, then you probably need to change physicians. Remember, the best medical care requires a healthy partnership (see the box "Patient's Bill of Rights").

One of the realities of medical care today is that physicians are often pressed for time. This makes it even more important that you prepare for the visit and use your time wisely.

Preparing for the Visit

• Before visiting your physician, make a written list of questions or concerns that you have. Also include notes about your symptoms (when they started, how long they last, what makes them worse or better, and so on). This list prepares you to clearly state your major concerns as well as concisely answer the questions your physician is likely to ask. Have you ever thought to yourself after you walked out of the office, "Why didn't I ask about . . ."? Limit your list to major concerns. At best, your physician is likely to have time to address only a few of your concerns at any one visit. *Be sure to state your concerns at the very beginning of the interview.* It is frustrating for physicians as well as patients when concerns are brought up at the end of a visit ("Oh, by the way could you . . . ") and there isn't time to properly address them.

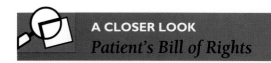
The American Hospital Association has developed a Patient's Bill of Rights with the expectation that observance of these rights will contribute to more effective patient care and greater satisfaction for the patient, the physician, and the hospital organization. The Association presents these rights in the expectation that they will be supported by the hospital on behalf of its patients as an integral part of the healing process. The traditional physician-patient relationship takes on a new dimension when care is rendered within an organizational structure. Legal precedent has established that the institution itself also has a responsibility to the patient. It is in recognition of these factors that these rights are affirmed.

1. Patients have the right to considerate and respectful care.

2. Patients have the right to obtain from their physicians complete current information concerning their diagnosis, treatment, and prognosis in terms patients can be reasonably expected to understand. When it is not medically advisable to give such information to patients, the information should be made available to an appropriate person on their behalf.

3. Patients have the right to receive from their physicians information necessary to give informed consent prior to the start of any procedure and/or treatment. Except in emergencies, such information should include but not necessarily be limited to the specific procedure and/or treatment, the medically significant risks involved, and the probable duration of incapacitation. Where medically significant alternatives for care or treatment exist, or when patients request information concerning the medical alternatives, patients have the right to such information.

4. Patients have the right to refuse treatment to the extent permitted by law and to be informed of the medical consequences of that action.

5. Patients have the right to every consideration of their privacy concerning their own medical care program. Case discussion, consultation, examination, and treatment are confidential and should be conducted discreetly.

6. Patients have the right to expect that all communications and records pertaining to their care be treated confidentially.

7. Patients have the right to expect that within its capacity a hospital must make reasonable response to the request of patients for services. The hospital must provide evaluation, service, and/or referral as indicated by the urgency of the case.

8. Patients have the right to obtain information about the relationship of their hospital to other health care and educational institutions insofar as their care is concerned. They also have the right to obtain information about any professional relationships among individuals who are treating them.

9. Patients have the right to be advised if the hospital proposes to engage in or perform human experimentation affecting their care or treatment. Patients have the right to refuse to participate in such research projects.

10. Patients have the right to expect reasonable continuity of care. They have the right to expect that the hospital will provide a mechanism whereby they are informed by their physician of the patients' continuing health care requirements following discharge.

11. Patients have the right to examine and receive an explanation of their bill regardless of the source of payment.

12. Patients have the right to know what hospital rules and regulations apply to their conduct as patients.

A hospital has many functions to perform, including the prevention and treatment of disease, the education of both health professionals and patients, and the conduct of clinical research. But all these activities must be conducted with an overriding concern for patients and, above all, the recognition of their dignity as human beings.

Adapted from The American Hospital Association, *Patient's Bill of Rights.*

- Bring a list of all medications (prescription and nonprescription) you are taking, or bring all these medications with you to the office so that your physician can review them. Also, if you have previous medical records or test results that might be relevant to your problems, bring them along.

During the Visit

- Try to be as open as you can in sharing your thoughts, feelings, and fears. If you are worried, try to

explain why: "I am worried that what I have is contagious; my father had similar symptoms before he died," and so on.

- Don't be afraid to ask what you may consider a "stupid" question. These questions can often indicate an important concern or misunderstanding.

- If you don't understand or remember something the physician said, admit that you need to go over it again.

- Give your physician feedback. If you don't like the

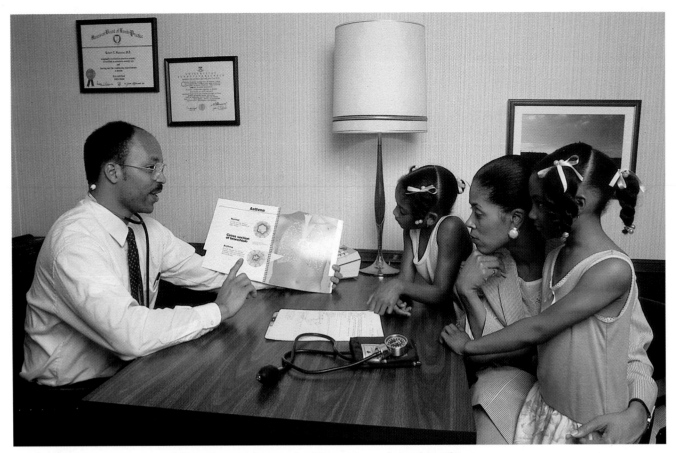

Good communication is a crucial factor in a satisfactory physician-patient relationship. This mother is learning about asthma, a condition that individuals can often manage successfully with medication and an inhaler.

way you have been treated by the physician or someone else on the health care team, let your physician know. If you have been unable to follow the physician's advice or had problems with a treatment, tell your physician so adjustments can be made. Also, most physicians very much appreciate compliments and positive feedback. So, if you are very pleased, let your physician know.

- When appropriate, ask your physician to write down instructions or recommend reading material for more information on a particular subject.

- If you have trouble remembering instructions, try taking notes during the visit or consider bringing along someone else to act as a second listener. Another set of eyes and ears may help you later recall some of the details of the visit or instructions.

After the Visit

- At the end of the appointment, briefly repeat back— in your own words—what you understood the physician to say about the nature of the problem and what you are supposed to do. This repetition helps

check your understanding and helps to ensure the best care.

- Make sure you understand what the next steps are. Should you return for a visit and, if so, when and why? Should you phone for test results? Are there any danger signs you should watch for and report back to your physician?

In addition to developing effective communication skills, understanding something about how a diagnosis is made, what treatment options are available, and what questions you should ask will help equip you to take a more active role in your own health care.

The Diagnostic Process

Solving a medical problem is sometimes like solving a mystery. The problem is presented, clues are discovered, evidence is sought, possibilities are tracked down, and finally (we hope) a correct diagnosis is made.

There are three main sources of clues and information on which to base a diagnosis. The first is the medical history, which is the patient's own description of what has happened. The second is the physical examination of the patient. The third is the results from various diagnostic tests and procedures. All this information is then evaluated to reach a diagnosis that names and explains the problem and guides treatment.

The Medical History: Telling It Like It Is

The most important part of medical diagnosis is the medical history. This is the description that you give the physician of your problem, concerns, and background. In well over 70 percent of cases, a careful history alone can lead to a correct diagnosis. Your ability to describe your illness clearly, concisely, and accurately is an essential first step in the diagnostic process. Depending on the nature of the problem, you may be asked about some or all of these areas.

- *The chief complaint.* To elicit the chief complaint, the physician may ask something like "What brings you here today?" Give the reason for your visit; and, if you have more than one concern, list them all briefly and concisely. Don't disguise any concerns (such as worries about cancer or sexual problems) or wait until the end of the visit to bring them up.

- *The present illness.* The physician will ask a series of questions to clarify the nature, character, and chronological course of your major symptom. Among them are "When did it begin?" "How long does it last?" "What brings it on or makes it worse?" Be concise but as specific as possible.

- *The past medical history.* You will be asked about your health in general and your medical history, including previous illnesses, hospitalizations, operations, immunizations, allergies, and medications. This information can provide clues to what is or is not causing your current symptoms. Report all medications you're taking and be specific about allergies to medications.

- *Review of systems.* The physician reviews symptoms you are experiencing in all your different body organs and physiological systems. Although the questions asked may not seem to be related to your chief complaint, your response may reveal information vital to managing your present illness or detecting unrecognized problems.

- *Social history.* The physician may ask questions about your job, living conditions, family, life stresses, and health habits like smoking and alcohol use. Clues that aid in the diagnosis might include exposure to toxic materials at work, a recent trip to a foreign country, and a family history of diseases.

Giving an accurate and concise medical history is critical to good medical care. You are the expert about how you feel and how you experience symptoms. You should know your body best and what's normal and abnormal for you. Through the medical history, you can share your expertise with the physician.

The Anatomy of a Physical Examination

The physician then proceeds to examine you. Depending upon your chief complaint, this examination may be a complete, head-to-toe exam or may be directed to certain areas or physiological systems.

Traditionally, the physical examination consists of inspection (looking), **palpation** (feeling), and **auscultation** (listening). The physician might examine:

- *Vital signs.* Pulse rate, breathing rate, temperature, and blood pressure may be measured.

- *Head, ears, eyes, nose, and throat.* The physician may look at the ear canal and eardrum with a lighted instrument (**otoscope**) for signs of infection or blockage. Your hearing may be tested by whispering, a ticking watch, a tuning fork, or an electronic device. The physician may inspect the external parts of the eye; redness may indicate an infection, paleness may suggest anemia. The pupil of the eye normally constricts when light shines in. The blood vessels, retina, and optic nerve at the back of the eye can be seen with a special lighted instrument called an **ophthalmoscope.** The physician may check the mucous membranes of your nose. A brisk tapping over the sinus cavities that causes pain may suggest infection. He or she may check your tongue, gums, mouth, and throat for abnormalities.

- *Neck.* The physician may feel your neck for the presence of swollen lymph nodes, indicating an infection, or for irregularities in the thyroid gland, which lies just below the Adam's apple. A stethoscope can help the physician detect abnormal sounds in the arteries of the neck, which may signal atherosclerotic blockage and risk of stroke.

- *Chest.* The physician may tap on your chest with his or her fingers to detect possible fluid accumulation or pneumonia. You will be asked to take deep breaths in and out through your mouth as your physician listens with a stethoscope. The stethoscope can also be used to detect irregularities in heart rhythm or abnormal clicks and **murmurs** as the heart valves open and close. Women's breasts are checked for lumps as a possible sign of breast cancer.

Palpation The act of feeling some organ or part of the body in order to make a diagnosis.

Auscultation The act of listening to sounds made by the body in order to make a diagnosis.

Otoscope A lighted instrument used to view inside the ear.

Ophthalmoscope A lighted instrument used to view the interior of the eye.

Murmur An abnormal sound heard over a blood vessel or the heart due to some blockage of blood flow.

TERMS

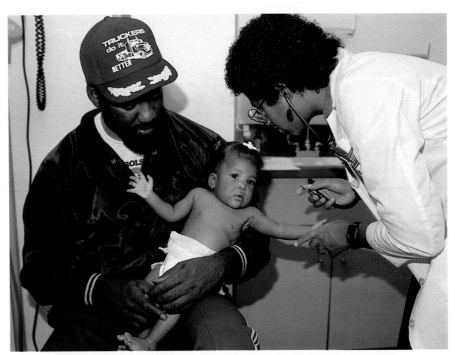

Physical examinations are particularly important for infants and are scheduled at regular intervals during the first few years of life. In addition to vaccinating the child against many diseases, the physician has the opportunity to spot any problems that may be developing, and the parents have the chance to discuss their concerns.

- *Abdomen.* The physician will use his or her fingers to probe your belly for tenderness or masses, checking your liver in the upper right side, your spleen in the upper left, your stomach in the upper middle, and intestines throughout. Your physician may also listen with a stethoscope to the sounds your intestines make.

- *Genitals.* In men, the penis and testicles will be checked for sores, tenderness, or growths. The physician may press a finger against the scrotal sac and lower abdomen to feel for a weakness in the abdominal wall. A bulge in the abdominal contents when you cough is a sign of a hernia. In women, a pelvic examination includes inspection, palpation, and a Pap test.

- *Rectum.* The physician may insert a gloved finger into your rectum to check for abnormal growths. In men, the prostate gland can be checked through the rectum for lumps, enlargement, or tenderness. In women, parts of the pelvic organs can also be felt through the rectum.

- *Extremities.* The physician may check your legs and feet for swelling, redness, or tenderness of the joints, suggesting arthritis. Painless but swollen ankles and feet may be a sign of heart, liver, or kidney disease. The pulses in your feet and wrists may be checked for adequate blood flow through the arteries. Your calves may be squeezed to check for blood clots in the veins.

- *Skin.* Your skin will be checked for sores, moles, lumps, and rashes. Paleness may suggest anemia; a yellow color (jaundice) may suggest a liver abnormality such as hepatitis.

- *Neurological signs.* Depending on your symptoms, the physician might check your nervous system. This check might include testing your muscle strength, balance, coordination, reflexes, and sensation. For example, tapping the tendon below your kneecap normally elicits a reflex contraction of a thigh muscle. This knee-reflex action brings many parts of the nervous system into play, and a malfunction can indicate problems in the nervous system and/or quadriceps muscle in the thigh.

If you notice any pain or unusual sensations during the examination, let your physician know. Your response may provide important information. Also, if you are curious about what is being done during the exam or why, ask your physician. (But not when the physician has the stethoscope in his or her ears!)

Medical Testing In addition to the medical history and physical examination, diagnostic testing now provides a wealth of new information to help solve medical problems. High-tech and high-cost medical testing now accounts for nearly a third of our national health bill. No body fluid, orifice, or cavity is beyond the reach of a medical probe: blood and urine tests, x-rays, biopsies, taps,

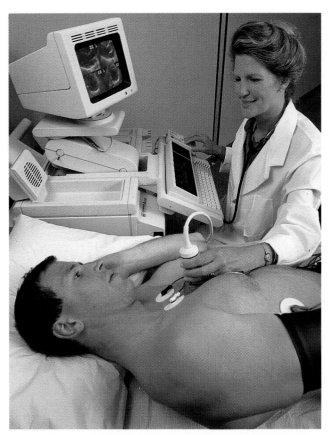

Physicians get information they need from medical tests, but patients have the right to know what the test is for, why they need it, what it will involve, and what the results will indicate. This man is undergoing an electrocardiogram to assess the condition of his heart and arteries.

scans, electronic monitors, and a bewildering array of **endoscopies** (bronchoscopy, arthroscopy, sigmoidoscopy, and so on), the scoping procedures that peer into nearly every part of the body.

More than 10 billion medical tests are done in the United States each year—over 40 tests per person—at a staggering cost of $140 billion, or $600 for each of us. Patients can no longer afford to take a passive role in this important phase of their medical care.

Careful scientific studies reveal that at least 25 percent of all medical tests are unnecessary. For example, one study showed that over half of the blood tests routinely ordered when a patient is admitted to the hospital for surgery were virtually useless, contributing little to patient care, but a lot to patient bills.

Of course, there are good reasons for ordering a medical test: to help your doctor diagnose symptoms accurately, monitor the progress of a known disease, or screen for a hidden one (see the box "Preventive Medicine for Healthy Adults"). Unfortunately, numerous tests are performed for other reasons. Many physicians may order tests to protect themselves from malpractice. Many physicians can earn more by ordering tests and doing diagnos-

tic procedures than by taking the same amount of time to question, examine, counsel, or think about a patient's problem.

Many patients feel that more tests mean better care. People often say, "My doctor is so thorough, he did nearly every test available." Although tests can provide a measure of reassurance, a diagnosis can be made 80 to 90 percent of the time with only a thorough history and physical examination. Also, the tests ordered may be the wrong ones.

Consider Anne, a 23-year-old woman complaining of a mild burning discomfort in her upper abdomen for about two weeks. Her physician asked her several brief questions, examined her abdomen, and ordered "a few tests": a urinalysis, a 12-test blood panel, a complete blood count, and an upper GI series (x-rays that outline the esophagus and stomach).

All these studies added extra costs to her bill but did little to change her suspected diagnosis of esophagitis—an inflamed esophagus caused by stomach acid backup. Nor did the tests affect her treatment—antacids. The most likely diagnosis and treatment could have been determined from her history without a lot of testing. In this respect, Anne was overtested. But she was also undertested. In the previous five years, she hadn't had a Pap test and pelvic exam, both cancer-screening tests generally recommended for women her age.

When you visit a physician you can help assure that you get the medical tests you need by asking some of the following questions. While it is not realistic to ask all these questions for every minor blood or urine test, you should consider such questions whenever an expensive, uncomfortable, or potentially risky test is recommended.

- *"Why do I need the test?"* Start by asking how the test will help diagnose your problem or change your treatment. A satisfactory answer might be "I'm recommending a barium enema because you've been passing blood in your stool. A previous test shows the blood isn't due to hemorrhoids, so we need to find the source of the bleeding. It may be quite harmless, but it could be a serious problem such as a bowel cancer that needs prompt treatment."

  Ask about alternatives. For example, if you have already had the proposed test, can those earlier results be used? To this end, it is wise to keep a record of all your medical tests—when and where they were done and the results.

  Then ask your physician about the risk of waiting

Endoscopies　Medical procedures in which a viewing instrument is inserted into body cavities or openings. The specific procedures are named for the area viewed: inside joints (arthroscopy), inside airways (bronchoscopy), inside the abdominal cavity (laparoscopy), and inside the lower portion of the digestive tract, called the *sigmoid colon* (sigmoidoscopy).

TERMS

Most people associate a visit to their physician with an illness or injury. But physicians can also play a crucial role in helping healthy people stay healthy. There are three primary components of preventive medical care: counseling about lifestyle and disease risks, appropriate immunizations, and screening tests for various diseases. Working together, you and your physician can help prevent many health problems and lessen the impact of any diseases you do develop. Preventive medicine is an important part of a healthy lifestyle.

Counseling

During periodic health checkups, your physician should counsel you about your disease risks, especially in areas where they are increased because of heredity, environment, or lifestyle. Your physician can reinforce the importance of many healthy behaviors, including eating a low-fat, high-fiber diet that contains adequate amounts of essential nutrients; controlling body fat; not smoking; using alcohol only in moderation and not in potentially dangerous situations; exercising regularly; practicing safer sex; avoiding unintended pregnancy (through abstinence or contraception); and not abusing drugs, illegal or prescription. Your physician might also advise you to wear a helmet while riding a motorcycle or bicycle, protect your back from injury on the job, or use sunscreen while outdoors. Although many of these behaviors are widely known as important parts of a healthy lifestyle, information and encouragement from a physician have been shown to be effective in motivating people to adopt healthy behaviors.

Immunizations

As discussed in earlier chapters, appropriate immunizations are an easy and effective way to protect yourself from certain infectious diseases. The need for immunization doesn't end with childhood. Everyone should receive a tetanus-diphtheria booster every 10 years. Anyone over age 65 should be immunized against influenza every year and receive a one-time pneumococcal vaccine. Physicians can help identify people in high-risk groups who may also need immunization against rubella, hepatitis B, or other diseases.

Screening Tests

Many tests are currently available to screen for early signs of disease. For a screening test to be truly useful, it must reliably detect a significant disease before symptoms develop, and the treatment for the disease must be more effective when begun before symptoms arise. A good example of a useful screening test is the Pap smear, which can identify cervical cancer before symptoms appear, when it is most easily cured. A test for an incurable form of lung cancer would not be a particularly useful test—if a person doesn't survive longer as a result of early diagnosis and treatment, it serves little purpose. The risk and cost of tests and treatment are also important issues to consider when evaluating screening tests.

Despite disagreements and limitations, some rough guidelines can be offered to help you select which medical tests to have and approximately how often they should be performed. These guidelines represent the minimum tests recommended for people *without symptoms*. If you have symptoms or are at risk for certain conditions, additional tests may be advised. Use the guidelines in the table below as a starting point, and discuss your particular needs with your physician. And remember, don't rely on medical testing to protect your health—a healthy lifestyle will do more to protect and promote your health than all the tests in the world.

Screening Test	Frequency
Medical and family history	Periodically
Total blood cholesterol	Every 5 years
Blood pressure	Every 2 years
Weight	Periodically
Sigmoidoscopy (a visual examination of the lower colon to detect colorectal cancer)	Every 5–10 years for anyone over age 50. Anyone at higher risk due to personal or family history should discuss appropriate screening with a physician.

and not testing. Monitoring the symptoms under a physician's supervision for a specific period of time may provide the necessary diagnostic clue, or the symptoms may simply resolve on their own.

- *"What are the risks?"* No test entirely lacks risks. Begin by weighing potential benefits against risks. Physical

risks vary, depending on the nature of the test, your age, past medical history, general state of health and ability to cooperate, and the skill and experience of your physician.

- *"How do I prepare for the test?"* For some tests, preparation is very important. Be sure to remind your

Screening Test	Frequency
Fecal occult blood test (a test for hidden blood in the stool to detect colon cancer)	Every 1–2 years. Anyone at increased risk for colon cancer due to personal or family history should discuss appropriate screening with a physician. (This test is of uncertain benefit for average-risk people age 50 and older.)
Skin examination	Periodically for anyone with history of excessive sun exposure or severe sunburns, skin cancer or precancerous skin conditions, family history of malignant melanoma.
Blood glucose (sugar) (a blood test for diabetes)	Periodically for anyone more than 50 pounds overweight, with a family history of diabetes or a history of diabetes during pregnancy, or of American Indian heritage.
Clinical breast exam (physical examination of breasts by health professional for breast cancer detection)	Every 1–2 years for all women over the age of 40; women at higher risk due to history of previous breast cancer or family history of breast cancer should have an exam every year beginning at age 35.
Breast self-exam (a self-examination for breast cancer detection)	Every month for all women over the age of 20
Mammogram (x-ray examination used to detect breast cancer)	Every 1–2 years for women age 50 to 75 who are of average risk (the test has less certain benefit between the ages of 40–50 and over age 75). Every year beginning at age 35 for women at higher risk due to personal or family history.
Pap test (an examination of the cells of the cervix for detection of cervical cancer)	Every 1–3 years for women ages 18–65 (less certain benefit after age 65 if previous tests normal)
Rubella antibodies (blood test for immunity to German measles)	Once for women of childbearing years who are fertile and do not know from previous blood tests if they are immune.
Sexually transmitted disease tests (gonorrhea, chlamydia, and syphilis)	Periodically for anyone with multiple sexual partners or history of other recent sexually transmitted diseases.
HIV testing (blood test for AIDS virus antibodies)	Periodically for anyone at risk (see Chapter 17).
Tuberculin skin test (PPD) (to detect infection with tuberculosis)	Periodically for anyone with close contact in the last two years with someone known to have tuberculosis or anyone who recently moved to the United States from Asia, Africa, Central America, South America, or Pacific Islands where TB is more common.
Testicular self-exam (a self-examination for testicular cancer)	Every month for men ages 18–45.

Recommendations adapted from U.S. Task Force Staff. 1989. *Guide to Clinical and Preventive Services: Report of the U.S. Preventive Services Task Force.* Baltimore: Williams and Wilkins.

physician about any allergies, especially to medications, anesthetics, or x-ray contrast materials. Mention medications you may be taking, bleeding problems, or whether you might be pregnant. Ask whether you should do anything special before the test, such as fasting or discontinuing medications.

• *"What will the test be like?"* Knowing how the test is done and how it will feel can decrease your anxiety and discomfort before and during a test. During and after the test, it is important to let the physician or assistants know what you are feeling. If you're uncomfortable, something can usually be done. Your sensations may provide the first clue to averting a developing complication.

- *"What do the results mean?"* No test is 100 percent accurate. When faced with an abnormal result, the natural tendency is to assume that you are sick. But the test result may be a **false positive;** that is, the test result itself may be wrong, indicating that you have a disease or condition when you really don't. Conversely, a test result may be a **false negative,** in which the test fails to accurately detect a disease or condition. For example, if a pregnancy test reads "negative" (no pregnancy) in a pregnant woman, this is a false negative.

Medical tests often give the impression of objectivity and precision. Yet some tests, such as x-rays, electrocardiograms, and scoping procedures, require subjective interpretation. A study of chest x-ray interpretation, for example, found that more than 70 percent of the reports contained disagreements among experienced radiologists; in 25 percent of the reports, the physicians missed important findings. Therefore, getting an experienced second opinion on diagnosis may be important, particularly when ominous symptoms are present or when risky therapies or procedures are prescribed on the basis of an abnormal test. Sometimes repeating the test can "cure" the disease.

Above all, remember that medical tests are only part of the diagnostic puzzle. Such clues must always be viewed in the context of other information about you: medical history, family, age, habits, medications, symptoms, and physical examination. Good physicians treat patients—not test results.

Medical and Surgical Treatments

Once a diagnosis is made, the treatment options can be considered. The treatments offered for diseases should reflect the wide variety of physical, chemical, and psychosocial factors that cause or aggravate the disease condition. Although some diseases can be cured or ameliorated by medical or surgical treatment, other diseases require no treatment at all or may be aggravated by attempts at therapy. Therefore, whenever a treatment is recommended, whether medication or an operation, it is important that you understand the reasons for treatments, options, risks, and expected benefits. Asking the following key questions may help ensure that you are getting the best possible care for yourself.

- *"What are my choices in treatments?"* Many conditions can be treated in a variety of ways, and your physician should be able to explain the alternative choices to you. In some cases, management with medication is a viable alternative to surgery. In other cases, lifestyle changes, including exercise, diet, and stress management, should be considered alongside

medication or surgery before making a choice. When any treatment is recommended, also ask what the consequences are likely to be if you postpone treatment.

- *"What are the risks, costs, and expected benefits of each treatment option?"* To make an informed choice about any treatment, you need to know what each of the options would cost you. No one can tell you which choice is right for you. However, to make an informed choice you need information about the treatment options. Informed *choice,* not merely informed *consent,* is an essential ingredient in quality medical care.

Prescription Medications Thousands of lives are saved each year by **antibiotics,** heart medications, insulin, and scores of other drugs. Pain medications and anesthetics make the unbearable bearable. Arthritis medications help preserve function for thousands of people. But we pay a price for having such powerful tools. Of all admissions to hospitals, nearly 5 percent are due primarily to drug reactions, and 20 percent of these patients are likely to have a second drug reaction during their hospital stay.

Part of the problem lies with physicians who overprescribe or misprescribe drugs. Mishaps also occur because patients do not receive adequate information about medications and often don't understand how to take them or fail to follow instructions given to them. Consumers should ask the following questions about their medications:

- *"Do I really need this medication?"* Some physicians often prescribe medications not because they are really necessary, but because they think that patients want and expect drugs. Ask about nondrug alternatives. Sometimes the best medication of all is no medication.

- *"What is the name of the medication, and what is it supposed to do?"* Your physician should tell you why the medication is being prescribed, how the prescription might be expected to help you, and how soon you can expect results.

- *"How and when do I take the medication, and for how long?"* Understanding how much of the medication to take and how often and how long to take it is frequently critical to its safe, effective use. For example, some medications you need take only until you feel better. To prevent a recurrence of illness, other medications, like antibiotics for bacterial infections, should be taken until you finish the entire prescription.

- *"What foods, drinks, other medications, or activities should I avoid while taking this medication?"* The presence of food in the stomach may help protect the stomach from some medications, but it can render

Dental diseases can be prevented through proper self-care and regular visits to the dentist. Follow these tips for healthy teeth and gums.

Brushing

Brushing the teeth removes plaque and food particles from the outer, inner, and biting surfaces of your teeth. Choose a soft brush with end-rounded or polished bristles. The size and shape of the brush should allow you to reach every tooth.

A number of different tooth-brushing methods are acceptable; the following is one effective way of removing plaque:

1. Place the head of your toothbrush beside your teeth, with the bristle tips at a 45-degree angle against the gumline.

2. Move the brush back and forth in short (half-a-tooth-size) strokes several times, using a gentle "scrubbing" motion.

3. Brush the outer surfaces of each tooth, upper and lower, keeping the bristles angled against the gumline.

4. Use the same method on the inside surfaces of all teeth, still using short back-and-forth strokes.

5. Scrub the chewing surfaces of the teeth.

6. To clean the inside surfaces of the front teeth, tilt the brush vertically and make several gentle up-and-down strokes with the "toe" (the front part) of the brush.

7. Brushing your tongue will help freshen your breath and clean your mouth by removing bacteria.

Flossing

Flossing removes plaque and food particles from between the teeth and under the gumline, areas where your toothbrush can't reach. When flossing, follow the instructions given to you by your dentist or dental hygienist. Here are some helpful suggestions:

1. Break off about 18 inches of floss, and wind most of it around one of your middle fingers.

2. Wind the remaining floss around the same finger of the opposite hand. This finger will "take up" the floss as you use it.

3. Hold the floss tightly between your thumb and forefingers, with about an inch of floss between them. There should be no slack. Using a gentle sawing motion, guide the floss between your teeth. Never "snap" the floss into the gums.

4. When the floss reaches the gumline, curve it into a C-shape against one tooth. Gently slide it into the space between the gum and the tooth until you feel resistance.

5. Hold the floss tightly against the tooth. Gently scrape the side of the tooth, moving the floss away from the gum.

6. Repeat this method on the rest of your teeth. Don't forget the back side of your last tooth.

Source: American Dental Association

---

other drugs ineffective. Other drugs you may be taking, even over-the-counter drugs and alcohol, can either amplify or inhibit the effects of the prescribed medication.

- *"What are the side effects, and what do I do if they occur?"* All medications have side effects. Some may be tolerable, minor annoyances while others may be life-threatening allergic reactions. You need to know what symptoms to look out for and what action to take should they develop. It is your responsibility to ask about precautions and possible side effects. If you have a drug allergy or another medical condition (such as diabetes or epilepsy) that may require special attention in the case of a medical emergency, it's important that you protect yourself by carrying a medical ID card or wearing a medical ID necklace or bracelet. For comprehensive emergency service, consider joining Medic Alert. This group provides a wallet ID card, a necklace or bracelet, and a 24-hour emergency phone hot line that can provide hospitals with your complete medical history. Call 1-800-ID-ALERT for more information.

- *"Can you prescribe an alternative or generic medication that is less expensive?"* Often there are several different medications that are equally safe and effective. You can sometimes save a lot of money by requesting the least expensive alternative.

- *"Is there any written information about the medication?"* Even if your physician takes the time to carefully

TERMS

False positive   When a test incorrectly detects a disease or condition in a healthy person.

False negative   When a test fails to correctly detect a disease or condition.

Antibiotic   A substance derived from a mold or bacteria that inhibits the growth of other microorganisms.

answer all your questions about medications, you will probably find it difficult to remember all this information. Fortunately, there are now many sources of information, from package inserts to pamphlets and books, where you can read more about the medications you are taking (see Appendix II, "Resources for Self-Care").

Remember, never share your prescription medication with anyone else, and never take someone else's. Store your drugs in a cool, dry place, out of direct light, and never use an old prescription for a new ailment.

Surgery   Americans are the most operated-on people in the world. Each year over 20 million operations are performed. About 20 percent of these operations are in response to an emergency such as a severe injury while 80 percent are **elective** surgeries, meaning the patient can generally choose when and where to have the operation if at all. The number of operations performed varies widely from country to country, city to city, and even surgeon to surgeon. The most important factor predicting rates of surgery in a given community is the number of surgeons, not the amount of disease. The more surgeons, the more surgery. All this suggests that you would do well to ask some questions when surgery is recommended for you or a family member to help ensure the operation is really necessary.

- *"Why do I need surgery at this time?"* Your physician should be able to explain to you the reason for the surgery, alternatives to surgery, and what is likely to happen if you don't have the operation. You should also ask about how the surgery is likely to benefit you.

  With most surgery, getting a *second opinion* is advised, and many health insurance plans now require a second opinion before all or certain elective operations. Studies show that when second opinions are required on elective surgical procedures, in 27 percent of cases the second surgeon does not agree that the recommended operation is necessary. Consulting a nonsurgeon may also be helpful in exploring alternatives to surgery. For more information about how to get a second opinion, you can call the second opinion hot line sponsored by the U.S. government at 1-800-638-6833.

  If your second opinion agrees with the recommendation for surgery, then you can feel more confident in proceeding. If the second opinion conflicts with the first, you may wish to have the physicians confer with each other to clarify the recommendations or you may want to get a third opinion. Disagreements among physicians are usually honest differences of opinion in gray areas of medical knowledge where an expert consensus has not yet been reached. In all cases, you yourself must weigh the opinions carefully, and make the final decision about your treatment.

  Although second opinions are most commonly sought for elective surgical procedures, you should also consider getting one for any treatment or diagnostic procedure with significant risk or cost.

- *"What are the risks and complications of the surgery?"* All surgical procedures carry some risk. The overall risk varies, depending on the type of operation performed, the surgeon, and your general state of health. You should ask about the **mortality rate** (risk of death) and **morbidity rate** (risk of nonlethal complications). You should also ask how often the surgeon has performed the operation and what his or her personal experience has been with the procedure. Studies show that surgical teams having more experience with an operation tend to have lower rates of complications. Some state governments and consumer organizations publish "report cards" on individual physicians or hospitals that show comparative complication rates for various surgical procedures or disease treatments.

  Sometimes an operation can be performed in several different ways, using different incisions, techniques, and anesthetics. Discuss these options with your surgeon so that you can better understand your choices.

  Blood transfusions may be required during some operations. If you need a transfusion, blood banks have adopted techniques that screen donor blood to ensure its safety. Nevertheless, if an elective operation is planned, ask if you can donate and store some of your own blood in the months preceding the surgery. Then if you need blood during surgery you can

TERMS

Elective surgery   A nonemergency operation that the patient can choose to schedule.

Mortality rate   The number of deaths occurring in a population of a given size in a given time period.

Morbidity rate   The number of illnesses or injuries occurring in a population of a given size in a given time period.

Autologous donation   A process in which a person can receive a transfusion of his or her blood that was previously withdrawn and stored.

Outpatient   A person receiving medical attention without being admitted to the hospital.

Vasectomy   Surgical cutting of the tubes that transport sperm (vasa deferentia), performed as a method of birth control.

Dilation and curettage (D&C)   Scraping of the interior of the uterus, usually performed to diagnose cancer or stop bleeding.

Tonsillectomy   Surgical procedure to remove the lymph tissue (tonsils) at the back of the throat.

Arthroscopic surgery   Examination of and surgery on a joint using a type of endoscope that is inserted into the joint through a small incision.

receive a transfusion of your own blood. This technique, known as **autologous donation**, reduces the risk even further of developing a transfusion reaction or contracting an infection such as viral hepatitis or HIV infection from infected donor blood.

- *"Can the operation be performed on an outpatient basis?"* More than 30 percent of all operations can now be safely performed on an **outpatient** (ambulatory) basis without requiring an overnight stay in the hospital. Ambulatory operative procedures are generally less complex and require less postoperative monitoring. Among the 200 different operations that can now be performed on an ambulatory basis are **vasectomies**, tubal ligations, some hernia repairs, breast biopsies, **dilation and curettage (D&C), tonsillectomies, arthroscopic** surgery, cataract surgery, some types of plastic surgery and orthopedic procedures, and scores of other minor surgical procedures.

  Outpatient surgery offers many advantages. In most cases, it is less than one-half the cost of comparable in-hospital operations. It prevents some of the family disruption and psychological trauma that often accompany hospitalization. And it decreases the opportunities for the patient to develop a hospital-acquired medical complication such as infection.

- *"What can I expect before, during, and after surgery?"* Knowing what to expect can help you prepare psychologically and physically for the operation. Preparation also appears to decrease postoperative discomfort and need for pain medications and to shorten postoperative hospital stays.

  You should also ask about how long it should take you to recover and what you can do to speed recovery. You should also be informed about what to expect after surgery in terms of symptoms and which symptoms might signal a complication and should be reported to your doctor.

You are an important part of the health care system; not only as a *consumer* of medical care but also as a primary health care *provider*. Managing common medical problems; knowing when and how to self-treat and when to seek professional care; communicating clearly and concisely with your physician; asking questions about medical tests, medications, and surgery; and knowing how to

Personal Insight People often feel overawed or intimidated by their physicians. Do you tend to accept everything your physician says? Do you assume he or she is always right? Do you feel comfortable saying that you would like to seek a second opinion? If not, what can you do to increase your feelings of partnership with your physician?

get more information on health topics are some of the essential skills for a health-wise consumer. Developing these skills will not only result in better health care but will also help you develop a real sense of competence and confidence about managing your health.

SUMMARY

- Easy access to health professionals, medical technology, and medications has led people to have less self-confidence in managing their health. On the other hand, the professional health care system would be overwhelmed if people stopped practicing self-care when appropriate.

Managing Medical Problems

- Self-care involves assessing the body for significant symptoms, which may indicate the need for professional assistance. Symptoms give clues about how well the body is managing an illness on its own.

- Home medical tests, one aspect of self-assessment, allow cost savings, convenience, privacy, an increased sense of control, and sometimes more comprehensive information.

- Informed self-care requires knowing how to evaluate symptoms so that you don't go to a physician too soon or too late. It's necessary to see a physician if symptoms are severe, unusual, persistent, and recurrent.

- Conditions that require emergency room treatment include major trauma or injury, such as broken bones or burns; uncontrollable or internal bleeding; intolerable or uncontrollable pain; severe chest pain; severe shortness of breath; and loss of consciousness.

- Because of the triage process, going to an emergency room when it's not an emergency means long waits for treatment as well as high costs.

- When professional advice is required, it's often possible to get it over the phone; visits can be arranged for a convenient time.

- Self-treatment doesn't necessarily require medication. The body can heal itself; or massage, ice or heat, exercises, and relaxation techniques can help.

- Over-the-counter drugs are a necessary and helpful part of self-care but should not be substituted for nondrug coping techniques. Effective use requires (1) reading drug labels and following directions, (2) not exceeding the recommended dose, (3) using caution regarding interaction with other medications, (4) selecting products with a single active ingredient, (5) trying to buy generic products, (6) never taking drugs from unlabeled containers, (7) not self-medicating when pregnant or nursing without consulting a physician, (8) disposing of expired medications, (9) storing medicines in a safe place, and (10) using special caution with aspirin for children and adolescents.

- A home medicine kit should contain small quantities of the medicines needed for an individual family as well as essential supplies.

Getting the Most Out of Your Medical Care

- Good communication with the physician and other members of the health care team is essential. The ideal relationship should be more like a partnership where the physician acts like a consultant and the patient actively participates.
- Preparation for a visit to a physician should include making a written list of questions or concerns and bringing a list of all medications.
- During the visit to the physician, it's important to be open, to ask questions, and request clarification. Repetition of the diagnosis and instructions to check understanding can help ensure good care.
- The medical history is a description of problems, concerns, and backgrounds. The physician asks questions that will elicit information on the chief complaint, the present illness, the past medical history, all bodily systems, and social history.
- Medical tests account for nearly a third of the national health bill. Physicians should not use tests as protection against malpractice or as a way to make money. Patients should ask questions about the need for the test, the risks, preparation, what the test will be like, and what the results mean.
- Treatments should reflect the wide variety of physical, chemical, and psychosocial factors that cause or aggravate the disease condition. Patients should understand the reasons for treatments, options, risks, and expected benefits. Patients should ask questions about other choices as well as about risks, costs, and expected benefits of the suggested treatment.
- Prescription medicines save lives but also cause problems from drug reactions. Patients should ask why they need medication, what the medication is supposed to do, how and when to take the medication, what to avoid when taking the medication, what the side effects are, whether a generic is available, and if any written information on the medication is available.
- When surgery is recommended, patients should ask whether it is necessary, what the alternatives are, and what the benefits are. A second opinion is advisable and is sometimes required by insurance companies.
- All surgical procedures carry risk. If elective surgery is planned, patients can arrange for autologous donation of blood. More operations can be performed on an outpatient basis, which reduces costs, family disruption, and psychological trauma.
- Knowing what to expect before surgery appears to decrease postoperative discomfort and the need for pain medications as well as to shorten hospital stays.

TAKE ACTION

1. Examine all the medications in your medicine cabinet. Discard any expired or unlabeled medications. Ask your physician or pharmacist whether you should keep any medications you are uncertain about. Compare the contents of your medicine cabinet with the list of medications in Table 21-1, and expand your supplies if you need to.

2. Before your next visit to your physician, prepare a written list of your concerns. Be prepared to ask questions. After the visit, review how it went—were your concerns satisfactorily addressed? Were you able to communicate your needs? Did you feel involved and in control? What aspects would you like to handle better the next time?

3. Review the box "Preventive Medicine for Healthy Adults." Are there any tests or immunizations you need to have done? If so, make an appointment at your clinic or medical office and have the test or immunization.

4. Ask your physician whether you have any medical condition that may require special attention in an emergency. If you do, complete a medical ID card for your wallet or obtain a medical ID bracelet or necklace. More complete emergency service can be obtained by joining Medic Alert (call 1-800-ID-ALERT for information).

JOURNAL ENTRY

1. Write a self-care medical profile of yourself in your health journal. Include your age and current weight and height; any conditions or diseases you have and the treatments or medications you take for them; any conditions or diseases that run in your family or that are common in your ethnic group; any surgery you have had and the date; the diseases against which you have been immunized and the dates of your last booster shots; and any drug or food allergies you have. Also include the names and telephone numbers of your health care practitioners and pharmacy; information about any prescriptions you take (including the prescription number, the number of refills remaining, and the phone number of the

pharmacy that filled each one); and information about your health insurance (including policy number and a telephone number for someone who can answer questions about it). Keep your self-care profile up-to-date and use it for reference.

2. *Critical Thinking:* Studies have shown that people often ignore the warnings and instructions on labels for over-the-counter drugs—they drive after taking an antihistamine that causes drowsiness or take more than the recommended dosage of a cold remedy or a stimulant. Do people have a responsibility to use medications as directed or do they have the right to choose any course of action affecting their own bodies or health, even if their choices have potential negative consequences for others, such as an automobile crash? In your health journal, write a brief essay outlining your opinion about individual responsibility for correct use of medications. Explain your reasoning.

BEHAVIOR CHANGE STRATEGY

COMPLYING WITH PHYSICIANS' INSTRUCTIONS

Even though we sometimes have to entrust ourselves to the care of medical professionals, that doesn't mean that we give up responsibility for our own behavior. Following medical instructions and advice often requires the same kind of behavior self-management that's involved in quitting smoking, losing weight, or changing eating patterns. For example, if you have an illness or injury, you may be told to take medication at certain times of the day, do special exercises or movements, or change your diet.

The medical profession recognizes the importance of patient adherence, or compliance, and encourages the use of different strategies to support it, such as the following:

1. Using reminders placed at home, in the car, at work, or elsewhere that improve follow-through in taking medication and keeping scheduled appointments.

2. Using a journal and other forms of self-monitoring to keep a detailed account of health behaviors, such as pill taking, diet, exercise, and so on.

3. Using self-reward systems so that desired behavior changes are encouraged, with a focus on short-term rewards (such as payment of a sum of money for each week of nonsmoking).

Communication is one of the key requirements of improved adherence. You as the patient must understand what needs to be done, and the physician or other medical staff member must listen to your concerns about the regimen. Sharing information and concerns contributes to a sense of shared responsibility for recovery. Successful

medical care involves more than following physicians' orders; it also has to accommodate the individual's habits and preferences. The next time you have to follow a treatment for an illness or injury, use the suggestions given here and in Chapter 1 to help you comply.

SELECTED BIBLIOGRAPHY

DeFriese, G. H., A. Woomert, P. A. Guild, A. B. Steckler, and T. R. Konrad. 1989. From activated patient to pacified activist: A study of the self-care movement in the United States. *Social Science and Medicine* 29(2):195–204.

Elliot-Binns, C. P. 1986. An analysis of lay medicine: Fifteen years later. *Journal of the Royal College of General Practitioners* 36:542–44.

Gartner, A., and F. Riessman. 1977. *Self-Help in the Human Services.* San Francisco, Calif.: Jossey-Bass.

Greenfield, S., S. Kaplan, and J. E. Ware. 1985. Expanding patient involvement in care: Effect on patient outcomes. *Annals of Internal Medicine* 102:520–28.

Guide to Clinical Preventive Services: Report of the U.S. Preventive Services Task Force. 1989. Baltimore, Md.: Williams and Wilkins.

Herman, P. G., D. E. Gerson, S. J. Hessel, and others. 1975. Disagreements in chest roentgen interpretation. *Chest* 68:278–82.

Kaplan, E. B., L. B. Sheiner, and others. 1985. The usefulness of preoperative laboratory screening. *Journal of the American Medical Association* 253:3576–81.

Levin, L. S., and E. L. Idler. 1981. *The Hidden Health Care System.* Cambridge, Mass.: Ballinger.

Lorig, K., R. G. Kraines, B. W. Brown, and N. Richardson. 1985. A workplace health education program that reduces outpatient visits. *Medical Care* 23:1044–54.

Robinson, J. S., M. M. Schwartz, K. S. Magwene, and others. 1989. The impact of fever health education on clinic utilization. *American Journal of Diseases of Childhood* 143:698–704.

Runkle, C., and C. Regan. 1985. The role of self-care in medical care. In *Patient Education and Health Promotion in Medical Care,* ed. W. Squyres. Palo Alto, Calif.: Mayfield.

Self-Medication: The New Era . . . A Symposium (condensation of papers and discussions). 1980 (March 31). Washington, D. C.: The Proprietary Association.

Vickery, D. M., T. J. Golaszewski, E. C. Wright, and H. Kalmer. 1988. The effect of self-care interventions on the use of medical service within a Medicare population. *Medical Care* 26(6):580–88.

Vickery, D. M., H. Kalmer, D. Lowry, M. Constantine, E. Wright, and W. Loren. 1983. Effect of a self-care education program on medical visits. *Journal of the American Medical Association* 250:2952–56.

Williamson, J. D., and K. Kanaher. 1978. *Self-Care in Health.* London: Croom Helm.

RECOMMENDED READINGS

See Appendix II of this chapter for annotated readings.

Self-Care Guide for Common Medical Problems

The following self-care guide will help you manage a dozen of the most common symptoms:

- Fever
- Sore throat
- Cough
- Nasal congestion
- Ear problems
- Nausea, vomiting, or diarrhea
- Heartburn and indigestion
- Headache
- Low back pain
- Strains and sprains
- Cuts and scrapes

Each symptom is described here in terms of what's going on in your body. Particular emphasis is given to the fact that most symptoms are part of the body's natural healing response and reflect your body's wisdom in attempting to correct disease. Self-care advice is also given, along with some guidelines as to when to seek professional advice. In most cases, the symptoms are self-limiting; that is, they will resolve on their own with time and simple self-care strategies.

No medical advice is perfect. You will always have to make the decision as to whether to self-treat or get professional help. This guide is intended to provide you with more information so that you can make better, more informed decisions. If the advice here differs from that of your physician, discuss the differences. In most instances, your physician will be best able to customize the advice to your individual medical situation.

The guidelines given here apply to *generally healthy adults*. If you are pregnant, nursing, or have a chronic disease, particularly one that requires medication, check with your physician for special self-care advice appropriate for you. For example, if you have a condition such as inflammatory bowel disease (colitis), your physician should give you specific advice on how to manage diarrhea and when to call for help. Also, if you have an allergy or suspected allergy to any recommended medication, please check with your physician before using it. For guidelines appropriate for children, see *Taking Care of Your Child: A Parent's Guide to Medical Care*, 1990, by R. H. Pantell, J. F. Fries, and D. M. Vickery (Reading, Mass.: Addison-Wesley).

If you have several symptoms, read about your main symptom first and then proceed to the lesser symptoms. Above all, use your common sense when determining self-care. If you are particularly concerned about a symptom or confused about how to manage it, call your physician to get more information.

FEVER

A fever is an abnormally high body temperature, usually over 100° F (37.7° C). It is most commonly a sign that your body is fighting an infection. Fever may also be due to an inflammation, an injury, or a drug reaction. Chemicals released into your bloodstream during an infection reset the thermostat in the hypothalamus of your brain. The message goes out to your body, "Quick, turn up the heat!" The blood vessels in your skin constrict, you curl up, and throw on extra blankets to reduce heat loss. Meanwhile, your muscles begin to shiver to generate enormous additional body heat. The resulting rise in body temperature is a fever.

Later when your brain senses that the temperature is too high, the signal goes out to increase sweating. As the sweat evaporates, it carries heat away from the body surface.

A fever may not be all bad; it may even help us fight infections by making the body less hospitable to bacteria and viruses. A high body temperature appears to bolster the immune system and may inhibit the growth of infectious microorganisms.

Most generally healthy people can tolerate a fever as high as 103–104° F (39.5–40° C) without problems. Therefore, if you are generally in good health there is little need to reduce a fever unless you are very uncomfortable. The elderly and those with chronic health problems such as heart disease may not tolerate the increased metabolic demand of a high fever, and fever reduction may be advised.

Most problems with fevers are due to the excessive loss of fluids from evaporation and sweating, which may cause dehydration.

Self-Assessment

1. If you are sick, take your temperature several times throughout the day. Oral temperatures should not be measured for at least ten minutes after smoking, eating, or drinking a hot or cold liquid. When using a glass thermometer, first clean it with rubbing alcohol or cool (hot water may break it) soapy water. Then grip the end opposite the bulb and shake vigorously as though trying to shake drops of water off the tip. Shake it down until it reads 95° F or lower. Place the oral thermometer under the tongue and keep your mouth tightly closed around it. Leave the thermometer in place for a *full three minutes*. If you leave it in for only two minutes, nearly one-third of temperature readings will be off by at least a half a degree.

    To read the glass thermometer, grip it at the end opposite the bulb and hold it in good light with the numbers facing you. Roll the thermometer slowly back and forth between your fingers until you see the silver or red reflection of the column. Note where the column ends, and compare it with the degrees marked in lines on the thermometer. Each long line is a full degree, and each short line counts for 0.2 (two-tenths) of a degree. Most thermometers have a special mark, usually an arrow, indicating a "normal" temperature of 98.6° F (36.8° C). Most thermometers for home use are calibrated in degrees Fahrenheit (F), but some may have the alternative scale of degrees Celsius (C). If you are using an electronic digital thermometer, follow the directions that came with it.

    "Normal" temperature varies from person to person, so it is important to know what is normal for you. Your normal temperature will also vary throughout the day, lowest in the early morning and rising by as much as a degree in the early evening. If you exercise or if it is a hot day, your temperature may normally rise. Also, a woman's body temperature typically varies by a degree or more through the menstrual cycle, peaking around the time of ovulation. Rectal temperatures normally run about 0.5° to 1° F higher than oral temperatures. If your recorded temperature is more than 1.0–1.5° F above your "normal" baseline temperature, you have a fever.

2. Look for signs of dehydration (excessive thirst; very dry mouth; infrequent urination with dark, concentrated urine; and light-headedness).

Self-Care

1. Drink plenty of fluids to prevent dehydration; at least 8 ounces of water, juice, or broth every two hours.
2. Sponge baths using lukewarm water will increase evaporation and help reduce body temperature naturally.

3. Don't bundle up. This decreases the body's ability to lose excess heat.
4. Take aspirin or aspirin substitute (acetaminophen or ibuprofen). For adults, two standard-size tablets every 4 to 6 hours can be used to reduce the fever and the associated headache and achiness. Do not use aspirin if you have a history of allergy to aspirin, ulcers, or bleeding problems. In addition, pediatricians warn that aspirin should usually not be used for fever in children and adolescents. This is because of the finding that some children with chickenpox, influenza, or other viruses have developed a life-threatening complication, Reye's syndrome, after taking aspirin.

When to Call the Physician

1. Fever over 103° F (39.5° C) [or 102° F (38.8° C) if over 60 years old]
2. Fever lasting more than five days
3. Recurrent unexplained fevers
4. Fever accompanied by rash, stiff neck, severe headache, cough with brown/green sputum, severe pain in flank or abdomen, painful urination, convulsions, or mental confusion
5. Fever with signs of dehydration
6. Fever after starting a new medication

SORE THROAT

A sore throat is caused by inflammation of the throat lining due to an infection, allergy, or irritation (especially from cigarette smoke). With an infection, you may also notice some hoarseness from swelling of the vocal cords and "swollen glands," which are enlarged lymph nodes that produce white blood cells to help you fight the infection. The lymph nodes, part of your body's defense system, may remain swollen for weeks after the infection subsides.

Most throat infections are caused by viruses. Your body knows how to fight virus infections, and antibiotics are not necessary or helpful with virus infections. However, about 20 to 30 percent of throat infections are due to streptococcal bacteria. This type of bacteria can cause complications such as rheumatic fever and rheumatic heart disease and therefore should be treated with antibiotics. Strep throat is usually characterized by very sore throat, high fever, swollen lymph nodes, a whitish discharge at the back of the throat, and the absence of other cold symptoms such as a cough and runny nose (which suggest a virus infection). Allergy-related sore throats are usually accompanied by running nose and watery, itchy eyes.

Self-Assessment

1. Take your temperature.
2. Look in a mirror at the back of your throat. Is there a whitish, puslike discharge on the tonsils or back of the throat?
3. Feel the front and back of your neck. Do you feel enlarged, tender lymph nodes?

Self-Care

1. If you smoke, stop smoking to avoid further irritation of your throat.
2. Drink plenty of liquids to soothe your inflamed throat.
3. Gargle warm salt water ($^1/_4$ tsp. salt in 4 oz. water) every one to two hours to help reduce swelling and discomfort.
4. Suck on throat lozenges, cough drops, or hard candies to keep your throat moist.
5. Use throat lozenges, sprays, or gargles that contain an anesthetic to temporarily numb your throat and make swallowing less painful.
6. Try aspirin or aspirin substitute to ease throat pain.
7. For an allergy-related sore throat, try an antihistamine such as chlorpheniramine.

When to Call the Physician

1. Great difficulty swallowing saliva or breathing
2. Sore throat with fever over 101° F (38.3° C), especially if you do not have other cold symptoms such as nasal congestion or cough
3. Sore throat with a skin rash
4. Sore throat with whitish pus on the tonsils
5. Sore throat and recent contact with a person who has had a positive throat culture for strep
6. Enlargement of lymph nodes lasting longer than three weeks
7. Hoarseness persisting longer than three weeks

COUGH

A cough is a protective mechanism of the body to help keep the airways clear. There are two types of cough: a dry cough (without mucus) and a productive cough (with mucus). Common causes of cough include infection (viral or bacterial), allergies, and irritation from smoking and pollutants. If you have a cold, the cough may be the last symptom to improve, because the airways may re-

main irritated for several weeks after the infection has resolved.

Your airways are lined with hairlike projections called *cilia,* which move back and forth to help clear the airways of mucus, germs, and dust. Infections and cigarette smoking paralyze and damage this vital defense mechanism.

Self-Assessment

1. Take your temperature.
2. Observe your mucus. A thick green, brown, or bloody mucus suggests a bacterial infection.

Self-Care

1. If you are a smoker, stop smoking. Smoking irritates the airways and undermines your body's defense mechanisms, leading to more serious infections and longer-lasting symptoms. Most people do not feel like smoking when they have a cold with a cough. If you want to quit, a cold may provide an excellent opportunity to do so.
2. Drink plenty of liquids (at least six 8-ounce glasses a day) to help thin mucus and loosen chest congestion.
3. Breathe steam through a vaporizer or in a hot shower to help loosen chest congestion.
4. Suck on cough drops, throat lozenges, or hard candy to keep your throat moist and help relieve a dry, tickling cough.
5. If you have a dry, nonproductive cough or the cough keeps you from sleeping, you can use a cough syrup or lozenge that contains the over-the-counter cough suppressant dextromethorphan. Since a cough that produces mucus is protective, it is generally not advised to suppress a productive cough.

When to Call the Physician

1. Cough with thick, green, brown, or bloody sputum
2. Cough with high fever—above 102° F (38.8° C)—and shaking chills
3. Severe chest pains, wheezing, or shortness of breath
4. Cough that lasts longer than two weeks

NASAL CONGESTION

Nasal congestion is most commonly caused by infection or allergies. With infection, the nasal passages become congested due to increased blood flow and mucus production. This congestion is actually part of the body's defense to fight infection. The increased blood flow raises the temperature of the nasal passages, making them less hospitable to germs. The nasal secretions are rich in white blood cells and antibodies to help fight and neutralize the invading organisms and flush them away. Nasal congestion associated with sore throat, cough, and fever usually indicates a virus infection.

Nasal congestion caused by allergies is often accompanied by a thin, watery discharge, sneezing, itchy eyes, and sometimes a seasonal pattern. In an allergic reaction, the offending allergen (pollen, dusts, molds, dander, and so forth) triggers the release of histamine and other chemicals from the cells lining the nose, throat, and eyes. These chemicals cause swelling, discharge, and itching. Antihistamine drugs block the release of these irritating chemicals.

Self-Assessment

1. Take your temperature.
2. Observe the color and consistency of your nasal secretions. A thick green, brown, or bloody discharge suggests a bacterial sinus infection.
3. Tap with your fingers over the sinus cavities above and below the eyes. If this causes increased pain, a bacterial sinus infection may be present.

Self-Care

1. If you smoke, stop smoking to prevent continuing irritation of the nasal passages.
2. Use moist heat from a hot shower or vaporizer to help liquefy congested mucus.
3. Use a decongestant nasal spray or drops to temporarily relieve congestion. However, if these decongestants are used for more than three days they can cause "rebound congestion" that actually creates more nasal congestion. As an alternative, use saltwater nose drops ($1/4$ tsp. salt in $1/2$ cup of boiled water).
4. Try an oral decongestant such as pseudoephedrine (60 mg every six hours) to help shrink swollen mucous membranes and open nasal passages. In some people, these medications can cause nervousness, sleeplessness, or heart palpitations. If you have uncontrolled high blood pressure, heart disease, or diabetes, check with your physician before using decongestants.

When to Call the Physician

1. Nasal congestion with severe pain and tenderness in the forehead, cheeks, or upper teeth and a high fever (above 102° F or 38.8° C)

2. Thick green, brown, or bloody nasal discharge
3. Nasal congestion and discharge unresponsive to self-care treatment and lasting longer than three weeks

EAR PROBLEMS

Ear symptoms include earache, discharge, itching, stuffiness, and hearing loss. They may be caused by problems in the external ear canal, eardrum, middle ear, or eustachian tube (the passageway that connects the middle ear space to the back of the throat). The ear canal can become blocked by excess wax, producing a sense of the ear being plugged and hearing loss. An infection of the external ear canal due to excessive moisture and trauma is often referred to as "swimmer's ear." It can cause pain, fullness, discharge, and itching. Congestion and blockage of the eustachian tube by a cold or allergy can result in pain, fullness, and hearing loss. A middle ear infection often produces severe pain, hearing loss, and fever.

Self-Assessment

1. Take your temperature. A fever may be a sign of infection.
2. Have someone look into the ear canal with a flashlight or otoscope. Look for wax blockage or a red, swollen canal indicating an external ear infection.
3. Wiggle the outer part of the ear. If this increases the pain, an infection or inflammation of the external canal is the likely cause.

Self-Care

1. If blockage of the ear canal with wax is the problem, first try a hot shower to liquefy the wax and use a wash cloth to wipe out the ear canal. You can also use a few drops of an over-the-counter wax softener and then flush the canal gently with warm water and a bulb syringe. Do not use sharp objects or cotton swabs; they can scratch the canal or push the wax in deeper.
2. To treat mild infections of the external ear canal, you must thoroughly dry the ear canal. A few drops of a drying agent (Burrow's solution) on a piece of cotton gently inserted into the canal can act as a wick to dry the canal.
3. To relieve congestion and blockage of the eustachian tube, try a decongestant like pseudoephedrine, a nasal spray (but for no longer than three days), or an antihistamine. Hot showers or a vaporizer may help loosen secretions, and yawning or swallowing may help open your eustachian tube. For a mild plugging

sensation without fever or pain, pinch your nostrils and blow gently to force air up the eustachian tube and "pop" your ears.

When to Call the Physician

1. Severe earache with fever
2. Puslike or bloody discharge from the ear
3. Sudden hearing loss, especially if accompanied by ear pain or recent trauma to the ear
4. Ringing in the ears or dizziness
5. Any ear symptom lasting longer than two weeks

NAUSEA, VOMITING, OR DIARRHEA

Nausea, vomiting, and diarrhea usually are defensive reactions of your body to rapidly clear your digestive tract of irritants. These symptoms are most commonly caused by the "stomach flu," a virus infection, but may also be caused by food poisoning, medications, or other types of infection. Vomiting dramatically ejects irritants from your stomach, and nausea discourages eating to allow the stomach to rest. In diarrhea, overstimulated intestines flush out the offending irritants.

The major complications of vomiting and diarrhea are dehydration from fluid losses and decreased intake and the risk of bleeding from irritation of the digestive tract.

Self-Assessment

1. Take your temperature. A fever is often a clue that an infection is causing the symptoms.
2. Observe the color and frequency of vomiting and diarrhea. This helps estimate severity of fluid losses and checks for bleeding (red, black, or "coffee grounds" material in stool or vomit).
3. Look for signs of dehydration: very dry mouth, marked thirst, infrequent urination with dark, concentrated urine, and light-headedness.
4. Look for signs of hepatitis, an infection of the liver that produces a yellow color in the skin and white parts of the eyes.

Self-Care

1. To replace fluids, take frequent, small sips of clear liquids such as water, non-citrus juice, broths, flat ginger ale, or ice chips.
2. When the vomiting and diarrhea have subsided, you can try nonirritating, constipating foods like the BRAT diet: bananas, rice, applesauce, and toast.
3. For several days avoid alcohol, milk products, fatty foods, aspirin, and other medications that might irritate the stomach. Do not stop taking regularly prescribed medications without discussing this change with your physician.
4. Medications are not usually advised for vomiting. For diarrhea, over-the-counter medications containing kaolin, pectin, or attapulgite may help thicken the stool. Loperamide, now available without a prescription, can be used to lessen diarrhea. Medications containing paregoric may help decrease painful intestinal spasms.

When to Call the Physician

1. Inability to retain any fluids for 12 hours, or signs of dehydration
2. Severe abdominal pains not relieved by the vomiting or diarrhea
3. Blood in the vomit (red or "coffee grounds-like" material) or in the stool (red or black, tarlike material)
4. Vomiting or diarrhea with a high fever (above 102° F or 38.8° C)
5. Yellow color in skin or whites of eyes
6. Vomiting with severe headache and history of recent head injury
7. Vomiting or diarrhea that lasts three days without improvement
8. Recurrent vomiting and/or diarrhea
9. If you are pregnant or have diabetes

HEARTBURN AND INDIGESTION

Indigestion and heartburn are usually a result of irritation of the stomach or the esophagus, the tube that connects the mouth to the stomach. The stomach lining is usually protected from stomach acids, but the esophagus is not. Therefore, if stomach acids "reflux" or back up into the esophagus, the result is usually a burning discomfort beneath the breastbone. The esophagus is normally protected by a muscular valve that allows food to enter the stomach but prevents stomach contents from flowing upwards into the esophagus. Certain foods (such as chocolate), medications, and smoking can loosen and open this protective sphincter valve. Overeating, lying down or bending over can also cause the stomach acids to gain access to the sensitive lining of the esophagus.

Self-Assessment

1. Look for a pattern in the symptoms. Do they occur after eating certain foods, taking certain medications,

or when you bend over or lie down? Does milk or an antacid relieve the symptoms?

2. Observe your bowel movements. Black tarlike stools may indicate bleeding in the stomach (iron tablets and Pepto-Bismol can also cause black stools).

Self-Care

1. Avoid irritants such as smoking, aspirin, ibuprofen, alcohol, caffeine (coffee, teas, colas), chocolate, onions, carbonated beverages, spicy or fatty foods, acidic foods (vinegar, citrus fruits, tomatoes), or anything else that you've noticed make your symptoms worse.

2. Take nonabsorbable antacids such as Maalox, Mylanta, or Gelusil every 1 to 2 hours and especially before bedtime.

3. Avoid tight clothing (belts and girdles).

4. Avoid overeating; eat smaller, more frequent meals.

5. Don't lie down for 1 to 2 hours after a meal. Elevate the head of your bed with 4- to 6-inch blocks of wood or bricks. Adding extra pillows usually makes things worse by creating a posture that increases pressure on the stomach. Using a waterbed also usually makes reflux worse.

6. If you are overweight in the abdominal area, weight loss may help. Abdominal obesity can increase pressure on the stomach when lying down.

When to Call the Physician

1. Stools that are black and tarlike or vomit that is bloody or contains material that looks like coffee grounds

2. Severe abdominal or chest pain

3. Pain that goes through to the back

4. No relief from antacids or milk

5. Symptoms lasting longer than three days

HEADACHE

Headache is one of the most common symptoms. There are three major types of headache: muscle tension (the most common type), vascular (related to the blood vessels), and sinus (involves blocked sinus cavities). Muscle tension headaches are often due to emotional stress or physical stress such as poor posture. The muscles in the neck, scalp, and jaws tighten, producing a dull, aching sensation or band of tension around the head. Vascular headaches, which include the common migraine, are due to a constriction and then dilation of blood vessels in the head. Vascular headaches are usually severe, one-sided,

throbbing headaches often associated with nausea, vomiting, and visual disturbances (flashing lights or stars). Sinus headaches are caused by blockage of the sinus cavities with resulting pressure and pain in the cheeks, forehead, and upper teeth. These headaches are often associated with nasal congestion. Sometimes a combination of these types of headaches will occur. Headache caused by elevated blood pressure is very uncommon and occurs only with very high pressures.

Self-Assessment

1. Take your temperature. The presence of fever may indicate a sinus infection. Fever, severe headache, and very stiff neck suggest meningitis, a rare, but serious infection around the brain and spinal cord.

2. Tap with your fingers over the sinus cavities in your cheeks and forehead. If this causes increased pain, it may indicate a sinus infection.

3. For recurrent headaches, keep a headache journal. Record how often and when your headaches occur, associated symptoms, activities that precede the headache, food and beverage intake.

Self-Care

1. Try applying ice packs or heat on your neck and head.

2. Gently massage the muscles of your neck and scalp.

3. Try deep relaxation or breathing exercises.

4. Take aspirin or aspirin substitute for pain relief.

5. If pain is associated with nasal congestion, try a decongestant medication like pseudoephedrine.

6. Try to avoid emotional stressors and physical stressors (like poor posture and eye strain).

7. Try avoiding certain foods that may trigger headaches. These include aged cheeses, chocolate, nuts, red wine, alcohol, avocados, figs, raisins, and any fermented or pickled foods.

When to Call the Physician

1. Unusually severe headache

2. Headache accompanied by fever and very stiff neck

3. Headache with sinus pain and tenderness and a fever

4. Severe headache following recent head injury

5. Headache associated with slurred speech, visual disturbance, numbness or weakness in face, arms, or legs

6. Headache persisting longer than three days

7. Recurrent unexplained headaches

8. Increasing severity or frequency of headaches

LOW BACK PAIN

Pain in the lower back is a very common condition that results in large part from our upright posture, which puts tremendous strain on our lower backs. The pain is most often due to a strain of the muscles and ligaments along the spine, which may or may not be triggered by bending, lifting, or other activity. Low back pain can also be due to bone growths (spurs) irritating the nerves as they leave the spine or to pressure from ruptured or protruding discs, the "shock absorbers" between the vertebrae. In addition to back pain, nerve irritation can produce lower leg pain, numbness, tingling, weakness, and loss of bowel or bladder control. Sometimes back pain is actually caused by an infection or stone in the kidney. Fortunately, however, simpler muscular strain is the most common cause of low back pain and can usually be effectively self-treated.

Self-Assessment

1. Take your temperature. Back pain with high fever may indicate a kidney or other infection.
2. Check for blood in your urine or frequent, painful urination, which may also indicate a kidney problem.
3. Observe for tingling or pain traveling down one or both legs below the knee with bending, coughing, or sneezing. These symptoms suggest a disc problem.

Self-Care

1. Lie on your back or in any comfortable position on the floor or on a firm mattress with knees slightly bent and supported by a pillow. Rest for 24 hours or longer if the pain persists.
2. Use ice packs on the painful area for the first 24 hours and then apply ice or heat.
3. Take aspirin or aspirin substitute for pain relief as needed.
4. After the acute pain has subsided, begin gentle back and stomach exercises. Practice good posture and lifting techniques to protect your back. To learn more about proper back exercises and use of your back, consult a physical therapist or your doctor.

When to Call the Physician

1. Back pain following a severe injury such as an accident or fall
2. Back pain radiating down the leg below the knee on one or both sides
3. Persistent numbness, tingling, or weakness in the legs or feet
4. Loss of bladder or bowel control

5. Back pain associated with high fever (above 101° F or 38.3° C), frequent or painful urination, blood in the urine, or severe abdominal pain
6. Back pain that does not improve after one week of self-care

STRAINS AND SPRAINS

Missteps, slips, falls, accidents, and athletic misadventures result in a variety of strains, sprains, and fractures. A strain occurs when you overstretch a muscle or a tendon (the connective tissue that attaches muscle to bone). Sprains are caused by overstretching or tearing of ligaments (the tough fibrous bands that connect bone to bone). Depending on the severity and location, a sprain may actually be more serious than a fracture because bones generally heal very strongly while ligaments may remain stretched and lax after healing. After a sprain, it may take six weeks for the ligament to heal.

After most injuries, you can expect pain and swelling. This is the body's way of immobilizing and protecting the injured part so that healing can take place. The goal of self-assessment is to determine whether you have a minor injury that you can safely self-treat or a more serious injury to an artery, nerve, or bone that should be treated by your physician.

Self-Assessment

1. Observe for coldness, blue color, or numbness in the limb beyond the injury. These may be signs of damage to artery or nerve.
2. Look for signs of a possible fracture, which would include misshapen limb, reduced length of the limb on the injured side compared to the uninjured side, inability to move or bear weight, grating sound with movement of injured area, extreme tenderness at one point along the injured bone as you press with your fingers, or a sensation of snapping at time of the injury.
3. Gently move the injured area through its full range of motion. Immobility or instability suggest a more serious injury.

Self-Care

1. Immediately immobilize, protect, and rest the injured area until you can bear weight on it or move it without pain. Remember, if it hurts, don't do it.
2. To decrease pain and swelling, immediately apply ice (cold pack or ice wrapped in a cloth) for 15 minutes every hour for the first 24 to 48 hours. Then apply ice or heat as needed for comfort.

3. Immediately elevate the injured limb above the level of your heart for the first 24 hours to decrease swelling.

4. Immobilize and support the injured area with an elastic wrap or splint. Be careful not to wrap so tightly as to cause blueness, coldness, or numbness.

5. Take aspirin or aspirin substitute for pain as needed.

When to Call the Physician

1. An injury that occurred with great force such as a high fall or motor vehicle accident

2. Hearing or feeling a snap at the time of the injury

3. A limb that is blue, cold, or numb

4. A limb that is bent, twisted, or crooked

5. Tenderness at specific points along a bone

6. Inability to move injured area

7. Wobbly, unstable joint

8. Marked swelling of the injured area

9. Inability to bear weight after 24 hours

10. Pain that increases or lasts longer than four days

CUTS AND SCRAPES

Cuts and scrapes are common disruptions of your body's skin. Fortunately, the vast majority of these wounds are minor and don't require stitches, antibiotics, or a physician's care. An abrasion involves a scraping away of the superficial layers of skin. Abrasions, though less serious, are often more painful than cuts because they disrupt more skin nerves. Cuts come in two varieties: lacerations (narrow slices of the skin) and puncture wounds (stabs into deeper tissues).

Normal healing of a cut or abrasion is a wondrous process. After the bleeding stops, small amounts of serum, a clear yellowish fluid, may leak from your wound. This fluid is rich in antibodies to help prevent an infection. Redness and swelling may normally occur as more blood is shunted to the area, bringing white blood cells and nutrients to speed healing. There may also be some swelling of nearby lymph nodes, which are another part of your body's defense against infection. Finally, a scab forms. This is "nature's Band-aid," which protects the area while it heals.

The main concerns about cuts are the possibilities of damage to deeper tissues and the risk of infection. Damage to underlying blood vessels may lead to severe bleeding as well as blueness and coldness to areas beyond the wound. Injured nerves may produce numbness and loss of ability to move parts of the body beyond the injured area. Damaged muscles, tendons, and ligaments can also result in inability to move areas beyond the cut.

Wound infection usually does not take place until 24 to 48 hours after an injury. Signs of infection include increasing redness, swelling, pain, pus, and fever. One of the most serious, though fortunately uncommon, complications of puncture wounds is tetanus ("lockjaw"). This bacterial infection thrives in areas not exposed to oxygen, so it is more likely to develop in deep puncture wounds or dirty wounds. Tetanus is not likely to develop in minor cuts or wounds caused by clean objects like knives. You need a tetanus shot following a cut under the following conditions:

- If you have never had the basic series of three tetanus immunization injections

- If you have a dirty or contaminated wound and it has been longer than five years since your last injection

- If you have a clean, minor wound and it has been longer than 10 years since your last injection

Self-Assessment

1. Look for warning signs of complications: persistent bleeding, numbness, inability to move injured area, or the later development of pus, increasing redness, and fever.

2. Measure the size of the cut. If your cut is shallow, less than an inch long, not in a high-stress area (such as a joint, which bends), and you can easily hold the edges of the wound closed, it probably won't need stitches.

Self-Care

1. Apply direct pressure over the wound until bleeding is stopped. The only exception is puncture wounds, which should be encouraged to bleed freely (unless spurting a large amount of blood) for a few minutes to flush out bacteria and debris.

2. Try to remove any dirt, gravel, glass, or foreign material from the wound with tweezers or by gentle scrubbing.

3. Wash the wound vigorously with soap and water, followed by an application of hydrogen peroxide solution as an antiseptic.

4. If it is an abrasion, cover the area with a sterile adhesive bandage until a scab forms. For minor lacerations, close the cut with a butterfly bandage or a sterile adhesive tape, drawing the edges close together but not overlapping. If there is an extra flap of clean skin, leave it in place for extra protection. Do not attempt to close puncture wounds. Instead soak puncture wounds in warm water for 15 minutes several times a day for several days. Soaking helps keep the wound open and thus prevents infection.

When to Call the Physician

1. Bleeding that can't be controlled with direct pressure
2. Numbness, weakness, or inability to move injured area
3. Any large, deep wound
4. A laceration in an area that bends and the edges of the cut cannot be easily held together
5. Cuts on the hands or face unless clean and shallow
6. Contaminated wound in which you cannot remove the foreign material
7. Any human or animal bite
8. If you need a tetanus immunization (see indications noted earlier)
9. Development of increasing redness, swelling, pain, pus, or fever 24 hours or more after the injury
10. If the wound is not healing well after three weeks

APPENDIX II

Resources for Self-Care

BOOKS

Bennett, W. I., S. E. Goldfinger, and G. T. Johnson, eds. 1987. *Your Good Health: How to Stay Well, and What to Do When You're Not.* Cambridge: Harvard University Press.

Benson, H., and E. M. Stuart. 1992. *The Wellness Book: The Comprehensive Guide to Maintaining Health and Treating Stress-related Illness.* New York: Birch Lane Press. *Combines relaxation response techniques with other behavioral medicine approaches, such as stress management, exercise, and nutrition, to provide the best practical guide to mind-body health now available.*

Consumer Reports Books. 1993. *The Complete Drug Reference.* Yonkers, N.Y.: Consumers Union. *A comprehensive reference book on medications from the United States pharmacopeia.*

Graedon, J., and T. Graedon. 1989. *The People's Pharmacy,* Rev. ed. New York: St. Martin's Press. *A lively and highly informative book discussing the pharmacology, profits, and politics that affect the drugs we use.*

Greenwood, S., B. Hasselbring, and M. Castleman. 1987. *The Medical Self-Care Book of Women's Health.* New York: Doubleday. *A well-written self-help consumer's guide to women's health issues.*

Griffith, H. W. 1989. *Complete Guide to Symptoms, Illness, and Surgery.* New York: Putnam. *A mammoth book discussing over 700 symptoms, 500 illnesses, and 160 surgeries.*

Griffith, H. W. 1992. *Complete Guide to Prescription and Nonprescription Drugs, 1993 edition.* New York: Putnam. *A comprehensive guide to side effects, warnings, and precautions for safe use of over 4,000 brand-name and generic drugs.*

Inlander, C. 1992. *150 Ways to Be a Savvy Medical Consumer.* Allentown, Penn.: The People's Medical Society. *Activist advice on how to save money and get excellent medical care.*

Inlander, C. B., and E. Weiner. 1991. *Take This Book to the Hospital with You,* Rev. ed. New York: Pantheon Books. *The lively and informative guide from The People's Medical Society on how to survive a hospital stay.*

Kemper, D. W., K. E. McIntosh, and T. M. Roberts. 1992. *Healthwise Handbook: A Self-Care Manual for You.* Boise, Idaho: Healthwise. (P.O. Box 1989, Boise, ID 83701). *Practical, straightforward guidelines on the best home care for a variety of common medical problems in adults and children.*

Kunz, Jeffrey R. M., ed. 1987. *The American Medical Association Family Medicine Guide,* Rev. ed. New York: Random House. *A comprehensive volume discussing more than 650 diseases. Contains question-and-answer charts to help evaluate common medical symptoms and decide when to see a physician.*

Larson, D. E., ed. 1990. *Mayo Clinic Family Health Book.* New York: William Morrow. *A comprehensive, thoroughly researched, and readable health reference book; abundant color photographs and illustrations bring alive more than 1,000 descriptions of diseases.*

Lewis, J. 1990. *So Your Doctor Recommended Surgery.* New York: Henry Holt. *A distinguished surgeon provides information you should know before you consent to surgery.*

Long, J. W. 1992. *The Essential Guide to Prescription Drugs.* New York: HarperCollins. *A comprehensive reference covering 300 medications; includes descriptions of how each drug works, possible side effects and adverse reactions, food and drug interactions, and other precautions.*

Madara, E. J., and A. Meese. 1992. *The Self-Help Sourcebook: Finding and Forming Mutual Aid Self-Help Groups.* Denville, N.J.: American Self-Help Clearinghouse (St. Claire's–Riverside Hospital, Pocono Road, Denville, N.J. 07834). *Provides a national listing of self-help groups and guidelines for anyone interested in forming a self-help group.*

Pantell, R. H., J. F. Fries, and D. M. Vickery. 1990. *Taking Care of Your Child: A Parent's Guide to Medical Care.* Reading, Mass.: Addison-Wesley. *An indispensable guide for common health problems of children, containing about 100 easy-to-use decision charts to help parents decide when to call the doctor and when to treat at home.*

Reader's Digest. 1992. *The Good Health Fact Book, 1992.* Pleasantville, N.Y.: The Reader's Digest Association. *Answers to over 1,000 health and medical questions; richly illustrated.*

Rees, A. M., and C. Hoffman. 1990. *Consumer Health Information Source Book.* Phoenix, Ariz.: Oryx Press. *An annotated bibliography of popular books and pamphlets on a wide variety of health topics as well as a listing of health-related clearinghouses, hot lines, and resource organizations.*

Simons, A., B. Hasselbring, and M. Castleman. 1992. *Before You Call the Doctor.* New York: Ballantine. *Safe, effective self-care for more than 300 common medical problems.*

Sobel, D. S., and T. Ferguson. 1985. *The People's Book of Medical Tests.* New York: Summit Books. *A consumer's guide that answers questions about 200 medical and home diagnostic tests.*

Stutz, D. R., and F. Feder. 1991. *The Savvy Patient.* New York: Consumer Reports Books. *Describes how patients can communicate effectively with their physicians and be active participants in their medical care.*

Tapley, D. F., ed. 1989. *The Columbia University College of Physicians and Surgeons Complete Home Medical Guide.* New York: Crown.

Vickery, D. M. 1986. *Taking Part: The Survivor's Guide to the Hospital.* Reston, Va.: Center for Corporate Health Promotion. *Using decision-making charts, this book offers a second opinion to help the patient decide whether hospitalization and surgery are necessary for the treatment of 20 common medical problems.*

Vickery, D. M., and J. F. Fries. 1992. *Take Care of Yourself: The Consumer's Guide to Medical Care,* 5th ed. Reading, Mass.: Addison-Wesley. *This excellent self-care guide includes over 100 easy-to-follow decision charts outlining when to see a physician and how to apply safe and effective home treatment.*

Wurman, R. S. 1985. *Medical Access.* Los Angeles: Access Press. *A travel guide to medical care containing descriptions of medical tests, surgical procedures, and the most commonly asked consumer health questions.*

Zimmerman, David R. 1992. *The Essential Guide to Nonprescription Drugs.* New York: HarperCollins. *The most comprehensive and authoritative review of the safety and effectiveness of over-the-counter products.*

NEWSLETTERS AND MAGAZINES

American Health Magazine. 28 West 23rd St., New York, NY 10010.

Consumer Reports on Health. 101 Truman Avenue, Yonkers, NY 10703-1057.

Harvard Health Letter. Harvard Medical School, Dept. of Continuing Education, 70 Garden St., Cambridge, MA 02138.

Healthline. C. V. Mosby Company, 11830 Westline Industrial Drive, St. Louis, MO 63146-3318.

Health Magazine. 301 Howard St., Suite 1800, San Francisco, CA 94105.

Mental Medicine Update. P.O. Box 381062, Boston, MA 02238-1062.

University of California at Berkeley Wellness Letter. P.O. Box 420149, Palm Coast, FL 32142-9821.

HEALTH INFORMATION CENTERS

Consumer Health Information Research Institute (3521 Broadway, Kansas City, MO 64111, 816-753-8850)

Consumer Information Center (Pueblo, CO 81009, or Room G142, 18th and F Streets, N.W., Washington, DC 20405, 202-501-1794)

National Health Information Center (P.O. Box 1133, Washington, DC 20013, 800-336-4797 or 703-522-2590 in Virginia)

Office of Minority Health Resource Center (P.O. Box 37337, Washington, DC 20013, 800-444-6472)

Planetree Health Resource Center (2040 Webster Street, San Francisco, CA 94115, 415-923-3680 or 415-923-3681)

SELF-HELP AND MUTUAL AID GROUPS

In the United States alone, more than 500,000 self-help groups and chapters of self-help organizations provide information and peer support for nearly every conceivable medical condition or problem. There are groups for diabetes, cancer, stroke, heart surgery, Alzheimer's disease, child abuse, drug abuse, infertility, asthma, cystic fibrosis, nursing mothers, blindness, epilepsy, DES (diethylstilbestrol) exposure, eating disorders, colitis, mental retardation, phobias, sleep disorders, sexual problems, women's health, and hundreds of others. You can look in the white pages of the telephone book for your local chapter or contact one of the following self-help clearinghouses for the names of self-help groups in your community.

American Self-Help Clearinghouse (St. Claire's–Riverside Medical Center, 25 Pocono Road, Denville, NJ 07834, 201-625-7101)

National Self-Help Clearinghouse (City University of New York, Graduate Center, Room 620, 25 West 43rd Street, New York, NY 10036, 212-642-2944)

The Self-Help Center (1600 Dodge Avenue, Suite 122, Evanston, IL 60201, 708-328-0470)

California Self-Help Center (2349 Franz Hall, 405 Hilgard Avenue, Los Angeles, CA 90024, 213-825-1799, or in California 800-222-5465)

Acquired Immune Deficiency Syndrome (AIDS): CDC AIDS Clearinghouse Hot Line, 800-342-AIDS, 800-344-SIDA (Spanish), 800-AIDS-TTY (hearing impaired); Information on clinical trials of AIDS drugs, sponsored by National Institutes of Health, 800-874-2572 (9:00 A.M.–7:00 P.M. ET); Project Inform—information on experimental drugs for AIDS, ARC, and HIV infection, 800-822-7422

Agoraphobia (fear of open spaces): The Agoraphobia and Anxiety Program of Temple University, Philadelphia, 215-667-6490

Alcohol: Al-Anon Family Group Headquarters, 800-344-2666; National Clearinghouse for Alcohol and Drug Information, 301-468-2600, 800-729-6686; National Council on Alcoholism and Drug Dependency, 800-NCA-CALL

Alzheimer's disease: Alzheimer's Disease and Related Disorders Association, 800-621-0379 (in Illinois, 800-572-6037), 24 hours

Anorexia and bulimia: National Association of Anorexia Nervosa and Associated Disorders, 708-831-3438

Arthritis: Arthritis Foundation Information Line, 800-283-7800

Asthma: Asthma and Allergy Foundation of America, 800-7-ASTHMA

Blindness: American Council of the Blind, National Legislative Hotline, 800-424-8666; American Foundation for the Blind, 800-232-5463; The National Library Service for the Blind (part of the Library of Congress), 800-424-8567 (in Washington, D.C., 202-287-5100)

Cancer: Cancer Information Service, part of the National Cancer Institute, 800- 4-CANCER (in Washington, D.C., 202-806-5700)

Cocaine: Cocaine Abuse Hot Line, 800-COCAINE, 7 days, 24 hours

Diabetes: Juvenile Diabetes Foundation, 800-223-1138 (in New York state, 212-889-7575); American Diabetes Association, 800-232-3472

Drugs, drug interactions and drug side effects: FDA Center for Drug Evaluation and Research, Legislative, Professional and Consumer Affairs Branch, 301-295-8012 (8:00 A.M.–5:00 P.M. ET)

Epilepsy: Epilepsy Foundation of America, 800-EFA-1000 (301-459-3700 in Maryland)

Food and cosmetics safety: The Consumer Inquiries Section of the Office of Consumer Affairs of the FDA, 301-443-3170 (8:00 A.M.–5:00 P.M. ET)

Headache: National Headache Foundation, 800-843-2256

Hearing problems: Dial-a-Hearing Screening Test, part of Occupational Hearing Services, 800-222-EARS

Infertility: Resolve National Phone Counseling Line, 617-623-0744 (M–Th, 9:00 A.M.–12:00 P.M., 1:00–4:00 P.M. EST)

Kidney disease: American Kidney Fund, 800-638-8299

Lung disease, respiratory disorders, asthma, allergies: Lung Line, sponsored by the National Jewish Center for Immunology and Respiratory Medicine in Denver, Colorado, 800-222-LUNG

Mental Health: National Mental Health Association, 800-969-6642

Premenstrual syndrome: PMS Access, 800-222-4PMS

Sexually Transmissible Diseases: STD Hotline, 800-227-8922

Sickle Cell Anemia: National Association for Sickle Cell Disease, 800-421-8453 (in California, 213-736-5455)

Spina bifida: Spina Bifida Association, 800-621-3141 (in Illinois, 708-960-2426)

Sports and sports injuries: Women's Sports Foundation, 800-227-3988

Sudden Infant Death Syndrome (SIDS): American Sudden Infant Death Syndrome Institute, 800-232-SIDS (in Georgia, 800-847-SIDS)

Surgery: Medicare Second Opinion Hotline, sponsored by the U.S. Government's Department of Health and Human Services, 800-638-6833

22

The Health Care System

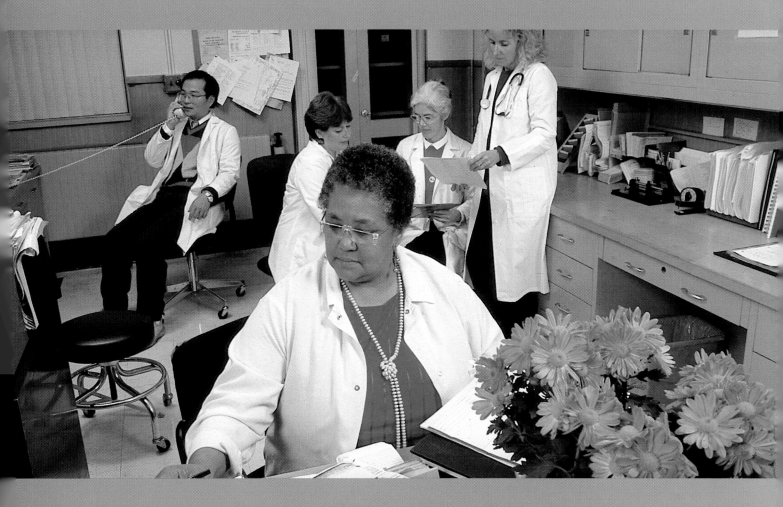

CONTENTS

BOXES

You saw a well-known celebrity on TV last night promoting a new "European formula" hair-replacement product. You're very concerned about your receding hairline and are eager to try any new treatments that promise to slow down hair loss. You're usually skeptical about such products, but since these claims were made on national TV by a well-known person, they must be true, right? Should you call the toll-free number and send in your check?

You decided to try a new physician who was recommended to you, and while you're waiting in the examination room you peruse the diplomas and certificates framed and hanging on the wall. After reading them all, you realize that this physician doesn't have an M.D. degree. Instead, he has a D.O.—doctor of osteopathy—degree. Is he a licensed practitioner who will give you reliable advice? Can you have confidence in his knowledge and skills? What should you ask him about his training when he comes in?

At your new job you're offered a choice between two different health insurance plans. One is described to you as a standard plan that pays 80 percent of most of your medical expenses, including some prescriptions and some office visits. The other one, which would involve a smaller payroll deduction for you, is described as a health maintenance organization based in a downtown clinic. Almost all of your medical expenses would be paid, but you would have to use the staff and facilities available at the clinic. How can you decide which of the two is better for you?

A friend of yours has been diagnosed as having a "systemic yeast infection" by a practitioner she refers to as a clinical ecologist. She says her symptoms were fatigue, fuzzy thinking, intestinal gas, a bloated feeling, and depression. You tell her that you have some of those symptoms on occasion and that you think probably everyone does. She suggests that maybe you have a yeast infection too and urges you to see her practitioner. Should you?

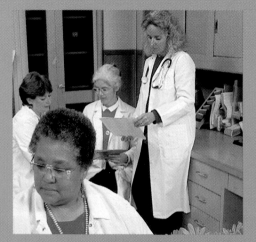

MAKING CONNECTIONS

Even when you take good care of yourself, sooner or later you're bound to have an illness or an injury that requires professional attention. To make the decisions that are right for you, you need to know which medical practices are legitimate, how to pay for them, and what to do when you encounter a questionable practice. In each of the scenarios presented on this page, all related to the health care system, individuals have to use information, make a decision, or choose a course of action. How would you act in each of these situations? What response or decision would you make? This chapter provides information about the health care system that can be used in situations like these. After finishing the chapter, read the scenarios again. Has what you've learned changed how you would respond?

When you seek medical care, how should you go about it? Should you go to a general practitioner? A specialist? A hospital emergency room? An urgent care center? Whom should you see? Of course, the best time to look for a physician is before you are ill.

Most experts believe it is best to have a primary physician who gets to know you and can treat you or coordinate referrals to specialists when needed. Physicians who are board-certified in family practice (for adults and children), internal medicine (for adults only), or pediatrics (for children only) are likely to be good choices because they have extensive training in the diagnosis and treatment of general medical problems.

Staff affiliation with a hospital connected with a medical school indicates that a physician is working with up-to-date colleagues and is apt to have up-to-date skills and information. Affiliation with a hospital that trains residents is also favorable. Less certain is affiliation with only privately owned hospitals—especially small ones—unless they are the only ones in the area. Lack of any hospital affiliation may be a sign of substandard care. Information on a physician's credentials may be obtainable from the physician's office, the local medical society, a local hospital, or a directory available at a medical or public library.

When choosing medical care, you should consider such factors as quality of care, cost, convenience, and whether follow-up care is available. Table 22-1 summarizes the advantages and disadvantages of various sources of medical care.

ORTHODOX PRACTITIONERS

Health professionals are regulated by state licensing laws. To become licensed, they must graduate from an accredited professional school, have additional clinical experience, and pass a licensing examination given by a state or national board. Competent professionals continue their education throughout their career by attending seminars, talking with colleagues, reading journals, and other activities. This section looks at five types of health professionals who are permitted by law to practice independently in the United States: medical doctors, osteopaths, podiatrists, optometrists, and dentists.

• Medical doctors are **independent practitioners** who hold an M.D. (doctor of medicine) degree from an accredited medical school. Once licensed, they are legally authorized to administer any type of medical or surgical treatment. What they actually do depends on their training, their inclinations, and the available facilities. Because the scope of medicine is so vast, most physicians take additional full-time training after graduation. (A partial list of medical specialties is given in the box "Common Names of Selected Medical Specialties.") Those choosing to become

specialists take three or more years of hospital-based specialty training, after which they can become "board-certified" by taking a stringent specialty examination. A few specialty boards require periodic recertification to ensure updated skills and knowledge. Some specialists require a referral by a primary physician, while others will also see patients without a referral. To work in a hospital, physicians must apply for staff privileges, which are based on training and experience and are reviewed annually.

• **Osteopathic physicians** are independent practitioners who have received a D.O. (doctor of osteopathy) degree. Osteopathy was founded more than a hundred years ago on an incorrect belief that the main cause of disease was mechanical interference with nerve and blood supply, correctable by spinal manipulation. But as medical science developed, osteopathy gradually incorporated all of its theories and practices. Today, osteopathic practice is virtually identical to medical practice except that osteopaths tend to have greater interest in musculoskeletal problems and manipulative therapy.

• **Podiatrists** are independent practitioners whose care is limited to problems of feet and legs. They are not medical doctors but hold a D.P.M. (doctor of podiatric medicine) degree. The length of their training is similar to that of physicians but emphasizes problems of the feet and legs. Podiatrists can prescribe drugs and do minor surgery in their offices. Those who wish to do major foot surgery must secure hospital privileges.

• **Optometrists** are independent practitioners who are trained to examine the eyes and related structures to detect vision problems, eye diseases, and other problems. They are not physicians but hold an O.D. (doctor of optometry) degree. All states allow them to use drugs for diagnostic purposes. If they detect eye disease, they are expected to refer the patient to an appropriate physician. However, about half of the states permit them to use drugs to treat minor ailments.

Independent practitioner A physician or other health professional who is legally permitted to provide health care services without supervision or direction from another health professional.

Osteopathic physicians Medical practitioners who have graduated from an osteopathic medical school. Osteopathy incorporates the theories and practices of scientific medicine but tends to focus on musculoskeletal problems.

Podiatrists Nonmedical practitioners whose practice is limited to the feet and legs.

Optometrists Nonmedical practitioners who primarily examine the eyes to detect vision problems and prescribe corrective lenses.

TABLE 22-1 Outpatient Health-care Facilities

Facility	Advantages	Disadvantages
Medical office	Maximum personal attention. Low cost per visit.	Limited hours
Multispecialty group practice	Low cost per visit. Consultations may be more readily available.	Same physician may not always be seen (varies with setup of group). May have less choice of consultants.
Student health service	Convenient location. Minimal cost.	Hours and scope of practice may be limited.
Emergicenter (urgent care center)	Costs less than hospital emergency room. Open long hours. Convenient appointment times.	Costs more than private office. May not be ideal setup for follow-up care. When care is episodic, physician does not get to know the patient as an individual.
Hospital emergency room	Open 24 hours a day. Able to handle serious emergencies. Sophisticated equipment available.	Highest cost. Nonemergency cases may not receive much attention. Follow-up care may be minimal. Care is episodic and less personal.
Hospital outpatient clinic	Fees may be reduced for individuals who cannot afford private care.	Patients may have to wait a long time to be seen. High staff turnover could mean different doctors may be seen.
Ambulatory surgical facilities	Surgery costs less than it would in a hospital.	Unsuitable for major surgery.

© 1988 Stephen Barrett, M.D.

• **Dentists** form another group of practitioners who can practice without medical supervision. They hold either a D.D.S. (doctor of dental surgery) or D.M.D. (doctor of medical dentistry) degree. Those who wish to become specialists complete two or more years of specialty training after graduation from dental school. Dentists are permitted to perform certain types of surgery and to prescribe a limited number of drugs within the scope of their training.

In addition to these independent practitioners, who make up a relatively small percentage of the total number of health care professionals in the United States, a large body of **allied health care providers** delivers care to mil-

lions of people. These trained practitioners include registered nurses (R.N.'s), licensed vocational nurses (L.V.N.'s), registered dietitians (R.D.'s), dental hygienists, physical therapists, occupational therapists, laboratory technicians, x-ray technicians, and many others.

Personal Insight   In general, how do you feel about the orthodox medical practices—confident, reverent, resigned, skeptical, suspicious, apprehensive? How about the unorthodox practices? Why do you think you feel the way you do?

Common Names of Selected Medical Specialties

Allergy and immunology Subspecialty of internal medicine that deals with allergies and other disorders of the immune system.

Anesthesiology Administration of drugs to prevent pain or to induce unconsciousness during surgical operations or diagnostic procedures.

Cardiology Subspecialty of internal medicine that deals with the heart and blood vessels.

Cardiovascular surgery Surgical treatment of diseases of the heart and blood vessels.

Dermatology Diagnosis and treatment of skin diseases.

Endocrinology and metabolism Subspecialty of internal medicine that deals with glandular and metabolic disorders.

Family practice General medical services for patients and their families.

Gastroenterology Subspecialty of internal medicine that deals with disorders of the digestive tract (esophagus, stomach, and intestine).

General surgery Surgery of parts of the body that are not in the domain of specific surgical specialties (some overlapping areas).

Geriatrics Subspecialty of family practice and internal medicine that deals with the medical problems of the elderly.

Hematology/oncology Subspecialty of internal medicine concerned with blood disorders and cancers.

Internal medicine Diagnosis and nonsurgical treatment of internal organs of the body of adults.

Nephrology Diagnosis and treatment of kidney diseases.

Neurology Diagnosis and nonsurgical treatment of diseases of the brain, spinal cord, and nerves.

Neurosurgery Diagnosis and surgical treatment of diseases of the brain, spinal cord, and nerves.

Nuclear medicine Use of radioactive substances for diagnosis and treatment.

Obstetrics and gynecology Care of pregnant women and disorders of the female reproductive system.

Ophthalmology Medical and surgical care of the eye, including the prescription of glasses.

Orthopedics Care of diseases of the muscles, and diseases, fractures, and deformities of the bones and joints.

Otolaryngology Care of diseases of the head and neck except for those of the eyes or brain.

Pathology Examination and diagnosis of organs, tissues, body fluids, and excrement.

Pediatrics Care of children from birth through adolescence. Subspecialties include allergy, cardiology, hematology/oncology, nephrology, and surgery.

Physiatry Treatment of convalescent and physically handicapped patients.

Plastic surgery Surgery to correct or repair deformed or mutilated parts of the body, or to improve facial or body features.

Proctology Medical and surgical treatment of disorders of the intestines and rectum.

Psychiatry Treatment of mental and emotional problems.

Pulmonary disease Subspecialty of internal medicine that deals with diseases of the lungs.

Radiology Use of radiation for the diagnosis and treatment of disease.

Rheumatology Subspecialty of internal medicine that deals with arthritis and related disorders.

Urology Treatment of male sex organs and urinary tract and female urinary tract.

UNORTHODOX PRACTITIONERS

The term *orthodox health care* as used in this chapter refers to the prevention, diagnosis, and treatment of disease based on currently accepted scientific information. Current medical beliefs are based on information gathered by practitioners and researchers throughout the world who share the results of their research and other careful observations. In contrast, the term *unorthodox practitioners* refers to individuals whose philosophy and methods either clash with accepted knowledge about health and disease or are both unproven and unlikely. Reliance on unscientific practitioners may delay effective care and often involves financial exploitation.

Dentists Nonmedical practitioners specializing in the prevention and treatment of diseases and injuries of the teeth, mouth, and jaws.

Allied health care providers Health care personnel who provide services under the supervision and/or control of independent practitioners.

TERMS

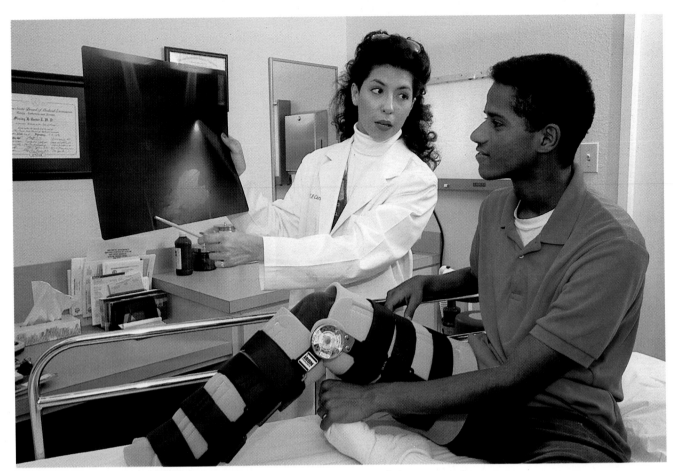

The health care system in the United States includes many different kinds of physicians and other health care workers. A physician can become a board-certified specialist in a particular field, such as orthopedics or radiology, by taking three or more years of special training and passing a stringent examination.

Common Unorthodox Practices

The 10 approaches to health care discussed in this section are based on theories that are unproven or rejected by the scientific community: chiropractic, applied kinesiology, homeopathy, naturopathy, acupuncture, iridology, reflexology, faith healing, chelation therapy, and "clinical ecology." The fact that an approach is unorthodox does not mean that its practitioners never help people or that everything they do should be considered quackery. Many people whose symptoms are bodily responses to tension (such as fatigue or headaches) may lose their symptoms following attention by anyone they believe in. Moreover, many of the practitioners described here might persuade patients to develop healthier living habits. Some also recognize their limitations and refer patients who need it for appropriate medical care.

Many of the practitioners described in this section refer to themselves as "holistic" (or "wholistic"), meaning that they treat the whole patient, giving attention to emotions and lifestyle in addition to physical problems. Good medical doctors have always practiced in this manner.

The holistic label is used by a few scientific practitioners who operate wellness clinics. But most "holistic" practitioners use a wide variety of unscientific methods of diagnosis and treatment, including high doses of vitamins.

Unorthodox methods are sometimes called "alternative" approaches to health care. However, this term can be misleading because it wrongly implies that the methods are *equivalent* or equally logical choices—which they are not.

- **Chiropractic** is based on the teachings of Daniel David Palmer, a "magnetic healer" who concluded in 1895 that the main cause of disease is misplaced spinal bones. He theorized that these partial dislocations interfere with the flow of "nerve energy" from the brain to the rest of the body and that spinal manipulation can restore the vertebrae to their proper places, enabling the body to heal itself. There is no scientific evidence to justify this belief.

  Chiropractors today are licensed in all 50 states, and most of their schools are accredited. They can be classified into two main groups, "mixers" and

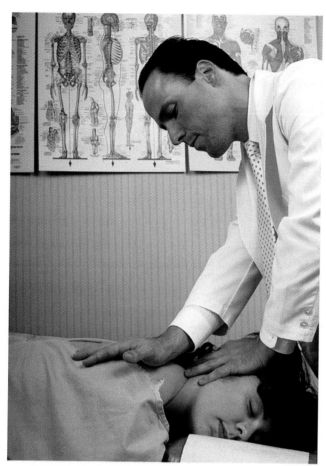

The primary treatment used by chiropractors is spinal manipulation. Properly applied, manipulation can benefit people with some types of musculoskeletal disorders.

"straights." Mixers, the larger group, acknowledge that germs, hormones, and other factors play a role in disease, but regard mechanical disturbances of the spine as the major underlying cause. In addition to manipulation, mixers use physical therapy methods and may prescribe food supplements. Straights still cling to Palmer's original doctrines and tend to confine themselves to manual manipulation of the spine. Some chiropractors completely reject Palmer's theories and limit their practice to musculoskeletal disorders; they are likely to work in tandem with medical doctors. Chiropractors are not licensed to prescribe drugs or perform surgery.

Most people who consult chiropractors suffer from backaches or other musculoskeletal disorders. Properly applied, manipulation can benefit people with back pain caused by lack of mobility of bony segments of the spine. Chiropractors often help people, but many of them encourage their patients to come weekly or monthly for "preventive maintenance" of their spine, a practice that has no medical justification. Chiropractors have also been criticized for inappropriately prescribing high doses of vitamins and for overuse of x-rays.

- **Applied kinesiology** is based on the notion that every organ dysfunction is accompanied by a specific weak muscle. Its proponents, most of whom are chiropractors, also claim that nutritional deficiencies, allergies, and other adverse reactions to food substances can be detected by placing substances in the mouth so that the patient salivates. "Good" substances will lead to increased strength in specific muscles, whereas "bad" substances will cause specific weaknesses. Treatment of muscles diagnosed as "weak" may include special diets, food supplements, acupressure, and/or spinal manipulation. These concepts do not conform to accepted scientific beliefs about the nature of health and disease, and critics believe that any apparent beneficial results are the result of patient suggestibility.

- **Homeopathy** is based on the theories of Samuel Hahnemann (1755–1843), a German physician. Hahnemann was justifiably alarmed about bloodletting, leeching, purging, and other medical procedures of his day that did far more harm than good. He was also critical of medications such as calomel (mercurous chloride), which was given in doses that caused mercury poisoning. Instead, he proposed his "law of similars"—that the symptoms of disease can be cured by substances that produce similar symptoms in healthy people. The word *homeopathy* is derived from the Greek words *homeo* ("similar") and *pathos* ("suffering" or "disease").

  Hahnemann believed that diseases represent a disturbance in the body's ability to heal itself and that only a small stimulus is needed to foster the healing process. After experimenting on himself and others, he concluded that the smaller the dose, the more powerful the effect—just the opposite of what pharmacologists believe today.

  Homeopathic remedies are plant products, minerals, or other substances diluted to an extreme degree. The dilution of some preparations is so great that no molecule of original substance remains. But Hahnemann believed that vigorous shaking with each step of dilution leaves behind a spiritlike essence that

Chiropractic   A system of health care based on the premise that misalignments of the vertebrae contribute to most diseases and ailments.

Applied kinesiology   A treatment method based on the theory that organ dysfunction is accompanied by muscle weakness that may be correctable by nutritional methods.

Homeopathy   A treatment method based on the theory that tiny doses of certain substances can exert powerful effects within the body.

TERMS

cures by restoring the body's "vital force" to normal.

As scientific drug use developed, homeopathy declined sharply, particularly in America, where its schools either closed or converted to modern methods. But a few hundred physicians trained in modern methods have kept the practice alive in this country by taking courses here or abroad or by training with a practicing homeopath.

Homeopathic remedies were recognized as drugs by the 1938 amendment to the Federal Food, Drug, and Cosmetic Act. Unlike most other drugs, homeopathic remedies have been allowed to remain on the market without proof of their effectiveness being presented to the FDA. They can be obtained from practitioners and are also available without a prescription from health food stores, pharmacies, and manufacturers. These products appeal primarily to people who are afraid of doctors or of taking more potent drugs.

- **Naturopathy** is based on the idea that disease is caused by a violation of nature's laws. Naturopaths say that diseases are the body's effort to purify itself and that cures result from "increasing the patient's vital force by ridding the body of toxins." Naturopathic treatment can include "natural food" diets, vitamins, herbs, tissue minerals, cell salts, manipulation, massage, remedial exercise, diathermy, colonic enemas, acupuncture, reflexology, hypnotherapy, and homeopathy. Radiation may be used for diagnosis but not for treatment. Drugs are forbidden except for compounds that are components of body tissues. Naturopaths, like many chiropractors, believe that most diseases are within the scope of their practice. Naturopaths are licensed in a few states, and one of their two schools is accredited.

- **Acupuncture,** a technique dating from ancient China, involves the insertion of needles into the skin, or muscles or tendons beneath, at one or more "acupuncture points." These points, said to represent various internal organs, are generally located along "meridians" on the surface of the body. Proponents claim that good health is produced by a harmonious mixture of yin and yang and that stimulation of acupuncture points can balance them so that internal organs can return to normal function. Similar claims are made for **acupressure (Shiatsu),** but no needles are used. (For a look at another system of treatment from China, see the box "Chinese Herbal Medicine.")

Acupuncture defines the body according to systems that have no relation to established facts about body physiology. "Meridians" and acupuncture points on the surface of the body cannot actually be seen or measured. They are part of the mystical ancient Chinese way of looking at the body, health,

disease, and nature. Although there is no evidence that acupuncture can affect the course of any physical illness, it may produce temporary pain relief. It probably works either by suggestion or by triggering release of the body's own morphinelike drugs, known as endorphins. The American Medical Association Council on Scientific Affairs has recommended that acupuncture for pain relief be regarded as experimental and performed only in medical research settings. However, some states license nonmedical acupuncturists.

- **Iridology** was devised more than a hundred years ago by Ignatz von Peczely, a Hungarian physician. It is based on the belief that each area of the body is represented by a corresponding area in the iris of the eye (the colored area surrounding the pupil). Iridologists claim that states of health and disease can be diagnosed from the color, texture, and location of various pigment flecks in the eye and that "imbalances" can be treated with vitamins, minerals, herbs, and similar products. According to a leading proponent, "Nature has provided us with a miniature television screen showing the most remote portions of the body by way of nerve reflex responses."

Iridologists use elaborate charts that supposedly show where various organs are represented in the eye. The American Medical Association Council on Scientific Affairs has noted that these charts are similar in concept to those used years ago in "phrenology," the pseudoscience that related protuberances of the skull to the mental faculties and character of the individual. Of course, medical doctors can diagnose a few conditions by examining the interior of the eye with an ophthalmoscope, but that is not what iridologists do.

- **Reflexology,** also known as "zone therapy," is based on the theory that pressing on certain areas of the hands or feet can help relieve pain and remove the underlying cause of disease in other parts of the body. Proponents claim that: (1) the body is divided into 10 zones that begin or end in the hands and feet, (2) each organ or part of the body is represented by an area on the hands and feet, (3) the practitioner can diagnose abnormalities by feeling the feet, and (4) massaging or pressing each area can stimulate the flow of energy, blood, nutrients, and nerve impulses to the corresponding body zone. Reflexologists also claim that their techniques have been effective against anemia, arthritis, asthma, cataracts, deafness, diabetes, heart disease, high blood pressure, kidney disease, and many other health problems.

Acupressure, iridology, and reflexology are utilized by some licensed practitioners (mainly chiropractors and naturopaths) as well as by bogus "nutritionists" and other unlicensed practitioners. In most states,

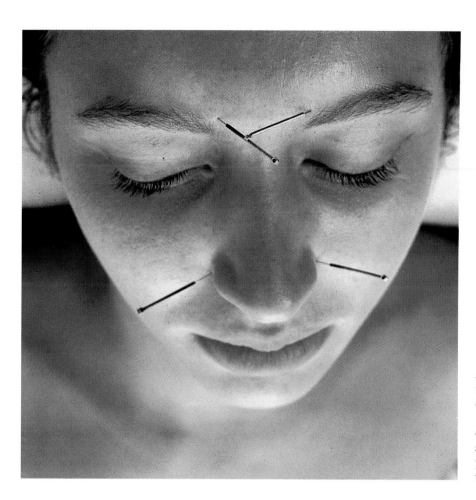

Acupuncture is based on the theory that illness results from an imbalance of vital energy flowing through the body along 12 meridians, each of which corresponds to a vital organ. The acupuncturist inserts needles at certain points and rotates them. This woman is undergoing treatment for hay fever.

unlicensed individuals who use these methods could be convicted of practicing medicine without a license, but few are ever prosecuted.

- **Faith healing,** a practice based on the belief that prayer and other rituals can heal, has existed since ancient times. The idea that demons cause disease was accepted by ancient practitioners; it still is prevalent today among segments of the American public. In the United States, several religions include faith healing as part of their dogma, and many evangelistic healers have attracted large followings.

  Few scientific attempts have been made to evaluate faith healing. Although testimonials abound, it is difficult and time-consuming to investigate such claims. Many cures attributed to faith healing are cases in which the ailment simply runs it natural course and the person recovers as he or she would have anyway. In one extensive study, Dr. William A. Nolen examined many people who had supposedly been "miraculously healed" and found that not one had been helped. A more recent investigation led by magician James Randi found that several prominent healers were outright frauds.

- **Chelation therapy** involves the injection of a synthetic amino acid called EDTA into the

bloodstream. Proponents claim that this treatment removes unwanted minerals from the body and is effective against heart disease, arthritis, emphysema, and many other serious diseases. However, no controlled study has shown that chelation therapy is an effective treatment for any of these conditions.

TERMS

Naturopathy   A treatment approach based on the belief that the basic cause of disease is violation of nature's laws.

Acupuncture   A technique based on the theory that insertion of needles into points on the skin can restore health.

Acupressure (Shiatsu)   A technique based on the theory that pressing on various body parts can restore health.

Iridology   A diagnostic method based on the theory that each area of the body is represented by a corresponding area in the eye.

Reflexology   A treatment method based on the theory that pressing on certain areas of the hands or feet can help relieve pain and remove the underlying cause of disease in other parts of the body.

Faith healing   Practices based on a belief that religious faith can bring about recovery or that prayer and faith in a healer can result in a cure through divine intervention.

Chelation therapy   An intravenous treatment claimed to provide various health benefits by removing unwanted substances from the body.

by Melinda J. Seid, California State University, Sacramento

When Americans think about medicine, they're likely to think of high-tech clinics, scientific labs, or prescriptions for the newest antibiotic or antihistamine. Other cultures have developed elaborate systems of medicine that are very different from this model. Such systems are often referred to as *traditional medicine*; they typically include a body of knowledge, passed down and recorded over the years; methods of training practitioners; and various standardized practices and treatments.

Chinese herbal medicine is probably the best known system of traditional medicine. It originated thousands of years ago as a collection of remedies that made use of the medicinal properties of plants. It also incorporated many principles of Chinese philosophy and religion. The system developed over the centuries, as knowledge about herbal remedies was compiled, updated, and standardized. The same system is in use today in China—alongside modern Western medical techniques—and in Chinese communities around the world.

Chinese herbal medicine does have some features in common with Western medicine, but there are also significant differences. Western pharmacology (the science of drugs) has its historical roots in herbal medicine. Aspirin, for example, was originally dervied from the willow bark; digitalis (a heart stimulant) from foxglove leaves; and penicillin from a fungus. Recently, taxol, a substance derived from the yew tree, has been found to combat ovarian cancer. Most drugs used in Western medicine are now produced synthetically in laboratories, but the search for plants with medicinal properties still goes on throughout the world.

Even when working with natural substances, however, Western medicine takes a different approach than does Chinese medicine. In Chinese medicine, whole plants and combinations of plants are used. Herbal prescriptions are believed to work because of the interactions among their ingredients. The use of whole herbs and herb blends also helps to buffer side effects. In Western pharmacology, on the other hand, the emphasis is on single, biologically active ingredients and their specific effects on the body. When Western scientists are investigating plants and other natural substances, they extract compounds and purify them to their barest molecular components. They then test these isolated active ingredients against tumors, viruses, and other disease agents.

Western and Chinese traditional medicine also differ in their ideas about treatment. In Chinese traditional medicine, herbal remedies are said to promote good health by restoring the body's balance and its natural ability to resist disease. From the Chinese point of view, the Western approach—administering drugs to destroy disease agents—controls symptoms but doesn't treat the underlying cause of the illness.

Antibiotics, for example, may kill bacteria, but they don't improve the body's resistance to infection; diuretics may rid the body of excess fluid, but they don't improve kidney function.

Diagnostic techniques and criteria also distinguish Chinese traditional medicine from Western medicine. Diagnosis is a central aspect of Chinese medicine. Four basic diagnostic methods are used: interviewing, observing, listening, and feeling. Data are collected on the pulse, the color of the complexion, the brightness of the eyes, the color and texture of the tongue, the condition of the internal organs, and the patient's dietary habits, emotional condition, and physical discomforts. Once the herbalist determines the nature and location of the disease through these techniques, he or she prescribes a specific herbal remedy.

Because each person is believed to respond in a unique way, herbal prescriptions tend to be customized—another way in which Chinese medicine differs from Western medicine. Different combinations of herbs are prescribed on a case-by-case basis. Western medicine, in contrast, focuses on standardized responses to drugs and treatments across broad populations. Research is conducted according to rigorous standards, and large-scale clinical trials are required before a drug can be approved for use.

The most fundamental differences between Chinese and Western medicine, however, are a function of their cultural contexts. Chinese medicine is embedded in the Chinese world view, which is very different from the Western world view. For example, diseases are classified into two broad categories—yin (cold) and yang (hot)—according to the patient's symptoms. The herbal medicines are also categorized as yin or yang. Using the principles of opposites and relative balance, Chinese herbalists treat what they consider yang illnesses with yin drugs and yin illnesses with yang drugs. Medicinal plants are further categorized by their "energies" and "tastes." The interrelatedness of energy and taste are important in determining which herbs should be prescribed for a particular illness. For example, ginger is sweet and warm and so is considered a suitable remedy for a cold.

Recently, scientists have begun analyzing Chinese medicinal plants to identify their active ingredients. Other scientists, inspired by the discovery of taxol, have renewed their search for anticancer substances in the natural world. Some observers think these activities signal a coming together of Chinese and Western medicine. But given the profound differences in the theories and philosophies on which they rest, it seems likely that the two systems will continue to be very different approaches to illness and health.

Sources: *A Barefoot Doctor's Manual*. 1990. (Philadelphia: Running Press); H. Beinfield and E. Korngold. 1991. *Between Heaven and Earth: A Guide to Chinese Medicine* (New York: Ballantine Books); D. P. Reid. 1992. *Chinese Herbal Medicine* (Boston: Shambhala); A. Emmett. 1992. "Where East does not meet West." *Technology Review* November/December.)

Chelation therapy is also expensive—thousands of dollars for a series of 20 to 50 injections—and has caused serious complications in some cases.

- **Clinical ecology** is practiced by a few hundred medical and osteopathic physicians. It is not a recognized specialty but is based on the notion that hypersensitivity to common foods and chemicals can cause depression, difficulty in thinking, headaches, muscle and joint pains, and many other common symptoms. Clinical ecologists speculate that the immune system is like a barrel that continually fills with chemicals until it overflows, leading to multiple symptoms. Much of their diagnosis is based on the provocation-neutralization test in which suspected substances are administered under the tongue or injected into the skin. If symptoms occur, the test is considered positive and the patient is diagnosed as suffering from **"environmental illness."** Steps are recommended to prevent or reduce contact with the substances involved—through dietary restriction and various environmental changes. Many clinical ecologists claim their patients are suffering from hypersensitivity to the common yeast *Candida albicans*. The American Academy of Allergy and Immunology, which is the nation's largest professional organization of allergists, considers clinical ecology a form of "poor medical practice" and regards the concepts of "environmental illness" and **candidiasis hypersensitivity** as "speculative and unproven."

Evaluating Unorthodox Practices

Given the relatively advanced state of medical science and the fairly high level of consumer awareness among Americans, why do unorthodox practices persist—and even thrive? Promoters of quackery appeal to people in many ways. They offer hope to people who feel desperate, including people with incurable diseases. They exploit any strains in the relationship between patient and physician, promising to cure those who are dissatisfied with the course of their treatment. They take advantage of current health threats—in another era it was typhoid fever; today it's HIV infection. They attack the medical establishment, suggesting that it is trying to suppress effective treatments or that physicians and scientists have other ulterior motives. They foster anxiety and doubt by suggesting that many people have problems that are actually uncommon, such as vitamin deficiencies and low blood sugar. And they promise new, quick, or easy ways to attain vitality, vigor, strength, energy, youthful looks, and much more.

How can you protect yourself against quackery? Most important is maintaining an appropriate level of suspicion. For example, don't assume that health claims made in advertisements or on radio or television talk shows must be true or would not have been allowed. This is not necessarily the case. To take advantage of the best that

medical science can offer and to avoid being led astray, it is necessary to make reasoned, informed decisions about what to believe. Many resources exist to help people assess the claims made for a product or treatment. You can consult a physician, registered dietitian, or other reputable professional; do some reading at a public library (preferably with some professional guidance); contact a consumer group or local health organization; or ask your insurance company whether they will pay for the treatment. The specific strategies listed in the box "Ten Ways to Avoid Being Quacked" will help you know what to do the next time you encounter a treatment that seems too good to be true.

Protection against quackery isn't just the individual's responsibility, of course. At the community, state, and national level, protection may be provided by various agencies; we turn to this topic next.

CONSUMER PROTECTION AGENCIES

Legal protection against health frauds and quackery is based on a framework of federal and state laws. Professional and voluntary agencies can sometimes apply pressure to wrongdoers. Educational information is available from many sources.

Federal Agencies

In addition to its mission to protect our food supply, the U.S. Food and Drug Administration (FDA) has jurisdiction over advertising of prescription drug products and labeling of nonprescription products and health devices. It is illegal to market a product without FDA approval (which usually means that the agency considers it safe and effective). When the FDA learns that a product is being marketed with unapproved claims, it can issue a warning letter, seize the product, or obtain an injunction. Criminal prosecution is also possible but rarely occurs.

The FDA has a very active public educational program. Its magazine, *FDA Consumer*, provides excellent coverage of health, nutrition, and safety issues. Its Office of Consumer Affairs distributes pamphlets, sponsors talks and conferences, and answers individual inquiries. Its field of-

---

Clinical ecology A treatment approach based on the concept that multiple symptoms can be triggered by hypersensitivity to common foods and chemicals when the immune system becomes "overloaded."

Environmental illness Fad diagnosis based on the unfounded idea that an overload of the immune system leads to multiple symptoms triggered by hypersensitivity to common foods and chemicals.

Candidiasis hypersensitivity A fad diagnosis based on the unscientific concept that hidden allergies to yeast can cause a wide spectrum of symptoms.

TERMS

Promoters of quackery know how to appeal to every aspect of human vulnerability. What sells is not the quality of their products but their ability to influence their audience. Here are 10 strategies to avoid being quacked:

- *Remember that quackery seldom looks outlandish.* Its promoters often use scientific terms and quote (or misquote) from scientific references. Some actually have reputable scientific training but have diverged from it.

- *Ignore any practitioner who says that most diseases are caused by faulty nutrition or can be remedied by taking supplements.* Although some diseases are related to diet, most are not. Moreover, in most cases where diet actually is a factor in a person's health problem, the solution is not to take vitamins but to alter the diet.

- *Be wary of anecdotes and testimonials.* If someone claims to have been helped by an unorthodox remedy, ask yourself and possibly your physician whether there might be another explanation. Most single episodes of disease recover with the passage of time, and most chronic ailments have symptom-free periods. Most people who give testimonials about recovery from cancer have undergone effective treatment as well as unorthodox treatment, but give credit to the latter. Some testimonials are complete fabrications.

- *Be wary of pseudomedical jargon.* Instead of offering to treat your disease, some quacks will promise to "detoxify" your body, "balance" its chemistry, release its "nerve energy," "bring it in harmony with nature," or correct supposed "weaknesses" of various organs. The use of concepts that are impossible to measure enables success to be claimed even though nothing has actually been accomplished.

- *Don't fall for paranoid accusations.* Unorthodox practitioners often claim that the medical profession, drug companies, and the government are conspiring to suppress whatever method they espouse. No evidence to support such a theory has ever been demonstrated. It also flies in the face of logic to believe that large numbers of people would oppose the development of treatment methods that might someday help themselves or their loved ones.

- *Forget about "secret cures."* True scientists share their knowledge as part of the process of scientific development. Quacks may keep their methods secret to prevent others from demonstrating that they don't work. No one who actually discovered a cure would have reason to keep it secret. If a method works—especially for a serious disease—the discoverer would gain enormous fame, fortune, and personal satisfaction by sharing the discovery with others.

- *Be wary of herbal remedies.* Herbs are promoted primarily through literature based on hearsay, folklore, and tradition. As medical science developed, it became apparent that most herbs did not deserve good reputations, and most that did were replaced by synthetic compounds that are more effective. Many herbs contain hundreds or even thousands of chemicals that have not been completely cataloged. While some may turn out to be useful, others could well prove toxic. With safe and effective treatment available, treatment with herbs rarely makes sense.

- *Be skeptical of any product claimed to be effective against a wide range of unrelated diseases—particularly diseases that are serious.* There is no such thing as a panacea or "cure-all."

- *Ignore appeals to your vanity.* One of quackery's most powerful appeals is the suggestion to "think for yourself" instead of following the collective wisdom of the scientific community. A similar appeal is the idea that although a remedy has not been proven to work for other people, it still might work for you.

- *Don't let desperation cloud your judgment.* If you feel that your physician isn't doing enough to help you, or if you have been told that your condition is incurable and don't wish to accept this fate without a struggle, don't stray from scientific health care in a desperate attempt to find a solution. Instead, discuss your feelings with your physician and consider a consultation with a recognized expert.

fices, located in major cities throughout the country, distribute educational materials, answer inquiries, and provide speakers.

The Federal Trade Commission (FTC) has jurisdiction over interstate advertising of all health products and services except for prescription drugs. However, it rarely takes action against licensed health practitioners because they are subject to supervision by state licensing boards. When the FTC becomes aware of wrongdoing, it can ob-

tain a cease-and-desist order, which, if violated, can trigger penalties up to $10,000 a day for each violation.

The U.S. Postal Service has jurisdiction over the sale of products or services by mail. When misleading mail-order promotions are detected, the agency can seek voluntary discontinuation or obtain administrative permission to intercept orders and return them to the senders. After a scheme has been stopped, a promoter who resumes similar activity can be fined up to $10,000 per day.

Although actions by federal agencies can be extremely powerful and put illegal operators out of business, federal enforcement has serious limitations. Some illegal schemes are never detected, while others are detected long after their promoter has done considerable harm. In some cases, offenders can remain in business for years by appealing to federal courts. Most important, the number of illegal schemes is so great that federal agencies don't have sufficient resources to act against all they detect.

State and Local Agencies

Licensed practitioners are regulated by state boards that can conduct investigations into alleged wrongdoing. When an offense takes place, the practitioner can be ordered to take corrective action and can be placed on probation or have his or her license suspended or revoked.

State attorneys general have jurisdiction over illegal health activities, such as illegal representations by unlicensed practitioners, marketing of unapproved drugs, and false advertising. In cases involving individual victims, local district attorneys may have primary jurisdiction.

The extent to which individual states protect their residents from quackery and health fraud depends on the strength of their laws and resources allotted to the problem. While some states conduct extensive investigations and prosecute many promoters of quackery, others do virtually nothing.

Professional and Voluntary Organizations

Professional groups such as state and local medical societies can often help individuals check the reputation of practitioners or products. These groups can also investigate accusations of unethical and unprofessional conduct and can sometimes persuade wrongdoers to take corrective action. Professional societies can reprimand or expel members. Hospital officials can reduce, suspend, or revoke a practitioner's privileges at their particular hospital. But practitioners who neither belong to a professional group nor work in a hospital are unlikely to be affected by the disciplinary efforts of these organizations.

Local Better Business Bureaus investigate unethical business practices but rarely get involved in disputes involving licensed practitioners. The National Council of Better Business Bureaus investigates and publishes occasional reports about quack products and their promotion. BBB's National Advertising Division investigates questionable product advertising and can sometimes persuade offending advertisers to stop.

The National Council Against Health Fraud is a membership organization of more than 1,000 persons concerned about quackery and health frauds. It sponsors meetings, publishes a newsletter and position papers, distributes other publications, helps victims obtain redress, and operates an information clearinghouse for individuals, government agencies, and media representatives. Information and advice are also available from many local, state, and national professional and voluntary organizations.

Table 22-2 lists places where you can obtain information or complain about questionable health matters. Remember that people who make appropriate complaints not only may help themselves, but also may help to protect others.

HEALTH INSURANCE

Health insurance enables people to budget in advance for health care costs that may otherwise be unpredictable and ruinously high. Hospital care costs hundreds of dollars a day, and surgical fees can cost thousands. So health insurance is important for everyone, especially as health care costs continue to rise (see the box "Health Care Costs in the United States").

Types of Policies

There are three basic types of health insurance coverage: basic, major medical, and comprehensive.

Basic protection includes expenses for hospital, surgical, and medical care. Hospital benefits may provide payment of a specific amount for a specified number of days, or full charges may be paid for daily room, board, routine nursing services, and intensive care up to a maximum number of days. Coverage may also be provided for various inpatient and outpatient services such as laboratory tests, x-ray films, medications, and physical therapy. Visits to physicians' offices are not usually covered.

Major medical insurance (also called "extended benefit" or "catastrophic coverage") is designed to help protect against medical expenses resulting from prolonged illness or serious injury. These contracts generally include a deductible clause, a co-insurance provision, high maximum limits, and coverage of a broad spectrum of services not included under basic coverage. Typically they pay 80 percent of covered services after a deductible that may range from $100 up to several hundred dollars. Psychiatric benefits are usually more limited than others. **Comprehensive major medical insurance** policies integrate basic and major medical insurance into one program.

Basic protection Insurance that includes hospital, surgical, and medical care.

Major medical insurance Insurance designed to help protect against medical expenses resulting from prolonged illness or serious injury.

Comprehensive major medical insurance Policies that combine basic and major medical insurance into one program.

TERMS

Health care costs continue to rise in the United States. This trend is increasingly seen as a threat to the country's economic health. It adds to the burden on businesses, which pay more than one-third of the country's medical bills; it tends to increase the federal budget deficit; and it swells the ranks of the uninsured, as more people and companies are forced out of the health insurance market.

Several factors contribute to the rise in health care costs, including the use of sophisticated, expensive equipment; the aging of the population; high earnings by many people in the health care industry; and costly treatments for some illnesses, such as cancer, heart disease, and HIV infection.

What are the dimensions of the health spending crisis? These are some of the facts:

Health Care Spending

- Total health spending in the United States in 1992 . . . $838.5 billion

- Projected health spending for 1993 . . . $939.9 billion

- Increase in health spending from 1992 to 1993 . . . 12 percent

- Projected increases in health spending each year from 1992 to 1996 . . . 12 to 13 percent

- Projected health spending for 1994 . . . over $1 trillion

Health Care Spending as a Proportion of GNP

- Proportion of GNP devoted to health spending in 1992 . . . 14 percent

- In 1991 . . . 13.2 percent

- In 1990 . . . 12.2 percent

- In 1981 . . . 9.6 percent

- Proportion of 1990 GNP devoted to health spending in Canada, France, Germany, and Sweden . . . 8–9 percent

- In Japan . . . 6.5 percent

- In Britain . . . 6.1 percent

Health Care Employment

- Total employment in the health care sector of the economy, 1992 . . . 10 million

- Total private employment, 1992 . . . 90 million

- Increase in health care employment, 1988–1992 . . . 43 percent

- Increase in private employment, 1988–1992 . . . 1 percent

The Uninsured

- Number of people without medical insurance in 1992 . . . 35.7 million

- In 1991 . . . 35.4 million

- In 1990 . . . 34.7 million

- Number of people who either lost their medical insurance or were added to Medicaid rolls between 1989 and 1991 . . . 7.7 million

- Proportion of all Latinos in the United States without medical insurance in 1991 . . . 32 percent

- Proportion of all African Americans without medical insurance in 1991 . . . 21 percent

Medicaid and Medicare

- Total federal spending on Medicaid, 1990 . . . $73 billion

- Increase in Medicaid spending, 1990–1991 . . . 29 percent

- Total federal spending on Medicare, 1990 . . . $113 billion

- Proportion of poor people's health care costs covered by Medicaid in 1992 . . . 42 percent

- Proportion of elderly people's health care costs covered by Medicare in 1992 . . . 40 percent

Who Pays?

- Total amount spent nationally on health care in 1990 . . . $666 billion

- Proportion of 1990 medical costs paid by private insurance companies . . . 33 percent

- By individual health care consumers (out-of-pocket expenses) . . . 20 percent

- By Medicare . . . 17 percent

- By Medicaid . . . 11 percent

- By other government programs . . . 14 percent

- By other private sources . . . 5 percent

Public Opinion Polls: Which Plan Do Americans Favor?

- National health plan run by government, financed by taxpayers, and covering all Americans . . . 44 percent

- Plan requiring employers to cover employees or contribute to federal fund covering all employees . . . 32 percent

- Current system of private insurance, Medicare, and Medicaid . . . 20 percent

- No opinion . . . 3 percent

Compiled from R. Pear. 1993. "Health-Care Costs Up Sharply Again, Posing New Threat." *The New York Times*, 5 January; "Medical Bills: Who Pays?" *Washington Post Health*, 21 July, 1992; and V. Cohn. 1992. "Moving on Health Care Reform." *Washington Post Health*. 21 January.

TABLE 22-2 Where to Complain or Seek Help

Problem	Agencies to Contact*
False advertising	FTC Bureau of Consumer Protection Regional FTC office National Advertising Division, Council of Better Business Bureaus Editor or station manager of media outlet where ad appeared
Product marketed with false or misleading claims	Regional FDA office State attorney general State health department Local Better Business Bureau Congressional representatives
Bogus mail-order promotion	Chief Postal Inspector, U.S. Postal Service Editor or station manager of media outlet where ad appeared
Improper treatment by licensed practitioner	Local or state professional society (if practitioner is a member) Local hospital (if practitioner is a staff member) State licensing board National Council Against Health Fraud Task Force on Victim Redress
Improper treatment by unlicensed individual	Local district attorney State attorney general National Council Against Health Fraud Task Force on Victim Redress
Advice needed about questionable product or service	National Council Against Health Fraud Local, state, or national professional or voluntary health groups

*Addresses
FTC Bureau of Consumer Protection, Washington, DC 20580. Tel. 202-326-2222.
National Advertising Division, Council of Better Business Bureaus, 845 Third Avenue, New York, NY 10022. Tel. 212-753-1358.
FDA, 5600 Fishers Lane, Rockville, MD 20857. Tel. 301-295-8024.
Chief Postal Inspector, U.S. Postal Service, Washington, DC 20260. Tel. 202-268-4267.
National Council Against Health Fraud, P.O. Box 1276, Loma Linda, CA 92354. Tel. 714-824-4690.
NCAHF Task Force on Victim Redress, P.O. Box 1747, Allentown, PA 18105. Tel. 215-437-1795.
For regional offices of federal agencies consult the telephone directory under U.S. Government.

© 1985, 1989, 1991, Stephen Barrett, M.D.

Health insurance policies may be sold to groups or individuals. Group policies generally offer more coverage and cost less than individual policies. Most people are insured through a group policy obtained through their place of employment. Because the extent and type of covered services vary widely from contract to contract, policies should be read carefully to understand what protection they provide.

Government Programs

In many states, certain categories of people who are unable to afford health care are eligible for **Medicaid**, a state-run, federally subsidized program that covers a broad spectrum of services.

Individuals who are chronically disabled or have reached age 65 are eligible for **Medicare**, a federal program composed of two parts. Part A provides hospital insurance financed through Social Security taxes. Part B helps pay for medical services and is financed through monthly premiums paid by those who wish to subscribe. Private insurance companies also sell "medigap" policies to supplement Medicare coverage.

Under Medicare, physicians who "accept assignment" are paid directly by the government and may not bill the patient for the difference between their usual fee and the amount the government pays (except for amounts that involve deductibles and co-insurance).

Medicaid Federally subsidized state-run plan of health care for indigent people.
Medicare Federal health insurance program for people 65 or older and for certain disabled younger people.

TERMS

Prepaid Group Plans

Most insurance contracts permit the policyholder complete freedom to decide where to obtain treatment. Because health care costs have been rising, insurance companies, hospitals, and private groups have been marketing plans aimed at controlling these costs. The physicians in these plans must agree to certain cost controls, and the patients are restricted in their choice of physicians.

Health maintenance organizations (HMOs) are comprehensive programs in which physicians agree to accept a monthly fee (**capitation**) per patient or to charge for actual services rendered according to a fee schedule that is usually lower than the physicians' standard fees. Many HMOs hold back a percentage of the fees until the end of the plan year. Then, if the plan meets its financial goals, the withheld funds will be distributed according to the agreement between the plan and the physicians. This type of arrangement is designed to encourage physicians to avoid unnecessary services. The physicians belonging to the HMO may be located in their own offices or at a central facility where the physicians are salaried. Under HMO programs, patients can choose their primary physician from a list of participating physicians and need a referral by the primary physician for services by specialists to be covered. However, the choice of physicians will be limited to those enrolled in the program.

Preferred provider organizations (PPOs) are programs in which participating physicians and hospitals agree to accept fixed fees that are usually 15 to 20 percent less than their usual fees. Patients can go to any provider, but use of nonparticipating providers results in considerably higher cost to the patient.

HMOs and PPOs are part of an increasing trend toward **managed care,** which includes measures to reduce the number of unnecessary services. In many plans, for example, special permission must be obtained from a plan administrator before a patient can be admitted to a hospital.

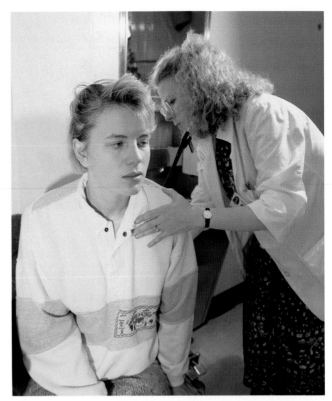

Physicians who work for a health maintenance organization usually receive a salary or monthly payment rather than fees from patients. The advantage of HMOs for patients is that their medical care is prepaid; the disadvantage is that the choice of physicians is narrowed.

Personal Insight   Do you believe that physicians and hospitals have a responsibility to treat and care for patients who can't pay? Do you think medical care is a right or a privilege? What is the basis for your beliefs and opinions?

Choosing a Policy

Choosing health insurance can be complicated because there are many types of plans and contracts can vary greatly from company to company and even within the same company. It's important for you to evaluate the services provided by different plans and choose the one that's best for you. (Refer to the box "Glossary of Health Insurance Terms" for help in understanding different policies.)

Colleges typically provide outpatient health services through a student health service. Some also require students to purchase additional insurance to cover hospitalization or other outside services. Students who are still covered under their family's policy may not be required to purchase additional insurance. It is usually most economical to remain covered under a family policy as long as possible rather than obtaining a separate policy of one's own.

TERMS

Health maintenance organization (HMO)   A prepaid health plan in which patients receive health care from designated providers.

Capitation   Payment to health providers according to number of patients they agree to serve rather than amount of service rendered.

Preferred provider organization (PPO)   A prepaid insurance plan in which providers agree to deliver services for discounted fees. Patients can go to any provider, but using nonparticipating providers results in higher costs to the patient.

Managed care   A health care system (such as HMO or PPO) that integrates the financing and delivery of services by using designated providers, utilization review, and financial incentives for following the plan's policies.

Because health insurance policies are legal contracts, they use precise legal language. Some of these terms appear in all policies, while others appear just in some. Understanding them will help you figure out how a policy works and what it actually covers. Following are terms not defined elsewhere in this chapter.

Assignment of benefits By signing a form (usually the insurance claim form), you authorize the insurance company to pay the physician directly. Otherwise, payment must be made directly to you. Most physicians will ask you to sign the form if you don't want to pay your bill before the insurance company pays its share.

Coinsurance An arrangement whereby you and the insurance company share costs. Typically, the insurer pays 75 to 85 percent of covered costs and you pay the rest. Some policies set an upper limit to co-insurance expense, after which the company pays all additional charges.

Conversion privilege A provision that enables those insured by group contracts to obtain an individual policy under various circumstances, such as leaving the job that provided the group coverage.

Coordination of benefits A provision that prohibits you from collecting identical benefits from two or more policies, thereby profiting when you are ill. After the primary company pays, other companies will calculate their coverage of the remainder. All group policies contain a coordination clause, but most individual policies do not.

Deductible The amount you must pay before the insurance company starts paying.

Endorsement or rider An attachment to the basic insurance policy that changes its coverage.

Exclusions Specified conditions or circumstances for which the policy does not provide benefits.

Grace period The number of days that you may delay payment of your premium without losing your insurance.

Guaranteed renewability A policy where the company agrees to continue insuring you up to a certain age (or for life) as long as you pay the premium. Under this provision, the premium structure cannot be raised unless it is raised for all members of a group or class of insured, such as all people living in your state with the same kind of policy.

Inpatient services Services received while hospitalized.

Notice of claim Written notice the company must receive when a claim exists. Typically it must be received within 20 days or as soon thereafter as reasonably possible.

Outpatient services Services obtained at a hospital by people who are not confined to the hospital.

Participating physician A physician who agrees to abide by the rules of a plan in return for direct payment by the insurance company. The agreement includes acceptance of a fixed fee schedule, a monthly fee per eligible patient, or other fee limitation.

Preexisting condition A health problem you had before becoming insured. Some policies exclude these conditions, while others do not.

Provider Any source of health care services, such as a hospital, physician, pharmacist, or laboratory.

Reasonable charge The amount a company will pay for a given service based on what most providers charge for it.

Waiting period A specified time between issuance of a policy and coverage of certain conditions. Typically there are waiting periods for preexisting conditions and maternity benefits.

After college it is usually best to see whether group coverage is available through work or membership in an organization. If you work for a large company, several plans may be available. If no group coverage is available, contact Blue Cross/Blue Shield and agents for several other insurance companies. After discussing your needs with them, obtain a copy of each policy that sounds suitable, read it carefully, and be sure you understand what it says. If you want both basic and major medical coverage, it is often best to get both from the same company to avoid gaps in coverage. However, your aim should be to insure mainly against the most serious types of losses. In the long run, it is more economical to absorb the cost of minor medical expenses as part of your overall budget. "Dread disease" policies that cover only one disease, such as cancer, are inadvisable, and other types of overlapping

policies should also be avoided. Mail-order policies that pay a daily amount generally have low limits and a waiting period, which make them unsuitable for basic coverage. The following questions are designed to help you choose the most appropriate insurance for you.

- What services are covered? Different policies may cover any of the following:

    Inpatient hospital costs

    Surgical costs, including anesthesia

    Inpatient medical services

    Physicians' office visits

    X-ray examinations

    Outpatient diagnostic tests

    Medications

Physical therapy

Maternity fees

Private-duty nursing

Psychiatric services

Skilled nursing home care

- Which of these services am I most likely to need?
- Are there exclusions for any preexisting conditions?
- How do the various policies compare in cost?
- Are the deductible and co-insurance provisions suitable?
- Are the maximum limits high enough?
- Will I be able to see the physicians I prefer?
- Does my present physician participate?

Most of the time, you can take care of yourself without personally consulting an expert. You can learn to manage stress, eat well, get adequate exercise, minimize contact with contagious disease, and so on. When you do need professional care—and Chapter 21 provides guidelines to help you identify those situations—you can continue to take responsibility for yourself by making reasoned decisions about the care and insurance you obtain.

Because so many people are involved in the health care field and because human knowledge has its limits, you are bound to have a frustrating or unpleasant experience now and then, as can happen in any area of your life. Take setbacks in stride and be persistent about getting what you need—within the bounds of practices based on scientific fact.

SUMMARY

- When seeking medical care, people usually should find a primary physician, who can refer them to specialists when necessary; in most cases, physicians should be affiliated with hospitals that are connected to medical schools or that train residents.

Orthodox Practitioners

- Medical doctors have degrees from accredited medical schools and are licensed to administer medical and surgical treatment; specialists have additional training and can become board-certified.
- Osteopathic practice has incorporated all of the theories and practices of medicine, though osteopaths usually have more interest in musculoskeletal problems and manipulative therapy.
- Podiatrists specialize in the care of feet and legs; they can prescribe drugs and do surgery.
- Optometrists examine the eyes to detect vision problems and eye diseases. They may use drugs for

diagnostic purposes but need to refer patients with eye disease to a physician.

- Dentists are permitted to perform certain types of surgery on the mouth and to prescribe certain drugs within the scope of their training.
- Other trained practitioners include registered nurses, licensed vocational nurses, dietitians, dental hygienists, physical therapists, occupational therapists, laboratory technicians, and x-ray technicians.

Unorthodox Practitioners

- Unorthodox practice consists of philosophies or methods that clash with accepted knowledge or are unproven and unlikely.
- Holistic practitioners pay attention to emotions and lifestyle as well as to physical problems; good medical practice has always been holistic.
- Chiropractic is based on the idea that the main cause of disease is misplaced spinal bones and that spinal manipulation can enable the body to heal itself.
- Applied kinesiology rests on the idea that every organ dysfunction is accompanied by a specific weak muscle.
- Homeopathy is based on the belief that the symptoms of disease can be cured by substances that produce similar symptoms in healthy people and that the smaller the dose, the more powerful the effect.
- Naturopathy is based on the idea that violations of nature's laws cause diseases, which are the body's effort to purify itself.
- Acupuncture involves the insertion of needles into the skin, muscles, or tendons at various points said to represent internal organs. Acupressure is a similar technique that doesn't use needles.
- Iridology is based on the belief that areas of the body are represented by corresponding areas in the iris of the eye and that diseases can be diagnosed from the color, texture, and location of various flecks in the eye.
- Reflexology is based on the theory that pressing on certain areas of the hands or feet can remove underlying causes of disease in other parts of the body.
- Faith healing is based on the belief that prayer and other rituals can heal; it is a part of some organized religions.
- Clinical ecology is based on the notion that hypersensitivity to common foods and chemicals can cause depression, headaches, and other symptoms.
- Promoters of unorthodox methods exploit others by offering hope to the desperate, taking advantage of

current health threats, attacking the medical establishment, fostering anxiety, and promising "quick fixes."

Consumer Protection Agencies

- The federal government offers protection against false advertising, mislabeling, and fraudulent mail-order schemes through the FDA, FTC, and U.S. Postal Service.

- State boards investigate alleged wrongdoing by licensed practitioners, and state attorneys general have jurisdiction over illegal health activities.

- Professional groups can help consumers check reputations and can investigate charges against members. Hospitals can restrict a practitioner's privileges. Better Business Bureaus and the National Council Against Health Fraud can provide information to consumers.

Health Insurance

- Basic health insurance includes expenses for hospital, surgical, and medical care. Coverage may include not only hospitalization but also laboratory tests, x-rays, medicines, and physical therapy.

- Major medical insurance protects against medical expenses resulting from prolonged illness or serious injury. These policies usually pay 80 percent of a broad range of services after a deductible has been paid.

- Comprehensive policies combine basic and major medical policies. Group policies usually offer more coverage and cost less than individual policies.

- Government programs include Medicaid, for the poor, and Medicare, for those who are 65 and over or chronically disabled.

- In health maintenance organizations (HMOs), physicians agree to accept a monthly fee per patient or to use a lower fee schedule than usual. With preferred provider organizations, participating physicians agree to accept lower fees.

- Group insurance usually offers the best coverage. Choice of a policy should depend on services covered, services needed, exclusions, deductibles, maximum limits, and choice of physicians.

TAKE ACTION

1. Visit the student health center on your campus or another health care facility. Evaluate the quality and kinds of services available. Consider such things as hours, waiting time, health literature available, scope of services, availability of specialists, and so on. Do

you think there is room for improvement? What recommendations would you make?

2. Talk to a practitioner of one or more of the unorthodox practices described in this chapter. Ask what training they have, what conditions they treat most often, how they make diagnoses, what treatments they give, and whether they have any pamphlets you can read. What questions do you have about these practices? Where would you go to find the answers?

JOURNAL ENTRY

1. Using the insurance guidelines in the chapter, evaluate your current coverage. In your health journal, make a list of the services it covers and does not cover; put a check mark next to the services that you are most likely to need. Examine the cost of the policy, including the deductibles and co-payments and the maximum limits on coverage. Also look at the rules governing your choice of physicians. Does your current plan meet your needs? Does it lack any services that are important for you or cover any unnecessary ones?

2. *Critical Thinking:* Examine and evaluate a TV or printed advertisement for a health-related product or service. What methods are used in the ad to make the product or service appeal to potential buyers? Does it contain any hidden messages? Are there any aspects of the ad that you feel are misleading? Write a short essay describing your findings.

SELECTED BIBLIOGRAPHY

American Academy of Allergy and Immunology. 1986. Position statement on "candidiasis hypersensitivity syndrome." *Journal of Allergy and Clinical Immunology* 78:271–73.

American Academy of Allergy and Immunology. 1986. Position statement on "clinical ecology." *Journal of Allergy and Clinical Immunology* 78:269–71.

American Heart Association. 1987. *Questions and Answers About Chelation Therapy.* Dallas: American Heart Association.

Barrett, S. 1990. Federal regulation of quackery: Improvement is needed. *Priorities* Fall, pp. 35–36.

Barrett, S. and the editors of Consumer Reports Books. 1990. *Health Schemes, Scams, and Frauds.* Yonkers, N.Y.: Consumer Reports Books.

Consumer Reports: Homeopathic remedies—These nineteenth-century medicines offer safety, even charm, but efficacy is another matter. 1987. *Consumer Reports.* January.

Cornacchia, H., and Barrett, S. 1993. *Consumer Health—A Guide to Intelligent Decisions,* 5th ed. St. Louis: Mosby Year Book.

Freedman, J. W. 1991. *Complete Guide to Dental Care.* Yonkers, N.Y.: Consumer Reports Books.

Fultz, O. 1992. Chiropractic: What can it do for you? *American Health,* April.

National Council Against Health Fraud. 1991. *Position Paper on Acupuncture.* Loma Linda, Calif.: National Council Against Health Fraud.

Harvard Heart Letter: Chelation therapy, risks without benefits? 1992. *Harvard Heart Letter* October.

Kenney, J. J. 1988. Applied kinesiology unreliable for assessing nutrient status. *Journal of the American Dietetic Association* 88:698–704.

National Council Against Health Fraud. 1991. *Position Paper on Acupuncture.* Loma Linda, Calif.: National Council Against Health Fraud.

Randi, J. 1989. *The Faith Healers.* Buffalo, N.Y.: Prometheus Books.

Raso, J. 1993. *Mystical Diets: Paranormal, Spiritual, and Occult Nutrition Practices.* Buffalo, N.Y.: Prometheus Books.

Stalker, D., and C. Glymour, eds. 1985. *Examining Holistic Medicine.* Buffalo, N.Y.: Prometheus Books.

Zwicky, J., A. Hafner, *et al.* 1992. *Reader's Guide to "Alternative" Health Methods: An analysis of more than 1,000 reports on unproven, disproven, controversial, fraudulent, and/or otherwise questionable approaches to solving health problems.* Chicago: American Medical Association.

RECOMMENDED READINGS

Barrett, S., and the editors of Consumer Reports Books. 1990. *Health Schemes, Scams, and Frauds.* New York: Consumer Reports Books. *A comprehensive discussion of current forms of quackery and how to avoid them.*

Barrett, S., and W. T. Jarvis (eds.). 1993. *The Health Robbers.* Buffalo, N.Y.: Prometheus. *A comprehensive look at quackery in America.*

Butler, K. 1992. *A Consumer's Guide to "Alternative Medicine."* Buffalo, N.Y.: Prometheus. *A critical look at homeopathy, acupuncture, faith healing, and many other unconventional treatments.*

Consumer Reports: Health Care in Crisis. 1992. *Consumer Reports,* July, August, September. *A three-part discussion of the high cost of health care and the need for a comprehensive national health insurance plan.*

Cornacchia, H., and S. Barrett. 1993. *Consumer Health—A Guide to Intelligent Decisions,* 5th ed. St. Louis: Mosby Yearbook. *A comprehensive guide to the health marketplace.*

Fultz, O. 1992. Chiropractic: What can it do for you? *American Health* April. *Discusses what happened when a reporter visited a chiropractor as a patient.*

Inglis, B., and R. West. 1983. *The Alternative Health Guide.* New York: Alfred A. Knopf. *Seventy "alternative" therapies from the viewpoint of two proponents.*

Jarvis, W. T. 1985. *Quackery and You.* Washington, D.C.: Review and Herald Publishing Association. *A 32-page booklet of basic facts about quackery.*

Lawrence, R. S., and others. 1989. *Guide to Clinical Preventive Services, Report of the U.S. Preventive Services Task Force.* Baltimore: Williams and Wilkins. *A comprehensive discussion of the periodic physical examinations, laboratory tests, immunizations, and other health services that are scientifically based and cost-effective.*

Vickery, D. and J. F. Fries. 1990. *Take Care of Yourself: Consumers' Guide to Medical Care.* Reading, Mass.: Addison-Wesley. *A practical manual with many flow sheets to help decide when medical care is needed.*

Young, J. H. 1992. *The Medical Messiahs.* Princeton, N.J.: Princeton University Press. *A social history of health quackery in twentieth-century America.*

Zwicky, J., A. Hafner, and others. 1992. *Reader's Guide to "Alternative" Health Methods.* Chicago: American Medical Association. *An analysis of more than 1,000 reports on questionable approaches to solving health problems.*

23

Injury Prevention and Control

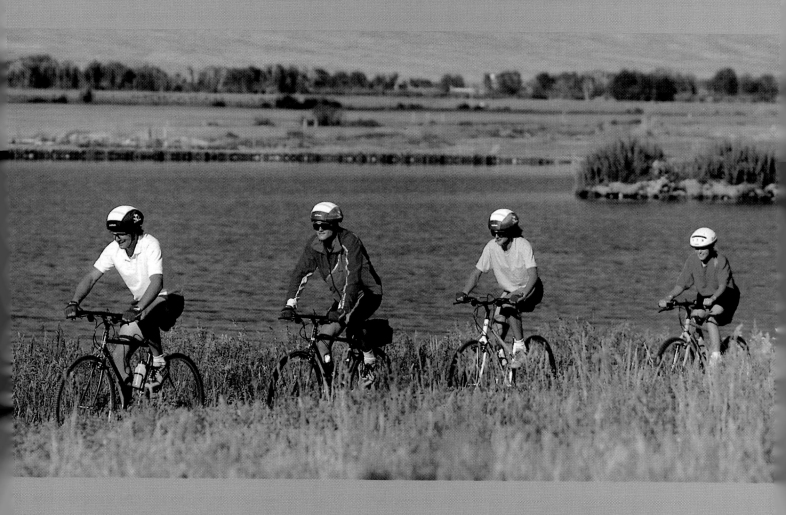

CONTENTS

▶ Your mother-in-law never wears a safety belt in her car or in anyone else's, even though most other people she knows do. She says she doesn't ever want to be trapped in a burning car or one that plunges into water. Is she right about the risks? Are people safer wearing these belts or not?

▶ You're driving home from school for Thanksgiving vacation in a freezing rain. As you're negotiating a curve in the road, the rear end of your car starts to fishtail, and then the rear wheels start skidding out to the left. One of your passengers says, "We're skidding—step on the brakes." The other one says, "No, steer into it—turn the wheel to the left." What should you do?

▶ You recently started jogging and have been following a popular jogging path around campus. Most of the route is along walking and bike paths, but in a few places it runs along main roads. You notice that some people jog with the traffic and some jog against it. Why? Which way should you jog?

▶ You've been enjoying a visit from your sister and her 2-year-old, who live in another state. While you're sitting out back drinking lemonade and talking, the toddler plays nearby and explores the shrubs and bushes. Suddenly he appears in front of you clutching a fistful of bright orange berries. There are orange stains around his mouth, too, and you realize he's been eating a plant he found in your yard. Your sister jumps up in alarm and asks you what kind of berries they are. You have no idea, but you tell her you're sure there wouldn't be anything dangerous growing in your yard. She's not reassured. Is there some action you should take?

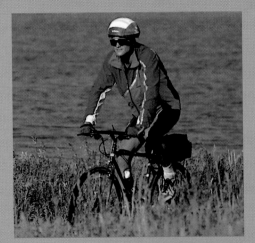

MAKING CONNECTIONS

Even the healthiest lifestyle can't protect you from the possibility of disability or premature death if you are injured. Luckily, most injuries are caused by recognizable and preventable factors, and there are many things you can do to avoid becoming an injury statistic. In each of the scenarios presented on this page, all related to injury prevention and control, individuals have to use information, make a decision, or choose a course of action. How would you act in each of these situations? What response or decision would you make? This chapter provides information about different types of injuries and how to prevent them that can be used in situations like these. After finishing the chapter, read the scenarios again. Has what you've learned changed how you would respond?

Injuries are the leading cause of death among Americans under age 45 and the fourth leading cause of death overall. Because injuries occur so often, especially among young people, they account for more **years of potential life lost** than cardiovascular disease and cancer combined. Injuries affect all segments of the population, but they are particularly common among minorities and people with low income, primarily due to social, environmental, and economic factors.

Not only are injuries common—affecting one out of every three Americans—but they are also costly. They result in loss of productivity due to premature death and disability, and they cause intense emotional suffering for injured people and their families, friends, and colleagues. Injuries also require a large allocation of medical resources for care, treatment, and rehabilitation. Last year alone, the cost of injuries in the United States was over $170 billion.

Injuries can be intentional or unintentional. An **intentional injury** is one that is purposely inflicted, either by oneself or another person; examples include homicide, suicide, and assault. If an injury occurs when no harm is intended, it is considered an **unintentional injury.** Motor vehicle crashes, falls, and fires often result in unintentional injuries. The term *accidents* was formerly used to describe unintentional injuries, but it is now considered inaccurate because it suggests events beyond human control. Most unintentional injuries are predictable outcomes of human and environmental factors that can be manipulated, controlled, or prevented.

Engineering, enforcement, and education have long been considered the three primary ways to prevent or reduce injuries. Engineering strategies include the design and production of products—such as auto safety belts with shoulder harnesses—as well as measures to minimize risks from the environment. Enforcement refers to compliance with the laws and regulations that have been passed for the safety and well-being of the population, such as the use by manufacturers of tamper-proof containers for over-the-counter medications. Education about potential risks can positively affect people's attitudes and skills, making it more likely they will act safely in the future. For example, education about driving while under the influence of alcohol can help eliminate or minimize injuries associated with this behavior. Together, engineering, enforcement, and education can help prevent injuries.

Ultimately, however, it is up to each individual to take responsibility for his or her actions and make appropriate choices about health and safety behaviors. Many injuries occur in situations or places where people usually feel safe—in motor vehicles, at work, at home, or during recreational activities (see the box "Facts About Injuries" for more information). Believing that injuries happen only to others, people increase their risks by ignoring safety precautions and taking chances. Many people these days are more aware of health issues and are taking better care of themselves, but this awareness has to extend to safety too. Many of the same sensible attitudes, responsible behaviors, and informed decisions that protect your health can improve your chances of avoiding injuries. This chapter explains how you can protect yourself and those around you from becoming the victims of serious or fatal injuries.

WHY DO INJURIES HAPPEN?

Injuries commonly result from risk-taking behaviors. How people perceive the relative risk associated with a situation influences their behavior. Many people are willing to engage in risk-taking behaviors if they perceive a reward, such as the admiration of their peers. Attempting a stunt on a dare or to show off in front of friends often involves behaviors risky to health and well-being. This type of risk-taking behavior is particularly common among people aged 15–24, the age group that has the highest percentage of deaths from injury in the United States. Attitudes toward risk-taking behavior need to change so that people will behave in ways that reduce the threat of intentional and unintentional injury.

Irresponsible attitudes are not the only cause of injuries. **Multiple causation theory** proposes that injuries are caused not by a single event or factor but by a combination of human and environmental factors working together in a dynamic interaction. Human factors are inner conditions or attitudes that lead to an unsafe state, whether physical, emotional, or psychological (Table 23-1). Environmental factors are external conditions and circumstances—poor visibility due to snow or fog, a defective tool or machine, a child running in the street, a poorly marked curve in the road. A person must be able to assess the risk in a given situation, consider the options or alternatives for action, and then act to minimize the risk.

Human Factors

Many different human factors can contribute to injuries. Physically, people have different levels of skill at different activities, and knowing one's own limits is an important step toward safe behavior. Sometimes injuries occur when

Years of potential life lost   The difference between an individual's life expectancy and his or her age at death.

Intentional injury   An injury that is purposely inflicted, either by oneself or another person.

Unintentional injury   An injury that occurs without anyone intending that harm be done.

Multiple causation theory   The theory that injury incidents are caused by several factors that interact dynamically.

TERMS

TABLE 23-1 Examples of Human and Environmental Factors in Injuries	
Human Factors	**Environmental Factors**
Physical incapability	Imperfect weather conditions
Poor visual acuity	Overcrowded conditions
Stress and fatigue	Defective equipment
False sense of security	Inadequate law enforcement
Distractibility	Nonsupportive social environment
Lack of knowledge	
Poor attitudes	Inadequate legislation
Bad habits	Lack of safety education programs

VITAL STATISTICS
Facts About Injuries

Did you know that . . .

- On the average there are about 10 injury deaths and 980 disabling injuries every hour during the year.
- A motor vehicle death occurs every 12 minutes.
- An injury occurs in the home every 10 seconds.
- Nearly 67 percent of all motor vehicle crashes involve improper driving, with speeding being the most common error.
- Use of safety belts can reduce the number of serious injuries and fatalities by 45 to 55 percent.
- Drinking alcohol is identified as a factor in about 50 percent of all fatal motor vehicle crashes.

Source: National Safety Council. 1992. *Accident Facts* (Chicago: National Safety Council).

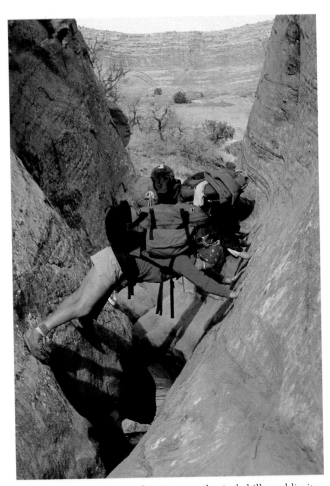

An accurate assessment of one's own physical skills and limitations is an important factor in injury prevention. Many people wouldn't want to try the tricky maneuver these climbers have mastered.

people try to do something beyond their capabilities, such as ride a bicycle on a busy street or swim across a lake. People also have natural physical limits in strength, endurance, sensory abilities, and so on. And as people age, physical abilities decline and vision and hearing often become impaired, sometimes without the individual's realizing the full extent of impairment. Older people may also have heart irregularities, balance problems, slower reflexes, and other conditions that can contribute to a fall or other type of injury.

Physical impairments are also produced by various drugs. Alcohol, a factor in at least half of all auto crashes, affects reason, judgment, and coordination. Marijuana affects perception, reaction time, and coordination. Cocaine initially enhances alertness and then, about 20 minutes later, lets the user down with a resulting loss of attention and judgment. One study revealed that almost one out of every four drivers between the ages of 16 and 45 who were killed in automobile crashes in New York City had taken cocaine. About half of those using cocaine had also used alcohol. Even legal drugs, both over-the-counter and prescription medications, can produce dizziness, drowsiness, distorted perceptions, and other potentially dangerous side effects. And, of course, people can be distracted by naturally occurring physical conditions like hunger, physical exhaustion, or illness.

Psychological factors—including knowledge, awareness, attitudes, beliefs, and emotions—can also play a role in injuries. Knowledge is critical. People need to know what is safe and what is unsafe, and, surprisingly, this is not always obvious. Sometimes people act on the basis of inadequate or inaccurate information. For example, a person who believes that safety belts trap people in

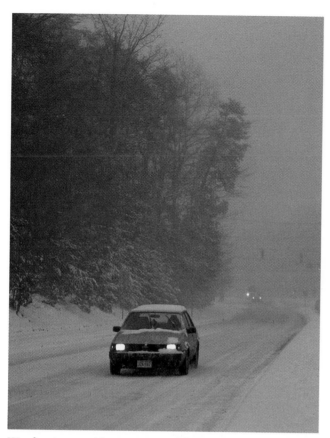

Weather is a crucial environmental factor in motor vehicle crashes. The slippery road surfaces and poor visibility of snowstorms require slower, more defensive driving.

another factor in injuries. An unsafe attitude common among many teenagers and young adults comes from the belief that they are special and that bad things happen only to others. They have a "personal fable" about themselves and believe they are exempt, immune, even immortal. They know that drinking impairs their ability to drive, for example, but they think that only other people have crashes. They know that engaging in horseplay around water can be dangerous, but they think that only others get hurt diving into pools. (Other common beliefs are that they can smoke without damaging their lungs and have unprotected sexual intercourse without getting pregnant.) Attitudes like these, by no means limited to adolescents, can lead to risk taking and ultimately to injuries.

Emotions and general psychological state also have a part in injuries. When you're angry or tired after work, impatient to finish mowing the lawn so you can watch your favorite television program, or stressed out by worry and lack of sleep, you may be easily distracted and unable to perceive events objectively and clearly. You may act on impulse or make a choice you would never make in a calmer frame of mind. Any or all of these "human, all-too-human" factors may be at work when an injury occurs.

Personal Insight Have you ever had a serious injury? If so, how did it change your feelings and behavior about safety?

cars when a crash occurs and who consequently decides not to wear a safety belt is acting on an inaccurate belief. No study has shown a higher incidence of injury for crash victims wearing safety belts than for those who don't wear safety belts, yet this misconception persists. Safety belts actually help a person retain control of the vehicle and reduce the likelihood of being thrown out of the car or against an object inside the car and knocked unconscious.

Awareness is another crucial ingredient in injuries and their prevention. Sometimes the potential for a serious injury exists, but a person is unaware of the danger. For instance, the role bicycle helmets play in preventing injury began receiving widespread publicity only in the last 10 years, and communities are just beginning to consider or pass laws mandating that children wear them. Adults who have ridden without helmets for years and have not been injured simply may not understand their necessity; the longer they ride without them, the more their unsafe behaviors and attitudes are reinforced. A false sense of security causes a rider to take even more risks, until eventually the combination of circumstances conspires to cause a crash and an injury.

Unsafe attitudes, often based on mistaken beliefs, are

Environmental Factors

Environmental factors play important roles in injuries too. They may be natural (weather conditions, an earthquake), societal (stop-and-go traffic, a drunk driver), work-related (defective equipment, unsafe facilities), or home-related (throw rugs, faulty wiring); or they might be caused by other dangerous conditions. Although changes in attitude and behavior are crucial to injury prevention, making the environment safer is also an important aspect of safety.

Sometimes, environmental hazards arise when new technological advances create unforeseen and unknown dangers. As knowledge and awareness increase, safety devices are developed and safety measures are introduced that control the dangers inherent in the technology. In some cases, however, people try to outsmart or bypass safety features, particularly in the workplace. They may fail to wear protective clothing because it impedes their movement or is uncomfortable, or they may figure out faster but more dangerous ways to operate machinery. The issue then arises of whether people have the right to act unsafely or whether they can be forced to be safe. In the workplace, employers have the responsibility to enforce safety regulations. In the public arena, laws requir-

VITAL STATISTICS

TABLE 23-2 Fatal and Disabling Injuries in the United States in 1991

	Deaths	% Change from 1990	Deaths per 100,000 People	Disabling Injuries
Motor vehicle	43,500	−7	17.2	1.6 million
Work	9,900	−7	3.9	1.7 million
Home	20,500	−2	8.1	3.1 million
Public	18,000	−3	7.1	2.3 million
All classes*	88,000	−5	34.9	8.6 million

Source: National Safety Council. 1992. *Accident Facts.* (Chicago: National Safety Council), p. 1.
*Deaths and injuries for the four separate classes total more than the "All classes" figures because of rounding and because some deaths and injuries are included in more than one class.

ing people to wear safety belts or helmets are based on the belief that the government has the right to demand a certain level of safety from the members of a society.

When an Injury Situation Occurs

When unsafe states (the human factors) and unsafe conditions (the environmental factors) interact, an injury is very often the result. At a critical moment, the individual must frequently make a decision that influences the outcome of the situation. If the decision is a good one, the injury may be avoided and the person may learn something from the experience. If the decision is not as good, or if the incident is unavoidable at this point, someone may be injured or killed.

Again, it is important to realize that injuries do not "just happen." With hindsight, we can almost always pinpoint the internal and external factors that combined to cause an injury situation. It may be a left-handed worker using a tool designed for a right-handed person and beginning a new job without adequate supervision. It may be an inexperienced driver maneuvering a tricky mountain road in a rainstorm. Or it may just be a distracted pedestrian thinking about what to buy for dinner and twisting an ankle on the curb. Knowing that hazards exist in everyday life is in itself an important step toward injury prevention.

Personal Insight Think back to the last time you were injured. What would you say caused the injury? Do you have a tendency to blame other people or environmental factors for things that happen to you?

PREVENTING UNINTENTIONAL INJURIES

Injury situations are generally categorized into four general classes, based on where they occur—motor vehicle injuries, home injuries, work injuries, and public injuries. The greatest number of deaths occur in motor vehicle crashes, but the greatest number of disabling injuries occur in the home (Table 23-2). In all of these arenas, the action you take can mean the difference between injury or death and no injury at all.

Motor-Vehicle Injuries

Incidents involving motor vehicles are the most common cause of death for people under 45 years of age. **Motor vehicle injuries** also result in the majority of cases of paralysis due to spinal injuries, and they are the leading cause of severe brain injury in the United States.

Driving Habits Nearly two-thirds of all motor vehicle crashes are caused by bad driving, especially speeding. Most people do not truly understand the safety implications of speeding. As speed increases, the motor vehicle's momentum and force of impact increase; simultaneously, the time allowed for the driver to react *decreases*. A car traveling at 30 miles per hour is traveling at 44 feet per second! If you are the driver, your **reaction time** must be within three-fourths of a second and you must react correctly in order to stop that vehicle within 80 feet. Moreover, these figures assume ideal conditions; wet pavement, decreased visibility, driving under the influence of drugs or when half asleep, and additional passengers in your car increase the stopping distance significantly.

Speed limits are posted to establish (1) the safest *maximum* speed limit (2) for a given area (3) under *ideal* con-

Myth   If I wore a seat belt, I might get trapped in my car if it caught on fire or were submerged in water.

Fact   In reality, only one-half of 1 percent of motor vehicle crashes involve fire or submersion. If that does happen, safety belts will help prevent you from being knocked unconscious, so you will have a better chance of escaping from your car.

Myth   I would be better off if I were thrown clear of the car in a crash.

Fact   The chances of being killed are 25 times greater if you're thrown out of the vehicle. Hitting a tree or the pavement can cause severe injuries, which won't occur if you stay buckled inside the car. Also, people who are thrown out of their cars are sometimes crushed or hit by their own vehicles or those of others.

Myth   I can brace myself in an accident, so I don't need to bother with a safety belt.

Fact   The force of an impact at just 10 mph can be equivalent to catching a 200-pound bag of cement thrown from a 10-foot ladder. At 35 mph the force of impact is even more brutal. There's no way your arms and legs can brace against that kind of force—even if you could react in time.

Source: National Traffic Safety Administration, Washington, D.C.

Myth   A safety belt couldn't possibly hold me in place during a sudden stop or collision. When I yank it by hand, it doesn't work.

Fact   Most safety belts are designed to lock automatically when the car stops suddenly or changes direction quickly. Belts normally expand and contract to allow freedom of movement.

Myth   I'm not going far or driving fast, so I don't need to wear a safety belt.

Fact   It is wise to wear a safety belt no matter where you are going since 75 percent of all crashes occur within 25 miles of home. Most deaths and injuries (80 percent) occur in automobiles traveling less than 40 mph. People have been killed in crashes at speeds of less than 12 mph.

Myth   Pregnant women are not supposed to wear safety belts.

Fact   According to the American Medical Association, both a pregnant woman and her unborn child are much safer with belts than without, provided the lap belt is worn as low as possible on the pelvic area.

Myth   I am a good driver, so I will never be in a crash. I don't need to wear a safety belt.

Fact   Safety belts are the most effective defense against a drunken driver. No matter how well you drive, you can't control what other drivers are going to do.

---

ditions. Such laws are meant to enhance safety, not infringe on your driving rights. If you consistently find that you need to speed to get where you're going on time, allow more time for traveling. By leaving 10 or 15 minutes earlier, you can relieve a lot of the pressure and compulsion to speed. Reduced speed also gives you control of your vehicle and increased time to react to any emergency situation.

Safety Belts and Air Bags   A second factor that contributes to injury and death in motor vehicle crashes is the decision not to wear safety belts. Failure to wear safety belts doubles your chances of being hurt in a crash. Using lap and shoulder safety belts could reduce the number of serious injuries and fatalities by 45 to 55 percent in motor vehicle mishaps. If you use a system that combines a lap and shoulder belt, your chances of survival are three to four times better than those of a person who rides beltless.

Safety belt systems may be passive, active, or a combination of both. Some cars have **automatic safety belts** that move into position when the door is closed or the car is started. These are considered passive systems because

no action is required by the occupants to engage them. In other cars, occupants must actively fasten their lap and shoulder belts. For cars with automatic shoulder belts and manual lap belts (a combination system), it's important that the lap belt be fastened to maximize safety. If the lap belt isn't fastened, the occupant may slide downward and out of the belt in a crash, a phenomenon known as "submarining."

Motor vehicle injuries   Injuries and deaths involving motor vehicles in motion, both on and off the highway or street. Examples of incidents causing motor vehicle injuries include collisions between vehicles and collisions with objects or pedestrians.

Reaction time   The time it takes for a person to react to what he or she has seen or heard. In a driving situation, the time required for the driver to release the accelerator and apply the brake.

Automatic safety belts   Motorized or nonmotorized safety belts that automatically engage when the door is shut or the engine starts; no action is required on the part of the user. Some systems have automatic shoulder and lap belts; others have only automatic shoulder belts.

TERMS

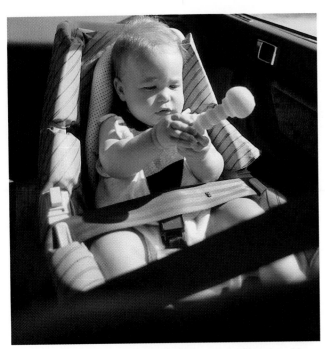

Buckling up is a habit that should begin in childhood and last a lifetime. Special car seats like this one, secured to the seat with the auto safety belt, are required for children 4 years old or younger.

Currently, most states and the District of Columbia have laws requiring the use of safety belts. Even in these states, however, rates of use vary from 85 percent down to 28 percent. Variations in rates reflect state and local factors such as public attitudes, enforcement practices, legal provisions, and public information or educational programs.

Most people who don't use safety belts don't understand their value (see the box "Myths About Safety Belts"). Safety belts work at the time of the "second collision." If a car is traveling at 55 mph and hits another vehicle, first the car must stop and then the occupants must stop because they are also traveling at the same speed. The **second collision** occurs when an occupant hits something inside the car, like the steering column, dashboard, or windshield. Using a safety belt helps prevent that second collision from occurring; the safety belt also spreads the stopping force over the body to reduce the likelihood of injury. (It also keeps occupants from being thrown out of the car.)

Relying solely on **air bags** is an unwise choice—they are intended to provide only supplemental protection. The air bags in most cars are designed to provide protection only in frontal collisions (not side, rear, or rollover crashes) and at speeds of at least 8 to 12 miles per hour or higher in some models (Figure 23-1). Most manufacturers do not provide air bags for the back seat, and air bags are not recommended for use in conjunction with child restraint systems. Because air bags deflate immediately af-

ter detonation, they are also less effective in multiple collisions. Air bags are most effective when used in combination with safety belts, reducing the risk of fatal or serious injury by 55 to 60 percent.

Developing the habit of buckling up puts you one step ahead. Taking three seconds for that one click can mean the difference, but you must take responsibility for that decision. Safety belts save lives—it's as simple as that.

Alcohol and Other Drugs Alcohol is identified as a factor in about half of all fatal motor vehicle crashes, and crashes involving alcohol are usually much more severe than other crashes. About two out of every five Americans will be involved in an alcohol-related crash at some time in their lives. Alcohol-impaired driving, defined by blood alcohol concentration (BAC), is illegal in all states. The legal limit of BAC in most states in 0.08 or 0.10 percent, but people are impaired at much lower BACs.

People who have a few drinks at a party may feel relaxed and less inhibited initially, but alcohol depresses the central nervous system. It affects reason and judgment first and then motor skills. Unfortunately, most people do not recognize that they are impaired. The impaired person who continues to drive is not in control and is taking a major risk. The same is true of the other psychoactive drugs. (Refer to Chapters 10 and 11 for full discussions of the effect of all these substances on users.)

Environmental Factors External influences such as weather and road type and condition also affect motor vehicle crashes. When weather deteriorates, you must drive more defensively. You need to increase the distance at which you follow another car in traffic and reduce speed to compensate for hazards. Of course, you also need to have your car in good working order. People typically take care of the obvious needs like tires, gas, and oil, but it's easy to forget the simple things like replacing windshield wipers, at least until it starts to rain and you find out they don't work. Regular inspection and maintenance checks make sense if you expect your vehicle to perform well.

Road type and location also influence the likelihood of injury or fatality in a crash. Many people travel on rural highways because they think they can drive at faster speeds without getting caught. Consequently, the fatality rates on rural highways are much higher. Contrary to common belief, interstate highways are much safer for a number of reasons; for example, visibility is increased, all travel is in one direction, and fewer incidents require driving adjustments. If you have a choice, it makes more sense to travel on the interstate. Moreover, about 75 percent of all motor vehicle crashes occur within 25 miles of home, where the driver is probably more familiar with the driving terrain and on roadways with speed limits of less than 40 miles per hour. Often the driver mistakenly believes that safety measures are not warranted for a quick

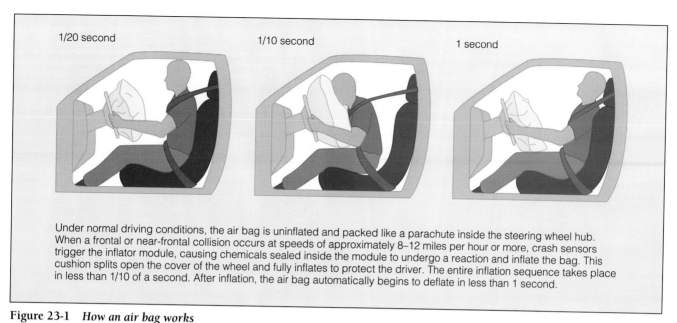

Under normal driving conditions, the air bag is uninflated and packed like a parachute inside the steering wheel hub. When a frontal or near-frontal collision occurs at speeds of approximately 8–12 miles per hour or more, crash sensors trigger the inflator module, causing chemicals sealed inside the module to undergo a reaction and inflate the bag. This cushion splits open the cover of the wheel and fully inflates to protect the driver. The entire inflation sequence takes place in less than 1/10 of a second. After inflation, the air bag automatically begins to deflate in less than 1 second.

Figure 23-1 *How an air bag works*

Source: U.S. Department of Transportation, National Highway Traffic Safety Administration, *Consumer Information*, November 1989.

trip to the store or for a short ride of a few blocks to a friend's house. The facts prove otherwise. To assess your driving skills and knowledge, take the quiz in the box "Do You Drive Like a Pro?"

Motorcycles and Mopeds   Motorcycles and mopeds are two types of motorized vehicles that are becoming more common on college campuses. Motorcycles are economical on gas, easy to park, and a fairly inexpensive investment. Unfortunately, motorcycles are also dangerous: About one out of every ten traffic fatalities among people aged 15 to 34 involves someone riding a motorcycle. Most motorcycle mishaps occur because the other driver did not see the motorcyclist. Another factor is lack of skill on the part of the motorcyclist, especially when it is necessary to take evasive action to avoid a collision. Skidding from either overbraking or improper braking is the most common problem associated with loss of control of the motorcycle. Alcohol is a prominent factor in more than half of all motorcycle mishaps.

Injuries from motorcycle collisions are generally more severe than those from automobile mishaps because motorcycles provide little, if any, protection. Head injuries are the major cause of death in motorcycle crashes, so use of a helmet is critical for rider safety. A helmet significantly reduces the risk of head injury from violent impact with other objects. Helmets should conform to acceptable safety standards established by the U.S. Department of Transportation, the American National Standards Institute, or the Snell Memorial Foundation. Helmets with full facial coverage provide the most protection. Helmet use is required by law in some states. Eye protection is also critical to the safety of a motorcyclist. Goggles, face shields,

or windshields protect the motorcyclist from wind, rocks, bugs, and other objects; regular eyeglasses do not provide adequate protection.

Motorcyclists should also do whatever they can to make themselves more conspicuous to others; such preventive measures include operating their headlight during both day and night, wearing light-colored clothing, and correctly positioning themselves in traffic. Most importantly, a motorcyclist should never assume that he or she has been seen by other drivers and should always drive defensively.

Moped operators should follow all of the advice for motorcyclists, but they should also remember that mopeds are not motorcycles. They usually have a maximum speed of 30–35 mph and have less power for maneuverability, especially in an emergency situation. Although not very fast in comparison to other vehicles, mopeds are still fast enough to result in injury if a mishap should occur. Moped users should use caution and take the time to develop the skills needed to handle the moped in traffic.

Along with safe cars, safety belts, air bags, and sobriety, driving skills are an important element in motor vehicle safety. Learn to drive defensively, avoiding dangerous situations and reacting intelligently in a crisis. To find out how well you drive already, try this defensive-driving quiz. (Some questions have more than one correct answer.)

1. The safest way to brake is:
   a. as fast as possible
   b. as far in advance as possible

2. In moderate town traffic, with another car at a safe distance in front of you, you're being tailgated. What do you do?
   a. Tap the brakes and start to slow down—gradually, keeping an eye on the rearview mirror.
   b. Increase your speed to the allowable limit.
   c. Try to pass the car in front of you.
   d. Pull over to the right.

3. You're heading toward a green light at an intersection. A woman (not in the crosswalk and walking against the light) steps off the curb and starts across without looking. Your first move is to:
   a. sound the horn loudly and maintain your speed
   b. change lanes to avoid her
   c. begin braking, anticipating a full stop if necessary, and sound the horn

4. Preparing to change lanes on a multilane highway, which of the following should you do?
   a. Check your rearview mirror.
   b. Check your side mirror.
   c. Take your eyes off the road momentarily and glance at the lane you're planning to move into.
   d. Turn on your directional signal.
   e. Be aware of what traffic in front of you is doing.

5. You've swerved to the right to avoid a collision on a two-way highway, and your right wheels drop off the pavement and are riding on the shoulder. To get back on the road you:
   a. accelerate, cutting the wheel to the left
   b. don't brake, but take your foot off the accelerator. Hold the wheel steady. When the car slows, check the traffic and steer back onto the pavement.
   c. brake sharply and try to pull off the road altogether. When you've got the car under control, pull onto the road again.

6. On a two-way highway, in what's clearly marked as a no-pass zone with limited visibility, a car pulls out to pass you. Your best move is to:
   a. speed up, hoping the car will move back behind you
   b. ignore the car—it's not your problem
   c. reduce your speed so the car can get around you faster

7. The most important factor in defensive driving is:
   a. quick reflexes
   b. anticipating trouble
   c. skill at vehicle handling
   d. strict observation of the law

8. You're most likely to go into a skid:
   a. in a steady downpour
   b. in the first few minutes of a light rain

9. Which of the following road conditions up ahead should tell you to reduce your speed?
   a. a deep pothole
   b. leaves on the pavement
   c. any bridge, when the temperature is just above freezing

10. Your rear wheel drive car is skidding (see diagram). What's the safest reaction?

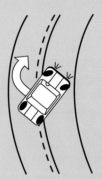

   a. Turn the wheel to the right.
   b. Turn the wheel to the left.
   c. Brake as hard as possible and avoid turning the wheel until you've stopped the car.

11. In two-way highway traffic, an oncoming car suddenly pulls into your lane. What action do you take?
   a. Brake hard and sound your horn.
   b. Move quickly into the left lane.
   c. Blow your horn, and head to the shoulder.

12. The best position for your hands on the steering wheel is:
   a. at 10 and 2 o'clock position
   b. at 8 and 4 o'clock
   c. wherever you're most comfortable
   d. at 9 and 3 o'clock

13. True or false: Underinflated tires are safer, particularly in hot weather.

14. You realize you're heading into a curve too fast. Therefore you should:
   a. brake sharply
   b. brake gradually
   c. avoid braking but take your foot off the accelerator

Answers

1. **(b)** A basic principle of defensive driving is never to get into a situation that calls for slamming on the brakes. This can throw you into a skid and injure you and your passengers. Good braking technique: pump the brakes, reapplying as you come to a full stop. However, according to Professor Donald Smith, Highway Traffic Safety Program, Michigan State University, if you are forced to brake fast and have disc brakes, "threshold" braking is the best technique: Push the brake just short of locking and hold it there.

2. **(a)** and **(d)**, depending on circumstances. If the tailgater is daydreaming, tapping your brakes (and activating the brake lights) should wake him or her up. If the driver is being aggressive, you've politely given a signal to let up. If the tailgating doesn't stop, pull over as soon as you can and let the other car pass.

3. **(c)** Always yield the right of way to pedestrians, even when they're in the wrong. Let them know you're there. A diversionary swerve could put you in the path of an oncoming car. Also, pedestrians might dart into your path.

4. **(all)** All steps are essential, but some people forget (c). You always have a blind spot (about a car length behind you on either side) and may not be able to see an overtaking vehicle in either mirror. Always glance over your shoulder before making your move. The signal light (turned on several seconds in advance) will help protect you as well.

5. **(b)** Braking hard or jerking the wheel can cause you to skid into oncoming traffic. Don't brake but do reduce your speed and stay on a steady course. Then, after checking traffic, make a sharp quarter turn to the left to put yourself back on the road, and then straighten out.

6. **(c)** Passing is always a cooperative venture. If this reckless driver has a head-on collision, you might be hurt, too.

7. **(b)** Obeying the law and vehicle-handling skills are all important. But anticipating trouble up ahead, and acting to prevent it, can make the speed of your reflexes far less important and thus may prevent many collisions.

8. **(b)** A little water plus the oil and dirt on the road form a slick film. A heavy rain will wash it clean. Be extra careful during the first half hour of a rainfall.

9. **(all)** The pothole may only jar you, but it could damage your car or even cause you to lose control. Leaves can send you into a skid. And even though there's no ice on the road, a bridge is about 6° F colder than a highway and may be hazardous when the road is not.

10. **(b)** Turn the wheel straight down your lane. That is, if your rear wheels are skidding left, as in the diagram, turn with the skid—that is, to the left. Don't brake; it increases skidding.

11. **(c)** Don't move left, which could put you in someone else's pathway. Always move right when heading off the road.

12. **(d)** And some expert drivers recommend that you hook your thumbs lightly over the horizontal spokes. This gives you a feel for the front tires and is a good way to get a quick grip if you strike a pothole.

13. **False.** An underinflated tire is more likely to skid, whether in hot weather or on wet or icy pavement. Because underinflation allows a tire to "flap" slightly and thus to create more heat, it's also likelier to blow out. Even for desert driving, keep tires at the recommended maximum air pressure, and check them weekly. The number should be printed on the side of the tires; or check the instruction manual if the car still has its original tires.

14. **(b)** Take your foot off the accelerator, and brake before you get into the curve, but gradually release brakes as you get into it. Once you're rounding the curve, accelerate. This will help you steer safely around it and onto the straightaway.

Adapted from "Driving Like the Pros." *University of California at Berkeley Wellness Letter,* October 1989.

Motor-Vehicle-Related Injuries

Injuries incurred by pedestrians and bicyclists are considered motor-vehicle-related injuries because motor vehicles are the primary cause of these injuries and deaths. Since most of us are pedestrians at some point during the day, and since bicycling is gaining in popularity, this is a growing area of concern.

Pedestrian Safety   Pedestrians are no match for the size, weight, and speed of motor vehicles. About one-fifth of all motor vehicle deaths each year involve pedestrians, and more than 100,000 pedestrians are injured each year. Males account for about 70 percent of the pedestrian fatalities in the United States. The highest rates of death and injury are for the very young and the elderly; inability to adequately judge vehicle distances and movements is often cited as a problem for these age groups. Most pedestrian injuries occur in urban settings, primarily after dark, and between intersections, where people may walk or dart into traffic. Alcohol plays a significant role in about half of all adult pedestrian fatalities, which have doubled in the past few years.

In most pedestrian injuries and deaths, poor decision making is the crucial factor, not the traffic situation itself. What can you do as a pedestrian to keep yourself safe? One key factor is visibility. You should follow traffic laws and do everything possible to make yourself visible. If you are walking along a roadway, always face the traffic; this helps make you more visible and allows you to react more quickly to any potential problems. Wearing light-colored and reflective clothing is recommended, particularly at night. Don't wear headphones for a radio or tape player—these may interfere with your ability to hear sounds or sirens from motor vehicles. This same advice also holds true for joggers. In addition, don't hitchhike—doing so may place you in a potentially dangerous situation.

Safe Cycling   Bicycling is now popular with over 125 million people, ranging from preschoolers to the elderly, who ride for transportation, recreation, and fitness. As more riders have entered the traffic flow, more unintentional deaths and injuries have occurred. Research indicates that these incidents are primarily the result of not knowing or misunderstanding the rules of the road, failure to follow laws and ordinances, and/or inexperience and lack of skill in traffic conditions. Over 90 percent of all bicycling deaths result from collision with motor vehicles; most injuries are due to falls. The highest bicycle death rates occur for people under 13 years of age. Alcohol plays a significant role in bicycle deaths and injuries for older groups.

A bicyclist can improve the safety situation by first of all realizing that bicycles are legally considered vehicles that must obey all local and state ordinances. Cyclists should always ride with the flow of traffic (not against it), know and use proper hand signals, ride defensively (never assume drivers see them), properly maintain their bike, and use the bicycle paths whenever available. Many injuries and deaths occur as a result of wrong-way riding, failure to look around and signal before turning, and failure to stop at a traffic light or stop sign. Wearing light-colored or reflective clothing can help increase visibility; pant clips or bands can prevent the potentially dangerous tangling of pants in the bicycle chain. All cyclists should also wear safety equipment, including helmets, eye protection, gloves, and proper footwear. Helmet use is a critical factor in reducing bicycle injuries and deaths, many of which result from head injuries (see the box "Bicycle Helmets" for more information).

Home Injuries

A person's place of residence, whether it be a house, an apartment, a trailer, or a dormitory, is considered home. Many people spend a majority of their time at home and feel that they are safe and secure there. However, home can be a dangerous environment. The most common fatal **home injuries** are falls, fires, poisoning, suffocation or asphyxiation, and unintentional firearm injuries. Everyone is at risk for home injuries, but males and the very young and very old are most likely to be injured (see the box "Special Precautions for the Young and Old"). Ongoing research indicates that alcohol may be a major contributing factor in many residential injuries.

Falls   Falls are second only to motor vehicle injuries in terms of causing deaths. About 85 percent of fatal falls involve people 45 years of age and older, but falls are the fifth leading cause of unintentional death for all people under 25. Most falls occur as a result of common activities in the home, with nearly two-thirds of the deaths occurring from falls at floor level rather than at a height. In most cases, a person falls because of difficulty in adjusting to different degrees of traction rather than because of the slipperiness of the surface. A rug, a bathtub, or some characteristic of the floor itself is often a factor in falls in the home. If you use rugs, large ones are better, but small rugs can be made safer with cork or rubber backing that helps reduce slippage. Avoid waxed floors, which can be dangerously slippery, and pick up objects from the floor. Children's toys often cause people to trip. You can prevent falls in the bathroom by using nonslip applications on the bottom of the tub or shower and by installing handrails on the walls. Outside the house, you should clear danger-

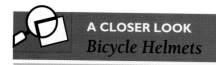
Every year, nearly 50,000 bicyclists suffer serious head injuries, and three out of four cyclists killed in crashes die as a result of head injuries. The brain is extremely sensitive to any impact, even bicycling at a very low speed. On a concrete surface, a fall from a distance of less than 1 foot can cause a concussion. A helmet can reduce your risk of serious head and brain injury by almost 90 percent should you be involved in a collision or fall. In addition to preventing injuries, helmets also provide other advantages:

- *Visibility.* You are easier to see with a white or yellow helmet on, especially at dusk, in rain or fog, or after dark. Putting reflective trim tape on the helmet makes you even more visible.

- *Climate protection.* A helmet will help keep your head dry in the rain or snow so that if you do have to cycle in bad weather, it will be more enjoyable.

- *Emergency data.* Put your name, address, and phone number and the name and number of an emergency contact on a piece of tape inside the brim of your helmet. If you have a medical emergency condition, include that information as well. Also, tape a quarter inside for an emergency phone call.

Helmets are designed to cushion a blow to your head and must pass special safety tests to be certified. A good helmet will have a hard outer shell to spread the force of a blow over a larger area and to shield against any sharp objects. A helmet should also have a crushable liner (usually polystyrene foam) to absorb the shock of a collision and a strong strap and buckle to keep the helmet securely on your head (see figure).

Every good bicycle shop carries a supply of helmets for adults and children. Ask someone who works at the shop to help you select a helmet that is right for you. It should be a bright color for visibility but should not interfere with your hearing or vision. Your helmet should have a label from either the Snell Memorial Foundation or American National Standards Institute (ANSI), certifying that it is safe for cyclists.

Adapted from Governor's Bicycle Task Force. 1990. "Get Into the Helmet Habit." Dover, Del.

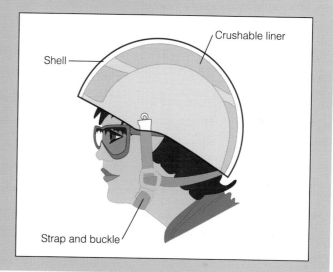

ous surfaces created by ice, snow, fallen leaves, or rough ground.

Ladders and stairs are also common sources of injuries in the home. People tend to get hurt using the stairs when the lighting is poor, a firm handrail for support is missing, or inappropriate footwear is worn. All of these potential problems are correctable. Height also becomes a concern when people stand on chairs or unstable objects rather than using stepladders or stepstools. When you use a stepladder, make sure the spreader brace is in the locked position and never stand higher than the third step from the top. If you use a straight ladder the "4 to 1" rule (setting the ladder base out one foot for every four feet of height) is also a safe procedure to follow. Use both hands when climbing a ladder and don't reach too far to either side.

Fire   Each year approximately 80 percent of fire deaths and 65 percent of fire injuries occur in the home. Most

people do not really appreciate or understand the dangers associated with fires. To burn, a fire requires (1) a source of ignition, (2) fuel, and (3) oxygen. If any one component can be eliminated, fire can be prevented.

Fire ignition of furniture, combustible liquid or gas, and bedding accounts for 60 percent of home fires. Most fires begin in the kitchen, living room, or bedroom. Many are caused by careless actions such as smoking in bed or leaving a cigarette burning in an ashtray. Misuse of electrical outlets and extension cords is another cause. When an outlet is overloaded, heat builds up in the wiring; this can eventually cause it to ignite. Extension cords can be-

Home injuries   Injuries and deaths that occur in the home and on home premises to occupants, guests, domestic servants, and trespassers. Examples of home injury incidents include falls, burns, poisonings, suffocations, unintentional shootings, drownings, and electric shocks.

TERMS

Anyone can be injured, but the very young and the very old are at special risk. Babies and children—especially inquisitive toddlers—easily get in trouble when the environment hasn't been adapted to their needs and limitations. About 4,000 children under 4 years of age die from injuries each year in the United States, the victims of falls, burns, chokings, poisonings, suffocation, and a variety of other dangers. Follow these guidelines to protect children in your home:

- Never leave a baby unattended on a bed or table or in a crib with the side down.

- Place gates at the tops and bottoms of stairs and in doorways to areas that are off limits to children. Place barriers around stoves, floor grates, and radiators. Install window guards (not just screens) to prevent children from falling out of windows.

- Keep all medicines, poisons, and household chemicals in locked cabinets or places inaccessible to children. Buy medications in the smallest available quantity, and keep purses out of children's reach.

- When driving, strap infants and toddlers into government-tested car seats. Never hold a child in your lap while a car is moving.

- Keep small objects out of reach of children under age 3, and don't give them raw carrots, hot dogs, nuts, popcorn, or hard candy. Balloons pose a serious choking hazard for young children.

- Inspect toys carefully for sharp edges, brittle materials, or small parts that could come loose and be put in the mouth.

- Inspect hand-me-down furniture to make sure it's free of lead-based paint and other hazards, such as spaces where a child's head could become stuck.

- Set your hot water heater no higher than 120° F and keep children out of the kitchen where they might be burned by spills.

- Keep electrical appliances away from a filled tub or sink. Use plastic covers over electrical outlets.

- Put pans on rear burners, and turn pot handles toward the back of the stove. Keep hot foods away from the edge of tables and counters, and not on a tablecloth that a small child can pull.

- Keep the number of the poison control center near your telephone, and keep a bottle of ipecac syrup on hand to induce vomiting if so instructed by the poison center or a physician.

At the opposite end of the spectrum, the elderly are also vulnerable to injuries, especially falls. Every year, about a quarter of all people over age 70 take a fall. Half of those hospitalized for a fall never regain their former level of independence.

Elderly people are at risk for falls for a variety of reasons. Many have become unsteady on their feet or have impaired vision, hearing, memory, mental status, or mobility. Some suffer from problems that affect balance. In some cases, medications cause problems, such as incoordination, weakness, light-headedness, or dizziness. Often, falls occur from a combination of infirmity and environmental hazards—poor vision and dim lighting, weak legs and ill-fitting shoes, uncertain balance and a loose rug.

Up to half of all falls can be prevented with some practical changes in the home environment. The following guidelines can help you make your home a safer place:

- Be sure stairs are well-lighted and have secure bannisters or handrails. Bright tape applied to the first and last steps can help a person with poor vision.

- Remove raised doorway thresholds or cover them with carpet. Fasten area rugs to the floor with tape or tacks, and don't use throw rugs. Rearrange furniture to keep electrical cords and furniture out of walking paths. Keep objects off the floor.

- Put a light switch by the door of every room (and by the bed in bedrooms) so that no one has to walk across a room to turn on a light. Plug night lights into electrical outlets in bedrooms, halls, and bathrooms.

- Install grab handles and nonskid mats inside and just outside the shower and tub and near the toilet. Shower chairs and bath benches minimize the risk of falling.

- Don't use difficult-to-reach shelves. Use nonskid floor wax, and wipe up floor spills immediately.

The best protection against a fall is to be in good overall health and aware of any potentially risky physical conditions. Elderly people should have their vision and hearing checked regularly, exercise, avoid alcohol, and discuss with their physician whether any medications they are taking may affect balance and coordination. Getting up slowly can help prevent dizziness from a drop in blood pressure. If a person sometimes feels dizzy, use of a cane or walker can help maintain balance; sturdy, low-heeled shoes with wide, non-slip soles are also recommended.

Adapted from J. Schickedanz, D. Schickedanz, K. Hansen, and P. Forsyth. 1993. *Understanding Children* (Mountain View, Calif.: Mayfield); "How to Prevent Falls." *Mayo Clinic Health Letter,* February 1993; and "30 Ways to Keep Children Safe." *University of California at Berkeley Wellness Letter,* April 1993.

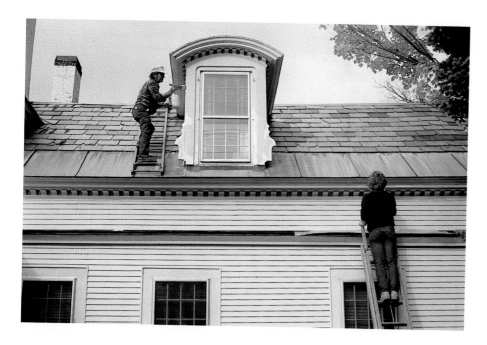

Home maintenance offers endless opportunities for injuries. These painters can reduce their risk of injury by positioning their ladders safely, moving in a cautious manner, and avoiding distractions.

come worn if they are placed under rugs, through doorways, or in areas where people usually walk. A worn or frayed extension cord is hazardous and should be replaced.

Heating equipment is a leading cause of home fires. Wire screens should be placed over wood stoves and fireplaces to prevent the escape of hot coals or sparks. Coals and ashes must be removed carefully and stored in airtight metal containers, not paper bags or plastic sacks. Flues and chimneys need annual cleaning. Portable kerosene heaters should be used only in areas with good ventilation; don't refuel a kerosene unit while it is in use. If you use portable heaters, keep them at least three feet away from curtains, bedding, towels, or anything else that might catch fire, and never leave them on when you're out of the room or sleeping. Furnaces also need preventive maintenance to ensure proper functioning.

Most people are inadequately prepared to handle fire-related situations. Such preparation includes planning escape routes, installing smoke-detection devices, and practicing using fire-extinguishing devices. Every resident should have an escape route planned; because smoke and flames can block a path of escape, plan two routes out of each room. Escape ladders or stairways may be needed for multistory buildings. As a group, residents should pick a place outside the home for everyone to meet. For practice, stage a home fire drill; do it at night, since that's when most deadly fires occur.

Smoke detectors should be installed on every level of your home. Your risk of dying in a fire is almost twice as high if you do not use them. (Heat detectors, which detect high or quickly rising temperatures, are more suited to industrial situations.) The batteries in smoke detectors should be tested once a month and replaced at least once a year. Clean the detectors monthly to get rid of dust and cobwebs. Be sure that all residents are familiar with the sound of the smoke detector's alarm.

When a fire occurs, the most important point to remember is to get out as quickly and safely as possible and go to the designated meeting place. Don't stop for a favorite keepsake or pet, and never hide in a closet or under a bed. Once outside, count heads to see if everyone is out and go to a nearby phone to call for help. If you think someone is still inside the burning building, tell the firefighters; don't go back in.

If you're trapped in a room, feel the door. If it is hot or if smoke is pouring in, don't open it; use your alternate escape route. Smoke is the largest single cause of death and injury in fires, so you should also know how to avoid smoke inhalation. The simplest method is to crawl along the floor away from the heat and smoke and cover your mouth, ideally with a wet cloth; taking short breaths is also helpful. If you can't get out of a room, go to the window and shout or wave for help. Get attention by hanging a sheet or towel out the window or waving a white cloth. Stay where you can be seen by firefighters. If your clothes catch fire, *do not run*. Drop to the ground, cover your face, and roll back and forth to smother the flames.

Fire extinguishers can be used to put out small fires, but you risk being trapped if you try for too long to fight a fire that is too large. Fires are classified into four categories—Class A (wood, cloth, and paper), Class B (flammable liquids such as greases, gasoline, and lubricating oils), Class C (electrical equipment), and Class D (combustible metals). Fire extinguishers labeled "ABC" are effective against the three kinds of fire you're likely to encounter in your home and are available in many stores. Standard procedures for using most fire extinguishers include breaking the seal and pulling the pin on the handle, squeezing the handle to make sure it works, aiming the

TABLE 23-3 Chemical Hazards in the Home

Product	Possible Hazards	Disposal Suggestions	Precautions and Substitutes
Aerosols	When sprayed, contents are broken into particles small enough to be inhaled. Cans may explode or burn.	Put *only* empty cans in trash. Do not burn. Do not place in trash compactor.	Store in cool place. Propellant may be flammable. Instead: use nonaerosol products.
Batteries: mercury button type	Swallowing one may be fatal if it leaks. *Toxicity 5**	Throw in trash.	No substitutes.
Bleach: chlorine	Fumes irritate eyes. Corrosive to eyes and skin. Poisonous if swallowed. *Toxicity 3**	Use up according to label instructions	*Never mix with ammonia!* Instead: use nonchlorine bleach or other laundry additive, sunlight, lemon juice.
Detergent cleaners	All are corrosive to some degree. Eye irritant. Toxicity varies. *Toxicity 2–4**	Use up according to label instructions or give away. May be diluted and washed down sink.	Instead: use the mildest product suitable for your needs. Liquid dishwashing detergent is mildest, laundry detergent is moderate, automatic dishwasher detergent is harshest.
Disinfectants	Eye and skin irritant. Fumes irritating. Poisonous if swallowed. *Toxicity 3–4**	Use up according to label instructions or dilute and pour down drain.	Some may contain bleach, others ammonia—*Do not mix!* Instead: use detergent cleaners whenever possible.
Drain cleaners	Very corrosive. May be fatal if swallowed. Contact with eyes can cause blindness.	Use up according to label instructions.	Prevention best; keep sink strainers in good condition. Instead: use plunger, plumber's snake, vinegar and baking soda followed by boiling water.
Flea powders, sprays, and shampoos	Moderately to very poisonous. *Toxicity 2–4**	Use up or save for hazardous waste collection day.	*Do not use dog products on cats.* Vacuum house regularly and thoroughly. Launder pet bedding frequently.
Insect and pest sprays	All are poisonous, some extremely so. May cause damage to kidneys, liver, or central nervous system. Toxicity varies from product to product.	Use very carefully and according to label instructions. Save for hazardous waste collection day.	Instead: do not attract insects; keep all food securely covered, practice good sanitation in kitchen and bathrooms, remove trash every night.
Medicines: unneeded or expired	Frequently cause child poisonings.	Take to a pharmacy.	Check contents of medicine chest regularly. Old medications may lose their effectiveness but not necessarily their toxicity.

discharge at the base of the flames, and then using a sweeping motion to cover the area that is burning. Remember always to leave yourself an escape route and never turn your back on a fire, even when you think it has been completely extinguished.

Poisoning The home is the site for about 80 percent of the deaths by poisonous solids and liquids and over 60 percent of those from poisonous gases and vapors. A majority of the cases involve children under age 5, although the 15–24 and 25–44 age groups have shown increased death rates in recent years. More than 2 million poisonings occur every year, with about 90 percent due to unintentional exposures.

Poisons come in many forms, some of which aren't typically thought of as poisons. For example, medications

TABLE 23-3 *Chemical Hazards in the Home (continued)*

Product	Possible Hazards	Disposal Suggestions	Precautions and Substitutes
Metal polishes	May be flammable. Mildly to very poisonous. *Toxicity 2–4**	Use up according to label instructions or give away.	Use only in well-ventilated area. Instead: substitute vinegar and salt or use baking soda on damp sponge.
Mothballs	Some are flammable. Eye and skin irritant, poisonous, may cause anemia in some individuals.	Use up according to label instructions or give away.	Do not use in living areas. Air out clothing and other items before use. Clean items before storage. Instead: use cedar shavings or aromatic herbs.
Oven cleaner	Corrosive. Very harmful if swallowed. Irritating vapors. Can cause eye damage. *Toxicity 2–4**	Use up according to label instructions or give away. Save for hazardous waste collection day.	Do not use aerosols, which can explode and are difficult to control. Instead: use paste. Or heat oven to 200 degrees, turn off, leave small dish of ammonia in oven overnight, then wipe oven with damp cloth and baking soda. Do not put baking soda on heating elements.
Toilet bowl cleaner	Corrosive. May be fatal if swallowed. *Toxicity 3–4**	Use up according to label instructions or wash down the sink or toilet with lots of water.	Ventilate room. Instead: use ordinary cleanser or detergent and baking soda.
Window cleaner	Vapor may be irritating. Slightly poisonous. *Toxicity 2**	Use up according to label instructions or give away.	Ventilate room. Instead: spray on vinegar, then wipe dry with newspaper.
Wood cleaners, polishes, and waxes	Fumes irritating to eyes. Product harmful if swallowed. Eye and skin irritant. Petroleum types are flammable.	Use up according to label instructions or save for hazardous waste collection day.	Do not use aerosols. Use only in well-ventilated areas. Instead: use lemon oil or beeswax.

*General Toxicity Ratings

Number rating	1	2	3	4	5	6
Toxicity rating	Almost nontoxic	Slightly toxic	Moderately toxic	Very toxic	Extremely toxic	Super toxic
Lethal dose for 150 lb. adult	More than 1 quart	1 pint to 1 quart	1 ounce to 1 pint	1 teaspoon to 1 ounce	7 drops to 1 teaspoon	Less than 7 drops

Source: National Safety Council

are safe when used as prescribed, but overdoses and incorrectly combining medications with another substance may result in poisoning. Your home may contain a multitude of potentially poisonous substances (Table 23-3). Solid and liquid forms include medications (prescription and over-the-counter drugs, vitamins and minerals), cleaning agents, petroleum-based products (kerosene, gasoline, antifreeze), insecticides and herbicides, and other household items (cosmetics, nail polish and remover, room deodorizers). Many plants have toxic parts that cause serious injury or death if eaten. Common plants that are potentially fatal if consumed include azalea, daffodil bulbs, hyacinth bulbs, mistletoe berries, oleander, poinsettia, rhododendron, wild mushrooms, and the seeds of apple, larkspur, morning glory, and wisteria; the green parts of potato, rhubarb, and tomato plants are

The single most important step you can take to prevent a poisoning injury or death is to go to the telephone book right now, look up the Poison Control Center located in your area, and write the number down where you will be able to find it in an emergency. Poison Control Centers exist in many areas of the United States to provide immediate and authoritative advice on how to handle poisonings. They are staffed by poisoning specialists who take calls 24 hours a day, 7 days a week. If you cannot locate a Poison Control Center, write down the number of the nearest hospital emergency room, physician, or paramedic service.

If you are faced with a case of poisoning, take the following emergency steps and then call the poison center or, preferably, have someone else call the poison center while you stay with the victim.

Swallowed poison

1. Do *not* follow emergency instructions on labels of containers; they may be old or incorrect.
2. Give water immediately, EXCEPT in these important cases: The person is unconscious, having convulsions, or cannot swallow; you don't know what the person swallowed; the person swallowed a strong acid or alkali (toilet bowl cleaner, rust remover, chlorine bleach, dishwasher detergent, etc.) or a petroleum product (kerosene, gasoline, furniture polish, lighter fluid, paint thinner, etc.)

Inhaled poison

1. Get the person to fresh air immediately.
2. Open doors and windows.

Poison on the skin

1. Remove contaminated clothing and flood skin with water for 10 minutes.
2. Wash skin gently with soap and water and rinse.

Poison in the eye

1. Flood the eye with lukewarm water poured from a glass held 2 or 3 inches from the eye. Continue for 15 minutes.
2. Have the person blink as much as possible while flooding the eye. Do not force the eyelid open.

When you contact the poison control center, be prepared to provide the following information: (1) the age and weight of the victim; (2) the name of the product involved; (3) how much was taken; and (4) when it was taken. The poison specialist may recommend that you induce vomiting. Keep a bottle of syrup of ipecac on hand in your home for this purpose. The poison center will tell you what dose to give. *Do not induce vomiting unless instructed to do so;* some products do more damage to the throat, esophagus, or lungs if they are vomited. If the person vomits, keep his or her head lower than the rest of the body so that choking on the vomit doesn't create another emergency.

If the victim is unconscious, maintain an open airway by tipping the head back or turning the person on his or her side. If the victim is having convulsions, loosen tight clothing but do not attempt to restrain him or her. In either of these cases, seek medical attention immediately by calling emergency rescue personnel for transportation to the hospital. Take the poison container with you to the hospital for inspection.

When someone has been poisoned, an immediate response can make the difference between life and death. Be sure that you know what to do, whom to call, and where to go before you find yourself in an emergency situation. More important, poison-proof your home and educate the members of your household, including small children, so that poisonings don't occur in the first place.

Adapted from *Emergency Action for Poisoning.* Central-Coast Counties Regional Poison Control Center, 751 S. Bascom Ave., San Jose, CA 95128.

---

also poisonous. The most common type of poisoning by gases is due to carbon monoxide poisoning, such as that emitted by motor vehicle exhaust. Other types commonly result from improper ventilation and incomplete combustion involving furnaces, kerosene heaters, and cooking appliances.

The introduction of childproof caps on many bottled products and medications has helped reduce the number of poisonings. Other strategies include keeping all medicines and dangerous household substances out of reach of children, leaving products in their original containers so the contents are known, and reading labels on all substances carefully before using them. To prevent poisoning by gases, never operate a vehicle in an enclosed space,

have your furnace inspected yearly, and use caution with any substance that produces potentially toxic fumes. Before purchasing plants, check to see which parts, if any, are toxic. If a poisoning occurs, it's important that you act quickly (see the box "What to Do in Case of Poisoning").

Suffocation and Choking Suffocation accounts for nearly 4,000 deaths annually in the United States. Young children, especially those under the age of 5, account for nearly half of these deaths. Children can suffocate if they put small items in their mouths, get tangled in their crib bedding, or get trapped in airtight appliances like old refrigerators or freezers. Elderly people have the highest death rate for suffocation; many die as a result of choking.

But, of course, anyone can choke on something if they fail to chew properly, eat hurriedly, or try to talk and eat at the same time.

Many choking victims can be saved with the **Heimlich maneuver** (Figure 23-2). Until 1986, the Red Cross recommended blows to the upper back for choking, but since then it has adopted the Heimlich maneuver (which it also calls "abdominal thrusts") as the easiest and safest thing to do when an adult is choking. Back blows administered in conjunction with chest thrusts are still an acceptable procedure for dislodging an object from the throat of an infant.

Unintentional Injury from Firearms

Firearms pose a significant threat to people between 15 and 24, with most fatalities involving males who are cleaning or handling guns they thought were unloaded. People who use firearms should (1) never point a loaded gun at something they do not intend to shoot; (2) store unloaded firearms under lock and key (in a place separate from the ammunition); (3) always inspect firearms carefully before handling; and (4) behave in the safe and responsible manner advocated in firearms safety courses.

Public Injuries

Recreational activities encompass a large part of our time, so it is not surprising that recreational injuries are a significant health problem in the United States. Significant problems with **public injuries** have been identified in the areas of drowning, boating, playground activities, the use of all-terrain vehicles (ATVs), and sporting events.

Drowning and Boating Injuries

Approximately 6,500 drownings occur annually in the United States. Males drown at a rate four times that of females; children under 5 years of age and people between 15 and 24 have the highest drowning rates. Between 40 and 45 percent of all drownings occur while the person is swimming. Most drownings occur during the summer; alcohol plays a significant role in many cases. Although most drownings are reported in lakes, ponds, rivers, and the ocean, more than half the drownings of young children take place in residential pools. Many of these incidents are attributed to a child's not understanding the consequences of being in deep water, although a majority occur when appropriate supervision is lacking. Pools not adequately secured with a fence can be a dangerous attraction for youngsters; a similar problem is now developing with the increasing presence of spas, hot tubs, and Jacuzzis. For adults the hazards increase when alcohol is introduced because prolonged use can lead to hypothermia-induced stupor and drowning.

Over 1,000 recreational boating fatalities and nearly 4,000 injuries are reported annually. Most injuries occur when a boat strikes another object, such as another boat, but most deaths occur when people fall overboard and drown. Most of these incidents occur on weekends, and between one-third and two-thirds of them involve alcohol. Studies show that the use of appropriate **personal flotation devices (PFDs)** would prevent many fatalities associated with boating incidents. Six types of PFDs have been recommended by the U.S. Coast Guard; each type is designed for particular water situations. For example, Type I is recommended for use in open water and in the ocean because it will float a person face up even if he or she is unconscious and in rough water.

Playground Injuries

More than 200,000 injuries occur on playgrounds each year. Schools and public playgrounds each account for about 25 percent of these incidents, but 40 percent involve residential playground equipment. Most of the injuries are not severe and don't require medical attention; deaths are usually the result of head injuries. Falls from the equipment to the ground are most often reported during emergency room visits, although striking a piece of equipment is also common. Analysis reveals that misuse of equipment is a common cause of injury. Equipment design, installation, and condition can also influence injuries on the playground, as can the surface beneath the equipment.

All-Terrain Vehicle Injuries

The use of **all-terrain vehicles (ATVs)** has caused a dramatic increase in fatalities and nonfatal injuries in the past decade. Most of the injuries associated with ATVs are head injuries, which account for approximately 70 percent of the deaths. Most injuries occur during recreational use; males under the age of 16 are those most often injured. Three-wheeled ATVs proved to be very unstable and contributed disproportionately to ATV injuries; manufacturers have recalled all unsold units (four-wheeled ATVs are still available). Just as in the case of motorcycle injuries, lack of experience, use of alcohol, and failure to use safety equipment like helmets are common contributors to ATV injuries.

Heimlich maneuver   A maneuver developed by Henry J. Heimlich, M.D., to help force an obstruction from the airway.

Public injuries   Injuries and deaths that occur in public places or places used in a public way, not involving motor vehicles. Most sports and recreation deaths and injuries are included. Examples of public injury incidents include falls, drownings, burns, and heat and cold stress.

Personal flotation devices (PFDs)   Devices designed to save a person from drowning by buoying up the body while in the water; also called life preservers.

All-terrain vehicles (ATVs)   A small open vehicle designed for recreational use on rugged terrain; most have three wheels and seat one person.

TERMS

American Red Cross

TO SAVE A LIFE

RESCUE BREATHING

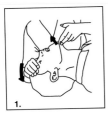

IF VICTIM APPEARS TO BE UN-CONSCIOUS, TAP VICTIM ON THE SHOULDER AND SHOUT "ARE YOU OKAY?"

1. Apply the major force with the hand on the forehead.
- Place fingertips under the bony part of the jaw.
- Support and lift the jaw with your fingertips. Avoid closing the mouth.
- Do not push the soft tissues of the throat; it may block the airway.

If necessary, pull the lower lip down slightly, with your open thumb to keep the mouth open.

2. Look, listen and feel for breathing for 3-5 seconds.

3.
- If the person is not breathing, pinch nose closed.
- Place your mouth tightly around victim's mouth and blow into his mouth.
- Give two full breaths

Stop blowing when victim's chest has expanded.
- Turn head and listen for exhalation.
- Give 1 breath every 5 seconds.

4. INFANTS AND SMALL CHILDREN
- Tilt head slightly.
- Cover & seal nose with your mouth.
- Blow shallow breaths.
- Give 1 breath every 3 seconds.

FIRST AID FOR CHOKING

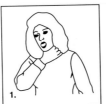

1. ASK: "ARE YOU CHOKING?"
If victim cannot breathe, cough, or speak...
GIVE THE HEIMLICH MANEUVER.
Stand behind the victim.
Wrap your arms around the victim's waist.

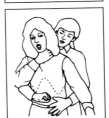

2. Make a fist with one hand; PLACE your FIST (thumb-side) against the victim's stomach in the midline just ABOVE THE NAVEL AND WELL BELOW THE RIB MARGIN.
Grasp your fist with your other hand.

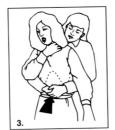

3. PRESS INTO STOMACH WITH A QUICK UP-WARD THRUST.
REPEAT IF NECESSARY.

4. IF A VICTIM HAS BE-COME UNCONSCIOUS: Sweep the mouth.

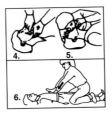

5. Attempt rescue breathing.

6. Give 6 - 10 abdominal thrusts.
Repeat Steps 4, 5, and 6 as necessary.

TO CONTROL BLEEDING

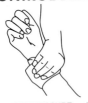

1. Apply DIRECT PRESSURE and elevate.

2. If bleeding continues, apply PRESSURE on the supplying artery.

Pressure on the brachial artery.

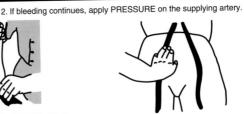

Hand pressure on the femoral artery.

Figure 23-2   *Rescue breathing, first aid for choking, and ways to control bleeding—procedures recommended by the Red Cross.*

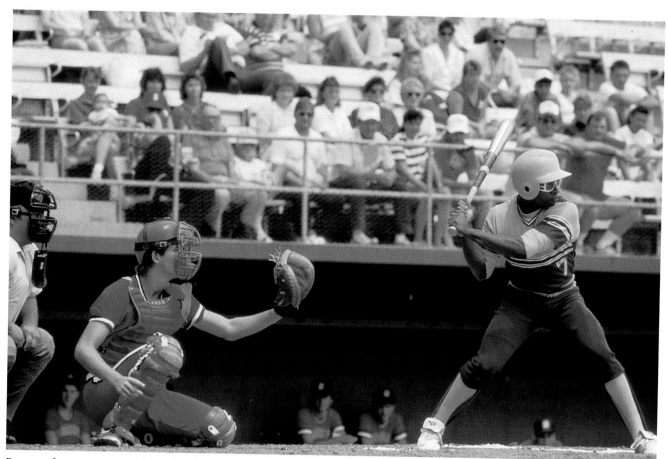

Proper safety equipment reduces the incidence of sport injuries. Head and face protection is the main concern for these baseball players.

Sports Injuries Sports also contribute to the public statistics on injury, especially since more people are participating in community, recreational, and intramural activities to improve their health and physical fitness. Regardless of the sport, following certain guidelines can reduce the incidence of injuries and deaths. They include developing the skills to enhance safer participation, recognizing and guarding against hazards associated with each activity, making sure facilities are safe, following the rules, and promoting good sportsmanship. It is also important to include appropriate exercises for conditioning, "warm up," and "cool down." Risks associated with endurance exercise include cramps, exhaustion, and heatstroke (see the box "Avoiding Heat Stress"). Another critical factor is the use of proper safety equipment (such as helmets for football, hockey, and baseball; eye protection for racquetball, handball, squash, and basketball; knee and elbow pads for volleyball, skateboarding, and soccer; mats for gymnastics and wrestling; appropriate footwear for each particular sport or activity). None of these suggestions will eliminate all dangers from sports and recreational activities (nor were they meant to), but these practices will enhance safety by encouraging self-responsibility for each participant.

Work Injuries

Since 1912, when industrial records were first kept in the United States, the work site has become a much safer place, as evidenced by a reduction in the unintentional death rate of nearly 76 percent. That figure becomes even more impressive when one realizes that the size of the work force has more than doubled and production has increased more than tenfold. One very significant factor to account for such a marked decline in **work injuries** has been the Occupational Safety and Health Act of 1970. As a result of that act, the Occupational Safety and Health Administration (OSHA) was created within the U.S. Department of Labor to ensure a safer and healthier environment for workers. Inspections, more detailed record keeping, and penalties for noncompliance have probably been most responsible for the changes.

> **Work injuries** Injuries and deaths that arise out of and in the course of gainful work. Examples of work injury incidents include falls, electric shocks, exposure to radiation and toxic chemicals, burns, cuts, back sprains, and loss of fingers or other body parts in machines.

TERMS

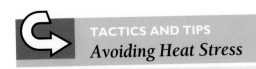
Excessive heat can subject your body to hazardous stress. Its potential toll ranges from mild discomfort to life-threatening heatstroke. You can protect yourself with commonsense approaches. But if heat stress strikes, be alert to its signs and act quickly to cool down.

How Your Body Cools Itself

Under typical conditions, your body maintains its normal temperature by radiating heat from its core outward to your skin's surface, where breezes help transfer it into the atmosphere. As air temperature rises, or when your body produces more heat during exertion, sweat production increases, which helps drive away heat through evaporation of the moisture. But if humidity exceeds 75 percent, evaporation of sweat diminishes rapidly, stopping completely when the humidity exceeds 90 percent.

When it's both hot and humid, it becomes more difficult for your body to release the heat that builds up. As a result, your body temperature can climb. Initially, you may be only mildly uncomfortable. You may feel dizzy, headachy, and tired.

Heat cramps represent the mildest form of heat stress. They are most often seen in poorly conditioned athletes who drink inadequate amounts of liquids before and during strenuous exercise. If relief from the heat is not obtained, heat exhaustion and heatstroke may follow.

Heat exhaustion results when your heart, circulatory system, and central nervous system fail to respond to heat stress. In the early stages, heat exhaustion causes nausea, vomiting, and muscle aches.

Heat exhaustion quickly can progress to *heatstroke*, a condition in which the temperature-regulating center in your brain shuts down. At this point, your body temperature soars. This can lead to severe, even fatal, brain, liver, or kidney damage.

Commonsense Approaches You Can Use to Beat the Heat

When the temperature pushes into the 90s or above and the humidity becomes oppressive, be alert for heat-related illness. Here are several suggestions:

- *Limit your activity.* Reserve vigorous exercise for the early morning or evening. If you participate in outdoor sports events, "acclimatize" yourself by gradually building up your tolerance to heat with exercise in similar conditions over five to six weeks.

- *Drink plenty of liquids.* Choose water or fruit or vegetable juices. Shun beverages containing alcohol or caffeine. A general rule: Drink at least 1½ times the amount that quenches your thirst.

- *Avoid the sun.* When outdoors, wear a wide-brimmed hat or carry an umbrella.

- *Keep rooms cool.* Open your windows on opposite sides of rooms to encourage cross-ventilation. Use fans to pull cooler air into rooms. Pull shades over sunny windows. If you have air conditioning, set the thermostat between 75° and 80° to both cool and help dehumidify the air. If you cannot cool your home, go to an air-conditioned public place such as a library or shopping mall.

- *Select the right clothing.* Wear lightweight, loose-fitting clothes that breathe. Light-colored clothes reflect heat. Take frequent cool showers or baths.

Another practical point to remember: On a hot day, *never* leave children or pets in a car with the windows rolled up. The temperature within the vehicle can quickly become life-threatening.

The table below provides a quick reference.

Condition	How to Recognize It	What to Do
Heat cramps	Painful muscle spasms, sweaty skin, normal body temperature.	1. Sit or lie down in the shade. 2. Drink cool water. 3. Stretching muscles may help. Do not massage.
Heat exhaustion	Profuse sweating, clammy or pale skin, dizziness, nausea, vomiting, headache, muscle aches, rapid pulse, thirst, normal or slightly elevated body temperature.	1. When mild, treat the same as for heat cramps. 2. If persistent headache and vomiting or confusion occur, gently apply wet towels and call for emergency help.
Heatstroke	Unconsciousness (or, if conscious: confused, staggered walk, agitated); hot, dry skin *or* (rarely) sweating; rapid pulse; body temperature of 105° F or higher.	1. Move person to a reclining position in the shade. 2. Call for emergency help. 3. If the person is conscious, offer sips of cool water. 4. Fan the person and sponge with cold water. An ice bath may be necessary.

Source: Mayo Clinic Health Letter, July 1989.

Almost everyone has to lift a heavy object at one time or another. Doing it the right way can protect your back from serious injury. Follow these simple rules:

- Know your strength and don't try to lift beyond it. Get help if necessary.

- Avoid bending at the waist. Try to remain in an upright—but not stiffly straight—position. If you need to lower yourself to grasp the object, crouch down. Bending at the knees and hips rather than at the waist is the key to safe lifting.

- Get a firm footing, with feet about shoulder width apart. Get a firm grip on the object with the palms of your hands. If the object or your hands are slippery, wipe them off.

- Lift gradually, keeping your arms straight. Avoid quick, jerky motions, which put a strain on your muscles. Lift by standing up or by pushing up with your leg muscles.

- Don't twist. Twisting is a common and dangerous cause of injury when you're moving something. If you have to turn with the object, change the position of your feet.

- Keep the object close to your body. Your ability to lift safely will be greatly increased.

- Put the object down gently, reversing the rules for lifting.

- Plan ahead. Make sure doors are open and your pathway is clear before you pick up the object.

Back injuries are among the most common, painful, and long-lasting of all the injuries you can sustain. If you hurt your back when you're young, you may have a "bad back" your whole life. It pays to take precautions to make sure your back will be there when you need it.

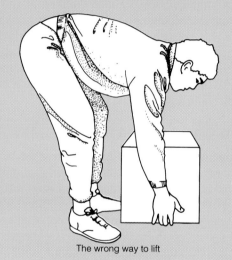

The wrong way to lift

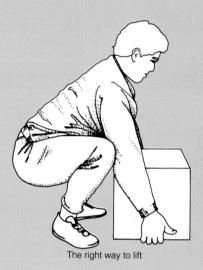

The right way to lift

The highest risk of injury or illness occurs among laborers. Although laborers make up less than half of the work force, they account for more than 75 percent of all work-related injuries and illnesses. Such jobs usually involve extensive manual labor and lifting, neither of which is addressed in OSHA safety standards. Consequently, back problems are the most frequently cited injury and account for over 20 percent of work injuries. For guidelines on safe lifting techniques, see the box "Protect Your Back When Lifting." Most fatal occupational injuries involve crushing injuries, severe lacerations, burns, and electrocutions. Experience may be a factor in these injuries, because more than 40 percent of work-related injuries and illnesses involve workers on the first year of a job. Advanced technology is making jobs more demanding and increasing the need for training and educational programs for workers.

Skin disorders account for nearly 40 percent of reported occupational illnesses. The introduction of more chemicals and hazardous materials at the worksite means that these disorders are of increasing concern. Examples include **asbestosis, contact dermatitis,** hearing loss, **silicosis,** and **Raynaud's phenomenon.**

New problems surfacing in the workplace are related

Asbestosis   A chronic, progressive lung disease caused by inhalation of asbestos particles.

Contact dermatitis   Skin irritation from direct exposure to chemicals or other substances.

Silicosis   A lung disease caused by inhalation of silica dust; the lungs become scarred and thickened, causing shortness of breath.

TERMS

to musculoskeletal injuries and disorders, particularly **cumulative trauma disorders (CTDs)**. CTDs are caused by repeated strain on the hand, arm, wrist, or any other part of the body. Twisting, vibrations, awkward postures, and other stressors may contribute to CTDs. **Carpal tunnel syndrome** is one type of CTD that has been brought to the attention of the public in recent years with the increased use of computer terminals, both at work and in the home. This condition is characterized by pain and swelling in the tendons of the wrists, and sometimes numbness and weakness. Permanent damage is possible unless the condition is recognized early. Computer users can protect themselves from carpal tunnel syndrome and other problems by maintaining good posture, positioning the computer screen at eye level, positioning the keyboard so that hands and wrists are straight, using a chair that provides support for the back, and placing the feet flat on the floor or on a foot rest. Periodic breaks are also recommended to lessen the cumulative effects of stressors. Whatever the working conditions, employees should make a conscious effort not to expose themselves to hazardous situations.

VIOLENCE AND INTENTIONAL INJURIES

Violence—the use of physical force with the intent to inflict harm, injury, or death upon oneself or another—is emerging as a major public health concern in the United States. The United States ranks first among industrialized nations in violent death rates, and deaths caused by violent and unintentional misuse of firearms exceed in number the combined total of the next 17 nations. Examples of types of violence include assault, homicide, sexual assault, domestic violence, suicide, and various forms of abuse. A violent crime occurs about every 19 seconds in this country, and at least 2.2 million Americans are victims of violent injury each year.

Violence-related Injuries and Deaths

Assault is the use of physical force by a person or persons to inflict injury or death on another; homicide, aggravated assault, and robbery are examples of assault. Research indicates that the victims of assaultive injuries and their perpetrators tend to resemble one another in terms of race, educational background, psychological profile, and reliance on weapons. In many cases, the victim actually magnifies the confrontation through the use of a weapon. Rates of injury from violent and abusive behavior are highest for males, African Americans, people aged 19 to 24 years, people who are separated or divorced, people of low income, and residents of inner cities. People under age 25 account for nearly half of the arrests for violent crimes in the United States and about 40 percent of the arrests for homicide.

Homicide is the tenth leading cause of death in the United States. Men, teenagers, young adults, and members of minority groups, particularly African Americans and Latinos, are most likely to be murder victims. Although homicide rates for African Americans have declined dramatically in the last 20 years, no cause of death so greatly differentiates African Americans from other Americans: In 1983 blacks made up 11.5 percent of the U.S. population but accounted for 43 percent of all homicide victims. Poverty has been identified as a very important factor in homicide, and this may account for the high rates of homicide among African Americans and other minority groups.

Most homicides are committed with a firearm, occur during an argument, and occur among people who know one another. Intrafamilial homicide, where the perpetrator and victim are related, accounts for about one out of every six homicides, primarily among young adults and African Americans. About half of family homicides are committed by spouses, usually following a history of physical and emotional abuse directed at the woman. Wives are more likely to be murdered than husbands, and when a wife kills a husband it is usually in self-defense.

Other forms of violence have been discussed in other chapters: child abuse (Chapters 4 and 5), domestic violence (Chapter 4), rape and sexual assault (Chapter 5), and suicide (Chapter 3).

Factors Contributing to Violence

Everyone gets angry sometimes, but few people translate their angry and aggressive impulses into action. Most intentional injuries and deaths are associated with an argument or the commission of another crime. The media play a major role in exposing audiences of all ages to violence as an acceptable and fairly effective means of solving problems; the consequences of violence, on both perpetrator and victim, are shown much less frequently. People may model their behavior on the acts of family members and peers as well as on what the media show. Studies have linked the male hormone testosterone to aggressive behavior, which may account in part for the high rates of violence among males. Prevailing cultural attitudes about male roles (men as dominant and controlling), as well as racism and discrimination, may also contribute to violence. Socioeconomic status is another significant risk factor—urban settings and poverty are primary determinants of violence. Alcohol and other drug intoxication, abuse, and dependence are consistently associated with interpersonal violence and suicide. Intoxication affects judgment and may increase aggression in some people, allowing a small argument to escalate into a serious physical confrontation.

Firearms and Intentional Injuries

Over 30,000 deaths and five times that number of injuries

occur each year as a result of firearms use. Firearms are used in more than 60 percent of the homicides in the United States, and studies reveal a strong correlation between the incidence of gun ownership and homicide rates for a given area of the country. Over half of all suicides involve the use of a firearm, and the increased presence of firearms in the home has been cited as a possible risk factor for this phenomenon. Men between the ages of 15 and 34 are at highest risk of death from homicide and suicide when guns are the weapon used.

Efforts are being made nationally to restrict the purchase of firearms except under certain conditions. Possible strategies include a waiting period for licensing and purchase and a limit on the number of firearms that can be purchased within a certain period. Some groups advocate a complete and universal federal ban on the manufacture, importation, sale, and possession of handguns.

PROVIDING EMERGENCY CARE

By following the safety guidelines described in this chapter and being aware of the potential risks associated with different activities, you can avoid many injuries on the road, at home, at work, and in public places. However, it's nearly inevitable that some injuries will occur. Therefore, it is also important that you take steps to prepare for those instances when you may need to provide emergency care for yourself or others. If you are prepared to provide help, you can improve someone else's chances of surviving or of avoiding the serious consequences of an injury. A course in **first aid,** such as one of those offered by the American Red Cross, can help you respond appropriately when someone is injured. One important benefit of first aid training is that you learn what *not* to do in certain situations. For example, a person with a suspected neck or back injury should not be moved unless other life-threatening conditions exist. A knowledgeable person can assess emergency situations accurately before acting. An emergency first aid guide is provided inside the back cover of this book.

Emergency rescue techniques can save the lives of people who are choking, who have stopped breathing, or whose hearts have stopped beating. As described earlier, the Heimlich maneuver is used when a victim is choking. Pulmonary resuscitation (also known as rescue breathing, artificial respiration, or mouth-to-mouth resuscitation) is used when a person is not breathing (see Figure 23-2). **Cardiopulmonary resuscitation (CPR)** is used when a pulse can't be found. Training is required before a person can perform CPR. Courses are offered by the Red Cross and the American Heart Association.

As a person providing assistance to someone, you are the first link in the **emergency medical services (EMS) system.** Your responsibility may be to render first aid as needed, provide emotional support for the victim, or just call for help. It is essential that you remain calm and act sensibly when an emergency occurs. Here are some tips for giving emergency care:

- Make sure the scene is safe for both you and the injured person. Don't put yourself in danger; otherwise, you may be of little help to the injured person.

- Try to find out exactly what happened. This information can help you give appropriate first aid and is crucial for medical personnel when they arrive or are contacted. Identify yourself to the victim, let him or her know that you are there to help, and ask what happened.

- Conduct a quick but thorough head-to-toe examination. Assess the victim's signs and symptoms, such as level of responsiveness, pulse, breathing, size of pupils, and the color, texture, and temperature of the skin. Look for bleeding and any indications of broken bones or paralysis due to a neck or spinal cord injury. An unconscious victim may make your assessment more difficult, but proper evaluation is probably even more critical.

- If the situation is life-threatening and requires immediate help, provide emergency first aid if you are trained to do so. Examples of life-threatening situations include absence of breathing, heart attack or stroke, heavy bleeding, poisoning, and shock. If you are alone, take care of the life-threatening situation first and then seek help immediately. If several people are available, one should go for help while the rest give first aid.

If you are injured yourself, you may need to instruct another person on how to help you, especially if that person has no first aid training or experience.

TERMS

Raynaud's phenomenon   A circulatory disorder affecting the hands or feet in which the blood supply to these parts is insufficient, causing numbness and pain. It can be caused by overexposure to prolonged vibration from a power tool.

Cumulative trauma disorders (CTDs)   Musculoskeletal injuries and disorders caused by repeated strain to the hand, arm, wrist, or other part of the body; also called repetitive stress injuries.

Carpal tunnel syndrome   Compression of the median nerve in the wrist, often caused by repetitive use of the hands (such as in computer use). It is characterized by numbness, tingling, and pain in the hands and fingers and can cause nerve damage.

First aid   Emergency care given to an ill or injured person until medical care can be obtained.

Cardiopulmonary resuscitation (CPR)   Emergency first aid procedure that combines artificial respiration and artificial circulation. It is used in first aid emergencies where breathing and blood circulation have stopped.

Emergency medical services (EMS) system   System designed to network community resources for providing emergency care.

Like other kinds of behavior, avoiding and preventing injuries and acting safely involve choices you make every day. If you perceive something to be a serious personal threat—whether physically or psychologically, socially or economically—you tend to take action to protect yourself. Ultimately, your goal is healthy, safe behavior. You can motivate yourself to act in the safest way possible by increasing your knowledge and level of awareness, by examining your attitudes to see if they're realistic, by knowing your capacities and limitations, by adjusting your responses when environmental hazards exist, and, in general, by taking responsibility for your actions. You can't eliminate all risks and dangers from your life—no one can do that—but you can improve your chances of avoiding injuries and living to a healthy, ripe old age.

Personal Insight How do you feel about being trained to handle emergency situations by taking courses in CPR or first aid? Does it make you feel more confident and in control to know you could help? Or does it feel like a possibly frightening responsibility? What is the basis for your feelings?

SUMMARY

Why Do Injuries Happen?

- According to the multiple causation theory, injuries are caused by a dynamic interaction of human and environmental factors. Risk-taking behavior is associated with a high rate of injury.

- Human factors in injuries include level of skill; use of psychoactive, prescription, and over-the-counter drugs; safety knowledge; awareness of risks; attitudes toward risk-taking behavior; and emotional and psychological states.

- Environmental factors may be natural, societal, work-related, or home-related. Environmental hazards can be the result of technological advances if safety features and equipment are used improperly.

- An injury is often the result of interaction between human factors and environmental factors. Sometimes an individual can make a decision that will help avoid an injury; the wrong decision can lead to injury or death.

Preventing Unintentional Injuries

- Bad driving, especially speeding, causes three-fourths of all motor vehicle crashes. Speed limits establish the safest *maximum* speed limit for a given area under *ideal* conditions.

- Safety belts prevent a second collision and spread the stopping force over the body. Air bags provide

protection only in frontal collisions; they are less effective in multiple collisions.

- Alcohol is a factor in about half of all fatal motor vehicle crashes.

- In bad weather, driving defensively and making sure the vehicle is well-maintained are especially important. Interstate highways are safer than rural roads.

- Motorcycle and moped crashes usually result from lack of visibility, lack of skill, and/or the use of alcohol and psychoactive drugs. Injuries can be prevented by driving defensively and wearing proper safety equipment, especially a helmet.

- Pedestrian injuries and deaths are usually the result of poor decision making, usually from inability to adequately judge vehicle distances or speeds. Lack of visibility, the use of headphones, and alcohol or drug intoxication are contributing factors.

- Bicyclists can improve safety by following all traffic laws, driving defensively, increasing visibility, and wearing proper safety equipment, especially a helmet.

- Most fall-related deaths are a result of falls at floor level, usually caused by difficulty in adjusting to degrees of traction. Stairs are a problem when lighting is poor, handrails are missing, or footwear is inappropriate.

- Being prepared for fire emergencies means planning escape routes, installing smoke detection devices, and knowing how to use fire-extinguishing devices. In a fire, smoke inhalation can be avoided by crawling along the floor and covering the mouth.

- Most home poisonings involve children under age 5. The home can contain many poisonous substances, including medications, cleaning agents, petroleum-based products, plants, and fumes from cars and appliances.

- Using the Heimlich maneuver can prevent deaths due to choking.

- Firearm injuries are particularly prevalent in the 15–24 age group, often as a result of cleaning a gun that is thought to be unloaded.

- Most drownings take place in summer; alcohol is a major factor in drownings among adults. Children more commonly drown in residential pools when there is no supervision. Use of personal flotation devices can help reduce boating injuries and deaths.

- Care in design, installation, maintenance, and use of playground equipment can reduce injuries.

- Most injuries associated with ATVs are due to instability of the vehicles, lack of experience, use of alcohol, and failure to use safety equipment.

- The risk of injuries and deaths in sports can be reduced by developing skills, recognizing hazards, making sure facilities are safe, promoting good sportsmanship, and using proper equipment.

- Most work-related injuries involve extensive manual labor and lifting. Back problems are most common, and skin disorders are increasing because of chemical and hazardous substances. Workers are especially at risk for injuries during their first year on the job.

Violence and Intentional Injuries

- The United States has the highest death rate from violence of all industrialized nations.
- Most homicides are committed with a firearm and occur during an argument among people who know one another.
- Factors contributing to violence include the influence of the media, cultural attitudes about sex roles, racism and discrimination, poverty, and alcohol and drug use and dependence.

Providing Emergency Care

- By taking first aid courses, people can learn how to help others who are injured in an accident. The Heimlich maneuver can be used for choking victims; pulmonary resuscitation and cardiopulmonary resuscitation can help save the lives of those who have stopped breathing or whose hearts have stopped beating.
- Steps in giving emergency care include making sure the scene is safe for you and the injured person, finding out exactly what happened, conducting a quick examination of the victim, giving emergency first aid in life-threatening situations, and seeking help.
- People make choices every day that help them avoid and prevent injuries.

TAKE ACTION

1. Contact your local fire department and obtain a checklist for fire safety procedures. What would you do if a fire started in your home? What types of evacuation procedures would be necessary? Do a practice fire drill at home to see what problems might arise in a real emergency.
2. Look up the nearest Poison Control Center in your telephone book and post the number near your telephone. Contact the center and ask them to send you information on poisonings. Read it carefully so you know what to do in case of poisoning.
3. Contact the Red Cross or American Heart Association in your area and ask about first aid and CPR classes. These courses are usually given frequently and at a variety of times and locations. They can be invaluable

in saving lives. Consider taking one or both of the courses.

JOURNAL ENTRY

1. In your health journal, list the positive behaviors that help you avoid injuries and keep yourself safe. What can you do to reinforce and support these behaviors? Then list the behaviors that keep you from following safety guidelines or that put you at risk of being injured. How can you change one or more of them?

2. *Critical Thinking:* Federal, state, and local governments have passed many regulations and laws to enforce a certain level of safety among citizens; examples of these include laws regulating seat belts, helmets, and firearms. Some people believe that government should not be involved in issues of individual safety and injury prevention; others feel the government has a right to demand certain behaviors for the public good. How do you feel about this issue? Write a brief essay outlining your opinion; be sure to explain your reasoning.

BEHAVIOR CHANGE STRATEGY

ADOPTING SAFER HABITS

Why do you get injured? What human and environmental factors contribute to injuries? Identifying those factors is one step toward making your lifestyle safer. Changing unsafe behaviors *before* they lead to injuries is an even better way of improving your chances.

For the next 7 to 10 days, keep track of any mishaps you are involved in or injuries you receive, recording them on a daily behavior record like the one shown in Chapter 1. Count each time you cut, burn, or injure yourself, fall down, run into someone, or have any other potentially injury-causing mishap, no matter how trivial. Also record any risk-taking behaviors, such as failing to wear your seat belt or bicycle helmet, drinking and driving, exceeding the speed limit, putting off home or bicycle repairs, and so on. For each entry (injury or incidence of unsafe behavior), record the date, time, what you were doing, who else was there and how you were influenced by him or her, what your motivations were, and what you were thinking and feeling at the time.

At the end of the monitoring period, examine your data. For each incident, determine both the human factors and the environmental factors that contributed to the injury or unsafe behavior. For example, were you tired? Distracted? Did you not realize this situation was dangerous? Did you take a chance? Did you think this incident couldn't happen to you? Was visibility poor? Were you using defective equipment? Then consider each contributing factor carefully, determining why it existed and how it could have been avoided or changed. Finally, consider what preventive actions you could take to avoid such incidents or change your behaviors in the future.

As an example, let's say that you usually don't use a safety belt when you run local errands in your car and that several factors contribute to this behavior—you don't really think you could be involved in a crash so close to home, you only go on short trips, you just never think to use it, and so on. One of the contributing factors to your unsafe behavior is inadequate or inaccurate knowledge. You can change this factor by obtaining accurate information about automobile crashes (and their usual proximity to a victim's home) from this chapter and from library research. Just acquiring information about automobile crashes and safety belt use may lead you to examine your beliefs and attitudes about safety belts and motivate you to change your behavior.

Once you're committed, you can use behavior change aids and techniques described in Chapter 1, such as completing a contract, asking family and friends for support, and so on, to build a new habit. Put a note or picture reminding you to buckle up in your car where you can see it clearly. Recruit a friend to run errands with you and remind you about buckling your safety belt. Once your habit is established, you may influence other people—especially people who ride in your car—to use safety belts all the time. By changing this behavior you have reduced the chances that you or your passengers will die or suffer a serious injury in a vehicle crash.

SELECTED BIBLIOGRAPHY

American National Red Cross. 1991. *First Aid: Responding to Emergencies.* St. Louis, Mo.: Mosby Year Book, 1991.

Bever, D. L. 1992. *Safety: A Personal Focus,* 3rd ed. St. Louis, Mo.: Mosby Year Book.

Bike helmets can save you more than headaches. 1991. *Healthline,* March.

Centers for Disease Control. 1988. Progress toward achieving the national 1990 objectives for injury prevention and control. *Morbidity and Mortality Weekly Report* 37:138–49.

Fire safety: Teach your children well. 1992. *Washington Post.* 28 April.

Florio, A. E., W. F. Alles, and G. T. Stafford. 1979. *Safety Education,* 4th ed. New York: McGraw-Hill.

It's fire time. 1993. *University of California at Berkeley Wellness Letter.* January.

Kraus, J. F. 1987. Homicide while at work: Persons, industries, and occupations at high risk. *American Journal of Public Health.* 77(10): 1285–89.

Lawson, D. C. 1992. *Wellness: Safety and Accident Prevention.* Guilford, Conn.: Dushkin.

National Highway Traffic Safety Administration. 1982. *The Automobile Safety Belt Fact Book.* Washington, D.C.: National Academy of Science.

National Research Council. 1985. *Injury in America: A Continuing Public Health Problem.* Washington, D.C.: National Academy Press.

National Safety Council. 1992. *Accident Facts.* Chicago: National Safety Council.

Rice, D. P., E. J. MacKenzie, and others. 1989. *Cost of Injury in the United States: A Report to Congress.* San Francisco, Calif.: Institute for Health and Aging, University of California, and Injury Prevention Center, Johns Hopkins University.

Rosenberg, M. L., and M. A. Fenley. 1991. *Violence in America.* New York: Oxford University Press.

Sleet, D., and others. 1984. Automobile occupant protection: An issue for health educators. *Health Education* 15(5): 25–66.

Sleet, D. A., A. Wagenaar, and P. Waller, eds. 1989. Drinking, driving and health promotion. *Health Education Quarterly,* vol. 16, no. 3.

U.S. Department of Health and Human Services. 1990. *Healthy People 2000.* Washington, D.C.: U.S. Government Printing Office, DHHS Publication No. (PHS) 91-50213.

U.S. National Committee for Injury Prevention and Control. 1989. *Injury Prevention: Meeting the Challenge.* New York: Oxford University Press. (Supplement to *American Journal of Preventive Medicine,* vol. 5, no. 3.)

RECOMMENDED READINGS

American Red Cross. 1991. *First Aid: Responding to Emergencies.* St. Louis, Mo.: Mosby Year Book. *Presents current, straightforward information essential for providing emergency care.*

Baker, S. B., B. O'Neill, M. Ginsburg, and G. Li. 1992. *Injury Fact Book,* 2nd ed. New York: Oxford University Press. *Contains current data on injuries.*

Baker, S. B., and S. P. Teret. 1981. Freedom and protection: A balancing of interests. *American Journal of Public Health* 71(3): 295–97. *Addresses the issue of freedom of choice in safety matters relative to the costs to society as a whole.*

Bever, D. L. 1992. *Safety: A Personal Focus,* 3rd ed. St. Louis, Mo.: Mosby Year Book. *Provides an overview of injury prevention, including automobile, fire, and recreational safety.*

Jagger, J., and P. Dietz. 1986. Deaths and injury by firearms: Who cares? *Journal of the American Medical Association.* 255:314. *Addresses the increasing number of deaths and injuries by firearms.*

Perin, M. J., W. L. Stohler, and W. G. Faraclas. 1984. *None for the Road.* Dubuque: Kendall/Hunt. *Discusses the problems associated with "driving under the influence" and recommends strategies for changing this pattern of behavior.*

Sweeting, R. L. 1990. *A Values Approach to Health Behavior.* Champaign, Ill.: Human Kinetics Books. *This textbook focuses on self-concept as the core of all health behavior, with specific reference in one chapter to examples pertinent to safety and security issues.*

U.S. Congress. Senate. 1992. *Bicycle Helmet Promotion Act: Report of the Senate Committee on Commerce, Science, and Transportation, on S. 3096.* Washington, D.C.: U.S. Government Printing Office. *Documents the need to promote the use of bicycle helmets.*

24

Environmental Health

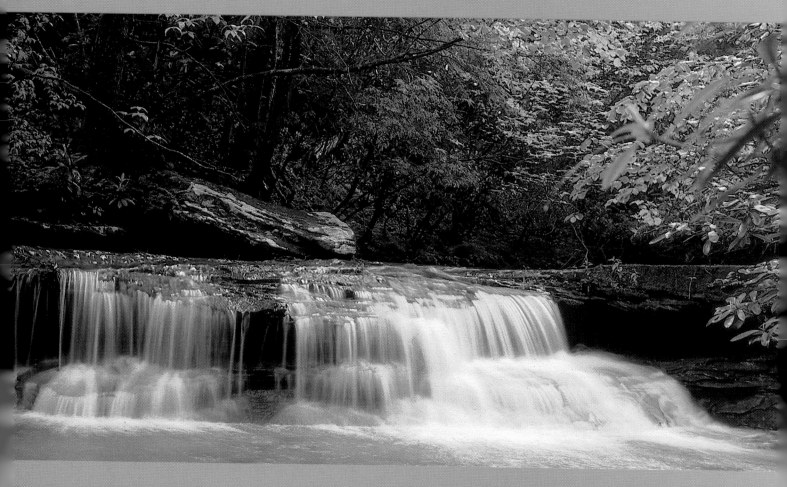

CONTENTS

▶ You're thinking about buying a car so you ask a friend to help you decide what type to get and what options to get with it. You'd like to have air conditioning, but your friend seems to think it's a bad idea. She says, "You don't really need air conditioning and, besides, it uses a lot of energy and makes the hole in the ozone layer worse." You like the comfort and convenience of automobile air conditioning. Is there something wrong with it? What does it have to do with ozone?

▶ You're moving out of your apartment and would like to get rid of a lot of the things you've accumulated under the sink for the past year—oven cleaner, bathroom tile cleaner, flea powder, bicycle chain lube, and several other items. A lot of the labels say you should dispose of empty containers by wrapping them in several layers of newspaper and throwing them in the trash, but they don't say what to do with half-full containers or leftover contents. Can you wrap them up and throw them in the trash anyway? Should you dump the liquids down the drain and then wrap and throw away the containers? How can you find out the best way to dispose of these products?

▶ Your roommate says his parents are doing some home improvements to lower the levels of radon inside their house. They're installing a ventilation system in their basement and resealing the basement walls and floor. Your roommate says they're worried about getting cancer by being exposed to radon in the soil, though he's not sure exactly what the connection is. Your parents live in the same state as his parents. Should they be making the same kinds of home improvements? How can they find out if radon is affecting their health?

▶ Your grandparents told you they would help you buy a car next year, and they'd like you to get a big high-powered model, which they think is safer. When you tell them you'd really like to get something a little more fuel-efficient, your grandfather says, "You don't need to worry about gasoline. A gallon of gas costs less than a gallon of milk." You know gas is available and inexpensive, but does that mean fuel efficiency isn't important?

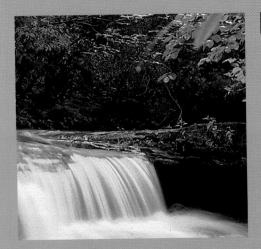

MAKING CONNECTIONS

Because of the intimate relationship between human beings and their environment, even the healthiest lifestyle can't protect a person from the effects of polluted air, contaminated water, or a nuclear power plant accident. Many of the health challenges of the next century will involve protecting the environment in order to maintain and improve the quality of life on earth. The individuals in the scenarios above have to use information, make a decision, or choose a course of action. How would you act in each of these situations? What response or decision would you make? This chapter provides information about environmental health that can be used in situations like these. After finishing the chapter, read the scenarios again. Has what you've learned changed how you would respond?

Current events constantly remind us of our intimate relationship with all that surrounds us—our environment. Although the planet supplies us with food, water, air, and everything else that sustains life, it also presents us with natural occurrences—earthquakes, hurricanes, drought, climate changes—that destroy life and disrupt society. In the past, human beings have frequently had to struggle against the environment to survive. Today, in addition to dealing with natural disasters, we also have to find ways to protect the environment from the by-products of our way of life.

Environmental health has historically focused on preventing infectious diseases spread by water, waste, food, rodents, and insects. Although these problems still exist, the focus of environmental health has expanded and become more complex, for several reasons. First, we now recognize that environmental pollutants contribute not only to infectious diseases but to many chronic diseases as well. Additionally, technological advances have increased our ability to affect and damage the environment. And finally, rapid population growth—which has resulted partly from past environmental improvements—means that far more people are consuming and competing for resources than ever before, magnifying the effect of humans on the environment (see the box "Environmental Index: The World").

Environmental health is therefore seen as encompassing all the interactions of humans with their environment and the health consequences of these interactions. Fundamental to this definition is a recognition that we hold the world in trust for future generations and for other forms of life. Our responsibility is to pass on to the next generation an environment no worse, and preferably better, than the one we enjoy today. Although many environmental problems are complex and seem beyond the control of the individual, there are many ways that people can make a difference in the future of the planet.

CLASSIC ENVIRONMENTAL HEALTH CONCERNS

The field of environmental health originally grew out of efforts to control communicable diseases. When certain insects and rodents were found to carry microorganisms that cause disease in humans, campaigns were undertaken to eradicate or control these animal *vectors*. It was also recognized that pathogens could live and be transmitted in sewage, drinking water, and food. These discoveries led to the development of such practices as systematic garbage collection, sewage treatment, filtration and chlorination of drinking water, food inspection, and the establishment of public health enforcement agencies.

These successful efforts to control and prevent communicable diseases changed the health profile of the developed world (see Chapter 1). Americans no longer worry about contracting **cholera**, typhoid fever, plague,

diphtheria, or any of the other diseases that once killed whole populations. But that doesn't mean that these diseases have been eradicated worldwide or that no efforts are required to keep them under control in the United States. Recently there have been more than a million cases of cholera in South and Central America, probably spread by contaminated seafood and poor sewage disposal. In the United States, a huge, complex health system is constantly at work behind the scenes attending to the details of these concerns. Every time this system is disrupted, danger recurs. Every time a flood, a hurricane, an earthquake, a tornado, or some other natural disaster damages a community, these areas again become of prime importance. And every time we venture beyond the boundaries of our everyday world, whether traveling to a less developed country or camping in a wilderness area, we are reminded of the importance of these basics—clean water, sanitary waste disposal, safe food, and insect and rodent control.

Clean Water

Few parts of the world have adequate quantities of safe, clean drinking water, and yet few things are as important to human health.

In the latter half of the nineteenth century, the United States and Great Britain both began building complex water systems that brought clean water to cities, right into buildings. Governments took on the role of inspecting water, and in most instances governments provided it too. As a result, the incidence of cholera, typhoid fever, and other water-borne diseases fell sharply by 1900 and remains virtually nil today in areas that have adequately treated water from municipal supplies.

Many cities still rely at least in part on wells that tap local groundwater, but often they have to find lakes and rivers to supplement wells. Because such surface water is more likely to be "dirty"—contaminated with both organic matter and disease-causing microorganisms—it is purified in water treatment plants before being piped into the community. At treatment facilities, the water is subjected to a variety of physical and chemical processes, including screening, filtration, and disinfection (often with chlorine), before it is introduced into the water supply system. In many communities, the water is also treated with fluoride (**fluoridation**), which reduces tooth decay by 20 to 40 percent. In most areas of the United States, water systems have adequate, dependable supplies, are

- Net increase in world population each hour: 11,000.

- Number of people who die each year from hunger and hunger-related diseases: 40 million.

- Proportion of the world's grain fed to livestock: 40 percent. In the United States: 70 percent.

- Time required to consume known reserves of oil at present rate of consumption: 40 years.

- Approximate rate of worldwide species extinction: 50–100 species per day.

- Proportion of the Pacific Northwest coast forest (the largest conifer forest on earth) that has been cut down: 60 percent.

- Amount of forest destroyed in Brazil each year: 5,335 square miles.

- Proportion of range and cropland in Australia that has

- turned to desert: 23 percent. In North America: 40 percent.

- Proportion of range and cropland in Central Asia that has been lost: 72 percent.

- Percentage decline in the total fish catch in the northwest Atlantic since the 1970s: 32 percent.

- Number of Americans who breathe unhealthy air: 150 million.

- Proportion of trees in the Czech Republic and Slovakia suffering from defoliation caused by air pollution: 71 percent.

- Estimated global pesticide sales in 1975: $5 billion. In 1990: $50 billion.

- Proportion of money that Americans spend on food that goes to packaging: 10 percent.

able to control water-borne disease, and provide water without unacceptable color, odor, or taste.

As we move toward the year 2000, water has once again become a worldwide environmental concern, although the reasons are different from those of a century ago. Water pollution from sewage and from many industrial sources has been controlled in the United States and some other countries, but many supplies of water, both on the surface and in the ground, are becoming polluted with hazardous chemicals. Manufacturing and agriculture are responsible for part of this toxic waste, but the accumulated hazardous waste from individual households also contributes to the problem. Increased incidence of cancer is just one of the health problems associated with chemical pollution of the water supply.

Water shortages are also a growing concern. Some parts of the United States are experiencing rapid population growth that outstrips the ability of local systems to provide adequate water to all. Many proposals are being discussed to relieve these shortages, including long-distance transfers, conservation, and the recycling of some water, such as that in office-building air conditioning towers.

According to the World Health Organization, only about 35 percent of the world's people have an adequate water supply. Groundwater pumping and the diversion of water from lakes and rivers for irrigation are further reducing the amount of water available to local communities. Groundwater is usually not replaced as quickly as it is removed, and the levels of rivers and lakes fluctuate in response to variations in levels of rain and snow (as California discovered in more than seven years of drought).

The Aral Sea, located in the former Soviet Republic of Kazakhstan and Uzbekistan, was once one of the largest inland seas in the world. Since the 1960s, it has lost two-thirds of its volume to irrigation, and people living around it have to deal with both a severe shortage of water and the health consequences of environmental degradation, including increased rates of respiratory disease and throat cancer linked to dust storms from the dry seabed. Although the United States has not experienced problems on this scale, the Colorado River is now diverted to the extent that it no longer flows into the ocean.

Problems of this scope obviously demand long-range solutions on both the national and the international level. Whatever the outcome of plans to address these problems, two actions are now being implemented. One involves minimizing pollution of all waters with hazardous substances. All freshwater supplies must be treated as if they will be needed as a source of drinking water in the future. In the United States, the Environmental Protection Agency (EPA) sets limits for the presence of contaminants in drinking water, and many countries regulate the discharge of industrial wastes into waterways.

The second action involves a rethinking of our water distribution system. Most cities usually have just one system that provides "treated" water to homes, industry, and agriculture alike. However, much of that water doesn't have to be made as pure and safe as drinking water. The water you use to wash a car or water a lawn doesn't have to meet the same standards as the water you drink. As treatment becomes more expensive and as the cleanest water becomes scarcer, conservation may have to be supplemented by a multilevel distribution system based on

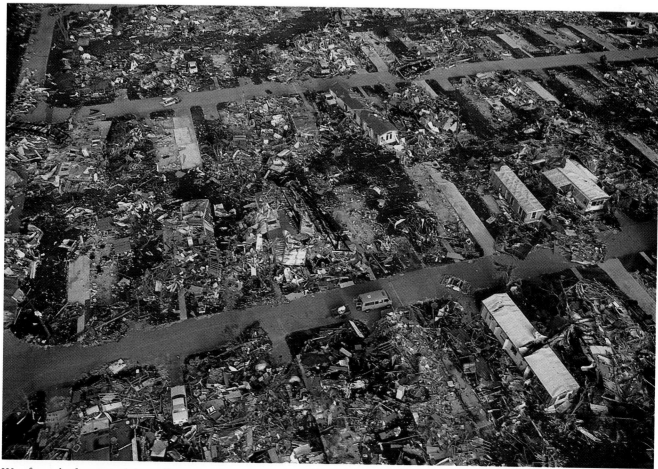

We often take for granted the well-organized system responsible for environmental health in our society, but natural disasters remind us of its fragility. In 1992, Hurricane Andrew disrupted essential services, including the delivery of clean drinking water.

intended use; such a system could be less costly than treating all water.

Waste Disposal

Humans generate large amounts of waste, which must be handled in an appropriate manner if the environment is to be safe and sanitary. Some of this waste is sewage composed of human excrement, some is garbage from food materials, and some is solid waste, a by-product of our "throw-away" society. This last category, consisting of packaging, newspapers, "junk mail," insulated fast-food wrappers, aluminum cans, and other trash, accounts for an ever-growing proportion of solid waste generated in the United States.

Sewage   Prior to the mid-nineteenth century, many people contracted diseases such as typhoid, cholera, and hepatitis A by direct contact with fecal matter, which was simply disposed of at random. Once the links between sewage and disease were discovered, practices began to change. People were taught how to build sanitary out-

houses and how to locate them so they wouldn't contaminate potential water sources. As plumbing moved indoors, sewage disposal became more complicated. In rural areas the **septic system,** a self-contained sewage disposal system for one family, worked quite well; today, many rural homes still rely on this system.

Different approaches became necessary as urban areas developed. Many early cities developed on rivers. The inhabitants got their drinking water upstream and dumped their sewage downstream. For small populations, this tended to work fairly well as long as the cities were sufficiently separated. If they are not overloaded by organic wastes, rivers and lakes can "clean themselves" fairly well through the processes of dilution and bacterial action. But as cities grew, governments began to regulate waste dis-

Septic system   A self-contained sewage disposal system for one family, often used in rural areas, in which waste material is decomposed by bacteria.

TERMS

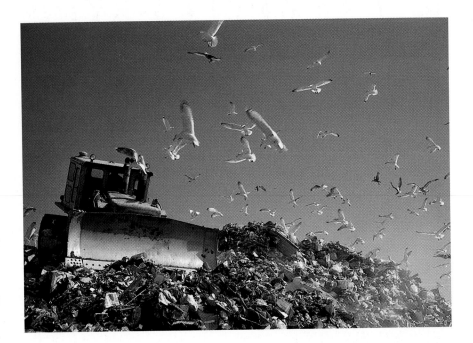

Many existing landfills are reaching their limits at the same time that people are becoming more resistant to the opening of new ones in their communities. The solution to the waste problem lies in less consumption of disposable items and more recycling.

posal just as they regulated water supplies. City and state health departments are responsible for these services in most areas in the United States today.

Most cities have sewage treatment systems that separate fecal matter from water in huge tanks and ponds and stabilize it so that it cannot transmit infectious diseases. Once treated and biologically safe, the water is released back into the environment. The sludge that remains behind may be spread on fields as fertilizer if it is free from **heavy metal** contamination, or it may be burned or buried. If incorporated into the food chain, heavy metals, such as lead, cadmium, copper, and tin, can cause illness and death. Recent studies indicate that even more care than once was thought necessary must be taken to prevent these chemicals from being released into the environment when sludge is burned or buried.

In addition to regulating industrial discharge, many cities have now begun to treat sewage further to remove heavy metals and other hazardous chemicals. This action has resulted from many studies linking exposure to such chemicals as mercury, lead, and **polychlorinated**

biphenyls (**PCBs**) with long-term health consequences, including cancer and central nervous system damage. Sewage treatment systems that collect and concentrate these chemicals from an entire city should not dump them back into the environment where they might contaminate a present or future water source. The technology to effectively remove heavy metals and chemicals from sewage is still developing, and the costs involved are immense.

Solid Waste   The bulk of the organic food garbage produced in American kitchens is now dumped in the sewage system by way of the mechanical garbage disposal. The garbage that remains is not very hazardous from the standpoint of infectious disease, since there is very little food waste in it, but it does represent an enormous disposal and contamination problem.

Since the 1960s much of this solid waste has been buried in **sanitary landfill** disposal sites. Careful site selection and daily management are an essential part of this approach to disposal. First, a thorough study is done of the site to make certain that it is not near groundwater, streams, or any other source of water that could be contaminated by leakage from the landfill. Soil composition under and around the site is studied to make certain that materials cannot leach, or seep, from the area. Sometimes protective liners are used around the site, and nearby monitoring wells are now required in most states. Layers of solid waste are covered with thin layers of dirt on a regular basis until the site is filled. Some communities then plant grass and trees and convert the site into a park. Landfill is relatively stable; almost no decomposition occurs in the solidly packed waste.

Burying solid waste in sanitary landfills has several disadvantages. Much of this waste contains chemicals, ranging from leftover pesticides to nail-polish remover to paints and oils, which should not be released indiscriminately into the environment. Despite precautions, buried contaminants do leak into the surrounding soil and groundwater. Burial is also expensive and requires huge amounts of space. Over two-thirds of the country's landfills have closed since the late 1970s, and one-third of those remaining will be full by 1994. At the same time that disposal is becoming more restricted, the amount of garbage is growing all the time. The average American produces more than one ton of solid waste per year, up 80 percent since 1960 and expected to rise another 20 percent by 2000. Our throw-away society uses ever more disposable products, ranging from plastic ketchup bottles to disposable diapers to overpackaged products of every kind.

The biggest single component of this trash (40 percent by weight) is paper products, a share fed by junk mail, glossy mail-order catalogs, and computer printouts. Yard waste is the next biggest source by weight (17.5 percent before recycling), followed by metals (8.5 percent). Plastics make up 8 percent of all trash by weight, but take up about 18 percent of landfill space. Most of this plastic waste is in the form of packaging, which accounts for about one third of the 6 million tons of plastics produced each year in the United States. Other significant sources of trash include food (7.3 percent by weight), glass (7 percent), and wood (3.5 percent). About 1 percent of the solid waste is toxic. Burning, as opposed to burial, reduces the bulk of this solid waste, but it may release hazardous material into the air. A partial solution to this problem is to reduce packaging and consume less.

Solid waste is not limited to household products. Manufacturing, mining, and other industries all produce large amounts of potentially dangerous materials that cannot simply be dumped. The experiences of communities like Love Canal near Buffalo, New York, and Times Beach, Missouri, demonstrated clearly the dangers of careless disposal of toxic wastes. At Love Canal, toxic industrial wastes had been dumped into a waterway for years until, in the 1970s, nearby residents began to suffer from associated birth defects and cancers. Human health was affected, government had to step in, people had to move from homes, and huge costs were incurred.

Because of the expense and potential chemical hazards posed by any form of solid waste disposal, many communities today encourage individuals and businesses to recycle their trash. Some cities offer curbside pickup of recyclables; others have recycling centers to which people can bring their waste. These materials are not limited to paper, glass, and cans but also include such things as discarded tires and used oils. By following recommended disposal procedures, participating in recycling, and buying goods in recycled containers and made from recycled materials, people can reduce the spread of chemical contamination, slow the rate at which natural resources are consumed, reduce the cost of solid waste disposal, and help the nation gain time to develop more environmentally efficient methods of disposal and packaging.

> **Personal Insight** Are you ever tempted to throw toxic substances down the drain or in the trash? If so, what do or can you tell yourself in order to resist?

Food Inspection

Today we take for granted that the food we buy in grocery stores and in restaurants is safe to consume. This has not always been the case. At the turn of the century, tremendous pressure was put on the government to set minimum standards in all areas of food preparation and handling, resulting in the Pure Food and Drug Act of 1906. Illness and death associated with food-borne disease and toxic food additives have decreased substantially ever since (although there have been increases in some bacterial illnesses associated with undercooked meat, fish, and poultry). However, we are now becoming more concerned with the long-term health consequences of the foods we eat, either because of chemical contamination or because of characteristics of the foods themselves (as discussed in Chapters 12, 15, and 16, on nutrition, cardiovascular disease, and cancer).

Most people would be surprised at the number of agencies that inspect food at the various points of production. On the federal level, the Department of Agriculture inspects grains and meats, and the Food and Drug Administration is responsible for ensuring the wholesomeness of foods and regulating the chemicals that can be used in food, drugs, and cosmetics. On the state level, public health departments inspect dairy herds, milking barns, storage tanks, tankers that transport milk, and processing plants. Local health departments inspect and license restaurants.

Considering the number of meals eaten outside the home and the number of meals prepared at home with purchased food, it is remarkable how few instances there are of food-borne illness or death. The food distribution system in the United States is very safe and efficient. Recalls of ice cream, cheese, and tuna in recent years have usually been based on a potential for illness because of processing error, not on actual illness or death. In fact, most food-associated illnesses are caused by contamination in the home, such as from salmonella bacteria or from **staphylococcus** poisoning (see Chapter 12). It is estimated that each person in the United States suffers an average of two to three episodes of food poisoning every year, although these episodes are usually assumed to be caused by a 24-hour virus.

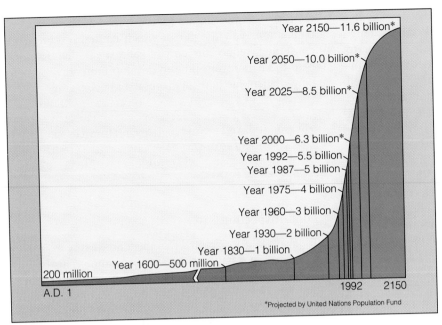

Insect and Rodent Control

A great number of illnesses can be transmitted to humans by animal and insect vectors. In recent years we have seen outbreaks of **encephalitis** transmitted by mosquitoes, **Lyme disease** from ticks in the Northeast, Midwest, and Pacific states (see Chapter 18), **Rocky Mountain spotted fever** from another type of tick in the Southeast, and **bubonic plague** from fleas on wild mammals in the West. Rodents carry forms of typhus, tapeworms, and even **salmonella**. Constant vigilance is necessary to minimize illness associated with insects and rodents. Disability and death from these diseases is prevented by spraying insecticides when necessary, wearing protective clothing, and exercising reasonable caution in infested areas.

POPULATION GROWTH

Throughout most of history, humans have been a minor pressure on the planet. About 200 million people were alive in A.D. 1; by the time Europeans were settling in the United States 1,600 years later, the world population had increased gradually to 500 million. But then it began rising exponentially—zooming to 1 billion by about 1830, more than doubling by 1950, and then doubling again in just 40 years (Figure 24-1). This rapid expansion of population, particularly in the last 50 years, is generally believed to be responsible for most of the stress humans put on the environment. A large and rapidly growing population makes it more difficult to provide the basic components of environmental health discussed earlier, including

clean and disease-free food and water; it is also a driving force behind many of the newer environmental health concerns, including chemical pollution, global warming, and thinning of the ozone layer of the atmosphere. (For more information on the relationship between population and land use, see the box "Indigenous Peoples and the Environmental Ethic.")

The world's population, currently about 5.5 billion people, is increasing at a rate of over a quarter of a million people a day. The United Nations now projects that even if fertility stabilizes at a replacement rate, world population will reach 10 billion by the year 2050 and level off at around 11.6 billion in about 2200. Most of this growth will take place in the developing world, where the population growth rates, although falling, are still double and even triple those of more affluent, developed countries. And the population of the developing world is young, with a greater potential for future growth: about 45 percent of Africans, 36 percent of Latin Americans, and 33 percent of Asians are under age 15, compared to about 20 percent in the developed nations. As a result, the developing countries are expected to account for about 85 percent of the world's population by 2025, up from their current level of 77 percent.

No one knows how many people the world can support, but most scientists agree that there is a limit. Factors that may eventually limit human population include the following:

- *Food.* Enough food is currently produced to feed the world's entire population, but economic and sociopolitical factors have led to food shortages and

DIMENSIONS OF DIVERSITY
Indigenous Peoples and the Environmental Ethic

At a time of increasing environmental problems, indigenous peoples could provide a model for a less exploitative relationship with the earth, according to a recent issue of *IDOC Internazionale,* an ecology-oriented magazine published in Rome.

"The technological advances of the last century have given many of us better health and longer life spans," writes editor Mary Judith Ress, "but in the process they have polluted our air, water, and soil. It is slowly dawning on us that technology has dulled our sense of affinity with the earth." Ress believes that it is time to take "a fresh look at indigenous people's view of the earth."

Indigenous peoples—the original inhabitants of a particular area—include Native Americans, aborigines in Australia, Maoris in New Zealand, Lapps in Scandinavian countries, and the native peoples of Greenland, Canada, and Alaska. Indigenous people are often national minorities, but they constitute the majority of the population in some countries, such as Bolivia, Guatemala, and South Africa. There are an estimated 200 million indigenous people in the world, approximately 4 percent of the total global population.

For most indigenous peoples, the land is the basis of existence. The earth is seen as a living entity from which life springs; as such, it must be respected and protected. The land is not something that can be accumulated or sold; even dividing it into plots may be viewed as akin to cutting and wounding it. Such views are being borne out in the Amazon rain forest. The native peoples who inhabit the Amazon see it as an intricate, harmoniously balanced world unto itself. Those who try to clear and cultivate Amazon lands find that the soil is poor and doesn't produce as expected. Once the natural balance is destroyed, the land dies, along with all it once supported.

A similar attitude is found toward human reproduction. Among the Desana, an indigenous people of the northwestern Amazon in Colombia, South America, humans have a responsibility to practice sexual and reproductive restraint in order to maintain a fragile equilibrium with the environment. In the Desana world view, all life draws on a vast, yet finite, reservoir of biological and reproductive energy. Every birth uses a small portion of the vital biological capacity upon which the entire natural world ultimately depends. Thus, human births, for all their personal pains and pleasures, do not take place in isolation. Each depletes the total energy available for the emergence of new life. The Desana build an ethical system around these views, designed to ensure that human beings respect the fundamental links between their own reproductive behavior and the fate of all other creatures.

The population ecologist may prefer to frame this idea differently—in terms of rising birth rates and falling death rates; in terms of the reduced capacities of pollution-degraded habitats to support animals, plants, and humans; or in terms of increased competition among species for fixed food resources. But the central message of the ecological scientist and the native are complementary, for both are rooted in the observations that life on earth is a vast interconnected system, that the fate of human beings is inextricably bound up with the fate of other species, and that nature is not inexhaustible.

Adapted from "Indigenous Peoples and the Environmental Ethic." *The Futurist,* May–June 1990; and D. Suzuki and P. Knudtson. 1992. *Wisdom of the Elders* (New York: Bantam Books), pp. 208–10.

---

famine. Food production can be expanded in the future, but better distribution of food will be needed to prevent even more widespread famine as the world's population grows. If all people are to receive adequate nutrition, the makeup of the world's diet may also need to change: Because animal products require more resources to produce, the world could support nearly twice as many vegetarians as people eating a typical American diet, which is based heavily on animal products.

• *Available land and water.* Rural populations rely on trees, soil, and water for their direct sustenance, and a growing population puts a strain on these resources—forests are cut for wood, soil is depleted, and water is withdrawn at ever-rising rates. These trends contribute to local hardships and to many global environmental problems, including habitat destruction and species extinction (see the box "Natural Ecosystems and Biodiversity").

• *Energy.* Currently, the majority of the world's energy comes from nonrenewable sources—oil, coal, natural gas, and nuclear power. As nonrenewable sources are depleted, the world will have to shift to renewable energy sources—hydropower, solar, geothermal,

---

Encephalitis An inflammation of the brain sometimes caused by insect-borne diseases.

Lyme disease A disease spread by a deer tick that can lead to fever and arthritis-like conditions if untreated.

Rocky Mountain spotted fever A wood-tick-borne disease causing high fevers and found primarily in the Southeast.

Bubonic plague A virulent infectious disease carried by fleas on wild mammals, marked by characteristic discolored swellings. One of the great plagues of the European Middle Ages.

Salmonella infection A bacterial infection often caused by eating food contaminated with fecal matter, such as improperly cleaned and cooked chicken.

TERMS

Our world supports an abundant variety of life. Scientists have identified about 1.4 million species, but they suspect that there are probably 10 to 80 million more. Different environments generate diverse life strategies, so that each ecosystem—from desert to tropical rain forest—contains a unique, close-knit community of organisms, linked together in a **food chain** or web. Plants use sunlight and soil for their needs. They, in turn, sustain herbivores (plant eaters), which may themselves succumb to predators. When predators and surviving herbivores die, they become food for scavengers, then insect larvae, and finally bacteria, which break them down into organic substances. These, drawn from the soil by plants, help to maintain the cycle. A similar system, based on plankton, exists in the oceans. Disruption at any point in this intricate, balanced cycle can alter or destroy an entire ecosystem.

Natural ecosystems provide humans with a wide variety of essential services. They maintain the climate and the composition of the atmosphere, cycle water and nutrients, produce food, dispose of organic wastes, generate and maintain soils, control pests, and pollinate crops; in addition, ecosystems support biological diversity (or **biodiversity**), represented by both the millions of different species on earth and the genetic diversity within these species. Biodiversity is critical, both as the basis for the future evolution of new species and as a genetic bank from which humans can draw useful genetic material and compounds. We have so far examined or used few of the available genetic resources, but those we have used have provided many benefits, including pest and disease resistance for crops and medicines. For example, species of wild rice in India and wild tomato in Peru have provided domestic species with the disease resistance they need to be productive, and many children with leukemia can now be saved due to drugs developed from the rosy periwinkle plant.

Human activity—driven by poverty and population growth in the developing world and excessive consumerism in the industrial nations—now threatens this biodiversity. Some species and populations are being lost through direct action, such as the overharvesting of whales, elephants, and certain fish. But the major danger comes indirectly, from habitat destruction: We are paving over, chopping down, digging up, draining, and poisoning many areas. The destruction of tropical rain forests, which are disappearing at the rate of an acre every second, is of particular concern. Rain forests cover only about 7 percent of the planet but are thought to harbor more than half the world's species. Extinction is irreversible, and species are disappearing far faster (50 to 100 a day) than they can be identified and assessed for useful properties. Some scientists fear that humans are precipitating a wave of mass extinction so great that the diminished stock of species will not be an adequate base on which natural selection can work to rebuild biodiversity. Even if adequate, it could take several million years for biodiversity to "bounce back." And because of the many ties between organisms and the physical environment, mass extinction could also threaten the functioning of the entire biosphere.

What can be done to maintain biodiversity? The United States has laws that protect specific (endangered) species, which by indirectly preserving natural communities help maintain biodiversity. International laws and conventions also protect certain rare species, although enforcement continues to be a problem. The Convention on Biological Diversity, signed by about 150 countries at the 1992 Earth Summit meeting in Rio de Janeiro, deals specifically with the issue of biodiversity. It commits countries to preserving and managing biological resources and to integrating plant and animal preservation into economic planning. It also allows countries that are rich in species but poor in cash to share in the profits from sales of medicines or other products derived from their biological resources. Although much still needs to be done to protect the biodiversity of our world, these actions are a step in the right direction.

---

wind, biomass, and ocean power. Supporting a growing population, maintaining economic productivity, and preventing further degradation of the environment will require greater energy efficiency and increased use of renewable energy sources.

- *Minimum acceptable standard of living.* The mass media have exposed the entire world to the American lifestyle and raised people's expectations of living at a comparable level. But the lifestyle in the United States is supported by levels of energy consumption that the earth cannot support on a worldwide basis. The United States has 5 percent of the world's population but uses 25 percent of the world's energy; India, with 16 percent of the population, uses only 3 percent of

the energy. An average American consumes 280 times the amount of energy that the average Ethiopian does. If *all* people are to enjoy a minimally acceptable standard of living, the population must be limited to a number that available resources can support.

Although it's apparent that population growth must be controlled, population trends are difficult to influence and manage. A variety of interconnecting factors fuel the current population explosion:

- *High fertility rates.* The combination of poverty, very high child mortality, and lack of social provisions of every type seen in the developing world are associated with high fertility rates. Perhaps families have to have more children to ensure that enough survive childhood to work for the household and to care for parents in old age.

- *Lack of family planning resources.* Half of the world's couples don't use any form of family planning, and 300 million couples worldwide say they want family planning services but cannot get them.
- *Lower death rates.* Although death rates remain relatively high in the developing world, they have decreased in recent years due to public health measures and improved medical care.

Changes in any of these factors can affect population growth, but the issues are complex. Increasing death rates through disease, famine, or war might slow population growth, but few people would argue in favor of this as a means of population control. Increased availability of family planning services is a crucial part of population management, but cultural, political, and religious factors also need to be considered (see Chapter 6 for more information on contraceptive use around the world).

To be successful, population management must change the condition of people's lives to remove the pressures for large families, especially poverty. Research indicates that the combination of improved health, better education, and increased literacy and employment opportunities for women works together with family planning to cut fertility rates. Unfortunately, in the fastest-growing countries, the needs of a rapidly increasing population use up financial resources that might otherwise be used to improve lives and ultimately slow population growth.

POLLUTION

As mentioned earlier, the classic environmental health concerns aren't just historical. They still have the potential to cause serious problems today under certain circumstances, and they take on added significance as our population grows. At the same time, new problems are arising, and some long-standing problems are gaining increased public attention. Many of these modern problems are problems of pollution. The term *pollution* refers to any unwanted contaminant in the environment that may pose a health risk. When we are talking about health risks, the level of concentration of a particular pollutant is very important. In typical concentrations, many environmental pollutants don't seem to harm our general health in the short term. The long-term effects are harder to evaluate.

Air Pollution

Air pollution is not a human invention or even a new problem. The air is "polluted" naturally with every forest fire, pollen bloom, and dust storm, as well as with count-

less other natural pollutants. To these natural sources, human beings have always contributed the by-products of their activities. During the Industrial Revolution, English cities had far more daily air pollution than we can observe or even imagine today. However, two recent developments have changed our attitudes toward air pollution. First, we are living long enough to experience both the short-term and the long-term consequences. Second, increased population growth, combined with more industrialization using old technologies, concentrates the problems and makes them more visible to the public and possibly more dangerous.

Air pollution can be more than just unsightly; it can cause illness and death if pollutants become concentrated for a period of several days or weeks. Public awareness of the dangers increased when London (1952) and New York City (1963) experienced air pollution disasters that made thousands ill and caused hundreds of premature deaths, primarily among those who already had respiratory problems. Increased amounts of carbon monoxide and air-borne acids and decreased amounts of oxygen all put excess strain on people suffering from **congestive heart failure** and **chronic obstructive pulmonary diseases**, such as chronic bronchitis or emphysema, as well as on the very young and the elderly.

Before an air pollution emergency can occur, three conditions must be present. First, there must be a source of pollution. Today, this is most frequently the burning of fossil fuels, such as coal in industry or gasoline in cars (Table 24-1). Second, there must be a topographical feature, such as a mountain range or a valley, that prevents the prevailing winds from pushing stagnant air out of the region. Third, there must be a weather event called a **temperature inversion**.

A temperature inversion occurs when there is little or no wind and a layer of warm air traps a layer of cold air next to the ground. Normally, the sun heats the earth, making the air closest to the ground warmer than that just above it. Warm air rises and is replaced by cooler air, which in turn is warmed and rises, thereby producing a

TERMS

Food chain   Transfers of food energy and other substances in which one type of organism consumes another.

Biodiversity   The variety of living things on earth, including all the different species of flora and fauna and the genetic diversity among individuals of the same species.

Congestive heart failure   A condition in which the heart cannot pump enough blood, leading to a buildup of fluid in the tissues.

Chronic obstructive pulmonary disease   A general term for respiratory diseases, such as emphysema and chronic bronchitis, in which airways are narrowed and oxygen intake is reduced.

Temperature inversion   A weather condition in which a cold layer of air is trapped by a warm layer so that pollutants cannot be dispersed.

TABLE 24-1 Sources and Effects of Common Air Pollutants

Pollutant	Sources	Effects
Sulfur dioxide (SO_2)	Burning of coal and fossil fuels	Irritates the respiratory tract; aggravates the symptoms of heart and lung disease; damages plants; (when mixed with water in the atmosphere) produces acid rain
Carbon monoxide (CO)	Combustion, especially fossil fuel combustion by motor vehicles	Deprives body of oxygen, causing headaches, fatigue, and impaired judgment; aggravates heart and vascular diseases
Nitrogen dioxide (NO_2)	Motor vehicles, power stations, industrial boilers, manufacture of fertilizers and other chemicals	Irritates the respiratory tract; causes bronchitis, pneumonia, and lowered resistance to respiratory infections; (when mixed with water in the atmosphere) produces acid rain
Particulates	Fossil fuel combustion	Carry heavy metals and carcinogens into the lungs; corrode metal; lessen visibility
Hydrocarbons (volatile organic compounds)	Incomplete fossil fuel combustion, evaporation of solvents and oil, natural sources	React with sunlight and other pollutants to form respiratory irritants and potential carcinogens
Ozone	Photochemical reactions (interaction of nitrogen oxides and hydrocarbons in the presence of sunlight)	Irritates mucous membranes; inflames eyes and respiratory tract; aggravates heart and lung diseases; damages plants and slows their growth

natural circulation. This circulation, combined with horizontal wind circulation, prevents pollutants from reaching dangerous levels of concentration.

When there is a temperature inversion, this replacement and cleansing action cannot occur. The effect is like covering an area with a dome that traps all the pollutants and prevents vertical dispersion. If this condition persists for several days, the buildup of pollutants may reach dangerous levels and threaten people's health. Many cities have plans for shutting down certain industries and even curtailing transportation if unsafe levels are approached. Most states and the federal government also have "clean air" legislation, which has improved air quality in the last 20 years in American cities.

The disasters of the 1950s and 1960s involved a human-made form of air pollution called smog. There are two types of smog, London-type smog and Los Angeles-type smog, distinguished primarily by the source of the pollution. **London-type smog** results from the burning of fossil fuels such as coal. At one time coal was the major source of heat for homes as well as the major energy source for factories. Now that many homes and factories use oil, steam, gas, and electricity, this source of pollution has been minimized in developed countries. However, coal burning is increasing in developing countries.

Los Angeles-type smog (also known as **photochemical smog**) is a more complex phenomenon. Here the source of pollution is primarily motor vehicle exhaust that contains oxides of nitrogen and hydrocarbons. When sunlight acts on these products (a photochemical reaction), the result is a characteristic brown smog. Large cities with a high ratio of cars to people and with poorly developed public transportation are more likely to experience Los Angeles-type smog. The health effects are very similar to London-type smog—eye irritation, impairment of respiratory and cardiovascular functioning in vulnerable individuals, and possibly cancers.

Concern about air pollution in the 1960s was one of several factors that led to the establishment of the U.S. Environmental Protection Agency (EPA), which has the task of setting standards and monitoring pollution levels. The EPA reports improved air quality as measured by decreased levels of smog and several airborne chemicals in many areas. How this improvement translates specifically into improved health status has yet to be determined.

In recent years, however, new atmospheric problems have surfaced that may have long-range effects on the planet, its climates, and its inhabitants. These are the "greenhouse effect," depletion of the ozone layer, and acid rain.

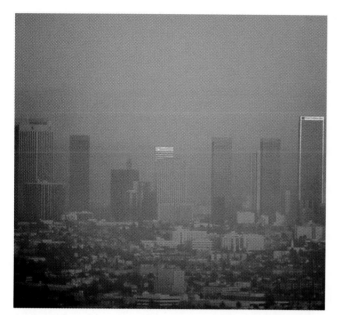

Smog tends to form over Los Angeles because of the natural geographical features of the area and because of the tremendous amount of motor vehicle exhaust in the air. The health effects of smog are most noticeable in people who already have some respiratory impairment.

The Greenhouse Effect and Global Warming The temperature of the earth's atmosphere depends on the balance between the amount of energy the earth absorbs from the sun (mainly as high-energy ultraviolet radiation) and the amount of energy radiated back into space as lower-energy infrared radiation. Key components of temperature regulation are carbon dioxide, water vapor, methane, and other "greenhouse gases"—so-called because, like a pane of glass in a greenhouse, they let through visible light from the sun but trap some of the resulting infrared radiation and reradiate it back to the earth's surface. This reradiation causes a buildup of heat that raises the temperature of the earth's lower atmosphere, a natural process known as the **greenhouse effect**. Without it, the atmosphere would be far cooler and considerably more hostile to life.

Human activity may be tipping this balance toward global warming. The concentration of greenhouse gases is increasing due to human activity, especially the combustion of oil, gasoline, coal, and natural gas. Carbon dioxide levels in the atmosphere have increased rapidly since the onset of the Industrial Revolution, and current levels are higher than at any time in the past 100,000 years. Deforestation, often by burning, also sends carbon dioxide into the atmosphere and reduces the number of trees available to convert carbon dioxide into oxygen. But energy use in the developed world is the primary cause of increases in the concentrations of greenhouse gases. The United States alone is responsible for over 20 percent of the world's total emission of greenhouse gases.

Many experts predict that this increase in greenhouse gases will cause temperatures on earth to rise and climates all over the planet to become warmer. Such a temperature rise, they say, may melt the polar ice caps, raise the level of the sea, and change ocean currents and weather patterns, affecting seacoasts and food-producing areas of the world. Some experts predict a rise of 4 to 7° F worldwide in the next 70 years; others predict a milder warming of 1 to 2° F. Whatever the outcome, the full implications of this type of climate change are unknown.

The Ozone Layer A second air pollution problem is the thinning of the **ozone layer** of the atmosphere—a fragile, invisible layer about 10 to 30 miles above the earth that shields the surface of the planet from the sun's hazardous ultraviolet (UV) rays. Since the mid-1980s, scientists have observed the seasonal appearance and growth of a "hole" in the ozone layer over Antarctica. More recently, thinning over the Arctic and other areas of the north, including Canada, Scandinavia, the northern United States, and parts of the former Soviet Union, has been noted.

The ozone layer is being destroyed primarily by **chlorofluorocarbons (CFCs)**, industrial chemicals used as coolants in refrigerators and in home and automobile air conditioners; as foaming agents in some rigid foam products, including insulation; as propellants in some kinds of aerosol sprays (most such sprays were banned in 1978); and as solvents. When CFCs rise into the atmosphere, winds carry them toward the polar regions. During winter, circular winds form a vortex that keeps air over Antarctica from mixing with air from elsewhere. Ice crystals form in the Antarctic clouds during the cold, sunless months; chemical reactions taking place on these crystals, which wouldn't take place in air, free chlorine atoms from CFCs. When stimulated by the reappearance of the sun, the chlorine atoms begin destroying ozone (Figure 24-2). When the polar vortex weakens in the summer, winds richer in ozone from the north replenish

TERMS

London-type smog An air pollution problem caused by coal burning.

Los Angeles-type smog An air pollution problem caused by the burning of transportation fuels in combination with sunlight.

Photochemical smog Another term for Los Angeles-type smog; caused by sunlight (hence "photo") reacting with transportation fuels (hence "chemical").

Greenhouse effect Warming of the earth due to a buildup of carbon dioxide and certain other gases.

Ozone layer A layer of oxygen molecules in the upper atmosphere that screens out ultraviolet rays from the sun.

Chlorofluorocarbons (CFCs) Chemicals used as spray-can propellants, refrigerants, and industrial solvents, implicated in the destruction of the ozone layer.

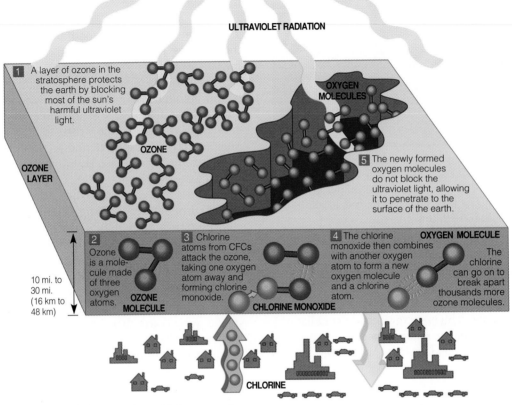

ULTRAVIOLET RADIATION

1 A layer of ozone in the stratosphere protects the earth by blocking most of the sun's harmful ultraviolet light.

OZONE LAYER

OZONE

OXYGEN MOLECULES

5 The newly formed oxygen molecules do not block the ultraviolet light, allowing it to penetrate to the surface of the earth.

10 mi. to 30 mi. (16 km to 48 km)

2 Ozone is a molecule made of three oxygen atoms. **OZONE MOLECULE**

3 Chlorine atoms from CFCs attack the ozone, taking one oxygen atom away and forming chlorine monoxide. **CHLORINE MONOXIDE**

4 The chlorine monoxide then combines with another oxygen atom to form a new oxygen molecule and a chlorine atom. **OXYGEN MOLECULE**

The chlorine can go on to break apart thousands more ozone molecules.

CHLORINE

Figure 24-2 *Destruction of the ozone layer of the atmosphere.*
Source: Time, 17 February 1992, p. 63.

the lost Antarctic ozone, but the ozone hole's growth each year may be contributing to the general thinning of the global ozone layer.

The ozone hole in the Antarctic in late 1992 was the largest to date—roughly equal to the size of North America. Scientists believe that in addition to the buildup of chlorine from CFCs and other chemicals, substances released by the 1991 volcanic eruptions of Mount Pinatubo in the Philippines and Mount Hudson in Chile accelerated the ozone depletion in 1992. Since 1979 about 15 percent of Antarctic ozone has been destroyed, although locally and seasonally up to 95 percent of the ozone disappears (forming the "hole"). In the Northern Hemisphere, ozone levels have declined 4 to 8 percent in the past decade, and certain regions may be temporarily depleted in late winter and early spring by as much as 40 percent.

The loss of ozone is of concern because without the ozone layer to absorb ultraviolet radiation from the sun, life on earth would be impossible. The potential effects of increased long-term exposure to UV light for humans include skin cancer, wrinkling and aging of the skin, cataracts and blindness, and reduced immune response. The United Nations Environmental Program predicts that a drop of 10 percent in overall ozone levels would cause a 26 percent rise in the incidence of nonmelanoma skin cancer. UV light may interfere with photosynthesis and cause lower crop yields; it may also kill phytoplankton and krill, which are the basis of the ocean food chain. And because heat generated by the absorption of UV rays in the ozone layer helps create stratospheric winds, the driving force behind weather patterns, a drop in the concentration of ozone could potentially alter the earth's climate systems.

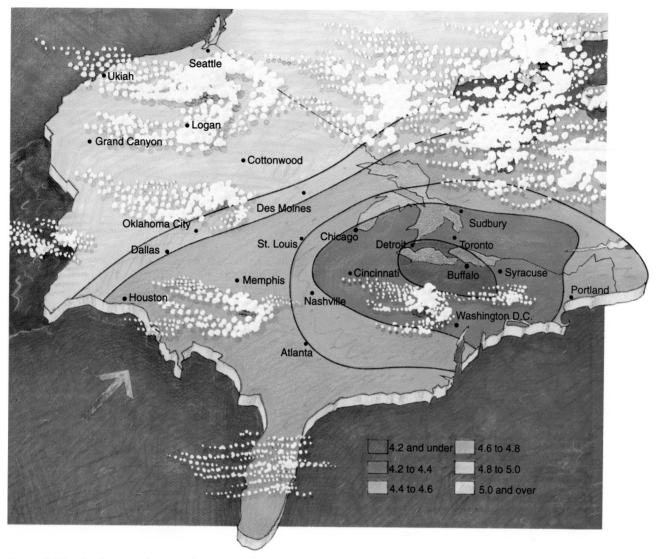

Figure 24-3 *Acid rain in the United States.*
On the 14-point pH scale of acidity and alkalinity, a perfectly neutral sample of water would
have a 7.0 rating. Unpolluted rainwater, which registers a pH of 5.6, may be described as
slightly acidic because of the combination of carbon dioxide with water vapor. A one-point
increase in acidity on this logarithmic scale means a tenfold boost in that critical measurement,
so a pH of 4.10, for example, indicates that rainfall is 31.6 times more acidic than normal.

Worldwide production and use of CFCs and other ozone-destroying substances has declined rapidly since the danger to the ozone layer was recognized. But even if all use of CFCs stopped today, future ozone losses are inevitable because CFCs can persist in the atmosphere for more than a century.

Acid Rain   A by-product of many industrial processes, **acid rain** occurs when atmospheric pollutants combine with moisture in the air and fall to earth as highly acidic rain or snow. It occurs especially when coal containing large amounts of sulfur is burned and sulfur dioxide, sulfur trioxide, nitrogen dioxide, nitric acid, and other chemicals are released into the atmosphere. These con-

centrations can be carried great distances by the prevailing winds and form a highly acidic mixture containing sulfuric acid and nitric acid. Most of the pollutants in acid rain are produced by coal-burning electric power plants. Other sources include motor vehicles and certain industrial activities, such as smelting.

Many trees and some aquatic life can tolerate only a very narrow range of acidity and are either weakened or killed by acid rain. Currently, acid rain seems to be affecting forests, lakes, and streams in Canada, the northeastern United States, southern Sweden, Norway, and parts of central Europe (Figure 24-3). Thousands of lakes in Sweden are now so acidified that fish stocks have been severely reduced, and in Bavaria and other areas of central

Although most people associate air pollution with the outdoors, your home may also harbor potentially dangerous pollutants. Some of these substances trigger allergic responses, while others have been linked to cancer. The EPA has reported that toxic chemicals found in the home are three times more likely to cause cancer than are outdoor airborne pollutants.

Radon is a naturally occurring radioactive gas produced by the breakdown of uranium. Virtually all soil contains some uranium and therefore some radon. Most radon enters a home by rising through the soil into the basement through dirt floors, cracks, and other openings; it can also enter via well water. When the breakdown products of radon are inhaled, they cling to lungs and bombard sensitive tissue with radioactivity, which can cause lung cancer. An elevated radon level in the home can be the cancer equivalent of smoking about 10 cigarettes a day.

Houses with elevated radon levels are usually found in areas where uranium-bearing rock formations are prevalent, such as in the Northeast and Midwest. However, there is great variation in radon levels from one house to another even in these areas. Kits for radon testing are available in many hardware stores; state or local health departments can usually provide lists of suppliers whose test kits meet EPA requirements.

Suggestions for reducing radon are described in free literature available from EPA offices or health agencies. A moderately high radon level can usually be reduced by sealing all basement floor and wall cracks and openings with caulking compound and covering openings to floor drains with airtight covers. Increasing basement ventilation is also helpful. High levels of radon require the skills of a qualified contractor, who usually must install pipes and fans that draw radon-laden air from under the basement floor to the outside.

Environmental tobacco smoke (ETS) has been classified as a human carcinogen by the EPA, and it also increases the risk for asthma, bronchitis, and cardiovascular disease. The solution to curbing this indoor air pollutant is a simple one: Don't smoke and don't allow others to smoke in your home or apartment. If that rule is too strict for your situation, limit smoking to a single, well-ventilated room.

Formaldehyde gas seeps from resins used in manufacturing particle board, plywood paneling, and some carpeting and upholstery. In the short term, it can cause eye, nose, and throat irritations; shortness of breath; headaches; nausea; and lethargy. Long-term exposure increases the risk of cancer. Mobile homes and newly built homes are most likely to be affected. Treatments for high levels of formaldehyde include removing or treating the sources, purifying the air, increasing ventilation, and avoiding new sources of the gas.

Asbestos and other mineral fibers, commonly used in insulation and building materials, can cause severe lung disease and cancer if they are released into the air and inhaled. About one quarter of existing American houses and apartment buildings are thought to contain some asbestos. Areas where it is most likely to be found include insulation around water and steam pipes, ducts, and furnaces; boiler wraps; vinyl flooring; floor, wall, and ceiling insulation; roofing and siding; textured paints made before 1978; and fireproof board.

Be cautious around suspected asbestos-containing materials in your house. Look for areas where asbestos has become damaged by water, dented, corroded, blistered, or otherwise changed in a fashion likely to release fibers into the air. An experienced contractor can pinpoint asbestos-containing materials in your home, which can be analyzed by a laboratory. If the sample tests positive, the asbestos should be sealed off, encapsulated, or removed by a professional.

Combustion by-products, including carbon monoxide, nitrogen dioxide, and sulfur dioxide, are produced when anything is burned; sources include wood stoves, fireplaces, candles, kerosene heaters and lamps, cigarettes, and gas ranges. If they build up in your house, they can cause chronic bronchitis, headaches, dizziness, nausea, fatigue, and even death. In most houses, pollution from combustion is not a serious problem, but appliances need to be properly installed, vented, and serviced. Having furnaces inspected regularly and chimneys cleaned once a year can help prevent problems.

Biological pollutants, including bacteria, dust mites, mold, and animal dander, can pollute indoor air and cause allergic reactions and other health problems. Two essential conditions to support biologic growth are nutrients and moisture, typically found in bathrooms, damp or flooded basements, humidifiers, air conditioners, and even some carpets and furniture. Techniques for ridding the home of biological pollutants include fixing leaks and moisture seepage, using exhaust fans in bathrooms and kitchens, venting clothes dryers to the outside, and using dehumidifiers. Keeping moist surfaces clean, washing bedding in hot water to kill dust mites, and dusting and vacuuming often can also help.

Some commonsense tips for controlling all indoor air pollution problems include the following:

- Keep your house adequately ventilated.
- Follow manufacturer's directions when using a product that emits pollutants.
- Keep paints, cleaning agents, and other chemical products in their original, tightly sealed containers and store them in cool, well-vented areas.
- Clean and service appliances regularly.
- Buy some houseplants, which have a natural ability to rid the air of harmful pollutants.

For more information about indoor air pollution, contact your local or state health department or the regional EPA office. Other sources of information include the Indoor Air Quality Clearing House (800-438-4318), the EPA Consumer Product Safety Commission hot line (800-638-2772), and the EPA Toxic Substances Control hot line (202-554-1404).

Europe, whole forests are dying. As for damage in the United States, the National Acid Precipitation Assessment Program found that acid rain has adversely affected aquatic life in about 10 percent of eastern lakes and streams, contributed to the decline of red spruce at high elevations by reducing its cold tolerance, and contributed to erosion and corrosion of buildings and materials. There is also concern that long-term exposure to acid rain could cause nutrient deficiencies in soil, endanger food chains, and activate heavy metals such as mercury, contaminating water supplies.

> *Personal Insight* If you found out you could get a smog certificate without having to get your car fixed, what would you do? Would the convenience be worth the pollution?

Chemical Pollution

Chemical pollution is by no means a new problem. The ancient Romans were plagued by lead poisoning, which damages the central nervous system, in part because they stored sugar solutions in lead containers. Two hundred years ago in Europe, the phrase "mad as a hatter" came from the hatters' practice of preparing felt hats with mercury—which also destroyed the central nervous system.

The difference today is that new chemical substances are constantly being created and introduced into the environment, whether as pesticides, herbicides, solvents, cleaning fluids, flame retardants, or any of hundreds of other products. We have many more chemicals, in more concentrated forms and in wider use, and larger numbers of people are exposed and potentially exposed to them than ever before.

Chemical pollutants have been responsible for several environmental disasters. The Hudson River in New York and the Housatonic River in Massachusetts have both been contaminated with polychlorinated biphenyls (PCBs), carcinogenic compounds used in the manufacture of electrical appliances. In 1984, thousands of people in Bhopal, India, were killed and injured when a powerful chemical used in manufacturing the insecticide Sevin was released from a plant. Catastrophes illustrate the short-term potential for disaster, but the long-term health consequences may be just as deadly. The following are brief descriptions of just a few current problems.

Asbestos A mineral-based compound, asbestos was widely used for fire protection and insulation in buildings until the late 1960s. When first introduced, asbestos was hailed as a great advance in fire safety. As long as it stayed where it was applied and its protective coating was not disturbed, there was no problem. However, microscopic asbestos fibers can be released into the air when this ma-

terial is applied or when it later deteriorates or is damaged. These fibers can lodge in the lungs, causing **asbestosis**, lung cancer, and other serious lung diseases. Similar conditions are risks in the coal mining industry, from exposure to coal dust (black lung disease), and in the textile industry, from exposure to cotton fibers (brown lung disease).

Media and public awareness led to a 1987 federal law requiring that asbestos be removed from schools under certain circumstances. Unfortunately, removal creates the very conditions in which asbestos is most dangerous, so it has to be done carefully by trained workers. Asbestos can also pose a danger in homes (for more information on asbestos and other hazards in the home, see the box "Indoor Air Pollution").

Lead Poisoning Lead poisoning continues to be a serious problem, particularly among children living in older buildings and adults who are exposed to lead in the workplace. When lead is ingested or inhaled, it can damage the central nervous system, cause mental retardation, hinder oxygen transport in the blood, and create digestive problems. Severe lead poisoning may cause coma or even death. Some symptoms of lead poisoning, including anemia, headaches, and abdominal pain, may cease if exposure stops, but neurological impairment can be permanent. Lead damage to the brain can start even before birth if a pregnant woman has elevated levels of lead in her body.

In 1991, the Centers for Disease Control lowered the standard of maximum safe lead exposure for children; they estimate that 3 million children under age 6 may have unsafe lead levels in their blood. Long-term exposure to low levels of lead can cause lead to build up in bones, where it may be released into the bloodstream in response to pregnancy or when bone mass is lost due to osteoporosis. Little is known about the effect of lead stored in or freed from bone.

Young children, who pick up dust and dirt on their hands and then put their hands in their mouths, can easily ingest lead from their environment. Lead-based paints are believed to be the chief culprit in lead poisoning of children. They were banned from residential use in 1978, but as many as 57 million American homes still contain lead paint. The use of lead in plumbing is now also banned, but some old pipes and faucets contain lead that can leach into drinking water. Lead gets into the air from

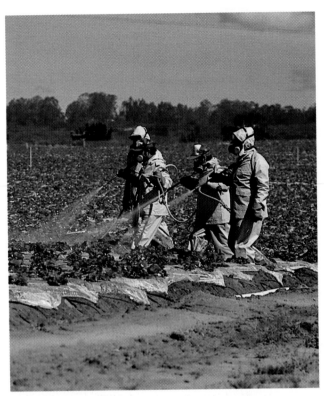

Although some pesticide residues may remain in or on produce when it reaches the consumer, the most serious health effects of pesticides are seen in agricultural workers. Special clothing and equipment help protect these workers from toxic chemicals as they spray strawberries.

industrial and vehicle emissions, from tobacco smoke and paint dust, and from the burning of solid wastes that contain lead. Levels of lead in the air have dropped sharply as leaded gas use declined, but many vehicles still use leaded fuel. Lead occurs naturally in soil, which also collects lead from the air and other sources. Other sources of lead include foods stored or served in lead-glazed pottery or lead crystal as well as processed foods sold in lead-soldered cans.

Pesticides   Pesticides are used primarily for two purposes—to prevent the spread of insect-borne disease and to maximize food production by killing insects that eat crops. Both uses have risks as well as benefits. Take, for example, the pesticide **DDT**. Recognized as a powerful pesticide in 1939, DDT was extremely important in efforts to control widespread insect-borne diseases in tropical countries and increase crop yields throughout the world. But in 1962, biologist Rachel Carson questioned the safety of DDT in her book *Silent Spring*, pointing out that the pesticide disrupts the life cycles of birds, fish, and reptiles. DDT also builds up in the food chain, increasing in concentration as larger animals eat smaller ones (a process known as **biomagnification**). DDT was banned in the United States in 1972 despite its effectiveness as a

pesticide because the costs associated with its use—to wildlife and potentially to human life—were too high. Most pesticide hazards to date have been a result of overuse and abuse, but there are concerns about the health effects of long-term exposure to small amounts of pesticide residues in foods.

The list of real and potential chemical pollution problems may well be as long as the list of known chemicals. To the preceding list we can add recent concern about mercury in fish, **formaldehyde** in synthetic building materials, and other by-products of our industrial age. As mentioned earlier, hazardous wastes are also found in the home and should be handled and disposed of properly. They include automotive supplies (motor oil, antifreeze, transmission fluid), paint supplies (turpentine, paint thinner, mineral spirits), art and hobby supplies (oil-based paint, solvents, acids and alkalis, aerosol sprays), insecticides, batteries, and household cleaners containing sodium hydroxide (lye) or ammonia. These chemicals are dangerous when inhaled or ingested, when they contact the skin or the eyes, or when they are burned or dumped. Many communities provide guidelines about approved disposal methods for household chemicals and have special hazardous waste collection days. (Refer to Table 23-3 in Chapter 23 for a summary of disposal guidelines for some hazardous wastes.)

Radiation

Many people are afraid of **radiation**; in part because they don't understand what it is. Basically, radiation is energy. It can come in different forms, such as ultraviolet rays, microwaves, or x-rays, and from different sources, such as the sun, uranium, and nuclear weapons. Although radiation can't be seen, heard, smelled, tasted, or felt, its health effects can include **radiation sickness** and death at high doses and chromosome damage, sterility, tissue damage, cataracts, and cancers at lower doses. Currently, health concerns about radiation center on nuclear weapons and nuclear energy, medical uses of radiation, and sources of radiation in the home and workplace.

Nuclear Weapons and Nuclear Energy   Nuclear weapons pose a health risk of the most serious kind to all species. Public health associations have stated that in the event of an intentional or accidental discharge of these weapons, both "health" and "public" would become meaningless words. In even the most conservative estimates of a "limited" nuclear war, the casualties would run into the hundreds of thousands or millions. Reducing these stockpiles is a challenge and a goal for the 1990s.

Power-generating plants that use nuclear fuel also pose health problems. When **nuclear power** was first developed as an alternative to oil and coal, it was promoted as clean, efficient, inexpensive, and safe. In general, this has

TABLE 24-2 Levels and Effects of Selected Sounds

Sound	Decibel (dB)	Effects
Normal conversation	50–65	Under 60 dB is comfortable listening.
Vacuum cleaner	70	More than 70 dB interferes with telephone use.
Lawn mower	85–90	More than 85 dB is very annoying. Hearing damage begins after 8 hours of exposure.
Power saw/chain saw	110	Regular exposure to more than 100 dB for longer than 1 minute risks permanent hearing loss.
Boom box—stereo with more than 120 watts	120	Threshold to produce vibration.
Jet takeoff	130	The threshold of pain is beyond 125 dB.
Shotgun firing	130	The threshold of pain is beyond 125 dB.
Rock concerts	110–140	The threshold of pain is beyond 125 dB.

Source: National Institute on Deafness and Other Communication Disorders

proven to be the case. Power systems in several parts of the world rely on nuclear generating plants. However, despite all the built-in safeguards and regulating agencies, accidents in nuclear power plants do happen, and the consequences of such accidents are far more serious than similar accidents in other types of power-generating plants. The accidents at Three Mile Island in 1979 and at Chernobyl in the former Soviet Union in 1986 demonstrated the potential for disaster that exists at nuclear plants.

An additional, enormous problem is disposing of the radioactive wastes these plants generate. They cannot be dumped in a sanitary landfill because the amount and type of soil used to cap a sanitary landfill is not sufficient to prevent radiation exposure. Deposit sites have to be developed that will be secure not just for a few years but for tens of thousands of years—longer than the total recorded history of human beings on this planet. To date, no storage method has been devised that can provide infallible, infinitely durable shielding for nuclear waste.

Medical Uses of Radiation
Another area of concern is the use of radiation in medicine, primarily the x-ray. The development of machines that could produce images of the internal bone structure was a major advance in medicine, and applications abounded. Chest x-rays were routinely given to screen for tuberculosis, and children's feet were even x-rayed in shoe stores to make sure their new shoes fit properly. But as is so often the case, this advance was not without a cost. As time passed, studies revealed that x-ray exposure is cumulative and that no exposure is absolutely safe.

Early x-ray machines are no longer used because of the high amounts of radiation they give off. Each "generation" of x-ray machines has used less radiation more effectively. From a personal health point of view, individuals should never have a "routine" x-ray examination. Each x-ray exam should have a definite purpose, and its benefits and risks should be carefully weighed. Many health professionals are beginning to recommend that records of all x-ray exposures be kept for every individual, the same way a record of vaccinations is kept.

Radiation in the Home and Workplace
Recently, there has been concern about the electromagnetic radiation associated with such common modern devices as microwave ovens, computer video display terminals (VDTs), microwave telephones, and even high-voltage power

TERMS

DDT A common insecticide now stringently controlled in the United States.

Biomagnification The accumulation of a substance in a food chain.

Formaldehyde A powerful disinfectant gas often used in solution for germ control but also given off by some synthetic building materials.

Radiation Energy transmitted in the form of rays, waves, or particles.

Radiation sickness An illness caused by excess radiation exposure, marked by low white blood counts and nausea; possibly fatal.

Nuclear power Use of controlled nuclear reactions to produce steam, which in turn drives turbines to produce electricity.

lines. We know that these forms of radiation do have effects on health. For example, new bone growth at the point of a fracture can be stimulated by a slight electric current. But current research is contradictory and inconclusive about the health effects of this type of radiation.

Another recent area of concern is **radon**, a form of radiation that is found in certain soils, rocks, and building materials. An unknown number of homes have been built on or with these substances. Well-insulated homes retain radon and allow higher concentrations to develop. Radon gas increases the incidence of lung cancer. Most state health departments can now test for radon gas concentrations, but the short- and long-term health consequences of radon are still unknown (for more on radon, see the box "Indoor Air Pollution").

Noise Pollution

We are increasingly aware of the health effects of loud or persistent noise in the environment. Concerns focus on two areas, hearing loss and stress. Prolonged exposure to sounds above 80–85 **decibels** (a measure of the volume of sound) can cause permanent hearing loss (Table 24-2). The scream of an infant, the noise in a machine shop, and freeway traffic sounds can all exceed the safe range. Two common potential sources of excessive noise are the workplace and large gatherings of people at sporting events, rock concerts, and so on. The Occupational Safety and Health Administration (OSHA) sets legal standards for noise in the workplace, but no laws exist regulating noise levels at rock concerts, which often exceed OSHA standards for the workplace.

Most hearing loss occurs in the first two hours of exposure, and hearing usually bounces back within two hours after the noise stops. But if exposure continues or is repeated frequently, hearing loss may be permanent. The employees of a club where rock music is played loudly are at much greater risk than the patrons of the club, who might be exposed for only two hours at a time. Another possible effect of exposure to excessive noise is **tinnitus**, a condition of more or less continuous ringing or buzzing in the ears.

Excessive noise is also an environmental stressor, producing the typical stress response described in Chapter 2—faster heart rate, increased respiration, higher blood pressure, and so on. A chronic and prolonged stress response can have serious effects on health. To prevent hearing loss and protect your general well-being, follow these key safety tips for dealing with noise:

- Wear ear protectors when working around noisy machinery.
- When listening on a headset with the volume numbered 1 through 10, keep the volume no louder than 4; your headset is too loud if you are unable to hear people around you speaking in a normal tone of voice.

- Avoid loud music. Don't sit or stand near speakers or amplifiers at a rock concert and don't play a car radio or stereo so high that you can't hear the traffic.
- Avoid any exposure to painfully loud sounds and avoid repeated exposure to any sounds above 80 decibels.

WHAT CAN YOU DO?

Faced with a vast array of confusing and complex ecological issues, you as an individual may feel overwhelmed. You may conclude that there isn't anything you can do about global problems. But this isn't true. If everyone made individual changes in his or her life, the impact would be tremendous. (To assess your current lifestyle, refer to the box "Environmental Health Checklist.")

At the same time, it's important to recognize that large corporations and manufacturers are the ones primarily responsible for environmental degradation. Many of them have jumped on the "environmental bandwagon" with public relations and advertising campaigns designed to make them look good, but they haven't changed their practices. To influence them, people have to become educated, demand changes in production methods, and elect people to office who consider both environmental concerns and business profits.

Large-scale changes and individual actions complement each other. What you do every day *does* count; the following is just a sampling of some of the ways that you can make a difference.

Conserving Energy, Improving the Air

- Cut back on driving. Ride your bike, walk, use public transportation, or carpool in a fuel-efficient vehicle.
- Keep your car tuned up and well-maintained. Use only unleaded gas and keep your tires inflated at recommended pressures. To save energy when driving, avoid jackrabbit starts, stay within the speed limit, don't use your air conditioner when opening the window would suffice, and don't let your car idle unless absolutely necessary.
- Use less electricity and less heat. Make sure your home is well-insulated; use insulating shades and curtains to keep heat in during winter and out during summer. Seal any openings in walls, floors, electrical outlets, and around doors and windows that are producing drafts. In cold weather, put on a sweater and turn down the thermostat. In hot weather, wear lightweight clothing and, whenever possible, use a fan rather than an air conditioner to cool yourself.
- Buy energy-efficient appliances and use them only when necessary. Run the washing machine, the dryer, and dishwasher only when you have full loads, and

The following list of statements relates to your impact on the environment. Put a check next to the statements that are true for you.

_____ I ride my bike, walk, carpool, or use public transportation whenever possible.

_____ I keep my car tuned up and well maintained.

_____ My residence is well insulated.

_____ Where possible, I use compact fluorescent bulbs instead of incandescent bulbs.

_____ I turn off lights and appliances when they are not in use.

_____ I avoid turning on heat or air conditioning whenever possible.

_____ I run the washing machine, dryer, and dishwasher only when they have full loads.

_____ I run the clothes dryer only as long as it takes my clothes to dry.

_____ I dry my hair with a towel rather than a hair dryer.

_____ I keep my car's air conditioner in good working order and have it serviced by a service station that recycles CFCs.

_____ I don't buy products that contain CFCs or methyl chloroform.

_____ When shopping, I choose products with the least amount of packaging.

_____ I choose recycled and recyclable products.

_____ I avoid products packaged in plastic and unrecycled aluminum.

_____ I store food in glass jars and waxed paper rather than plastic wrap.

_____ I take my own bag along when I go shopping.

_____ I recycle newspapers, glass, cans, and other recyclables.

_____ When shopping, I read labels and try to buy the least toxic products available.

_____ I dispose of household hazardous wastes properly.

_____ I take showers instead of baths.

_____ I take short showers and switch off the water when I'm not actively using it.

_____ I do not run the water while brushing my teeth, shaving, or hand-washing clothes.

_____ My sinks have aerators installed in them.

_____ My shower has a low-flow showerhead.

_____ I have a water displacement device in my toilet.

_____ I snip or rip plastic six-pack rings before I throw them out.

_____ When hiking or camping, I never leave anything behind.

Statements that you have not checked can help you identify behaviors that you can change to improve environmental health.

---

do laundry in warm or cold water instead of hot; don't overdry your clothes. Clean refrigerator coils and the clothes dryer lint screens frequently. Dry your hair with a towel instead of an electric dryer.

- Replace incandescent light bulbs with compact fluorescent bulbs (not fluorescent tubes). They cost more initially but save you money over the life of the bulb. They produce a comparable light, last longer, and use about one-third to one-quarter of the energy of a regular bulb. By using less electricity, they contribute to lower carbon dioxide emissions from electric power plants.

- Plant and care for trees in your own yard and neighborhood. Because they recycle carbon dioxide, trees work against global warming. They also provide shade and cool the air, so less air conditioning is needed.

Saving the Ozone Layer

- Keep your car's air conditioner in good working order and have it serviced by a service station that recycles CFCs. (Auto air conditioners are a major source of CFC emissions in the United States.)

- Check labels on aerosol cans and avoid those that contain CFCs (some products, including VCR-head cleaners and drain plungers, are still allowed to contain CFCs). Also, avoid products containing methyl chloroform, also called 1,1,1-trichloroethane, which also depletes the ozone layer. Bug sprays, fabric protectors, spot removers, and a variety of other consumer products typically contain methyl chloroform.

- Don't use foam plastic insulation in your home, unless it is made with ozone-safe agents. Buy an energy-efficient refrigerator and keep it in good working order. Don't buy a halon fire extinguisher for

---

TERMS

Radon A naturally occurring radioactive gas that is emitted from rocks and natural building materials and that can become concentrated in insulated homes, causing lung cancer.

Decibel A unit for expressing the relative intensity of sounds; 0 is least perceptible, and 130 is the average pain level.

Tinnitus Ringing in the ears, a condition that can be caused by excessive noise exposure.

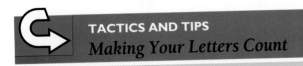

It takes only a few minutes to write to an elected official, but it can make a difference on an environmental issue you care about. When elected officials receive enough letters on a particular issue, it will influence their votes—they want to be reelected and your vote counts!

To help give your letter the greatest possible impact:

- Use your own words and your own stationery.

- Be concise, but try to write more than just one or two sentences. A one-page letter is a good length.

- Identify your subject clearly—refer to legislation by its name or number.

- Discuss only one issue in each letter—different issues are handled by different staff members, so stick to one subject to ensure your letter goes to the right person.

- Ask the legislator to do something specific—to vote a particular way on a particular bill, request hearings, cosponsor a bill, etc.

- Ask for a reply.

- Try not to use form letters.

- Don't be unnecessarily critical. Never threaten or insult.

To find out the current status of legislation pending in the House or Senate, call the legislative status line: 202-225-1772.

Your phone book has addresses of all state and local representatives. United States senators and representatives can be reached at the following addresses:

The Honorable _____
United States Senate
Washington, DC 20510

Dear Senator_____:

The Honorable_____
U.S. House of Representatives
Washington, DC 20515

Dear Representative _____:

Adapted from R. Wild, ed. 1990. *The Earth Care Annual 1990.* Emmaus, Penn.: National Wildlife Federation and Rodale Press.

---

home use (halons are as much as 10 times more destructive to ozone than are CFCs).

Reducing Garbage

- Buy products with the least amount of packaging you can, or buy products in bulk. For example, buy large jars of juice, not individually packaged juice drinks. Buy products packaged in glass, paper, or metal containers; avoid plastic and aluminum (unless it's recycled). Reuse glass containers to store products bought in bulk or other household items.

- Buy recycled or recyclable products. Avoid disposables; instead use long-lasting or reusable products such as refillable pens and rechargeable batteries.

- When shopping, take along your own bag. Reuse paper and plastic bags.

- Don't buy or use products stored or served in polystyrene foam. Avoid using foam or paper cups and plastic stirrers by bringing your own china coffee mug and metal spoon to work or wherever you buy and drink coffee or tea.

- To store food, use glass jars and reusable plastic containers rather than plastic wrap.

- Recycle your newspapers, glass, cans, paper, and other recyclables. If your sanitation department doesn't pick up recyclables, take them to a local recycling center. If you receive something packaged with foam pellets, take them to a commercial mailing center that accepts them for recycling.

- Start a compost pile for your organic garbage (non-animal food and yard waste) if you have a yard. If you live in an apartment, you can create a small composting system using earthworms or take your organic wastes to a community composting center.

Reducing Chemical Pollution and Toxic Wastes

- When buying products, read labels and try to buy the least toxic ones available. Choose nontoxic, nonpetrochemical cleansers, disinfectants, polishes, and other personal and household products.

- Dispose of your household hazardous wastes properly. If you're not sure whether something is hazardous or don't know how to dispose of it, contact your local environmental health office or health department. Don't burn trash.

- Buy organic produce or produce that is in season and has been grown locally. Consider eating less meat; animal products require more pesticides, fertilizer, water, and energy to produce.

Saving Water

- Take showers, not baths, to cut water consumption. Don't let water run when you're not actively using it while brushing your teeth, shaving, or hand-washing clothes. Don't run a dishwasher or washing machine until you have a full load.

- Install sink faucet aerators and water-efficient showerheads, which use two to five times less water with no noticeable decrease in performance.

- Put a displacement device in your toilet tank to reduce the amount of water used with each flush. A plastic bottle or bag filled with water works well.

Preserving Wildlife and the Natural Environment

- Snip or rip plastic six-pack rings. When seabirds and animals get them stuck on their necks or bills, they can strangle or starve to death.

- Don't buy products made from endangered species, such as furs or ivory. Avoid tropical hardwoods.

- When you're hiking or camping, don't leave anything behind, not even soapsuds in lakes or streams.

Beyond Individual Actions . . .

- Make sure your friends and family are informed and knowledgeable about environmental issues. Share what you learn.

- Join, support, or volunteer your time to organizations working on environmental causes that are important to you.

- Contact your elected representatives and communicate your concerns. For guidelines on how to be heard, see the box "Making Your Letters Count."

These are just a few of the steps you can take to improve the quality of the environment. Assuming responsibility for your actions in relation to the environment isn't very different from assuming responsibility for your own health behaviors. It involves knowledge, awareness, insight, motivation, and commitment. You can also use the same strategies to change your behaviors in relation to the environment that you use to change your health behaviors. And as with personal health behaviors, the crucial step is to get started, today. Let the size and scope of the problems be a call to action, not an excuse for apathy.

Personal Insight Do you recycle? If you don't, why don't you? How convenient would it have to be to get you to recycle?

Classic Environmental Health Concerns

- In the nineteenth century, controlling communicable diseases was more important than controlling pollution. This concern led to government involvement in garbage collection, sewage treatment, water protection, and food inspection.

- Water used in municipal systems must be purified because it's likely to be contaminated with organic matter and disease-causing microorganisms.

- Concerns with water today center on hazardous chemicals from industry and households as well as on shortages.

- Although rivers and lakes can purify themselves when not overloaded, population growth has made sewage treatment necessary. Sewage treatment must also deal with heavy metals and hazardous chemicals.

- The sanitary landfills that are used today for solid waste disposal are subject to careful site selection and daily management.

- The amount of garbage is growing all the time, and paper is the biggest component. Burning can reduce bulk but may release hazardous material into the air. Recycling can help solid waste disposal problems.

- Illness and death associated with food-borne disease and toxic food additives have decreased substantially. Concern today centers on long-term health consequences because of chemical contamination or the characteristics of the foods themselves.

- Disability and death from diseases transmitted by insects and rodents can be prevented by spraying insecticides, wearing protective clothing, and avoiding or taking care in infested areas.

Population Growth

- The world's population is increasing rapidly and is expected to reach 10 billion by 2050. Most of this increase will occur in the developing world.

- Factors that may eventually limit human population include food, availability of land and water, energy, and minimum acceptable standard of living.

- Many factors influence population growth, including high fertility rates, lack of family planning resources, and decreasing death rates. Successful population management requires elimination of the pressures for large families.

Pollution

- In terms of health risks, the level of concentration of a particular pollutant is very important. Long-term effects of pollutants are difficult to evaluate.

- People today live long enough to experience the long-term consequences of air pollution, and increased population and industrialization make the problems more visible and dangerous.

- Increased amounts of air pollutants are especially stressful to those with heart and lung problems. Air pollution emergencies occur when (1) fossil fuels are burned, (2) a topographic feature prevents prevailing winds from pushing stagnant air away, and (3) a temperature inversion exists.

- Temperature inversions prevent the vertical circulation of air that, along with horizontal wind circulation, prevents pollutants from building up.

- Smog is human-made air pollution caused by burning fossil fuels (London-type) or by motor vehicle exhausts containing oxides of nitrogen (Los Angeles-type).

- Carbon dioxide and other natural gases act as a "greenhouse" around the earth, increasing the temperature of the atmosphere. Levels of these gases are rising through human activity; as a result, the world's climate could change.

- The ozone layer shields the earth's surface from the sun's ultraviolet rays, but a "hole" over Antarctica has been found seasonally since the 1980s. One cause is the release of chlorofluorocarbons, which break down into chlorine in the atmosphere; chlorine destroys ozone molecules.

- Acid rain or snow occurs when certain atmospheric pollutants combine with moisture in the air. Because many trees and aquatic life can tolerate only a very narrow range of acidity, they are damaged or killed by acid rain.

- Asbestos can protect against fire, but if its fibers are released into the air, they can cause serious lung damage. Ingestion of lead can damage the central nervous system and hinder oxygen transport in the blood.

- Pesticides prevent the spread of insect-borne diseases and kill insects that eat crops; hazards are usually a result of overuse or abuse.

- Radiation can cause radiation sickness, chromosome damage, and cancers, among other health risks.

- Millions of casualties would occur as a result of even a limited nuclear exchange. Accidents at nuclear power plants are potentially disastrous, and disposal of their radioactive waste is another major problem, so far not resolved. Exposure to medical x-rays is cumulative, and no exposure is absolutely safe.

- Radon, found in certain soils, rocks, and building materials, can concentrate in homes; it increases the incidence of lung cancer.

- Loud or persistent noise can lead to hearing loss and/or stress; two common sources of excessive noise are the workplace and rock concerts.

What Can You Do?

- Most health advances today must come from lifestyle changes and improvements in the global environment. The impact of personal changes made by every concerned individual could be tremendous.

TAKE ACTION

1. Do an inventory to find out what hazardous chemicals you have in your household. Read the labels for disposal instructions. If there aren't any instructions, call your local health department and ask how to dispose of specific chemicals. Also ask if there are hazardous waste disposal sites in your community or special pickup days. If possible, get rid of some or all of the hazardous wastes in your home.

2. Investigate the recycling facilities in your community. Find out how materials are recycled and what they are used for in their recycled state. If recycling isn't available in your community, contact your local city hall to find out how a recycling program can be started.

3. Junk mail is an environmental hazard coming and going—millions of trees are cut down to produce the paper it's printed on, and millions of pieces of junk mail clog the nation's landfills. Keep your name from being sold to any more mailing list companies by writing to Mail Preference Service, Direct Marketing Association, 6 East 43rd Street, New York, NY 10017. Recycle the junk mail you still get; newspaper can be recycled with newspapers, paper and envelopes (without windows) with paper.

4. Keep track of exactly how many bags (or gallons) of trash your household produces per week. Is it more or less than the national weekly average of 6.73 bags (87.5) gallons per three-person household? In either case, try to reduce it by recycling, composting, and buying and using fewer disposable products.

JOURNAL ENTRY

1. In your health journal, list the positive behaviors that help you protect the environment. What can you do to reinforce and support these behaviors? Then list the behaviors that may harm the environment. How can you change one or more of them?

2. *Critical Thinking:* Some developing nations want to "catch up" with the West in terms of economic

development and standard of living by using the same kinds of industrial practices that developed nations have used to get where they are. They are cutting down forests to raise cattle for beef, using pesticides that have been banned in the developed nations on export crops, and polluting their water and air with industrial and agricultural wastes. Do you think it's fair to expect them to be environmentally conscious when the developed nations weren't? Do they have a right to the same standard of living that Americans have, no matter what the environmental costs? Write a short essay that makes a case for or against their continuing use of these practices.

SELECTED BIBLIOGRAPHY

Allison, M. 1992. Lead poisoning: Not just for kids. *Harvard Health Letter,* May.

Clark, S. L. 1991. *Fight Global Warming: 29 Things You Can Do.* New York: Consumer Reports Books.

Cohen, J. 1992. How many people can earth hold? *Discover,* November, pp. 114–19.

Easterbrook, G. 1990. Everything you know about the environment is wrong. *The New Republic,* 20 April.

Ehrlich, P. R., and A. H. Ehrlich. 1991. *Healing the Planet: Strategies for Solving the Environmental Crisis.* Reading, Mass.: Addison-Wesley.

Elmer-Dewitt, P. 1992. Summit to save the earth: Rich vs. poor. *Time* 1 June, pp. 42–58.

Freed, V. H. 1986. Hazards in the physical environment. *The Oxford Textbook of Public Health,* vol. 1, ed. V. W. Holland, R. Detels, and G. Knox. Oxford: Oxford University Press.

Hidden home pollutants. 1992. *Healthline,* July.

How we're killing our world. 1990. *San Jose Mercury News,* 8 April.

Hunter, L. M. 1989. *The Healthy Home: An Attic-to-Basement Guide to Toxin-Free Living.* Emmaus, Penn.: Rodale Press, pp. 69–103.

Lemonick, M. D. 1992. The ozone vanishes. *Time,* 17 February, pp. 60–68.

Monastersky, R. 1991. Antarctic ozone hole sinks to a record low. *Science News* 140:244–45.

Myers, N., ed. 1993. *Gaia: An Atlas of Planet Management,* Rev. ed. New York: Anchor Books.

Naar, J. 1990. *Design for a Livable Planet: How You Can Help Clean Up the Environment.* New York: Harper and Row, pp. 85–89.

News about noise. 1992. *Healthline,* March.

Okun, D. A. 1986. Water and waste disposal. In *Public Health and Preventive Medicine,* 12th ed., ed. Maxcy-Rosenau. Norwalk, Conn.: Appleton-Century-Crofts.

Polar "ozone hole" grows to record size. 1992. *Facts on File,* 1 October.

ReVelle, P., and C. ReVelle. 1984. *The Environment: Issues and Choices for Society.* Boston: Willard Grant Press.

Roberts, L. 1991. How bad is acid rain? *Science* 251:1303.

Rubin, E. S., and others. 1992. Realistic mitigation options for global warming. *Science* 257:148–49, 261–66.

Sadik, N. 1991. Healthy people—in numbers the world can support. *World Health Forum* 12:347–55.

The science and politics of ozone depletion. 1992. *Star Tribune,* 28 June.

Stevens, W. K. 1992. Humanity confronts its handiwork: An altered planet. *The New York Times,* 5 May, pp. B5–B7.

Too much, too fast. 1992. *Newsweek,* 1 June, pp. 34–35.

Waldron, H. A. 1986. The control of the physical environment. In *The Oxford Textbook of Public Health,* vol. 2, ed. W. W. Holland, R. Detels, and G. Knox. Oxford: Oxford University Press.

Warde, J. 1992. Home improvement: Cleaning up the air inside your home. *The New York Times,* 26 November.

World Resources Institute. 1992. *The 1993 Information Please® Environmental Almanac.* Boston: Houghton Mifflin.

RECOMMENDED READINGS

The Bennet Information Group. 1990. *The Green Pages: Your Everyday Shopping Guide to Environmentally Safe Products.* New York: Random House. *A practical guide covering over 900 items by brand name, including detergents, cleansers, shampoo, paper towels, flea collars, and many more.*

Carson, R. 1962. *Silent Spring.* Boston: Houghton Mifflin. *The classic that awakened people to the dangers of wide-scale insecticide spraying.*

Dubos, R. 1986. *Man, Medicine, and Environment.* New York: Praeger. *A landmark book, written by a highly respected scientist, that focused scientific concern on environmental issues.*

The Earth Works Group. 1989. *50 Simple Things You Can Do to Save the Earth.* Berkeley, Calif.: Earthworks Press. *Full of useful information, practical advice, sources, and resources, this slim volume is an indispensable guide to improving the environment. Includes names and addresses of organizations that can provide further information on specific issues. Several other similar books are also available.*

Ehrlich, P. R. 1990. *The Population Explosion.* New York: Ballantine Books. *An update of Ehrlich's landmark 1971 book calling attention to the problems associated with population growth.*

Goldman, B. A. 1991. *The Truth About Where You Live: An Atlas for Action on Toxins and Mortality.* New York: Times Books/Random House. *The results of a five-year project to transform governmental data on environmental and health conditions into a usable format. Charts, tables, maps, and descriptions of health issues ranging from childhood cancers to industrial toxins are presented in atlas format.*

Martin, D. L., and G. Gershuny, eds. 1992. *The Rodale Book of Composting: Easy Methods for Every Gardener.* Emmaus, Penn.: Rodale Press. *Contains easy-to-follow instructions for making and using compost, including helpful tips for apartment dwellers and suburbanites.*

Moeller, D. W. 1992. *Environmental Health.* Cambridge: Harvard University Press. *New survey text by a Harvard professor who has taught environmental health for 25 years.*

Myers, N., ed. 1993. *Gaia: An Atlas of Planet Management,* Rev. ed. New York: Anchor Books. *A beautifully illustrated and informative guide to environmental problems and possible solutions.*

Schneider, S. H. 1990. *Global Warming: Are We Entering the Greenhouse Century?* New York: Vintage/Random House. *A thorough review of the greenhouse effect written by a recognized expert on climate.*

There are many national and international organizations working on environmental health problems. For information about these organizations, call their local chapter or national headquarters or consult the *Conservation Directory,* published yearly by the National Wildlife Federation. A few of the largest and most well-known environmental organizations are listed below.

Greenpeace, USA, Inc.
1436 U Street NW
Washington, DC 20009
202-462-1177

National Audubon Society
700 Broadway
New York, NY 10003
212-979-3000

National Wildlife Federation
1400 16th Street NW
Washington, DC 20036
202-797-6800

The Nature Conservancy
1815 North Lynn Street
Arlington, VA 22209
703-841-5300

Sierra Club
730 Polk Street
San Francisco, CA 94109
415-776-2211

Index

Boldface numbers indicate pages on which glossary definitions appear.

"*t*" indicates that the information is in a table.

Dilation and curettage (D&C), **178**, **580**
Dilation and evacuation (D&E), **178**
Disabled individuals and exercise, 380
Discrimination
    and cardiovascular disease, 417
    and stress, 36
Distillation, **251**
Distress, **28**
Disulfiram (Antabuse), 252, 264
Diuretics, **419**
Diverticulitis, 310
Divorce, 90
DNA (deoxyribonucleic acid), **437**
    and cancer, 446–448
Douche, **147**
Drowning, 633
Drugs
    abuse, **277**; *see also* Addiction/dependency;
        Psychoactive drugs
    advertising, 567
    antianxiety, 283–284
    anti-inflammatory, 510, **511**
    antihypertensive, 112*t*, **419**
    definition, **275**
    "designer," **291**–292
    dose-response function, **279**
    generic vs. brand-name, 566
    home pharmacy, 568*t*, 569
    and injuries, 618
    intelligent use of, 566–569
    labels of, 567
    legalization of illicit, 293
    over-the-counter (OTC), 566–568, **567**
    pharmacological properties, **279**
    physical dependence, **277**
    and pregnancy, 204, 207*t*, 281
    psychoactive; *see* Psychoactive drugs
    questions to ask about, 578–580
    testing (for abusive drugs), 293–294
    time-action function, **279**
DTs (delirium tremens), **263**
Dying; *see* Death/dying
Dysmenorrhea, 106–107

Ear problems, self-treatment, 587–588
Eastern European Jews, risk of Tay-Sachs
    disease, 190
Eating disorders, **358**, 362–366, 368
Eclampsia, **209**
Ectopic pregnancy, 208–**209**
Education attainment and smoking rates, 227,
    229*t*
Ejaculation, 110, **138**, 139
    disorders of, 113–114
Electrical impedance analysis, 351–352
Electrocardiogram (EKG or ECG), 381, 422,
    423
Electroconvulsive treatment (ECT), 64
Electroencephalogram (EEG), 424, **425**, **539**
ELISA test, **471**
Embalming, 552, **553**
Embolus, **423**
Embryo, **199**
Emergencies, 421, 565
Emergency medical services (EMS), **639**
Emphysema, 232–**233**
Encephalitis, 650, **651**
Endocrine glands, **102**, 103
Endocrine system, **35**
Endometriosis, 113, 193
Endometrium, **199**, 442, 443
Endorphins, **29**, 35, 378
Endoscopies, **575**
Energy conservation, 662–663

Environmental health issues, 645–668
    acid rain, 657, **659**
    air pollution; *see* Air pollution
    chemical waste disposal, 649, 664
    citizen action on, 662–665
    environmental carcinogens, 452–453, 452*t*
    food safety, 329–332, 650
    garbage disposal, 648–649, 664
    global warming, 655
    groups concerned with, 668
    insect and rodent control, 650
    noise pollution, 661*t*, 662
    nuclear waste disposal, 661
    ozone destruction, 655–657, 662–663
    and population growth, 650–653
    radiation, 453, 658, 660–**661**
    sewage disposal, 647–648
    tobacco smoke, 223, 235–237, 658
    water-related issues, 645–647, 665
"Environmental illness," **605**
Environmental Protection Agency (EPA), 236,
    646, 654, 658
Environmental tobacco smoke (ETS), **223**,
    235–237, 407, 437, 658
Enzymes, **493**
Epididymitis, **478**
Epinephrine (adrenaline), **29**, 378, **379**
Episiotomy, **212**
Epithelial layer, 434, **435**
Epstein-Barr virus, 481, **505**, 507
Erectile dysfunction, **113**, 114
Erikson, Erik, 54, 55, 116
Erogenous zones, **110**
Erotic fantasy, 118–**119**
Erotica, **124**, 125
Erythropoietin, 457
Essential hypertension, **419**
Essential nutrients, **305**; *see also* individual nu-
    trients
Estimated Safe and Adequate Daily Dietary In-
    takes (ESADDIs), 316–317, 318*t*
Estrogens, 102, 103, 132, **133**
    for osteoporosis, 316
Ethnicity; *see* Race/ethnicity
Euphoria, 282–**283**
Eustress, **28**
Euthanasia
    active, 548–**549**
    passive, **547**–548
Exercise, 373–402
    aerobic, **377**
    and aging, 520–521
    benefits of, 6, 375–381, 376*t*, 390–391*t*
    calories burned during, 390–391*t*
    cardiorespiratory endurance, **377**,
        383–385
    cooling down from, 389
    cross-training, 397
    and diet, 393
    for disabled individuals, 380
    equipment, 392
    for flexibility, 385, 386–387
    and fluid requirements, 393–394
    and heart disease, 375
    and immunity, 512
    injuries, 375, 395–397
    intensity of, 383–384
    isokinetic, 388, **389**
    isometric, 388, **389**
    isotonic, 388–**389**
    and mental health, 378, 379
    muscle-strengthening, 385, 388–389
    and osteoporosis, 381
    and pregnancy, 206–208, 210–211

program design, 381, 383*t*, 385, 397,
    399–401
    periodization of training, 384, **385**
    resistive, **385**, 388–389
    skill training, 389
    strength training, 385, 388–389
    and stress reduction, 36–37, 377–378
    warming up for, 389
    and weight control; *see under* Weight manage-
        ment
    weight training; 385, 388–389
Exhibitionism, 120
Exposure therapy, **67**
External stimuli (cues), **11**

Faith healing, **603**
Fallopian tubes (oviducts), 99–100
Family health tree, 192
Family life, 90–94
Fast foods, 337–340
Fats, 306–308
    blood; *see* Cholesterol; Triglycerides
    body, measurement of, 351–352
    dietary, and cancer, 450
    dietary, and heart disease, 411
    intake, calculation of, 309
    reduction of dietary, 322, 344, 345
    sources, 307–308, 308*t*
    types, 306–308
Fellatio, 119
Fermented substance, **251**
Fertility, **135**, 189–191, 193–196
Fertilization, 192, **193**
    in vitro, 194–**195**
Fertilized egg, 190, **191**
Fetal alcohol syndrome (FAS), **206**, 258–260,
    259
Fetal development, 199–203
    agents that can influence, 207*t*
Fetal monitoring, **212**
Fetishism, 120
Fetus, **188**
Fever, self-care, 584–585
Fiber
    and cancer protection, 310, 450
    cholesterol-binding, 310, 412
    in diet pills, 360
    excess, problems from, 311
    insoluble, 310, **311**
    soluble, 310, **311**
Fight-or-flight reaction, **29**
Firearms, role in injuries, 633, 638–639
Fires, 627, 629–630
First aid, 634, **639**
Fish oils, 308, 412
Fitness clubs, 396
Fitness; *see* Physical fitness
Flashbacks, 290
Flexibility, exercises for, 385, 386–387
Flukes, **508**
Fluoridation, **645**
Folic acid, 188–189, 311*t*, 319*t*
Follicle-stimulating hormone (FSH), **105**, 106,
    107
Follicles (ovarian), **188**, 189
Food
    additives, 330–332
    basic components, 305–315
    chain, 652, **653**
    enrichment, 330
    ethnic, 326–328
    "fast," 337–340
    fat content of, 308*t*, 322
    fortification, 330

panic disorder, **61–62**
phobias, 60–61
postraumatic stress disorder, 62
professional help, 66, 70–72
psychosis, **288**
self-help, 69
schizophrenic, **61**, 65–66
social anxiety, 61
Mescaline, 291
Metabolism, **253**, 308, **309**, **346**
and energy balance, 355
Metastasis, **433**
Methadone maintenance, 294–295
Mexican Americans
angina risk among, 415
Día de los muertos celebration among,
541–542
diabetes risk among, 191
hypertension risk among, 415
see also Latinos
Middle Eastern American diet, 327
"Midlife crisis," 108
Midwives, 211–212
Minerals, **305**, 315
functions and food sources, 317t
Miscarriage, **209**
Mononucleosis, infectious, 505, 507
Monosodium glutamate (MSG), 332
Monounsaturated fats, **307**
Mood disorders, 62–65
Moped safety, 624
Morbidity rate, **580**
"Morning after" pills, 137–138, 174
"Morning sickness," 196
Mortality rate, **580**
infant, **209**–210
Motor vehicle injuries, 618–625, 620t, **621**
air bags and, 621–622, **623**
alcohol and other drugs and, 255–257, 258,
622
driving habits and, 620–621
environmental factors and, 622–623
mopeds, 623
motorcycles, 623
safety belts and, 621–622
second collision and, 622, **623**
Motorcycle safety, 623
Mourning, 210–210
Murmur (bruit), **573**
Muscle strengthening, 385, 388–389
Mutagens, **447**
Mycoplasma, **503**–504
Myocardial infarction, 230, **231**, **421**
Myocardium, 230, **231**
Myotonia, **110**

Narcotic drugs (opiates), 282–283, 291
Narcotics Anonymous, 295
National Cholesterol Education Program
(NCEP), 408–409, 411
Native Americans
access to health care among, 9
alcoholism among, 191
attitudes toward aging among, 534
diabetes among, 9, 191, 312
diversity among, 9
health status of, 8–9
lactose intolerance among, 191
patterns of alcohol abuse and treatment
among, 262
smoking rates of, 229t
drug abuse treatment programs for, 294
Natural killer cells, **495**
Naturopathy, 602, **603**

Nausea
in pregnancy, 196
self-treatment, 588
Negative reinforcers, **14**
Neoplasm, malignant, **433**
Neuron, **519**
Neuropeptides, 35
Neurotransmitters, 378, **379**, 527
Neutrophil, **494**
Nicotine, **223**
addiction, 223–224
physiologic effects, 229–230
poisoning, 229
Nicotine gum, 241–242
Nicotine patches, 242
Nitrates/nitrites, 330–331, 449t, 452
Nitrogen dioxide, 654t
Nitrosamines, **452**
Nocturnal emissions, **116**
Noise pollution, 661t, 662
Nonoxynol-9, 140, 474, **475**
Nonspecific vaginitis (NSV), 113
Norepinephrine, **29**, 378, **379**
Normality, **51**
Norplant, 135–137
Northern European ancestry
lactose intolerance and, 191
osteoporosis and, 191, 316
Nuclear magnetic resonance (NMR), **423**
Nuclear power, 660–**661**
Nuclear waste disposal, 661
Nursing homes, 531
Nutrition, 303–340
advice, sources of, 329
basic food components, *see under* Food
behavior change strategies, 322, 334–335,
412t, 429, 460–461
defined, **305**
dietary guidelines, 316, 317, 319–322
essential nutrients, **305**
prenatal, 204, 205t
self-assessment of diet, 323
and stress, 37–38
vegetarian eating; *see* Vegetarian diets
See also Diet(s); Food(s); Vitamin(s); Weight
management

Obesity
adverse health effects, 353, 413, 458
and aging, 518
causes, 354–357
in childhood, 354–355
defining, **343**, 352–353
eating triggers, 356–357
prevalence, 343
and socioeconomic status, 357
See also Weight management
Obsessions, 62
Oedipus complex, 117
Omega-3 fatty acids, 308, **309**, 412
Oncogenes, **447**–449
Oncologist, 434, **435**
Ophthalmoscope, **573**
Opiates, 282–283, 291
Opportunistic diseases, 498, **499**
Optometrists, **597**
Oral contraceptives, 132-135, 136t
definition, **133**
Organ donation, 551, 552
Orgasm, **109**, 110-112
Orgasmic dysfunction, 114, **115**
Orthodox practitioners, 597–599
Osteopathic physicians, **597**
Osteoporosis, 108, 191, **316**–317, **381**, **518**

Other-directed personality, **52**, 53
Otoscope, **573**
Outpatient, 580
Ovary, 100, **188**, 189
Over-the-counter (OTC) drugs, 566–568, **567**
Overfat, 352–353; *see also* Obesity; Weight
management
Overload, 388, **389**
Overweight, 352–353; *see also* Weight manage-
ment
Oviducts (fallopian tubes), 99–100, 190, **191**
Ovulation, 106, 132–**133**
Ozone layer, 444, **655**–657, 662–663

Pacemaker, **406**
Palliative care, 545
Palpation, 439, **573**
Panic disorder, **61**–62
Pap test (Papanicolaou test), 135, **442**, 576, 577
Papillomavirus, human, 442, 480–**481**
Paranoid thinking/behavior, **264**
Paraphilia, **120**
Parasitic infections, 505, 508
Parasympathetic nervous system, **30**
Parenthood, preparation for, 187–188
Parenting, 90–92
Paresis, **477**
"Passive smoking," 407, 437
Pasteur, Louis, 499
Pathogens, **493**
Pathologist, **442**
Patient's Bill of Rights, 571
PCP (phencyclidine), 291
Pedestrian safety, 626
Pedophilia, 120
Pelvic inflammatory disease (PID), 113, **138**,
139, 193, **479**–480
Penicillin, 504, **505**
Penis, 101
Pension, **523**
Peptic ulcer, 313
Percutaneous transluminal angioplasty (PCTA),
422–**423**
Periodontitis, 518
Personal flotation devices (PFDs), **633**
Personality
healthy characteristics, 52–53
and heart disease, 413, 414
inner-directed vs. other-directed, 53
stages of psychological development, 54–55
Pesticides, 660
Phencyclidine (PCP), 291
Phenylpropanolamine (PPA), 360
Pheromones, **109**
Phobias, 60–61
Phrenology, 602
Physical examination, 521, 573–574
Physical fitness, 375–376
and aging, 520–521
assessment, 394–395
components, 375
See also Exercise
Physicians; *see Medical care*
Pipe smoking, 231, 235
Pituitary gland, **28**, **102**, 103
Placebo effect, **281**
Placenta, **199**–200, 215
Planned Parenthood, 157
Plaque (atherosclerotic), 230, **231**, 415, 419
Platelets, **406**, 407
PMS (premenstrual syndrome), **106**–107
Pneumocystis carinii, 470, **471**, 474
Podiatrists, 597
Podophyllin, 481

strains and sprains, 590–591
  See also Self-examination
Self-concept, **52**, 56
Self-contracts, 15–16
Self-esteem, **52**, 55–56, **79–80**
Self-image, **79–80**, 366–367
Self-examination
  breasts, 440–441, 577
  genitals (for STDs), 486
  testicles, 113, 446, 577
Self-help groups, 20, 295, 593
Self-medication, 566–569; *see also* Self-care
Self-talk, 57–58, 348–349
Selye, Hans, 28, 31
Semen, 102, 110
Seminiferous tubules, 101–102
Septic system, **647**
Seroconversion, 472, **473**
Serotonin, 345–**346**
Set (expectations), **281**
Set point theory, 354
Sewage disposal, 647–648
Sex/sexuality, 97–128
  abuse, child, 120–121
  adolescent, 116
  adult, 116–117
  and aging, 107–108, 519
  attitudes toward, 154–155
  bisexuality, **116**, 117
  childhood, 116, 120–121
  coercive, 119–**120**; *see also* Rape
  definitions, **99**
  disorders, **113**
  dysfunction, **113**–114
  education, 156
  gender identity, **115**
  heterosexuality, **116**, 117
  homosexuality, **116**, 117
  hormones, **99**, 105–108
  and intimacy, 80–82
  knowledge, self-test of, 102
  and love, 80–82
  masturbation; *see* Masturbation
  orientation, roots of, 117-118
  during pregnancy, 198
  premarital, 116, 154–155
  reproductive organs, 99–103
  responsible, 125
  sex therapy, 114
  sexual responses, 109–113
  stages of arousal, 110–111
  variations, **120**
Sex chromosomes, 104–**105**
Sex offenders, **120**
Sex organs
  female, 99–100, 105–106
  male, 100–102, 107
Sexual assault, **122**, 123–125
Sexual harassment, **120**, 121–112
Sexual intercourse, 108, **109**, 119
Sexual orientation, **85**, **116**, 117–118
Sexually transmissible diseases (STDs), 131,
    463–490
  AIDS; *see* AIDS; HIV infection
  candidiasis, **483**, **507**
  chlamydia, **477**–478, 479
  defined, **131**, **465**
  diagnosis, 485, 577
  education about, 483–485
  genital warts, 480–**481**
  gonorrhea, 478–**479**
  hepatitis, 206, **475**–476
  herpes, **481**–482
  infertility from, 113, 479

myths about, 478
nonspecific vaginitis (NSV), 113
pelvic inflammatory disease (PID), **479**–480
prevalence, 465; *see also* individual STDS
prevention, 125, 139, 140–141, 484, 486–488
pubic lice ("crabs"), **483**
risk self-assessment, 484
scabies, **483**
self-examination guide, 486
syphilis, 476–**477**
telling partner about, 485
trichomoniasis, 113, 482
Shiatsu; *see* Acupressure
"Shock treatment," 64
Shyness, 61, 74
Sickle-cell anemia, 9, 190, 417
Sidestream smoke, 235
Sigmoidoscope, **439**
Silicosis, **637**
Singlehood, 85–86
Skin
  aging, 444
  cancers; *see* Cancer, skin
Skinfold measurement, 351
Sleep, stages, 32
Sleeping sickness, African, **508**
Smallpox, 498–499, 505
Smog
  London-type, 654, **655**
  Los Angeles type (photochemical), 654–**655**
Smoke detectors, 629
Smokeless tobacco, 234–235, 445, 458
  promotion, 239
  warning label, 238
Smoking
  and absenteeism, 234
  and appetite, 230
  benefits of quitting, 234, 242, 243*t*
  and cancer, 223, 231, 437, 442, 443, 445,
    446, 457–458
  cigar, 231, 235
  cost of, 232
  and fires, 627
  health hazards to nonsmokers, 235–237,
    407, 437
  health hazards to smoker, 230–234, 416
  and heart disease, 230–231
  low tar/nicotine cigarettes, 229
  mainstream smoke, **235**
  Nonsmoker's Bill of Rights, 240
  physiological effects, 229–230
  pipe, 231, 235
  and pregnancy, 206, 237
  premature deaths from, 223
  prevalence, 225, 227, 228
  prohibition during air travel, 235
  quitting, 239, 241–242, 245–247
  reasons for, 225–227
  sidestream smoke, **235**
Snuff, 234
Social anxiety, 61
Social Security, **528**, 529, 532, 534–535
Social workers, 70
Socioeconomic status
  abortion rates and, 175
  eating disorders and, 363
  obesity and, 357–358
Somatic nervous system, 33
Sonogram, 202, **203**
Sore throat, self-care, 585–586
"Spanish fly," 112*t*
Specialties, medical, 599
"Speedball" drug mixtures, 286
Sperm cell, 99, 101, 190–**192**, 194

Spermicides, **140**, 146–147, 474–475
Sphygmomanometer, 418–**419**
Spiritual health, 4
Spirochetes, 502–503; *see also* Lyme disease;
    Syphilis
Sponge, contraceptive, **145**–146
Spontaneous abortion, **209**
Sprains, self-treatment, 590–591
Squamous cell carcinoma, 444, **445**
"Squeeze technique," 114
Staphylococci, 502, **503**, 648, 649
State dependency, **286**, 287–288
STD hot line, 484
STDs; *see* Sexually transmissible diseases
Sterilization, **151**–154
  reversible, 154
  tubal, 152–**153**
  vasectomy, 151–152, **580**
Steroids, anabolic, **385**, 388
Stimulants, **255**, 285
Stimuli, **67**
  external, **11**
  internal, **11**
Stool tests for blood, 438, 456*t*, 577
Strains, self-treatment, 590–591
Strength training, 385, 388–389
Strep throat, 425, 503
Streptococci, 502, **503**
Stress, 25–48
  and aging, 521
  body response to, 28–32, 34–35
  and caffeine, 38
  definition, **27**, 28
  emotional responses to, 31, 33–34
  exercise and, 36–37, 377–378
  and exhaustion, 30–31
  and high blood pressure, 34
  hormones, 28–29
  and immune system, 34, 512
  management techniques, 35–44, 349
  mobilization for, 28–30
  and nutrition, 37–38
  post-traumatic, 62
  relaxation techniques, 40–43, 47
  role in disease, 34–35, 413, 417, 447
  self-assessment questionnaire, 39
  signs, 33
  and social support systems, 36
  sources, 27–28
  stages; *see* General adaptation syndrome (GAS)
  and time management, 38–40
  test anxiety, 46–48
Stress response, **28**
Stress test (for heart disease), 422
Stressors, **28**, 37
Stroke, 231, 406, 407, 422, **423**–424
Students Against Driving Drunk (SADD), 269
Sudden infant death syndrome (SIDS), **210**
Sugar, 321, 344
Suicide, 63–64, 542–**543**
  danger signals, 63–64
  myths about, 63
  reasons for, 542–543
Sulfites, 331
Sulforaphane, **450**, 451
Sulfur dioxide, 654*t*
Sunscreens, 444, **445**
Supplementation, nutritional, 38, 325
  during pregnancy, 328
  possible need for, 327–329
Suppressor gene, **449**–450
Surgery, 580–581
  arthroscopic, **580**
  cardiovascular, 423